Nutrition
in
Exercise
and Sport

NUTRITION in EXERCISE and SPORT

Editor, Ira Wolinsky

Nutrition
in
Exercise
and Sport

Third Edition

Edited by

Ira Wolinsky, Ph.D.

Professor of Nutrition
University of Houston
Houston, Texas

CRC Press
Boca Raton   New York

Acquiring Editor: Marsha Baker
Project Editor: Debbie Didier
Cover Design: Dawn Boyd
PrePress: Greg Cuciak

Library of Congress Cataloging-in-Publication Data

Nutrition in exercise and sport / edited by Ira Wolinsky. — 3rd ed.
       p. cm. — (Nutrition in exercise and sport)
    Includes bibliographical references and index.
    ISBN 0-8493-8560-1
    1. Athletes—Nutrition.   2. Exercise—Physiological aspects.
  I. Wolinsky, Ira. II. Series.
    [DNLM: QT N976 1997]
  TX361.A8N88   1997
  613.2′024′796—dc21
  DNLM/DLC   97-8495
  for Library of Congress   CIP

© 1998 by CRC Press LLC

No claim to original U.S. Government works
International Standard Book Number 0-8493-8560-1
Library of Congress Card Number 97-8495
Printed in the United States of America   2 3 4 5 6 7 8 9 0
Printed on acid-free paper

The wise, for cure, on exercise depend
          (Epistle to John Driden of Chesterton, 92)

               John Dryden 1631–1700

Respectful of the past, this volume is dedicated to the memories of my forefathers who knew no sport and whose only exercise was work.

PREFACE

The *CRC Series on Nutrition in Exercise and Sport* is designed to provide the setting for in-depth exploration of the many and varied aspects of nutrition and exercise, including, of course, sport. The topic of sports nutrition gained heightened interest among physiologists in the 1960s, and, since then, numerous scientific studies have focused on the healthful benefits of good nutrition and exercise. As we move foward in time scientists will continue to search for the elusive "optimum" nutritional preparation. As they try to unlock nature's secrets, we must remember that there must be a range of diets that will support excellent physical performance. Inevitably there will be attempts by scientists and laymen alike to distill the diets to some common denominator — a formula for success. The *CRC Series on Nutrition in Exercise and Sport* is dedicated to providing a stage upon which to explore these issues. Each volume provides a detailed and scholarly examination of some aspect of this topic. The Series provides a set of authoritative volumes for consultation by scientists, physicians, and a broad range of health care providers and individuals who participate in exercise and sport, whether for recreation, competition, or therapy.

The third edition of *Nutrition in Exercise and Sport* is respectfully submitted to the Series. The first and second editions of this volume were very well received and praised by many sports nutritionists and health professionals. It is being used as a primary college text. This third edition is an updated and expanded contribution to keep pace with the latest developments in the rapidly burgeoning field of sport nutrition. All topics have been updated. It contains chapters on subjects not included before: the history of sports nutrition, antioxidants, vegetarianism, the young athlete, the older athlete, the diabetic athlete, the disabled athlete, sports-specific nutrient requirements, body composition changes. Some of these chapters were suggested by readers and workers in the field. I would welcome further suggestions for possible future editions. We hope this volume, as we aspired for the prior editions, will be useful to the scientific, athletic, and lay communities in evaluating the existing body of knowledge on exercise and sports nutrition and will facilitate the recommendation of dietary allowances and appropriate food choices.

Ira Wolinsky, Ph.D.
University of Houston
Houston, Texas
Editor

THE EDITOR

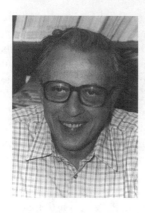 **Ira Wolinsky, Ph.D.,** is Professor of Nutrition at the University of Houston. He received his B.S. degree in chemistry from the City College of New York in 1960 and his M.S. (1965) and Ph.D. (1968) degrees in biochemistry from Kansas University. He has served in research and teaching positions at the Hebrew University (both the Medical School and the Faculty of Agriculture), the University of Missouri, and Pennsylvania State University. He has also conducted research at NASA research centers and served as official consultant in India, the U.S.S.R., Hungary, and Bulgaria.

Dr. Wolinsky is a member of the American Society for Nutritional Sciences and the American Society for Clinical Nutrition, among other scientific organizations. He is the editor of the CRC Series on Modern Nutrition, the CRC Series on Nutrition in Exercise and Sport, and co-editor of the CRC Series on Methods in Nutrition Research and the CRC Series on Exercise Physiology.

Dr. Wolinsky has contributed numerous nutrition papers in the open literature, co-authored a book on the history of the science of nutrition, and co-edited the CRC volumes *Nutritional Concerns of Women* and also *Sports Nutrition, Vitamins and Trace Elements*. His current major research interests include the nutrition of bone and calcium and sports nutrition.

CONTRIBUTORS

Doron Aaronson, M.D.
Metabolism Section
Joslin Diabetes Clinic
Harvard Medical School
Boston, Massachusetts

John J. B. Anderson, Ph.D.
Department of Nutrition
University of North Carolina School of
  Public Health
Chapel Hill, North Carolina

Eldon W. Askew, Ph.D.
Division of Foods and Nutrition
University of Utah
Salt Lake City, Utah

Terry L. Bazzarre, Ph.D., F.A.C.S.M.
National Center
American Heart Association
Dallas, Texas

Lindsay Bishop, M.P.H.
Department of Nutrition
University of North Carolina
Chapel Hill, North Carolina

Luke R. Bucci, Ph.D., C.C.N., C.N.S.
Weider Nutrition International
Salt Lake City, Utah

Jennifer Bunger, M.Ed.
Health, Physical Education, and Recreation
  Department
Southwest Texas State University
San Marcos, Texas

Elsworth R. Buskirk, Ph.D.
Noll Physiological Research Center
Pennsylvania State University
University Park, Pennsylvania

Priscilla M. Clarkson, Ph.D.
Department of Exercise Science
University of Massachusetts
Amherst, Massachusetts

Elyse A. Cohen, M.S., L.N.
Nutrition Department
General Mills, Inc.
Minneapolis, Minnesota

Amy B. Duckett, B.S.P.H., R.D.
Department of Nutrition
University of North Carolina
Chapel Hill, North Carolina

James A. Freeman, Ph.D.
English Department
University of Massachusetts
Amherst, Massachusetts

Tracy A. Gautsch, M.S.
Division of Nutritional Sciences
University of Illinois
Urbana, Illinois

Ann C. Grandjean, Ed.D.
International Center for Sports Nutrition
Omaha, Nebraska

Susan M. Groziak, Ph.D., R.D., L.D.
National Dairy Council
Rosemont, Illinois

G. Harley Hartung, Ph.D., F.A.C.S.M.
Department of Medicine
Cardiology Service
Tripler Army Medical Center
Honolulu, Hawaii

Emily M. Haymes, Ph.D.
Department of Nutrition, Food, and
  Movement Sciences
Florida State University
Tallahassee, Florida

Laurie Hoffman-Goetz, Ph.D., M.P.H.
Department of Health Studies and
  Gerontology
University of Waterloo
Waterloo, Ontario, Canada

Craig A. Horswill, Ph.D.
Gatorade Sports Science Institute
Exercise Physiology Laboratory
Barrington, Illinois

Catherine G. Ratzin Jackson, Ph.D.
Department of Kinesiology
California State University
Fresno, California

Jayanthi Kandiah, Ph.D., R.D., C.D.
Department of Family and Consumer
  Sciences
Ball State University
Muncie, Indiana

Mitchell M. Kanter, Ph.D.
Gatorade Sports Science Institute
Exercise Physiology Laboratory
Barrington, Illinois

Frank I. Katch
Department of Exercise Science
University of Massachusetts
Amherst, Massachusetts

Victor L. Katch
Department of Kinesiology
University of Michigan
Ann Arbor, Michigan

Donald K. Layman, Ph.D.
Department of Foods and Nutrition
University of Illinois
Urbana, Illinois

Michael Liebman, Ph.D.
Department of Family and Consumer
  Sciences
University of Wyoming
Laramie, Wyoming

Henry C. Lukaski, Ph.D.
United States Department of Agriculture
Agricultural Research Service
Grand Forks Human Nutrition Research
  Center
Grand Forks, North Dakota

Leonard F. Marquart, Ph.D., R.D.
Nutrition Department
General Mills, Inc.
Minneapolis, Minnesota

William D. McArdle
Department of Family, Nutrition, and
  Exercise Science
Queens College
Flushing, New York

Robert G. McMurray, Ph.D.
Department of Physical Education, Exercise
  and Sport Science
University of North Carolina
Chapel Hill, North Carolina

Gregory D. Miller, Ph.D., F.A.C.N.
National Dairy Council
Rosemont, Illinois

Robert Murray, Ph.D.
Gatorade Sports Science Institute
Exercise Physiology Laboratory
Barrington, Illinois

Tinker D. Murray, Ph.D.,
  F.A.C.S.M.
Department of Health, Physical Education,
  and Recreation
Southwest Texas State University
San Marcos, Texas

Gregory L. Paul, Ph.D.
Quaker Oats Company
Barrington, Illinois

Susan M. Puhl, Ph.D.
State University of New York at Cortland
Cortland, New York

Rosemary A. Ratzin, Ed.D.
Department of Health, Physical Education
  and Recreation
Frostburg State University
Frostburg, Maryland

Elliott Rayfield, M.D.
Department of Internal Medicine
Mount Sinai Medical Center
New York, New York

Kristin J. Reimers, M.S., R.D.
International Center for Sports Nutrition
Omaha, Nebraska

Cheryl L. Rock, Ph.D., R.D.
Department of Family and Preventive
  Medicine
University of California at San Diego
  Cancer Prevention and Control
La Jolla, California

Pamela Rondano, M.P.H., R.D.
Department of Nutrition
University of North Carolina
Chapel Hill, North Carolina

Jaime S. Ruud, M.S., R.D.
Nutrition Consultant
Nutrition Link
Lincoln, Nebraska

Leo C. Senay, Jr., Ph.D.
Department of Pharmacological and
  Physiological Science
St. Louis University Medical School
St. Louis, Missouri

**Sarah H. Short, Ph.D., Ed.D., R.D.,
  F.A.D.A.**
Department of Nutrition and Food
  Management
Syracuse University
Syracuse, New York

Eric Small, M.D., F.A.A.P.
Sports Medicince Department
Blythedale Children's Hospital
Valhalla, New York
and
Pediatrics
Mount Sinai Medical Center
New York, New York

**William G. Squires, Jr., Ph.D.,
  F.A.C.S.M.**
Department of Biology
Texas Lutheran University
Seguin, Texas

Mark Stender, M.D.
Department of Sports Medicine
Student Health Services
University of North Carolina
Chapel Hill, North Carolina

John G. Wilkinson, Ph.D.
School of Physical and Health Education
University of Wyoming
Laramie, Wyoming

CONTENTS

EXERCISE NUTRITION: FROM ANTIQUITY TO THE TWENTIETH CENTURY AND BEYOND*

Frank I. Katch
William D. McArdle
Victor L. Katch
James A. Freeman

CONTENTS

I.   PREFACE

This chapter consists of two parts. Part 1 presents an historical overview of those individuals from antiquity to our century whose experiments have demonstrated the intimate connection of medicine, physiology, exercise, and nutrition. Building on these seminal linkages, Part 2 urges the creation of a cross-disciplinary academic field to be known as Exercise Nutrition.

The important accomplishments on the time line of Part 1 provide a powerful rationale for developing an integrated subject. We believe it requires the new name Exercise Nutrition to gain acceptance. The currently popular name, sports nutrition, falls short because it restricts itself almost exclusively to athletics. Faculty governance bodies might be concerned that programs with sports in the title lack sufficient academic rigor.

Our proposal for a new field updates the notion that sports nutrition is a subset of nutrition. Exercise Nutrition should develop its own core courses, blending knowledge from traditional fields like biochemistry, chemistry, exercise physiology, medicine, nutrition, and physiology.

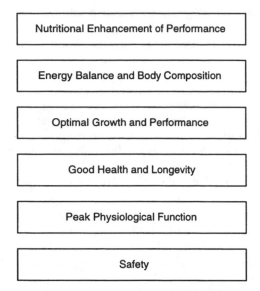

Nutritional Enhancement of Performance
Energy Balance and Body Composition
Optimal Growth and Performance
Good Health and Longevity
Peak Physiological Function
Safety

FIGURE 1 Model for a discipline of Exercise Nutrition. The six areas constitute the core of the discipline.

This new program, independent of umbrella departments like nutrition, exercise science (kinesiology), or public health, would fit logically with other life sciences and benefit them all.

A cross disciplinary field like Exercise Nutrition enlarges the scope of current offerings. Today, sports nutrition concentrates on athletic performance. We differ. Our six-component model includes both athletes and non-athletes (nutritional enhancement of performance, energy balance and body composition, optimal growth and performance, good health and longevity, peak physiological function, safety, Figure 1). Thus, it emphasizes breadth, not exclusivity, for studying nutrition and human physical activity.

People seldom implement new ideas without trauma. However, modern exercise nutritionists should refine and expand the enormous wealth of data bequeathed to us by the pioneers whose contributions follow. Just as they synthesized previous knowledge, modern researchers can consolidate data from even wider sources.

II. PART 1. ANTIQUITY TO THE TWENTIETH CENTURY

Nutrition as applied to exercise and sports originated before the Golden Age of Greece. Concerns about physical exertion, proper food, and general health occupied thinkers in Sumeria, India, Egypt, China, Persia, and other ancient civilizations. Early nomads subsisted on foods available from the environment such as fish, animal meats, nuts, beans, grains, and wild fruits. The most physically able of the group, who traveled long distances over sometimes hostile and unfamiliar terrain to capture and retrieve food for the tribe, were indeed the first "athletes." After hunter gatherers settled, they could devote time in their towns to games interspersed with manual labor. Early medicine men knew what elements to combine to make soaps, curatives, unguents, and emetics. Even at the dawn of systematized knowledge, Egyptian scribes passed on medical knowledge by mixing dyes and inks to illustrate their papyrus records. The records describe sedatives for pain and cures for stomach disorders and forms of blindness. The versatile Imhotep (ca. 2650 B.C.) not only constructed the giant Step Pyramid at Saqqara but also treated workers injured during its construction. The colossal complex, which was nearly 500 feet tall and required 2.5 million blocks of stone weighing up to 15 tons (15,000 kg) each, caused accidents to uncounted numbers of laborers. The records validate Imhotep's reputation as a medical practitioner when they describe crude surgical operations.

In addition, the Egyptians realized the importance of diet. Herotodus (ca. 440 B.C.), the Greek historian and traveler, said:[1]

> ... there is an inscription in Egyptian characters on the pyramid which records the quantity of radishes, onions, and garlic consumed by the labourers who constructed it, and I perfectly well remember that the interpreter who read the writing to me said that the money expended in this way was 1600 talents of silver. If this then is a true record, what a vast sum must have been spent on the iron tools used in the work, and on the feeding and clothing of the labourers.

In the ancient view, no particular diet made one strong or wholesome. Overindulgence in food and drink could lead to discomforts like diarrhea, constipation, and disease. Although physicians understood the general dangers of excess, a tomb inscription found near the Great Pyramid of Cheops describes a wealthy landowner who could receive nourishment from cows, oxen, calves, goats, asses, sheep, and poultry, as well as the bread and beer he produced.[2] Insights about food, work, and well-being from such early records link the ancient world to our modern era.

Our tour of the history of Exercise Nutrition continues with the early Greek philosophers and physicians who provided a conceptual framework about the workings of the human body. Many of their ideas about physiology were erroneous; nevertheless, they governed medical practice for 17 centuries. Not until human dissection and more sophisticated scientific instruments became commonplace could researchers challenge, verify, and discover the true roles that exercise and nutrition play in health. As the famous French physiologist Claude Bernard (1813–1878) said[3] when he reused the words of a medieval philosopher:

> We stand upon the intellectual shoulders of the medical giants of bygone days and, because of the help they afford us, we are able to see more clearly than they were able to do.

III.   THE EARLY GREEK PHILOSOPHERS AND PHYSICIANS

Greek thinkers utilized "scientific" ideas about food, medicine, and treatment of sickness that came from Egypt and other cultures. The earliest philosophers believed that the supernatural governed the human realm. Gradually, logic and observation emphasized the physical workings of the body. Although the ethos of the time suppressed dissection of humans, animal vivisection routinely determined their internal structures and bodily functions. Such knowledge of animal anatomy encouraged analogous conclusions about human systems. Of course, many early biological notions turned out to be incorrect. For example, blood vessels and nerves do not originate from the umbilicus; the sternum does not contain seven segments; there are no pores between the left and right chambers of the heart to transport blood; the nerves are not hollow and carry no air; blood does not circulate through the body only fifty times daily. Still, each philosopher focused on questions essential to understanding bodily functions.

Empedocles (ca. 500–c. 430 B.C.), a pupil of the famous mathematician Pythagoras (born ca. 582 B.C.) and a contemporary of Alcmaeon of Crotona (ca. 500 B.C.), was one of the first Greeks to write about "modern" medicine. Alcmaeon believed that disease resulted from an imbalance of the body's four humors. Such notions differed from theological beliefs that hostile gods caused sickness. Empedocles went beyond the work of Alcmaeon by dissecting animals. He discovered the nerves leading from the brain to the eyes and the canal

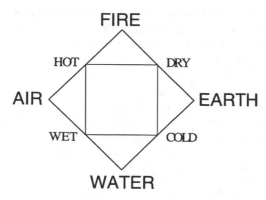

FIGURE 2   The four elements Empedocles proposed — earth, air, fire, and water — and their four qualities of cold, hot, dry, and wet.

leading from the throat to the middle ear.* He also espoused the religious notion (paralleled by Deuteronomy xii.23) that a mysterious "innate heat" or essential life factor, resided in the blood. Consequently, the heart (and thus the soul) served as the center of the body. Contemporary theory claimed blood vessels transported this innate heat from the heart throughout the body. However naive, the heat-transfer belief explained how circulatory and respiratory systems functioned until challenged by Aristotle (384–322 B.C.) and the later Athenian School.[4]

Empedocles contributed another legacy. Figure 2 illustrates the four elements he proposed — earth, air, fire, and water — and their four qualities of cold, hot, dry, and wet. His idea of four elements makes rational an ancient Egyptian faith in the magical power of the number four. The figure shows how the four elements oppose each other — they also interconnect. Thus, hot and dry characterize fire, cold and dry signify earth, cold and wet typify water, and hot and wet identify air. Varying proportions of these elements govern all physical phenomena. Accordingly, man developed from the fire that sprang from the earth, forming shapes that eventually took on life forms; growth took place from a warming of the body, and cold debilitated humans as they aged. Melancholy or "Black Bile," for example, caused by dry and cold humors or elements, could be treated by using their opposites, wet and hot. Physical conditions like health and disease and emotional states like Love and Strife resulted from the interaction of humors. An imbalance in the four humors could cause anger, melancholy, sluggishness, or vigor. Overeating (as practiced by wrestlers and boxers) was treated with hot baths and drugs made from mixtures of dry powders that would soothe the dyspepsia. Linking disease and diet in the sixth century demonstrates the antiquity of "sports nutrition."

Hippocrates (b. 460 B.C.), a physician from the island of Cos, and his contemporaries dealt more scientifically with their patients. They applied inductive reasoning to discern facts and then applied solutions based on logic and experience. The followers of the "Hippocratic Method" listened carefully to patients; they connected cause and effect and espoused a rational approach to healing without relying on oracles or divine intervention. The Hippocratic scholars kept meticulous records so that others could treat similar ailments. Their writings deal with health and nutrition.[5]

---

* In 1562, the Italian anatomist Bartolemeo Eustachio rediscovered these minute structures that connect the middle ear to the back of the throat; they bear his name, Eustacian tubes.

Growing bodies have the most innate heat; they therefore require the most food, for otherwise their bodies are wasted. In old persons the heat is feeble, and therefore they require little fuel, as it were, to the flame, for it would be extinguished by much. On this account, also, fevers in old persons are not equally acute, because their bodies are cold.

In the Golden Age of Greece (384–322 B.C.), Aristotle, the young pupil of Plato (427–347 B.C.), advanced scientific thought by teaching that biology and anatomy should be acquired from logic and examination, not myth. However, some of his medical teachings were mistaken. Aristotle taught that the heart, not the brain, controlled life and intelligence. This concept remained valid until the 18th century. Aristotle also believed that the brain secreted a fluid, phlegm, that cooled the heart. In addition, Aristotle refined the system of the four elements originally posited by Empedocles. According to Singer,[6] the doctrine of the four elements contributed to Jewish, Christian, and Moslem theology and remained unquestioned until the 17th century.

Erasistratus of Chios (fl. ca. 280 B.C.), often called the father of physiology, investigated bodily functions, particularly those of arteries, veins, and nerves. A student at the famous medical school at Alexandria, Erasistratus experimented on the brain and its main nerve branchings. He also attempted to discover where in the body air became transformed into the "vital spirit." According to Garrison,[7] Erasistratus devised the first respiration apparatus. He placed fowls into a jar, then weighed them and their excreta before and after they consumed food. This type of metabolic experiment, which attempted to reconcile energy input and output, was not to be repeated for another 2000 years by Santorio. Erasistratus hypothesized that the blood and its vital spirit reached the brain, where it was transformed into "animal spirit" and dispersed by hollow nerves throughout the body. The physiological ideas developed by Erasistratus were incorporated in the writings of Galen.

Five centuries after Hippocrates, perhaps the most well known physician that ever lived, Claudius Galenus or Galen (129–201 A.D.), left a mark on medicine and health practices that remained intact for almost 1300 years. The son of a wealthy architect, Galen was born in the city of Pergamon and began studying medicine at about age 16. Over the next 50 years, he enhanced the current thinking about health and hygiene, areas that some might consider applied exercise physiology. Throughout his life, Galen taught and practiced the "laws of health" — breathe fresh air, eat proper foods, drink the right beverages, exercise, get adequate sleep, have a daily bowel movement, and control one's emotions. A prolific writer, he produced at least 80 sophisticated treatises (and perhaps as many as 500 essays) on numerous topics. Many concerned human anatomy and physiology, nutrition, growth and development, the beneficial effects of exercise and deleterious consequences of sedentary living, as well as a variety of diseases and their treatment. One of the first "bench physiologists," Galen conducted original experiments in physiology, comparative anatomy, and medicine, including dissections on goats, pigs, cows, monkeys, horses, elephants, and other beasts from the gladiatorial games. As physician to the gladiators, Galen treated torn tendons and muscles by using surgical procedures he invented. He developed rehabilitation therapies and exercise regimens. Following the Hippocratic school of medicine, Galen believed that science must be grounded in experimentation and observation. For example, Galen first traced the main arteries accurately and proved that they carry blood, not air.

However, Galen's ideas about the function of the heart and circulatory system were physiologically incorrect because his information about human physiology came from animal dissections. Galen postulated that three kinds of spirits — natural, vital, and animal — ebbed and flowed throughout the body by means of hollow nerve channels. These beliefs remained essentially unchallenged for the next 13 centuries until experimental anatomists of the early 16th and 17th centuries discovered from post-mortem dissections on humans how physiological function matched anatomical observation.

Galen described "swift" and vigorous exercises, including their proper quantity and duration. He also wrote extensively about maintenance of good health, including proper diet. His words, quoted below from the first complete English translation by Green[8] of *Hygiene* (*De Sanitate Tuenda*), combined with later medical discoveries, paved the way for the new discipline of Exercise Nutrition.

The uses of exercise, I think are twofold, one for the evacuation of the excrements, the other for the production of good condition of the firm parts of the body. For since vigorous motion is exercise, it must needs be that only these three things result from it in the exercising body — hardness of the organs from mutual attrition, increase of the intrinsic warmth, and accelerated movement of respiration. These are followed by all the other individual benefits which accrue to the body from exercise; from hardness of the organs, both insensitivity and strength for function; from warmth, both strong attraction for things to be eliminated, readier metabolism, and better nutrition and diffusion of all substances, whereby it results that solids are softened, liquids diluted, and ducts dilated. And from the vigorous movement of respiration the ducts must be purged and the excrements evacuated.

Now, in the matter of diet, it must be considered whether dyspepsia has occurred more or less frequently than usual; or whether the patient ingested a surfeit of indigestible foods, or whether he drank sweet instead of aged wine, or thick or turbid instead of thin; or whether he has switched completely from wine-drinking to water-drinking, not once or twice changing in either of the aforesaid, but continuously and for a long time.

And for the same reason, it is not suitable for those having the excess of their raw juices in the primary veins to exercise, or move at all, or even to bathe. For all such activities drive these juices into the whole body. Therefore one must keep the patients at total rest, and give them food and drink and drugs that thin and cut and reduce the thickness of the juices, without warming appreciably; for the greatly warmed juices go everywhere through the body. Therefore, you should feed them chiefly with oxymel, giving also a little barley and black barley sometimes. And most of them get along on this thin diet, using the excess of undigested juices, which they gradually digest, for the sustenance of the body. And since the hypochondrium in all such patients becomes swollen and distended, and whatever they take turns easily to gas, it would be better to give some long pepper with the food; for this dissolves the thickness of the flatulent gas, and also pushes towards the lower abdomen what is sluggishly arrested in the hypochondrium, and contributes to the digestion of food, according to the common property of all peppers. But if long pepper is not available, white pepper should be used; for it a better tonic for the abdomen than both the other kinds of peppers. ... And after this you should purge with a drug which is most suitable for indigestion. But when only digestion exists without excess of blood, it is necessary to proceed to that catharsis which is appropriate to the offending excrement. This may be either yellow bile, or black bile, or phlegm, either alkaline or acid, and each of these may be either serous or thick or intermediate in its consistency, concerning whose diagnosis let us now speak ...

But if this is not available, the best black pepper should be used, and this is the heaviest. But it is better to use the so-called drug of Diospolis. And this compounded in two ways: sometimes of equal parts of cummin and pepper and springwort and nitre, and thus it is more solvent for the abdomen; and sometimes an equal part of each of the other constituents is mixed with an equal half total weight of nitre. Soften the cummin in acetic acid or vinegar, then immediately rub it, or first chill it moderately in an earthen vessel that has been thoroughly baked in the oven. For a vessel that has been merely dried is more porous than earthenware, and absorbs some of their property from the drugs. The springwort leaves also should be only moderately dried; for, if they are dried too much, they become acrid and bitter and warmer than is desirable; but, if not dried at all, they contain some excrementary moisture not yet completely converted, as a result of which they do not become wholly free from gas. To these four, foamless honey is sometimes added, sometimes not, but they are mixed alone without the honey, and added to the barley-broth and to whatever other food seems most suitable.

Why did Galen's ideas about biology and medicine persist for so long? Singer[6] reminds us that Galen's writings survived despite widespread destruction of other manuscripts. They were translated into Latin, Egyptian, Spanish, Indian, Syriac, Arabic, Persian, and Hebrew. Some writers ascribed their own work to Galen. Before the mid-15th century and the advent of mechanical printing, each manuscript required tedious copying by hand. Thus, Galen's ideas were perpetuated, sometimes accurately, sometimes mistakenly.

Copyists were not always accurate, and sometimes would improve manuscripts by omitting parts with which they did not agree, or by inserting their own ideas when the opportunity was presented. ... People in other locations, or at a later period of time, ... had to start from the beginning and reaccumulate the same information. Thus there was little chance for the survival and accretion of a culture.[9]

IV.   THE FIRST SPORTS NUTRITIONISTS — THE PHYSICIANS OF THE ANCIENT OLYMPIC GAMES

The Olympics lasted from 776 B.C. to 393 A.D. when the Christian Byzantine Emperor Theodosius I abolished them. During this period, paidotribes (trainers or private coaches) advised their athletes about food and exercise. Paidotribes owned their own palaestrai, or they coached athletes in the public gymnasia. Early distinguished paidotribes included Iccus of Tarentum, who won the pentathlon at an early Olympic festival, and Melesias, who trained 30 wrestling champions.

Paidotribes taught young athletes general skills, but more specialized trainers (gymnaste) instructed elite athletes.[10,11] The trainers, well versed in practical medicine, treated injuries from wrestling, boxing, and chariot racing. Trainers quarreled with physicians because the latter regarded trainers as unscientific quacks.[12]

From ancient scrolls and vase pictures, we learn that athletes followed strict regimens of exercise, rest, massage, bathing, and diet for 10 consecutive months prior to the games. Paidotribes prescribed large quantities of food for boxers and wrestlers. About 480 B.C., Dromeus of Stymphalus, a two-time Olympic champion in the long race, advocated an innovative diet of meat.[10] Herodicus of Selymbria, a sickly contemporary of Socrates, modified his diet to improve his own health.

In general, according to Gardiner,[13]

The diet of the old athletes had been, like that of most Greek country folk, mainly vegetarian, consisting of figs, fresh cheese from the baskets, porridge, and meal cakes with only occasional meat as a relish, and wine. The frequently repeated statement that the athlete's diet was regulated by the law of the Games, and that he was not allowed to drink wine is entirely groundless. But shortly after the Persian Wars a change took place. A meat diet was introduced by some trainers.

The object of a meat diet was to produce the bulk and strength supposed to be necessary for the boxer and wrestler. In Greece classification by weight was unknown, and in boxing and wrestling the heavyweight has a natural advantage. Therefore, to produce bulk, the trainer prescribed enormous quantities of meat, which had to be counteracted by excessive exercise. Eating, sleeping, and exercise occupied the athlete's whole time and left little leisure for other pursuits.

When athletes were not training, they ate frugally like common citizens. Gardiner[12] quotes the poet Lynceus:

One brings in a great dish in which are five smaller ones; the first contains garlic, the second two sea-urchins, the third a sweet meal-cake, the fourth ten oysters, the fifth a little sturgeon. While I eat one, my neighbor makes another disappear; while he eats one, I despatch another. Gladly, my friend, would I partake of both, but my wish is not attainable, as my mouth is not fivefold.

The typical Athenian ate three meals daily.[12] An early morning meal consisted of bread dipped in unmixed wine (in contrast, athletes drank wine diluted with three to five parts water); a "light" later morning meal between 9 a.m. and noon; and a more substantial meal at sundown that offered choices from red, white, and yellow wines (often mixed with resin), and portions of fish and sometimes meats. Desserts included nuts, olives, figs, cheese, and sweet cakes.

In addition,[12]

The staple of their food was porridge made of barley, and bread, for which their city was famous, together with their native figs, olives, and honey, cheese which they imported especially from Sicily, and a number of herbs, mallows, cabbages, beans, lupines, and the like. In addition to these, every Athenian who could afford it ... ate oysters or fresh or salt fish. Fresh fish was caught in large quantities in the Phaleric roads; salt fish and oysters came mostly from the Propontis and the Euxine; all were excessively cheap at Athens. Sometimes, for a variety, sausages or black puddings, or a haggis would be purchased, and the wealthier classes would get the eels of the Copaic lake, or hares and thrushes; even the flesh of lambs or goats. ... The custom prevailed of using oil in cooking most dishes.

Cereal food could be taken in three forms: (1) as a sort of barley-broth or porridge; (2) as a sort of thin pancake, lightly baked over a charcoal fire and rolled up; (3) as regular loaves made with yeast. No doubt the luxurious in cities usually ate leavened bread; but in country places, and in early times, ... the soft pancake form was usual.

Learning from observation and intuition, these early trainers understood that food affected athletic performance.

V. POST-HIPPOCRATIC MEDICINE AND NUTRITION

The eight books of *De Medicina*,[14] attributed to the Roman Aulus Cornelius Celsus (born about 24 A.D. during the reign of the Emperor Tiberius), contains sage advice even by today's standards:

A man in health, who is both vigorous and his own master, should be under no obligatory rules, and have no need, either for a medical attendant, or for a rubber and anointer. His kind of life should afford him variety; he should be now in the country, now in town, and more often about the farm; he should sail, hunt, rest sometimes, but more often takes exercise; for whilst inaction weakens the body, work strengthens it; the former brings on premature old age, the latter prolongs youth.

It is well also at times to go to the bath, at times to make use of cold waters; to undergo sometimes inunction, sometimes to neglect the same; to avoid no kind of food in common use; to attend at times a banquet, at times to hold aloof; to eat more than sufficient at one time, at another no more; to take food twice rather than once a day, and always as much as one wants provided one digests it. But whilst exercise and food of this sort are necessaries, those of the athletes are redundant; for in the one class any break in the routine of exercise, owing to necessities of civil life, affects the body injuriously, and in the other, bodies thus fed up in their fashion age very quickly and become inform.

The weak, however, among whom are a large portion of townspeople, and almost all those fond of letters, need greater precaution, so that care may re-establish what the character of their constitution or of their residence or of their study detracts. Anyone therefore of these who has digested well may with safety rise early; if too little, he must stay in bed, or if he has been obliged to get up early, must go to sleep again; he who has not digested, should lie up altogether, and neither work nor take exercise nor attend to business. He who without heartburn eructates undigested food should drink cold water at intervals and none the less exercise self-control.

He can tell that his body is sound, if his morning urine is whitish, later reddish; the former indicates that digestion is going on, the latter that digestion is complete. On waking one should lie still for a while, then, except in winter time, bathe the face freely with cold water; when the days are long the siesta should be taken before the midday meal, when short, after it. In winter, it is best to rest in bed the whole night long; if there must be study by lamp-light, it should not be immediately after taking food, but after digestion. He who has been engaged in the day, whether in domestic or on public affairs, ought to keep some portion of the day for the care of the body. The primary care in this respect is exercise, which should always precede the taking of food; the exercise should be ampler in the case of one who has labored less and digested well; it should be lighter in the case of one who is fatigued and has digested less well.

Celsus continues with contemporary-sounding advice about exercise and eating.

Useful exercises are: reading aloud, drill, hand-ball, running, walking; but this is not by any means most useful on the level, since walking up and down hill varies the movement of the body, unless indeed the body is thoroughly weak; but it is better to walk in the open air than under cover; better, when the head allows of it, in the sun than in the shade; better under the shade of a wall or of trees than under a roof; better a straight than a winding walk. But the exercise ought to come to an end with sweating, or at any rate lassitude, which should be well this side of fatigue; and sometimes less, sometimes more, is to be done. But in these matters, as before, the example of athletes should not be followed, with their fixed rules and immoderate labor. The proper sequel to exercise is: at times an anointing, whether in the sun or before a brazier; at times a bath, which should be in a chamber as lofty, well lighted and spacious as possible. However, neither should be made use of invariably, but one of the two the oftener, in accordance with the constitution. There is need of a short rest afterwards.

Coming to food, a surfeit is never of service, excessive abstinence is often unserviceable; if any intemperance is committed, it is safer in drinking than in eating. It is better to begin a meal with savouries, salads and such-like; and after that meat is to be eaten, best either when roasted or boiled. All preserved fruits are unserviceable for two reasons, because more is taken owing to their sweetness, and even what is moderate is still digested with some difficulty. Dessert does no harm to a good stomach, in a weak one it turns sour. Whoever then in this respect has too little strength, had better eat dates, apples and such-like at the beginning of the meal. After many drinkings which have somewhat exceeded the demands of thirst, nothing should be eaten; after a surfeit, of food there should be no exertion. Anyone who has had his fill digests the more readily if he concludes the meal with a drink of cold water, then after keeping awake for time has a sound sleep. When a full meal is taken midday, after it there should be no exposure to cold, heat or fatigue, which do not harm the body so easily when it is empty as when it is full. When from whatever causes there is prospective want of food, everything laborious should be avoided.

Celsus discusses remedies for gastrointestinal distress. He also warns that purging and vomiting endanger the thin or infirm, the precursor of modern concerns about anorexia nervosa and bulimia nervosa.

But as I have mentioned, a vomit and a purge among thinning measures, there are some things to be said in particular concerning them. ... A vomit is more advantageous in winter than in summer, for then more phlegm and severer stuffiness in the head occur. It is unsuitable for the thin and for those with a weak stomach, but suitable for the plethoric, and all who become bilious, whether after overeating or imperfect digestion. For if the meal has been larger than can be digested, it is not well to risk its corruption; and if it has already become corrupted, nothing is more to the purpose than to eject it by whatever way its expulsion is first possible. When, therefore, there are bitter eructations, with pain and weight over the heart, recourse should be had at once to a vomit, which is likewise of service to anyone who has a heartburn and copious salivation or nausea, or ringing in the ears or watering of the eyes, or a bitter taste in the mouth. ... No one who wants to keep well, and live to old age, should make it a daily habit. He who after a meal wants to vomit, if he does so easily should first take tepid water by itself; when there is more difficulty, a little salt or honey should be added. To cause a vomit on getting up in the morning, he should first drink some honey or hyssop in wine, or eat a radish, and after that drink tepid water as described above. The other emetics prescribed by the ancient practitioners all disturb the stomach. After a vomit, when the stomach is weak, a little suitable food should be taken, and for drink, unless the vomiting has made the throat raw, three cupfuls of cold water.

The second volume of *De Medicina*[15] describes various drugs. Celsus lists agglutinants for wounds, caustics of varying strengths, emollients, styptics, and substances to induce healing, relieve irritation, and encourage the growth of new "flesh." He also inventories prescriptions and their quantities, including anodynes, antidotes, draughts, dusting powders, gargles, liniments, ointments, pastils, pessaries, plasters, poultices, and pills.

Celsus summarized for his generation the wisdom of Hippocrates and Alexandrian physicians. *De Medicina* no doubt assisted Roman trainers to prescribe medications for their athletes, formulate diets, diagnose injuries, and treat ailments.[9] Although eminently practical in its day, Celsus' work went largely unnoticed until its rediscovery in 1478.

VI. RENAISSANCE PERIOD TO THE TWENTIETH CENTURY

New ideas formulated during the Renaissance exploded almost every idea inherited from antiquity. Johannes Gutenberg's (ca. 1400–1468 A.D.) printing press disseminated both classic and newly acquired knowledge. The common man could learn about local and world events. Education became more available because universities sprang up in such centers as Oxford, Cambridge, Cologne, Heidelberg, Prague, Paris, Angiers, Orleans, Vienna, Padua, Bologna, Siena, Naples, Pisa, Montpellier, Toulouse, Valencia, Lisbon, and Salamanca. Art broke with past forms emphasizing spatial perspective and realistic depictions of the human body.

Although the supernatural still influenced discussions of physical phenomena, many people turned from dogma to experimentation as a source of knowledge. For example, medicine had to confront the new diseases spread by commerce with distant lands. Plagues and epidemics decimated at least 25 million people throughout Europe in just 2 years (1348 to 1350). New towns and expanding populations in confined cities led to environmental pollution and pestilence, forcing authorities to cope with new problems of community sanitation and care for the sick and dying. Science had not yet solved the medical problems brought on by disease carriers such as insects or rats.

As populations multiplied throughout Europe and elsewhere, medical care became more important for all levels of society. But medical knowledge failed to keep pace with need. For roughly 12 centuries, little advance had been made over Greek and Roman medicine.[16] The writings of physicians like Celsus had either been lost or preserved only in the Arab world. Thanks to the prestige of classical authors, Hippocrates and Galen still dominated medical education until the end of the 15th century. Renaissance discoveries greatly modified their theories, however. New anatomists went beyond simplistic notions of four humors when they discovered the complexities of the circulatory, respiratory, and excretory mechanisms.

Once rediscovered, these new ideas caused turmoil. The Vatican seemed to ban human dissections with the papal bull (*De Sepulturis*) of Pope Boniface VIII (ca. 1300), but a number of medical schools continued to conduct them. This training helped physicians to solve legal questions about the circumstances of a person's death. In 1316, the first book of human anatomy, *Anathomia*, was published in Latin by Mondino de Luzzio (ca. 1275–1326), professor of anatomy at Bologna. He based his teaching on human cadavers, not Greek and Latin authorities or studies of animals. The 1513 edition of *Anathomia* presented the same drawing of the heart with three ventricles as the original edition, a tribute to his accuracy.

In the sections that follow, we briefly note key discoveries that bridged the years between the ancients and the early 20th century. These advances in medicine, physiology, metabolism, and nutrition form the historical base for a new field of Exercise Nutrition.

A. LEONARDO DA VINCI (1452–1519)

Da Vinci dissected cadavers at the hospital of Santa Maria Nuova in Florence and made detailed anatomical drawings. Accurate as the sketches were, they still preserved Galenic ideas. Although he never saw the pores in the septum of the heart, he included them, believing they existed because Galen had "seen" them. Da Vinci first accurately drew the heart's inner structures and constructed models of valvular function that showed how the blood passed in only one direction. This observation contradicted Galen's notion about the ebb and flow of blood between the heart's chambers. Because many of da Vinci's drawings were lost for nearly two centuries, they did not influence later anatomical research.

Da Vinci's work built upon and led to discoveries by two fellow artists. Leon Battista Alberti (1404–1472), an architect, perfected three-dimensional perspectives which influenced da Vinci's concepts of internal relationships. Da Vinci's drawings no doubt inspired the incomparable Flemish anatomist Andreas Vesalius (1514–1564). The three exemplary Renaissance anatomists empowered physiologists to understand the systems of the body with technical accuracy, not theoretical bias.

B. ALBRECHT DÜRER (1471–1528)

Dürer, a German contemporary of da Vinci, extended the Italian's concern for ideal dimensions as depicted in the famous "Quadrate Man" by illustrating age-related differences in body segment ratios. Dürer's work inspired Behnke[17] in the 1950s to quantify body proportions into reference standards to evaluate body composition in men and women.

C. MICHELANGELO BUONARROTI (1475–1564)

Michelangelo, like da Vinci, was a superb anatomist. Body segments appear in proper proportion in his accurate drawings. The famous "David" clearly shows veins, tendons, and muscles enclosing a realistic skeleton. Although frescos on the Sistine ceiling often exaggerate musculature, they still convey a scientist's vision of the human body.

D. ANDREAS VESALIUS (1514–1564)

Vesalius learned Galenic medicine in Paris, but, after making careful human dissections, rejected the Greek's ideas about bodily functions. At the start of his career, Vesalius authored books on anatomy, originally relying on Arabic texts, but then incorporating observations from his own dissections. His research culminated in the exquisitely illustrated text first published in Switzerland in 1543, *De Humani Corporis Fabrica* (*On the Fabric of the Human Body*). The same year, he published *Epitome*, a popular version of *De Fabrica* without Latin text.

Some physicians and clergymen became outraged, fearful that the new science was overturning Galen's time-honored speculations. Vesalius' treatise accurately rendered bones, muscles, nerves, internal organs, blood vessels, and the brain, but he differed from Galenic tradition by ignoring what he could not see.

Despite his attempt at accuracy, some of Vesalius' drawings contain curious inaccuracies. For example, he drew the inferior vena cava as a continuous vessel; he inserted an extra muscle to move the eyeball; and he added an extra neck muscle, present only in apes. Despite these minor discrepancies, Vesalius attempted to connect form with function. He showed that a muscle contracted when a longitudinal slice was made along the muscle's belly, but a transverse cut prevented contraction. Vesalius substantiated that nerves controlled muscles and stimulated movement.

Vesalius' two texts profoundly influenced medical education. They demolished traditional theories about human anatomy and emboldened later researchers to explore circulation and metabolism unburdened by past misconceptions. The illuminating work of Vesalius hastened the next important discovery in physiology.

E. SANTORIO SANTORIO (1561–1636)

A friend of Galileo and professor of medicine at Padua, Santorio used innovative mechanisms for his research. He recorded changes in daily body temperature with the first air thermometer. He also measured pulse rates with Galileo's pulsilogium (pulsiometer). Ever inventive, Santorio studied digestion by constructing a wooden frame that supported a chair, bed, and work table. Suspended from the ceiling with scales, the frame recorded changes in weight.

For 30 years, Santorio slept, ate, worked, and made love in the weighing contraption to record how much his weight changed as he ate, fasted, or excreted. He invented the term "insensible perspiration" to account for differences in body weight because he believed that weight was gained or lost through the pores or during respiration. Often depriving himself of food and drink, Santorio determined that the daily change in body mass approached 1.25 kg. Santorio's book of medical aphorisms, *De Medicina Statica Aphorismi* (1614), drew worldwide attention (J. Davis made the first English translation, followed in 1712 by John Quincy's).[16] Although he did not explain the role of nutrition in weight gain or loss, Santorio nevertheless inspired later researchers in metabolism, especially during the eighteenth century.

F. WILLIAM HARVEY (1578–1657)

Harvey discovered that blood circulates continuously in one direction and, like Vesalius, overthrew 2000 years of medical dogma. Animal vivisection disproved the ancient supposition that blood moved from the right to left side of the heart through pores in the septum — pores that even da Vinci and Vesalius acknowledged. Harvey announced his discovery during a three-day dissection-lecture at the Royal College of Physicians in London on April 16, 1616. Twelve years later, he published the details in a 72 page monograph, *Exercitatio Anatomica de Motu Cordis et Sanguinis in Animalibus* (*An Anatomical Treatise on the Movement of the Heart and Blood in Animals*).

By combining the new technique of experimentation on living creatures with mathematical logic, Harvey deduced that, contrary to received standard opinion, blood flowed in only one direction — from the heart to the arteries and from the veins back to the heart. It then traversed to the lungs before completing a circuit and re-entering the heart. Harvey publicly demonstrated the one-way flow of blood by placing a tourniquet around a man's upper arm that constricted arterial blood flow to the forearm and stopped the pulse. By loosening the tourniquet, Harvey allowed some blood into the veins. Applying pressure to specific veins forced blood from a peripheral segment where there was little pressure into the previously empty veins. Thus, Harvey proved that the heart pumped blood through a closed, unidirectional system, from arteries to veins and back to the heart. As he put it,

> It is proved by the structure of the heart that the blood is continuously transferred through the lungs into the aorta as by two clacks of a water bellows to raise water. It is proved by a ligature that there is a passage of blood from the arteries to the veins. It is therefore demonstrated that the continuous movement of the blood in a circle is brought about by the beat of the heart.[9]

Harvey's experiments with sheep proved mathematically that the mass of blood passing through the sheep's heart in a fixed time was greater than the body could produce, a conclusion identical to that concerning the human heart. Harvey reasoned that if a constant mass of blood exists, then the large circulation volumes would require a one-way, closed circulatory system. Harvey did not explain why the blood circulated, only that it did. However, he correctly postulated that circulation might distribute heat and nourishment throughout the body.

Despite the validity of Harvey's observations, distinguished scientists criticized them. Jean Riolan, an ardent Galenist who chaired the anatomy and botany departments at the University of Paris in the 1640s, maintained that if anatomical findings differed from Galen's, then the body in question must be abnormal and the results faulty.[18] Nevertheless, Harvey's discovery governed subsequent research on circulation.

G.   GIOVANNI ALFONSO BORELLI (1608–1679)

Borelli, a protégé of Galileo and mathematician at the University of Pisa, used mathematical models to explain how muscles enabled animals to walk, fish to swim, and birds to fly. His ideas explaining how air entered and exited the lungs, though equally important, were less well known. Borelli's accomplished student, Marcello Malpighi (1628–1694), described how he had observed blood flowing through microscopic structures (capillaries) around the lung's terminal air sacs (alveoli). Borelli observed that lungs filled with air because chest volume increased as the diaphragm moved downward. He concluded that air passed through the alveoli and into the blood, a sharp contrast to Galen's notion that air in the lungs cooled the heart and an advance on Harvey's general observation concerning blood flow.

H.   ROBERT BOYLE (1627–1691)

Working at Gresham College, London, with his student Robert Hooke (1635–1703), Boyle devised experiments with a vacuum pump and bell jar to show that combustion and respiration required air. Boyle partially evacuated air from the jar containing a lit candle. The flame soon died. When he removed air from a jar containing a rodent or bird, it became unconscious; recirculating air back into the jar often revived the animal. Compressing the air produced the same results; animals and flames lived longer.

Boyle removed the diaphragm and ribs from a living dog and forced air into the lungs with a bellows. Although the experiment did not prove that air was essential for life, it demonstrated that air pressure alternately contracted and expanded the lungs. He repeated the experiment, this time pricking the lungs so air could escape.[9] Boyle kept the animal alive by forcing air into its lungs, proving that chest movement maintained air flow and disproving the earlier assertion that lungs effected circulation.

Scientific societies and journals broadcast these discoveries. Boyle belonged to the Royal Society of London which Charles II had chartered in 1662. Four years later in France, Louis XIV sponsored the Académie Royale des Sciences so its salaried members could conduct a variety of studies. Both societies established journals (*Philosophical Transactions of the Royal Society* and *Journal des Scavans*) to disseminate information in chemistry, physics, medicine, nutrition, and metabolism to scientists and an educated lay public.

I. STEPHEN HALES (1677–1761)

A renowned English plant physiologist and Fellow of the Royal Society, Hales amassed facts from his experiments with animals about blood pressure, the heart's capacity, and velocity of blood flow. His *Vegetable Statics: Or, an Account of Some Statical Experiments on the Sap in Vegetables...Also, a Specimen of an attempt to Analyze the Air* (1727) contains a section titled *Haemastaticks*. Guerlac[19] describes Hales' experiments:

> He tied a live mare on her back and ligating one of her femoral arteries, inserted a brass cannula; to this he fixed a glass tube nine feet high; when he untied the ligature, the blood rose to the height of more than eight feet. Detaching the tube at intervals, he allowed a measured quantity of blood to flow out, noting how the pressure changed during exsanguination. He succeeded in recording, by the same method, the venous pressure of a number of animals including an ox, a sheep, a fallow doe, three horses, and several dogs. ... His interest in the mechanics of the circulation now enhanced, Hales turned his attention to the chief factors that must maintain the blood pressure: the output of the heart per minute and the peripheral resistance in the small vessels. He made a rough estimate of cardiac output by multiplying the pulse rate of an animal by the internal volume of its left ventricle, of which he made a cast in wax after the animal had been killed. He noted that the pulse was faster in smaller animals than in large ones, and that the blood pressure was proportional to the size of the animals. ... Hales next studied peripheral resistance with perfusion experiments. Injecting various chemical substances (brandy, decoction of the Peruvian bark, various saline solutions), he compared the rate of flow of the perfusate and showed that certain substances had a pronounced effect on the rate at which the blood could flow through an isolated organ. He attributed this to changes in the diameter of the capillaries and so — although he did not observe the phenomenon directly — discovered vasodilatation and vasoconstriction.

Hales also analyzed air. *Vegetable Staticks* tells how water absorbed air when phosphorus and melted brimstone (sulfur) burned in a closed glass vessel. Hales measured the volume of air released or absorbed and demonstrated that air was a constituent of many common substances. His experiments proved that chemical changes occurred in solids and liquids upon calcination (oxidation during combustion).

In addition, Hales developed an idea suggested by Newton in 1713 and provided the first experimental evidence that the nervous system played a role in muscular contraction.[19]

Hales' experiments, translated into French, Dutch, German, and Italian, influenced chemists. Lavoisier may have read a French version of Hales' book,[19] thus becoming familiar with the works of Black, Priestley, and Cavendish. The work of these chemists was summarized at length in Lavoisier's first important book, *Opuscles Physiques et Chemiques* (1774).

J. JAMES LIND (1716–1794)

Trained in Edinburgh, Lind entered the British Navy as a surgeon's mate in 1739. During an extended trip on the *Salisbury* (1747), Lind carried out a decisive experiment that changed the course of naval medicine. He knew that scurvy ("the great sea plague") often killed two-thirds of a ship's crew. Their diet included 1 lb. (0.45 kg) and 4 oz. (113.4 g) of cheese bisquits daily, 2 lb. (0.90 kg) salt beef twice weekly, 2 oz. (56.7 g) dried fish and butter three times weekly, 8 oz. (226.8 g) peas four days a week, and one gallon (3.79 l) of beer daily. Deprived of vitamin C, sailors fell prey to scurvy. By adding fresh fruit to their diet, Lind fortified their immune systems so that British sailors no longer perished. Krehl[20] quotes from Lind's *Treatise on the Scurvy* (1753):

> On the 20th of May, 1747, I selected 12 patients in the scurvy, on board the Salisbury at sea. Their cases were as similar as I could have them. They all in general had putrid gums, the spots and lassitude, with weakness of their knees. They lay together in one place, being a proper

apartment for the sick in the fore-hold: and had one diet common to all, viz, water-gruel sweetened with sugar in the morning; fresh mutton-broth oftentimes for dinner; at other times light puddings, boiled biscuit with sugar, etc., and for supper, barley and raisins, rice and currants, sago and wine, or the like. Two of these were ordered each a quart of cyder a day. Two other took 25 drops of elixer of vitriol 3 times a day, upon an empty stomach; using a gargle strongly acidulated with it for their mouths. Two others took 2 spoonfuls of vinegar 3 times a day, upon an empty stomach; having their gruels and their other food sharpened with vinegar, as also the gargle for their mouth. Two of the worst patients, with the tendons in the ham quite rigid (a symptom none of the rest had) were put under a course of sea water. Of this they drank half a pint every day, and sometimes more or less, as it operated, by way of gentle physic. Two others had each two oranges and one lemon given them every day. These they ate with greediness, at different times, upon an empty stomach. They continued but six days under this course, having consumed the quantities that could be spared. The 2 remaining patients took the bigness of a nutmeg 3 times a day, or an electary recommended by an hospital-surgeon, made of garlic, mustard-seed, horse-radish, balsam of Peru, and gum myrh; using for common drink barley-water boiled with tamarinds; by which, with the addition of cream of tartar, they were gently purged 3 or 4 times during the course.

The consequence was, that the most sudden and visible good effects were perceived from the use of oranges and lemons; one of those who had taken them, being at the end of 6 days fit for duty. The spots were not indeed at that time quite off his body, nor his gums sound; but without any other medicine than a gargle for his mouth he became quite healthy before we came into Plymouth which was on the 16th of June. The other was the best recovered in his condition; and being now pretty well, was appointed nurse to the rest of the sick.

Next to oranges, I thought the cyder had the best effects. It was indeed not very sound. However, those who had taken it, were in a fairer way of recovery than the others at the end of the fortnight, which was the length of time all these different courses were continued, except the oranges. The putrification of their gums, but especially their lassitude and weakness, were somewhat abated, and their appetite increased by it.

An early innovator in "food technology," Lind obtained pure drinking water from the condensate in steam during cooking with sea water. He also described how to preserve citrus juice.

Let the squeezed juice of these fruits be well cleared from the pulp and depurated by standing for some time; then poured off from the gross sediment; or, to have it stay purer, it may be filtered. Let it them be put into any clean oven vessel of china or stoneware which should be wider at the top than at the bottom. so that there may be the largest surface above to favor the evaporation. ... Into this pour the purified juice: and put it into a pan of water come almost to a boil and continue nearly in the state of boiling ... until the juice is found to be the consistency of a thick syrup when cold. ... It is then when cold, to be corked up in a bottle for use. Two dozen of good oranges weighing 5 pounds 4 ounces, will yield 1 pound 9 ounces and a half of depurated juice; and when evaporated there will remain about 5 ounces of the rob or extract; which in bulk will be equal to less than 3 ounces of water. So that thus the acid, the virtues of 12 dozens of lemons or oranges, may be put into a quart bottle, and preserved for several years.

Lind published two books: *An Essay on Preserving the Health of Seamen in the Royal Navy* (1757) and *Essay on Diseases Incidental to Europeans in Hot Climates* (1768). Easily available, his books were translated into German, French, and Dutch. Lind's landmark emphasis on the crucial importance of dietary supplements antedates modern practices. Despite the efficacy of the remedy, 50 years had to pass before the British Admiralty required fresh citrus fruit on all ships, another sad example of damage done when politics neglects science.

K. JOSEPH BLACK (1728–1799)

After graduating from the medical school in Edinburgh, Black became professor of chemistry at Glasgow. *Experiments Upon Magnesia Alba, Quicklime, And Some Other Alcaline Substances* (1756) determined that air contained carbon dioxide gas.[6] He observed that carbonate (lime) lost half its weight after burning. Black reasoned that removing air from lime treated with acids produced a new substance he named "fixed air," or carbon dioxide ($CaCO_3 = CaO + CO_2$). Black's discovery that gas existed either free or combined with other substances encouraged later experiments on the chemical composition of gases.

L. JOSEPH PRIESTLEY (1733–1804)

Although Priestley discovered oxygen by heating red oxide of mercury in a closed vessel, he stubbornly clung to the phlogiston theory which misled other scientists. Dismissing Lavoisier's (1743–1794) proof that respiration produced carbon dioxide and water, Priestley continued to believe in an immaterial constituent (phlogiston) that supposedly escaped from burning substances. He told the Royal Society about oxygen in 1772 and published *Observations on Different Kinds of Air* in 1773. Priestley recounts:[19]

> ... I proceeded to examine, by the help of it (as a burning glass), what kind of air a variety of substances, natural and factitious, would yield. ... But what surprised me more than I can well express, was a candle burns in this air with more splendour and heat...than in the other airs. ... Who can tell, but that, in time, this pure air may become a fashionable article in luxury. Hitherto only two mice and myself have had the privilege of breathing it.

Elated by his discovery, Priestley failed to grasp two facts that later research confirmed: a body needs oxygen, and respiration produces carbon dioxide.

M. CARL WILHELM SCHEELE (1742–1786)

In one of history's coincidences, Scheele, a Swedish pharmacist, discovered oxygen independently of Priestley. Scheele noted that heating mercuric oxide released "fire-air" (oxygen), and burning other substances in fire-air produced violent reactions. When different mixtures contacted air inside a sealed container, the air volume decreased by 25% and could not support combustion. Scheele named the gas that extinguished fire "foul air." In a memorable experiment, he added two bees to a glass jar immersed in limewater containing fire-air. After a few days, the bees remained alive but the level of limewater had risen in the bottle and became cloudy. Scheele concluded that fixed air replaced the fire-air to sustain the bees. At the end of eight days, however, the bees died despite ample honey inside the container. Scheele blamed their demise on phlogiston, which he felt was hostile to life. What Scheele called foul-air (phlogisticated air in Priestley's day) was later identified as nitrogen.

Scheele, like Priestley, refused to accept Lavoisier's explanations about respiration. In 1783, Scheele wrote:

> Is it impossible to convince Lavoisier that his system will not find universal acceptance? The idea of nitric acid from nitrous air and pure air, of carbonic acid from carbon and pure air, of sulphuric acid from sulphur and pure air, of lactic acid from sugar and pure air! Can one believe such things?[22]

Although Scheele adhered to the phlogiston theory, he discovered, in addition to oxygen, chlorine, manganese, silicon, glycerol, silicon tetrafluoride, hydrofluoric acid, and copper arsenite (known as Scheele's green).[22]

N. HENRY CAVENDISH (1731–1810)

Cavendish and his contemporaries, Black and Priestley, began to identify the constituents of carbohydrates, lipids, and proteins. *On Factitious Air* (1766) describes a highly flammable substance, later identified as hydrogen, that was liberated when acids combined with metals. *Experiments in Air* (1784) showed that "inflammable air" (hydrogen) combined with "deflogisticated air" (oxygen) produced water.

O. ANTOINE LAURENT LAVOISIER (1743–1794)

Lavoisier ushered in modern concepts in metabolism, nutrition, and exercise physiology. More has been written about Lavoisier than of his worthy contemporaries, Black, Priestley, Cavendish, and Hales[21] for one simple reason: his discoveries in respiration chemistry and human nutrition were as essential as William Harvey's were to circulatory physiology and medicine. A Paris monument summarizes Lavoisier's contributions:

> Analysis and Synthesis of Air — Composition of Oxides and Acids — Composition of Water — Theory of Combustion — Respiration and Animal Heat — Permanence of Weight of Matter and Simple Substances — Imponderable Nature of Heat and Its Role in Chemistry

The accomplishments most germane to Exercise Nutrition pertain to respiratory chemistry and exercise metabolism. Lavoisier knew of Scheele's experiment with bees from correspondence in 1774. Three years later, Lavoisier used accurate balance scales* to determine what Scheele, Priestly, and others could not explain: an animal in a closed chamber consumed "air eminently respirable" (oxygéne) and produced "aëriform calcic acid" (carbon dioxide). Lavoisier noted:[22]

> ... that if after an animal had perished in a confined space and the carbon dioxide in the atmosphere was absorbed by alkali the "foul air" remaining was the same kind of air as that found after metals had been calcined in air in an inclosed space. All the former qualities of this air could be restored by adding to it "air eminently respirable."

Lavoisier's respiration experiments invalidated the phlogiston theory despite protestations from Priestley and Scheele. Lavoisier collaborated with French mathematician Pierre Simon de Laplace (1749–1827) on problems in respiration chemistry. Their vital experiments with guinea pigs in 1780 first quantified the oxygen consumed and carbon dioxide produced by metabolism. Over a ten-hour period, they collected approximately 3.33 g of carbonic acid from an animal breathing oxygen. In a second experiment, they placed a guinea pig into a wire cage, which in turn was placed into a double-walled container. Ice packed into the double walls of the outer container maintained a constant temperature; ice between the cage and the inner wall of the container melted because of the animal's body heat. During 24 hours, 13 oz. (368.6 g) of ice melted. Lavoisier and Laplace concluded that the total heat produced by the animal equaled the amount of heat required to melt ice. In their own words:**

> Thus, one can look at heat produced during respiration by the transformation of humid air into dry air, as the principle cause of animal heat conservation and if other causes intervene, their effect is negligible.

---

* A collection of Lavoisier's instruments are in the *Conservatoire des Arts et Métiers* in Paris. One of the balances could weigh 600 mg to ±5 mg, and another was accurate to the nearest ±0.1 mg.

** Translation provided by Pierre P. Lagasse, Ph.D., Division of Kinesiology, Department of Social and Preventive Medicine, University of Laval, Québec, Canada.

Respiration is thus a very slow combustion phenomenon, very similar to that of coal; it is conducted inside the lungs, not giving off light, since the fire matter is absorbed by the humidity of the organs of the lungs. Heat developed by this combustion goes into the blood vessels which pass through the lungs and which subsequently flow into the entire animal body. Thus, air that we breathe is used to conserve our bodies in two fashions: it removes from the blood fixed air, which can be very harmful when abundant; and heat which enters our lungs from this phenomenon replaces the heat lost in the atmosphere and from surrounding bodies.

… animal heat conservation is thus largely attributable to heat produced by the combination of humid air inspired by the animals and dry air in the blood vessels.

With his colleague, the chemist Armand Séguin (1767–1835), Lavoisier studied the influence of muscular work on metabolism. A contemporary painting shows the seated Séguin as he depresses a pedal while a copper mask captures the expired air. A physician takes Séguin's pulse to determine the separate effects of exercise and food consumption. (For several hours before the experiment, Séguin had abstained from food.) Resting energy metabolism without food in a cold environment increased by 10%; it increased 50% due solely to food; 200% with exercise; and 300% by combining food intake with exercise.

Lavoisier and Séguin also observed that oxygen consumption, pulse rate, and respiratory rate increased during work.

Consequently, from the experiments conducted on Mr. Séguin, it results that a fasted man in a state of rest and in 26 degrees of temperature, divided into 80 parts, consumes 1210 cubic inches (24.002 litres) of vital air; it also results that this consumption increases in a cold environment and that the same man, fasted and resting, in 12 degrees of temperature, consumes 1344 cubic inches (26.600 litres) of vital air.

During digestion, this process is increased to 1,800 or 1,900 cubic inches (37.689 litres). All these values are increased during movement and exercise. Mr. Séguin, fasted and carrying a weight of 15 pounds (7.343 kg) on a distance of 613 feet (199.776 metres), consumed 800 cubic inches of air, e.g., 3200 cubic inches (63.477 litres) per hour.

Lastly, when the same exercise was done during digestion, the quantity of vital air consumed reached a value of 4600 cubic inches (91.248 litres). The exercise performed by Mr. Séguin involved carrying a 15 pound weight (7.343 kg) over a distance of 650 feet (211.146 metres) during 15 minutes.[22]

Lavoisier and Séguin connected two essential components of physiology — external respiration and internal combustion (heat production). This linkage proved that oxidative processes (combustion) were affected not only by food intake, but also by temperature and mechanical work. Atmospheric air provided oxygen for animal respiration. Furthermore, the "caloric" (now known as heat) was liberated in metabolism. Formerly, a "vital flame" was said to burn within the heart itself; now respiration, the "substance of the animal itself," provided the necessary ingredients for combustion.

In 1837, the German physiologist Heinrich Gustave Magnus (1802–1870) first analyzed blood and corrected one flaw in Lavoisier's explanation. The Frenchman assumed that hydrogen and carbon were oxygenated in the lungs. Magnus argued that combustion must occur throughout the body and not just in the lungs. His famous experiments showed that both carbon dioxide and oxygen existed in arterial and venous blood. Because there was more oxygen in arterial blood, Magnus deduced that the lungs could not be the primary site of combustion.

In addition to studying respiration, Lavoisier conducted research in nutrition.[23] Already knowing that animal tissues contained nitrogen, he investigated the composition of isolated plant fractions and concluded that combinations of carbon, hydrogen, and oxygen alone constituted sugars, gums, and starches.

Noting that France's food supplies were becoming depleted, Lavoisier reported in 1778 to the Academy of Sciences on practical methods to measure wheat and flour. He wrote:

> It has to be accepted that other grains such as barley and oats, which do not contain gluten, are also nutritious. Starch must therefore be nutritious, but Parmentier seems to us to go too far in singling out starch as the only nutritive element in wheat. It seems obvious that gluten, with its chemical properties, is more "animalized" and therefore eminently nutritive.

Lavoisier paved the way for future studies of energy balance by recognizing for the first time that the elements involved in metabolism (carbon, hydrogen, nitrogen, and oxygen) appeared neither suddenly nor disappeared mysteriously. Rather, they reconfigured themselves in a predictable sequence during combustion. He supplied basic truths: only oxygen participates in animal respiration, and the "caloric" liberated during respiration is itself the source of the combustion.

These discoveries, fundamental to modern concepts of energy balance, could not protect Lavoisier from the intolerance of his revolutionary countrymen. He was beheaded by the Jacobin tribunal in 1794. Yet once more, thoughtless resistance to innovative science temporarily delayed the triumph of truth.

P.   LAZZARO SPALLANZANI (1729–1799)

An accomplished Italian physiologist, Spallanzani debunked spontaneous generation and studied fertilization and contraception in animals. In a famous study of digestion, he refined regurgitation experiments similar to those of the French scientist, René-Antoine Fercault de Réaumur (1683–1757), again demonstrating the international interest in physiology. Réaumur's *Digestion in Birds* (1752) told how he recovered partially digested food from the gizzard of a kite. Spallanzani swallowed a sponge tied to the end of a string and then regurgitated it. He found that the sponge had absorbed a substance that dissolved bread and various animal tissues, thus indirectly observing how gastric juices function. His animal experiments showed that the tissues of the heart, stomach, and liver consume oxygen and liberate carbon dioxide, even in creatures without lungs.

Spallanzani's idea that respiration and combustion took place within the tissues was novel and appeared posthumously in 1804. A century later this phenomenon would be called internal respiration.

VII.   NINETEENTH CENTURY METABOLISM AND PHYSIOLOGY

The untimely death of Lavoisier did not terminate fruitful research in nutrition and medicine. During the next half century, scientists discovered the chemical composition of carbohydrates, lipids, and proteins and further clarified the energy balance equation.

A.   CLAUDE LOUIS BERTHOLLET (1748–1822)

A French chemist and contemporary of Lavoisier, Berthollet identified the "volatile substances" associated with animal tissues. One of these "substances," nitrogen, was produced when ammonia gas burned in oxygen. Berthollet showed that normal tissues did not contain ammonia. He believed that hydrogen united with nitrogen during fermentation to produce ammonia.[23] In 1865, Berthollet took exception to Lavoisier's ideas concerning the amount of heat liberated when the body oxidized an equal weight of carbohydrate or fat. According to Berthollet, "the quantity of heat liberated in the incomplete oxidation of a substance is equal to the difference between the total caloric value of the substance and that of the products formed."[23] Barthollet was so highly regarded as a chemist that during the winter of 1797, Napoleon attended his lectures and invited him to tour Egypt with other distinguished scientists.

B. JOSEPH LOUIS PROUST (1755–1826)

Proust proved that a pure substance isolated in the laboratory or found in nature would always contain the same elements in the same proportions. Known as the "Law of Definite Proportions," Proust's ideas about the chemical constancy of substances provided an important milestone for future nutritional explorers, helping them analyze the major nutrients and calculate energy metabolism as measured by oxygen consumption.

C. HUMPHREY DAVEY (1778–1829)

Best known for his pioneering work in electrochemistry, Davey contributed to nutritional chemistry by experimenting with oxygen and blood. In 1799, he obtained arterial blood from the carotid artery of a calf and then heated it. Oxygen escaped from the blood before it completely coagulated and turned black. Heating the venous blood also formed carbon dioxide. Davey concluded that oxygen, in combination with heat and light, formed a new compound he called "phosoxygen." He believed venous blood absorbed phosoxygen in the absence of light, changing color from dark red to bright vermillion.[22] Davey also proved that the oxides of new metals he had isolated (magnesium, potassium, calcium, barium, strontium, boron, silicon, and sodium) were alkalis. In 1810, Davey refined Lavoisier's belief that oxygen constituted all acids. *Elements of Agricultural Chemistry* (1813) consolidated for the first time all of the chemical data related to nutrition. In addition he coined the term *element*. Davey used electricity to dissolve alkaline and alkali substances, isolating 47 elements which he defined:

> All the varieties of material substances may be resolved into a comparatively small number of bodies, which, as they are not capable of being decomposed, are considered in the present state of chemical knowledge as *elements*.[6]

D. LOUIS-JOSEPH GAY-LUSSAC (1778–1850)

In 1810, Gay-Lussac, a pupil of Berthollet, analyzed the chemical composition of 20 animal and vegetable substances. He placed the vegetable substances into one of three categories depending on their proportion of hydrogen to oxygen atoms. One class of compounds — called saccharine (later identified as carbohydrate) — was accepted by Prout (1785–1850) in his classification of the three basic macronutrients.[24]

E. WILLIAM PROUT (1785–1850)

Following up the studies of Lavoisier and Séguin on muscular activity and respiration, the Englishman Prout measured the carbon dioxide exhaled by men exercising to fatigue (*Annals of Philosophy*, 2, 328, 1813). Moderate exercise such as walking raised carbon dioxide to a plateau. This observation heralded the modern concept of steady-state gas exchange kinetics in exercise. Although Prout could not determine the exact amount of carbon dioxide respired because there were no instruments to measure respiratory rate, he nevertheless observed that carbon dioxide in expired air reduced dramatically during fatiguing exercise.*

Prout extolled milk as the perfect food in *Treatise on Chemistry, Meteorology, and the Function of Digestion* (1834) because

> ... even in the utmost refinements of his luxury, and in his choicest delicacies, the same great principle is attended to; and his sugar and flour, his eggs and butter, in all their various forms and combinations, are nothing more or less, than disguised imitations of the great alimentary prototype MILK, as furnished to him by nature.

F. FRANÇOIS MAGENDIE (1783–1855)

In 1821, Magendie founded the first journal for the study of experimental physiology (*Journal de Physiologie Expérimentale*), a field he literally created. The next year, he showed that anterior spinal nerve roots control motor activities, while posterior roots control sensory functions.

Magendie's accomplishments, however, were not limited to neural physiology. He had a strong interest in experimental pharmacology. His first publication in 1809 dealt with the properties of strychnine; he later studied morphine, iodides, and bromides. As early as 1816 his *Précis élémentaire de Physiologie* categorized foods into nitrogenous and non-nitrogenous. Unlike others who claimed that the tissues derived their nitrogen from the air, Magendie argued that food provided the nitrogen. To prove his point, he studied animals subsisting on nitrogen-free diets. Magendie described his 1836 experiment:[27]

> ... I took a dog of three years old, fat, and in good health, and put it to feed upon sugar alone, and gave it distilled water to drink: it had as much as it chose of both. ... It appeared to thrive very well in this way of living the first 7 or 8 days; it was brisk, active, ate eagerly, and drank in its usual manner. It began to get meagre upon the second week, though it had always a good appetite, and took about 6 or 8 ounces of sugar in 24 hours. ... In the third week its leanness increased, its strength diminished, the animal lost its liveliness, and its appetite was much lessened. At this period there was developed, first upon one eye, and then upon the other, a small ulceration in the center of the transparent cornea; it increased very quickly, and in a few days it was more than a line in diameter; its depth increased in the same proportion; the cornea was very soon entirely perforated, and the humours of the eye ran out. This singular phenomenon was accompanied with an abundant secretion of the glands of the eyelids.

> It, however, became weaker and weaker, and lost its strength; and though the animal took from 3 to 4 ounces of sugar every day, it became at length so weak that it could neither chew nor swallow; for the same reason every other motion was impossible. It expired the 32nd day of the experiment. I opened it with every suitable precaution; I found a total want of fat; the muscles were reduced by more than five-sixths of their ordinary size; the stomach and the intestines were also much diminished in volume, and strongly contracted.

---

* In addition to Prout, other scientists investigated the relation between nutrient-energy metabolism and muscular work. Benedict and Cathcart[25] point out that beginning about 1850 (following the classic calorimetric work of Despretz and Dulong in France in 1822), German and French scientists like Vierordt, Valentin, Doyère, Apjohn, Menzies, Berthollet, Fyfe, Hirn, Jurine, Meyer, and Scharling studied muscular work. They preceded Liebig, Pettenkoffer, and Voit. Guggenheim[34] mentions the work of J. Pereira (1804–1853), who advocated a well-balanced diet to promote good health. Cathcart's 1912 book[26] about the physiology of protein metabolism includes 430 citations, mostly to the German literature through 1910, dealing with topics related to metabolism.

The excrements, that were also examined by M. Chevreul, contained very little azote (nitrogen), whilst they generally present a great deal. ... A third experiment produced similar results, and thence I considered sugar incapable of supporting dogs of itself.

Magendie's *Précis* advocated good nutrition for society's well being.[27]

The useful object of cookery is to render aliments agreeable to the senses, and of easy digestion; but it rarely stops here: frequently with people advanced in civilization its object is to excite delicate palates, or difficult tastes, or to gratify vanity. Then, far from being a useful art, it indeed exerts a great social influence, and contributes somewhat to the comfort and improvement of society; but oftener becomes a real scourge, which occasions a great number of diseases, and has frequently brought premature death.

Lesch[28] spotlights Magendie's centrality as the one who demonstrated that experimental physiology is a science. For example, he taught Claude Bernard (1813–1878), perhaps the greatest physiologist of the 19th century.

G. WILLIAM BEAUMONT (1785–1853)

One of the most fortuitous experiments in medicine began on June 6, 1822 at Fort Mackinac on the upper Michigan peninsula. As fort surgeon, Beaumont tended the accidental shotgun wound that perforated the abdominal wall and stomach of an 18-year-old French Canadian, Alexis St. Martin, a voyageur for the American Fur Company. The wound healed after 10 months, but continued to provide new insights concerning digestion. Part of the wound formed a small natural "valve" that led directly into the stomach. Beaumont turned St. Martin on his left side, depressing the valve, and then inserted a tube the size of a large quill five or six inches into the stomach. He began two kinds of experiments on the digestive processes from 1825 to 1833. First, he observed the fluids discharged by the stomach when different foods were eaten (*in vivo*); second, he extracted samples of the stomach's content and put them into glass tubes to determine the time required for "external" digestion (*in vitro*).

Beaumont revolutionized concepts about digestion. For centuries, the stomach was thought to produce heat that somehow "cooked" foods. Alternatively, the stomach was imaged as a mill, a fermenting vat, or a stew pan.*

Beaumont published the first results of his experiments on St. Martin in the *Philadelphia Medical Recorder* for January, 1825, and full details in his *Experiments and Observations on the Gastric Juice and the Physiology of Digestion* (1833).[29] Beaumont ends his treatise with a list of 51 inferences based on his 238 separate experiments. Although working away from the centers of medicine, Beaumont used findings from Spallanzini, Carminiti, Viridet, Vauquelin, Tiedemann and Gmelin, Leuret and Lassaigne, Montegre, and Prout. Even with their information, he still obeyed the scientific method, basing all his inferences on direct experimentation.

With respect to the agent of chymification, that principle of life which converts the crude aliment into chyme, and renders it fit for the action of the hepatic and pancreatic fluids, and final assimilation and conversion into the fluids, and the various tissues of the animal organism — no part of physiology has, perhaps, so much engaged the attention of mankind, and exercised the ingenuity of physiologists. It has been a fruitful source of theoretical speculation, from the

---

* Jean Baptise van Helmont (1577–1644), a Flemish doctor, is credited with being first to prescribe an alkaline cure for indigestion.[21] Observing the innards of birds, he reasoned that acid in the digestive tract could not alone decompose meats and that other substances ("ferments") must break down food. Today we refer to the ferments as digestive enzymes.

father of medicine down to the present age. It would be a waste of time to attempt to refute the doctrines of the older writers on this subject. Suffice it to say, that the theories of Concoction, Putrefaction, Trituration, Fermentation and Maceration, have been prostrated in the dust before the lights of science, and the deductions of experiment.

I had opportunities for the examination of the interior of the stomach, and its secretions, which has never before been so fully offered to any one. This most important organ, its secretions and its operations, have been submitted to my observation in a very extraordinary manner, in a state of perfect health, and for years in succession. I have availed myself of the opportunity afforded by concurrence of circumstance which probably can never again occur, with a zeal and perseverance proceeding from motives which my conscience approves; and I now submit the result of my experiments to an enlightened public, who I doubt not will duly appreciate the truths discovered, and the confirmation of opinions which before rested on conjecture.

I submit a body of facts which cannot be invalidated. My opinions may be doubted, denied, or approved, according as they conflict or agree with the opinions of each individual who may read them; but their worth will be best determined by the foundation on which they rest — the incontrovertible facts.

Beaumont concluded:

I think I am warranted, from the result of all the experiments, in saying, that the gastric juice, so far from being "inert as water," as some authors assert, is the most general solvent in nature, of alimentary matter — even the hardest bone cannot withstand its action. It is capable, *even out of the stomach*, of effecting perfect digestion, with the aid of due and uniform degrees of heat, (100 Fahrenheit,).

The fact that alimentary matter is *transformed*, in the stomach, into chyme, is now pretty well conceded. ... Without pretending to explain the exact *modus operandi* of the gastric fluid, yet I am impelled by the weight of evidence, afforded by the experiments, deductions and opinions of the ablest physiologists, but more by direct experiment, to conclude that the change effected by it on aliment is *purely chemical*. We must, I think, regard this fluid as a chemical agent, and its operation as a chemical action.

The decay of the dead body is a chemical operation, separating it into its elementary principles — and why not the solution of aliment in the stomach, and its ultimate assimilation into fibrine, gelatine and albumen? Matter, in a natural sense, is indestructible. It may be differently combined; and these combinations are chemical changes. It is well known that all organic bodies are composed of very few simple principles, or substances, modified by excess or diminution of some of their constituents.

The gastric juice appears to be secreted from numberless vessels, distinct and separate from the mucous follicles. These vessels, when examined with a microscope, appear in the shape of small lucid points, or very fine papillae, situated in the interstices of the follicles. They discharge their fluid only when solicited to do so, by the presence of aliment, or by mechanical irritation.

Pure gastric juice, when taken directly out of the stomach of a healthy adult, unmixed with any other fluid, save a portion of the mucus of the stomach with which it is most commonly, and perhaps always combined, is a clear, transparent fluid; inodorous; a little saltish; and very perceptibly acid. Its taste, when applied to the tongue, is similar to thin mucilaginous water, slightly acidulated with muriatic acid. It is readily diffusible in water, wine or spirits; slightly effervesces with alkalis; and is an effectual solvent of the *materia alimentaria*. It possesses the property of coagulating albumen, in an eminent degree; is powerfully antiseptic, checking the putrefaction of meat; and effectually restorative of healthy action, when applied to old, fetid sores, and foul, ulcerating surfaces.

TABLE 1a Top Mean Time of Digestion of Different Foods
***In Vivo* (in the Stomach) and *In Vitro* (in Vials)**

| | Mean Time of Chymification | | | |
| | In Stomach | | In Vials | |
Articles of Diet	Preparation	h, min	Preparation	h, min
Tapioca	domestic	2 00	domestic	3 20
Milk	domestic	2 00	domestic	4 15
Gelatine	boiled	2 30	boiled	4 45
Brains, animal	domestic	1 45	domestic	4 30
Spinal marrow, animal	boiled	2 00	domestic	5 25
Codfish, cured dry	boiled	2 00	boiled	5 00
Trout, salmon, fresh	broiled	1 30	broiled	3 30
Beef, steak	broiled	3 00	chewed	8 15
Suet, beef, fresh	boiled	5 30	entire piece	12 00
Apple, sour hard	raw	2 50	entire piece	18 00

TABLE 1b Temperature of the Interior of the Stomach During
Different Seasons of the Year and at Various Times
of Day (5 PM to Midnight)

| | | | Empty | Chymification |
Date/Year	Wind/Weather	Time	Rest/Exer	Rest/Exer
Dec 6, 1829	S/Cloudy and damp	63	98	
Dec 4, 1832	NW/Snowing	35	—/101	
Jan 31, 1833	NE/Rainy	45	101.25/101.5	101.25/—
Feb 1, 1833	NW/Clear	28	101/—	—/102

From Beaumont, W., *Experiments and Observations on the Gastric Juice and the Physiology of Digestion*, 1833, reprint 1959, pp. 269–270, 273.

Table 1 reproduces Beaumont's data for the "time of Chymification" in both the stomach and in vials.

Beaumont's important experiments quickly reached an international audience. Within 15 years, Calvin Cutter's popular *Anatomy and Physiology Designed for Academies and Families* (1848)[30] included Beaumont's mean times for digesting foods. Claude Bernard cited Beaumont's work in his 1865 *Introduction to the Study of Experimental Medicine*. Bernard may have learned about it from a German translation published in 1834 or from Beaumont's own 1825 paper from the *Philadelphia Medical Recorder* that was abstracted both in a German magazine (1826) and a French medical journal (1828; *Archives generales de Médecine*, Paris). In any case, Bernard created fistulas in animals to observe how the pancreas and small intestines functioned in digestion.

Beaumont's accomplishment is even more remarkable because the United States, unlike England, France, and Germany, provided no research facilities for experimental medicine. Little was known about the physiology of digestion. Yet Beaumont, a "backwoods physiologist,"[31] inspired future studies of gastric emptying, intestinal absorption, electrolyte balance, rehydration, and nutritional supplementation with "sports drinks."

H. MICHEL EUGENE CHEVREUL (1786–1889)

During his long life as a chemist, Chevreul carried on a 200-year family tradition of studying chemistry and biology. His *Chemical Investigations of Fat* (1823) described different fatty acids. In addition, Chevreul separated cholesterol from billiary fats, coined the term margarine, and was the first to show that lard consisted of two main fats (a solid he called *stearine*, the other a liquid called *elaine*). He also showed that sugar from a diabetic's urine resembled cane sugar.

I.   JEAN BAPTISTE BOUSSINGAULT (1802–1884)

Boussingault, often credited as the father of "scientific agriculture," published his first scientific paper at age 19.[32] Shortly thereafter, he taught chemistry at the school of mines in Bogotá, Colombia.[33] For 10 years he researched nutritional problems of the Colombians. He provided them with iodine to counteract goiter. In turn, the government insisted that iodine be combined with salt. Boussingault's instincts proved correct because by the end of the 19th century iodine was known to be an essential mineral component of the thyroid-gland hormone, thyroxine.

Boussingault's studies of animal nutrition paralleled later studies of human nutrition. He calculated the effect of calcium, iron, and nutrient intake (particularly nitrogen) on energy balance. Boussingault also turned his attention to plants. He showed that the carbon within a plant came from atmospheric carbon dioxide. He also determined that a plant derived most of its nitrogen from the nitrates in the soil, not from the atmosphere, as previously believed.

> … I am far from believing that nitrogeneous substances alone are sufficient for nutrition; but it is a fact that a highly nitrogenous vegetable food is usually accompanied by other organic and inorganic constituents, useful or indispensable to nutrition (*Économie Rurale*, ii, 263, Paris, 1851).

J.   GERARDUS JOHANNIS MULDER (1802–1880)

Professor of chemistry at Utrecht, Mulder analyzed albuminous substances that he called "proteine."[34] He postulated a general protein radical identical in chemical composition to plant albumen, casein, animal fibrin, and albumen. This protein would contain substances other than nitrogen available only from plants. Because animals consume plants, substances from the vegetable kingdom, later called amino acids, build up their tissues. Unfortunately, an influential German chemist, Justis von Liebig (1803–1873), attacked Mulder's theories about protein so vigorously that they fell out of favor.

Despite the academic controversy, Mulder strongly advocated society's role in promoting quality nutrition. He asked, "Is there a more important question for discussion than the nutrition of the human race?"[35] Mulder urged people to observe the golden mean by eating neither too little nor too much food. He established minimum standards for his nation's food supply that he believed should be compatible with *optimum* health. In 1847, he gave these specific recommendations: laborers should consume 100 g of protein daily; those doing routine work about 60 g. He prescribed 500 g of carbohydrate as starch, and included "some" fat without specifying an amount.

Mulder's 1854 *Assay on General Physiological Chemistry, 1843–1850* established him as a founder of this branch of chemistry. He researched the composition of bile and caffeine (then known as theine). Mulder promoted the idea that soil regulates a plant's reaction to fertilizer, not the plant alone, so that soil should receive primary attention in farming. Mulder used Boussingault's animal experiments (1844) on nitrogen in feed to determine what foods lead to optimal productivity. Because he believed so strongly in practical experiences for students, he secured funds to build chemistry laboratories in schools. Today, the Netherlands honors Mulder as the founder of modern chemical education.[23]

K.   JUSTUS VON LIEBIG (1803–1873)

After studying in France with Gay-Lussac, Liebig became Professor of Chemistry at the University of Giessen when he was only 21. He dominated both organic chemistry and, after 1840, agricultural chemistry. In later years, however, his ideas about the proper constituents of fertilizers were criticized because the benefits could not be substantiated. Like other innovators, he fought with influential chemists[23] such as Jean Baptiste Dumas, whom he accused of plagiarism.[24]

Although embroiled in professional controversies, Liebig established a large, modern chemistry laboratory that attracted numerous students. He developed unique equipment to analyze inorganic and organic substances. Liebig restudied protein compounds (alkaloids discovered by Mulder) and concluded that muscular exertion by horses or humans required mainly proteins, not just carbohydrates and fats. Liebig's influential *Animal Chemistry* (1842) communicated his ideas about energy metabolism:[23]

> The turnover of proteinaceous foods by adult animals, as shown by the continued excretion of urea even when none of these materials is consumed, is explained by muscles consuming themselves when they exert their muscular force. This force is released by the molecule breaking into two fragments.

> The breakdown of muscle that occurs during the day is compensated for by re-formation of tissues during sleep, and the "force" or vitality of the muscles is regained. For an active adult, 7 hours of sleep are required. An old man, who is necessarily less active, requires only 3.5 hours. In each case "waste is in equilibrium with supply." However, in the infant who sleeps 20 hours and is awake for only 4, there is an excess supply, and this explains the child's ability to gain weight and grow.

> Since only those substances that are capable of conversion to blood can properly be called nutritious, or considered to be food, the protein elements of food are the only true nutrients, that is, the only ones capable of forming or replacing active tissue.

> Someone who feels cold is induced to engage in physical activity. This stimulates respiration, part of which is needed for the breakdown of muscle fibers, but it admits more oxygen, which also results in more combustion of the non-nitrogenous protectors and, thus, in more heat production.

Because he dominated chemistry, Liebig's theoretical pronouncements about the relation of dietary protein to muscular activity were generally accepted without review by other scientists until the 1850s. Guggenheim[34] emphasizes the surprising fact that Liebig never carried out a physiological experiment or performed nitrogen balance studies on animals or humans. Liebig looked down on physiologists, believing them incapable of commenting on his theoretic calculations unless they themselves achieved his level of expertise.

By mid-century, physiologist Adolf Fick (1829–1901) and chemist Johannes Wislicenus (1835–1903) challenged Liebig's dogmatic pronouncements about the role of protein in exercise. Their simple experiment measured changes in urinary nitrogen during a mountain climb. The protein that broke down could not have supplied all the energy for the their hike. The result discredited Liebig's principle assertion about the role of protein metabolism in exercise (refer to page 31, top).

Although erroneous, Liebig's notions about protein as a primary exercise fuel worked their way into popular writings. By the turn of the 20th century, an idea that survives today seemed unassailable: athletic prowess requires a large protein intake. He lent his name to two commercial products; *Liebig's Infant Food*, advertised as a replacement for breast milk, and *Liebig's Fleisch Extract* (meat extract), which supposedly conferred special benefits to the body. Liebig argued that consuming his extract and meat would help the body perform extra "work" to convert plant material into useful substances.[36,37] Even today, fitness magazines tout protein supplements for peak performance with little except anecdotal confirmation.[23] Whatever the merit of Liebig's claims, debate continues, building on the metabolic studies of W. O. Atwater (1844–1907), F. G. Benedict (1870–1957), and R. H. Chittenden (1856–1943) in the United States and M. Rubner (1854–1932) in Germany.

L.   HENRI VICTOR REGNAULT (1810–1878)

With his colleague Jules Reiset (1811–?) at the University of Paris, Regnault, professor of chemistry and physics, used closed-circuit spirometry to determine the respiratory quotient (VCO_2/VO_2) in dogs, insects, silkworms, earthworms, and frogs (1849). Animals were placed into a sealed, 45-liter bell jar surrounded by a water jacket. A potash solution filtered the carbon dioxide gas produced during respiration. Water rising in a glass receptacle forced oxygen into the bell jar to replace the quantity consumed during energy metabolism. A thermometer recorded temperature, and a manometer measured variations in chamber pressure. For dogs, fowl, and rabbits deprived of food, the respiratory quotient was less than when the same animals consumed meat. Regnault and Reiset reasoned that starving animals subsist on their own tissues. Foods were never completely destroyed during their metabolism because urea and uric acid were recovered in the urine.

Regnault's 1868 monograph did not cite the earlier research by German physiologists Friedrich Bidder (1810–1894) and Carl Schmidt (1822–1894; student of Liebig) who used the Pettenkofer-Voit respiration apparatus to define the conditions for basal metabolism.[22] Nevertheless, Regnault established relationships between different body sizes and metabolic rates. These ratios preceded the Law of Surface Area[38,39] and allometric scaling procedures now used in exercise science.[40,41] Regnault and Reiset related oxygen consumption to heat production and body size in animals:[22]

> The consumption of oxygen absorbed varies greatly in different animals per unit of body weight. It is ten times greater in sparrows than in chickens. Since the different species have the same body temperature, and the smaller animals present a relatively larger area to the environmental air, they experience a substantial cooling effect, and it becomes necessary that the sources of heat production operate more energetically and that respiration increase.

M.   CLAUDE BERNARD (1813–1878)

Bernard, generally acclaimed as the greatest physiologist of all time, succeeded Magendie as Professor of Medicine at the Collège de France. Bernard interned in medicine and surgery before serving as laboratory assistant (*préparateur*) to Magendie in 1839. Three years later, he followed Magendie to the Hôtel-Dieu hospital in Paris. For the next 35 years, Bernard discovered fundamental properties about physiology. He participated in the explosion of scientific knowledge in the mid-century. Following Darwin's *The Origin of Species* (1859), Louis Pasteur (1822–1895) refuted spontaneous generation between 1860 and 1865 and stimulated the growth of microbiology. In 1865, Gregor Mendel (1822-1884) promulgated the laws of heredity. Artists too experimented with technique (Corbet, Courbet, Degas, Daumier, Manet, Millet, Monet, Renoir, and Rodin). Philosophers (de Tocqueville, Comte, Bergson, Proudhon) and writers (Balzac, Baudelaire, Dumas, Hugo, Flaubert, Maupassant, and Stendhal) boldly explored new frontiers. Radical individualism that fostered science and art also encouraged social turmoil: coups, two revolutions (1848, 1870), and two wars against Austria and Prussia. Reflecting on this unrest, Marx and Engels drafted the *Communist Manifesto* in Paris in 1848.

Bernard remained oblivious to all except his "physico-chemical science." Mayer[42] writes about Bernard's approach to science:

> Bernard combined with a capacity for hard and prolonged work in the laboratory his appreciation of the importance of leisure spent in quiet meditation. His adherence to exact truth was absolute, and he was always ready to recognize the limitations or the error of what had seemed

like a promising idea until tested in the laboratory. His technical skill was superb, both as an experimental surgeon and as a biochemist. Yet essential as these characteristics were, they are not sufficient to explain his unequaled series of fertile discoveries.

Bernard, first of all, believed strongly in the necessity of always having a working hypothesis, derived from perusal of the literature and observation of natural phenomena, before starting on the experiment proper. He used to say: "He who does not know what he is looking for will not lay hold of what he has found when he gets it."

But imagination is not equivalent to genius unless it is joined to what was perhaps Bernard's outstanding characteristic, the ability to devise the single, definitive crucial experiment which will test a far-reaching hypothesis. Bernard, like a great general who maps and executes a campaign by striking at the vital points of the enemy hosts, and takes only those positions which have to be taken to bring decisive victory, never wasted any time on experiments which were not essential to his progress. And, of course, his skill allowed him to perform these experiments in a minimum of time and with a maximum of precision.

Bernard had an extraordinary capacity for extracting from his results the most general and far-reaching conclusions that could be solidly supported by them; hence, his role as a progenitor in so many branches of the biological sciences.

Bernard indicated his single-minded devotion to research by producing an M.D. thesis (1843) on gastric juice and its role in nutrition (*Du sac gastrique et de son rôle dans la nutrition*). Ten years later, he received the Doctorate in Natural Sciences for his study entitled *Recherches sur une nouvelle fonction du foie, consideré comme organe producteur de matière sucrée chez l'homme et les animaux* (Research on a new function of the liver as a producer of sugar in man and animals). Prior to his seminal research, scientists assumed that only plants could synthesize sugar and sugar within animals must be derived from ingested plant matter. Bernard disproved these notions by documenting the presence of sugar in the hepatic vein of a dog whose diet lacked carbohydrate.

Bernard's experiments changed medicine.[43]

1. The discovery of the role of the pancreatic secretion in the digestion of fats (1848).
2. The discovery of a new function of the liver — the "internal secretion" of glucose into the blood (1848).
3. The induction of diabetes by puncture of the floor of the fourth ventricle (1849).
4. The discovery of the elevation of local skin temperature upon section of the cervical sympathetic nerve (1851).
5. The production of sugar by washed excised liver (1855) and the isolation of glycogen (1857).
6. The demonstration that curare specifically blocks motor nerve endings (1856).
7. The demonstration that carbon monoxide blocks the respiration of erythrocytes (1857).

Bernard's work also influenced other sciences. His discoveries in chemical physiology spawned physiological chemistry and biochemistry, which in turn created molecular biology. His contributions to regulatory physiology helped the next generation understand how metabolism and nutrition affect exercise.

Despite the importance of Bernard's discoveries, the French government barely supported scientific research. Germany, Russia, and England provided laboratories in universities and hospitals, while Bernard's predecessors, Magendie and Bert, worked in small rooms, poorly lit and inadequately ventilated.[19] Bernard spoke out against his government's neglect of science. Still, he continued to experiment.

Bernard's influential *Introduction à l'étude de la médecine expérimentale* (The Introduction to the Study of Experimental Medicine, 1865; translated 1927)[44] illustrates the self control that enabled him to succeed despite external perturbations. It requires researchers to vigorously observe, hypothesize, and test their hypothesis. In the last third of the book, Bernard shares his strategies for verifying results. His disciplined approach remains valid and would be required reading for Exercise Nutritionists.

His life inspired appreciative works by the Cambridge physiologist Sir Michael Foster[45] (1836–1907) and historian Grmek[46.] A few days after his death, Bernard's friend and colleague Paul Bert wrote[44] the following poignant eulogy:

> Nothing in his pure and harmonious life was turned aside from its chief aim. Enamored of literature, art and philosophy, Claude Bernard as a physiologist lost nothing by these noble passions; on the contrary, they all helped in developing the science with which he identified himself, and of which he is the highest and most complete embodiment. He as a physiologist such as no man had been before him. "Claude Bernard," said a foreign scientist, "is not merely a physiologist, he is physiology."

> His very death seems to mark a new era in science. For the first time in our country, a man of science will receive those public honors hitherto reserved for political and military celebrities. … And one phrase … sums up all that we have said: "The light, which has just been extinguished, cannot be replaced."

N. EDWARD SMITH (1819–1874)

Smith, a physician, public health advocate, and social reformer, advocated better living conditions for Britain's lower classes, including prisoners. He believed they were maltreated because they received no additional food while toiling on the exhausting "punitive treadmill." In 1863, the first government sponsored survey of food consumption in low income families, supervised by Smith, proved the inadequacy of their diet. Carpenter[23] summarizes Smith's data: bread was the staple (19.1 lb [8.7 kg] per adult per week), followed by potatoes (2.4 lb; 10.9 kg), milk, (16 oz.; 453.6 g), meats (0.8 lb; 362.9 g), sugar (0.5 lb; 0.23 kg), and fats (0.3 lb; 0.14 kg). A daily food intake of 2,190 kcal (9167 kJ) consisted of 370 g of carbohydrate, 53 g of fat, and 55 g of protein. Smith argued that prisoners consuming a diet consisting of 93% carbohydrate would become ill. Diet thus had social consequences. Disabled by weakness, prisoners would not be able to perform hard labor after release and would more likely resort to crime.

Smith had observed prisoners climbing up a treadwheel, whose steps resembled the side paddle wheels of a Victorian steamship. Prisoners climbed for 15 minutes, after which they were allowed a 15-minute rest, for a total of four hours work three times a week. To overcome resistance from a sail on the prison roof attached to the treadmill, each man traveled the equivalent of 1.43 miles up a steep hill.

Curious about this strenuous exercise, Smith conducted studies on himself. He constructed a closed-circuit apparatus (face mask with inspiratory and expiratory valves) to measure carbon dioxide production while climbing at Brixton prison.[23] He expired 19.6 more grams of carbon while climbing for 15 minutes and resting for 15 minutes than he expired while resting. Smith estimated that if he climbed and rested for 7.5 hours, his total daily carbon output would increase 66%. Smith analyzed the urine of 4 prisoners over a three week period, showing that urea output related to the nitrogen content of the ingested foods, while carbon dioxide related to intensity of exercise.[47]

Smith inspired two German researchers to validate the prevailing idea that protein alone powered muscular contraction. Adolf Eugen Fick (1829–1901), a physiologist at the University of Zurich,* and Johannes Wislicenus (1835–1903), professor of chemistry at Zurich, questioned whether the oxidation of protein or of carbohydrates and fats supplied energy for muscular work. In 1864,[48] they climbed Mt. Faulhorn in the Swiss Alps. Prior to the climb, they eliminated protein from their diet, reasoning that non-protein nutrients would have to supply them energy. They collected their urine three times: before and immediately after the ascent, and the following morning. They calculated the external energy equivalent of the 1,956-m climb by multiplying their body mass by the vertical distance. This external energy exceeded protein catabolism reflected by nitrogen in the urine.* Therefore, they concluded that the energy from protein breakdown hardly contributed to exercise energy requirement ("... since the muscle-machine can undoubtedly be heated by means of the non-nitrogenous fuel, this fuel is in all cases that best suited for it." Reference 48, p. 502).

Fick's brother-in-law,[49] Edward Frankland (1825–1899), a London chemist trained in Germany, confirmed Fick and Wislicenus' conclusions about how protein fuels exercise. By measuring heat production during the complete oxidation of various foods and urea, Frankland proved that carbohydrate and fat, not protein, provided energy for the climb. Similar results were reported by German chemist M. Traube (1826–1894) whose 1861 paper cited by Guggenheim[34] declared that muscle tissue did not provide the fuel for exercise and that muscular force could not be assessed by urea production. Thus, the experiments by Smith, Fick and Wislicenus, Frankland, and Traube nullified Liebig's claim that protein served as the primary source of muscular power.

O. EDWARD HITCHCOCK, JR. (1828–1911)

Hitchcock[50] graduated from Amherst College (1849) and Harvard Medical School (1853). He served as Professor of Hygiene and Physical Education in 1861, a position he held continuously to 1911. From 1861 to 1888, Hitchcock measured almost every Amherst student for 6 segmental heights, 23 girths, 6 breadths, 8 lengths, 8 measures of muscular strength, lung capacity, and pilosity (amount of hair on the body). In 1889, Hitchcock published a 37-page anthropometric manual that included five tables of anthropometric statistics of students. This compendium described how to take physical measurements, test eyes, and examine lungs and heart before testing muscular strength. The first of its kind to analyze anthropometric and strength data, it influenced Yale, Harvard, Wellesley, and Mt. Holyoke to include anthropometric measurements as part of their physical education and hygiene curriculum.

Early anthropometrists wondered whether daily, vigorous exercise improved fitness. Hitchcock studied anthropometry at college while the military measured Civil War soldiers.[51] The government tried to determine relationships among anthropometric, demographic, and anthropological statistics. Even now, studies of obesity and energy balance require assessment of body composition.

Hitchcock also set the stage for academic research involving body composition in medicine, physiology, and exercise physiology. By 1928, when anthropometric measurements were made of athletes at the Amsterdam Olympic Games, Hitchcock's visionary ideas had obviously taken hold. Today, many of his methods assess the relation of physique to exercise performance. Modern anthropometry, defined as kinanthropometry at the International

---

* Fick contributed to hemodynamics by determining cardiac output by multiplying oxygen consumption by the arterio-venous oxygen difference. Developed in 1870, this principle is known as Fick's law. Fick also developed techniques of blood flow plethysmyography, studied heat generation during muscle shortening and lengthening, built an apparatus to measure work output, and studied the effects of electrical stimulation on neural phenomena.

* James Prescott Joule (1818–1899) and others had shown that the energy needed to raise a weight of 423 kg against the force of gravity by a height of one meter equaled the heat required to raise one kg of water by one degree centigrade (1 kcal), provided that all of the energy dissipated as friction.[52]

Congress of Physical Activity Sciences in conjunction with the 1976 Montreal Olympic Games,[53] was restated in 1980[54] as follows:

> Kinanthropometry is the application of measurement to the study of human size, shape, proportion, composition, maturation, and gross function. Its purpose is to help us to understand human movement in the context of growth, exercise, performance, and nutrition. We see its essentially human-enobling purpose being achieved through applications in medicine, education, and government.

P.   EDUARD PFLÜGER (1829–1910)

Pflüger, a German physiologist, published a "turning point" experiment in human respiratory physiology in 1872. Until his work, blood flow (with its content of oxygen and carbon dioxide) was thought to maintain "life" in the body's tissues. Pflüger proved that minute changes in the partial pressure of blood affected the rate of oxygen release and transport across capillary membranes. Thus, cellular dynamics in the tissues, not simply blood flow, govern the tissues' oxygen uptake. Because of Pflüger, the cell became the central controlling mechanism that dictated how much oxygen would be delivered to sustain it. He wrote, "For oxygen must go everywhere in the body where there is life, and life is everywhere."[52] Pflüger's work on tissue dynamics terminated age-old conjectures that blood was some vital force superintending life.

Q.   CARL VON VOIT (1831–1908)

After graduating as a medical doctor in 1854, Voit then studied chemistry with Max Joseph von Pettenkofer (1818–1901),* attended lectures by Liebig at Munich, spent an additional year studying chemistry in Gottingen, and became an assistant in anatomy and physiology to physiologist Theodor Bischoff (1807–1882) at Munich's Physiological Institute. Voit was appointed Professor of Physiology at the University of Munich.

Over the next 30 years, he teamed with Bischoff and Pettenkofer* to study metabolism in animals and humans. At the time of Voit's research, Liebig still claimed that protein was the primary fuel for muscle contraction. In contrast, Voit and Bischoff's carefully conducted nitrogen balance experiments on dogs disproved Liebig's view. In some experiments, dogs fed on different foods ran on an exercise wheel. To the researcher's surprise, urea output (which reflects protein breakdown) failed to increase in proportion to the intensity or duration of exercise. Protein catabolism could not provide energy required for the work. Liebig and Voit debated in the scientific literature, with Voit eventually triumphing.

Beginning in 1861, Voit and Pettenkofer used Pettenkofer's respiration chamber to study energy balance. Fresh air was pumped into the sealed chamber and exhausted air sampled for carbon dioxide. Newer versions of the machine could measure water vapor in the expired air. By perfecting respiration calorimetry, Voit and Pettenkofer determined how much fat and carbohydrate contributed to metabolism during rest and exercise, health and disease. Their subjects repeatedly turned a hand crank, increasing their energy expenditure without relying on the breakdown of tissue protein. Oxidation of carbohydrate and fat (the non-nitrogenous

---

* Pettenkofer is best known for more than 200 publications in scientific hygiene,[55] a field he founded. He experimented on air quality, soil composition and ground water, moisture content of structures, building ventilation, functions of clothing, spread of disease, and water quality. Pettenkofer discovered creatinine, an amino acid in urine. He founded two journals, *Zeitschrift für Biologie* (1865; Voit was a co-founder) and *Zeitschrift für Hygiene* (1885). An English translation[56] of one of Pettenkofer's monographs shows his design for a chamber to measure human respiration during exercise.

substances) fueled muscular effort. Voit and Pettenkofer corrected Leibig's view concerning the role of protein in exercise. A student of Voit, Max Rubner, worked on metabolism through the beginning of the 20th century.

Voit influenced Americans at the turn of the 20th century. His former student, Wilbur Olin Atwater (1844–1907), devised the elegant respiration calorimeters at Wesleyan University. Graham Lusk (1866–1932), another Voit protégé, also made contributions to nutrition.[57-60] Holmes[61] provides original and secondary German resources about Voit; Lusk[22] gives personal insights about his mentor's life and scientific works.

R.   AUSTIN FLINT, JR., (1836–1915)

Flint was professor of physiology and physiological anatomy at New York's Bellevue Hospital Medical College and chair of the Department of Physiology and Microbiology from 1861 to 1897. In 1866, he published a series of five classic textbooks, the first entitled *The Physiology of Man; Designed to Represent the Existing State of Physiological Science as Applied to the Functions of the Human Body. Vol. 1; Introduction; The Blood; Circulation; Respiration.* Eleven years later, Flint published *The Principles and Practice of Medicine,* a synthesis of his first five textbooks that consisted of 987 pages of meticulously organized material with supporting documentation. The text included 4 lithographs and 313 woodcuts detailing the body's major systems.

The American Medical Association awarded a prize to Flint for basic research on the heart based on his medical school thesis "The Phenomena of Capillary Circulation" (which appeared in the *American Journal of the Medical Sciences,* 1878). Flint admired other scholars such as William Harvey and Claude Bernard; he owned a copy of Beaumont's book, as well as a photograph of Alexis St. Martin.[29]

Flint wrote about topics important to the emerging science of exercise physiology and the future science of Exercise Nutrition. In 1877, he wrote:[62]

1. Influence of posture and exercise on pulse rate (p. 52–53)

> It has been observed that the position of the body has a very marked influence upon the rapidity of the pulse. Experiments of a very interesting character have been made by Dr. Guy and others, with a view to determine the difference in the pulse in different postures. In the male, there is a difference of about ten beats between standing and sitting, and fifteen beats between standing and the recumbent posture. In the female, the variations with position are not so great. The average given by Dr. Guy is, for the male — standing, 81; sitting, 71; lying, 66; and the female — standing, 91; sitting, 84; lying, 80. This is given as the average of a large number of observations.

> *Influence of age and sex.* In both the male and female, observers have constantly found a great difference in the rapidity of the heart's action at different periods of life.

> During early life, there is no marked and constant difference in the rapidity of the pulse in the sexes; but, toward the age of puberty, the development of the sexual peculiarities is accompanied with an acceleration of the heart's action in the female, which continues even into old age.

> *Influence of Exercise, etc.* It is a fact generally admitted that muscular exertion increases the frequency of the pulsations of the heart; and the experiments just cited show that the difference in rapidity, which is by some attributed to change in posture (some positions, it is fancied, offering fewer obstacles to the current of blood than others), is mainly due to muscular exertion. Every one knows, indeed, that the action of the heart is much more rapid after violent exertion, such as running, lifting, etc. Experiments on this point date from quite a remote period. Bryan Robinson, who published a treatise on the "Animal Economy" in

1734, states, as the result of observation, that a man in the recumbent position has 64 pulsations per minute; sitting, 68; after a slow walk, 78; after walking four miles in one hour, 100; and 140 to 150 after running as fast as he could. This general statement, which has been repeatedly verified, shows the powerful influence of the muscular system on the heart. The fact is so familiar that it need not be farther dwelt upon.

2. Influence of muscular activity on respiration (p. 150–151)

Nearly all observers are agreed that there is a considerable increase in the exhalation of carbonic acid during and immediately following muscular exercise. In insects, Mr. Newport has found that a greater quantity is sometimes exhaled in an hour of violent agitation than in twenty-four hours of repose. In a drone, the exhalation in twenty-four hours as 0.30 of a cubic inch, and during violent muscular exertion the exhalation in one hour was 0.34. Lavoisier recognized the great influence of muscular activity upon the respiratory changes. In treating of the consumption of oxygen, we have quoted his observations on the relative quantities of air vitiated in repose and activity.

The following results of the experiments of Dr. Edward Smith on the influence of exercise are very definite and satisfactory:

In walking at the rate of two miles an hour, the exhalation of carbonic acid during one hour was equal to the quantity produced during 1 $^4/_5$ hour of repose with food, and 2 $^1/_2$ hours with, and 3 $^1/_2$ hours without food.

One hour's labor at the tread-wheel, while actually working the wheel, was equal to 4 $^1/_2$ of rest with food, and 6 hours without food.

The various observers we have cited have remarked that, when muscular exertion is carried so far as to produce great fatigue and exhaustion, the exhalation of carbonic acid is notably diminished.

3. Influence of muscular exercise on nitrogen elimination (p. 429–430)

We have had an opportunity of settling definitely the vexed question of the influence of muscular exercise upon elimination of nitrogen. In 1871, we made an exceedingly elaborate series of observations upon Mr. Weston, the pedestrian. Of these we can only give here a brief summary. Mr. Weston walked for five consecutive days as follows: First day, 92 miles; second day, 80 miles; third day, 57 miles; fourth day, 48 miles; fifth day, 40.5 miles. The nitrogen of the food was compared with the nitrogen excreted for three periods; viz, five days before the walk, five days walking, and five days after the walk. A trusty assistant was with Mr. Weston day and night for the fifteen days; the food was weighted and analyzed; the excreta were collected; and other observations were made during the entire period. The analyses were made independently, under the direction of Prof. R.O. Doremus, who had no idea of the results until we had classified and tabulated them. The conclusions were most decided, and, as far as possible, all the physiological conditions were fulfilled. As regards the proportion of nitrogen eliminated to the nitrogen of the food, the general results were as follows:

> For the five days before the walk, with an average exercise of about eight miles daily, the nitrogen eliminated was 92:82 parts for 100 parts of nitrogen ingested. For the five days of the walk, for every hundred parts of nitrogen ingested, there were discharged 153:99 parts. For the five days after the walk, when there was hardly any exercise, for every hundred parts of nitrogen ingested, there were discharged 84:63 parts. During the walk, the nitrogen excreted was in direct ratio to the amount of exercise; and, what was still more striking, the excess of nitrogen eliminated over the nitrogen of food almost exactly corresponded with a calculation

of the nitrogen of the muscular tissue wasted, as estimated from the loss of weight of the body.

S. NATHAN ZUNTZ (1847–1920)

Zuntz studied with physiologist Edourd Pflüger at the University of Bonn. His thesis for the medical degree studied carbonic acid in blood and this acid's movement between red blood cells and plasma. Zuntz initiated the idea that carboxy hemoglobin freely diffused and easily permeated tissue membranes. He served as Professor of Anatomy at the University of Bonn (1874–1880) and established a new scientific laboratory at the Agricultural College in Berlin with an interdisciplinary focus among chemistry, physiology, and metabolism. A prolific scientist, Zuntz produced 430 articles concerning blood and blood gases, circulation, mechanics and chemistry of respiration, general metabolism and metabolism of specific foods, energy metabolism and heat production, and digestion. In addition, Zuntz proved that carbohydrates were precursors for lipid synthesis. He maintained that fats and carbohydrates should not be consumed in equal quantities in the diet.

Zuntz believed discoveries concerning oxygen consumption and production of carbon dioxide and water would reveal secrets of tissues' energy metabolism. For such experiments, Zuntz modified the Pettenkofer respirometer that simultaneously measured oxygen and carbon dioxide. To improve portability, he switched from the cumbersome wet-spirometer to a smaller and lighter dry gas meter. Zuntz and his students used the portable respirometer to measure respiratory exchange (energy expenditure) in livestock and in humans at sea level and at high altitude.

Zuntz formulated standards to measure basal metabolism. In 1893, one of Zuntz's students (Magnus-Levy) used the portable spirometer to make the first detailed measurements of resting metabolism in patients with hyperthyroidism, obesity, acromegaly, cancer, diabetes, gout, and pernicious anemia. Magnus-Levy's experiments confirmed results of a German physician. Friedrich Müller had reported that hyperthyroidism accelerated metabolism in a patient who lost 24 kg of body mass despite consuming adequate calories to maintain body mass.

The data from Zuntz and Shaumburg's 1901 experiments (displayed in *Exercise Physiology. Energy, Nutrition, and Human Performance*, Table 8.1[50]) quantified the relative contributions of carbohydrate and fat to energy metabolism based on the ratio of carbon dioxide expired to oxygen consumed (respiratory quotient). Their studies also provided a basis for determining the caloric value for oxygen consumption from the metabolic mixture. Zuntz studied fuel utilization during exercise; he discovered protein played a minor role in the total exercise energy requirement.

Aware that science should reach everyone, Zuntz wrote popular articles in sports journals, attempting to convey technical information for a mass audience. A biography[63] summarizes his many studies of exercise in humans and animals such as the effects of training (and mode of training) on energy metabolism. Specializing in the relationships among metabolism, nutrition, and exercise, Zuntz would make an ideal professor in a modern Department of Exercise Nutrition.

T. WILBUR OLIN ATWATER (1844–1907)

Atwater received his Ph.D. from Yale in 1869 for studies on the chemical composition of corn. Studying in Berlin and Leipzig, he became familiar with Voit, Rubner, and Zuntz. As Professor of Chemistry at Wesleyan, he studied the effects of fertilizers in farming and established the first agricultural experimental station in the United States at Wesleyan in 1875 (which in 1877 became part of the famous Sheffield Scientific School at Yale). From 1879 to 1882, Atwater determined the chemical composition and nutritive values of fish and animal tissues. Returning to Germany in 1882–83, Atwater studied the metabolism of mammals in Voit's laboratory.

Atwater's familiarity with German techniques for measuring respiration and metabolism helped him to conduct human nutrition studies: food analysis, dietary evaluations, energy requirements for work, digestibility of foods, and economics of food production. He helped to convince the U.S. Government to fund studies of human nutrition. Atwater directed various studies at agricultural experiment stations throughout the country that resulted in the 1896 publication of 2,600 chemical analyses of American foodstuffs. An additional 4,000 analyses were completed in 1899, including another 1,000 analyses done under Atwater's supervision. The 1906 re-issue of the original report included the maximum, minimum, and average values for water, protein, fat, total carbohydrates, ash, and a food's "fuel value" calculated using Rubner's methods. Modern databases of food composition in the United States still employ these values.

Atwater compared the data about food evaluation from the United States to European data. Although Voit and other agricultural chemists advocated a minimum protein intake of more than 100 grams per day, Atwater felt this amount to be excessive. He recommended controlled dietary studies to determine how nutrient intake affected metabolism and muscular effort. After reviewing his dietary studies, Atwater worried that the population consumed too much food, particulary fats and sweets, and did not exercise enough.[64]

> It is a fair question whether the results of these things have induced among us in a large class of well-to-do people, with little muscular activity, a habit of excessive eating and may be responsible for great damage to health, to say nothing of the purse.

Perhaps the metabolic studies Atwater began just before the turn of the century contributed most to the emerging science of human nutrition and exercise. He and E. B. Rosa (Professor of Physics at Wesleyan and later chief physicist of the National Bureau of Standards) perfected over a 12-year period the most accurate respiration calorimeter to study human metabolism. Accounting for almost 100% of the heat produced and substrates metabolized, this system allowed them to quantify the dynamics of energy metabolism, directly measure the balance between food (energy) intake and energy output, and evaluate the effects of diet and muscular activity on metabolism. The classic papers of Atwater and Rosa,[65] Atwater and Benedict,[66] and Benedict and Carpenter,[67] with their meticulous technical detail and experimental procedures, should be studied by all who are interested in Exercise Nutrition. Before Atwater died in 1907, he had completed more than 500 energy balance experiments. Maynard[64] believes that Atwater's most valuable contributions concerned human energy balance. They confirmed that the law of conservation of energy governed transformation of matter in both the human body and inanimate world. Penned in 1895,[68] Atwater's comments sound contemporary:

> Food may be defined as material which, when taken into the body, serves to either form tissue or yield energy, or both. This definition includes all the ordinary food materials, since they both build tissue and yield energy. It includes sugar and starch, because they yield energy and form fatty tissue. It includes alcohol, because it is burned to yield energy, though it does not build tissue. It excludes creatin, creatininin, and other so-called nitrogeneous extractives of meat and likewise thein or caffein of tea and coffee, because they neither build tissue nor yield energy, although they may, at times, be useful aids to nutrition.

U. MAX RUBNER (1854–1932)

During the 1870s, Rubner studied in Munich with Carl von Voit. He researched the body's energy exchange from nitrogen loss in the urine and feces. Using bomb calorimetry,

Rubner explained how the heat values of foods were interchangeable, an insight later known as the Isodynamic Law. To quote Rubner: "the food-stuffs may under given conditions replace each other in accordance with their heat-producing value." The calorific values from his 1878 experiments are essentially the same as those used today: 4.1 kcal per g for protein and carbohydrate; 9.3 kcal per g for lipids. Using these energy values, Rubner determined the basal metabolism of animals and humans. He measured heat production in different species and developed the Surface Area Law which states that during rest, heat production is proportional to body surface area.

In 1885, Rubner established his own laboratory at Marburgh, where within four years he built the world's most accurate respiration calorimeter. It showed how closely body heat lost in the calorimeter agreed with heat produced by combustion estimated from gas exchange using indirect calorimetry. In 1894, Rubner validated the conservation of energy principle originally proposed by German chemist J. R. Mayer (1814–1878) in 1842 and 1845, and the 1861 experiments of German physiologist Hermann Helmholtz (1821–1894). Rubner showed that the heat of combustion of food consumed by a dog equaled the heat of combustion of its excreta plus heat loss. The results were spectacular. During 45 days in the calorimeter, the dog produced the caloric equivalent of 17,349 kcal (72,623 kJ). Based on respiratory data and nitrogen excretion, total heat production equaled 17,406 kcal — a difference of only 1.27 kcal (5.3 kJ) per day! Rubner's experiments with humans further confirmed the theory of conservation of matter.

Rubner complemented his success in the laboratory with success in the classroom. In 1891, Rubner became Professor of Hygiene at the University of Berlin, and then Professor of Physiology in 1909 until his retirement in 1924. He influenced W.O. Atwater. Another of Rubner's distinguished pupils, Graham Lusk (1866–1932), became Professor of Physiology at Cornell University Medical College. Using experience gained in Rubner's laboratory, Lusk constructed his own respiration calorimeter at Cornell to do key research in nutrition and metabolism.[69]

At his retirement, Rubner reflected on his main accomplishments:[70]

> … discovery of the surface area law that applied in man, birds, aquatic animals, amphibians, and reptiles, that the surface area law did not apply during starvation, discovery of the isodynamic law and the caloric basis of metabolism, the physical regulation of body temperature, and the specific dynamic action or SDA phenomenon (increased heat production after consuming fat, protein, and carbohydrate).

Rubner's SDA experiments indicated that metabolism increased 45% above rest when a fasting man worked. When the man consumed a high protein diet without working, metabolism increased an average 27%. Combining a high protein intake with exercise augmented the SDA effect on metabolism to 78%. Rubner believed that the SDA effect was partitioned between the energy needed for normal cell function and an additional energy required to "fuel" intermediary metabolism.

V.   RUSSEL HENRY CHITTENDEN (1856–1943)

Chittenden excelled in chemistry at Yale's Sheffield Scientific School, where his senior project investigated why leftover scallops tasted sweeter when recooked. Chittenden discovered that muscle tissue contained large amounts of free glycogen. With encouragement from his mentor, Chittenden published his paper in the *American Journal of Science* (1875; republished in a British and German journal).[71]

After graduation, Chittenden traveled to Heidelberg, where he worked with the notable enzyme chemist Kühne. Surprisingly, Kühne had read Chittenden's article on glycogen in scallops. In his memoirs, Chittenden recalled:

The atmosphere had changed, and my spirits rose accordingly, reaching a still higher level when Kühne remarked that he would find a place for me in the laboratory at once. ... After a month in the laboratory, Kühne asked me if I would like to serve as his assistant in the lecture demonstrations.

Chittenden attended classes in advanced chemistry (given by Professor Bunsen), anatomy, surgery, and pathology, and visited German laboratories where he met distinguished researchers. The year's experience at Heidelberg resulted in three publications and influenced his approach to science. In 1880, Chittenden received the first Ph.D. degree in physiological chemistry from an American university (Yale). Two years later, he became Professor of Physiological Chemistry at Sheffield, a post he held for the next 40 years.

Chittenden published 144 scientific papers, including *Physiological Economy In Nutrition, With Special Reference To The Minimal Proteid Requirement Of The Healthy Man. An Experimental Study.*[72] It refocused attention on man's minimal protein requirement while resting or exercising, and influenced future research in nutrition and exercise physiology. After studying laborers who consumed approximately 3100 kcal (12,977 kJ) daily, the Germans Rubner and Voit maintained that protein intake should be either 118 g per day (Voit) or 127 g per day (Rubner); the American Atwater recommended a protein intake similar to Rubner's. Recommendations for protein intake were even higher for soldiers doing hard physical labor (Voit 145 g; Rubner 165 g; Atwater 150 g). In contrast, Chittenden's experiments contradicted these figures because they showed that no debilitation occurred in normal and athletic young men (including himself) subsisting on low protein diets.

Chittenden's[72] data included daily dietary and urine histories to determine nitrogen excretion (protein utilization). For nine months, he recorded his own body weight. Although it decreased from 65 to 58 kg, and his daily protein intake was two-thirds less than Voit recommended to maintain nitrogen equilibrium, Chittenden's health remained excellent without compromising physical vigor or muscular tone. In a year-long study, athletic men in excellent health on a low protein diet (less than one g per kg daily) likewise suffered no deterioration of health or ability to perform arduous physical tasks. Chittenden's data proved that, even without a large protein intake, individuals could maintain their health and fitness. Chittenden summarized his findings:

> In presenting the results of the experiments, herein described, the writer has refrained from entering into lengthy discussions, preferring to allow the results mainly to speak for themselves. They are certainly sufficiently convincing and need no superabundance of words to give them value; indeed, such merit as the book possesses is to be found in the large number of consecutive results, which admit of no contradiction and need no argument to enhance their value. The results are presented as scientific facts, and the conclusions they justify are self-evident.

W. FREDERICK GOWLAND HOPKINS (1861–1947)

Hopkins did not rise to prominence in the early 20th century by following normal academic channels. Beginning work at 17 for an insurance company and then a railroad, he eventually enrolled in the Royal School of Mines and assisted in a private chemistry laboratory. Hopkins qualified for membership in the Institute of Chemistry by attending lectures at London's University College. While studying medicine, he worked as a chemistry assistant at Guy's Hospital. Following graduation, Hopkins became a demonstrator in physiology at London University. Sir Michael Foster, Professor of Physiology at Cambridge University, invited Hopkins to develop a research and teaching program in chemical physiology.

By 1901, Hopkins had devised new methods to isolate uric acid (thought to be related to protein breakdown); subsequent experiments showed how to make pure (crystalline) preparations of this compound. In France, Magendie had already demonstrated that an animal would die if fed a single foodstuff such as carbohydrate. Hopkin's breakthrough discovery isolated and identified the structure of the amino acid tryptophan, for which he shared the 1929 Nobel Prize in Medicine or Physiology. Hopkin's experiments proved that "unidentified accessory food factors" prevented the development of deficiency diseases. Rats sickened and died on a purified diet of sufficient energy but thrived when fed a supplement of either 3 ml of milk (less than 4% of the whole food eaten) or an alcoholic extract of milk. Hopkins first proved that the "accessory food factor" (later called vitamins) had organic properties indispensable for maintaining good health. He stated:

> It is possible that what is absent from artificial diets and supplied by such addenda as milk and tissue extracts is of the nature of an organic complex (or of complexes) which the animal body cannot synthesize. But the amount which seems sufficient to secure growth is so small that a catalytic or stimulative function seems more likely.[73]

In 1906,[73] Hopkins shared his ideas about the need for supplementary nutrients to promote health:

> … no animal can live on a mixture of proteins, carbohydrates, and fats, and even when the necessary inorganic material is carefully supplied the animal still cannot flourish. The animal body is adjusted to live either on plant tissues or the tissues of other animals, and these contain countless substances, other than the proteins, carbohydrates, and fats.

> Physiological evolution, I believe, has made some of these well-nigh as essential as are the basal constituents of diet. Lecithin, for instance, has been repeatedly shown to have a marked influence upon nutrition, and this just happens to be something already familiar, and a substance that happens to have been tried. The field is almost unexplored; only is it certain that there are many minor factors in all diets, of which the body takes account.

> In diseases such as rickets, and particularly in scurvy, we have had for long years knowledge of a dietetic factor; but though we know how to benefit these conditions empirically, the real errors in the diet are to this day quite obscure. They are, however, certainly of the kind which comprises these minimal qualitative factors that I am considering.

> I can do no more than hint at these matters, but I can assert that later developments of the science of dietetics will deal with factors highly complex and at present unknown.

Hopkins both produced pioneering studies in nutritional biochemistry and collaborated with physiologist Walter Morley Fletcher (mentor to A. V. Hill) to study muscle chemistry. Their classic 1907 paper in experimental physiology employed new methods to isolate lactic acid in muscle. Prior studies of stimulated muscle showed large concentrations of lactic acid in both stimulated and non-exercised muscle. Fletcher and Hopkins' chemical methods reduced the muscle's enzyme activity prior to analysis to isolate the reactions. They found that a muscle contracting under low oxygen conditions produced lactic acid at the expense of glycogen.[74] Conversely, oxygen in muscle suppressed the formation of lactic acid. The researchers deduced that lactic acid forms from a non-oxidative (anaerobic) process during contraction; during recovery in a non-contracted state, an oxidative (aerobic) process removes lactic acid with oxygen present. A. V. Hill (1886–1965), Nobel Prize recipient (1922), credited this experiment as the catalyst to subsequent research in muscle chemistry through 1925.[75]

Hopkins won honors — first professor of biochemistry at Cambridge; knighthood (1925); Copley Medal of the Royal Society (1926); President of the Royal Society (1931); Order of Merit (1935; highest civilian prize) — and actively researched until his retirement,[76,77] an admirable exemplar for Exercise Nutrition.

X.   FRANCIS GANO BENEDICT (1870–1957)

A chemist, Benedict assisted Atwater in the Department of Chemistry at Wesleyan University. Over a 12-year period, they conducted more than 500 experiments concerning rest, exercise, and diet using the Atwater-Rosa respiration calorimeter. Their results appeared in six bulletins of the Office of Experiment Stations of the U.S. Department of Agriculture under the general title *Experiments on the Metabolism of Matter and Energy in the Human Body.* In addition, Benedict published studies on the physiological action of alcohol (which proved to be controversial and were opposed by the temperance organizations) and the effects of muscular exercise and mental effort on energy metabolism. When Atwater died in 1907, Benedict became Director of the Nutrition Laboratory (Boston), a post he held for 30 years until retirement.

Relocating from Wesleyan to Boston provided Benedict with ready access to outstanding medical facilities. His work in respiratory metabolism complemented that of scientists in allied health fields such as renowned endocrinologist Elliot P. Joslin (*Metabolism in Diabetes Mellitus*, Carnegie Institution of Washington, Washington, D.C., no. 136, 1912). Benedict studied metabolism in newborn infants, growing children and adolescents, starving people, athletes, and vegetarians. He also investigated the effects of diet, temperature regulation, and exercise on metabolism. Traveling to Christian Bohr's laboratory in Copenhagen in 1907, he met August Krogh (1874–1943; 1920 Nobel Prize in Physiology or Medicine). The next summer, Benedict accompanied Krogh to Greenland to measure excretion of Eskimos.[78]

In 1919, Harris and Benedict published their influential "metabolic standards" tables based on sex, age, height, and weight to compare normals and patients. In addition, Benedict published extensively on animal and agricultural nutrition. Collaborative research with E. C. Ritzman, University of New Hampshire at Durham, determined fat and carbohydrate usage relative to energy metabolism from the smallest mouse to an 1800-kg elephant. By modifying the respiratory apparatus, Benedict could accommodate lizards, turtles, birds, and snakes. His last monograph, *Vital Energetics, A Study In Comparative Basal Metabolism* (Carnegie Institution Monograph no. 503, 1938), refers to many of his approximately 400 publications. Maynard[79] chronicles Benedict's accomplishments, and a biography[80] lists 300 of his publications. However, Benedict's work was not without detractors. Kleiber[39] disparaged Benedict's method for expressing metabolic rate in wild and domesticated animals.

Y.   AUGUST KROGH (1874–1949)

Krogh began his career in the laboratory of the noted Christian Bohr (1855–1911), who himself had been trained by physiologist Carl Ludwig in Leipzig. Bohr had already clarified the dynamics of muscle contraction and solubility of oxygen in different fluids including blood. His studies of oxygen influenced Krogh's early experiments of tissue respiration in animals. Krogh devised equipment to measure respiratory gas exchange in snails, frogs, and fishes. Krogh's *An Account of the Structure and Function of the Lungs and Air Sacks of Birds*, the equivalent of a master's thesis (1899), proved oxygen diffused rapidly through the thin pulmonary membranes, while the skin eliminated carbon dioxide. Subsequent experiments in gas transport corrected the prevailing view that lungs were gland-type structure that *secreted* oxygen and carbon dioxide. Krogh's highly accurate equipment analyzed respiratory gases and established that pulmonary gas was exchanged by the mechanism of diffusion, not secretion. Krogh stated:

> The cutaneous absorption of oxygen cannot be regulated at all by the organism, hence I am of the opinion that with a probability almost amounting to certainty it is affected by plain physical powers — diffusion.

Krogh determined to win the prestigious Seegan Prize* by solving the problem of whether or not free nitrogen or nitrogenous gases were released from the body as a normal by-product of metabolism. In 1906, he proved that gaseous nitrogen remained constant and won the prize. His original approach using respiratory methods to quantify nitrogen dynamics also won fame. It succeeded without using the traditional German method of Liebig, Rubner, and their students who measured nitrogen in ingested food and fluid and excreted nitrogen in feces and urine. In 1905, Krogh married Marie Jorgensen, a promising medical student and scientist in her own right.** The husband-wife team researched transport of carbon dioxide in the lungs, metabolism of Eskimos (with Benedict), and insulin's role in the body. Together, they published seven important papers known as the "seven little devils." Their experiments disproved the oxygen secretion hypothesis championed by Krogh's early mentor, Christian Bohr. Krogh invented the microtonometer, indispensable for quantifying gas transport in blood. Krogh earned enough money from selling equipment to support his laboratory.

Krogh published nearly 300 research papers,[78] many of which we consider "classics" in exercise physiology. For example, he and Johannes Lindhard (1870–1947) studied regulation of respiration and circulation during exercise and recovery. Krogh devised a bicycle ergometer with magnets and weights to quantify exercise intensity. He perfected a method that used nitrous oxide gas to estimate exercise cardiac output. He found that tissues extracted more oxygen during exercise; concurrently, circulation and ventilation increased. Interested in how a muscle receives oxygen, he studied capillary blood flow, as well as oxygen's pressure and diffusing capacity through tissues.[78]

Krogh won the 1920 Nobel Prize in Physiology or Medicine for discovering the mechanism that controlled capillary blood flow in resting and active muscle (in frogs).[81-83] He chronicled his research in 1922.[84] Although there are brief reviews of his career,[85,86] a biography by August Krogh's daughter (Bodil Schmidt-Nielsen[78]) furnishes the most "up-close and personal" information about the lives of both August and Marie Krogh.

August Krogh's research links exercise physiology with nutrition and metabolism. Experiments in comparative zoology (zoophysiology) and cardiovascular physiology inspired experiments in exercise physiology. Krogh interacted with distinguished physiologists A. Keys, Abbey H. Turner, E. M. Landis, E. H. Christensen, F. G. Kovian, A. M. Hemmingsen, H. H. Ussing, and T. W-Fogh. He influenced the next generation of scientists in exercise physiology, particularly those in Nordic countries and the United States. They in turn taught others to investigate human nutrition during acute and chronic physical activity.

Z. OTTO FRITZ MEYERHOF (1884–1951)

The distinguished biochemist Meyerhof contributed to muscle physiology, muscle chemistry, and nutrition. Trained as a physician in Heidelberg, he maintained close contact with established chemists. His early studies of metabolism in sea urchins eventually led to discoveries about cellular events during muscular activity. At age 39, Meyerhof shared the 1922 Nobel Prize in Physiology or Medicine with A.V. Hill for elucidating the cyclic characteristics of intermediary cellular energy transformation processes. Meyerhof's interests in cellular metabolism linked heat produced in metabolism to energy liberated in combustion of the macronutrients, ideas grounded in earlier work by Liebig, Voit, Rubner, Atwater, and Cathcart.

---

* Established by the Imperial Academy of Sciences in Vienna with a cash award of four thousand kroner.
** In 1914, she became the fourth Danish woman to earn a scientific doctoral degree in medicine (Dr. med.).

Meyerhof focused on the way cells utilized energy within food. Dedicating himself for more than four decades to unlocking secrets of intermediary metabolism, he published about 400 papers, particularly on skeletal muscle. Some of Meyerhof's contributions:[87]

1. Showed that without oxygen, muscle glycogen precedes lactic acid formation. With oxygen, some of the lactic acid formed during the anaerobic contraction became oxidized but did not account for all of the lactic acid.
2. Confirmed Pasteur's assumption that less carbohydrate is consumed in the presence of oxygen than in its absence. Depression of glycolysis by respiration is known as the Pasteur-Meyerhof effect.
3. Explained heat production from analyzing the glycogen-lactic acid cycle in relation to respiration.
4. Discovered the glycolytic enzyme system in muscle (the catalysts responsible for converting glycogen to lactic acid), thereby explaining cellular glycolysis.
5. Discovered the high-energy content of ATP and phosphocreatine.
6. Discovered that ATP breakdown preceded phosphocreatine; thus, explaining that ATP served as the primary energy source for muscle contraction.
7. Discovered that lactic acid production and phosphocreatine breakdown participate indirectly in muscle contraction by resynthesis of ATP during muscular activity.
8. Discovered that ATP is involved in the energy transfer reactions of all cells. Furthermore, interconversion occurred between different forms of energy (mechanical, osmotic, light, electrical during different bodily processes.
9. Coined the term "energetic coupling" between oxidation and phosphorylation to explain the mechanism of ATP through oxidation-reduction reactions of glycolysis.

Meyerhof published 350 articles in German journals up to 1939. After the Germans invaded France, he escaped to the United States and became Research Professor of Physiological Chemistry at the School of Medicine, University of Pennsylvania. There, he published another 50 papers on intermediary metabolism. A list of publications appears in his scientific biography.[87]

AA. ARCHIBALD VIVIAN HILL (1886–1977)

A brilliant student at Trinity and Kings Colleges, Cambridge, England, Hill attracted the notice of two eminent physiologists. W. M. Fletcher and (Sir) F. G. Hopkins (Nobel Prize in Physiology or Medicine, 1923) convinced Hill to pursue advanced studies in physiology rather than mathematics. Hill's early experiments researched the effects of electrical stimulation on nerve function, the mechanical efficiency of muscle, energy processes in muscle during recovery, the interaction between oxygen and hemoglobin, and quantitative aspects of drug kinetics on muscle. Hill used his background in mathematics to explain the results. Later, Hill devised mathematical models describing heat production in muscle and applied kinetic analysis to explain the time course of oxygen uptake during both exercise and recovery. Hill combined aspects of physics and biology, a discipline which he championed as bio-physics.

During World War I, Hill directed a laboratory and published technical reports on anti-aircraft defense.[88] After the war, Hill achieved international acclaim for research in muscle physiology. In 1920, he left Cambridge to Chair the Physiology Department at Manchester University. In newly refurbished laboratories, Hill expanded his work on muscle physiology in animals which resulted in a book on muscular activity (1924).[75] Hill shared the Nobel Prize in Physiology or Medicine (1922) with German chemist Otto Meyerhof for discoveries about the chemical and mechanical events in muscle contraction.

While Hill's research is best known in physiology and exercise physiology, he was also acclaimed by nutritionists. G. Lusk's *Lectures on Nutrition* [58] (based on a series of lectures given at the Mayo Foundation and five universities) contains chapters by Hill on muscular activity and carbohydrate metabolism. (Other prominent scientists, F. G. Benedict, E. F. DuBois, E. V. McCollum, H. M. Evans, and Lusk, lectured about nutrition-related topics). The opening paragraph of Hill's lecture connects muscle physiology with nutrition:

It has long been discussed whether the breakdown of carbohydrate, rather than of other substances, is primarily responsible for the provision of energy in muscular contraction. It is known and accepted that work may be done, in the general melting-pot of the body, by the use of any kind of foodstuff. We are now concerned, however, specifically with the *primary* process of muscular contraction. In the complete chain of processes involved in long-continued exercise, this primary process may be disguised, or even apparently obliterated, by simultaneous transformations that take place between the different food constituents. Considering the internal combustion engine, it is obvious that petrol and benzole may be used indiscriminately for providing power and driving the machinery. In the same way, however, as we ask whether carbohydrate is the specific fuel of muscle, or whether fat may be used in an identical manner, so we might query whether petrol or coal can be used in an internal combustion engine. The obvious answer is that coal must be prepared beforehand by distillation, before it can be used in the engine, while petrol can be used directly; and that in the preparation of coal to form benzole for use in the engine, a considerable proportion of the energy of the coal is wasted, as regards its work-producing power. Putting our problem in terms of the modern theory of muscular activity and assuming that the initial process in contraction — that which causes the mechanical response — is an entirely non-oxidative one, consisting of the formation of lactic acid from glycogen, we are asking now whether the recovery process by which the lactic acid is restored to its precursor can go on at the expense of *any* oxidation, or *only* of that of carbohydrate. *May the recovery mechanism, so to speak, be driven by any kind of combustion, as a steam engine may be, or is it necessary specifically to combust carbohydrate?*

An avid sportsman, Hill became interested in recovery from exercise after himself experiencing fatigue during track meets. He coined the term "oxygen debt" based on experiments in the early 1920s.[89-92] He maintained that the amount of oxygen consumed above resting in recovery represented the oxidation of approximately one-fifth of the lactic acid produced during exercise and provided the necessary energy to resynthesize the remaining lactic acid to glycogen.

Hill's more important scientific achievements included:[88] discovery and measurement of heat production associated with the nerve impulse; improved analysis of heat development accompanying active shortening in muscle; application of thermoelectric methods to measure vapor pressure above minute fluid volumes; analysis of physical and chemical changes associated with nerve excitation; and excitation laws for animal tissue. Hill wrote popular articles about science,[93] a practice he continued after retiring in 1951.[94,95]

VIII. PART 2. EXERCISE NUTRITION FOR THE FUTURE: CREATING AN ACADEMIC DISCIPLINE

In Part 1, we reviewed important discoveries from two millennia in chemistry, exercise, metabolism, nutrition, and physiology to bolster our argument that history now requires a utilitarian synthesis which we have titled Exercise Nutrition. So far as we know, no university in the United States or Canada grants a graduate degree in it. Some universities sponsor a concentration in sports nutrition by offering courses from several departments, typically, Nutrition or Health Science and Exercise Science or Kinesiology. Students graduate from one of the departments without benefit of a diploma titled Exercise Nutrition.

Our proposal for an academic major breaks with the traditional approach in two ways. First, we recommend a change in name from sports nutrition to Exercise Nutrition. The term exercise includes more than the word sports and better reflects the new academic content. Second, Departments of Exercise Nutrition should be housed neither in a Department of Nutrition nor a Department of Exercise Science or Kinesiology. Rather, the new department that embraces both disciplines deserves a unique identity within a larger administrative structure. A logical home would be a College of Life Sciences. Such an arrangement would neuter control issues between competing departments and allow a Department of Exercise Nutrition to chart its own course. Figure 1 presents six areas that constitute Exercise Nutrition; Table 2 lists specific topics within each area.

The focus of a Department of Exercise Nutrition is cross-disciplinary. It synthesizes knowledge from the separate but related fields of nutrition and of exercise. A number of existing fields are cross-disciplinary. Biochemists do not receive in-depth training as chemists or biologists. Instead, their training as biochemists makes them more competent biochemists than more narrowly focused chemists or biologists. The same inclusivity characterizes a biophysicist, radio astronomer, molecular biologist, and geophysicist.

Part 1 provided historical precedents for linking two kinds of studies: those involving nutrition and those involving exercise. The chemist Lavoisier, for example, employed exercise to study respiration, probably not thinking that his discoveries would impact fields other than chemistry. A. V. Hill, a competent mathematician and physiologist, won a Nobel Prize in Physiology or Medicine, not for his studies of mathematics or physiology per se, but for his integrative work with muscle that helped to unravel secrets about the biochemistry of contraction.

In the cross-discipline of Exercise Nutrition, students specialize neither in exercise nor nutrition. Instead, they are trained in aspects of *both* exercise and nutrition. Our concept of an academic discipline agrees with Henry's.[96] It is an organized body of information collectively embraced in a formal course of instruction. Acquiring knowledge without demanding practical application is a worthy goal in itself. The content of this curriculum, theoretical and scholarly, distinguishes it from technical and professional ones. This generalization does not imply that the latter are unworthy. Achieving mechanical competence in a particular task should not be confused with mastering the core components of the academic field. Using a computer to calculate calories for candy bars, for instance, does not mean that the operator understands energy metabolism. August Krogh, a Nobel Laureate, became proficient at glass blowing and soldering to build the instruments his research demanded. Yet their mechanical intricacies were merely means to an end and not an essential part of respiratory physiology.

Exercise Nutrition synthesizes data from physiology, exercise physiology, and nutrition. The renal physiologist studies the kidney as an isolated organ to determine its functions. The exercise scientist measures the effects of exercise on the kidney. Here the researcher emphasizes exercise physiology more than physiology. By contrast, the exercise nutritionist would investigate how diet impacts kidney functions in general and in specific circumstances like physical activity.

The discipline of Exercise Nutrition uses data from chemistry, exercise physiology, nutrition, biochemistry, medicine, and physiology. Graduates of Exercise Nutrition may not be full-fledged chemists, exercise physiologists, or nutritionists; however, their cross-disciplinary training will give them a broader and more appropriate perspective to advance their discipline. With the salutary example of Krogh in mind, we assert that Exercise Nutrition does not need to immediately apply its composite knowledge. No doubt practical applications will follow.

For the present, we urge the establishment of a separate discipline to unite previously disparate fields. Like children standing on the backs of giants, we hope that progressive faculty and administrators share our vision and implement this plan for the 21st century.

TABLE 2   Selected Topics Within Each Area of the Proposed Model for Exercise Nutrition

Nutritional Enhancement of Performance

- Optimal nutrition vs. optimal nutrition for exercise
- Athletic competition
- Environmental stressors
- Individual differences
- Special military and environmental applications
- Spaceflight

Peak Physiological Function

- Protein, carbohydrate, and lipid requirements
- Oxidative stress
- Fatigue and staleness
- Tissue repair and growth
- Micronutrient needs
- Reproductive interactions

Good Health and Longevity

- Eating patterns
- Exercise patterns
- Nutrition-exercise related interactions
- Reproductive interactions
- Mortality and morbidity

Safety

- Disordered eating
- Ergogenic/ergolytic substances
- Thermal stress and fluid replacement
- Nutrient abuse
- Exercise-stress-nutrient interactions
- Synthetic substances

Energy Balance and Body Composition

- Metabolism
- Exercise performance
- Body proportions
- Assessment
- Weight control/obesity
- Body size and shape

Growth and Performance

- Normal and abnormal
- Bones, muscle, other tissues
- Children
- Effects on cognitive behaviors
- Effects of chronic exercise
- Sport specific problems

ACKNOWLEDGMENTS AND COMMENT

Dr. Pierre LaGasse, Division of Kinesiology, Department of Social and Preventive Medicine, Laval University, Québec, Canada, kindly translated original passages from Lavoisier into English. After completing our article, we became aware of Simmons, J., *The Scientific*

100. A Ranking of the Most Influential Scientists, Past and Present, Citadel Press Books, Secaucus, New Jersey, 1996. Simmons profiles six of the individuals we highlighted: Lavoisier, Bernard, Vesalius, Liebig, Harvey, and Hopkins.

REFERENCES

1. Rawlinson, G., Translation from Herodotus, *Histories,* Book II; http://the-tech.mit.edu/Classics/Herodotus/history.ii.html.
2. Breasted, J. H., The rise of man, *Science*, 74, 639, 1930.
3. Cathcart, E. P., The early development of the science of nutrition, in, Bourne, G. H. and Kidder, G. W., Eds., *Biochemistry and Physiology of Nutrition*, Vol. 1, Academic Press Inc., New York, 1953, 1.
4. Furley, D. J. and Wilkie, J. S., *Galen on Respiration and the Arteries*, Princeton University Press, Princeton, 1984.
5. Clagett, M., *Greek Science in Antiquity*, Books for Library Series, Freeport, ME, 1955.
6. Singer, C., *A Short History of Scientific Ideas to 1900*, Oxford University Press, Oxford, 1959.
7. Garrison, F. H., *An Introduction to the History of Medicine*, 4th ed., Saunders, Philadelphia, 1929.
8. Green, R. M., *A Translation of Galen's Hygiene (De Sanitate Tuenda)*, Charles C. Thomas Publisher, Springfield, IL, 1951.
9. Gardner, E. J., *History of Biology*, 3rd ed., Burgess Publishing Company, Minneapolis, 1972.
10. Robinson, R. S., *Sources for the History of Greek Athletics*, Revised, Ares Publishers, Chicago, 1955, 118.
11. Gardiner, E. N., *Greek Athletic Sports and Festivals*, Macmillan and Co. Limited, London, 1910.
12. Gardner, P. and Jevons, F. B., *A Manual of Greek Antiquities*, Charles Scribner's and Sons, New York, 1895, 327.
13. Gardiner, E. N., *Athletics of the Ancient World*, Clarendon Press, Oxford, 1930.
14. Celsus, *De Medicina, Volume I,* English translation by Spencer, W. G., Harvard University Press, Cambridge, MA, 1935.
15. Celsus, *De Medicina, Volume II,* English translation by Spencer, W. G., Harvard University Press, Cambridge, MA, 1938.
16. Guerlac, H., *Essays and Papers in the History of Modern Science*, The John Hopkins University Press, Baltimore, 1977.
17. Behnke, A. R. and Wilmore, J. H., *Regulation of Body Build and Composition*, Prentice-Hall, Englewood Cliffs, NJ, 1974.
18. Knight, B., *Discovering the Human Body*, Bloomsbury Books, London, 1992.
19. Guerlac, H. G., *Essays and Papers in the History of Modern Science*, The Johns Hopkins University Press, Baltimore, 1977.
20. Krehl, W. A., James Lind, M.D., *J. Nutr.,* 50, 3, 1953.
21. Harré, R., *Great Scientific Experiments*, Phaidon Press Limited, Oxford, 1981.
22. Lusk, G., A history of metabolism, in, Barker, L., Ed., *Endocrinology and Metabolism*, D. Appleton and Company, New York, 1922, 3.
23. Carpenter, K. J., *Protein and Energy: A Study of Changing Ideas in Nutrition*, Cambridge University Press, London, 1994.
24. Gillispie, C. C., Ed., *Dictionary of Scientific Biography*, Volume V, Charles Scribner's and Sons, New York, 1965, 317.
25. Benedict, F. G. and Cathcart, E. P., *Muscular work. A metabolic study, with special reference to the efficiency of the human body as a machine*, Carnegie Institute of Washington, Washington, D.C., 1913.
26. Cathcart, E. P., *The Physiology of Protein Metabolism*, Longmans, Green and Co., New York, 1912.
27. Fenton, P. F., François Magendie, *J. Nutr.*, 43, 3, 1951.
28. Lesch, J. E., *Science and Medicine in France. The Emergence of Experimental Physiology, 1790–1855*, Harvard University Press, Cambridge, 1984.
29. Beaumont, W., *Experiments and Observations on the Gastric Juice and the Physiology of Digestion,* Dover Publications, Inc., New York, 1959.
30. Cutter, C., *Anatomy and Physiology Designed for Academies and Families*, Benjamin B. Mussey and Co., Boston, 1848.
31. Smith, A. H., William Beaumont, *J. Nutr.*, 44: 3, 1951.
32. Cowgill, G. R., Jean Baptiste Boussingault-A Biographical Sketch, *J. Nutr.*, 84, 3, 1964.
33. Huntress, E. H., Biographical digests. IV. Centennials and polycentennials during 1952 with interest for chemists and physicists, *Proc. Am. Acad. Arts Sci.*, 81, 43, 1952.
34. Guggenheim, K. Y., *Nutrition and Nutritional Diseases*, Collamore Press, Lexington, MA, 1981.
35. Brouwer, E., Gerrit Jan Mulder, *J. Nutr.,* 46, 3, 1952.

36. Holmes, F. L. Justus von Liebig, *Dictionary of Scientific Biography*, Volume VIII. Charles Scribner's and Sons, New York, 1973, 329.
37. Shenstone, W. A., *Justus von Liebig: His Life and Work (1803–1873)*, Macmillan, New York, 1895.
38. Lusk, G., *Nutrition*, Hafner Publishing Company, New York, 1964, 87.
39. Kleiber, M., Body size and metabolic rate, in, Catlett, R. H., Ed., *Readings in Animal Energetics*, MSS Information Corporation, New York, 7, 600, 1973.
40. Vanderburgh, P. M., Katch, F. I., Balabinis, C., and Elliot, R., Multivariate allometric scaling of men's world indoor rowing championship performance, *Med. Sci. Sports Exerc.*, 28, 626, 1996.
41. Vanderburgh, P. M. and Katch, F. I., Ratio scaling of VO$_2$max penalizes women with larger percent body fat, not lean body mass, *Med. Sci. Sports Exerc.*, 28, 1204, 1996.
42. Mayer, J., Claude Bernard, *J. Nutr.*, 45, 3, 1951.
43. Fruton, J. S., Claude Bernard the scientist, in, Robin, E. D., Ed., *Claude Bernard and the Internal Environment. A Memorial Symposium*, Marcel Dekker, Inc., New York, 1979.
44. Bernard, C., *The Introduction to the Study of Experimental Medicine* (translated by H. C. Greene), Henry Schuman, Inc., New York, 1927.
45. Foster, M., *Claude Bernard*, Longmans, Green & Co., New York, 1899.
46. Grmek, M. D., Claude Bernard, in *Dictionary of Scientific Biography*, Volume II, Charles Scribner's and Sons, New York, 1971, 24.
47. McCollum, E. M., *A History of Nutrition*, Houghton Mifflin Company, Boston, 1957, 124.
48. Fick, A. and Wislicenus, J., On the origin of muscular power, *Phil. Mag. & J. Sci.*, London (4th ser., No. 212), 31, 485, 1866.
49. Brock, W. H., Edward Frankland, in *Dictionary of Scientific Biography*, Vol. V, Charles Scribner's and Sons, New York, 1972, 124.
50. McArdle, W. D., Katch, F. I., and Katch, V. L., *Exercise Physiology. Energy, Nutrition, and Human Performance*, 4th ed., Williams & Wilkins, Baltimore, 1996, xxiii, 147.
51. Gould, B. A., *Investigations in the Military and Anthropological Statistics of American Soldiers*, Published for the U.S. Sanitary Commission, Hurd and Houghton, New York, 1869.
52. Coleman, W., *Biology in the Nineteenth Century. Problems of Form, Function, and Transformation*, Cambridge University Press, Cambridge, 1971.
53. Ross, W. D., Kinanthropometry: an emerging scientific technology, in, Landry, F. and Orban, W. A. R., Eds., *Biomechanics of Sports and Kinanthropometry*, Book 6, Symposia Specialists, Inc., Miami, 1978, 269.
54. Ross, W. D., Drinkwater, D. T., Bailey, D. A., Marshall, G. W., and Leahy, R. M., Kinanthropometry: traditions and new perspectives, in, Ostyn, M., Ed., *Kinanthropometry II*, University Park Press, Baltimore, 1980, 3.
55. Dolman, C. E., Max Joseph von Pettenkofer, in *Dictionary of Scientific Biography*, Volume X, Charles Scribner's and Sons, New York, 1974, 556.
56. Brook, A. T., Description of apparatus for testing the results of perspiration and respiration in the Physiological Institute of Munich, *Smithsonian Report for 1864*, Washington, D.C., 235–239, 1865.
57. Lusk, G., The *Fundamental Basis of Nutrition*, Yale University Press, New Haven, 1914.
58. Lusk, G., *Lectures on Nutrition, 1924–1925,* W. B. Saunders Company, Philadelphia, 1925.
59. Lusk, G., *Nutrition*, Clio Medica Series, Hafner Publishing Company, New York, 1933.
60. Lusk, G., *The Elements of the Science of Nutrition*, 2nd ed., W. B. Saunders Company, Philadelphia, 1909.
61. Holmes, F. L., Carl von Voit, in *Dictionary of Scientific Biography*, Volume XIV, Charles Scribner's and Sons, New York, 1976, 63.
62. Flint, A., Jr., *A Text-Book of Human Physiology; Designed for the Use of Practitioners and Students of Medicine,* D. Appleton, New York, 1877.
63. Forbes, R. M., Nathan Zuntz, *J. Nutr.*, 57, 3, 1955.
64. Maynard, L. A. and Wilbur O., Atwater — a biographical sketch, *J. Nutr.*, 78, 3, 1962.
65. Atwater, W. O. and Rosa, E. B., *Description of a New Respiration Calorimeter and Experiments on the Conservation of Energy in the Human Body*, Bulletin 63, U.S. Department of Agriculture, Office of Experiment Stations, Government Printing Office, Washington, D.C., 1899.
66. Atwater, W. O. and Benedict, F. G., *A Respiration Calorimeter with Appliances for the Direct Determination of Oxygen*, Carnegie Institute of Washington, Washington, D.C., 1905.
67. Benedict, F. G. and Carpenter, T. M., *Respiration Calorimeters for Studying the Respiratory Exchange and Energy Transformations of Man*, Bulletin 123, U.S. Department of Agriculture, Office of Experiment Stations, Government Printing Office, Washington, D.C., 1910.
68. Atwater, W. O., *Methods and Results of Investigations on the Chemistry and Economy of Food*, Bulletin 21, U.S. Department of Agriculture, Office of Experiment Stations, Government Printing Office, Washington, D.C., 1895.
69. Deuel, H., Jr., Graham Lusk, *J. Nutr.*, 41, 3, 1959.
70. Chambers, W. H., Max Rubner, *J. Nutr.*, 48, 3, 1952.
71. Vickery, H. B., Russel Henry Chittenden, *Biographical Memoirs*, XXIV, National Academy of Sciences, Washington, D.C., 1947.

72. Chittenden, R. H., *Physiological Economy In Nutrition, With Special Reference To The Minimal Proteid Requirement of the Healthy Man. An Experimental Study*, Frederick A. Stokes Company, New York, 1904.

73. Hopkins, F. G., The analyst and the medical man, *The Analyst*, 31, 386, 1906.

74. Fletcher, W. M. and Hopkins. F. G., Lactic acid in amphibian muscle, *J. Physiol.*, 35, 247, 1907.

75. Hill, A. V., *Muscular Activity*, Herter Lectures. Sixteenth Course. Williams & Wilkins Company, Baltimore, 1926.

76. Baldwin, E., Frederick Gowland Hopkins, in *Dictionary of Scientific Biography*, Volume VI, Charles Scribner's and Sons, New York, 1972, 498.

77. Baldwin, E. and Needham, J., Eds., *Hopkins and Biochemistry*, W. Heffer, Cambridge, England, 1949.

78. Schmidt-Nielsen, B., *August & Marie Krogh. Lives in Science*, American Physiological Society, Oxford University Press, New York, 1995.

79. Maynard, L. A., Francis Gano Benedict — a biographical sketch, *J. Nutr.*, 98, 1, 1969.

80. DuBois, E. and Riddle, O., Biographical memoirs, *Nat. Acad. Sci.*, XXXII, 67, 1958.

81. Krogh, A., The rate of diffusion of gases through animal tissues with some remarks on the coefficient of invasion, *J. Physiol.*, 52, 1919.

82. Krogh, A., The number and distribution of capillaries in muscles with calculations of the oxygen pressure head necessary for supplying the tissue, *J. Physiol.*, 52, 1919.

83. Krogh, A., The supply of oxygen to the tissues and the regulation of the capillary circulation, *J. Physiol.* (London), 52, 457, 1919.

84. Krogh, A., *The Anatomy and Physiology of Capillaries*, Yale University Press, New York, 1922.

85. Liljestrand, G., August Krogh, *Acta Physiol. Scand.*, 20, 109, 1950.

86. Snorrason, E., Krogh, Shack August Steenberg, in *Dictionary of Scientific Bibliography*, Volume VII, Charles Scribner's and Sons, New York, 1973, 501.

87. Nachmanson, D., Ochoa, S., and Lipmann, F. A., Otto Meyerhof, Biographical Memoirs, *National Academy of Sciences*, XXXIV, Columbia University Press, New York, 1960.

88. Katz, B., Archibald Vivian Hill, *Dictionary of National Biography*, Oxford University Press, Oxford, 1986, 406.

89. Hill, A. V., Long, C. N. H., and Lupton, H., Muscular exercise, lactic acid and the supply and utilization of oxygen. Pt. I–III, *Proc. Roy. Soc. B*, 96, 438, 1924.

90. Hill, A. V., Long, C. N. H., and Lupton, H., Muscular exercise, lactic acid and the supply and utilization of oxygen. Pt. IV–VI, *Proc. Roy. Soc. B*, 97, 84, 1924.

91. Hill, A. V., Long, C. N. H., and Lupton, H., Muscular exercise, lactic acid and the supply and utilization of oxygen. Pt. VII–IX, *Proc. Roy. Soc. B*, 97, 155, 1924.

92. Hill, A. V. and Lupton, H., Muscular exercise, lactic acid, and the supply and utilization of oxygen, *Quart. J. Med.*, 16, 135, 1923.

93. Hill, A. V., The scientific study of athletics, *Sci. Amer.*, April, 224, 1926.

94. Hill, A. V., *The Ethical Dilemma of Science, and Other Writings*, Rockefeller Institute Press, New York, 1960.

95. Hill, A. V., *Trails and Trials in Physiology. A Bibliography, 1909–1964; With Reviews of Certain Topics and Methods and a Reconnaissance for Further Research*, E. Arnold, London, 1965.

96. Henry, F. M., Physical education: an academic discipline, *J. Hlth, Phys. Educ. Rec.*, 35, 32, 1964.

Chapter 2

OVERVIEW: NUTRITION IN EXERCISE AND SPORT

John J. B. Anderson
Robert G. McMurray

CONTENTS

I. INTRODUCTION TO NUTRITION IN EXERCISE AND SPORT

The relationship between nutrition and physical fitness/performance continues to develop in terms of knowledge base and understandings. Nevertheless, the general principles of sound nutritional practices have changed very little over the years. Significant progress, however, has been made in the fine tuning of information relating the consumption of specific nutrients and fluids to athletic performance. This introductory chapter attempts to provide a sound nutritional background for the readership as well as highlight several of the major research findings on this topic that have been reported over the last five years.

II.   GENERAL NUTRITION CONCEPTS

Sound nutrition is based on the wise selection of foods and beverages according to the stage of the life cycle of the individual and, therefore, the nutrient needs of the individual (see below under Basic Food Guide or Pyramid). In this section, information on the nutritional needs of adult and growing athletes is provided. Additional information on this topic is also presented in the chapters that follow.

A.   NUTRITION FOR TISSUE MAINTENANCE

Exercise per se contributes to damage of tissues used in physical activities, namely, muscles, tendons, and ligaments. Depending on the severity of tissue damage, repair can be quite rapid, i.e., within minutes to a few hours, or much longer, i.e., within days to weeks. Good nutrition, including the consumption energy, protein, and micronutrients from foods, provides the sources for tissue recovery. No magic supplements or herbals have been identified yet to enhance the renewal of damaged tissues other than a good supply of nutrients from the wise selection of foods and beverages.

B.   NUTRITION AND GROWTH

Athletes who have not completed their growth in height need to assure adequate intakes of energy, protein, and micronutrients to allow for exercise and at the same time permit the normal skeletal growth process to continue. Suspension of growth by some types of young athletes, such as wrestlers and gymnasts, has been reported because of periods of undernutrition, but this practice is not recommended.

Meeting the nutrient needs of growing children and adolescents who are also athletes may not be so difficult if restrictions on weight-gain are not placed on any individual. The Basic Food Guide or Pyramid should be the best resource for getting the balance of nutrients in the appropriate amounts from the different food groups (see below). Typically, appetite is the best guide for growing youngsters, but ensuring adequate energy intake from carbohydrates (and not so much from fats) may be more difficult without good meal planning by a parent or guardian or by the athletes themselves. It should be recognized that children have specific nutrient needs that are different from adults. Therefore, young growing athletes typically need special guidance by adults in the appropriate selection of foods that provide the required nutrients to meet the requirements of growth and performance (see Chapter 18 for an expanded review of this topic).

In addition to energy, adequate intakes of protein and micronutrients also may be much more critical for individuals who have marginal intakes of iron and calcium, and possibly of other micronutrients. Protein-rich foods, such as dairy foods (other than butter) and meats, provide the bulk of the calcium and iron, respectively, from the vast array of foods in all the other groups. This pattern of marginal consumption of protein-rich foods may occur among some, but not all, vegetarian athletes who have inadequate nutrition knowledge of foods and who could benefit from nutrition education (see below and Chapter 17).

C. NUTRITION AND IMMUNE FUNCTION

An emerging area of significant research is the relationship of immune function to athletic performance. The physical stress on body tissues of athletic performance may require efficient immunologic defense mechanisms in order to protect against the development of infections from bacteria and viruses. Much research over recent decades has established the importance of adequate nutrient intakes, especially of the micronutrients, for support of host defense against the invasion and multiplication of microorganisms. Only recently have sports nutritionists and related scientists begun to investigate the roles of specific nutrients in supporting the immune system of athletes. This area of investigation holds great promise. Again, the consistent message being reported by scientists is that good overall nutrition helps better than any other known approach, i.e., supplements of one type or another, to maintain the immune defense mechanisms. A review of this topic is presented in Chapter 26 of this volume.

III. BASIC FOOD GUIDE OR PYRAMID

The numbers of recommended servings, according to the Basic Food Guide or Pyramid, are set for moderately active people, not for athletes or vegetarian athletes (Figure 1). Therefore, athletes must increase the numbers of servings to meet, first, their energy requirements from carbohydrates and other macronutrients and, secondly, to satisfy their requirements of other nutrients.

This issue of increased numbers of servings is probably not so critical for athletes with respect to getting enough energy and protein from foods because they typically eat according to "hunger" or appetite and therefore obtain sufficient amounts of the macronutrients. Where they may fall short is in the micronutrients, simply because of not being careful to select the minimum numbers of servings in all the food groups. For example, iron and calcium are two micronutrients found most often to be deficient in the diets of female athletes. The reasons for inadequate intakes have been clearly established: female athletes typically consume too few servings of foods from the meat (iron) and dairy (calcium) groups each day. Therefore, the minimal numbers of servings is most critical for getting the dietary balance that provides all the nutrients, both macronutrients and micronutrients, on a daily basis (see Chapters 8 and 9). Wise eating patterns should be established as part of an athlete's overall preparation for events or games, and this healthy eating practice should then hold for the lifetime of the individual.

Use of the Basic Food Guide/Pyramid can be enhanced by the satisfactory understanding of the Nutrition Facts Panel now used in food labeling. The Panel gives the amount (in grams) of a serving of food, plus information on the amounts of the macronutrients (except for protein) and energy (in Calories, the equivalent of kilocalories) in a serving. In addition, the Panel provides the percent daily value (% DV) of the major nutrients in each serving, based on a 2000 kcal diet. For many breakfast cereals, information is given for a serving of cereal combined with a half cup of milk. When these figures are factored into the total day's food consumption, individuals can have a better estimate of their needs for calories and the major micronutrients. In addition, the new labeling emphasizes the amounts of fat, saturated fat, sugar, and sodium consumed in a serving of food for the purpose of reducing the amounts of these potential health-risk nutrients (see items numbered 4–6 below under Dietary Guidelines for Americans). Food typically high in these nutrients are referred to as low-nutrient density foods because they contain energy (as fat or sugar) with very little nutritional value from the critical micronutrients. Examples of these foods, which should be consumed rarely, include rich desserts, candies, and select types of snack foods.

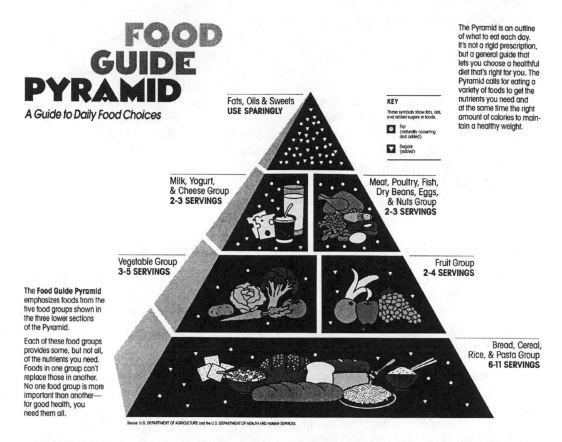

FIGURE 1   Basic Food Guide or Pyramid. The recommended servings per day from each of the food groups for adults. At the base of the Pyramid are the grains and then the vegetables and fruits, all plant food sources, which should be consumed in the greatest amounts each day. Then, near the top are the animal foods, which should be consumed in lesser amounts, and on the tip the miscellaneous foods for which no recommendation is made. Athletes typically need to consume at the higher end of each range of recommended numbers of servings, with males generally needing more servings per food group than females on a daily basis. (Courtesy: National Cattlemen's Beef Association.)

IV.   DIETARY GUIDELINES FOR AMERICANS

The newest edition of the *Dietary Guidelines for Americans* (4th ed., 1995),[1] issued jointly by the U.S. Department of Agriculture (USDA) and the U.S. Department of Health and Human Services (USHHS), is not appreciably different from earlier editions, but a few new emphases on the diet are highlighted herein because they apply to athletes as well as to nonathletes.

The seven Dietary Guidelines are as follows:

1. Eat a variety of foods.
2. Balance the food you eat with physical activity — maintain or improve your weight.
3. Choose a diet with plenty of grain products, vegetables, and fruits.
4. Choose a diet low in fat, saturated fat, and cholesterol.
5. Choose a diet moderate in sugars.
6. Choose a diet moderate in salt and sodium.
7. If you drink alcoholic beverages, do so in moderation.

The first Dietary Guideline is extremely important — many different foods a day, i.e., variety, enable an athlete to consume virtually all of the micronutrients and non-nutrient molecules from plant foods. The second Dietary Guideline relating to weight regulation has almost no meaning for practically all athletes because they are in topnotch physical condition for high-level performance. Therefore, this guide is intended primarily for less physically active adults and children. The other Dietary Guidelines are designed to assure adequate intakes of complex carbohydrates, dietary fiber, and micronutrients, but not too much sugar, salt, fat, and cholesterol. A new aspect presented in the Dietary Guidelines is the recognition that vegetarian diets can be consistent with the seven specific guidelines. These accepted views about food choices are very appropriate for athletes as they are for other individuals.

V. NUTRITIONAL NEEDS OF ATHLETES RELATED TO COMPETITION

The nutritional needs of competitive athletes are considered herein with respect to the three major time periods surrounding and including an event, namely, pre-competitive and post-competitive meals and the need for energy and fluids during a competition.

A. PRE-COMPETITION MEAL

The purpose of the pre-competition meal is to maximize glycogen stores, especially in skeletal muscles, and to provide adequate hydration, while minimizing gastric distress, hunger, and digestion during the competition. What an athlete eats before competition can do more to hinder than to enhance competitive performance. However, no single menu appears best for pre-competition meals, as any drastic change from the normal diet can result in gastric distress, diarrhea, or even lethargy. Therefore, if an athlete normally consumes a high fat/protein diet and decides to switch to a high carbohydrate/sugar diet before competition, a strong likelihood exists for the occurrence of diarrhea during competition.[2] Similarly, the consumption of spicy foods immediately prior to competition for an athlete that normally eats a bland diet could increase gastric distress and intestinal gas. The literature suggests four important constructs with regard to pre-competition meals: (1) timing; (2) amount; (3) components of the meal; and (4) fluids. Each of these aspects is briefly reviewed.

The timing of the meal is important. Research has indicated that glycogen stores depleted by training cannot be replenished by a pre-competition meal; however, there is limited ability of the muscle to generate glycogen stores when the meal is ingested 4–6 hours before competition.[3] The 4–6 hour period prior to competition also insures that blood insulin levels have returned to normal at the start of competition. Conversely, an individual who eats within a couple hours prior to competition may have elevated insulin levels at the start of exercise. Hyperinsulinemia reduces β-oxidation and causes a greater reliance on muscle glycogen stores than desirable.[4] Therefore, during prolonged exercise glycogen stores would be more likely to be prematurely depleted. The 4–6 hour timing of the pre-competition meal also would insure that the majority of digestion was complete and that the stomach would be relatively empty at the onset of exercise. Thus, blood needed for digestion would be diverted to the muscle for exercise.

The amount of food can also affect exercise performance. Too small a meal can leave the person with low blood glucose levels during prolonged competition. Conversely, too large a meal can leave the person lethargic. In addition, large meals take longer to digest which can diminish blood flow to skeletal muscles and lead to gastric distress (nausea, bloating, intestinal gas) or diarrhea during prolonged competition, such as a soccer game, long-distance running or cycling.

The meal should consist mainly of carbohydrates, and typically lesser amounts of proteins and lipids than in regular meals. Research has suggested 75–150 g of moderate glycemic-index carbohydrates.[5] Moderate and high glycemic-index carbohydrates should be completely digested and insulin normalized prior to the start of competition. A carbohydrate content of less than 75 g may not be adequate to replenish glycogen stores, whereas a larger amount could result in insulin rebound and hunger during exercise. Moderate glycemic-index foods would include breads, rice, spaghetti, potatoes, bananas, raisins, beets, corn, and many cereals like shredded wheat or oatmeal.[6,7] High glycemic-index foods have the potential to produce insulin-rebound hypoglycemia prior to the onset of exercise, and this reduction in blood glucose may increase the risk of gastric distress. High glycemic-index foods would include honey, corn flakes, glucose, and sweets. The protein in the meal reduces the risk of hunger during exercise and also may reduce the potential for rebound hypoglycemia during the postprandial period. Low fat content of pre-competition meals is important, since fats slow gastric emptying and thereby prolong the duration of digestion and absorption for up to 8 hours. Therefore, blood that could be used by the skeletal muscles for exercise would be diverted, at least in part, to the digestive tract. The ingestion of a high fat meal has been shown to increase free fatty acid metabolism and conserve glycogen stores.[2] A high-fat intake, however, could be of potential benefit for prolonged exercise. Other published research reports, unfortunately, do not support this contention.[8,9] Therefore, a high carbohydrate (60–70%), moderate protein (10–20%), and low fat (10–25%) pre-competition meal appears to be best for athletes.

Some foods should be avoided as they may be difficult to digest and thereby produce gastric distress, flatulence. Other foods may contain too much bulk, i.e., dietary fiber, which could stimulate a defecation response at an undesirable time. Depending upon the normal diet of the person, the pre-competition meal should include food sources that are not high in fiber, cellulose, roughage, and seedy vegetables which would add bulk and produce gastric distress. Also, this meal should not contain the following: spicy ingredients that may cause heartburn and flatulence; greasy foods that slow digestion; or a large amount of simple sugars that could cause diarrhea. As stated above, if the athlete is accustomed to eating these foods, it is best not to radically change his/her diet.

Finally, animal research has suggested that fasting prior to exercise can enhance performance.[10] Human studies, however, do not agree with this conclusion. Dohm et al.[11] and Loy et al.[12] have independently shown that 24 hours of fasting prior to exercise reduces the endurance of cycling or running performers. The reduction in exercise capacity appears to be related to the fasting-induced muscle glycogen stores, prior to the onset of exercise. Therefore, fasting prior to competition should not be recommended for athletes.

The final consideration of a pre-competition meal is hydration. Athletes should ingest sufficient fluid to start the competition hydrated but not in a state of diuresis. Initiating hydration 4–6 hours prior to exercise helps to ensure that fluid balance is re-established and that dehydration, even a moderate fluid imbalance, is prevented. At the same time any diuretic response would be abated. The source of fluids at this time does not appear to matter. However, a high fructose drink may result in some gastrointestinal distress because of its low glycemic index.[2,13] In addition, the ingestion of large amounts of caffeinated beverages at this time could lead to diuresis and incomplete hydration at the onset of exercise.

B. ENERGY DURING COMPETITION

The need for exogenous sources of energy during exercise is dependent upon the duration of exercise. In general for unconditioned athletes, body stores of carbohydrate are sufficient to last for approximately 90 minutes of exercise. The stores of carbohydrates of highly trained athletes, however, should last for at least 120 minutes of moderate to high-intensity exercise.[12] Therefore, exercise lasting longer than 90 minutes should benefit from an additional supply of carbohydrate provided during the period of exercise. Similarly, if the athlete starts exercise with depleted stores of glycogen, an exogenous supply of carbohydrate could prove beneficial for shorter durations of activity than 90 minutes. Davis et al.[15] has shown that the ingestion of a 6% glucose/sucrose solution better maintained blood glucose levels during 2 hours of cycling. Coyle et al.[12] found that the ingestion of a glucose polymer solution (1 g/kg body weight) at 20-minute intervals during cycling to exhaustion improved ride times by 17%. Similarly, Williams[16] also found improvement in running time to exhaustion of athletes who ingested a carbohydrate solution during exercise. More recently, Tsintzas et al.[17] have shown that the ingestion of a 5.5% carbohydrate solution during 60 minutes of exercise resulted in a 28% reduction in glycogen use. Therefore, the ingestion of carbohydrate solutions appears to be beneficial during prolonged exercise. The use of fructose as the source of carbohydrate, however, may not be as beneficial as other carbohydrate sources, since one report has indicated that fructose is less readily available for oxidation and may cause diarrhea.[13]

The published data suggesting an enhancement of short-term exercise performance by the ingestion of carbohydrate solutions, however, is equivocal. Nishibata et al.[18] found that the use of a glucose solution had no significant effect on exercise performance during 60 minutes of cycling at 73% of maximal capacity, even when the exercise was completed on three successive days. Conversely, Lambert et al.[19] demonstrated that performance during resistance training (weight lifting) was significantly improved by the ingestion of a glucose polymer solution. This topic is discussed at greater length in Chapter 14 of this volume.

C. POST-COMPETITION MEAL

The purposes of this meal are: to replenish as much glycogen as possible prior to the next exercise session; to rehydrate; and to replace electrolytes lost during prolonged sweating. The post-game/competition meal should include more food than any other meal of that day. Glycogen stores are best replenished by a high-carbohydrate diet. The original research suggested that complex carbohydrates were best for replacing glycogen stores.[20,21] More recent research, however, has shown that simple sugars are also an effective source of carbohydrate, especially during the first 24 hours after exercise.[22]

The exerciser needs to consume sufficient amounts of fluid to re-establish water balance. The source of fluid may not be important, but sports drinks that contain about 10–12% sugar and electrolytes may be of benefit because they enhance rehydration, replacement of electrolytes, and glycogen replenishment. Simply replacing glycogen and fluids, however, does not assure complete recovery from exhaustive exercise.[23] Recall that overall good nutrition according to the basic food guide or pyramid is critical for tissue repair and maintenance. These guidelines are applicable to athletes participating in strenuous and prolonged training sessions as well as for post-competition meals.

VI. SPECIAL NUTRITIONAL CONSIDERATIONS FOR ATHLETES

Both female and male athletes may have special nutritional needs because of either physiological changes or sport specificity. The special consideration of females will be covered first and then of males, and in the next section the needs of athletes in specific sports are briefly noted.

Young female athletes undergo significant physiological, reproductive, and psychological changes that can potentially have adverse impacts on both performance and injuries and even possibly on optimal physical development. Dietary practices often change as girls begin the path toward womanhood, and concerns about body composition and conformation often become predominant. Among female athletes, weight control often emerges as a major reason for altering food habits, but also many young female athletes adopt a partial or total vegetarian diet. In extreme cases, female athletes may skip meals with sufficient frequency to develop eating disorders.[24-28]

In addition to potential eating disorders relating to general undernutrition, female athletes also commonly have marginal intakes of iron or calcium, and sometimes both, despite adequate consumption of total energy and protein from foods. The more marginal status of iron deficiency, not accompanied by anemia, is prevalent among female athletes, especially in menstruating athletes.[29-32]

Inadequate intake of iron-rich animal products (except for dairy foods that are iron-poor) are primarily responsible for iron deficiency. More severe inadequacy of iron consumption leads to iron-deficiency anemia (see case of female athlete triad with iron deficiency anemia in Chapter 9). Women diagnosed with severe iron deficits will, in virtually all cases, require iron supplementation for a period of several months,[31] but not all female athletes apparently benefit from iron supplements.[33] Vegetarian athletes, or those who exclude red meats in their diets, frequently develop iron deficiency despite amenorrhea.[30-34]

Two major factors contribute to bone loss in otherwise healthy female athletes: too little calcium in the diet and amenorrhea. Low calcium consumption nearly always results from insufficient ingestion of dairy products, although other calcium-rich foods may also be neglected in the typical diets of female athletes. Although osteopenia, or too little bone mass, may occur because of diets inadequate in calcium-rich foods,[35-37] amenorrhea secondary to intensive physical training is a major contributor to low bone mass.[35-36] Use of oral contraceptive agents by amenorrheic adolescent and young adult athletes may actually improve their bone mass without detracting from their athletic performance.[38,39] The potential adverse consequences of amenorrhea-induced osteopenia, complicated by low calcium intake, include leg injuries and stress fractures, that are especially common in distance runners and ballerinas.[40,41] Calcium supplements may help amenorrheic young female athletes retain more skeletal mineral if milk and related foods cannot be consumed in adequate amounts.

Female athletes also have been reported to display deficiencies in other micronutrients besides iron and calcium that may place them in jeopardy of diminished performance levels and increased injury rates. In the latter regard, females seem to experience greater disability from these micronutrient deficits than do males because of lower total caloric intakes. Male athletes usually have little difficulty consuming enough energy and protein from foods, but unlike most weight-conscious females they generally have far too high consumption of fat.

In contrast to females, male athletes have had no known reports of problems of eating disorders and any associated undernutrition. Similarly, calcium and iron deficiencies have been less commonly diagnosed in males, but iron deficits may be under-recognized, especially in rapidly growing adolescent athletes whose requirements for iron are increased because of continued muscle growth.

In general, male athletes tend to have irregular eating habits, including much snacking. While such practices do not necessarily lead to inadequate intakes of macronutrients, they may contribute to micronutrient insufficiencies because of a limited number of food choices. In most males restricted consumption of fruits and vegetables, except for fries and other forms of potatoes, is common.[42] Because fruits and vegetables provide many of the B vitamins, vitamin C, and many trace elements, athletic males can easily develop marginal nutritional status with respect to several vitamins and trace minerals. They can also become iron deficient if they do not consume enough meats and other high-iron foods.[32]

More than anything else, male athletes need to broaden their choice of foods and select more fruits and vegetables and whole-grain breads and cereals, that assure a greater percentage of complex carbohydrates of their total energy intake and also provide greater amounts of micronutrients and dietary fiber. Fruits and vegetables contain good amounts of potassium, the electrolyte critical for the function of muscle and other tissues. Enough sodium is usually consumed from many of the other foods in a balanced diet, especially meats and dairy products, and most processed foods contain large amounts of added sodium. The high-fiber foods should, of course, be largely consumed in the bigger meal of the day after any daily sports activities have been concluded (see section above on Post-competition meals).

VII. POTENTIAL NUTRITIONAL PROBLEMS OF SPECIFIC TYPES OF ATHLETES

Several sports and related activities, including dance, contribute to less than satisfactory nutritional status. The suboptimal nutritional status not only affects performance but probably increases the likelihood of injuries related to these activities. The specific sports focused on here are gymnastics, wrestling, long-distance running, and ballet dancing. The contact and collision sports also contribute to both exertional dehydration and mineral losses in sweat, which can hasten the loss of mental concentration and thereby increase the chance of injury in these sports.

Performance in gymnastics and certain other sports requires physical attributes that are based on a low percentage of body fat and, conversely, a relatively high percentage of skeletal muscle. Female gymnasts typically consume too little energy from foods, which translates to inadequate consumption of nearly all of the micronutrients.[43,44] Vitamin-mineral combination supplements can be recommended for these underconsuming female athletes,[45] but it is advisable first to have a physical examination by a physician and a nutritional assessment by a dietitian/nutritionist.[46]

Wrestlers typically reduce their energy consumption from foods to meet the upper limits of body weight for specific competitive classes.[47,48] Although such underconsumption by young, growing wrestlers and female gymnasts will temporarily suspend their physical growth, they later catch-up in development, and growth normally follows when energy and protein intakes of athletes are normalized. These athletes may also experience dehydration because of food and fluid restriction.[47-49] Unbalanced diets and fluid restriction are frequently accompanied by common colds, other infections, and nagging minor injuries, and occasionally by more serious injuries (see below, Nutrition and Injury Prevention).

Long-distance runners, especially females, typically have low-calorie diets despite their tremendous expenditure of energy in training and competitive events.[44,50,51] Like female gymnasts, female runners are potentially amenorrheic (either secondary or primary), which places them at increased risk for stress fractures and other injuries. Female runners, whether or not they are taking oral contraceptive agents, should make certain that they consume adequate amounts of calcium, i.e., at or approaching the Recommended Dietary Allowance (RDA) level for their age. They should consume low-fat (0.5 or 1.0% fat content) milks because they provide so many other essential nutrients in good amounts. They may also benefit from a daily micronutrient supplement containing iron, if their typical food patterns do not provide minimum servings from each of the basic food groups. Male long-distance runners should follow the same guidelines as females.

Female ballet dancers, and possibly other types of dancers, represent another class of athletes with generally inadequate nutrient intakes. Because of the physical demands of training and performance, ballerinas need to be light and lean. The notoriously poor intakes of ballerinas put them at high risk of injuries, including the legs, feet, and joints of the lower extremities. They tend to suffer from the same problem as female gymnasts and, thus, they should take a one-a-day type of micronutrient supplement and assure that they have adequate intakes of calcium from foods and/or supplements, i.e., RDA amounts.[24,44,52,53]

VIII. NUTRITION AND INJURY PREVENTION

This important area of knowledge has been under-investigated. Probably as high as 50% of injuries in non-contact sports can be prevented, and a large fraction of these may potentially be prevented by the consumption of healthy diets. Although precise recommendations cannot yet be made, several general ones are reasonable in light of epidemiologic studies of sports injuries.

The most important nutrient deficit associated with athletic injuries is that of water. Dehydration contributes to injuries in all sports and dance, but it is especially important in football, wrestling, and other sports in which a reduction in mental function may greatly contribute to injuries. Water replacement during games/events and practices cannot be over-emphasized as one of the most critical factors in preventing tissue sprains, muscle pulls, contusions, and even more serious injuries. Water replacement also helps to prevent problems such as heat cramps, heat exhaustion, and heat stroke. Under conditions of high temperature and high humidity, water replacement is absolutely essential if practices and games are to take place. Under extremely adverse weather conditions when excessive losses of electrolytes occur through sweat, electrolyte drinks may be needed to replace both fluids, energy, and the important electrolytes. A more in-depth discussion of water and electrolytes during physical activity can be found in Chapter 11 in this volume.

Severe deficiencies or even modest underconsumption of macro- or micronutrients remain more difficult to link directly to injuries in sports. Chronic low energy intakes, of course, have been shown to limit work output in various activities, but micronutrient deficits generally have to be greatly reduced to demonstrate an adverse effect on physical function. Nevertheless, poor nutritional status, as evidenced by low glycogen stores, iron deficiency, or insufficiency of other micronutrients, has been demonstrated to result in substandard performance or reduced endurance. Injuries rates are greater in female athletes and dancers who are either amenorrheic [52-56] or anorexic.[57,58] Lower extremity injuries are especially common in aerobic dancers[59] and young athletes[60] from overuse. Specific nutrient deficiencies have been reported for athletes in diverse sports with injuries.[61]

The general nutritional guidelines for injury prevention are listed in Table 1. Nutrient supplements may be recommended for specific individuals, especially females, in order to assure an adequate amount of all nutrients, but remember that foods, particularly plant foods, provide non-nutrient molecules in addition to nutrients. All of these molecules may be important for healthy living. Strict vegetarian athletes may have difficulty obtaining sufficient amounts of calcium, iron, zinc, vitamin D, and a few other micronutrients, in addition to vitamin B_{12} (cobalamin) that is totally absent in plant foods.

IX. NUTRITION EDUCATION FOR ATHLETES

Competitive athletes in general, not just elite athletes, need much more nutrition knowledge than they are assimilating at school from teachers and coaches and also from magazines and the electronic media. Athletes need to understand the basic concepts of nutrition (outlined in Section II above) and they need to be able to put these concepts into their everyday practice of selecting foods and beverages wisely. This area of knowledge is too frequently neglected in sports programs around the nation (see Chapter 23).

X. SUMMARY

This introduction to the third edition of *Nutrition in Exercise and Sport* presents a broadly based background on the principles of sound nutrition for individuals who exercise and

TABLE 1   Nutritional Guidelines for Injury Prevention

1. Eat according to the Pyramid every day or practically every day.
2. Establish a healthy eating pattern that begins with a breakfast meal and limits snacks to nutrient-rich or dense foods rather than nutrient-poor choices.
3. Drink plenty of fluids, but limit the types of beverages largely to low-fat dairy products, citrus drinks, other fruit juices, and water. Use soft drinks, cola beverages, and coffee sparingly. Tea is an acceptable beverage on occasion.
4. Try to distribute calories within three meals and one or more snacks a day, but limit the "big" meal of the day to post-athletic events or training periods.

Adapted from Anderson, J. J. B., in *Prevention of Athletic Injuries: The Role of the Sports Medicine Team, Mueller, F. O. and Ryan, A. J., Eds., F. A. Davis, Philadelphia, 1991, 230.*

participate in athletic competition. The responsibility of nutrition educators is to provide sound information about eating foods and obtaining the necessary nutrients and energy to permit optimal physical performance in activities, according to the current interpretations of research, both current and past. Major recommendations highlighted herein are the importance of the following: the maintenance of optimal glycogen stores in skeletal muscle; the provision of fluids to maintain adequate hydration and water balance; and the appropriate selection of foods during pre- and post-competition meals. Also, new emphasis in this chapter is placed on the provision of carbohydrate solutions during prolonged exercise, such as running and cycling, as well as in other running sports such as soccer that cover extended periods of time. Finally, good nutrition and adequate hydration are unquestionably important for the prevention of athletic-related injuries.

REFERENCES

1. U.S. Department of Agriculture and U.S. Department of Health and Human Services, *Nutrition and Your Health: Dietary Guidelines for Americans*, 4th ed., Home and Garden Bulletin No. 232, U.S. Government Printing Office, Washington, D.C., 1995.
2. Sherman, W. M., Simonsen, J., Wright, D. A., and Dernbacj, A., Effects of carbohydrate in four hour pre-exercise meals, *Med. Sci. Sports Exercise*, 20, S157, 1988.
3. Coyle, E. F., Coggan, A. R., Hemmert, M. K., Lowe, R. C., and Walters, T. J., Substrate usage during prolonged exercise following a pre-exercise meal, *J. Appl. Physiol.*, 59, 429, 1985.
4. Hedge, G. A., Colby, H. D., and Goodman, R. L., *Clinical Endocrine Physiology*, Saunders, Philadelphia, 1987, 272.
5. Jandrain, B., Krzentowski, G., Pirnay, F., Mosora, F., Lacroix, M., Luyckx, A., and Lefebvre, P., Metabolic availability of glucose ingested three hours before prolonged exercise in humans, *J. Appl. Physiol.*, 56, 1314, 1984.
6. Jenkins, D. J. A., Wolever, T. M. S., Taylor, R. H., Barker, H., Fielden, H., Baldwin, J. M., Bowling, A. C., Newman, H. C., Jenkins, A. L., and Goff, D. V., Glycemic index of foods: a physiological basis for carbohydrate exchange, *Am. J. Clin. Nutr.*, 34, 362, 1981.
7. Guezennec, C. Y., Satabin, P., Duforez, F., Koziet, J., and Antoine, J. M., The role of type and structure of complex carbohydrates response to physical exercise, *Int. J. Sports. Med.*, 14, 224, 1993.
8. Costill, D. L., Coyle, E. F., Dalsky, G., Evans, W., Fink, W., and Hoopes, D., Effects of elevated plasma FFA and insulin on muscle glycogen use during exercise, *J. Appl. Physiol.*, 43, 695, 1977.
9. Decombaz, J., Arnaud, M. J., Milton, H., Moesch, H., Philippossian, G., Thelin, A. L., and Howald, H., Energy metabolism of medium-chained triglycerides versus carbohydrates during exercise, *Eur. J. Appl. Physiol.*, 52, 9, 1983.
10. Dohm, G. L., Tapscott, E. B., Barakat, A., and Kasparek, G. J., Influence of fasting on glycogen depletion in rats during exercise, *J. Appl. Physiol.*, 55, 830, 1983.
11. Dohm, G. L., Beeker, R. T., Israel, R. G., and Tapscott, E. B., Metabolic response to exercise after fasting, *J. Appl. Physiol.*, 61, 1363, 1986.
12. Loy, S. F., Conlee, R. K., Winder, W. W., Nelson, A. G., Arnall, D. A., and Fisher, A. G., Effects of 24-hour fast on cycling endurance time at two different intensities, *J. Appl. Physiol.*, 61, 654, 1986.
13. Massicotte, D., Peronnet, F., Brisson, G., Bakkouch, K., and Hillaire-Marcel, C., Oxidation of a glucose polymer during exercise: comparison with glucose and fructose, *J. Appl. Physiol.*, 66, 179, 1989.

14. Coyle, E. F., Hagberg, J. M., Hurley, B. F., Martin, W. H., Ehsani, A. A., and Holloszy, J. O., Carbohydrate feeding during prolonged strenuous exercise can delay fatigue, *J. Appl. Physiol.*, 55, 230, 1983.
15. Davis, J. M., Lamb, D. R., Pate, R. R., Slentz, C. A., Burgess, W. A., and Bartoli, W. P., Carbohydrate-electrolyte drinks: effects on endurance cycling in the heat, *Am. J. Clin. Nutr.*, 48, 1023, 1988.
16. Williams, C., Nute, M. G., Broadbank, L., and Vinall, S., Influence of fluid intake on endurance running performance, *Eur. J. Appl. Physiol.*, 60, 112, 1990.
17. Tsintzas, O.-K., Williams, C., Boobis, L., and Greenhaff, P., Carbohydrate ingestion and glycogen utilization in different muscle fiber types in man, *J. Physiol. (Lond.)* , 489, 243, 1995.
18. Nishibata, I., Sadamoto, T., Mutoh, Y., and Miyashita, M., Glucose ingestion before and during exercise does not enhance performance of daily repeated endurance exercise, *Eur. J. Appl. Physiol.*, 66, 65, 1993.
19. Lambert, C. P., Flynn, M. G., Boone, J. B., Michaud, T. J., and Rodriguez-Zayas, J., Effects of carbohydrate feeding on multiple-bout resistance exercise, *J. Appl. Sport Sci. Res.*, 5, 192, 1991.
20. Costill, D. L., Sherman, W. N., Fink, W. J., Marsch, C., Witten, M., and Miller, J. M., The role of dietary carbohydrates in muscle glycogen resynthesis after strenuous running, *Am. J. Clin. Nutr.*, 34, 1831, 1981.
21. Newsholme, E. A. and Leech, T., *The Runner*, Walter L. Maegher, Roosevelt, NJ, 1983, 64.
22. Roberts, K. M., Noble, E. G., Hayden, D. B., and Taylor, A. W., Simple and complex carbohydrate-rich diets and muscle glycogen content of marathon runners, *Eur. J. Appl. Physiol.*, 57, 70, 1988.
23. Keizer, H. A., Kuipers, H., van Kranenburg, G., and Geurten, P., Influence of liquid and solid meals on muscle glycogen resynthesis, plasma fuel hormone response, and maximal physical work capacity, *Int. J. Sports Med.*, 8, 99, 1986.
24. Hamilton, L., Brooks-Gunn, J., and Warren, M., Nutritional intake of female dancers: a reflection of eating problems, *Int. J. Eating Disorders,* 5, 925, 1986.
25. Weight, L. and Noakes, T., Is running an analog of anorexia? A survey of the incidence of eating disorders in female distance runners, *Med. Sci. Sports Exer.,* 19, 213, 1987.
26. Thornton, J., Feast or famine: eating disorders in athletes, *Phys. Sportsmed.,* 18, 116, 1990.
27. Leon, G., Perry, C., Mangelsdorf, C., and Tell, G., Adolescent nutritional and psychological patterns and risk for development of an eating disorder, *J. Youth Adolesc.,* 18, 273, 1989.
28. Leon, G., Eating disorders in female athletes, *Sports Med.,* 12, 219, 1991.
29. Brown, R., McIntosh, S., Seabolt, V., and DaNiel, W., Jr., Iron status of adolescent female athletes, *J. Adolesc. Health Care,* 6, 349, 1985.
30. Snyder, A., Dvorak, L., and Roepke, J., Influence of dietary iron source on measures of iron status among female runners, *Med. Sci. Sports Exer.,* 21, 7, 1989.
31. Rowland, T., Iron deficiency in the young athlete, *Pediatr. Clin. North Am.,* 37, 1153, 1990.
32. Risser, W. and Risser, J., Iron deficiency in adolescents and young adults, *Phys. Sportsmed.,* 18, 87, 1990.
33. Selby, G., When does an athlete need iron?, *Phys. Sportsmed.,* 19, 96, 1991.
34. Slavin, J., Lutter, J., and Cushman, S., Amenorrhea in vegetarian athletes, *Lancet,* 1, 1474, 1984 (letter).
35. Drinkwater, B., Nelson, K., Chesnut, C., III, Bremner, W., Shainholtz, S., and Southworth, M., Bone mineral content of amenorrheic and eumenorrheic athletes, *New Engl. J. Med.,* 311, 277, 1984.
36. White, C. and Hergenroeder, A., Amenorrhea, osteopenia, and the female athlete, *Pediatr. Clin. North Am.,* 37, 1125, 1990.
37. Henderson, R., Bone health in adolescence: anorexia and athletic amenorrhea, *Nutr. Today,* 26, 25, 1991.
38. Quadagno, D., Faquin, L., Lim, G.-N., Kurrunka, W., and Maffatt, R., The menstrual cycle: does it affect athletic performance?, *Phys. Sportsmed., 19,* 121, 1991.
39. Schelkun, P., Exercise and "the pill," *Phys. Sportsmed.,* 191, 143, 1991.
40. Myburgh, K., Grobler, N., and Noakes, T., Factors associated with shin soreness in athletes, *Phys. Sportsmed.,* 16, 129, 1986.
41. Lloyd, T., Triantafyllou, S., and Baker, E., Woman athletes with menstrual irregularities have increased musculoskeletal injuries, *Med. Sci. Sports Exer.,* 18, 374, 1986.
42. Short, S. H. and Short, W. R., Four-year study of university athletes' dietary intake, *J. Am. Diet. Assoc.,* 82, 632, 1983.
43. Loosli, A., Benson, J., Gillien, D., and Bourdet, K., Nutrition habits and knowledge in competitive adolescent female gymnasts, *Phys. Sportsmed.,* 14, 118, 1986.
44. Loosli, A. and Benson, J., Nutritional intake in adolescent athletes, *Pediatr. Clin. North Am.,* 37, 1143, 1990.
45. Sirota, L., Vitamin requirements and deficiencies: theoretical and practical considerations for athletes, *J. Phys. Educ. Recreat. Dance,* 62 (No. 8), 57, 1991.
46. Slavin, J., Assessing athletes' nutritional status, *Phys. Sportsmed.,* 19, 79, 1991.
47. Tipton, C., Commentary: physicians should advise wrestlers about weight loss, *Phys. Sportsmed.,* 15, 160, 1987.
48. Steen, S. and McKinney, S., Nutrition assessment of college wrestlers, *Phys. Sportsmed.,* 14, 100, 1986.
49. Maughan, R. and Noakes, T., Fluid replacement and exercise stress: a brief review of studies on fluid replacement and some guidelines for the athlete, *Sports Med.,* 12, 16, 1991.
50. Clark, N., Nelson, M., and Evans, W., Nutrition education for elite runners, *Phys. Sports Med.,* 16, 124, 1988.

51. Nelson, M., Fisher, E., Catsos, P., Meredith, C., Turksoy, R., and Evans, W., Diet and bone status in amenorrheic runners, *Am. J. Clin. Nutr.,* 43, 910, 1986.

52. Warren, M., Brooks-Gunn, J., Hamilton, L., Warren, L., and Hamilton, W., Scoliosis and fractures in young adult ballet dancers: relation to delayed menarche and secondary amenorrhea, *New Engl. J. Med.,* 314, 1348, 1986.

53. Benson, J., Geiger, C., Eiserman, P., and Wardlaw, G., Relationship between nutrient intake, body mass index, menstrual function, and ballet injury, *J. Am. Diet. Assoc.,* 89, 58, 1989.

54. Cann, C., Martin, M., Genant, H., and Jaffe, R., Decreased spinal mineral content in amenorrheic women, *J. Am. Med. Assoc.,* 251, 626, 1984.

55. Marcus, R., Cann, C., Madvig, P., Minkoff, J., Goddard, M., Bayer, M., Martin, M., Gaudiani, L., Haskell, W., and Genant, H., Menstrual function and bone mass in elite women distance runners endocrine and metabolic features, *Ann. Int. Med.,* 102, 158, 1985.

56. Drinkwater, B., Bruemner, B., and Chesnut, C., III, Menstrual history as a determinant of current bone status in young athletes, *J. Am. Med. Assoc.,* 263, 545, 1990.

57. Rigotti, N., Nussbaum, S., Herzog, D., and Neer, R., Osteoporosis in women with anorexia nervosa, *New Engl. J. Med.,* 311, 1601, 1984.

58. Brooks-Gunn, J., Warren, M., and Hamilton, L., The relation of eating problems and amenorrhea in ballet dancers, *Med. Sci. Sports Exer.,* 19, 41, 1987.

59. Kovan, J. R. and McKeag, D. B., Lower extremity overuse injuries in aerobic dancers, *J. Musculoskel. Med.,* 9, 43, 1992.

60. Maffulli, N. and Baxter-Jones, A. D. G., Common skeletal injuries in young athletes, *Sports Med.,* 19, 137, 1995.

61. Anderson, J. J. B., Nutrition and injury prevention, in *Prevention of Athletic Injuries: The Role of the Sports Medicine Team,* Mueller, F. O. and Ryan, A. J., Eds., F. A. Davis, Philadelphia, 1991, 230.

Chapter 3

CARBOHYDRATE METABOLISM IN SPORT AND EXERCISE

John G. Wilkinson
Michael Liebman

CONTENTS

I. INTRODUCTION

Carbohydrates are an important energy source for human metabolism. Skeletal muscle glycogen and liver-derived blood glucose are readily available carbohydrates which are used as primary sources of fuel during both anaerobic and aerobic exercise. The breakdown of muscle glycogen or blood-borne glucose to lactic acid contributes to muscular fatigue during high intensity exercise. The dietary manipulation of carbohydrate intake prior to, during, and after exercise can improve exercise performance largely through optimizing muscle and liver glycogen stores or through the maintenance of blood glucose homeostasis. Recent research on carbohydrate metabolism during exercise has established that:

1. Blood glucose becomes an increasingly important energy source as prolonged moderate exercise continues beyond two hours.
2. Carbohydrate metabolism during exercise is regulated by a complex interaction of hormonal and local control.
3. Glucose transport into muscle appears to regulate glucose utilization and glycogen synthesis during and following exercise, respectively.
4. The effectiveness of carbohydrate supplementation during exercise is dependent upon the rate of gastric emptying and the type, timing, and rate of carbohydrate ingestion.
5. Post-exercise glycogen resynthesis is also dependent upon type, timing, and amount of carbohydrate ingested following exercise.

The purpose of this chapter is to review these topics related to carbohydrate metabolism and to provide practical guidelines for carbohydrate nutrition and optimal exercise performance.

II. CARBOHYDRATE INTAKE AND METABOLISM

A. DIET, DIGESTION, AND STORAGE

Carbohydrates are the most abundant and readily available source of energy for human nutrition. The 1989 Recommended Dietary Allowance (RDA) subcommittee recommended that more than half the energy requirement beyond infancy be provided by carbohydrate.[1] Important dietary carbohydrates have the general formula $(CH_2O)_n$ and include sugars and complex carbohydrates. Commonly consumed sugars can be subdivided into monosaccharides, such as glucose and fructose, and disaccharides such as sucrose, maltose, and lactose (milk sugar). Dietary polysaccharides, or complex carbohydrates, include the glucose polymer, starch, and a number of indigestible plant cell wall materials (cellulose, hemicellulose, pectins) which are classified as components of dietary fiber. In terms of discussing the relationship between dietary carbohydrates and carbohydrate metabolism in exercise, this section will focus only on "available" carbohydrates — i.e., those that can be hydrolyzed by human digestive enzymes and absorbed in the small intestine.

Based on the 1989–91 Continuing Survey of Food Intakes by Individuals,[2] average daily carbohydrate intake in the United States for adult males and females was 257 and 190 g, respectively. After a decline in total carbohydrate intake (expressed as percent of energy) from the 1930s to the 1960s, intake began to rise in the late 1960s such that intake in the late 1980s was 46% of caloric intake.[3] An average of 41% of daily carbohydrate intake came from grain products and 23% from fruits and vegetables. Monosaccharides and disaccharides, found primarily in fruits, milk (lactose), and processed foods containing added sweeteners, account for about half of the total digestible carbohydrate intake in the United States.[1]

Dietary carbohydrates are hydrolyzed in the stomach and small intestine to monosaccharides, with glucose typically predominating. Both glucose and galactose are absorbed by an active transport mechanism whereas fructose is absorbed by facilitated diffusion.[4] The fact that the rate of glucose absorption is more than twice that of fructose[5] has important implications with respect to the comparative value of ingesting these monosaccharides during exercise. Absorbed monosaccharides are transported to the liver via the hepatic portal vein. The maintenance of minimal plasma fructose and galactose levels even in the fed (postprandial) state supports the role of the liver as a "sink" with respect to these monosaccharides. Fructose is primarily metabolized via the triose phosphate stage of the glycolytic pathway to pyruvate thereby contributing to the hepatic pool of acetyl CoA which can serve as a substrate for fatty acid and triglyceride synthesis. Fructose-derived triose phosphates can also serve as gluconeogenic precursors which ultimately provide substrate for glycogen synthesis.[4]

Glycogen is the major storage form of carbohydrate in animals. In addition to α-1,4 glycosidic linkages which produce the straight chain polymer of glucose, glycogen has branch points produced by α-1,6 bonds. Thus, the structure of glycogen resembles that of the branched chain component of starch (amylopectin) rather than the straight chain component (amylose).[4] Glycogen molecules are effectively trapped in cells by virtue of their large size. Due to the hydrophilic nature of carbohydrates, glycogen is stored with 3 g water/g glycogen. This yields an energy density of 4.2 kJ/g (1 kcal/g), thereby imposing definite limits on the amount of energy stored in the form of glycogen.[6]

Overall storage of carbohydrate in the body as glycogen is small. Glycogen in liver and muscle, the two primary storage sites, accounts for about 1–2% of the total substrate reserves of the body. The greatest potential source of fuel is triglyceride stored predominantly in adipose tissue (80% of substrate reserves). The only other potentially significant source is body protein (17% of energy reserves).[4] However, amino acids derived from body protein will be used primarily for protein synthesis and other anabolic functions in the well-fed individual who has adequate stores of carbohydrate and lipid. Estimates of the contribution of amino acids as a fuel during exercise have ranged from 1–3% of total energy expenditure.[7] Thus, it is clear that lipid and carbohydrate constitute the two most physiologically important energy substrates in individuals consuming normal diets. This generalization holds true not only during the fasting (postabsorptive) state when the body must rely totally on endogenous stores of energy but also during the prolonged exercise situation in which glucose and fatty acids are oxidized to provide the fuel needed for contracting skeletal muscle.

There is a higher concentration of glycogen in liver (typically ranging from 4% after an overnight fast up to 8% after meals) compared to skeletal muscle. Glycogen in muscle typically has a concentration of less than 1.5% and requires deliberate carbohydrate loading to approach and exceed 3%.[8] However, the average total amount of glycogen stored in muscle (300–400 g) is greater than that in liver (80–90 g) due to the substantially greater overall mass of skeletal muscle.[9] There appears to be an even distribution of glycogen within skeletal muscle fibers although slightly more is stored in fast- than in slow-twitch fibers.[10] When taken together, hepatic and muscle glycogen stores combined with circulating blood glucose (approximately

20 g) represent only about 1800 kcal, an energy level which would not be sufficient to support the total daily caloric expenditure of most adults for even one 24-hr period.[9]

B. CARBOHYDRATE METABOLISM
1. Postabsorptive State

Muscle glycogen provides a readily available source of glucose for glycolysis only within muscle itself because of absence of the enzyme glucose-6-phosphatase. In contrast, presence of this enzyme in liver allows hepatocytes to play a predominant role in mobilizing stored glycogen for maintenance of the blood glucose level, particularly during the postabsorptive state. Via the stimulation of the glycogenolytic pathway and the pathway by which glucose is synthesized from non-carbohydrate precursors (gluconeogenesis), the liver is the sole contributor of glucose to maintain glucose homeostasis, except during prolonged fasting, when an enhancement of gluconeogenesis in the kidney also contributes to maintenance of normal blood glucose levels.[11]

Both muscle and hepatic glycogen levels are dependent on nutritional status. Fasting will essentially deplete hepatic glycogen stores within 24 to 48 hr post-meal ingestion.[12] In this case, gluconeogenesis will be activated to ensure adequate circulating blood glucose concentrations, which requires the release of 100 mg/min to replace glucose used by the nervous system.[6] Thus, blood glucose homeostasis is achieved during fasting by hepatic release of glucose at rates equal to those of tissue utilization. Hypoglycemia can lead to brain dysfunction and severe hypoglycemia can result in coma and death.[11]

In the first few hours during the transition from the fed to the fasted state, release of glucose from liver is largely met via glycogenolysis. After an overnight fast, approximately 65–75% of basal hepatic glucose release is derived from glycogenolysis and the remainder (25–35%) from gluconeogenesis.[12] As the fast continues, increased reliance on gluconeogenesis for blood glucose homeostasis parallels the decreased reliance on glycogenolysis as hepatic glycogen stores become progressively depleted. Physiologically important gluconeogenic precursors in liver are lactate, alanine, pyruvate, glycerol, and a number of other amino acids.[11] Lactate, formed by the glycolytic catabolism of glucose in skeletal muscle and by erythrocytes, can be transported to the liver for glucose resynthesis. The use of lactate produced in extrahepatic tissues as a gluconeogenic precursor in liver is called the Cori (or lactic acid) Cycle[11] (Figure 1). There is also evidence to support the existence of a glucose-alanine cycle analogous to the Cori Cycle.[13,14] In skeletal muscle, glucose is oxidized to pyruvate, followed by transamination to alanine. Alanine is transported to liver and after removal of the amino group is converted to glucose via the gluconeogenic pathway (Figure 1). Figure 2 also indicates reactions catalyzed by key gluconeogenic enzymes in liver by highlighting reactions which differ between glycolysis and gluconeogenesis. There are three irreversible reactions in glycolysis due to their highly exergonic nature, i.e., those catalyzed by hexokinase/glucokinase, phosphofructokinase, and pyruvate kinase. It is at these three points that specific gluconeogenic enzymes are required. For example, pyruvate carboxylase and PEP carboxykinase are required to circumvent the pyruvate kinase reaction of glycolysis.[4]

A summary of the predominant carbohydrate-related metabolic pathways during the postabsorptive state is given in Figure 3. These general metabolic alterations also occur during endurance exercise although there is a significantly greater dependence on glucose oxidation for energy production during exercise. During the fasting, resting state, fatty acids ultimately derived from triglycerides stored in adipose tissue provide the major energy substrate for skeletal muscle thus sparing glucose for tissues with obligatory glucose requirements.

In terms of carbohydrate utilization during the postabsorptive state for energy production, glycogen can be degraded to glucose-1-phosphate by action of the enzyme phosphorylase, after which it is converted to glucose-6-phosphate by the enzyme phosphoglucomutase.

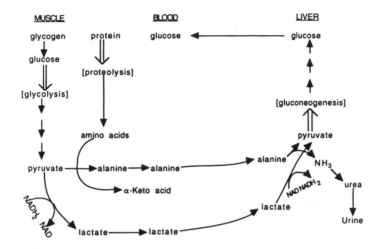

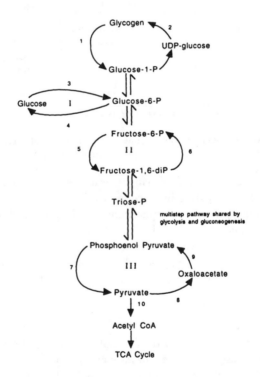

FIGURE 1 Use of lactate and alanine as gluconeogenic precursors in liver.

Points of divergence between glycolysis and gluconeogenesis (I, II, III) indicated
Key enzymes: 1 Phosphorylase, 2 Glycogen Synthase, 3 Hexokinase,
4 Glucose-6-phosphatase, 5 Phosphofructokinase,
6 Fructose-1,6-diphosphatase, 7 Pyruvate Kinase,
8 Pyruvate Carboxylase, 9 PEP Carboxykinase,
10 Pyruvate Dehydrogenase

FIGURE 2 Hepatic glucose metabolism indicating key glycolytic and gluconeogenic enzymes.

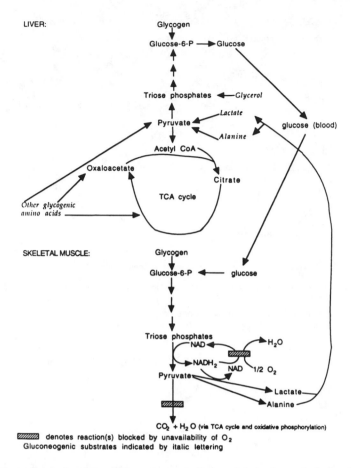

FIGURE 3 Carbohydrate-related metabolic pathways in liver and skeletal muscle during the postabsorptive state; similar metabolic alterations occur during endurance exercise.

Although this degradative pathway also involves a debranching mechanism, the step catalyzed by phosphorylase is rate-limiting in glycogenolysis.[4]

In skeletal tissue, glucose-6-phosphate can also be produced by the action of hexokinase on free glucose obtained from blood. Thus, this compound constitutes a merge point for glucose units derived from glycogen and those transported across the cell membrane from blood. Due to inability of phosphorylated glucose molecules to diffuse out of tissues, glucose-6-phosphate produced in skeletal muscle will invariably be metabolized via the glycolytic pathway.

2. Postprandial State

In the postprandial state, absorbed macronutrients are used for energy, structural repletion of tissues, and in the case of glucose and fatty acids, stored for use during the postabsorptive state, especially during the overnight fast. Thus, pathways ultimately dependent on the availability of glucose are activated in the fed state. These include glycogen synthesis (glycogenesis), glycolysis, and in adipose tissue, lipogenesis, where glucose is required to provide the α-glycerol phosphate backbone needed for triglyceride formation. It follows that glycogenolysis and lipolysis would be minimally active in this situation. After a few hours of fasting, there is essentially a total reversal as pathways activated in the fed state slow down and those depressed after food ingestion are stimulated. The production of glucose from glycogenolysis and from peripheral precursors (amino acids, lactate, glycerol) becomes an important function of the liver when dietary glucose is not available.

With glucose ingestion after a period of fasting, there is no longer a net production of glucose by hepatocytes but rather a net synthesis and storage of glycogen. Glycogen may be synthesized by a direct pathway (glucose $\rightarrow$ glucose-6-P $\rightarrow$ glycogen) or via an indirect pathway (glucose $\rightarrow$ C_3 compound $\rightarrow$ glucose-6-P $\rightarrow$ glycogen).[15] In accord with the indirect pathway, a significant proportion of dietary glucose may bypass hepatic tissue, is metabolized to lactate in extrahepatic tissues such as skeletal muscle, and lactate recycles back to liver for conversion to glycogen via a still-active gluconeogenic pathway.[16,17] Based on a 1988 review of studies which estimated contributions of the direct and indirect pathways to glycogen formation, the most important factor was size of the glucose load. The indirect pathway made a greater contribution with smaller glucose loads whereas the direct pathway dominated with higher glucose loads and more marked hyperglycemia.[15]

A possible advantage of the so-called "indirect pathway" for glycogen synthesis in liver is that skeletal muscle and peripheral tissues with obligatory glucose requirements (e.g., central nervous system, red blood cells, kidney medulla) would be provided with substrate in the form of glucose for oxidation or for restoration of glycogen reserves (in the case of skeletal muscle) prior to repletion of glycogen reserves in the liver. If only limited carbohydrate is provided by diet, the higher priority of providing peripheral tissues with glucose can be met if this indirect pathway operates to the extent suggested by some investigators.[16,17]

In the postprandial state, much of the fructose and galactose absorbed from the small intestine would be converted to glucose in the liver.[4] Fructose enters the glycolytic sequence at the triose phosphate stage and thus provides intermediates for glucose synthesis. Humans have been shown to deposit more than two times as much liver glycogen when given fructose as compared to glucose.[18] Flatt[6] recently estimated that after a typical meal, one-quarter to one-third of the carbohydrate is converted to liver glycogen, one-third to one-half to muscle glycogen, with the remainder oxidized during the postprandial hours.

3. Glycolysis

The ability of glycolysis to generate adenosine triphosphate (ATP) in the absence of oxygen is of physiological significance because it provides useful energy to working skeletal muscle even when aerobic oxidation is limited. This ATP production also enables tissues with significant glycolytic capacity to survive hypoxic episodes. Tissues with poor glycolytic ability (e.g., cardiac muscle) are characterized by poor survival under conditions of ischemia.[19]

Although glycolysis can be discussed in terms of anaerobic and aerobic phases, relative availability of oxygen does not alter in any way the actual sequence of reactions in glycolysis but rather is a primary determinant of the metabolic fate of pyruvate produced from glycolysis. Under normal conditions, with an adequate supply of oxygen, most pyruvate is transported into the mitochondria for terminal oxidation to carbon dioxide and water via the tricarboxylic acid cycle and respiratory chain. When oxygen is limiting, reoxidation of reduced nicotinamide adenine dinucleotide (NADH) formed from NAD during glycolysis by transfer of reducing equivalents through the respiratory chain to oxygen is impaired. In this situation, oxidation of NADH to NAD can be coupled to reduction of pyruvate to lactate, a reaction catalyzed by lactate dehydrogenase (Figure 3). Thus, glycolysis can proceed under anaerobic conditions but the amount of energy liberated per mole of glucose oxidized (2 or 3 ATP for glucose derived from blood or from glycogen, respectively) is severely limited compared to the amount generated when glucose is completely oxidized in the mitochondria to carbon dioxide and water (38 ATP).

It is an oversimplification to imply that oxygen status of the cell is the sole determinant of the metabolic fate of pyruvate. During periods when there is high glycogenolytic activity (e.g., during the early stages of aerobic exercise), pyruvate can be reduced to lactate even under conditions of adequate oxygen supply. This occurs via a mass action reaction of lactate dehydrogenase when excess pyruvate is produced in the cell.[19]

III. ENERGY SOURCES FOR EXERCISE

ATP is the common energy currency used for all cellular biological work. Energy gained following the breakdown of ATP to adenosine diphosphate (ADP) and inorganic phosphate (Pi) is used for skeletal muscle contraction during exercise. In addition to ATP, skeletal muscle has another high-energy phosphate, creatine phosphate (CP), which can be used for the resynthesis of ATP. Prolonged endurance activity such as cross-country skiing may require ATP energy production 20 to 30 times above rest, while the energy demand of skeletal muscle during high-intensity sprinting may be 120 times greater than at rest.[8] The three energy systems that supply and produce ATP during different types of exercise are: 1) the ATP-CP System, 2) the Lactic Acid System, and 3) the Aerobic System (Figure 4).[20-22]

The ATP-CP (phosphagen) system uses both ATP and CP stored in skeletal muscle fibers. There are very limited ATP stores within skeletal muscle, enough to perform maximal exercise for a few seconds, while the concentration of CP in skeletal muscle is three to five times greater than that of ATP. Therefore, there is only enough stored high energy phosphate for about 8–10 sec of all-out exercise.[21] Performance of short duration, high intensity exercise such as 100 meter sprint, weightlifting, football, and field events in track are reliant upon this energy system.

The lactic acid system is an anaerobic system in which ATP is produced in skeletal muscle via glycolysis. It involves the incomplete breakdown of glucose to 2 molecules of lactic acid (hence the name "lactic acid system"). ATP is generated for high intensity exercise from the breakdown of either glucose derived from the circulation or more importantly from muscle glycogen stores. This system is engaged when oxygen supply is inadequate or the energy demands of exercise are greater than the capacity of the aerobic system to provide ATP. The lactic acid system is operative with the onset of all-out exercise, however, it only becomes the predominant energy system as muscle CP stores become depleted. Thus, the lactic acid system is critically important for high intensity anaerobic power events which last 20 s to 2 min, such as 200, 400, and 800 meter sprinting and 100 and 200 meter swimming events (Figure 4).[21,22]

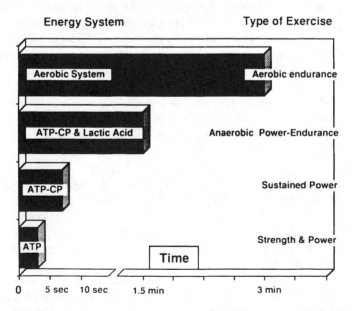

FIGURE 4 Energy systems used and performance times for different types of exercise. (Modified from McArdle, W. D., Katch, F. I., and Katch, V. I., *Exercise Physiology: Energy, Nutrition, and Human Performance,* Lea & Febiger, Philadelphia, 1991.)

The aerobic system involves the catabolism of carbohydrates, fats, and protein and subsequent degradation to CO_2 and H_2O via the tricarboxylic acid cycle and the electron transport system. However, it should be reemphasized that in the first hour of exercise the most important source of glucose for aerobic energy production is stored muscle glycogen and as discussed previously, the aerobic system is far more efficient than the lactic acid system. Maximal oxygen consumption or maximal aerobic power ($\dot{V}O_2$ max) is the upper limit of an individual's ability to consume oxygen. It involves pulmonary ventilation, oxygenation of blood, cardiovascular system circulation to exercising skeletal muscle, and oxygen utilization in skeletal muscle mitochondria. The aerobic system is the predominant energy system used in exercise that lasts longer than 3 min (Figure 4). There are many examples of this so-called endurance or aerobic exercise such as 3000 meter to marathon running, road cycling, soccer, and cross-country skiing. For additional information on the energy systems used for exercise, see Chapter 6, Brooks et al.,[8] McArdle et al.,[21] and Wilmore and Costill.[22]

IV. FUEL SOURCES DURING EXERCISE

It is generally acknowledged that oxidation of amino acids makes only a minor contribution to the total amount of ATP synthesized by exercising muscle.[7] Thus, the four major energy sources during exercise are muscle glycogen, blood glucose, plasma fatty acids, and intramuscular triglyceride.[23] Key factors dictating the relative contribution and absolute quantity of these substrates oxidized are intensity and duration of exercise, level of exercise training, initial muscle glycogen levels, and carbohydrate supplementation during exercise. How the fuel mixture is affected by each of these factors will be discussed.

Skeletal muscle glycogen stores and circulating blood glucose originating in liver from glycogenolysis or gluconeogenesis represent the primary sources of carbohydrate used for energy production by exercising muscle. Triglycerides stored in adipose tissue and muscle provide most of the free fatty acids (FFA) oxidized during exercise. Although these triglyceride stores represent a tremendous energy reserve, fatty acid oxidation is limited thus necessitating heavy reliance on carbohydrate oxidation to provide energy for exercise of at least moderate intensity.[24]

The relative amount of carbohydrate to fat utilized by humans can be indirectly assessed from ventilatory exchange by computation of the non-nitrogen R-value or respiratory exchange ratio (RER). RER is the ratio of volume of expired CO_2 to volume of oxygen absorbed by the lungs per unit of time. The predominance of carbohydrate or fat as energy substrate is indicated by a RER near 1.00 or 0.7, respectively. Transition from resting to the exercise state is characterized by a shift from almost exclusive dependence on fatty acids to heavy dependence on glucose as an energy substrate for skeletal muscle.

A. EXERCISE INTENSITY

The relative contribution of carbohydrate and fat to the energy mixture during exercise is largely determined by exercise intensity. Relative contribution of carbohydrate oxidation to total metabolism increases as a curvilinear function of exercise intensity up until approximately the point of $\dot{V}O_2$ max, at which time glucose essentially becomes the sole energy substrate.[20]

During light exercise (30–50% $\dot{V}O_2$ max) there is a gradual increase in the absolute amount of fat oxidized as aerobic endurance exercise progresses. In this situation, fatty acids derived from lipolysis in adipocytes serve as the primary fuel source[24,25] which allows very prolonged activity, such as walking, even in the fasted state. Maximal utilization of fatty acids in the untrained individual may occur at around 50% $\dot{V}O_2$ max. With higher exercise intensities, reliance on fatty acids decreases such that there is a reciprocal relationship between the substrate contribution of fat and carbohydrate during exercise.[26] Romijn et al.[23] demonstrated a progressive decrease in plasma FFA as exercise intensity was increased from 25–85% $\dot{V}O_2$ max. The finding that a high rate of adipocyte lipolysis was maintained as exercise intensity increased suggested that fatty acids become trapped in adipose tissue. This could be attributed to a reduced fatty acid transport from adipose cells into the systemic circulation[27] which could in turn be related to reduced adipocyte blood flow or inadequate supply of the FFA carrier albumin.[28] At moderate exercise intensity (65% $\dot{V}O_2$ max), the increase in total fat oxidized despite a reduced plasma FFA concentration was attributed to increased oxidation of fatty acids derived from intramuscular triglyceride. At this intensity, fat and carbohydrate are approximately equal contributors to the total fuel mixture.[23]

With high-intensity exercise (>85% $\dot{V}O_2$ max), carbohydrate oxidation provides at least two-thirds of the energy needs with the remainder provided by plasma FFA and intramuscular triglycerides. At this intensity, delivery of fatty acids from adipocyte triglyceride stores to muscle is very low, thus necessitating a heavy reliance on muscle glycogenolysis for energy needs.[24] Even at relatively high exercise intensities, fatty acids serve as an important secondary fuel. This spares muscle glycogen thereby prolonging the exercise time before glycogen depletion and exhaustion occur.[29] Depletion of muscle glycogen is invariably associated with reduced exercise output and eventual discontinuation of strenuous exercise.[30,31] Thus, muscle glycogen plays a primary role in determining exercise capacity, even when other energy substrates are available.

There is a direct relationship between exercise intensity and dependence on muscle glycogen as an energy substrate. During low intensity exercise (<50% $\dot{V}O_2$ max), muscle glycogen is used slowly; sedentary individuals will not become exhausted at this exercise intensity.[20] Price et al.[32,33] demonstrated that muscle glucogen falls to a new steady-state value after several hours of low-intensity exercise and then remains constant despite continued exercise. The leveling off of muscle glycogen content was attributed to the ability of human gastrocnemius muscle to degrade and synthesize glycogen simultaneously during prolonged low-intensity exercise and appeared to be regulated locally in individual muscle fibers.

A linear relationship between exercise intensity and reductions in muscle glycogen was documented by Hermansen and co-workers.[31] These investigators showed that muscle glycogen was reduced by only 20% after two hr of cycling at low intensity, whereas glycogen was essentially depleted when subjects performed at near maximal effort. In addition, exercise intensities corresponding to 50, 75, and 100% $\dot{V}O_2$ max have been demonstrated to produce glycogenolysis rates of 0.7, 1.4, and 3.4 mmol/kg/min, respectively.[20] At very high exercise intensities, oxygen transport to working muscle may not adequately meet demands of oxidative metabolism, thus necessitating a greater reliance on carbohydrate for energy. At intensities above 90% $\dot{V}O_2$ max, exhaustion typically occurs before muscle glycogen depletion. Thus, the strong relationship between muscle glycogen depletion and exhaustion occurs only at exercise intensities corresponding to approximately 60–85% $\dot{V}O_2$ max.[34]

Exercise intensity is also directly related to glucose uptake from the circulation by muscle as well as liver glucose output.[35] The progressive increase in blood glucose turnover with increasing exercise intensity appears to offset the progressive decline in FFA turnover.[23] The rise in RER with increased exercise intensity results from an augmented rate of both muscle and liver glycogenolysis.[36] Increased glucose uptake by contracting muscle can be attributed to increases in muscle blood flow and in efficiency of muscle glucose extraction. Blood flow to working muscle is linearly related to intensity of exercise.[37] The approximately two- to three-fold increase in fractional glucose extraction can be attributed to a greater demand for glucose by each active muscle fiber and/or an increase in number of active muscle fibers.[38] Increased arteriovenous glucose difference has been suggested to play a relatively minor role compared to the dramatic rise in muscle blood flow in mediating the exercise-induced stimulation of glucose uptake.[39]

B. EXERCISE DURATION

At the onset of exercise, muscle glycogen declines rapidly.[31,40,41] After the 5–20 min of exercise, use of muscle glycogen slows as stores become partially depleted. This decrease in use of muscle glycogen-derived glucose is associated with an increased utilization of blood glucose.[42,43] The inverse relationship between glucose uptake by skeletal muscle and rate of glycogen utilization may be mediated by the smaller extracellular downhill gradient for glucose uptake when significant cellular glucose is being derived from glycogenolysis.[20] Accumulation of glucose-6-phosphate, which is likely to occur with rapid glycogenolysis, is negatively correlated with rate of plasma glucose uptake during exercise.[38]

At 65% $\dot{V}O_2$ max, there is a progressive increase in reliance on plasma FFA and glucose as exercise duration increases. The relative constancy of total fat and carbohydrate oxidation over time suggested that there is a progressive decrease in the utilization of intramuscular triglycerides and glycogen as energy substrates.[23]

Wahren et al.[35] demonstrated that during moderate to strenuous cycling exercise, net glucose uptake by leg muscles increases ten- to twenty-fold above the resting value. With continuing exercise, there is an increase in plasma glucose utilization while total carbohydrate oxidation remains constant or decreases. Thus, use of plasma glucose represents an increasing percentage of both total energy expenditure and total carbohydrate oxidation during prolonged exercise and can account for 70–100% of total carbohydrate oxidation after 2–3 hr of exercise, provided that plasma glucose availability is maintained.[38]

Heavy reliance on blood glucose as an energy substrate is associated with a concomitant increase in hepatic glucose output, primarily by means of augmented glycogenolysis, in order to maintain euglycemia.[35] The markedly greater reliance on glycogenolysis compared to gluconeogenesis for hepatic glucose production is more pronounced during early phases of exercise and at higher exercise intensities. The relative contribution of gluconeogenesis to total liver glucose output increases with increased duration of exercise and may provide between 20–50% of total glucose release at the end of prolonged exercise.[38]

Prolonged endurance exercise beyond 2.5 hr, such as ultra-endurance cycling, nordic skiing, 100 km runs, and triathlon place particular stress on the whole body carbohydrate stores. An average male athlete has between 1850 and 2000 kcal (7744 and 8372 kJ) of energy stored as carbohydrate when combining muscle and liver glycogen and blood glucose.[11] Considering that a marathon (42 km) requires approximately 2800 kcal (11,721 kJ) for a 70 kg man and ultra-endurance events may require between 5000 and 10,000 kcal per day (20,930 and 41,860 kJ), stored triglycerides and hepatic gluconeogenesis become increasingly important as exercise duration increases.[44,45] In addition, carbohydrate loading and feeding before, during, and after exercise all become important strategies for maintaining carbohydrate stores in endurance and ultra-endurance athletes (see section VI, Dietary Manipulation of Carbohydrate Intake).

In humans, blood glucose levels are typically maintained within a narrow range due to a close coupling between peripheral tissue utilization of blood-borne glucose and hepatic output of glucose.[20] However, glucose production from gluconeogenesis is relatively limited such that decreases in plasma glucose may occur once hepatic glycogen stores are severely depleted.[46,47] This can occur during prolonged exercise, with rate of blood glucose decrease partially dictated by exercise intensity.[46-48] Decreases in blood glucose to approximately 2.5 mmol/L (45 mg/dl) can precipitate symptoms related to hypoglycemia-induced neuroglucopenia (lightheadedness, lethargy, nausea)[34] and can thus be an important contributing factor to the onset of fatigue during prolonged exercise. Although there is evidence that less than 50% of individuals exercising at 60–70% $\dot{V}O_2$ max for 2.5–3.5 hr will exhibit symptoms of hypoglycemia,[47,49] it has been clearly established that carbohydrate supplementation during prolonged exercise of at least 2 hr duration can increase plasma glucose availability and thus improve performance (see section VI.C, Carbohydrate Supplementation During Exercise).

In summary, as prolonged exercise continues, RER typically decreases indicating a shift from carbohydrate to fat oxidation while at the same time the quantitative importance of blood glucose compared to endogenous muscle glycogen as an energy source for muscle oxidation increases. Plasma glucose is clearly an important energy substrate as it can supply between 20 and 50% of the total oxidative energy production during submaximal exercise.[38] For additional information regarding the effects of exercise intensity and duration on carbohydrate utilization, see Saltin and Gollnick,[20] Romijn et al.,[23] Coyle,[24] Coggan,[38] and Björkman and Wahren.[39]

C. EFFECTS OF TRAINING

Endurance training enhances an individual's ability to perform more aerobically at the same absolute exercise intensity. This appears to be related to an increased mitochondrial volume density within trained muscle and the corresponding increase in respiratory capacity.[20] Muscle oxidative enzyme activities were 100% greater in endurance trained than in untrained subjects during exercise at 65% $\dot{V}O_2$ max.[50]

After endurance training, increased utilization of fat as an energy source during submaximal exercise may be attributed to the adaptive increase in mitochondrial enzymes required for fatty acid oxidation. In skeletal muscle, FFA oxidation appears to inhibit glucose uptake, glycolysis, and glycogenolysis.[51] This carbohydrate-sparing effect of increased fat oxidation results in slower depletion of muscle glycogen and decreased utilization of plasma glucose during exercise.[52]

Depletion of muscle glycogen is associated with cessation of exercise or a decrease in exercise intensity.[26] Thus, the glycogen-sparing effect of increased lipid oxidation appears to largely account for the training-induced increase in endurance for prolonged exercise. Lower plasma FFA combined with evidence of decreased adipose tissue lipolysis has been reported in trained vs. untrained individuals during submaximal exercise of similar absolute intensity. This suggests that intramuscular triglyceride stores, rather than triglyceride stored in adipose cells, are the primary source of additional fatty acids used.[29,50]

Increased capacity for glycogen storage in muscle also occurs as a result of endurance training. Thus, the trained athlete is likely to have higher glycogen stores at the onset of exercise which are depleted at a slower rate during exercise.[53]

D. INITIAL GLYCOGEN LEVELS

It has been long appreciated that the relative proportion of carbohydrate and fat oxidized during an exercise session is markedly affected by the dietary carbohydrate and initial muscle glycogen content.[36] For example, a standard 30-min exercise test at 74% $\dot{V}O_2$ max was associated with less muscle glycogen oxidation when subjects consumed a fat-protein diet compared to a mixed or high-carbohydrate diet.[54]

The ability to sustain prolonged moderate to heavy exercise is largely dependent on the starting glycogen content in the skeletal muscles. Bergstrom et al.[30] demonstrated that an initial glycogen content of 1.75 g/100 g wet muscle allowed subjects to tolerate a standard work load for 114 min. When the carbohydrate content of the diet was altered to produce initial glycogen levels of 0.63 or 3.31 g/100 g, work times to exhaustion were 57 min and 167 min, respectively. Thus, high muscle glycogen levels allow exercise to continue longer at a given submaximal workload. Even in the absence of carbohydrate loading, there is typically a strong correlation between initial glycogen level and time to exhaustion and/or overall performance during strenuous exercise lasting for at least 1 hr,[55-57] although not all studies have documented this relationship.[58,59] Saltin and Gollnick[20] suggested that the importance of initial glycogen stores is related to the inability of glucose and fatty acids to cross the cell membrane rapidly enough to provide adequate substrate for mitochondrial respiration.

As indicated above, initial muscle glycogen levels can clearly affect performance during prolonged moderate to heavy exercise. In contrast, exercise performance appears to be unrelated to starting level of intramuscular glycogen during short-term single bouts of high-intensity exercise,[60,61] provided glycogen is not extremely low which could compromise performance.[62] With this type of activity, glycogen availability is not likely to limit performance since exhaustion typically precedes glycogen depletion. Vandenberghe et al.[61] recently demonstrated that with adequate initial glycogen stores, regulation of glycogenolysis during high-intensity exercise is not influenced by the pre-exercise intramuscular glycogen level. The high and normal glycogen conditions were associated with similar rates of lactate accumulation and blood pH changes during exercise and with similar exercise times to exhaustion.

Rate of muscle glycogenolysis also appears to be affected by body hydration status. Hargreaves et al.[63] demonstrated a 16% reduction in net muscle glycogen utilization during 2 hr of cycling exercise (67% $\dot{V}O_2$ max) in association with fluid ingestion. Proposed mechanisms were an attenuation of the normal exercise-induced increase in epinephrine and lowered muscle temperature.

Coggan[38] summarized a number of studies which suggested that alterations in carbohydrate intake can affect the utilization of plasma glucose during exercise. Most work in this area has demonstrated that the contribution of plasma glucose to the total fuel mixture is inversely related to the utilization of FFA and directly related to the dietary carbohydrate level, at least when it is varied over the range of low to normal. However, the percentage plasma glucose contribution to total carbohydrate oxidation is lowered when muscle glycogen levels are increased by high carbohydrate ingestion.[42]

As stated previously, hepatic glucose production during exercise results from a combination of glycogenolysis and gluconeogenesis. With restricted carbohydrate intakes, liver glycogen is largely depleted which necessitates a greater reliance on gluconeogenesis during exercise. Increased glucose production from gluconeogenesis, however, cannot totally compensate for reduced hepatic glycogenolysis thus increasing the likelihood of hypoglycemia during prolonged exercise.[38] In contrast, exercise-induced reductions in plasma glucose are less likely after the ingestion of high carbohydrate diets because higher reliance on muscle glycogenolysis to provide glucose reduces the relative contribution of plasma glucose oxidation to total carbohydrate oxidation.[42] In addition, the relatively greater contribution of glycogenolysis (compared to gluconeogenesis) to liver glucose production allows a closer coupling between utilization of blood-borne glucose by exercising muscle and hepatic output of glucose.[30,64]

E. CARBOHYDRATE SUPLEMENTATION DURING EXERCISE

The ingestion of carbohydrate during exercise does not appreciably alter the pattern of energy substrate usage described in the previous sections. As stated earlier, skeletal muscles rely heavily on blood glucose for energy 2 hr into exercise.[24] Thus, a major effect of carbohydrate ingestion during exercise is to exert a liver glycogen-sparing effect and cause a reduction in gluconeogenesis, two alterations which can delay the onset of hypoglycemia.[42] Although carbohydrate ingestion allows the oxidation of exogenous carbohydrate to partially spare hepatic glycogen stores, the rate of utilization of muscle glycogen is unchanged.[43,65] During prolonged exercise at 70% $\dot{V}O_2$ max, reductions in RER and total carbohydrate oxidation occurred despite the ingestion of carbohydrate during the exercise trial.[42,65]

F. LACTATE PRODUCTION

As alluded to earlier, the breakdown of glycogen to lactate with the production of some ATP is of physiological significance because it allows skeletal muscle to perform very high intensity exercise even when oxygen transport to muscle is limited. Lactate production occurs in muscle even under aerobic conditions and accelerates when oxygen supply is limited.[20] Lactate production under aerobic conditions results from a mismatch between rate of pyruvate production from glycolysis and rate of pyruvate transport into mitochondria for the terminal reactions of its oxidative metabolism. The lactate dehydrogenase reaction is an equilibrium reaction and will thus favor the production of lactate whenever pyruvate and NADH are available to the enzyme.

During exercise, lactate production is directly related to intensity of exercise. A minor fraction of the lactate produced appears to serve as a gluconeogenic precursor thereby playing a role in maintenance of blood glucose. More importantly, much of this lactate is shuttled via the interstitium and vasculature to areas of high cellular respiration. Thus, lactate provides the vehicle by which more glycolytic fibers within a working muscle bed can shuttle oxidizable substrate to neighboring muscle fibers with higher respiratory rates[66] or to the myocardium which preferentially uses lactate over glucose and FFA.[67] Brooks[66] summarized a number of animal and human studies which support this concept of a lactate shuttle and suggested that lactate may be a quantitatively important oxidizable substrate during exercise.

It is clear that lactate production and oxidation contribute to energy-producing capacity of muscle. However, excessive lactate production can adversely affect muscle fibers by dissociating into lactate and H^+ ions thereby lowering their pH. Lowering muscle pH may exert a negative effect on processes involved in excitation-contraction coupling[68] and thus appears to be a contributing factor to development of muscular fatigue.[69]

Decreased lactate production at a given absolute exercise intensity after physical training can be directly attributed to smaller buildup of pyruvate and NADH to fuel the lactate dehydrogenase reaction. Due to increased FFA oxidation, there is decreased reliance on glycolysis and thus less pyruvate formation after training. In addition, a greater percentage of pyruvate formed from glycolysis is transported into mitochondria because of their increased volume density in trained muscle.[20]

V. REGULATION OF CARBOHYDRATE METABOLISM DURING EXERCISE

Glycogen stores are the most important supplier of glycolytic substrate in muscle during exercise which lasts less than an hour. Glucose tracer studies, which typically underestimate glucose utilization, have demonstrated that blood glucose may provide 20–50% of the energy substrate used in muscle during prolonged submaximal exercise. The previous section indicated that a number of factors affect carbohydrate utilization during exercise including state of training, initial muscle glycogen concentration, and intensity and duration of exercise. This section briefly reviews the factors which regulate muscle glycogenolysis, glycogenesis, hepatic glucose production, and glucose utilization by muscle during exercise. For additional information on regulation of carbohydrate metabolism see Brooks et al.,[8] Saltin and Gollnick,[20] Coggan,[38] Björkman and Wahren,[39] Stanley and Connett,[70] Ren and Hultman,[71] Bonen et al.,[72] and Wasserman.[73]

A. SKELETAL MUSCLE GLYCOGENOLYSIS AND GLYCOGENESIS

The rate of glycogenolysis in exercising skeletal muscle is dependent upon initial muscle glycogen and activation of the enzyme glycogen phosphorylase (PHOS).[21,74] PHOS b, the inactive form, is converted via a phosphorylation reaction to PHOS a, the active form, in the presence of catecholamines, cyclic adenosine monophosphate (AMP), Ca^{++}, and increased muscle pH. It should also be noted that PHOS b can be activated in the presence of AMP and inosine monophosphate (IMP), while PHOS a does not require AMP to be active. Pi, a byproduct of CP and ATP breakdown, also works synergistically with PHOS a to increase glycogenolysis during exercise. In addition, accumulation of glucose-6-phosphate (G-6-P) in muscle provides direct feedback inhibition of PHOS. Thus, control of glycogenolysis occurs via neural-muscle activation (Ca^{++}), endocrine (catecholamine, cyclic-AMP), and metabolic (AMP, G-6-P, IMP, Pi, and pH) mechanisms.[70,72]

Skeletal muscle stimulation is accompanied by a release of Ca^{++} from the sarcoplasmic reticulum and a rise in free cytosolic Ca^{++}. Free Ca^{++} in turn activates phosphorylase kinase, which is responsible for the phosphorylation, activation, and conversion of PHOS b to PHOS a.[11] Apparently this initial activation is only transient during exercise and PHOS reverts back to the inactive form within minutes.[72,75] Epinephrine reactivates the enzyme and stimulates glycogen catabolism in contracting muscle via adrenergic stimulation and the cyclic AMP-phosphorylase kinase second messenger system. This method of PHOS activation provides continuous control of glycogenolysis coupled with exercise-induced sympathetic hormone changes and appears to act synergistically with cellular Ca^{++} control. During different types of exercise, one mechanism of PHOS activation may predominate. For example, it has been suggested that Ca^{++} activation predominates during short-term high-intensity exercise and during heavy resistance exercise when muscle blood flow is restricted. Prolonged exercise, on the other hand, may require sympathetic stimulation of PHOS.[20]

AMP and IMP stimulate PHOS b activity while IMP and Pi have both been shown to be positive allosteric modulators of PHOS a. Since these metabolites are products of CP and ATP hydrolysis, there is potential for excessive glycogenolytic flux following the initial activation during exercise. However, metabolic control of glycogenolysis during exercise is established either directly through G-6-P negative feedback inhibition of PHOS or indirectly by control of glycolysis. G-6-P accumulates in muscle with the onset of exercise due to rapid increases in glucose uptake and glycogenolysis.[20,76] In this way, increases in G-6-P may regulate skeletal muscle glucose utilization and glycogenolysis via inhibition of hexokinase and PHOS, respectively.

Other indirect intracellular regulatory mechanisms affect the rate of glycolysis and therefore the rate of glycogenolysis. The most important are metabolic controls which influence phosphofructokinase (PFK), the rate limiting enzyme of glycolysis. PFK is regulated by many allosteric modulators including activation by ADP, AMP, Pi, fructose-6-phosphate, and NH$_3$ and inhibition by ATP, H$^+$, and citrate.[20,70,72] Thus, glycolytic flux and G-6-P concentration can be tightly controlled by PFK activity. It has also been shown that glycogen synthesis continues under conditions of net glycogen breakdown during skeletal muscle contraction.[77-79] Glycogenolysis and glycogenesis are dynamic processes which are occurring at all times. Consequently, the degree of glycogen usage depends upon the difference between their relative rates.[71,72]

The activation of glycogen synthase (GS), the rate-limiting enzyme in the formation of glycogen, plays an important regulatory role in glycogen synthesis. GS has two forms. The less active D-form is phosphorylated and activated by G-6-P, while the active I-form of GS is dephosphorylated and its activity is independent of G-6-P. Both exercise and insulin stimulate glycogen synthesis by increasing the proportion of I-form GS. Similarly, when muscle glycogen is depleted a dephosphorylation enzyme catalyses the conversion of synthase D to the I-form.[80,81] Therefore, there is normally an inverse relationship between muscle glycogen content and GS I activity. Although the muscle glycogen level itself plays a key role in regulating glycogenesis, other factors such as G-6-P formation, insulin sensitivity, and glucose transport may be equally important.[80]

Friedman et al.[80] suggested that glucose transporter activity is the fundamental regulatory mechanism which controls both glucose utilization and glycogen resynthesis. Since glucose transporter activity can increase without an increase in insulin activity, increases in exercise-induced glucose transport during recovery from exercise may be important for glycogen resynthesis post-exercise.[82] The sensitivity of glucose transport to insulin also increases 5- to 10-fold following acute endurance exercise.[83-86] The synergistic effects of exercise- and insulin-mediated glucose transport are discussed more fully in the section on glucose transport.

B. HEPATIC GLUCOSE PRODUCTION

The liver provides virtually all of the glucose entry into the circulation during exercise either by glycogenolysis or gluconeogenesis. During the early phases of exercise of moderate intensity (35–50 min), glucose production occurs predominantly by glycogenolysis and this dominance increases with higher exercise intensity.[73,87] Even with exercise lasting 4 hr, the contribution of hepatic gluconeogenesis only rises to 45% of the overall hepatic glucose output.[39]

Hepatic glucose production is stimulated by increases in glucagon, catecholamines, and cortisol and by decreases in insulin. The magnitude of these hormone changes is greater with increasing intensity and duration of exercise. Plasma insulin concentration decreases with endurance exercise which may account for up to 55% of increased glucose production via indirect stimulation of hepatic glycogenolysis. Although plasma glucagon is not altered during mild exercise, a basal level is required for normal hepatic glucose production. Glucagon rises during heavy and/or prolonged exercise and may be responsible for 60% of the exercise-induced increase in glucose production during this type of exercise.[73] Both insulin and glucagon secretion appear to be regulated by sympathetic activity during exercise rather than by plasma glucose, because blood glucose concentration does not change or may even increase in the first hour of exercise.[38,39] Epinephrine and, more importantly, norepinephrine seem to stimulate pancreatic glucagon output while inhibiting insulin release.[88]

Increases in glucagon are not the only stimulus for an exercise-induced rise in hepatic glycogenolysis.[39] Catecholamines also seem to play an important regulatory role in hepatic glucose production along with reciprocal stimulation/inhibition by glucagon and insulin, respectively.[89,90] Presumably, either direct sympathetic stimulation of hepatocytes[91] and/or circulating levels of catecholamines influence liver glycogenolysis during exercise. Epinephrine is not an important factor in hepatic glucose production during short term moderate exercise, but controls a significant portion of glucose production after 120 min of exercise and during ultra-endurance events. Growth hormone is also involved in the regulation of hepatic glucose production, but its role appears to be minor during exercise.

Hepatic gluconeogenesis becomes quantitatively more important as endurance exercise progresses beyond an hour. Splanchnic fractional extraction and uptake of gluconeogenic precursors such as lactate, pyruvate, and alanine increases with exercise duration. The fractional extraction of glycerol, another gluconeogenic precursor, is very high at rest and changes little with exercise. Nevertheless, the contribution of glycerol to gluconeogenesis increases during endurance exercise because of the steady rise in arterial glycerol concentration.[38]

Maximal hepatic glucose production is ultimately dependent on liver glycogenolysis because hepatic gluconeogenesis is not able to maintain glucose production as liver glycogen becomes depleted. Therefore, hypoglycemia occurs more readily after hepatic glycogen depletion. Gluconeogenesis is regulated in part by glucagon, catecholamines, cortisol, and growth hormone. The role of cortisol in this regard may be more pronounced during ultra-endurance events.[73] However, the relative importance of these hormones during exercise is still in question.[92] In addition, much of this endocrine research has been conducted in dogs, a species which appears to differ from humans with respect to the regulation of hepatic glucose production.

In summary, both hepatic glycogenolysis and gluconeogenesis appear to be under redundant multiple hormone regulatory control. Even though increased plasma glucagon and catecholamines along with reduced insulin are of primary importance in the regulation of hepatic glucose production during exercise, other circulating hormones and plasma glucose may be involved.[38,39,73]

C. SKELETAL MUSCLE GLUCOSE TRANSPORT

Both glycogen synthesis and glucose utilization by muscle are primarily controlled by glucose delivery and subsequent transport into muscle cells. As stated previously, skeletal muscle glycogen depletion during exercise coincides with increased glucose uptake into muscle. Blood glucose uptake is also important for glycogen resynthesis following prolonged exercise,[80] as discussed in the last section of this chapter. Insulin plays an important role in regulating glucose transport into skeletal muscle.[92] However, muscle contraction alone appears to increase glucose transport into muscle fibers.[93-95] This section briefly reviews the roles of insulin and contractility in regulating muscle glucose transport and uptake during exercise. For additional information on skeletal muscle glucose transport, see Wasserman,[73] Friedman et al.,[80] and Bonen et al.[95]

Glucose is transported across the muscle membrane down a concentration gradient by carrier-mediated (glucose transporter protein) facilitated diffusion. The glucose uptake capacities of different skeletal muscle fiber types are quite diverse. Slow-oxidative muscle fibers exhibit greater glucose uptake capacity at rest compared to fast-glycolytic fibers.[96-98] This is due to greater insulin sensitivity and responsiveness in oxidative muscle fibers. These differences are also apparent during exercise and are likely due to differential insulin binding, glucose transporter (GT) availability, blood flow to individual fibers, and contraction-induced changes in sarcolemmal permeability. Wasserman[73] suggested that glucose transport dictates glucose uptake and oxidation during exercise. Resultant exercise adaptations in turn are manifest by increases in the number, turnover, and/or availability of GTs. However, exercise and insulin likely signal GT translocation from different intracellular pools by separate physiological mechanisms.[73]

1. Muscle Contractility and Glucose Transport

Early experiments by Berger et al.[99] and Vranic et al.[100] suggested that glucose uptake into muscle was dependent upon small quantities of insulin. However, more recently, it has been shown that glucose uptake increases during and after exercise in the absence of insulin.[93,94,97,98,101,102] Vranic and Lickley[92] questioned the physiological significance of these findings because insulin is never totally absent in muscle. In addition, Nesher et al.[103] reported that contractile activity exerted an additive effect on glucose uptake in the presence of insulin. Both insulin and contractility appear to stimulate GT recruitment in muscle.[101,103,104] Exercise stimulates translocation of GTs from intracellular storage sites to the plasma membrane, and appears to increase the activity of these GTs.[70]

At least two GTs are expressed in muscle. GLUT-1, the insulin independent form is minimally present in skeletal muscle. GLUT-4 is the major transporter species found in muscle and is responsible for insulin-dependent glucose transport.[80] Several studies have reported that both insulin and exercise increase the concentration and translocation of insulin-dependent transporter GLUT-4 in skeletal muscle.[101,105-107] Contraction-stimulated uptake of glucose into rat muscle appears to be directly related to GLUT-4 protein concentrations.[108] However, in human muscle, contraction-stimulated uptake of glucose is dependent on protein concentration, activity of each transporter, and movement of the GLUT-4 transporters to the sarcolemma.[109,110]

2. Insulin-Dependent Glucose Transport

There is still some question whether glucose transport into muscle can be augmented by muscle contractions alone. Vranic and Lickley[92] suggested that insulin plays a pivotal role in the control of glucose uptake by skeletal muscle *in vivo*. This is because of the difficulty in proving that insulin has been completely removed from *in situ* experiments and because insulin-like growth factors could still be present. In addition, Björkman and Wahren[39] noted that although exercise is accompanied by a fall in plasma insulin, insulin delivery to working muscle may actually increase because of the rise in muscle blood flow during exercise.

Research has focused on the characterization and translocation of GTs in skeletal muscle and their regulation by insulin.[95,111] Insulin-dependent glucose uptake into muscle does not seem to be a function of increased insulin binding to skeletal muscle receptors.[97] Similarly, while phosphorylation of the insulin receptor via tryosine kinase activity was once thought to regulate insulin receptor activity, there is no conclusive evidence that this mediates insulin-dependent glucose transport.[112] Bonen and co-workers[95] indicated that there is at least circumstantial evidence to suggest the following: 1) GTs are activated in both the presence and absence of insulin, 2) GT affinity and activity can be altered by contractile activity, and 3) GT differences between muscle fiber types likely exist. They also suggested that fast-glycolytic muscle fibers, which are quite unresponsive to insulin, can still exhibit marked increases in glucose uptake during exercise. This may be mediated by a contraction-induced rise in cytosolic Ca^{++} which increases GT translocation and affinity.[70]

VI. CARBOHYDRATE INTAKE AND EXERCISE

A. PRE-EXERCISE DIET

The importance of high carbohydrate diets to promote glycogen storage in days preceding an exhaustive endurance event is well established. Individuals who exercise regularly should routinely consume a diet which provides 4.5–6.0 g carbohydrate/kg body weight or 55–70% of total calories. Endurance athletes and those who train exhaustively on successive days are likely to require 65–75% of calories from carbohydrate to optimize performance.[113] Glycogen depletion during training can be prevented by a high carbohydrate diet and periodic rest days to allow muscles time to rebuild glycogen stores. Feelings of tiredness associated with overtraining could be partially related to lowered glycogen stores.[114]

There is also evidence that compared to high-fat diets, high-carbohydrate diets can increase time to exhaustion with short-term intense exercise. For example, Larson et al.[115] used ^{31}P-magnetic resonance spectroscopy to demonstrate that increased time to exhaustion was associated with more potent ATP production when carbohydrate made a greater contribution to the energy substrate mixture.

Foods rich in complex carbohydrates are preferable to those high in refined sugars, because they are more nutrient dense in terms of absolute levels of vitamins, minerals, and fiber and tend to be very low in fat. Numerous selections of grains, legumes, fruits, and vegetables will ensure sufficient glucose absorption for the maintenance of adequate glycogen stores. Specific guidelines regarding the design of diets with appropriate emphasis on carbohydrates can be found in a number of publications.[53,116-118]

Liver glycogen is markedly reduced by an overnight fast, and muscle glycogen levels will be suboptimal if the daily diet has not been high in carbohydrate.[34] Pre-exercise meals emphasizing easily digested high-carbohydrate foods can increase liver and muscle glycogen concentrations, thereby delaying the time at which carbohydrate reserves become depleted and improving performance.[24,119] A typical recommendation is that the meal should be light (approximately 300 Kcal or 1256 kJ), consist primarily of low-fiber carbohydrate containing foods, and include a moderate amount of protein.[118] For prolonged exercise, a relatively large pre-exercise meal containing more than 200 g carbohydrate appears to improve performance by allowing the athlete to oxidize carbohydrates at a higher rate late in exercise.[24] Consumption of the pre-exercise meal at least 2–3 hr before the exercise session will typically allow for complete gastric emptying and minimize the possibility of exercise-induced gastrointestinal upset.[53]

1.   Timing of Carbohydrate Intake

Some controversy exists regarding optimal timing of the last meal/snack ingested prior to an endurance exercise event. It has been clearly established that performance can be improved when a relatively large carbohydrate-rich meal is consumed 3–4 hr prior to prolonged exercise compared to fasting during the same period.[24] Improved performance may be related to the "topping off" of muscle and liver glycogen stores or to the provision of exogenous carbohydrate from the small intestine during the exercise session.[120]

Ingestion of a carbohydrate snack or beverage from 15 min to 1 hr before the exercise bout can lead to hypoglycemia during exercise[121,122] and in two studies exerted a negative effect on performance.[123,124] Post-ingestion increases in insulin at the start of and during exercise could lower blood glucose due to increased reliance on glucose as an energy substrate and suppression of hepatic glucose output.[121] Increased glucose utilization would be expected to result from the antilipolytic effect of insulin on adipose cells (i.e., an inhibition of triglyceride mobilization) and increased uptake and utilization of glucose by insulin-sensitive tissues.[122] In addition, carbohydrate ingestion-induced hyperinsulinemia can act synergistically with contracting skeletal muscle to accentuate plasma glucose uptake during exercise.[120]

Even when a high carbohydrate meal was ingested 4 hr before exercise, thereby allowing a return of plasma insulin to fasting levels during the 2 hr immediately preceding exercise, a decrease in blood glucose during the first hour of exercise and a suppression of the normal exercise-induced increase in plasma FFA and glycerol were observed.[125] These data suggested a persistent effect of insulin may have been responsible for the observed decreases in blood glucose and in adipocyte lipolysis.

In contrast to the above-stated findings, work performance may not be adversely affected and can be actually improved by the pre-exercise ingestion of carbohydrate within 1 hr of exercise.[24,126] Carbohydrate ingested prior to exercise can be oxidized by active muscle. Improvements in exercise performance, when observed, may result from a delay in the normal decline in blood glucose since pre-exercise carbohydrate ingestion has been suggested to aid in maintaining hepatic glycogen reserves[127] but does not appear to affect rate of muscle glycogen utilization.[119]

A number of studies support the assertion that ingestion of carbohydrate within 1 hr of start of exercise can improve cycling performance.[128-131] Gleeson et al.[128] reported that cyclists rode an average of 13 min longer after ingesting 1 g glucose/kg body weight 45 min before cycling to exhaustion. Neufer et al.[129] demonstrated a 10% mean increase in work output during 15 min of cycling preceded by 45 min of cycling at 80% $\dot{V}O_2$ max when subjects consumed either 45 g of a glucose polymer solution or a solid carbohydrate confectionary bar 5 min before exercise.

Sherman et al.[130] used trained cyclists and a cycling time-trial performance to simulate athletic competition. Exercise performance was improved by 12.5% when 1.1 or 2.2 g of liquid carbohydrate/kg body weight was ingested 60 min before 90 min of cycling at 70% $\dot{V}O_2$ max followed by a 45 min cycling-performance trial. Compared to the placebo treatment, carbohydrate ingestion produced markedly higher serum insulin and markedly lower FFA levels at the onset of exercise and was associated with a 12% greater amount of carbohydrate oxidation. The authors suggested that improved performance was related to greater carbohydrate availability which most likely resulted from continued gastric emptying of pre-exercise carbohydrate during exercise.

Anantaraman et al.[131] recently examined whether a 10% glucose polymer solution (30 g glucose polymer) consumed 2 min pre-exercise, as compared to consumption both before and during exercise, enhances endurance performance when subjects perform high-intensity cycle ergometry for 1 hr. Compared to placebo, pre-exercise glucose ingestion resulted in significantly greater total work due to less power decrement with no further benefit accrued from ingestion of the same amount of glucose every 15 min during exercise. These results support the contention that for high-intensity exercise of 1 hr duration or less, consumption of carbohydrate 0–15 min pre-exercise should improve performance, but further ingestion of carbohydrate during exercise will not exert an additional ergogenic effect.[132]

It must be acknowledged that not all studies have reported positive effects of pre-exercise carbohydrate ingestion on exercise performance.[122-124,133,134] Individual responses to pre-exercise carbohydrate feedings may vary considerably which could be partially related to differences in susceptibility and sensitivity to a transient lowering of blood glucose. Thus, individual athletes should experiment to determine whether their performance can be improved.

2. Type of Carbohydrate Intake

It has been suggested that fructose might be superior to glucose as a pre-exercise carbohydrate source due to lower post-ingestion increases in serum insulin and glucose.[122,135] However, no differences in endurance performance after ingestion of glucose compared to fructose have been observed.[122,133] Thus, there appears to be little rationale for recommending use of fructose for pre-exercise feeding especially in light of the possibility of incomplete absorption, cramps, and diarrhea resulting from the ingestion of even moderate (50 g) fructose doses.[136]

A recent area of investigation has been to determine whether there are specific advantages to the pre-exercise ingestion of low glycemic compared to high glycemic index foods. The relative glycemic potency, or propensity to raise blood glucose, of many carbohydrate-containing foods have been compared to a standard (typically white bread), and these data have been published in the form of a glycemic index (GI).[137] Differences in glycemic response primarily relate to the rate at which carbohydrates are digested which in turn is affected by factors such as food form, particle size, nature of the starch or saccharide, food processing, and presence of antinutrients. Incorporation of low GI foods into diets has been associated with reduced blood glucose, insulin, and lipid levels.[138]

Since plasma glucose is a key determinant of the insulin response, the potential advantage of concentrating on low GI foods would be lower pre-exercise insulin levels. For reasons previously indicated, a blunted post-ingestion increase in insulin could decrease reliance on glucose as an energy substrate thereby improving performance by delaying the time at which carbohydrate reserves become depleted.

Guezennec et al.[139] examined the metabolic 2 hr cycling exercise bout at 60% $\dot{V}O_2$ max. The low GI foods (rice or spaghetti) were associated with lowest insulin responses, highest blood glucose, and lowest RER levels after 30 min of exercise compared with coresponding levels after ingestion of foods with a relatively high GI (glucose, potatoes, or bread). In a similarly designed study, Thomas et al.[140] compared biochemical and physiological responses of trained cyclists to equal carbohydrate portions of a low GI food (lentils) and two high GI foods (glucose and potato) ingested 1 hr before cycling to exhaustion. Compared to the consumption of glucose or potato, lentil ingestion produced: lower plasma glucose and insulin for 30–60 min post-ingestion, higher FFA levels and lower total carbohydrate oxidation during exercise, and an endurance time which averaged 9 min and 20 min longer than the corresponding times for glucose and potato, respectively.

Glycemic response can be markedly altered by levels of protein, fat, and dietary fiber provided by a given food.[141] Jarvis et al.[142] investigated some of these so-called "food matrix" effects on carbohydrate utilization during exercise by comparing ingestion of 70 g liquid glucose, 30 min prior to exercise, to the pre-exercise ingestion of three test meals (a refined hot cereal with or without a water soluble fiber and an oat bar). The test meals decreased the initial glycemic and insulinemic responses compared to glucose alone and slowed down the rate of exogenous carbohydrate utilization. The exercise protocol, 4 hr of walking at an intensity corresponding to 40% $\dot{V}O_2$ max, did not allow a comparative assessment of endurance performance. However, it appears unlikely that any performance-related advantages would have accrued from ingestion of the test meals compared to glucose alone since neither the cumulative 4 hr utilization of exogenous or endogenous carbohydrate was significantly altered by their ingestion.

Similar results were recently obtained by Paul et al.[143] who assessed metabolic and physical performance responses to ingestion of pre-exercise meals with different macronutrient and fiber profiles. Compared with corn and wheat, oat ingestion was associated with decreased plasma insulin levels and a decreased carbohydrate oxidation rate 60 min after meal ingestion. During exercise, which was initiated 90 min post meal ingestion, glucose decreased from pre-exercise levels only when wheat and corn was ingested. Although performance ride times did not differ among treatments, the different metabolic responses observed could be attributed to the lower carbohydrate and higher protein, fat, and soluble fiber content of oat cereal compared with corn and wheat.

Improved performance in association with pre-exercise consumption of low compared to high glycemic index foods has not been a consistent finding. Differing exercise intensity may provide a partial explanation for these divergent results as improved performance was noted when exercise was conducted below[140] but not above[143,144] the anaerobic threshold.

In summary, improvements in endurance performance following pre-exercise carbohydrate ingestion may result from promotion of liver and muscle glycogen synthesis and/or via a direct contribution to the pool of blood glucose which is ultimately oxidized by working muscle. Pre-exercise carbohydrate feedings can be provided as a solid or liquid, and recommended dosage is between 1–5 g/kg body weight, depending on meal timing.[126] The likelihood of gastrointestinal distress is decreased if the carbohydrate content of the meal is reduced as ingestion time before exercise decreases. Liquid meals may be better tolerated than regular meals close to competition because of their shorter gastric emptying time.[53] For additional information regarding pre-exercise carbohydrate intake and endurance performance, see Coyle,[24] Sherman and Wimer,[34] Costill and Hargreaves,[114] Sherman,[119] Walberg-Rankin,[145] and Williams.[146]

B. CARBOHYDRATE SUPERCOMPENSATION

As stated earlier, depletion of muscle glycogen results in a decrease in exercise energy output followed by cessation of exercise.[26] Thus, use of carbohydrate supercompensation (loading) to maximize muscle glycogen stores at the onset of exercise may be beneficial for athletes engaged in continuous exercise for more than 90–120 min. There is also evidence that under certain conditions, carbohydrate loading can improve high-intensity, short-duration exercise performance.[147]

The initially proposed so-called "classical" method of carbohydrate supercompensation included glycogen depletion followed by loading.[30] Glycogen-depleted muscles become supersaturated in a proportional response to high (500–600 g) carbohydrate intakes.[113] This method involves the depletion of glycogen by exhaustive exercise and consumption of a low carbohydrate diet and then a supercompensation phase in which a very high carbohydrate diet (>90% of total kcal) is consumed (Figure 5).[148] This is no longer the preferred method for most athletes because the three day low carbohydrate feeding period may cause hypoglycemia, irritability, and chronic fatigue. In addition, the two bouts of exhaustive exercise only a few days before the event could result in injury, soreness, and fatigue.[81]

A modified version, also depicted in Figure 5, entails the "tapering down" of exercise during the 6 d prior to the event. At the same time, daily carbohydrate intake is progressively increased from an initial level of approximately 350 to 550 g or 70% of total kcal (whichever is larger) during the last 72 h preceding competition.[53,116] Sherman et al.[149] demonstrated that this modified version is as effective as the classical glycogen supercompensation regimen. This regimen will increase muscle glycogen stores 20–40% above normal.[24]

The ingestion of at least 550 g of carbohydrate is typically achieved by the consumption of large quantities of pasta, rice, and/or bread, which may cause a minor degree of gastrointestinal fullness and discomfort in some athletes. Lamb and Synder[150] demonstrated that partial substitution of a low residue, high-calorie, maltodextrin-rich drink for most of the pasta and

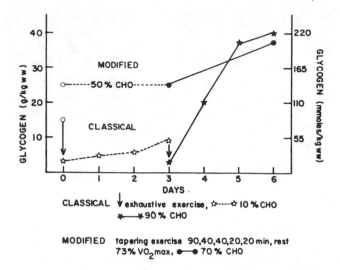

FIGURE 5 Schematic representation of the "classical" and modified methods of carbohydrate loading. (From Sherman, W. M. and Costill, D. L., *Am. J. Sports Med.*, 12, 44, 1984. With permission.)

rice commonly used in glycogen loading diets was at least as effective as a pasta/rice diet in improving glycogen stores and running performance in 14 well-trained males. Ten of the runners reported less gastrointestinal discomfort when consuming the liquid carbohydrate supplement compared to the pasta/rice diet and 90% indicated that they would be more likely to use the supplemented diet for glycogen loading. Thus, a viable option for glycogen loading appears to be a carbohydrate supplement drink which is consumed with normal high carbohydrate meals and as a snack between meals.

Tarnopolsky et al.[151] recently demonstrated a sex difference in ability of similarly trained male and female endurance athletes to increase muscle glycogen in response to an increase in carbohydrate intake from 55–60 to 75% of energy intake. The men and women increased muscle glycogen concentration by 41 and 0%, respectively, in response to the 4 d high carbohydrate period and only males exhibited a significant increase in exercise endurance time. Since lower concentrations of muscle glycogen are a stimulus for glycogen repletion,[152] the higher muscle glycogen response observed in men may be partly attributed to a greater post-exercise glycogen depletion prior to the carbohydrate loading phase of the experimental period. The authors also suggested that absolute amount of carbohydrate ingested may be more important than relative amount (i.e., 75% of energy intake) with respect to carbohydrate loading. The men and women had increased their carbohydrate intake to 614 and 370 g, respectively.

In summary, normal carbohydrate intake and glycogen reserves are generally adequate for exercise that lasts less than 60 min,[153] although carbohydrate loading may improve high intensity, short duration exercise performance under certain conditions.[147] Carbohydrate loading can increase high-intensity exercise time (duration) but will not usually affect pace during the first hour of an event.[53] Due to the approximately 3 g of water stored with each extra gram of glycogen, increasing glycogen stores from 15–40 g/kg in 20 kg muscle would represent an increase in glycogen and water of 1 and 3 lb, respectively. This high degree of glycogen supercompensation and associated weight gain may create a feeling of heaviness or stiffness that could contribute to muscular cramping and premature fatigue.[153] Thus, athletes who use this procedure should experiment to determine the pre-event dietary and exercise modifications which produce an optimal degree of glycogen supercompensation for endurance performance.

C. CARBOHYDRATE SUPPLEMENTATION DURING EXERCISE

It has been well established that initial muscle glycogen stores directly influence prolonged endurance exercise performance. As previously discussed, daily carbohydrate intake and pre-exercise carbohydrate feeding clearly affect these skeletal muscle glycogen stores. When muscle glycogen is depleted during exercise, blood glucose utilization becomes increasingly important as a function of both intensity and duration of exercise. In the last decade, numerous studies have evaluated the efficacy of ingesting carbohydrate during prolonged exercise. This section reviews the current literature on this subject. It also provides some practical guidelines with regard to the volume, composition, temperature, rate, and timing of carbohydrate supplements taken during exercise. For additional information on this topic, see Coyle,[24,155] Williams,[146] Coggan and Coyle,[154] Maughan and Noakes,[156] Maughan,[157] and Noakes et al.[158]

1. Ingestion, Utilization, and Glycogen Status

Carbohydrate ingestion during low-intensity exercise (30% $\dot{V}O_2$ max) increases blood glucose and insulin concentrations, which results in a two-fold increase in glucose uptake into skeletal muscle. This leads to increased use of blood glucose and decreased use of plasma FFA during exercise.[154] Carbohydrate ingestion during moderate-intensity exercise (50–75% $\dot{V}O_2$ max) seems to result in smaller changes in blood glucose and insulin compared to those observed during low-intensity exercise. This is likely due to greater glucose utilization by muscle and increased sympathetic inhibition of pancreatic insulin secretion. The ability of carbohydrate ingestion to increase blood glucose turnover and glucose oxidation during moderate exercise (70% $\dot{V}O_2$ max) has been associated with improved performance in cyclists.[155] Coyle[155] also estimated that blood glucose utilization accounted for almost all of the carbohydrate oxidized between 3 and 4 hr of moderate-intensity exercise. Thus, it is now accepted that blood glucose can be oxidized at very high rates during low, moderate, and prolonged exercise, and ingested carbohydrates make a significant contribution to the energy substrate used by skeletal muscle.[154,155]

It was initially hypothesized that carbohydrate ingestion during prolonged exercise improved performance by sparing muscle glycogen. This reduction in skeletal muscle glycogenolysis purportedly delayed the onset of fatigue and increased exercise time to exhaustion. However, direct measurements of muscle glycogen before and after endurance exercise, with and without carbohydrate feedings have disproved this hypothesis.[159-161] Coyle et al.[162] also demonstrated that muscle glycogen utilization was unchanged during moderate-intensity exercise even when hyperglycemia was maintained by continuous glucose infusion. This lent support to the notion that carbohydrate ingestion during continuous moderate-intensity exercise does not reduce muscle glycogen utilization. One caveat to this conclusion still exists for other types of exercise. Several authors have observed that glycogen synthesis is ongoing during low-intensity and intermittent exercise. Carbohydrate feeding, which seems to promote glycogen synthesis and may limit muscle glycogenolysis could therefore, spare muscle glycogen under these specific exercise conditions.[77,163,164]

Both the rate of hepatic glycogenolysis and gluconeogenesis are reduced with carbohydrate ingestion during low-intensity exercise.[154] It is also well established that carbohydrate ingestion helps to maintain blood glucose concentration in the third and fourth hour of prolonged moderate-intensity exercise.[155] McConell et al.[165] observed increased skeletal muscle glucose uptake and suppression of hepatic glucose production with carbohydrate ingestion during 2 hr of cycling exercise at 69% of $\dot{V}O_2$ max. Similar results were reported by Bosch et al.[65] including delayed hypoglycemia, when cyclists ingested a 10% carbohydrate drink during 3 hr of cycling. However, no muscle glycogen-sparing effect was observed. In a subsequent study of glucose ingestion during exercise, Bosch and co-workers[42] found that glucose oxidation and glycogen depletion rate were dependent on initial carbohydrate loading status.

2.   Ingestion, Performance, and Fatigue

Early studies yielded conflicting evidence concerning the effects of carbohydrate ingestion on performance during prolonged endurance exercise. Investigations published in the 1980s demonstrated that endurance performance could be improved by carbohydrate ingestion.[154] This was somewhat surprising because no differences in glycogen utilization were reported.[155] Fatigue seemed to be associated with the onset of hypoglycemia rather than glycogen depletion. This led to the hypothesis and observation that carbohydrate feeding delayed fatigue and improved endurance performance by helping to maintain euglycemia.[166] During the first 2 hr of moderate-intensity exercise, substrate utilization is similar with and without carbohydrate ingestion. Beyond 2 hr, if glycogen is depleted and no carbohydrate has been consumed, blood glucose concentration may decline to a critical level (2.5–3.0 mmol/L) which promotes fatigue due to inadequate skeletal muscle glucose uptake and oxidation.[154] Coyle[155] further suggested that carbohydrate feedings do not prevent fatigue during moderate-intensity exercise, but only delay it for 30–60 min. There also appears to be an upper limit of the intensity of prolonged exercise (75% $\dot{V}O_2$ max) that can be sustained with carbohydrate supplements.[155]

Carbohydrate and electrolyte ingestion during prolonged exercise decreased plasma cortisol and suppressed activation of the hypothalamic-pituitary-adrenal axis.[167] Thus, glucose receptors in the hypothalmus and liver may modulate cortisol response to exercise and in turn delay the onset of hypoglycemia. Hargreaves et al.[63] reported that fluid ingestion during endurance exercise reduces muscle glycogen depletion, which may partially account for the reduction in fatigue and performance enhancement observed with the use of carbohydrate drinks. While these studies provide a partial explanation for the delay in fatigue with carbohydrate ingestion, further investigation will be needed to elucidate the overall mechanisms.

Maughan et al.[168] demonstrated that fluid carbohydrate supplementation improved performance in shorter duration (70–90 min) exercise, and Below and co-workers[169] recently reported that both fluid replacement and a 6% CHO feeding improved 50 min cycling performance. Several studies have evaluated the effects of carbohydrate feeding during running events lasting between 6 and 14 min. While the results were not completely consistent, enhanced performance was generally observed.[170-173] Improvement of shorter duration exercise performance with carbohydrate ingestion is not well understood, but Maughan and Noakes[156] speculated that it may be linked to a supplementation-induced increase in blood glucose levels.

3.   Ingestion and Gastric Emptying

The most important barrier to the availability of ingested fluid and carbohydrate is the rate of gastric emptying. Gastric emptying controls the rate at which fluids are delivered to and absorbed from the small intestine. The rate of gastric emptying is primarily determined by the volume and composition of the fluid ingested.[156,158] Noakes et al.[158] emphasized that volume, and therefore the pattern of drinking during exercise, is a major factor which regulates the rate of gastric emptying. The volume of ingested water is particularly important in maintaining euhydration during prolonged exercise. Water volume affects carbohydrate availability because carbohydrates are usually ingested in the form of a sports drink. Gastric emptying follows an exponential time course and decreases rapidly as volume remaining in the stomach decreases. Therefore, maintenance of high stomach volume with repeated drinking seems to improve gastric emptying and carbohydrate availability.[174-176]

Glucose concentration, caloric density, and electrolyte content of ingested solutions all seem to influence gastric emptying. Dilute glucose solutions (5% or less) are emptied from the stomach more quickly than concentrated solutions. Therefore, if optimal hydration is the primary goal, dilute glucose-electrolyte solutions should be ingested.[156] In contrast, greater net glucose absorption occurs with increased glucose concentrations in sport drinks. It has also been suggested that sodium should be a constituent of glucose-electrolyte drinks due to its stimulation of rapid absorption of carbohydrate and water in the small intestine.[156] However, a recent study did not report any effect of adding varying Na^+ concentrations to fluid-carbohydrate replacement beverages.[177]

Osmolality seems to delay the rate of glucose gastric emptying. Therefore, glucose polymers, such as maltodextrin, should theoretically be emptied more rapidly than glucose solutions, because of their lower osmolality.[158] Additional research will be required to determine why this glucose polymer effect on gastric emptying has not been consistently demonstrated.[175,178,179] Palatability has been suggested to be a significant advantage of glucose polymer solutions, because they are not nearly as sweet tasting as glucose solutions of the same concentration.[174] Another interesting recent finding was that multiple substrate carbohydrate solutions were absorbed more quickly than solutions with only one substrate, when osmolarity was held constant.[180]

Exercise intensity appears to affect gastric emptying, particularly at higher exercise work loads.[158] The inhibitory effect on gastric emptying is quite small up to an intensity of 70% $\dot{V}O_2$ max and then becomes more important at intensities greater than 80% $\dot{V}O_2$ max.[181] This intensity-related reduction in gastric emptying may be due to sympathetic inhibition of blood flow and/or gastric motility and may be partially responsible for the existence of an exercise intensity threshold (75% $\dot{V}O_2$ max) above which carbohydrate feeding has little effect.

Other factors cited as regulators of gastric emptying include temperature and carbonation. Costill and Saltin[182] originally reported that 5°C solutions were absorbed twice as quickly as 35°C solutions. However, Maughan and Noakes[156] reported that while cool drinks are more palatable, temperature seems to have little effect on gastric emptying. Similarly, while it was once thought that carbonation would improve gastric emptying of water and carbohydrate, a recent study found little or no effect.[183]

4. Type, Timing, and Rate of Ingestion

Compared to glucose, sucrose, and glucose polymers, fructose is absorbed less rapidly across the gut, promotes less water uptake, and is metabolized in the liver rather than directly by muscle. Fructose ingestion during exercise results in lower insulin concentrations and lower carbohydrate oxidation than levels reported for other sugars. Since carbohydrate supplements during exercise do not seem to spare glycogen, the lower carbohydrate oxidation may explain why improvements in performance have not been observed with fructose ingestion.[173,184] In addition, liquid carbohydrate feeding seems to improve endurance performance to a greater extent than feeding of semi-solids during exercise.[185]

Both the timing and rate of carbohydrate ingestion during exercise can influence performance. Carbohydrate supplementation throughout prolonged endurance exercise or provided at least 35 min before the onset of fatigue are both effective in delaying fatigue.[155] Coggan and Coyle[154] suggested that ingesting carbohydrate throughout prolonged exercise may be of greater advantage because of the potential for glycogen resynthesis. Blood glucose concentration is well maintained by supplying supplemental glucose at a rate of 45 g/hr during moderate-intensity exercise.[166,186] If the supplementation is provided prior to fatigue during prolonged exercise, the carbohydrate solution should be more concentrated. Murray and co-workers[187] found no difference in performance after feeding carbohydrate at rates of 26, 52 and 78 g/hr during 2 hr of moderate intensity exercise. They concluded that a dose-response relationship does not exist between total carbohydrate ingested and exercise performance. Nevertheless, Coggan and Coyle[154] recommended that carbohydrate supplementation be sufficient to provide a minimum of 45–60 g of total carbohydrate for exercise performance to be improved.

D. POST-EXERCISE DIET

Replenishment of liver and muscle glycogen reserves after strenuous physical activity is critical in terms of ability to perform subsequent endurance exercise. This section will discuss the various nutritional factors, including amount, type, and timing of post-exercise carbohydrate ingestion, which influence glycogen resynthesis. It should be recalled from section II of this chapter that only a portion of dietary glucose is initially metabolized in the liver. Thus, it appears that a greater percentage of the glucose provided in the postprandial state is converted to muscle glycogen than to liver glycogen.[6]

Blood glucose is the primary precursor for muscle glycogen synthesis and thus must initially be transported across the cell membrane. With the cessation of exercise, the major pathway of glucose disposal in muscle is glycogen synthesis.[80] In 1967, Bergstrom and Hultman[188] reported that the highest rates of glycogen synthesis occur in muscle depleted of its glycogen stores. Work in the early 1970s suggested that following exhaustive exercise, a period greater than 1 day may be required for restoration of glycogen levels to normal.[189,190] However, more recent work demonstrated that increasing carbohydrate consumption from between 188–648 g/day resulted in proportionately greater muscle glycogen resynthesis during the 24 hr post-exercise period. Muscle glycogen levels could be normalized within 24 hr with a carbohydrate intake of 525–648 g.[191]

1.   Timing of Carbohydrate Intake

There appears to be an upper level of carbohydrate intake, ranging from 500–600 g/day, above which little additional contribution to glycogen storage or enhancement of athletic performance occurs.[192] Basing carbohydrate intake recommendations on a specific percentage of total energy intake can lead to daily intakes well above this recommended range when overall energy intakes are particularly high. These considerations led to the recommendation that the amount of carbohydrate consumed by athletes is more appropriately based either on total daily consumption (g/day) or, to account for differing body sizes of athletes, total daily consumption per unit body weight (g/kg/day).[34]

A number of studies, summarized by Ivy[193] and Friedman et al.[80] have estimated the upper limit of glycogen synthesis rate for subjects fed varying amounts of carbohydrate immediately following exercise. Overall results suggested that providing 0.7–1.5 g glucose/kg body weight every 2 hr, for up to 6 hr after exhaustive exercise, will maximize glycogen resynthesis rate at 5–8 mmol/kg wet weight of muscle/hr.[80,193]

The rapid resynthesis of muscle glycogen to near pre-exercise levels within 24 hr has been partially attributed to a glycogen depletion-induced increase in percentage of activated I-form of glycogen synthase. Glycogen synthase catalyses the transfer of glucose from uridine diphosphate-glucose onto the glycogen skeleton which is thought to be the rate-limiting step in glycogen synthesis.[194] As previously discussed, the percentage of synthase in the I-form has been shown to be inversely related to the amount of glycogen present in muscle.[152,195] Other critical factors appear to be increases in the permeability of the muscle cell membrane to glucose and in muscle's sensitivity to insulin resulting from contractile activity in muscle.[81]

For maximal glycogen resynthesis, carbohydrate intake must be high enough to ensure sufficient blood glucose for muscle glucose uptake and sufficient insulin to keep a high percentage of glycogen synthase in the active form. However, there appears to be both insulin-dependent and insulin-independent phases of post-exercise human muscle glycogen resynthesis. With gastrocnemius muscle glycogen depletion to levels <35 mM, glycogen synthesis was not affected by low insulin, whereas at >35 mM, there was no glycogen synthesis without insulin.[196] These results supported earlier work in rats which suggested that glycogen-depleting exercise can stimulate glycogen synthesis independent of insulin.[197]

To determine the effect of relative muscle glycogen depletion on subsequent rate of resynthesis, Zackwieja et al.[152] used one- and two-legged cycling exercise to induce high and low muscle glycogen levels in cyclists. Glycogen resynthesis rate and glycogen synthase activity were higher in the more glycogen depleted leg. Since both legs were exposed to a similar glucose load, these data suggested glycogenic drive within muscle, largely dictated by degree of glycogen depletion, was a primary determinant of rate of glycogen resynthesis during post-exercise.

The rate of glycogen resynthesis appears to be most rapid in the first 2 hr immediately following exercise.[152,195,198] In addition to the glycogen-depletion-induced activation of glycogen synthase, this phenomena may be partially mediated by an increased rate of glucose transport as control of glucose transport across the sarcolemma appears to play a key role in the overall regulation of glycogen synthesis.[80,199] However, waiting 2 hr before consuming carbohydrate does not appear to decrease muscle glycogen replenishment during the post-exercise 24 hr recovery period,[200] especially when high GI carbohydrates are consumed.[201]

Pascoe and Gladden[199] recently described differences in post-exercise muscle glycogen resynthesis between prolonged exercise; short-term, high intensity exercise; and resistance exercise. As indicated earlier, maximum rates of glycogen resynthesis following prolonged exercise range from 5–8 mmol/g/h. Corresponding rates following resistance exercise are in a similar range, whereas markedly higher rates (15.1–33.6 mmol/kg/h) have generally been reported following short-term, high-intensity exercise. Contributing factors to the high rate of glycogen resynthesis in this latter case likely include higher post-exercise plasma glucose and insulin levels, higher muscle glucose and glycolytic intermediates, higher muscle and blood lactate levels, and greater recruitment of fast-twitch glycolytic muscle fibers.[199]

Of interest is the finding that carbohydrate ingestion during a 2 hr cycling trial at 70% $\dot{V}O_2$ max had little effect on post-exercise muscle glycogen resynthesis. Since post-exercise muscle glycogen levels did not differ between the carbohydrate and control exercise trials, there was an equal glycogen depletion-induced stimulus for glycogen resynthesis between trials.[200] These results support the assertion that degree of glycogen depletion is a primary determinant of rate of glycogen resynthesis during post-exercise.

2. Type of Carbohydrate Intake

The type of carbohydrate consumed following exercise can also affect rate of muscle glycogen resynthesis. This effect is likely mediated by differential glycemic and insulinemic responses to different carbohydrates. For example, fructose ingestion is associated with markedly lower blood glucose and insulin levels compared to those resulting from glucose or sucrose ingestion.[201,202] This is consistent with the finding by Blom et al.[203] that glucose and sucrose ingestion were significantly more effective than fructose in promoting post-exercise muscle glycogen synthesis. Fructose infusion has led to greater restoration of liver glycogen[18] which follows from the fact that fructose metabolism is largely confined to the liver.[4]

Potential differences between simple and complex carbohydrates on muscle glycogen resynthesis have also been investigated.[191,204,205] Costill et al.[191] reported that a starch-based diet was more effective than glucose in promoting glycogen synthesis during the second day of recovery from exercise. No differences were observed during the first day nor were any differences observed between simple and complex carbohydrates in the study by Roberts et al.[204] In contrast, simple carbohydrates were demonstrated to promote a greater increase in muscle glycogen content compared to complex carbohydrates during the first 6 hr after exercise but, by 20 hr post-exercise, the two diets had produced similar muscle glycogen concentrations.[205]

In terms of maximizing rate of muscle glycogen resynthesis, it may be advantageous to consider the glycemic index classification of carbohydrate-containing foods. The "simple" vs. "complex" carbohydrate classification can be misleading because there are numerous exceptions to the generalization that simple carbohydrates are characterized by the highest GI (e.g., fructose is a low GI carbohydrate). In support of this concept is the finding that consumption of carbohydrates with a high GI (i.e., foods which produce relatively high glycemic and insulinemic responses) in the 24 hr after prolonged exercise resulted in greater glycogen synthesis compared to ingestion of an equivalent amount of low GI carbohydrate foods.[206]

Based on these considerations, maximum glycogen resynthesis should occur when athletes consume carbohydrate soon after exercise, strive to consume the equivalent of 0.7–1.5 g glucose/kg body weight every 2 hr during the initial 6 hr post-exercise,[203,207] and ingest approximately 600 g of carbohydrate or close to 10 g/kg body weight during the 24 hr post-exercise period.[114] High-carbohydrate foods or beverages such as fruits, fruit juices, or commercially available carbohydrate drinks, especially those with a high GI, are likely to be good choices for the initial post-exercise feedings. Solid and liquid carbohydrates appear to be similarly effective in promoting muscle glycogen synthesis after exercise.[208] There is also evidence that combining protein with carbohydrate ingestion can increase the rate of post-exercise glycogen resynthesis, which was attributed to the synergistic interaction of carbohydrate and protein on insulin secretion.[209]

3. Muscle Damage and Glycogen Resynthesis

Friedman et al.[80] recently summarized several studies which demonstrated that muscle glycogen resynthesis is impaired following certain types of exercise which commonly produce muscle damage and soreness. Decreased glycogen resynthesis occurs after both eccentric exercise,[210,211] characterized by forced lengthening contraction of muscle, and exhaustive running.[212] Decreased availability of glucose for glycogen resynthesis may be attributed to damage to the sarcolemma and subsequent interference with glucose transport.[80] A reduced level of GLUT4 after eccentric exercise has been reported.[213]

In addition, the inflammatory response to muscle damage results in significantly greater glucose oxidation by white blood cells and promotes release of a factor that stimulates glucose oxidation by the surrounding muscle cells.[211] Thus, Costill et al.[211] suggested that emphasis on high carbohydrate intakes may be of even greater importance after eccentric exercise and exhaustive running because of the potential for this dietary regimen to partially overcome the muscle damage-induced depression of glycogen resynthesis. For additional information regarding the effect of post-exercise diet on glycogen resynthesis, see Coyle,[24] Sherman and Wimer,[34] Friedman et al.,[80] Ivy,[81] Sherman,[119] and Williams.[146]

VII. SUMMARY

The preferential use of carbohydrate over fat as an energy substrate for exercising muscle is directly related to exercise intensity and initial glycogen levels and inversely related to duration of aerobic exercise and level of physical conditioning.[23,24] Skeletal muscle glycogen stores and circulating blood glucose originating in liver from glycogenolysis or gluconeogenesis represent the primary sources of carbohydrate used for energy production by muscle.[73] Glucose derived from muscle glycogen is the most important substrate used during high intensity anaerobic exercise and during the first 2 hr of aerobic exercise. As prolonged exercise continues, the quantitative importance of blood glucose compared to endogenous muscle glycogen as an energy source for muscle oxidation increases. Plasma glucose oxidation can supply 20–50% of the total oxidizable substrate during submaximal exercise.[38]

Although plasma glucose is clearly an important energy substrate during prolonged submaximal exercise, it should be emphasized that initial skeletal muscle glycogen stores are the primary determinant of one's ability to sustain prolonged moderate to heavy exercise. Glycogen storage in muscle is largely dependent on level of exercise training and both the long-term and acute state of carbohydrate nutriture. Trained skeletal muscles have greater glycogen stores which are depleted at a slower rate during exercise.[53]

   The dietary manipulation of carbohydrate intake prior to, during, and after exercise can improve exercise performance largely through optimizing muscle and liver glycogen stores or through the maintenance of blood glucose homeostasis.[24,73] Improved performance is generally associated with maintenance of carbohydrate availability and a high rate of carbohydrate utilization during exercise. Specific recommendations and conclusions related to carbohydrate intakes are as follows:

1. Individuals who exercise regularly should routinely consume a diet which provides 55–70% of the total calories from carbohydrate or 4.5–6.0 g carbohydrate/kg body wt/day.
2. The consumption of pre-exercise meals consisting primarily of low-fiber carbohydrate (solid or liquid) foods, ingested at least 2–3 hr before the exercise session, can improve performance during endurance-type events.
3. Pre-exercise carbohydrate ingestion less than 1 hr before exercise can improve work performance although some individuals may experience a transient lowering of blood glucose and associated fatigue.
4. Pre-exercise feedings should contain 1–5 g carbohydrate/kg body weight. Liquid carbohydrate intakes at the lower end of this range are better tolerated than solid meals and higher intakes when consumed close to competition because of shorter gastric emptying time.
5. For prolonged exercise, a relatively large pre-exercise meal containing more than 200 g carbohydrate appears to improve performance.
6. There appears to be no advantage of pre-exercise ingestion of fructose over glucose. Improved performance in association with pre-exercise consumption of low compared to high glycemic index foods has been reported but is not a consistent finding.
7. Carbohydrate supercompensation can improve endurance performance in individuals engaged in continuous exercise for more than 90 min.
8. Carbohydrate ingestion of at least 45–60 g during exercise can delay fatigue and improve endurance performance by helping to optimize blood glucose availability.
9. Dilute glucose solutions (5% or less) should be ingested during exercise for optimal hydration because they are emptied from the stomach more quickly than concentrated solutions. However, greater net glucose absorption occurs with increased glucose concentrations in sports drinks.
10. The use of glucose polymer solutions during exercise may be advantageous because of their lower osmolality and potential for more rapid gastric emptying. In contrast, fructose is not the preferred source of carbohydrate because of its relatively slow absorption and its primarily hepatic site of metabolism.
11. Replenishment of liver and muscle glycogen reserves after strenuous physical activity can occur within 24 hr and is critical in terms of ability to perform subsequent endurance exercise.
12. Maximum glycogen resynthesis occurs when individuals ingest carbohydrate soon after exercise, strive to consume the equivalent of 0.7–1.5 g glucose/kg body weight every 2 hr during the initial 6 hr post-exercise, and ingest approximately 600 g of carbohydrate or close to 10 g/kg body weight during the 24 hr post-exercise period.
13. Post-exercise ingestion of fructose compared to glucose induces more liver glycogen synthesis but less muscle glycogen synthesis.
14. High-carbohydrate foods or beverages such as fruits, fruit juices, or commercially available carbohydrate drinks, especially those with a high glycemic index, appear to be good choices for promoting post-exercise glycogen resynthesis.

REFERENCES

1. National Research Council, *Recommended Dietary Allowances*, 10th ed., National Academy Press, Washington, D.C., 1989, chap. 4.
2. U.S. Department of Agriculture, *Food and Nutrient Intake by Individuals in the United States, 1 Day, 1989–91*, Continuing Survey of Food Intakes by Individuals, 1989-91, Nationwide Food Surveys Rep. No. 91-2, 1995.
3. Stephan, A. M., Sieber, G. M., Gerster, Y. A., and Morgan, D. R., Intake of carbohydrate and its components — international comparisons, trends over time, and effects of changing to low-fat diets, *Am. J. Clin. Nutr.*, 62, 851S, 1995.
4. Berdanier, C. D., *Advanced Nutrition: Macronutrients,* CRC Press, Boca Raton, FL, 1995, chap. 5.
5. Cori, C. F., The fate of sugar in the animal body. I. The rate of absorption of hexoses and pentoses from the intestinal tract, *J. Biol. Chem.*, 66, 691, 1925.
6. Flatt, J. P., Use and storage of carbohydrate and fat, *Am. J. Clin. Nutr.*, 61(suppl), 952S, 1995.
7. Hood, D. A., and Terjung, R. L., Amino acid metabolism during exercise and following endurance exercise, *Sports Med.*, 9, 23, 1990.
8. Brooks, G. A., Fahey, T. D., and White, T. P., *Exercise Physiology: Human Bioenergetics and Its Applications,* Mayfield Publishing Co., Mountain View, CA, 1996, chaps. 3, 5, 9, and 28.
9. Murray, R. K., Granner, D. K., Mayes, P. A., and Rodwell, V. W., *Harper's Biochemistry*, 22nd ed., Appleton & Lange, Norwalk, CT, 1990, chap. 20.
10. Saltin, B. and Gollnick, P. D., Skeletal muscle adaptability: Significance for metabolism and performance, in *Handbook of Physiology*, Peachy, L. D., Adrian, R. H., and Geiger, S. R., Eds., Williams & Wilkins, Baltimore, 1983, 555.
11. Murray, R. K., Granner, D. K., Mayes, P. A., and Rodwell, V. W., *Harper's Biochemistry*, 22nd ed., Appleton & Lange, Norwalk, CT, 1990, chap. 21.
12. Nilsson, L. H. and Hultman, E., Liver glycogen in man: the effect of total starvation or a carbohydrate-poor diet followed by carbohydrate refeeding, *Scand. J. Clin. Lab. Invest.*, 32, 325, 1973.
13. Felig, P., Pozefsky, T., Marliss, E., and Cahill, G.F., Alanine: key role in gluconeogenesis, *Science*, 167, 1003, 1970.
14. Felig, P. and Wahren, J., Amino acid metabolism in exercising man, *J. Clin. Invest.*, 50, 2703, 1971.
15. Landau, B. R. and Wahren, J., Quantification of the pathways followed in hepatic glycogen formation from glucose, *FASEB J.*, 2, 2368, 1988.
16. Foster, D.W., From glycogen to ketones — and back, *Diabetes*, 33, 1188, 1984.
17. McGarrey, J. D., Kuwajima, M., Newgard, C. B., and Foster, D. W., From dietary glucose to liver glycogen: the full circle round, *Ann. Rev. Nutr.*, 7, 51, 1987.
18. Nilsson, L. H. and Hultman, E., Liver and muscle glycogen in man after glucose and fructose infusion, *Scand. J. Clin. Lab. Invest.*, 33, 5, 1974.
19. Murray, R. K., Granner, D. K., Mayes, P. A., and Rodwell, V. W., *Harper's Biochemistry*, 22nd ed., Appleton & Lange, Norwalk, CT, 1990, chap. 19.
20. Saltin, B. and Gollnick, P. D., Fuel for muscular exercise: role of carbohydrate, in *Exercise, Nutrition and Energy Metabolism*, Horton, E. S. and Terjung, R. L., Eds., Macmillan Publishing Co., New York, 1988, chap. 4.
21. McArdle, W. D., Katch, F. I., and Katch, V. I., *Exercise Physiology: Energy, Nutrition, and Human Performance*, Lea & Febiger, Philadelphia, 1991, Chap. 7.
22. Wilmore, J. H. and Costill, D. L., *Physiology of Sport and Exercise*, Human Kinetics Publishers, Champaign, IL, 1994, Chap. 5.
23. Romijn, J. A., Coyle, E. F., Sidossis, L. S., Gastaldelli, A., Horowitz, J. F., Endert, E., and Wolfe, R. R., Regulation of endogenous fat and carbohydrate metabolism in relation to exercise intensity and duration, *Am. J. Physiol.,* 265, E380, 1993.
24. Coyle, E. F., Substrate utilization during exercise in active people, *Am. J. Clin. Nutr.,* 61(suppl), 968S, 1995.
25. Phinney, S. D., Bistrian, B. R., Evans, W. J., Gervino, E., and Blackburn, G. L., The human metabolic response to chronic ketosis without caloric restriction: preservation of submaximal exercise capacity with reduced carbohydrate oxidation, *Metabolism*, 32, 769, 1983.
26. Gollnick, P. D. and Saltin, B., Fuel for muscular exercise: role of fat, in *Exercise, Nutrition and Energy Metabolism*, Horton, E. S. and Terjung, R. L., Eds., Macmillan Publishing Co., New York, 1988, chap. 5.
27. Hodgetts, V., Coppack, S. W., Frayn, K. N., and Hockaday, D. R., Factors controlling fat mobilization from human subcutaneous adipose tissue during exercise, *J. Appl. Physiol.*, 71, 445, 1991.
28. Bulow, J. and Madsen, J., Influence of blood flow on fatty acid mobilization from lipolytically active adipose tissue, *Pflügers Arch.*, 390, 169, 1981.
29. Holloszy, J. O., Utilization of fatty acids during exercise, in *Biochemistry of Exercise VII*, Taylor, A. W., Gollnick, P. D., Green, H. J., Ianuzzo, C. D., Noble, E. G., Métivier, G., and Sutton, J. R., Eds., Human Kinetics Publishers, Champaign, IL, 1990, 319.

30. Bergstrom, J., Hermansen, L., Hultman, E., and Saltin, B., Diet, muscle glycogen and physical performance, *Acta Physiol. Scand.*, 71, 140, 1967.

31. Hermansen, L., Hultman, E., and Saltin, B., Muscle glycogen during prolonged severe exercise, *Acta Physiol. Scand.*, 71, 129, 1967.

32. Price, T. B., Rothman, D. L., Avison, M. J., Buonamico, P., and Shulman, R. G., ^{13}C-NMR measurements of muscle glycogen during low-intensity exercise, *J. Appl. Physiol.*, 70, 1836, 1991.

33. Price, T. B., Taylor, R., Mason, G. F., Rothman, D. L., Shulman, G. I., and Shulman, R. G., Turnover of human muscle glycogen with low-intensity exercise, *Med. Sci. Sports Exer.*, 26, 983, 1994.

34. Sherman, W. M. and Wimer, G. S., Insufficient dietary carbohydrate during training: does it impair athletic performance?, *Int. J. Sport Nutr.*, 1, 28, 1991.

35. Wahren, J. P., Felig, P., Ahlborg, G., and Jorfeldt, L., Glucose metabolism during leg exercise in man, *J. Clin. Invest.*, 50, 2715, 1971.

36. Hickson, R. C., Carbohydrate metabolism in exercise, in *Ross Symposium on Nutrient Utilization During Exercise*, Fox, E. L., Ed., Ross Laboratories, Columbus, OH, 1983, 1.

37. Jorfeldt, L. and Wahren, J., Leg blood flow during exercise in man, *Clin. Sci.*, 41, 459, 1971.

38. Coggan, A. R., Plasma glucose metabolism during exercise in humans, *Sports Med.*, 11, 102, 1991.

39. Björkman, O. and Wahren, J., Glucose homeostasis during and after exercise, in *Exercise, Nutrition and Energy Metabolism*, Horton, E. S. and Terjung, R. L., Eds., Macmillan Publishing Co., New York, 1988, chap. 7.

40. Ahlborg, B., Bergstrom, J., Ekelund, L., and Hultman, E., Muscle glycogen and muscle electrolytes during prolonged physical exercise, *Acta Physiol. Scand.*, 70, 129, 1967.

41. Baldwin, K. M., Reitman, J. S., Terjung, R. L., Winder, W. W., and Holloszy, J. O., Substate depletion in different types of muscle and in liver during prolonged running, *Am. J. Physiol.*, 225, 1045, 1973.

42. Bosch, A. N., Weltan, S. M., Dennis, S. C., and Noakes, T. D., Fuel substrate kinetics of carbohydrate loading differs from that of carbohydrate ingestion during prolonged exercise, *Metabolism,* 45, 415, 1996.

43. Coyle, E. F., Coggan, A. R., Hemmert, M. K., and Ivy, J. L., Muscle glycogen utilization during prolonged strenuous exercise when fed carbohydrates, *J. Appl. Physiol.*, 61, 165, 1986.

44. Davies, C. T. M. and Thompson, M. N., Physiological responses to prolonged exercise in ultra marathon athletes, *J. Appl. Physiol.*, 61, 611, 1986.

45. Kreider R. B., Physiological considerations in ultra endurance performance, *Int. J. Sports Med.*, 1, 3, 1991.

46. Ahlborg, G., Felig, P., Hagenfeldt, L., Hendler, R., and Wahren, J., Substrate turnover during prolonged exercise in man: splanchnic and leg metabolism of glucose, free fatty acids, and amino acids, *J. Clin. Invest.*, 53, 1080, 1974.

47. Ahlborg, G. and Felig, P., Lactate and glucose exchange across the forearm, legs, and splanchnic bed during and after prolonged leg exercise, *J. Clin. Invest.*, 69, 45, 1982.

48. Pruett, E. D. R., Glucose and insulin during prolonged work stress in men living on different diets, *J. Appl. Physiol.*, 28, 199, 1970.

49. Coyle, E. F., Hagberg, J. M., Hurley, B. F., Martin, W. H., Ehsani, A. A., and Holloszy, J. O., Carbohydrate feeding during prolonged strenuous exercise can delay fatigue, *J. Appl. Physiol.*, 55, 230, 1983.

50. Jansson, E. and Kaijser, L., Substrate utilization and enzymes in skeletal muscle of extremely endurance-trained men, *J. Appl. Physiol.*, 62, 999, 1987.

51. Holloszy, J. O., Metabolic consequences of endurance exercise training, in *Exercise, Nutrition and Energy Metabolism*, Horton, E. S. and Terjung, R. L., Eds., Macmillan Publishing Co., New York, 1988, chap. 8.

52. Coggan, A. R., Kohrt, W. M., Spina, R. J., Bier, D. M., and Holloszy, J. O., Endurance training decreases plasma glucose turnover and oxidation during moderate-intensity exercise in men, *J. Appl. Physiol.*, 68, 990, 1990.

53. Coleman, E., Carbohydrates: the master fuel, in *Sports Nutrition for the 90s*, Berning, J.R. and Steen, S.N., Eds., Aspen Publishers, Inc., Gaithersburg, MD, 1991, chap. 3.

54. Gollnick, P. D., Piehl, K., Saubert, C. W., Armstrong, R. B., and Saltin, B., Diet, exercise, and glycogen changes in human muscle fibers, *J. Appl. Physiol.*, 33, 421, 1972.

55. O'Keeffe, K. A., Keith, R. E., Wilson, G. D., and Blessing, D. L., Dietary carbohydrate intake and endurance exercise performance of trained female cyclists, *Nutr. Res.*, 9, 819, 1989.

56. Simonsen, J. C., Sherman, W. M., Lamb, D. R., Dernbach, A. R., Doyle, J. A., and Strauss, R., Dietary carbohydrate, muscle glycogen, and power output during rowing training, *J. Appl. Physiol.*, 70, 1500, 1991.

57. Lamb, D. R. and Snyder, A. C., Muscle glycogen loading with a liquid carbohydrate supplement, *Int. J. Sport Nutr.*, 1, 52, 1991.

58. Sherman, W. M., Doyle, J. A., Lamb, D. R., and Strauss, R. H., Dietary carbohydrate, muscle glycogen, and exercise performance during 7 days of training, *Am. J. Clin. Nutr.*, 57, 27, 1993.

59. Costill, D. L., Bowers, R., Branam, G., and Sparks, K., Muscle glycogen utilization during prolonged exercise on successive days, *J. Appl. Physiol.*, 31, 834, 1971.

60. Symons, J. D. and Jacobs, I., High-intensity exercise performance is not impaired by low intramuscular glycogen, *Med. Sci. Sports Exer.*, 21, 550, 1989.

61. Vandenberghe, K., Hespel, P., Eynde, B. V., Lysens, R., and Richter, E. A., No effect of glycogen level on glycogen metabolism during high intensity exercise, *Med. Sci. Sports Exer.*, 27, 1278, 1995.

62. Sahlin, K., Broberg, S., and Katz, A., Glucose formation in human skeletal muscle, *Biochem. J.*, 258, 911, 1989.

63. Hargreaves, M., Dillo, P., Angus, D., and Febbraio, M., Effect of fluid ingestion on muscle metabolism during prolonged exercise, *J. Appl. Physiol.*, 80, 363, 1996.

64. Hultman, E., Regulation of carbohydrate metabolism in the liver during rest and exercise with special reference to diet, in *Biochemistry of Exercise III*, Landry, F. and Orban, W. A. R., Eds., Symposia Specialists, Miami, 1977.

65. Bosch, A. N., Dennis, S. C., and Noakes, T. D., Influence of carbohydrate ingestion on fuel substrate turnover and oxidation during prolonged exercise, *J. Appl. Physiol.*, 76, 2364, 1994.

66. Brooks, G. A., The lactate shuttle during exercise and recovery, *Med. Sci. Sports Exer.*, 18, 360, 1986.

67. Stainsby, W. N. and Brooks, G. A., Control of lactic acid metabolism in contracting muscles and during exercise, in *Exercise and Sport Sciences Reviews*, Vol. 18, Pandolf, K.B., Ed., Williams & Wilkins, Baltimore, 1990, 29.

68. Donaldson, S. K. B. and Hermansen, L., Differential, direct effects of H^+ on Ca^{2+}-activated force of skinned fibers from the soleus, cardiac and adductor magnus muscles of rabbits, *Pflügers Arch.*, 376, 55, 1978.

69. Fitts, R. H. and Metzger, J. M., Mechanisms of muscular fatigue, in *Principles of Exercise Biochemistry*, Poortmans, J.R., Ed., Karger, Basel, Switzerland, 1988, 212.

70. Stanley, W. C. and Connett, R. J., Regulation of muscle carbohydrate metabolism during exercise, *FASEB J.*, 5, 2155, 1991.

71. Ren, J. M. and Hultman, E., Regulation of glycogenolysis in human skeletal muscle, *J. Appl. Physiol.*, 76, 2243, 1989.

72. Bonen, A., McDermott, J. C., and Hutber, C. A. Carbohydrate metabolism in skeletal muscle: an update of current concepts, *Int. J. Sports Med.*, 10, 385, 1989.

73. Wasserman D. H., Regulation of glucose fluxes during exercise in the postabsorptive state, *Annu. Rev. Physiol.*, 57, 191,1995.

74. Richter, E. A. and Galbo, H., High glycogen levels enhance glycogen breakdown in isolated contracting skeletal muscle, *J. Appl. Physiol.*, 61, 827, 1986.

75. Conlee, R.K., McLane, J.A., Rennie, M.J., Winder, W.W., and Holloszy, J.O., Reversal of phosphorylase activation in muscle despite continued contractile activity, *Am. J. Physiol.*, 237, R291, 1979.

76. Katz, A., Broberg, S., Sahlin, K., and Wahren, J., Leg glucose uptake during maximal dynamic exercise in humans, *Am. J. Physiol.*, 251, E65, 1986.

77. Hutber, C. A. and Bonen, A., Glycogenesis in muscle and liver during exercise, *J. Appl. Physiol.*, 66, 2811, 1989.

78. Kuipers, H., Keizer, H. A., Brouns, F., and Saris, W. H. M., Carbohydrate feeding and glycogen synthesis during exercise in man, *Pflügers Arch.*, 410, 652, 1987.

79. Kuipers, H., Saris, W. H. M., Brouns, F., Keizer, H. A., and Bosch, C., Glycogen synthesis during exercise and rest with carbohydrate feeding in males and females, *Int. J. Sports Med.*, 10, S63, 1989.

80. Friedman, J. E., Neufer, P. D., and Dohm, G. L., Regulation of glycogen resynthesis following exercise, *Sports Med.*, 11, 232, 1991.

81. Ivy, J. L., Muscle glycogen synthesis before and after exercise, *Sports Med.*, 11, 6, 1991.

82. Friedman, J. E., Sherman, W. M., Reed, M. J., Elton, C. W., and Dohm, G. L., Exercise training increases glucose transporter protein (GLUT 4) in skeletal muscle of obese Zucker (fa/fa) rats, *FEBS Lett.*, 268, 13, 1990.

83. Cartee, G. D., Young, D. A., Sleeper, M D., Zierath, J., and Wallberg-Hendriksson, H., Prolonged increase in insulin stimulated glucose transport in muscle after exercise, *Am. J. Physiol.*, 256, E494, 1989.

84. Richter, E. A., Garetto, L. P., Goodman, M. N., and Ruderman, N. B., Muscle glucose metabolism following exercise in the rat: increased sensitivity to insulin, *J. Clin. Invest.*, 69, 785, 1982.

85. Richter, E. A., Hanson, S. A., and Hanson, B. F., Mechanisms limiting glycogen storage in muscle during prolonged insulin stimulation, *Am. J. Physiol.*, 255, E621, 1988.

86. Zorzano, A., Balon, T. W., Goodman, M. N., and Ruderman, N. B., Additive effects of prior exercise and insulin on glucose and AIB uptake by rat muscle, *Am. J. Physiol.*, 252, E21, 1986.

87. Stanley, W. C., Wisneski, J. A., Gertz, E. W., Neese, R. A., and Brooks, G. A., Glucose and lactate interrelations during moderate-intensity exercise in humans, *Metabolism*, 37, 850, 1988.

88. Kjaer, M., Engfred, K., Fernandes, A., Secher, N., and Galbo, H., Influence of sympathoadrenergic activity on hepatic glucose production during exercise in man, *Med. Sci. Sports Exer.*, 22, S81, 1990.

89. Hoelzer, D. R., Dalsky, G. P., Clutter, W. E., Shah, S. D., Schwartz, N. S., and Holloszy, J. O., Glucoregulation during exercise: hypoglycemia is prevented by redundant glucoregulatory systems, sympathochromaffin activation, and changes in islet hormone secretion, *J. Clin. Invest.*, 77, 212, 1986.

90. Hoelzer, D. R., Dalsky, G. P., Schwartz, N. S., Clutter, W. E., Shah, S. D., and Holloszy, J. O., Epinephrine is not critical to prevention of hypoglycemia during exercise in humans, *Am. J. Physiol.*, 251, E104, 1986.

91. Freude, K. A., Sandler, L. S., and Zieve, F. J., Electrical stimulation of the liver cell: activation of glycogenolysis, *Am. J. Physiol.*, 240, E226, 1981.
92. Vranic, M. and Lickley, H. L. A., Hormonal mechanisms that act to preserve glucose homeostasis during exercise, in *Biochemistry of Exercise VII*, Taylor, A. W., Gollnick, P. D., Green, H. J., Ianuzzo, C. D., Noble, E. G., Métivier, G., and Sutton, J. R., Eds., Human Kinetics Publishers, Champaign, IL, 1990, 279.
93. Plough, T., Galbo, H., and Richter, E. A., Increased muscle glucose uptake during contraction: no need for insulin, *Am. J. Physiol.*, 247, E276, 1984.
94. Wallberg-Henriksson, H. and Holloszy, J. D., Contractile activity increases glucose uptake by muscle in severely diabetic rats, *J. Appl. Physiol.*, 57, 1045, 1984.
95. Bonen, A., McDermott, J. C., and Tan, M. H, Glucose transport in skeletal muscle, in *Biochemistry of Exercise VII*, Taylor, A. W., Gollnick, P. D., Green, H. J., Ianuzzo, C. D., Noble, E. G., Métivier, G., and Sutton, J. R., Eds., Human Kinetics Books, Champaign, IL, 1990, 295.
96. Bonen, A., Tan, M. H., and Watson-Wright, W. M., Insulin binding and glucose uptake differences in rodent skeletal muscles, *Diabetes*, 30, 702, 1981.
97. Bonen, A., Tan, M. H., and Watson-Wright, W. M., Effects of exercise on insulin binding and glucose metabolism in muscle, *Can. J. Physiol. Pharmacol.*, 62, 1500, 1984.
98. James, D. E., Kraegen, E. W., and Chisholm, D. J., Muscle glucose metabolism in exercising rats: comparison with insulin stimulation, *Am. J. Physiol.*, 248, E575, 1985.
99. Berger, M., Hagg, S., and Ruderman, N. B., Glucose metabolism in perfused skeletal muscle: interaction of insulin and exercise on glucose uptake, *Biochem. J.*, 146, 321, 1975.
100. Vranic, M., Kawamori, R., Pek, S., Kovacevic, N., and Wrenshall, G. A., The essentiality of insulin and the role of glucagon in regulating glucose utilization and production during strenuous exercise in dogs, *J. Clin. Invest.*, 57, 245, 1976.
101. Goodyear, L. J., King, P. A., Hirshman, M. F., Thompson, C. M., Horton, E. D., and Horton, H. S., Contractile activity increases plasma membrane glucose transporters in absence of insulin, *Am. J. Physiol.*, 258, E667, 1990.
102. Richter, E. A., Plough, T., and Galbo, H., Increased muscle glucose uptake after exercise: no need for insulin during exercise, *Diabetes*, 34, 1041, 1985.
103. Nesher, R., Karl, I. E., and Kipnis, D. M., Dissociation of effects of insulin and contraction on glucose transport in rat epitrochlearis muscle, *Am. J. Physiol.*, 249, C226, 1985.
104. Holloszy, J. O., Constable, S. H., and Young, D. A., Activation of glucose transport in muscle by exercise. *Diabetes Metab. Rev.*, 1, 409, 1986.
105. Douen, A. G., Ramial, T., Klip, A., Young, D. A., Cartee, G. D., and Holloszy, J. O., Exercise-induced increase in glucose transporter in plasma membranes of rat skeletal muscle, *Endocrinology*, 124, 449, 1989.
106. Douen, A. G., Ramial, T., Rastogi, S., Bilan, P. J., Cartee, G. D., Vranic, M., Holloszy, J. O., and Klip, A., Exercise induces recruitment of the "insulin-responsive glucose transporter," *J. Biol. Chem.*, 265, 13427, 1990.
107. Klip, A., Ramial, T., Young, A., and Holloszy, J. O., Insulin-induced translocation of glucose transporters in rat hindlimb muscles, *FEBS Lett.*, 224, 224, 1987.
108. Hendriksen, E. J., Bourey, R. E., Rodnick, J., Koranyi, L., Permutt, M. A., and Holloszy, J. O., Glucose transporter protein content and glucose transport capacity in rat muscles, *Am. J. Physiol.*, 259, E593, 1990.
109. McConnell, G., McCoy, M., Proietto, J., and Hargraves, M., Skeletal muscle GLUT-4 and glucose uptake during exercise in humans, *J. Appl. Physiol.*, 77, 1565, 1994.
110. Kristiansen S., Hargraves, M., and Richter, E. A., Exercise-induced increase in glucose transport, GLUT-4, and VAMP-2 in plasma membrane from human muscle, *Am. J. Physiol.*, 270, E197, 1996.
111. Klip, A. and Paquet, M. R., Glucose transport and glucose transporters in muscle and their metabolic regulation, *Diabetes Care*, 13, 228, 1990.
112. Treadway, J. L., James, D. E., Burcel, E., and Ruderman, N. B., Effect of exercise on insulin receptor binding and kinase activity in skeletal muscle, *Am. J. Physiol.*, 256, E138, 1989.
113. Sherman, W., Carbohydrates, muscle glycogen and muscle glycogen supercompensation, in *Ergogenic Aids in Sports*, Williams, M. H., Ed., Human Kinetics Publishers, Champaign, IL, 1983, 3.
114. Costill, D. L. and Hargreaves, M., Carbohydrate nutrition and fatigue, *Sports Med.*, 13, 86, 1992.
115. Larson, D. E., Hesslink, R. L., Hrovat, M.I ., Fishman, R. S., and Systrom, D. M., Dietary effects on exercising muscle metabolism and performance by ³¹P-MRS, *J. Appl. Physiol.*, 77, 1108, 1994.
116. Hoffman, C. J. and Coleman, E., An eating plan and update on recommended dietary practices for the endurance athlete, *J. Am. Diet. Assoc.*, 91, 325, 1991.
117. Coleman, E., *Eating for Endurance*, Bull Publishing Co., Palo Alto, CA, 1988, chap. 4.
118. Clark, N., *Nancy Clark's Sports Nutrition Guidebook: Eating to Fuel Your Active Lifestyle*, Leisure Press, Champaign, IL, 1990.
119. Sherman, W. M., Carbohydrate feedings before and after exercise, in *Ergogenics — Enhancement of Performance in Exercise and Sport*, Lamb, D. R. and Williams, M. H., Eds., Benchmark Press, Dubuque, IA, 1991, 1.

120. Coggan, A. R. and Swanson, S. C., Nutritional manipulations before and during endurance exercise: effects on performance, *Med. Sci. Sports Exer.,* 24(suppl), S331, 1992.

121. Costill, D. L., Coyle, E., Dalsky, G., Evans, W., Fink, W., and Hoopes, D., Effects of elevated plasma FFA and insulin on muscle glycogen usage during exercise, *J. Appl. Physiol.,* 43, 695, 1977.

122. Koivisto, V. A., Karvonen, S., and Nikkilä, E. A., Carbohydrate ingestion before exercise: comparison of glucose, fructose, and sweet placebo, *J. Appl. Physiol.,* 51, 783, 1981.

123. Foster, C., Costill, D. L., and Fink, W. J., Effects of pre-exercise feeding on endurance performance, *Med. Sci. Sports,* 11, 1, 1979.

124. Keller, K. and Schwarzkopf, R., Pre-exercise snacks may decrease exercise performance, *Phys. Sportsmed.,* 12, 89, 1984.

125. Coyle, E. F., Coggan, A. R., Hemmert, M. K., Lowe, R. C., and Walters, T. J., Substrate usage during prolonged exercise following a pre-exercise meal, *J. Appl. Physiol.,* 59, 429, 1985.

126. Sherman, W. M. and Wright, D. A., Pre-event nutrition for prolonged exercise, in *The Theory and Practice of Athletic Nutrition: Bridging the Gap,* Grandjean, A. C. and Storlie, J., Eds., Report of the Ross Symposium, Ross Laboratories, Columbus, OH, 1989, 30.

127. Costill, D. L., Carbohydrate for athletic training and performance, *Contemporary Nutr.,* 15, 9, 1990.

128. Gleeson, M., Maughan, R. J., and Greenhaff, P. L., Comparison of the effects of pre-exercise feeding of glucose, glycerol and placebo on endurance and fuel homeostasis in man, *Eur. J. Appl. Physiol.,* 55, 645, 1986.

129. Neufer, P. D., Costill, D. L., Flynn, M. G., Kirwan, J. P., Mitchell, J. B., and Houmard, J., Improvements in exercise performance: effects of carbohydrate feeding and diet, *J. Appl. Physiol.,* 62, 983, 1987.

130. Sherman, W. M., Peden, M. C., and Wright, D. A., Carbohydrate feeding 1 hr before exercise improves cycling performance, *Am. J. Clin. Nutr.,* 54, 866, 1991.

131. Anantaraman, R., Carmines, A. A., Gaesser, G. A., and Weltman, A., Effects of carbohydrate supplementation on performance during 1 hour of high-intensity exercise, *Int. J. Sports Med.,* 16, 461, 1995.

132. Gisolfi, C. V. and Duchman, S. M., Guidelines for optimal replacement beverages for different athletic events, *Med. Sci. Sports Exer.,* 24, 679, 1992.

133. Hargreaves, M., Costill, D. L., Fink, W. J., King, D. S., and Fielding, R. A., Effect of pre-exercise carbohydrate feedings on endurance cycling performance, *Med. Sci. Sports Exer.,* 19, 33, 1987.

134. Devlin, J. T., Calles-Escandon, J., and Horton, E. S., Effects of pre-exercise snack feeding on endurance cycle exercise, *J. Appl. Physiol.,* 60, 980, 1986.

135. Decombaz, J., Sartori, D., Arnaud, M. J., Thelin, A.L., Schurch, P., and Howard, H., Oxidation and metabolic effects of fructose or glucose ingested before exercise, *Int. J. Sports Med.,* 6, 282, 1985.

136. Ravich, W. J., Bayless, T. M., and Thomas, M., Fructose: incomplete intestinal absorption in humans, *Gastroenterology,* 84, 26, 1983.

137. Foster-Powell, K. and Miller, J. B., International tables of glycemic index, *Am. J. Clin. Nutr.,* 62, 871S, 1995.

138. Wolever, T. M., The glycemic index, *World Rev. Nutr. Diet.,* 62, 120, 1990.

139. Guezennec, C. Y., Satabin, P., Duforez, F., Koziet, J., and Antoine, J. M., The role of type and structure of complex carbohydrates response to physical exercise, *Int. J. Sports Med.,* 14, 224, 1993.

140. Thomas, D. E., Brotherhood, J. R., and Brand, J. C., Carbohydrate feeding before exercise: effect of glycemic index, *Int. J. Sports Med.,* 12, 180, 1991.

141. Hollenbeck, C. B. and Coulston, A. M., The clinical utility of the glycemic index and its application to mixed meals, *Can. J. Physiol. Pharmacol.,* 69, 100, 1991.

142. Jarvis, J. K., Pearsall, D., Oliner, C. M., and Schoeller, D. A., The effect of food matrix on carbohydrate utilization during moderate exercise, *Med. Sci. Sports Exer.,* 24, 320, 1992.

143. Paul, G. L., Rokusek, J. T., Dykstra, G. L., Boileau, R. A., and Layman, D. K., Oat, wheat or corn cereal ingestion before exercise alters metabolism in humans, *J. Nutr.,* 126, 1372, 1996.

144. Anderson, M., Bergman, E. A., and Nethery, V. M., Pre-exercise meal affects ride time to fatigue in trained cyclists, *J. Am. Dietet. Assoc.,* 94, 1152, 1994.

145. Walberg-Rankin, J., Dietary carbohydrate as an ergogenic aid for prolonged and brief competitions in sport, *Int. J. Sport Nutr.,* 5, S13, 1995.

146. Williams, C., Macronutrients and performance, *J. Sports Sci.,* 13, S1, 1995.

147. Pizza, F. X., Flynn, M. G., Duscha, B. D., Holden, J., and Kubitz, E. R., A carbohydrate loading regimen improves high intensity, short duration exercise performance, *Int. J. Sport Nutr.,* 5, 110, 1995.

148. Sherman, W. M. and Costill, D. L., The marathon: dietary manipulation to optimize performance, *Am. J. Sports Med.,* 12, 44, 1984.

149. Sherman, W. M., Costill, D. L., Fink, W. J., and Miller, J. M., The effect of exercise and diet manipulation on muscle glycogen and its subsequent utilization during performance, *Int. J. Sports Med.,* 2, 114, 1981.

150. Lamb, D. R. and Snyder, A. C., Muscle glycogen loading with a liquid carbohydrate supplement, *Int. J. Sport Nutr.,* 1, 52, 1991.

151. Tarnopolsky, M. A., Atkinson, S. A., Phillips, S. M., and MacDougall, J. D., Carbohydrate loading and metabolism during exercise in men and women, *J. Appl. Physiol.,* 78, 1360, 1995.

152. Zachweija, J. J., Costill, D. L., Pascoe, D. D., Robergs, R. A., and Fink, W. J., Influence of muscle glycogen depletion on the rate of resynthesis, *Med. Sci. Sports Exer.*, 23, 445, 1991.

153. McArdle, W. D., Katch, F. I., and Katch, V. I., *Exercise Physiology: Energy, Nutrition, and Human Performance*, Lea & Febiger, Philadelphia, 1991, Chap 23.

154. Coggan, A. R. and Coyle, E. F., Carbohydrate ingestion during prolonged exercise: effects on metabolism and performance, *Exerc. Sport Sci. Rev.*, 19, 1, 1991.

155. Coyle, E. F., Carbohydrate supplementation during exercise, *J. Nutr.*, 122, 788, 1992.

156. Maughan, R. J. and Noakes, T. D., Fluid replacement and exercise stress, *Sports Med.*, 12, 16, 1991.

157. Maughan, R. J., Carbohydrate-electrolyte solutions during prolonged exercise, in *Ergogenics-Enhancement of Performance in Exercise and Sport*, Lamb, D. R. and Williams, M. H., Eds., Benchmark Press, 1991, 35.

158. Noakes, T. D., Rehrer, N. J., and Maughan, R. J., The importance of volume in regulating gastric emptying, *Med. Sci. Sports Exer.*, 23, 307, 1991.

159. Flynn, M. G., Costill, D. L., Hawley, J. A., Fink, W. J., Neufer, P. D., Fielding, R. A., and Sleeper, M. D., Influence of selected carbohydrate drinks on cycling performance and glycogen use, *Med. Sci. Sports Exer.*, 19, 37, 1987.

160. Mitchell, J. B., Costill, D. L., Houmard, J. A., Fink, W. J., Pascoe, D. D., and Pearson, D. R., Influence of carbohydrate dosage on exercise performance and glycogen metabolism, *J. Appl. Physiol.*, 67, 1843, 1989.

161. Noakes, T. F., Lambert, E.V ., Lambert, M. I., McArthur, P. S., Myburgh, K. H., and Benade, A. J. S., Carbohydrate ingestion and muscle glycogen depletion during marathon and ultramarathon racing, *Europ. J. Appl. Physiol.*, 57, 482, 1988.

162. Coyle, E. F., Hamilton, M. T., Alonso, J. G., Montain, S. J., and Ivy, J. L., Carbohydrate metabolism during intense exercise when hyperglycemic, *J. Appl. Physiol.*, 70, 834, 1991.

163. Kuipers, H., Keizer, H. A., Brouns, F., and Saris, W. H. M., Carbohydrate feeding and glycogen synthesis during exercise in man, *Pflügers Arch.*, 410, 652, 1987.

164. Kuipers, H., Saris, W. H. M., Brouns, F., Keizer, H. A., and Bosch, C., Glycogen synthesis during exercise and rest with carbohydrate feeding in males and females, *Int. J. Sports Med.*, 10, S63, 1989.

165. McConell, G., Fabris, S., Proietto, J., and Hargraves, M., Effect of carbohydrate on glucose kinetics during exercise, *J. Appl. Physiol.*, 77, 1537, 1994.

166. Coggan, A. R. and Coyle, E. F., Reversal of fatigue during prolonged exercise by carbohydrate infusion or ingestion, *J. Appl. Physiol.*, 63, 2388, 1987.

167. Denster, P. A., Singh, A., Hofmann, A., Moses, F. M., and Chronsos, G. C., Hormonal responses to ingesting water or a carbohydrate beverage during a 2 h run, *Med. Sci. Sports Exer.*, 24, 72, 1992.

168. Maughan, R. J., Leiper, J. B., and McGaw, B. A., Effects of exercise intensity on absorption of ingested fluids in man, *Exper. Physiol.*, 75, 419, 1990.

169. Below, P. R., Mora-Rodriguez, R., Gonzalez-Alonso, J., and Coyle, E. F., Fluid and carbohydrate ingestion independently improve performance during 1 h of intense exercise, *Med. Sci. Sports Exer.,* 27, 200, 1995.

170. Coggan, A. R. and Coyle, E. F., Effect of carbohydrate feedings during high-intensity exercise, *J. Appl. Physiol.*, 63, 2388, 1988.

171. Mitchell, J. B., Costill, D. L., Houmard, J. A., Fylnn, M. G., Fink, W. J., and Beltz, J. D., Effects of carbohydrate ingestion on gastric emptying and exercise performance, *Med. Sci. Sports Exer.*, 20, 110, 1988.

172. Murray, R., The effects of consuming carbohydrate-electrolyte beverages on gastric emptying and fluid absorption during and following exercise, *Sports Med.*, 4, 322, 1987.

173. Murray, R., Paul, G. L., Seifert, J. G., Eddy, D. E., and Halaby, G. A., The effect of glucose, fructose and sucrose ingestion during exercise, *Med. Sci. Sports Exer.*, 21, 275, 1989.

174. Rehrer, N. J., Beckers, E., Brouns, F., Ten Hoor, F., and Saris, W. H. M., Exercise and training effects on gastric emptying of carbohydrate beverages, *Med. Sci. Sports Exer.*, 21, 540, 1989.

175. Rehrer, N. J., Brouns, F., Beckers, E., Ten Hoor, F., and Saris, H. M., Gastric emptying with repeated drinking during running and bicycling, *Int. J. Sports Med.*, 11, 238, 1990.

176. Mitchell, J. B. and Voss, K. W., The influence of volume of fluid ingested on gastric emptying and body fluid balance, *Med. Sci. Sports Exer.*, 22, S90, 1990.

177. Gisolfi, C. V., Summers, R. D., Schedl, H. P., and Bleiler, T. L., Effect of sodium concentration in a carbohydrate-electrolyte solution on intestinal absorption, *Med. Sci. Sports Exer.*, 27, 1414, 1995.

178. Mitchell, J. B., Costill, D. L., Houmard, J. A., Fink, W. J., Robergs, R. A., and Davis, J. A., Gastric emptying: influence of prolonged exercise and carbohydrate concentration, *Med. Sci. Sports Exer.*, 21, 269, 1989.

179. Sole, C. C. and Noakes, T. D., Faster gastric emptying for glucose-polymer and fructose solutions than for glucose in humans, *Europ. J. Appl. Physiol.*, 58, 605, 1989.

180. Xiacoai, S., Summers, R. W., Schedl, H. P., Flanagan, S. W., Chang, R., and Gisolfi, C. V., Effects of carbohydrate type and concentration and solution osmolarity on water absorption, *Med. Sci. Sports Exer.*, 27, 1607, 1995.

181. Foster, C., Gastric emptying during exercise. Influence of carbohydrate concentration, carbohydrate source, and exercise intensity, in *Fluid Replacement and Heat Stress*, National Academy of Science, Washington, D.C., 1990, chap. 6.

182. Costill, D. L. and Saltin, B., Factors limiting gastric emptying during rest and exercise, *J. Appl. Physiol.*, 37, 679, 1974.

183. Zachwieja, J. J., Costill, D. L., Widrick, J. J., Anderson, D. E., and McConell, G. K., Effects of drink carbonation on the gastric emptying characteristics of water and flavored water, *Int. J. Sport Nutr.*, 1, 45, 1991.

184. Massicotte, D., Peronnet, F., Brisson, G., Bakkouch, K., and Hilliare-Marcel, C., Oxidation of a glucose polymer during exercise: comparison of glucose and fructose, *J. Appl. Physiol.*, 66, 179, 1989.

185. Peters, H. P. F., Schelven, P. A., de Boer, R. W., Erich, W.B.M., van der Togt, C. R., and de Vries, W. R., Exercise performance as a function of semi-solid and liquid carbohydrate feeding during prolonged exercise, *Int. J. Sports Med.*, 16, 105, 1995.

186. Murray, R., Seifert, J. G., Eddy, D. E., Paul, G. L., and Halaby, G. A., Carbohydrate feeding and exercise: effect of beverage carbohydrate content, *Europ. J. Appl. Physiol.*, 59, 152, 1989.

187. Murray, R., Paul, G. L., Seifert, J. G., and Eddy, D. E., Responses to varying rates of carbohydrate ingestion during exercise, *Med. Sci. Sports Exer.*, 23, 713, 1991.

188. Bergstrom, J. and Hultman, E., Muscle glycogen synthesis after exercise: an enhancing factor localized to the muscle cells in man, *Nature*, 210, 309, 1966.

189. Piehl, K., Time course for refilling of glycogen stores in human muscle fibers following exercise-induced glycogen depletion, *Acta Physiol. Scand.*, 90, 297, 1974.

190. Costill, D. L., Bowers, R., Branam, G., and Sparks, K., Muscle glycogen utilization during prolonged exercise on successive days, *J. Appl. Physiol.*, 31, 834, 1971.

191. Costill, D. L., Sherman, W. M., Fink, W. J., Maresh, C., Witten, M., and Miller, J. M., The role of dietary carbohydrates in muscle glycogen resynthesis after strenuous running, *Am. J. Clin. Nutr.*, 34, 1831, 1981.

192. Lamb, D. R., Rinehardt, K. F., Bartels, R. L., Sherman, W. M., and Snook, J. T., Dietary carbohydrate and intensity of interval swim training, *Am. J. Clin. Nutr.*, 52, 1058, 1990.

193. Ivy, J. L., Carbohydrate supplementation for rapid muscle glycogen storage in the hours immediately after exercise, in *The Theory and Practice of Athletic Nutrition: Bridging the Gap*, Grandjean, A. C. and Storlie, J., Eds., Report of the Ross Symposium, Ross Laboratories, Columbus, OH, 1989, 47.

194. Soderling, T. R. and Park, C. R., Recent advances in glycogen metabolism, in *Advances in Cyclic Nucleotide Research*, Vol. 4, Greengard, P. and Robinson, G. A., Eds., Raven Press, New York, 1974, 283.

195. Conlee, R. K., Hickson, R. C., Winder, W. W., Hagberg, J. M., and Holloszy, J. O., Regulation of glycogen resynthesis in muscles of rats following exercise, *Am. J. Physiol.*, 235, R145, 1978.

196. Price, T. B., Rothman, D. L., Taylor, R., Avison, M. J., Shulman, G. I., and Shulman, R. G., Human muscle glycogen resynthesis after exercise: insulin-dependent and independent phases, *J. Appl. Physiol.*, 76, 104, 1994.

197. Wallberg-Henriksson, H., Constable, S. H., Young, D. A., and Holloszy, J. O., Glucose transport into rat skeletal muscle: interaction between exercise and insulin, *J. Appl. Physiol.*, 65, 909, 1988.

198. Ivy, J. L., Katz, A. L., Cutler, C. L., Sherman, W. M., and Coyle, E. F., Muscle glycogen synthesis after exercise: effect of time of carbohydrate ingestion, *J. Appl. Physiol.*, 64, 1480, 1988.

199. Pascoe, D. D. and Gladden, L. B., Muscle glycogen resynthesis after short term, high intensity exercise and resistance exercise, *Sports Med.*, 21, 98, 1996.

200. Zachwieja, J. J., Costill, D. L., and Fink, W. J., Carbohydrate ingestion during exercise: effects on muscle glycogen resynthesis after exercise, *Int. J. Sport Nutr.*, 3, 418, 1993.

201. Febbraio, M. A., Parkin, J. M., Martin, I. K., Stojanovska, L., and Carey, M. F., The effect of timing of ingestion of high glycemic index food on muscle glycogen storage following prolonged exercise, *Clin. Sci.*, 87(suppl.), 48A, 1994.

202. Vrana, A. and Fabry, P., Metabolic effects of high sucrose or fructose intake, *Wld. Rev. Nutr. Diet.*, 42, 56, 1983.

203. Blom, P. C. S., Hostmark, A. T., Vaage, O., Kardel, K. R., and Maehlum, S., Effect of different post-exercise sugar diets on the rate of muscle glycogen synthesis, *Med. Sci. Sports Exer.*, 19, 491, 1987.

204. Roberts, K. M., Nobel, E. G., Hayden, D. B., and Taylor, A. W., Simple and complex carbohydrate-rich diets and muscle glycogen content of marathon runners, *Eur. J. Appl. Physiol.*, 57, 70, 1988.

205. Kiens, B., Raben, A. B., Valeur, A. K., and Richter, E. A., Benefit of dietary simple carbohydrates on the early post-exercise muscle glycogen repletion in male athletes, *Med. Sci. Sports Exer.*, 22, S88, 1990.

206. Burke, L. M., Collier, G. R., and Hargreaves, M., Muscle glycogen storage after prolonged exercise: effect of the glycemic index of carbohydrate feedings, *J. Appl. Physiol.*, 75, 1019, 1993.

207. Ivy, J. L., Lee, M. C., Brozinick, J. T., and Reed, M. J., Muscle glycogen storage after different amounts of carbohydrate ingestion, *J. Appl. Physiol.*, 65, 2018, 1988.

208. Coleman, E., Update on carbohydrate: solid versus liquid, *Int. J. Sport Nutr.*, 4, 80, 1994.

209. Zawadzki, K. M., Yaspelkis, B. B., III, and Ivy, J. L., Carbohydrate-protein complex increases the rate of muscle glycogen storage after exercise, *J. Appl. Physiol.*, 72, 1854, 1992.

210. O'Reilly, K. P., Warhol, M. J., Fielding, R. A., Frontera, W. R., Meredith, C. N., and Evans, W. J., Eccentric exercise-induced muscle damage impairs muscle glycogen repletion, *J. Appl. Physiol.*, 63, 252, 1987.

211. Costill, D. L., Pascoe, D. D., Fink, W .J., Robergs, R. A., Barr, S. I., and Pearson, D., Impaired muscle glycogen resynthesis after eccentric exercise, *J. Appl. Physiol.*, 69, 46, 1990.
212. Blom, P. C. S., Costill, D. L., and Vollestad, N. K., Exhaustive running: inappropriate as a stimulus of muscle glycogen supercompensation, *Med. Sci. Sports Exer.*, 19, 398, 1987.
213. Asp, S., Daugaard, J. R., and Richter, E. A., Eccentric exercise decreases glucose transporter GLUT4 protein in human skeletal muscle, *J. Physiol.*, 482, 705, 1995.

Chapter **4**

EFFECTS OF DIET AND EXERCISE ON LIPIDS AND LIPOPROTEINS

Tinker D. Murray
William G. Squires, Jr.
G. Harley Hartung
Jennifer Bunger

CONTENTS

0-8493-8560-1/97/$0.00+$.50
© 1998 by CRC Press LLC

I . INTRODUCTION

Dietary therapy and recommendations for increased physical activity or exercise have been used as effective strategies to positively influence plasma lipids and lipoproteins for more than 40 years. For example, as early as 1961, an ad hoc committee of the American Heart Association (AHA) released an updated report about the possible relation of dietary fat to heart attacks and stroke.[1] The report included the following recommendations:

1. Overweight persons should decrease their caloric intake and attempt to achieve a desirable body weight.
2. The composition of the diet should be altered by reducing intakes of total fats, saturated fats, and cholesterol and by increasing intakes of polyunsaturated fats.
3. Weight reduction should be facilitated by regular moderate exercise.
4. Men at increased risk for coronary heart disease should pay particular attention to dietary alteration.
5. For those at high risk, dietary changes should be carried out with medical supervision.[1]

Followup reports by the AHA on dietary guidelines to reduce coronary heart disease (CHD) risk were released in 1965, 1968, 1973, 1978, 1986, 1988, and 1990. The National Heart, Lung, and Blood Institute in 1985 began the National Cholesterol Education Program (NCEP)[2] which reinforced the AHA's position statements (linking cholesterol and CHD) at the national and international levels. Together, these two developments firmly planted the seed of cholesterol awareness in the public's mind at the beginning of the 1990s. In 1994, the NCEP and the AHA revised their initial guidelines for the detection, evaluation, and treatment of high blood cholesterol in adults.[3] The 1994 NCEP/AHA guidelines include the following new features as compared to the 1988 report:

1. An increased emphasis on CHD risk status as a guide to type and intensity of cholesterol lowering therapy.
2. More attention to high density lipoproteins (HDL) as a CHD risk factor.
3. An increased emphasis on weight loss and physical activity as components of the dietary therapy of high blood cholesterol.

With the increased public awareness of the importance of controlling lipids and lipoproteins, manufacturers have eagerly made nutritional and exercise claims about how their products help reduce or control cholesterol levels. These claims are often reported in various media formats and may or may not be accurate in regards to cholesterol reduction. The manipulation of lipids and lipoproteins has become the major established treatment modality for atherosclerosis in the 1990s.[4] Major advances have occurred in the past 10 to 20 years which have expanded our knowledge about lipid and lipoprotein metabolism. Yet, numerous unresolved issues remain about how changes in diet and/or exercise patterns can favorably alter lipid and lipoprotein levels.[5]

Previously, we reviewed studies that emphasized the effects of plasma lipids and lipoproteins and their effects on optimal health and/or athletic performance.[6,7] We summarized the following findings from the relevant literature:

1. Lipids are a major fuel source for exercise.[8]
2. Plasma lipids and lipoproteins are associated with the etiology of CHD.[9-12]
3. Dietary factors have various effects on plasma lipids and lipoproteins.[13]
4. Lipid metabolism is influenced by physical training.[14]

The purpose of this third review is to update what is currently known and unknown about dietary and exercise influences on lipids and lipoproteins. The review will focus on research findings which have implications for the acquisition and maintenance of health and physical fitness in adults.

II. OVERVIEW OF THE CHARACTERISTICS OF PLASMA LIPIDS, LIPOPROTEINS, AND APOLIPOPROTEINS

Lipids are a heterogeneous group of chemicals that include free fatty acids (FFA) and substances found naturally in chemical association with them.[15] The major lipids found in humans are FFA, triglycerides (TG), steroids, phospholipids, prostaglandins, fat-soluble vitamins, provitamins, and lipoproteins. The function of lipids are:[15]

1. To provide fuel
2. To serve as insulation
3. To provide protective padding for organs and structures
4. To supply building blocks for other chemicals
5. To provide essential fatty acids
6. To serve as components of cell membranes and other cell structures.

A brief description of how plasma lipids and lipoproteins function in the body will provide the basic framework for the remainder of this chapter. More detailed reviews of lipid metabolism are available elsewhere.[16-21]

TG are the chief lipid ingested and are stored within the body. They consist of three FFA combined with glycerol. The digestion of TG, cholesterol, and phospholipids originates in the small intestine and concludes with the entry of the chylomicrons into the thoracic duct. Small amounts of FFA are also absorbed directly by the liver via the portal circulation. Triglycerides are stored in the body in adipose tissue, the liver, and skeletal muscle.[22]

The major plasma lipids, including cholesterol (a fatlike pearly substance) and TG, are transported in the form of lipoprotein complexes. The plasma lipoproteins transport both endogenously synthesized products and exogenously ingested dietary lipids. The plasma lipoporteins contain both free and esterified cholesterol, TG, phospholipid, and protein.[23] Lipoproteins are classified into six major classes by their gravitional density as follows:

1. Chylomicrons (primarily exogenous TG, density < 0.96 g/ml)
2. Very low-density lipoprotein cholesterol (VLDL-C) (primarily endogenous triglycerides, density = 0.96–1.006)
3. Intermediate-density lipoprotein cholesterol (IDL-C) (low-density lipoprotein cholesterol [LDL-C] precurser, density = 1.006–1.019)
4. LDL-C (approximately 50% cholesterol transport, 60–75% of the total plasma cholesterol, density = 1.019–1.063).
5. Lipoprotein (a) or Lp (a) (similar to LDL-C but has both lipoprotein and blood clotting properties, density = 1.055–1.120)
6. High-density lipoprotein cholesterol (HDL-C) (often identified as HDL_2 and HDL_3 subfractions, normally transports 20–25% of the total plasma cholesterol; HDL_2 density = 1.063–1.125 and HDL_3 density = 1.125–1.210

Four major enzymes that significantly influence lipid metabolism are lipoprotein lipase (LPL), hepatic lipase (HL), cholesteryl ester transfer protein (CETP), and lecithin cholesterol acetyltransferase (LCAT). Lipoprotein lipase is a lipolytic enzyme that controls TG hydrolysis and is the rate-limiting step in the uptake of lipoprotein, TG, and FFA into adipose tissue and muscle.[24,25] Hepatic lipase interacts with lipoproteins in the liver and may play a role in the reconversion of HDL-C$_2$ to HDL-C$_3$.[26] Cholesteryl ester transfer protein has been linked to HDL particles and is one of several transfer proteins that mediates the transfer of esterified cholesterol from HDL-C$_2$ to VLDL and is involved in the formation of HDL-C$_3$.[27] The enzyme LCAT catalyzes esterified cholesterol while binding to HDL-C$_3$ and moves it into the HDL-C core.[28]

Apoliproproteins are also important to the understanding of plasma lipid and lipoprotein metabolism. The apoplipoproteins regulate biochemical reactions by stabilizing lipoprotein particles, providing recognition sites for cell membranes and by acting as co-factors for enzymes. The apolipoproteins determine the structure and regulatory functions of lipoproteins. Most apolipoproteins are synthesized by the liver or intestine. Some like apo B-100 and apo A-I are produced by both. The major apolipoproteins and their primary functions are as follows:[23,29]

1. Apo A-I: activates LCAT.
2. Apo A-II: inhibits LCAT or activates heparin-releasable hepatic triglyceride hydrolase.
3. Apo A-IV: associated with chylomicrons.
4. Apo B-48: syhtesizes chylomicrons.
5. Apo B-100: involved in LDL receptor binding.
6. Apo (a): similar to plasminogen and may promote thrombotic effects.
7. Apo C-I: activates LCAT.
8. Apo C-II: activates LPL.
9. Apo C-III: inhibits LPL.
10. Apo D: acts as a core lipid transfer protein.
11. Apo E: functions in the catabolism of chylomicron, VLDL, and HDL.

The sequence of the metabolism of lipids and lipoproteins begins when the TG of chylomicrons are hydrolyzed by LPL into monoglycerides and FFA in the capillaries of adipose tissue and skeletal muscle. The FFA are re-esterified or oxidized by adipose or muscle cells. The remnants of the chylomicrons are cleared by the liver.[30]

The VLDL-C originates in the liver and small intestine and is increased with excess carbohydrate-rich diets. VLDL-C is hydrolyzed to IDL-C by LPL. The IDL-C remnants are further hydrolyzed to LDL probably by LPL and hepatic triglyceride lipase (HTGL).[19,31] Some of the IDL-C is cleared from plasma by hepatic LDL receptors that bind apolipoprotein E in the liver. The residual IDL-C forms LDL-C with apolipoprotein B-100 on its surface. Apolipoprotein B-100 is recognized by the hepatic and extrahepatic LDL receptors. The plasma LDL-C levels are influenced by LDL-C receptor number and each cell's need for cholesterol. When the need is low, cells make fewer receptors and LDL-C is removed at lower rates. When this occurs plasma LDL-C rises. Elevated LDL-C levels can accelerate the rate of atherosclerosis increasing CHD risk.[19,32]

The LDL-C supplies cholesterol to extrahepatic cells where it is used for cell membrane and steroid hormone synthesis. Some of the LDL-C is degraded by scavenger cells which help control high plasma concentrations. The liver removes the remaining circulating LDL-C. Thus, the LDL-C concentration depends upon the balance between the liver's production of VLDL-C, the partitioning of VLDL-C between hepatic removal, and conversion to LDL-C, as well as the activity of LDL-C receptors.[19,32]

It is thought that HDL-C serves as the cholesterol acceptor in reverse transport and excretion of cholesterol from the tissues.[33,34] Direct production of HDL-C occurs in both the liver and the intestine. The HDL-C binds unesterified cholesterol and delivers cholesteryl esters to the liver and VLDL-C. Some of the cholesterol is delivered to the liver by HDL-C and is excreted into the gallbladder as bile. High-density lipoprotein cholesterol can be subdivided into 15 subfractions.[35] Two of the major subfractions include HDL_2-C and a more dense HDL_3-C. Mature HDL (HDL_3-C converted to HDL_2-C) is formed by the addition of surface components derived from chylomicron and VLDL-C metabolism.[20]

Low levels of HDL-C (<35 mg/dl) are as predictive for coronary heart disease (CHD) as high blood pressure, cigarette smoking, or diabetes.[2,4,5] The major causes of reduced HDL-C include: cigarette smoking, obesity, lack of exercise, androgenic and related steroids (androgens, progestional agents, and anabolic steroids), beta-adrenergic blocking agents, hypertriglyceridemia, and genetic factors (i.e., hypoalphalipoproteinemia).[2,4]

A variety of genetic disorders in lipoprotein metabolism have been identified. These include abnormal functions with all the apolipoproteins and enzymes, as well as certain cell surface receptors that bind apolipoproteins. Genetic abnormalities have been found for gene encoding of LDL-C receptors, defective deregulation of LDL-C receptor synthesis, apo-B 100 structure abnormalities, and defects in VLDL-C metabolism which overproduces LDL-C.[4] Most of these disorders are fairly rare, but they are of clinical significance because they can produce severe hyperlipdemia and predispose individuals to premature CHD.[36]

The aging process itself decreases the activity of LDL-C receptors and causes the TC and LDL-C plasma levels to rise.[4] The mechanism for these increases as we get older are presently unknown, but may be due to cellular aging or a decrease in the body's overall metabolic rate.[4]

III. PLASMA LIPID/LIPOPROTEIN LEVELS AND CHD RISK

Interest in lipids and lipoproteins greatly intensified in the 1980s and 1990s due to findings that elevated cholesterol levels are causally linked to an increased risk of CHD.[2,4] Total cholesterol (TC), LDL-C, and HDL-C are all strong predictors of CHD risk.[37] Increased levels of plasma of TC and LDL-C are positively linked to CHD risk, while increased levels of HDL-C are negatively linked to CHD risk. High plasma levels of HDL_2-C are inversely related to the extent of coronary artery disease, and HDL_2-C predicts CHD risk better than HDL-C or HDL_3-C.[38] There is also evidence that smaller LDL-C particles are more atherogenic than larger LDL-C particles.[39]

The plasma lipid and lipoprotein profile may be more useful for estimating CHD risk than a single value.[11] The combination of a moderately high plasma total cholesterol level, elevated HDL-C, and low LDL-C is not as atherogenic as the same total cholesterol with low HDL-C and high LDL-C values. The HDL-C/total cholesterol and HDL-C/LDL-C ratios (or reciprocals) have been reported to be more powerful predictors of CHD than total cholesterol alone.[37] Although the lipid/lipoprotein ratios are important for predicting CHD risk, the National Cholesterol Education Program's Adult Treatment Panel[2] recommends that plasma TC and HDL-C be measured first (serum cholesterol multiplied by 0.97 = plasma values). Total cholesterol and HDL-C are more commonly available and usually less expensive to assess than LDL-C. If the TC is higher than 240 mg/dl, then a person is classified as having high blood cholesterol unless they have elevated levels of HDL-C ($\geq$60 mg/dL) which is protective against CHD. A LDL-C level of 130–159 mg/dl places an individual at borderline high risk, while a level of $\geq$160 mg/dl is indicative of high risk for CHD. When the HDL-C is below 35 mg/dl CHD is significantly increased.[2,4]

Elevated plasma TG levels are associated with increased risk for CHD. However, the association often disappears when adjustments are made for other risk factors like TC and HDL-C.[3,40] One report suggests that TG concentration is a marker of increased CHD risk, especially in subjects with high LDL-C/HDL-C ratios.[41] The measurement of plasma TG is positively related to LDL-C and inversely related to HDL-C, particularly HDL_2-C. Although the measurement of TG levels may not be the best current indicator to help monitor CHD risk, they do allow one to estimate LDL-C, if TC and HDL-C are known.[36] Most clinical laboratories can measure TC, HDL-C, and TG, thus, from the Friedwald equation:[42]

$$LDL\text{-}C = TC\text{-}[HDL + (TG/5)]$$

The equation allows the simple prediction of LDL-C as long as TG are less than 400 mg/dl.[35]

The serum apolipoproteins have been used as specific markers of CHD risk. Apolipoproteins A-I (apo A-I, associated with HDL-C) and B (apo B, associated with LDL-C) have also been used individually and as ratios (AI:B) to assess CHD risk.[36] Apo B has frequently been found to be elevated, compared to LDL-C, in patients with vascular disease. Apo AI correlates highly with HDL-C and has been a consistent predictor of coronary artery disease. It has been suggested that HDL-C subfractions containing apo AI and apo AII may be better markers of CHD risk than HDL-C alone. However, Stampfer et al.[43] found that neither apolipoprotein levels, nor HDL_2-C of HDL_3-C added significantly to predicting CHD, compared to the predictive power of measures of LDL-C and HDL-C. Although the ability to routinely obtain accurate and reliable measures of the apolipoproteins has improved significantly in the past 5 years these techniques are still beyond the capability of most clinical laboratories.[29,36,44]

IV. RATIONALE FOR INTERVENTION: DIET MODIFICATION AND EXERCISE

Lipid/lipoprotein metabolism is regulated by a variety of physiological variables that can affect the synthesis and catabolism of the various particles. These variables include: aging, genetics, hormones, diet composition, calorie intake, alcohol consumption, cigarette smoking, medication, body composition, and exercise.[2-4,23]

Diet modification and regular exercise are typically recommended as the first step for adults, by physicians, to lower TC (and thus LDL-C) prior to drug intervention.[2,4,45] The rationale for this advice is based on epidemiological evidence, which indicates that there is a direct correlation between TC levels and CHD rates.[46-49] The relationship is continuous throughout the range of TC levels based on CHD mortality.[50] When TC exceeds 240 mg/dl, an individual has approximately a two-fold increase in CHD risk.[2,4]

Clinical trials using single or multifactor interventions have shown that lowering LDL-C in men can reduce CHD incidence and actually slows or produces regression of coronary atherosclerosis.[50] This has been found in primary and secondary CHD prevention trials.[51]

Women are also at high CHD risk when LDL-C levels are elevated, but prior to menopause their LDL-C levels are lower than those found for men. Following menopause, their risk of CHD increases due to loss of estrogen-stimulated LDL receptor activity.[4] The data for clinical trials on LDL-C lowering are mainly available only in middle-aged men with initially high cholesterol levels.[4]

When TC levels are lowered by 1%, there is a 2–3% reduction in CHD rates.[4,11,51] It does appear that at least an 8–9% reduction in TC is needed to significantly reduced CHD mortality. But, if individuals could lower their TC by 10–15% with diet and exercise, they should reduce their CHD risk by 20–30%.[2]

For individuals that have multiple risk factors for CHD, lowering TC (and LDL-C) can have even greater effects.[4,52,53] Grundy[46] has shown that there is a hypothetical level (60% of coronary artery with raised plaque) which predicts the severity of atherosclerosis by age, at various cholesterol levels in relationship to other established CHD risk factors. If individuals

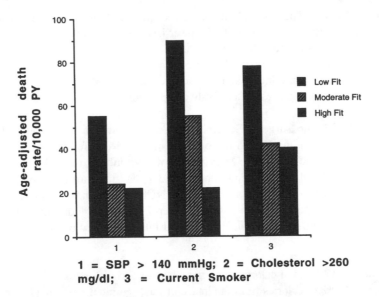

FIGURE 1 The relationship between fitness and all-cause mortality in men with high levels of other risk factors. Men in the moderate-fitness category have much lower death rates than the lower-fitness men in each of the other risk factor groups. (From Blair, S. N., *Gatorade Sports Sci. Exch.*, 3, 3, 1990. With permission.)

have a TC level of 200 mg/dl, they would most likely become high risk for CHD at age 70, in the absence of other risk factors. If smoking is added, the critical stage is reached at 60. The addition of hypertension and diabetes to the risk profile would drop the ages for significantly increased CHD risk to 50 and 40, respectively. Thus, attention should be placed on managing all CHD risks in concert with controlling one's lipid/lipoprotein levels.

Blair et al.[54] have shown that men who are moderately active (based on treadmill fitness measures) have lower CHD mortality rates than inactive males, even when other risks for CHD are present (Figure 1). Men who had levels of TC >240 mg/dl and were moderately active had significantly reduced mortality for CHD than men who were less fit. These relationships also appear to apply to to women, but the data is based on fewer subjects than that for males.

Dietary modification and regular exercise (which can raise HDL-C) provide the foundation for the initial intervention for hyperlipidemia, because they can have significant positive affects on lipid and lipoprotein metabolism.[55,56] For most Americans, diet modification and regular exercise can help reduce cholesterol-CHD risk, even when they are used as adjunct therapy to medication.[4,19] Diet modification and exercise are also more economical than medication therapy.

V. DIETARY FACTORS

A. DIETARY GOALS

It has been reported that the most significant factor influencing hypercholesterolemia is diet.[2,4,5] A variety of dietary strategies can be utilized to lower TC and LDL-C. The cholesterol-lowering response to dietary intervention is variable and depends on several factors including the following:

1. composition of the diet (high saturated fat intake, high dietary cholesterol intake, or both),

2. the initial TC level (people with the highest levels usually have the greatest decrease per mg/dl, but even those with initially lower levels see a similar percent change),
3. the responsiveness of the individual,
4. acceptance and compliance with diet,
5. balance between caloric intake and expenditure, and
6. changes in body weight (especially body composition changes)[2,4,23]

The AHA, NCEP, The Surgeon General's Report on Nutrition and Health, the National Academy of Sciences Diet and Health Report, the National Research Council, the American Diabetes Association, and the U.S. Departments of Agriculture (USDA) and Health and Human Services (HHS) all recommend similar guidelines in regard to dietary composition to control lipid and lipoprotein levels.[2,4,5,57] These NCEP guidelines for the Step 1 (eating pattern recommeded for general population) and Step 2 (for those individuals already on the Step 1 diet who need further reductions in saturated fat and dietary cholesterol) diet include the following:

1. Consume >55% of total calories from the intake of carbohydrates.
2. Consume ≤30% of calories from the intake of fats; saturated fats should comprise no more than 8–10% of the total fat intake in Step 1 and <7% in Step 2, with up to 10% coming from polyunsaturated fats and up to 15% coming from monounsaturated fats.
3. Protein should represent approximately 15% of the dietary intake.
4. To achieve these dietary composition goals, the diet should contain a variety of nutrients and be palatable.
5. The diet should contain less than 300 mg/day intake of cholesterol in Step 1 and <200 mg/day in the Step 2.
6. The total number of calories should be balanced toward the achievement or maintenance of desirable body weight.

Several detailed reviews of the effects of diet on lipids and lipoproteins can be found in the professional literature.[2,4,5,13,19,23,45,47,58-61] These studies form the basis for our chapter, which will summarize the following dietary issues related to lipids/lipoproteins: total dietary fat, cholesterol intake, saturated vs. unsaturated fats, carbohydrate intake, fiber intake, vegetarianism, vitamins, alcohol consumption, and obesity (weight gain).

B. TOTAL FAT INTAKE

Americans consume 36–37% of their total calories from fat.[4] As mentioned above, many professsional organizations like the AHA recommend that there should be no more than 30% total daily calories from fat. The rationale to reduce total fat in the diet is based on the concept that it will decrease saturated fatty acids (SF) intake, decrease the total calories in the diet, and promote weight reduction. However, it has been reported that excessive reduction of fat intake can increase TG levels and lower HDL-C.[3,58,62,63] Two primary methods of lowering SF intake include substituting carbohydrates for fat intake (by balancing caloric intake) thereby, reducing LDL-C level or by replacing SF intake without caloric replacement which can promote weight loss.[4] Reducing the fat intake below 30% of the total dietary calories is not necessary to reduce CHD risk for most individuals, although there can be benefits for high risk sub-groups within the population.[64] When total fat intake is reduced to the 20–25% level it is important to insure adequate intake of calcium and iron are maintained.[4] It should also be noted that low fat diets (below 30% of the the total calories) are not very palatable and may not be accepted well by many individuals. There are data that demonstrate that fat quality has a more significant affect on plasma lipid/lipoprotein response than fat quantity.[23]

Lowering total fat in the diet will reduce SF intake and can be facilitated further when unsaturated fatty acids (UF) are substituted for SF.[23,58]

C. DIETARY CHOLESTEROL

In metabolic ward studies, the cholesterol-raising action of dietary cholesterol is a consistent finding.[4,58] However, individuals vary in their responsiveness from treatment to treatment. In free-living setting studies, increased dietary cholesterol has variable effects on individuals, but LDL-C is generally increased. American men consume about 400 mg/day on average, while women consume about 300 mg/day.[23] Raising cholesterol intake from a baseline level of 200–400 or 500 mg/day will increase TC 5–10 mg/dl.[19,46,65] Mechanisms that cause this increase appear to be related to the suppression of LDL-C receptor synthesis with a secondary increase in hepatic cholesterol content.[19,66] The plasma lipid response to dietary cholesterol will be affected by baseline intake and the type of fat in the diet.

D. SATURATED FATTY ACIDS

The U.S. diet contains about 14% of the total calories as SF, where many nutritionists have recommended that intake should be 7% or less.[2,19] Saturated fats are those found in animal fats, coconut, palm kernel oil, and palm oil. The hypercholesterolemic effects of SF have been studied for more than 40 years and can be predicted.[23,66,67] The extra 7% of SF in the average person's diet increases TC by about 20 mg/dl, most of which is LDL-C. Generally, for every 1% increase of SF intake, TC increases about 2.7 mg/dl.[23] Increased SF intake decreases LDL-C receptor activity by several possible mechanisms.[19] It has been reported that some of the longer-chain SF (like stearic acid) may be less hypercholesterolemic than medium-chain SF, but more research is needed to determine the relative effects of different SF on lipid/lipoprotein levels.[19,61]

E. POLYUNSATURATED FATTY ACIDS

If SF are reduced in the diet they must be replaced by other sources of fats including polyunsaturated fats (PF). Americans consume approximately 7% of their total calories in the form of PF.[4,23] One source of PF includes linoleic acid (an Omega-6 fatty acid) which is consumed as vegetable oils, like corn oil, soybean oil, sunflower oil, etc. It has been shown that a 1% increase of linoleic acid in the diet decreases TC by 1.4 mg/dl.[23,65] Increasing PF intake is routinely recommended as a substitute to SF intake.[4,5] The mechanism by which linoleic acid lowers TC and LDL-C may be due to increased LDL-C receptor activity or simply because it replaces SF content in the diet. However, when PF intake in the form of linoleic acid exceeds 10% of the total calories, it has been reported that there is a lowering of HDL-C, supression of the immune system, increased risk for cholesterol gallstones, promotion of carcinogensis, and increased LDL-C oxidation (which is associated with rendering LDL-C atherogenic).[4,5,68-72]

Omega-3 fatty acids (O3FA) are another type of PF, and they are found in fish and fish oils. The O3FA have been promoted as an alternative replacement for SF instead of linoleic acid.[23,73] The most consistent finding of O3FA on lipids/lipoproteins is the reduction of TG, which occurs with high doses.[46,74] They do not appear to lower TC or LDL-C any more than other UF. There are reports that O3FA have also been found to be anti-thrombotic, because they reduce platelet aggregation and are anti-imflammatory.[75] It is prudent to encourage fish consumption as a substitute for meats that are high in SF, which may help reduce CHD risk. However, not all fish are rich in O3FA even though they are low in fat. Fish oil supplements (which are commercially available without a prescription) are not recommended either to lower TC or LDL-C levels or CHD risk.[4]

F. MONOUNSATURATED FATTY ACIDS

Monounsaturated fatty acids (MF) have been shown to lower LDL-C as much as PF.[4,63,76] Americans consume approximately 14–16% of their total calories from MF. Sources of MF (oleic acid) include animal (the majority of the American diet) and vegetable sources (i.e., olive oil and canola oil). It is recommended by the AHA and NCEP that MF should comprise up to 15% of the total dietary intake and vegetable sources should be emphasized.[2,4,75] None of the side effects found for lioleic acid have been found for oleic acid, and therefore this form of MF may be the preferred replacements for SF.[5] Substituting MF at higher levels than recommended by the AHA or NCEP may promote weight gain, if indeed, the total fat intake exceeds 30% of the total calories. Thus, the diet should be balanced according to the specific fatty acid guidelines for each nutrient.

G. HIGH CARBOHYDRATE DIETS

Carbohydrates should make up ≥55% of the total calories in the diet. It is recommended that at least half the dietary carbohydrate should come from complex carbohydrates in the form of vegetables, fruits, and grains.[4] When carbohydrates are substituted for saturated fat in the diet LDL-C levels fall similar in nature to increasing PF or MF ingestion. By increasing carbohydrates in the diet there will be a reduction of total fat intake and this may promote weight loss. However, high intakes of carbohydrates can stimulate hepatic synthesis of TG and raise VLDL-C levels.[4,5,77,78] There is currently disagreement as to the importance of these changes.[4]

H. DIETARY FIBER

The effects of dietary fiber consumption on lipids/lipoproteins has received widespread media attention and has confused consumers due to the release of reports with conflicting conclusions. Much of the confusion is caused by different study designs, different study populations, and the evaluation of different types of fiber. Dietary fiber which is water soluble (oats, fruits, beans, rice, peas, etc.) have been shown in epidemiological studies to lower TC by 5–15%, while water-insoluble fiber (cellulose, lignin, wheat bran, etc.) consumption shows no TC lowering effect.[2,4,23] There is evidence that water-soluble fiber can bind bile acids and increase fecal bile acid exertion.[79-81] It is recommended that dietary fiber intake for adults should be 20–30 g/day with 6 g coming from soluble sources.[4,82] However, the use of excessively large fiber intake can cause abdominal discomforts, decreased nutrient absorption, diarrhea, and other negative side effects. These same side effects can occur, when one decides to increase their dietary fiber intake, unless they do so gradually over time.[23]

I. VEGETARIAN DIETS

Vegetarian diets are low in total fat, SF, cholesterol, and high in fiber. Vegetarians have been found to have lipid/lipoprotein profiles which are consistent with reduced CHD risk.[23,83,84] Vegetarian diets, which limit red meat consumption and reduce the consumption of animal by-products to control SF intake, are often recommended to patients with hypercholesterolemia to control TC and LDL-C. If one decides to adopt a vegetarian type of diet, one should make sure that one consumes a variety of foods to insure proper nutrient balance.

J. VITAMINS

It has been shown that when LDL-C in aterial walls is oxidized it increases atherogenicity.[85] Vitamins like vitamin C, vitamin E, and beta carotene have been shown to have antioxidant properties and are speculated to be involved in the prevention of atherosclerosis.[4,86] Some experts have recommended that adults should take antioxidant vitamin supplements, but there is insufficient evidence to support this concept presently. The AHA and the NCEP recommend that adults consume five or more servings of fresh fruits and vegetables a day to insure the consumption of the appropriate amount of vitamins required.[87]

K. ALCOHOL CONSUMPTION

Moderate alcohol consumption has been shown to be associated with reduced CHD risk and increased HDL-C.[6,88] The increases in total HDL-C may be due to increases in HDL$_3$-C vs. HDL$_2$-C which some investigators have suggested would not be as desirable as the opposite effect.[13] Hartung et al.[89] found that alcohol consumption in habitual male exercisers increased HDL-C, HDL$_2$-C, HDL$_3$-C, and Apo A-I. However, the manipulation of alcohol intake in premenopausal exercising women does not appear to have any significant influence on the same variables.[90] The average intake of alcohol in the U.S. diet is approximately 5% of the total calories, although this value varies greatly.[4] It is recommended that alcohol consumption should not exceed more than two drinks for men and one drink for women per day.[4,91] It is not presently known if the increase in HDL-C from alcohol consumption prevent or protect against CHD. Therefore, at this time, alcohol intake cannot be recommended to favorably change lipid/lipoprotein profiles.

L. OBESITY (WEIGHT GAIN)

Obesity (9–13.6 kg or more over desirable body weight; body mass index ≥27.8 for men and ≥27.3 for women) may be the most underestimated cause of hypercholesterolemia.[5,61] Diet composition changes are usually recommended prior to weight reduction in those with clinically elevated lipid/lipoprotein levels.[5,92] American adults increase their weight by 9–13.6 kg on average from age 20 to age 50.[19] It has been reported that the weight gain is associated with increases in TC that average 25 mg/dl. The increase in TC is mainly due to LDL-C increases and partly due to VLDL-C increases. High-density lipoprotein cholesterol levels are usually reduced in obese individuals.[46] Grundy[19] has summarized two metabolic effects that obesity has on lipid/lipoproetin metabolism and they are:

1. Obesity promotes hepatic output of apo B-lipoproteins, which enhances the conversion of VLDL-C to LDL-C, and
2. Whole-body synthesis of cholesterol is increased by obesity, expanding the hepatic cholesterol pool and this supresses LDL-C receptor synthesis.

Thus, obesity may be the number one nutritional factor responsible for increased CHD risk in the United States.[5,57,61] Controlling obesity is also important in reducing CHD risk for those individuals with elevated lipids/lipoproteins that have related chronic disease processes like hypertension, hyperinsulinemia, and diabetes mellitus. The effects of weight loss on lipid/lipoprotein levels will be discussed in the next section of the review which highlights exercise as an intervention.

M. SUMMARY

In summary, dietary factors can have a significant impact on modifying plasma lipids/lipoproteins (see Table 1).[13] Health-care professionals, who provide diet modification advice to individuals for the control of lipid/lipoprotein levels, should consider the following prudent recommendations:

1. Implement diet strategies which parallel those published by organizations like the AHA, the NCEP, the USDA, and HHS.

2. Provide flexibility in diet planning, particularly for individuals with multiple CHD risk factors or other hyperlidemia-related disorders (i.e., hypertension, diabetes mellitus, etc.).

3. Encourage and instruct individuals about how to attain and maintain desirable body weight.

TABLE 1   Effects of Dietary Modification on Plasma Lipids and Lipoproteins

	Decrease in Fat	Decrease in Cholesterol	Increase in Polyunsaturated/ Saturated	Increase in Carbohydrates[a]	Increase in Alcohol
Total cholesterol	–	–	–	–, 0	0
Triglyceride	–, +	–, +	–	+	+
LDL-C	–	–	–	–	–
HDL-C	–, 0	–, 0	–, 0	–	+
HDL-C/total cholesterol	–, 0	–, 0	0	–	+

Note: + = increase; – = decrease; 0 = no change.

[a]   Carbohydrates, especially simple sugars.

Data from Hartung, G. H., *Sports Med.*, 1, 413, 1984.

VI.   EXERCISE

A.   EXERCISE GOALS

Hyperlipidemic individuals are usually encouraged by health-care professionals to increase their physical activity levels, engage in more exercise, or improve their physical fitness levels as part of a prudent risk factor modification plan. Although the terms physical activity, exercise, and physical fitness are used synonymously, they are defined by epidemiologists differently and can confound the interpretations of lipid/lipoprotein lowering investigations.[3,93] In this review, the term "exercise" will be used as all encompassing, to include references from the relevant lipid/lipoprotein literature which have evaluated high vs. low physical activity levels, exercise training volumes, or physical fitness levels.

The AHA, NCEP, USDA and HHS all recommend that regular exercise should be part of an effective lipid/lipoprotein lowering strategy.[2,4,87,89,91] Generally, exercise is encouraged by these groups due to the positive associations with weight reduction, fat weight loss, and increased caloric expenditure. Although low levels of exercise (walking 3.23 km in 30 min, 4–5 times per week) have been found to lower all-cause mortality in men and women, higher intensities, durations, and frequencies of exercise training may be required for significant and specific exercise-related lipid/lipoprotein changes.[54,94-96] In the past, the AHA and the American College of Sports Medicine (ACSM) have recommended that adults should be encouraged to exercise 3–5 times per week, for 30–40 min, at an intensity of 60–90% of maximal heart rate reserve or 50–80% of maximal oxygen consumption, for the maintenance of good cardiovascular health.[94,95,97] More recently, the ACSM, the Centers for Disease Control and Prevention (CDC), and the U.S. Surgeon General's Office have promoted the fact that health benefits can be acquired by engaging in moderate physical activity, but greater health benefits can be achieved by increasing the amount (duration, frequency, or intensity) of physical activity.[98,99]

In our previous reviews,[6,7] we reported that favorable alterations in lipid/lipoprotein levels may require jogging the equivalent of about 13–20 km/week or greater than 1000 kcal/week (or 4,186,000 J/week) of caloric expenditure involving endurance exercise over a 9–52 week period.[100-102] The specific effects of exercise training on plasma lipids and lipoproteins are illustrated in Table 2[13] and are discussed in the following sections.

TABLE 2   Effects of Exercise Training on Plasma Lipids and Lipoprotein

	Cross-Sectional Studies		Longitudinal Studies	
	Men	Women	Men	Women
Total cholesterol	–, 0	–, 0	–, 0	–, 0
Triglyceride	–	–	–	–, 0
LDL-C	–	–	–	–
HDL-C	+	+, 0	+, 0	+, 0
HDL-C/total cholesterol	+	+, 0	+	+, 0

Note: + = increase; – = decrease; 0 = no change.

Data from Hartung, G. H., *Sports Med.*, 1, 413, 1984.

The effects of exercise on blood lipids/lipoproteins have been reviewed extensively by several authors prior to 1990.[6,13,26,103-106] Other reviews have appeared in the literature since then.[3,7,29,100,101,107,108] The focus of this review will be to summarize the cross-sectional and longitudinal effects of exercise on blood lipids/lipoproteins by highlighting the following issues: endurance vs. resistance (strength) training influences, acute exercise training influences, influences on men vs. women, influences on lipid metabolism enzymes and particle size, and the influences of the interaction of exercise vs. weight loss effects.

B. ENDURANCE EXERCISE

Endurance exercise includes sustained aerobic exercise over time (training) like that required by brisk walking (5.65–7.26 km/hr), jogging (7.26–9.68 km/hr), running (>9.68 km/hr), cross-country skiing, tennis, soccer, or vigorous occupations (e.g.. lumberjacks).[6,7] Cross-sectional studies involving endurance exercise, with few exceptions, have shown that in large epidemiological samples, as well as small study sub-groups, exercise increases HDL-C (or its subfractions) and decreases TG, while VLDL-C changes are inversely related to those of HDL-C.[20,29,89,100,101,110,111]

Hartung et al.[112] analyzed data from 10 cross-sectional studies and found that for every 10 km/week run or jogged, the HDL-C was approximately 3.0 mg/dl higher in both men and women. The correlation between physical activity level and HDL-C was 0.81 for men and 0.89 for women. HDL_2-C was found to be 1.5 mg/dl higher in men and 2.7 mg/dl higher in women for every 10 km covered. The correlation between physical activity and HDL_2-C was 0.78.

The cross-sectional evidence of the effects of exercise training on TC and LDL-C is mixed, with usually no effect found on TC, while LDL-C may drop due to increases in HDL-C or its subfractions or the confounding influences of weight loss, plasma volume expansion, or dietary intake changes.[3,29,113] Some cross-sectional studies have reported higher Apo A-I levels for endurance-trained men and women, but Apo A-II levels are not typically different between endurance-trained vs. untrained individuals.[29] Lipoprotein (a) which may mimic plasminogen and promote thrombotic effects does not appear to be influenced by exercise in cross-sectional studies.[113,114]

In longitudinal studies, endurance exercise is generally associated with no significant change in TC, decreases or no change in LDL-C and VLDL-C, increases in HDL-C (or its subfractions), and decreases in TG.[3,29,100,101,115-119] The effects of exercise in longitudinal studies for women are usually less than those observed for men (at least for HDL-C) and will be discussed in another section.

The positive longitudinal benefits of exercise on HDL-C levels for men have been reported in numerous studies, and it appears that an exercise dosage of the equivalent of 13–20 km/week of jogging for 4–6 months is required for significant benefit.[3,29,100,101] Apo A-I levels have been shown to increase or not change with longitudinal endurance training.[120,121] The conflicting longitudinal training results related to Apo A-I levels may be related to body weight changes, caloric intake, or body composition changes. Apo A-II levels are not influenced by longitudinal endurance training.[29] Longitudinal training studies also indicate that Lipoprotein (a) does not appear to be influenced significantly.[29,122]

C.   RESISTANCE (STRENGTH) EXERCISE

The reports from cross-sectional studies which have evaluated lipid/lipoprotein profiles in strength-trained individuals have produced conflicting results.[100,101,107] This may be due to the lack of control of various factors in the study designs, which have been shown to confound the lipid/lipoprotein levels. In longitudinal resistance (strength) training studies prior to 1990, investigators generally found favorable changes in blood lipid/lipoprotein levels. However, the conclusions of these studies are weakened by the following study design flaws: lack of control for day-to day variation in lipids/lipoproteins, body composition changes, use of anabolic steroids, dietary factors, acute vs. chronic training effects, and plasma volume shifts.[107,123-125] When these methodological concerns were controlled, strength training for 20 weeks did not alter plasma lipid/lipoprotein profiles or regulatory enzymes that influence TG and HDL-C in men that were at risk for CHD.[126]

More recently, it has been recognized that different resistance training regimens are used and include powerlifting, Olympic weightlifting, and body building. Powerlifters and Olympic weightlifters usually work against high resistance, do few repetitions, and have long rest intervals. Body builders use less resitance, do more repetitions, and have short rest intervals. Thus, body builders have more favorable lipid and liporpoteins profiles.[29] Generally, the results of the cross-sectional and longitudinal resistance training studies concerning lipids and lipoproteins have produced conflicting results. For example, HDL-C has been shown to increase in several studies,[100] not change in others,[100] and be lower in men and women who were stronger than their cohorts.[127]

Resistance training individuals who use anabolic steriods have been found to have significant reductions in their HDL-C levels while their LDL-C are elevated.[128-130] It has been reported that the mean HDL-C level for weightlifters on anabolic steriods was 26 mg/dl while a control group of weightlifters not on anabolic steriods had a mean HDL-C of 50 mg/dl.[131] In one recent longitudinal study it was reported that male competitive body builders who used self-administered anabolic androgenic steriods significantly reduced their HDL-C to LDL-C lipid ratio while producing a significant reduction in their serum Lipoprotein (a) level.[132] The method by which lipoprotein (a) was reduced and the clinical significance of the lipoprotein (a) reduction is currently unclear.

D.   ACUTE EXERCISE

Durstine and Haskell,[29] in 1994, reported that there were more than 70 published journal articles and abstracts concerned with the effects of single bouts of exercise of varying modes, intensities, and duration on changes in lipids and lipoproteins. Several factors may influence the results of acute exercise interventions on lipids and lipoproteins. These include and are not limited to the following: pre-exercise lipoprotein levels, total amount of work completed, timing of blood sampling, length of followup, adjustments for changes in plasma volume, and the training state of the subjects' populations.[29]

If acute bouts of exercise are to postively influence TC, TG, VLDL-C, LDL-C, HDL-C, or HDL-C subfractions, the exercise must be prolonged and require sufficient energy expenditure.[29,100,101] The best estimates for an energy expenditure threshold to produce postive lipid and lipoprotein changes is an exercise durtion of 1.5 hours with more than 1000 kilocalories (or 4,186,000 J/week) of energy expenditure.[29,133,134] The acute exercise changes observed in lipids and lipoproteins may be delayed for 24–48 hr following an intervention.[29,100,135] Acute exercise increases HDL-C and HDL$_2$-C subfraction in most studies.[100,101] The largest and most pervasive changes in HDL-C and HDL$_2$-C have been found following single moderate-to-high intensity, long-duration exercise bouts such as marathon runs.[100,101] Acute exercise has been shown to raise HDL-C in women, but there are inconsistent findings for temporal changes and changes in HDL-C subfractions.[136]

E. INFLUENCES ON MEN VS. WOMEN

Exercise tends to have the same effects on lipid/lipoprotein levels in men and women (see Table 2), except that HDL-C and TG changes in women are not usually as significantly altered, unless there are large increases in exercise intensity and duration.[100,101] Women, prior to menopause, usually have higher HDL-C levels compared to men, and their HDL-C levels may be more difficult to modify by any means.[100,101,137] The effects of exercise training on HDL-C in women remains controversial because there have not been any long-term random-ized controlled studies conducted.[5,100]

Postmenopausal women tend to show greater responsiveness to increases in HDL-C with endurance exercise than premenopausal women.[138] HDL-C levels can also vary due to when lipid and lipoprotein measures are taken in relationship to phases of the menstrual cycle.[136]

Williams[139] has recently reported that the mean HDL-C concentrations in women who ran more than 64 km/week were significantly higher than for women who ran less than 48 km/week. He also reported that HDL-C levels increased significantly in relationship to the number of kilometers ran per week in premenopausal women who were not using oral contraceptives and in postmenopausal women, whether they were receiving estrogen-replace-ment therapy or not. In fact, a dose-response relationship was noted for HDL-C in relation to the number of kilometers ran. However, this amount of running (>64 km/week) by women may increase their risks for reproductive and musculoskeletal problems compared to more moderate levels of physical activity.[140]

F. INFLUENCES ON LIPID METABOLISM, ENZYMES, AND PARTICLE SIZE

Exercise training may influence the following lipid metabolism regulating enzymes: LPL, HL, CETP, and LCAT (see section II). Exercise has a significant postive impact on all these regulating enzymmes which enhances metabolism of triglyceride-rich lipoproteins and reverse cholesterol transport.[29,101,141] Lipoprotein lipase catabolizes triglyceride-rich lipoproteins releasing free fatty acids and making surface cholesterol compoenets avaiable for the HDL-C particle, thus increasing HDL-C.[142] It has been reported in most studies that LPL is higher in physically active subjects and increases with exercise training.[3,100,141,142]

Hepatic lipase is thought to help in the removal of lipid from HDL-C facilitating its removal by the liver. The HL activity in inactive subjects has been found to be lower than in physically active groups.[100,142] LCAT which helps convert HDL-C$_3$ to HDL-C$_2$ and its activity has been found to increase following acute exercise and with training in some studies.[100,142] However, other reports have indicated that LCAT activity does not change with training or detraining.[100,135]

Lower CETP levels promote increased concentrations of HDL-C.[101] Marathon runners have been found to have lower CETP levels than inactive individuals,[143] and cyclists have been found to have lower CETP activity following a 230 km race.[144] The dosages of exercise necessary to create favorable changes in these enzymes are currently unknown.

The particle sizes of various lipoproteins have also been reported to be influenced by exercise.[3,26] Smaller LDL-C mass particles are considered to be more atherogenic than larger LDL-C particles, and exercise has been reported to lower small mass LDL-C particles.[3,35,145,146]

Specific HDL-C particles (HDL$_2$-C) have been reported to increase in endurance runners compared to non-exercising controls and have been found to be inversely correlated to increased CHD risk.[145,146]

G. THE INFLUENCE OF EXERCISE VS. WEIGHT LOSS

The precise relationship between the influence of exercise on lipids/lipoproteins has been difficult to interpret due to a variety of interacting variables like: age, initial lipid/lipoprotein levels, length of training, training intensity, level of aerobic fitness, and weight loss (particularly when expressed as percent body fat).[29,100,101,147] It has been reported that plasma lipid/lipoprotein changes are associated more with fat weight reduction than exercise training itself.[3,121,148] These findings suggest that specific thresholds of exercise training and/or fat weight loss must be obtained prior to the observation of favorable changes in HDL-C and TG.[3] The following discussion summarizes what is currently known about the exercise vs. fat weight loss influences on lipids/lipoproteins.

Williams et al.[149] was one of the first to find that weight loss was strongly associated with HDL-C and HDL$_2$-C during exercise training in middle-aged men. In a longitudinal study which compared runners (8 miles/week) and controls, Wood et al.[121] found that significant changes in HDL-C and HDL$_2$-C were significantly correlated with changes in body fat and caloric intake.

When overweight men were studied in a 1 year trial, fat loss acquired by either diet or exercise was equally effective in raising HDL-C.[148] Changes in LDL-C and TC were not significantly influenced for the full trial, and an increase in aerobic capacity ($\dot{V}O_2$ max) was associated with decreases in TG for exercisers only. Wood et al.[148] concluded that fat loss was the key to raising HDL-C, whether an individual achieved the results via dieting or exercise.

The issue of exercise vs. weight loss influence on lipids/lipoproteins has been evaluated more recently by Wier et al.[150] These investigators studied more than 1500 men, of varying age and fitness levels, cross-sectionally, and they also followed-up on a sub-set of 156 men longitudinally (for 3 years), to assess the effects of exercise and weight loss on TC, LDL-C, TG, and HDL-C. In the cross-sectional data — age, fat weight, fat-free weight, and $\dot{V}O_2$ max — were independently related to TC and HDL-C. Triglycerides were related to age, fat weight and $\dot{V}O_2$ max, while LDL-C was related to age and $\dot{V}O_2$ max only. In the longitudinal sample, TC, LDL-C, and TG were only related to changes in weight (LDL-C) or changes in fat weight and changes in fat-free weight (TC and TG) and not $\dot{V}O_2$ max. Changes in both $\dot{V}O_2$ max and fat weight were significantly related with changes in HDL-C.

The authors concluded that their cross-sectional and longitudinal data indicated that:

1. when one assesses changes in lipids/lipoproteins, body composition should be the focus for TC and TG;
2. LDL-C is not influenced much by exercise-related changes in body composition or $\dot{V}O_2$ max; and
3. favorable changes in HDL-C are most responsive to changes in both body composition and $\dot{V}O_2$ max.

It is important to note that a 1 mg/dl increase in HDL-C is associated with a 2% decrease in CHD risk for men and a 3% decrease in women.[151] In order to raise the HDL-C by 5 mg/dl, Wier et al.[150] predicted that fat weight would have to fall 5 kg and $\dot{V}O_2$ max would have to be increased by 9 ml · kg^{-1} · min^{-1} in their subjects. For a man weighing 79 kg, with 20% body fat and a $\dot{V}O_2$ max of 37 ml · kg^{-1} · min^{-1}, he would have to reduce his body fat to 14.6% and raise his $\dot{V}O_2$ max to 46 ml $\cdot$ kg^{-1} $\cdot$ min^{-1}, to achieve the 5 mg/dl HDL-C increase. Although these fitness changes would require significant attention to increasing exercise habits (particularly if one is sedentary), this predictive example is consistent with the threshold of exercise training reported by others,[3,6,7,100-102] to yield beneficial changes in HDL-C.

In contrast to the above findings, other investigators have confirmed that exercise training without weight loss can result in increased HDL-C levels.[100,152,153] In fact Sopko et al.[154] found that the effects of exercise with weight constant and weight loss without exercise on HDL-C were independent and additive in obese men. It has also been reported that young men, who participated in exercise training for 20 weeks and who had significant weight and fat loss with significant gains in $\dot{V}O_2$ max, did not increase their HDL-C levels.[155]

Williams has recently reported that exercise was related to increases in HDL_{2a}-C and HDL_{3a}-C subfractions while weight loss was related to increased HDL_2-C mass and HDL_{2b}-C subfractions.[156] The exercise vs. weight loss controversy regarding lipids/lipoproteins remains unresolved, while the specific mechanisms by which exercise increases HDL-C and its subfractions remains unknown and requires further investigation.

VII. SUMMARY

The NCEP has recommended that every adult over the age of 20 should know what his or her plasma TC level is, because the measurement of TC is a simple and inexpensive CHD risk screening tool.[2,4] In primary prevention, if the TC level is below 200 mg/dl, LDL-C is ≤130, and the HDL-C is >35 mg/dl, the person has a desirable lipid and lipoprotein profile and they should be encouraged to follow the AHA prudent diet guidelines and have their TC evaluated in 5-year intervals.[4,36] If the TC, LDL-C, or HDL-C levels are not at desirable levels then the person should be given dietary modification information, encouraged to engage in physical activity, and have followup lipid and lipoprotein measures conducted every 1–2 years.[4,36]

Recently the American College of Physicians (ACP) proposed new guidelines for cholesterol testing for the prevention of CHD in adults which differ substantially from those of the NCEP and the AHA.[157-159] The ACP guidelines recommend (not require) only screening for TC in men 35–65 years and women 45–65 years of age. The ACP guidelines would thus exclude many people over 65 and men and women younger than 35 and 45 years, respectively.[159] HDL-C sreening is not recommended by the ACP. The ACP guidelines have subsequently been labeled incorrect and misguided,[59] yet clinicians and consumers may be faced with continued conflicting messages about cholesterol screening.[159]

In conclusion, based upon our previous reviews[6-7] and the current relevant literature, we feel that the combined effects of a healthy diet, maintenance of desirable body weight and appropriate levels of endurance/resistance exercise can favorably influence lipid/lipoprotein profiles and reduce CHD risk in adults, as part of a primary prevention benefit.[29,36,100,101] In individuals with diagnosed CHD, the benefit of controlling lipid/lipoprotein levels is much larger than even that found for primary prevention.[146]

ACKNOWLEDGMENT

This chapter is again dedicated to the memory of Laurette Nichols who typed our original manuscript for the first edition of this publication and who was recognized as an outstanding employee at Southwest Texas State University during 1991.

REFERENCES

1. Gotto, A. M., Preface, *Circulation*, 80 , 716, 1989.
2. National Cholesterol Education Program, Report of the Expert Panel on detection, evaluation, and treatment of high blood cholesterol in adults, *Arch. Intern. Med.*, 148, 36, 1988.
3. Superko, H. R., Exercise training, serum lipids, and lipoprotein particles: is there a change threshold?, *Med. Sci. Sports Exer.*, 23, 677, 1991.
4. National Cholesterol Education Program, Report of the Expert Panel on detection, evaluation, and treatment of high blood cholesterol in adults. (Adult Treatment Panel II), *Cirulation*, 89, 1333, 1994.
5. Grundy, S. M., Cholesterol and coronary disease: future directions, *J. Amer. Med. Assoc.*, 264, 3053, 1990.
6. Murray, T. D., Squires, W. G., and Hartung, G. H., Regulation of lipids and lipoproteins by diet and exercise, in *Nutrition in Exercise and Sport*, Hickson, J. F. and Wolinsky, I., Eds., CRC Press, Boca Raton, FL, 1989, 63.
7. Murray, T. D., Squires, W. G., and Hartung, G. H., Putative effects of diet and exercise on lipids and lipoproteins, in *Nutrition in Exercise and Sport*, 2nd ed., Wolinsky, I. and Hickson, J. F., Eds., CRC Press, Boca Raton, FL, 1994, 65.
8. Bowers, R. W. and Fox, E. L., Eds., *Sports Physiology*, 3rd ed., William C. Brown, Dubuque, IA, 1988.
9. Gordon, T., Castelli, W. P., Hjortland, M. C., Kannel, W. B., and Dawber, T. R., High density lipoprotein as a protective factor against coronary disease. The Framingham Study, *Am. J. Med.*, 62, 707, 1977.
10. Castelli, W. P., Doyle, J. T., Gordon, T., Hames, C. G., Hjortland, M. C., Hulley, S. B., Kagan, A., and Zukel, W. J., HDL cholesterol and other lipids in coronary disease. The cooperative lipoprotein phenotyping study, *Circulation*, 55, 767, 1977.
11. Lipid Research Clinics Program, The Lipid Research Clinics Coronary Primary Prevention Trial Results II. The relationship in incidence of coronary heart disease to cholesterol lowering, *J. Amer. Med. Assoc.*, 251, 365, 1984.
12. Miller, G. J. and Miller, N. E., Plasma high density lipoprotein concentration and development of ischemic heart-disease, *Lancet*, 1, 16, 1975.
13. Hartung, G. H., Diet and exercise in the regulation of plasma lipids and lipoproteins in patients at risk of coronary disease, *Sports Med.*, 1, 413, 1984.
14. Dufax, B., Assman, G., and Hollman, W., Plasma lipoproteins and physical activity: a review, *Int. J. Sports Med.*, 3, 123, 1982.
15. Lewis, B., Ed., *The Hyperlipidemias: Clinical Laboratory Practice*, Blackwell Scientific, Oxford, 1976, chap. 1.
16. Goldstein, J. L. and Brown, M. S., The low density lipoprotein pathway and its relation to atherosclerosis, *Ann. Rev. Biochem.*, 46, 897, 1977.
17. Gotto, A. M., High-density lipoproteins: biochemical and metabolic factors, *Am. J. Cardiol.*, 52, 2B, 1983.
18. Brown, M. S. and Goldstein, J. L., A receptor-mediated pathway for cholesterol homeostasis, *Science*, 232, 34, 1986.
19. Grundy, S. M., Multifactorial etiology of hypercholesteroemia: implications for prevention of coronary heart disease, *Arteriosclerosis and Thrombosis*, 11, 1619, 1991.
20. Breslow, J. L., Genetics of lipoprotein disorders, *Circulation*, 87 (Suppl III), III161, 1993.
21. Brewer, H. B., Greg, R. E., Hoeg, J. M., and Fojo, S. S., Apolipoproteins and lipoproteins in human plasma: an overview, *Clin. Chem.*, 34(8), (Suppl B), B4, 1988.
22. Brooks, G. A. and Fahey, T. D., *Exercise Physiology:Human Bioenergetics and Its Applications*, 2nd ed., Mayfield, Mountain View, CA., 1995.
23. Kris-Etherton, P. M., Krummel, D., Dreon, D., Mackey, S., Borchers, J., and Wood, P. D., The effects of diet on plasma lipids, lipoproteins, and coronary heart disease, *J. Am. Dietetic Assoc.*, 88, 1374, 1988.
24. Marniemi, J., Dahlstorm, S., Kvist, M., Seppanen, A., and Hietanen, E., Dependence of serum lipid and lecithin: cholesterol acytltransferase levels on physical training of young men, *Eur. J. Appl. Physiol.*, 49, 25, 1982.
25. Kinnunen, P. K., Virtanen, J. A., and Vainio, P., Lipoprotein lipase and hepatic endothelial lipase: their roles in plasma lipoprotein metabolism, *Atherosclerosis Rev.*, 11, 65, 1983.
26. Superko, H. R. and Haskell, W. L., The role of exercise training in the therapy of hyper-lipoprotenemia, in *Exercise and the Heart*, Vol. 5, No. 2, Hanson, P., Ed., W. B. Saunders, Philadephia, 1987.
27. Tall, A. R., Plasma Plasma lipid transfer proteins, *J. Lipid Res.*, 27, 361, 1986.
28. Tikkanen, M. J., Plasma lipoproteins and atherosclerosis, *J. Diabetes Complications*, 4, 35, 1990.
29. Durstine, J. L. and Haskell, W. L., Effects of exercise training on plasma lipids and lipoproteins, in *Exercise and Sport Sciences Reviews*, Holloszy, J. O. , Ed., Williams and Wilkins, Baltimore, 477, 1994.
30. Eisenberg, S. and Levy, R. I., Lipoprotein metabolism, *Adv. Lipid Res.*, 13, 1, 1976.
31. Levy, R. and Rifkind, B. M., The structure and metabolism of high density lipopoteins: a status report, *Circulation*, 62, IV-4, 1980.
32. Shepard, J., Lipoprotein metabolism: an overview, *Ann. Acad. Med.*, 21, 106, 1992.
33. Glomset, S. A., The plasma lecithin cholesterol acyltransferase reaction, *J. Lipid Res.*, 9, 155, 1968.

34. Carew, T. E., Kroschinsky, T., Hayes, S. B., and Steinberg, D., A mechanism by which high-density lipoporoteins may slow the atherogenic process, *Lancet*, 1, 1315, 1976.
35. Williams, P. T., Krauss, R. M., Wood, P. D., Lindgren, F. T., Giotas, C., and Vranizan, K. M., Lipoprotein subfractions of runners and sedentary men, *Metabolism*, 35, 45, 1986.
36. Brown,W. V., Lipoproteins: what, when, and how often to measure?, *Heart Dis. Stroke*, 1, 21, 1992.
37. Gordon, T., Kannel, W. B., Castelli, W. B., and Dawber, T. R., Lipoproteins, cardiovascular disease and death: the Framingham Study, *Arch. Intern. Med.*, 141, 1128, 1981.
38. Miller, N. E., Hammett, F., Saltissi, S., Van Zeller, H., Coltart, J., and Lewis, B., Relation of angiographically defined coronary artery disease to plasma lipoprotein subfractions and apolipoproteins, *Br. Med. J.*, 282, 1741, 1981.
39. Williams, P. T., Krauss, R. M., Kindel-Joyce, S., Dreon, D. M., Vranizan, K. M., and Wood, P. D., Relationship of dietary fat, protein, cholesterol, and fiber intake to atherogenic lipoproteins in men, *Am. J. Clin. Nutr.*, 44, 788, 1986.
40. Hartung, G. H., Squires, W. G., and Gotto, A. M., Effect of exercise training on plasma high-density lipoprotein cholesterol in coronary disease patients, *Am. Heart J.*, 101,181, 1981.
41. Manninen, V., Tenkanen, L., Koskinen, P., Huttunen, J. K., Manttari, M., Heinonen, O. P., and Frick, M. H., Joint effects of serum triglyceride and LDL cholesterol concentrations on coronary heart disease risk in the Helsinki Heart Study: implications for treatment, *Circulation*, 85, 37, 1991.
42. Friedwald, W., Levy, R., and Fredrikson, D., Estimation of the concentration of low-density lipoprotein cholesterol in plasma, without use of the preparative ultracentrifuge, *Clin. Chem.*, 18, 499, 1972.
43. Stampfer, M. J., Sacks, F. M., Salvini, S., Willet, W. C., and Hennekens, C. H., A prospective study of cholesterol, apolipoproteins, and the risk of myocardial infarction, *N. Eng. J. Med.*, 325, 373, 1991.
44. Vega, G. L. and Grundy, S. M., Does measurement of Apolipoprotein B have a place in cholesterol management?, *Arteriosclerosis*, 10, 668, 1990.
45. McBride, P. E., Plane, M. B., and Underbakke, G., Hypercholesterolemia: the current educational needs of physicians, *Am. Heart J.*, 123, 817, 1992.
46. Grundy, S. M., Cholesterol and coronary heart disease: a new era, *J. Amer. Med. Assoc.*, 256, 2849, 1986.
47. Kannel, W. B., Castelli, W. P., and Gordon, T., Serum cholesterol lipoproteins and risk of coronary disease: the Framingham Study, *Ann. Intern. Med.*, 74, 1, 1971.
48. Final Report of the Pooling Project Research Group, Relationship of blood pressure, serum cholesterol, smoking habit, relative weight and ECG abnormalities to incidence of major coronary events, *J. Chronic Dis.*, 31, 201, 1978.
49. Goldbourt, V., Holtzman, E., and Neufeld, H. N., Total and high density lipoprotein cholesterol in the serum and risk of mortality: evidence of a threshold effect, *Br. Med. J.*, 290, 1239, 1985.
50. Stamler, J., Wentworth, D., and Neaton, J., Is the relationship between serum cholesterol and risk of death from coronary disease continuous and graded?, *J. Amer. Med. Assoc.*, 256, 2823, 1986.
51. Holme, I., An analysis of randomized trials evaluating the effect of cholesterol reduction on total mortality and coronary heart disease incidence, *Circulation*, 82, 1916, 1990.
52. Stamler, J., Major coronary risk factors before and after myocardial infarction, *Postgrad. Med.*, 57, 34, 1975.
53. Stamler, J., Primary prevention of coronary heart disease: the last 20 years, *Am. J. Cardiol.*, 47, 722, 1981.
54. Blair, S. N., Kohl, H. W., Paffenbarger, R. S., Clark, D. G., Cooper, K. H., and Gibbons, L. W., Physical fitness and all-cause mortality: a prospective study of healthy men and women, *J. Amer. Med. Assoc.*, 262, 2395, 1989.
55. Conner, W. E. and Conner, S. L., The dietary prevention and treatment of coronary heart disease, in *Coronary Heart Disease*, Conner, W. E. and Bristow, J. D., Eds., J. B. Lippincott, Philadelphia, 1984.
56. LaRosa, J. C., Cholesterol agonistics, *Ann. Intern. Med.*, 124, 505, 1996.
57. U.S. Departments of Agriculture and Health and Human Services, Nutrition and Your Health: Dietary Guidelines for Americans, 4th ed., Washington D.C.: Home and Garden Bulletin No. 232, 1995.
58. Grundy, S. M., Brown, W. V., Dietschy, J. M., Ginsberg, H., Goodnight, S., Howard, B., La Rosa, J. C., and McGill, H. C., Workshop III, Basis for Dietary Treatment, AHA Conference Report on Cholesterol, *Circulation*, 80, 729, 1989.
59. U.S. Department of Health and Human Services, *Healthy People 2000*, National Health Promotion and Disease Prevention Objectives, DDHS Publication No. (PHS) 91-50212, U.S. Government Printing Office, Washington, D.C., 1991.
60. Foreyt, J. P. and Goodrich, G. K. Impact of behavior therapy on weight loss, *Am. J. Health Promot.*, 8, 466, 1994.
61. Blair, S. N., Horton, E., Leon, A. S., Lee, I.-M., Drinkwater, B. L., Dishman, R. K., Mackey, M., and Kienholz, M. L., Physical activity, nutrition, and chronic disease, *Med. Sci. Spts. Exer.*, 28, 335, 1996.
62. Grundy, S. M., Comparsion of monosaturated fatty acids and carbohydrates for lowering plasma cholesterol, *N. Eng. J. Med.*, 314, 745, 1986.
63. Mensink, R. P. and Katan, M. B., Effect of monosaturated fatty acids versus complex carbohydrates in high-density lipoproteins in healthy men and women, *Lancet*, 1, 122, 1987.

64. Hartung, G. H., Reeves, R. S., Sigurdson, A. S., Traweek, M. S., Foryet, J. P., and Blocker, W. P., Effect of a low-fat diet and exercise on plasma lipoproteins and cardiac dysrhythmia in middle-aged men, *Circulation*, 68 (Part 2), III-226, 1983.

65. Keys, A., Anderson, J. T., and Grande, F., Serum cholesterol response to changes in the diet: II. The effect of cholesterol in the diet, *Metabolism*, 14, 759, 1965.

66. Socri-Thomas, M., Wilson, M. D., Johnson, F. L., Williams, D. L., and Rudel, L. L., Studies on the expression of genes encoding apolipoproteins B100 and B48 and the low density lipoprotein receptor in primates, *J. Biol. Chem.*, 264, 9039, 1989.

67. Hegsted, D. M., McGandy, R. B., Meyers, M. L., and Stare, F. J., Quantitative effects of dietary fat on serum cholesterol in man, *Am. J. Clin. Nutr.,* 17, 281, 1965.

68. Shepard, J., Packard, C. J., Patsch, J. R., Gotto, A. M., and Taunton, O. D., Effects of dietary polyunsatuurated and saturated fat on the properties of high-density lipoprotein and the metabolism of apolipoprotein AI, *J. Clin. Invest.,* 61, 1582, 1978.

69. Weymen, C., Berlin, J., Smith, A. D., and Thompson, R. S. H., Linoleic acid as an immunosuppressive agent, *Lancet,* 2, 33, 1975.

70. Strurdevant, R. A. L., Pearce, M. L., and Dayton, S., Increased prevalence of cholelithiasis in men ingesting a serum-cholesterol-lowering diet, *N. Eng. J. Med.,* 288, 24, 1973.

71. Reddy, B. S., Amount and type of dietary fat and colon cancer: animal model studies, *Prog. Clin. Biol. Res.,* 222, 295, 1986.

72. Parthasarathy, S., Khoo, J. C., Miller, E., Barnett, J., and Witztum, J. L., Low-density lipoprotein rich in oleic acid is protected against oxidative modification: implications for dietary prevention of atherosclerosis, *Proc. Natl. Acad. Sci.,* 87, 3894, 1990.

73. Simons, L. A., Hickie, J. B., and Balasubramaniam, S., On the effects of dietary omega-3 fatty acids (Max EPA) on plasma lipids and lipoproteins in patients with hyperlipidemia, *Atherosclerosis,* 54, 75, 1985.

74. Phillipson, B. E., Rothbrock, D. W., Conner, W. E., Harris, W. S., and Illingworth, D. R., Reduction of plasma lipids, lipoproteins, and apoproteins by dietary fish oils in patients with hypertriglyceridemia, *N. Eng. J. Med.*, 312, 1210, 1985.

75. National Dietary Council, Nutrition and health effects of unsaturated fatty acids, *Dairy Council Dig.*, 59, 1, 1988.

76. Mensink, R. P. and Katan, M. B., Effects of dietary fatty acids on serum lipids and lipoproteins: a meta analysis of 27 trials, *Arterioscler. Thromb.*, 12, 911, 1992.

77. Grundy, S. M., Comparison of monounsaturated fatty acids and carbohydrates for lowering plasma cholesterol, *N. Eng. J. Med.*, 314, 745, 1986.

78. Grundy, S. M., Florentin, L., Nix, D., and Whelan, M. F., Comparison of monounsaturated fatty acids and carbohydrates for reducing raised levels of plasma cholesterol in man, *Am. J. Clin. Nutr.*, 47, 965, 1988.

79. West, C. E., Sullivan, D. R., Katan, M. B., Halferkamps, I. N., and van der Torre, H. W., Boys from populations with high-carbohydrate intake have higher fasting triglyceride levels than boys from populations with high fat intake, *Am. J. Epidemiol.*, 131, 271, 1990.

80. Kay, R. M. and Truswell, A. S., Effect of citrus pectin on blood lipids and fecal steroid excretion in man. *Am. J. Clin. Nutr.*, 30, 171, 1977.

81. Kay, R. M., Dietary fiber, *J. Lipid Res.*, 23, 221, 1982.

82. Pilch S.M., Ed., *Physiological Effects of Health Consequences of Dietary Fiber*, Life Sciences Research Office, Federation of American Societies for Experimental Biology, Bethesda, MD, 1987.

83. Sacks, F. M., Castelli, W. F., Donner, A., and Kass, E. H., Plasma lipids and lipoproteins in vegetarians and controls, *N. Eng. J. Med.*, 292, 1148, 1975.

84. Zetts, R. A., Avent, H. H., Murray, T. D., and Squires, W. G., Comparison of high density lipoprotein levels (HDL) between vegetarian and non-vegetarian females, *Med. Sci. Sports Exer.*, 17, 285, 1985.

85. Steinberg, D., Parthasarathy, Carew, T., Khoo, J., and Witztum, J., Beyond cholesterol: modification of low density lipoprotein that increases its atherogenicity, *N. Eng. J. Med.*, 322, 147, 1990.

86. Kagan, V. E., Spirichev, V. B., Serbinova, E. A., Witt, E., Erin, A. N., and Packer, L., The significance of vitamin E and free radicals in physical exercise, in *Nutrition in Exercise and Sport*, 2nd ed., Wolinsky, I. and Hickson, J. F., Eds., CRC Press, Boca Raton, FL, 1994, 185.

87. U.S. Department of Health and Human Services, *Five a Day for Better Health*, National Institutes of Health, DDHS Publication No. (PHS) 92- 3248, U.S. Government Printing Office, Washington, D.C., 1991.

88. Hartung, G. H. and Foreyt, J. P., The effect of alcohol intake on high-density lipoprotein cholesterol and coronary heart disease, *Cardiovasc. Rev. Rep.*, 5, 678, 1984.

89. Hartung, G. H., Foreyt, J. P., Reeves, R. S., Krock, L. P., Patsch, W., Patsch, J. R., and Gotto, A. M., Effect of alcohol dose on plasma lipoprotein subfractions and lipoplytic enyzme activity in active and inactive men, *Metabolism*, 39, 81, 1990.

90. Hartung, G. H., Reeves, R. S., Foreyt, J. P., Patsch, W., and Gotto, A. M., Effect of alcohol intake and exercise on plasma high-density lipoprotein subfractions and apolipoprotein A-I in women, *Am. J. Cardiol.*, 58, 148, 1986.

91. U.S. Department of Agriculture and U.S. Department of Health and Human Services, *Nutrition and Your Health: Dietary Guidelines for Americans,* 3rd ed., Home and Garden Bulletin, 232, 1995.

92. Kannel, W. B., Gordon, T., and Castelli, W. P., Obesity, lipids, and glucose intolerance: the Framingham Study, *Am. J. Nutr.,* 32, 1238, 1979.

93. Casperson, C. J., Physical activity epidemiology: concepts, methods, and applications to exercise science, in *Exercise and Science Reviews,* 17, 423, Pandolf, K. P., Ed., Williams & Wilkins, Baltimore, 1989.

94. American College of Sports Medicine, Position Stand, The recommended quantity and quality of exercise for developing and maintaining cardiorespiratory and muscular fitness in healthy adults, *Med. Sci. Sports Exer.,* 22, 265, 1990.

95. American College of Sports Medicine, *Guidelines for Exercise Testing and Perscription,* 5th ed., Williams & Wilkins, Baltimore, MD, 1995.

96. Leon, A. S. and Norstrom, J., Evidence of the role of physical activity and cardiorespiratory fitness in the prevention of coronary heart disease, *Quest,* 47, 311, 1995.

97. American Heart Association, *1990 Heart and Stroke Facts,* National Center, Dallas, 1994.

98. Pate, R. R., Pratt, M., Blair, S. N., Haskell, W. L., Macera, A. A., Bouchard, C., Buchner, D., Ettinger, W., Health, G. W., King, A. C., Kriska, A., Leon, A. S., Marcus, B. H., Morris, J., Paffenbarger, R. S., Jr., Patrick, K., Pollock, M. L., Rippe, J. M., Sallia, J., and Wilmore, J. H., Physical activity and public health: a recommendation from the Centers for Disease Control and Prevention and the American College of Sports Medicine, *J. Am. Med. Assoc.,* 273, 402, 1995.

99. U.S. Department of Health and Human Services, Physical activity and health: a report of the Surgeon General, *US Department of Health and Human Services, Centers for Disease Control and Prevention,* National Ceneter for Chronic Disease Prevention and Health Promotion, Atlanta, GA, 1996.

100. Hartung, G. H., High density lipoprotein cholesterol and physical activity: An update — 1983–1993, *Ital. J. Sport Sci.,* 1, 7, 1994.

101. Hartung, G. H., Physical activity and high density lipoprotein cholesterol, *J. Sports Med. Phys. Fitness,* 35, 1, 1995.

102. Superko, H. R., Haskell, W. L., and Wood, P. D., Modification of plasma cholesterol through exercise: rationale and recommendations, *Postgrad. Med.,* 78, 64, 1985.

103. Wood, P. D., Williams, P. T., and Haskell, W. L., Physical activity and high-density lipoproteins, in *Clinical and Metabolic Aspects of High-Density Lipoproteins,* Miller, N. E. and Miller, G. J., Eds., Elsevier Science Publishers, New York, 1984.

104. Haskell, W. L., The influence of exercise training on plasma lipids and lipoproteins in health and disease, *Acta Med. Scandinavica,* Suppl. 711, 23, 1986.

105. Goldberg, A. P., Aerobic and resistive exercise modify risk factors for coronary heart disease, *Med. Sci. Sports Exer.,* 21, 669, 1989.

106. Hurley, B. F., Effects of resistive training on lipoprotein-lipid profiles: a comparsion to aerobic exercise training, *Med. Sci. Sports Exer.,* 21, 689, 1989.

107. Kokkinos, P. F. and Hurley, B. F., Strength training and lipoprotein-lipid profiles: a critical analysis and recommendations for further study, *Sports Med.,* 9, 266, 1990.

108. Verrill, D., Shoup, E., McElveen, G., Witt, K., and Bergey, D., Resistive exercise training in cardiac patients, *Sports Med.,* 13, 171, 1992.

109. Schieken, R. M., Effect of exercise on lipids, *Ann. N.Y. Acad. of Sci.,* 623, 269, 1991.

110. Marti, B., Knobloch, M., Riesen, W. F., and Howald, H., Fifteen-year changes in exercise, aerobic power, abdominal fat, and serum lipids in runners and controls, *Med. Sci. Sports Exer.,* 23, 115, 1991.

111. Stray-Gundersen, J., Denkee, M. A., and Grundy, S. M., Influence of lifetime cross-country skiiing on plasma lipids and lipoproteins, *Med. Sci. Sports Exer.,* 23, 695, 1991.

112. Hartung, G. H., Lally, D. A., Prins, J., and Goebert, D. A., Relation of high-density lipoprotein cholesterol to physical activity levels in men and women, *Med. Exer. Nutr. Health,* 1, 293, 1992.

113. Superko, R. M., Exercise, lipoproteins, and coronary artery disease, *Circulation,* 79, 1143, 1989.

114. Hubinger, L., Traeger, L., and Lepre, F., Lipoprotein (a) (Lp(a)) levels in middle-age male runners and sedentary controls, *Med. Sci. Sports Exer.,* 27, 490, 1995.

115. Baker, T, Allen, D., Lei, K. Y., and Willcox, K. K., Alterations in lipid and protein profiles of plasma lipoproteins in middle-aged men consequent to an aerobic exercise program, *Metabolism,* 35, 1037, 1986.

116. Thompson, P. D., Cullinane, E. M., Sady, S. P., Flynn, M. M., Bernier, D. N., Kanter, M. A., Saritelli, A L., and Herbert, P. N., Modest changes in high-density lipoprotein concentration and metabolism with prolonged exercise training, *Circulation,* 78, 25, 1988.

117. Ratliff, R., Knehans, A., and McCarthy, M., Effects of frequency of exercise training on plasma lipids and lipoproteins, *Med. Sci. Sports Exer.,* 22, S48, 1990.

118. Marti, B., Suter, E., Riesen, W. F., Tschopp, A., Wanner, H. U., and Gutzwiller, F., Effects of long-term, self-monitored exercise on the serum lipoprotein and apolipoprotein profile in middle-age men, *Atherosclerosis,* 81, 19, 1990.

119. Rubinstein, A., Burstein, R., Lubin, F., Chetrit, A., Dann, E. J., Levtov, O., Geter, R., Deuster, P. A., and Dolev, E., Lipoprotein profile changes during intense training of Israeli military recruits, *Med. Sci. Sports Exer.*, 27, 480, 1995.

120. Kiens, B., Jorgenson, I., Lewis, S., Jensen, G., Lithell, H. et al., Increased plasma HDL cholesterol and Apo A-I in sedentary middle-aged men after physical conditioning, *Eur. J. Clin. Invest.*, 10, 203, 1980.

121. Wood, P. D., Haskell, W. L., Blair, S. N., Williams, P. T., Krauss, R. M., Lindgren, F. T., Albers, J. J., Ho, P. H., and Farquhar, J. W., Increased exercise level and plasma lipoprotein concentrations: a one-year randomized, controlled study in sedentary, middle-aged men, *Metabolism*, 32, 31, 1983.

122. Israel, R. G., Sullivan, M. J., Marks, R. H. L., Cayton, R. S., and Chenier, T. C., Relationship between cardiorespiratory fitness and lipoprotein (a) in men and women, *Med. Sci. Sports Exer.*, 26, 425, 1994.

123. Hurley, B. F., Hagberg, J. M., Goldgerg, A. P., Seals, D. R., Ehsani, A. A., Brennan, R. E., and Holloszy, J. O., Resistance training can reduce coronary risk factors without altering VO_2 max or percent body fat, *Med. Sci. Sports Exer.*, 20, 150, 1988.

124. Kokkinos, P. F., Hurley, B. F., Vaccaro, P., Patterson, J. C., Gardner, L. B., Ostrove, S. M., and Goldberg, A. P., Effects of low- and high-repetition resistive training on lipoprotein-lipid profiles, *Med. Sci. Sports Exer.*, 20, 50, 1988.

125. Kokkinos, P. F., Hurley, B. F., Smutok, M. A., Farmer, C., Reece, C., Shulman, R., Charabogos, C., Patterson, J., Will, S., Devane-Bell, J., and Goldgerg, A.P., Strength training dose not improve lipoprotein-lipid profiles in men at risk for CHD, *Med. Sci. Sports Exer.*, 23, 1134, 1991.

126. Manning, J. M., Dooley-Manning, C. R., White, K., Kampa, I., Silas, S., Kesselhaut, M., and Ruoff, M., Effects of a resistance training program on lipoprotein-lipid levels in obese women, *Med. Sci. Sports Exer.*, 23, 1222, 1991.

127. Kohl, H. W., Gordon, N. F., Scott, C. B., Vaandrager, H., and Blair, S. N., Musculoskeletal strength and serum lipid levels in men and women, *Med. Sci. Sports Exer.*, 24, 1080, 1992.

128. Costill, D. L., Pearson, D. R., and Fink, W. J., Anabolic steriod use among athletes: changes in HDL-C levels, *Phys. Sportsmed.*, 12, 112, 1984.

129. Hurley, B. F., Seals, D. R., Hagberg, J. M., Goldberg, A. C., Ostrone, S. M., Holloszy, J.O., Wiest, W. G., and Goldberg, A. P., High density lipoprotein cholesterol in body builders vs. power lifters. Negative effects of androgen use, *J. Amer. Med. Assoc.*, 252, 507, 1984.

130. Webb, O. T., Laskarzewski, P., M., and Glueck, C. J., Severe depression of high density lipoprotein cholesterol levels in weight lifters and body builders by self-administered exogenous testosterone and anabolic-androgenic steriods, *Metabolism*, 33, 971, 1984.

131. Kantor, M. A., Bianchini, A., Bernier, D., Sady, S. P., and Thompson, P. D., Androgens reduce HDL2 cholesterol and increase hepatic triglyceride lipase activity, *Med. Sci. Sports Exer.*, 17, 462, 1985.

132. Cohen, L. I., Hartford, C. G., and Rogers, G. G., Lipopreotein (a) and cholesterol in body builders using anabolic androgenic steriods, *Med. Sci. Sports Exer.*, 28, 176, 1996.

133. Durstine, J. L., Miller, W., Farrell, S., Sherman, W. M., and Ivy, J. L., Increases in HDL-cholesterol and the HDL/LDL cholesterol ratio during prolonged endurance exercise, *Metabolism*, 32, 993, 1983.

134. Davis, P. G., Bartoli, W. P., and Durstine, J. L., Effects of acute exercise intensity on plasma lipids and apolipoproteins in trained runners, *J. Appl. Physiol.*, 72, 914, 1992.

135. Pronk, N. P., Short term effects of exercise on plasma lipids and lipoproteins in humans, *Sports Med.*, 16, 431, 1993.

136. Krummel, D., Etherton, T. D., Peterson, S., and Kris-Etherton, P. M., Effects of exercise on plasma lipids and lipoproteins of women, *Proc. Soc. Exp. Biol. Med.*, 204, 123, 1993.

137. Lokey, E. A. and Tran, Z. V., Effects of exercise training on serum lipid and lipoprotein concentrations in women: a meta-analysis, *Int. J. Sports Med.*, 10, 424, 1989.

138. Douglas, P. S., Clarkson, T. B., Flowers, N. C., Hajjar, K. A., Horton, E., Klocke, F. J., LaRosa, J., and Shively, C., Exercise and atherosclerotic heart disease in women, *Med. Sci. Sports Exer.*, 24, S266, 1992.

139. Williams, P. T., High-density lipoprotein cholesterol and other risk factors for coronary heart disease in female runners, *N. Eng. J. Med.*, 334, 1298, 1996.

140. Manson, J. E. and Lee, I. M., Exercise for women — how much pain for optimal gain?, *N. Eng. J. Med.*, 334, 1325, 1996.

141. Podl, T. R., Zmuda, J. M., Yurgalevitch, S. M., Fahrebach, M. C., Bausserman, L. L., Terry, R. B., and Thompson, P. D., Lipoprotein lipase activity and plasma triglyceride clearance are elevayed in endurance-trained women, *Metabolism*, 101, 43, 1994.

142. Berg, A., Frey, I., Baumstark, M. W., Halle, M., and Keul, J., Physical activity and lipoprotein disorders, *Sports Med.*, 17, 6, 1994.

143. Serrat-Serrat, J., Ordonez-Llanos, J., Serra-Grima, R., Gomez-Gerique, J. A., Pellicer-Thoma, E., Payes-Romero, A., and Gonzalez-Sastre, F., Marathon runners presented lower serum cholesterol ester transfer activity than sedentary subjects, *Atherosclerosis*, 101, 43, 1993.

144. Foger, B., Wohlfarter, T., Ritsch, A., Lecheitner, M., Miller, C. H., Diensi, A., and Patsch, J. R., Kinetics of lipids, apolipoproteins, and cholesteryl ester transfer protein in plasma after a bicycle marathon, *Metabolism*, 43, 633, 1994.

145. Wirth, A. C., Diehm, C., Hanel, W., Welte, J., and Vogel, I., Training-induced changes in serum lipids, fat tolerance, and adipose tissue metabolism in patients with hypertriglyceridemia, *Atherosclerosis*, 54, 263, 1985.

146. LaRosa, J. C. and Cleeman, J. I., Cholesterol lowering as a treatment for established coronary heart disease, *Circulation*, 85, 1229, 1992.

147. Tran, Z. V., Weltman, A., Glass, G. V., and Mood, D. P., The effects of exerise on blood lipids and lipoproteins: a meta analysis of studies, *Med. Sci. Sports Exer.*, 15, 393, 1983.

148. Wood, P. D., Stefanick, M. L., Dreon, D. M., Frey-Hewitt, B., Gary, S. C., Williams, P. T., Superko, H. R., Fortmann, S. P., Albers, J. J., Vranizan, K. M., Ellsworth, N. M., Terry, R. B., and Haskell, W. L., Changes in plasma lipids and lipoproteins in overweight men during weight loss through dieting as compared to exercise, *N. Eng. J. Med.*, 319, 1173, 1988.

149. Williams, P. T., Wood, P. D., Haskell, W. L., Krauss, R. M., Vranizan, K. M., Blair, S. N., Terry, R., and Farquhar, J. W., Does weight loss cause the exercise-induced increase in plasma high density lipoproteins?, *Atherosclerosis*, 47, 173, 1983.

150. Weir, L. T., Jackson, A. S., and Pinkerton, M. B., Effects of body composition and VO$_2$ max on HDL-C: cross-sectional and longitudinal analyses, *Med. Sci. Sports Exer.*, 23, S50, 1991.

151. Gordon, D .J., Probstfield, J. L., Garrison, R .J., Neaton, J. D., Castelli, W. P., Knoke, J. D., Jacobs, D. R., Bangdiwala, S., and Tyroler, H. A., High-density lipoprotein and cardiovascular disease: four prospective American studies, *Circulation*, 79, 8, 1989.

152. Higuchi, M., Hashimoto, I., Yamakawa, K., Tsuji, E., Nishimuta, M., and Suzuki, S., Effect of exercise training on plasma high-density lipoprotin cholesterol at constant weight, *Clin. Physiol.*, 4, 125, 1984.

153. Kiens, B., Lithell, H., and Vessby, B., Further increase in high density lipoprotein in trained males after enhanced training, *Eur. J. App. Physiol.*, 52, 426, 1984.

154. Sopko, G., Leon, A. S., Jacobs, D. R., Foster, N., Moy, J., Kuba, K., Anderson, J. T., Casal, D., McNally, C., and Frantz, I., The effect of exercise and weight loss on plasma lipids in young obese men, *Metabolism*, 34, 227, 1985.

155. Despres, J.-P., Bouchard, C., Savard, R., Tremblay, A., and Allard, C., Lack of relationship between changes in adiposity and plasma lipids following endurance training, *Atherosclerosis*, 54, 135, 1985.

156. Williams, P. T., Krauss, R. M., Stefanick, M. L., Vranizan, K. M., and Wood, P. D., Effects of low-fat diet, caloric restriction, and running on lipoprotein subfraction concentrations in moderately overweight men, *Metabolism*, 43, 655, 1994.

157. Garber, A. M. and Browner, W. S., American College of Physicians guidelines for using serum cholesterol, high density lipoprotein cholesterol, and triglycerides as screening tests for the prevention of coronary heart disease in adults, *Ann. Intern. Med.*, 124, 515, 1996.

158. Garber, A. M., Browner, W. S., and Hulley, S. B., Cholesterol screening in asymptomatic adults, revisited, *Ann. Intern. Med.*, 124, 518, 1996.

159. Grundy, S., Balady, G. J., Criqui, M., Fletcher, G., Greenland, P., Hiratzka, L., Houston-Miller, N., Kris-Etheron, P., Krumholz, H. M., LaRosa, J., Ockene, I. S., Pearson, T., Reed, J., and Washington, R. L., Cholesterol sreening in asymtomatic adults: no cause to change, *Circulation*, 93, 1067, 1996.

Chapter 5

AMINO ACID AND PROTEIN METABOLISM DURING EXERCISE AND RECOVERY

Gregory L. Paul
Tracy A. Gautsch
Donald K. Layman

CONTENTS

0-8493-8560-1/97/$0.00+$.50
© 1998 by CRC Press LLC

I. AMINO ACID METABOLISM ASSOCIATED WITH EXERCISE

Amino acid metabolism is a key component of the body's ability to grow, adapt, and perform in an ever-changing environment. Twenty amino acids are essential for life as the building blocks for proteins which provide for structure and mobility and for enzymes that regulate all body processes. Amino acids are also precursors for numerous other molecules including hormones, neurotransmitters, nucleic acids, and polyamines. This diversity and essential nature of amino acids make them critical to any understanding of metabolic regulation and performance capabilities.

Of the 20 amino acids required by the body, 9 must be furnished in the diet and are termed "essential" or "indispensable." The designation as indispensable means that the body lacks the ability to synthesize the basic carbon chain of the amino acid. Requirements for these amino acids are dependent upon body size and physiological conditions.

Understanding of amino acid metabolism and dietary needs for amino acids requires review of regulations at the molecular level within tissues and organelles and also at interorgan and whole body levels. Individual amino acids play key metabolic roles in specific tissues such as skeletal muscle, liver, and kidney and under specific physiological conditions such as exercise and food intake. This chapter explores the effects of exercise and food intake on utilization of amino acids for energy and synthesis of new proteins; examines the regulation of protein synthesis in skeletal muscle; and reviews current information defining protein requirements for exercise and performance.

A. IMPACT OF AMINO ACIDS ON ENERGY METABOLISM AND PHYSICAL PERFORMANCE

Exercise produces extensive metabolic changes. Short-term responses are aimed at energy balance and regulation of nitrogen metabolism while long-term responses provide for adaptation of genetic expression of proteins. Long-term adaptations derive from needs for changes in mobility or performance, changes in body composition, and metabolic potential.

Exercise produces changes in carbohydrate, lipid, and amino acid metabolism. Carbohydrates and lipids have been studied most because of their primary roles as energy substrates.[1] Amino acids have received much less attention because they account for a relatively small percentage of energy use. On the other hand, recent studies suggest that changes in amino acid metabolism may be key to understanding regulation of metabolic adaptations that occur during exercise.

There are numerous reviews that summarize the role of amino acids as energy substrates for exercise and of the effects of exercise on protein or amino acid requirements.[2-6] In summary, amino acids account for 12–20% of the American diet. During non-growth conditions, amino acids consumed in excess of that needed to maintain normal physiological functions will move directly to energy. For athletes, the protein requirement has been reported at 1.4–1.8 g/kg/d for strength athletes and 1.2–1.4 g/kg/d for endurance athletes compared with the RDA of 0.8 g/kg/d for the mean of the American population.[5-7] These requirements are based on needs for tissue building and replacement as well as energy metabolism determined from nitrogen metabolism and losses.

This review focuses on recent developments in amino acid metabolism, interorgan amino acid exchange, the translational regulation of skeletal muscle protein synthesis, and current knowledge about the effects of exercise on nutritional requirements for protein or amino acids. New information expands our understanding of the roles and interactions of the amino acids leucine, alanine, and glutamine with glucose, insulin, and insulin-like growth factors (IGFs) in the control of muscle protein synthesis and glucose and nitrogen metabolism. These developments help us to understand the unique role of skeletal muscle in whole body metabolic processes and the potential need for specific nutritional supplements associated with extensive exercise. Our recent studies have helped to elucidate the metabolic changes that occur during endurance exercise and during the recovery period after exercise.[4,8-10] These findings provide new information about the regulation of protein synthesis and the potential importance of post-exercise nutrition.

We have limited our discussion to short-term metabolic regulations in skeletal muscle including changes in amino acid flux, metabolic pathways, the effects of amino acids on protein synthesis, and the impact of exercise on protein requirements. Data from our laboratory elucidate an important role for leucine in muscle protein synthesis and unique interactions among leucine, insulin, pyruvate, and alanine.[4,10] Based on these data, we provide speculation as to potential mechanisms for the interrelationships of hormones, amino acids, and energy in the translational control of skeletal muscle protein synthesis.

B. FATES OF AMINO ACIDS: FREE POOLS AND FLUX

The vast majority of the amino acids in the body are in protein structures. Only 0.5–1.0% of the total amino acids in the body are present as free amino acids in plasma or intracellular and extracellular space.[11] However, the relatively small amounts of amino acids present in the "free pools" are responsible for the metabolic or substrate influences of all amino acids.

Plasma and tissue amino acid concentrations for selected amino acids are presented in Table 1. The amino acids in highest concentration in the plasma and tissues are the dispensable amino acids glutamine, glycine, and alanine. Among the indispensable amino acids, the ones present in the highest concentrations are lysine, threonine, and the branched-chain amino acids (BCAA), valine, leucine, and isoleucine.[12] In most cases, amino acids are transported into tissues by active transports, which assures that even relatively small changes in plasma concentrations will be reflected in tissue levels.[13]

While the free amino acid pool is small and relatively stable in size, amino acid concentrations change in response to food intake or exercise, but they change within relatively narrow limits. However, the free pool is highly active. Changes in plasma concentrations are not reflective of the movement or flux of amino acids through the free pool. To appreciate the "real size" of the amino acid pool, one must consider both the amino acid concentration

TABLE 1 Amino Acid Concentrations in Serum and Muscle (μmol/dl)

Amino Acid	Serum	Muscle
Dispensable		
Alanine	32.6	110
Glutamate	12.0	826
Glutamine	65.2	1038
Glycine	33.6	62
Indispensable		
Lysine	38.0	93.0
Threonine	20.3	33.0
Phenylalanine	6.9	5.9
Leucine	16.6	11.2
Valine	18.8	14.7
Isoleucine	10.8	6.8

Adapted from Morgan et al., *J. Biol. Chem.*, 246, 2152, 1971.

TABLE 2 Amino Acid Pool Size and Flux

	Rat	Man
Free amino acids[a] (mmol/kg)	4.0	2.4
Amino acid flux (mmol/kg/d)	200	12
Half-life of free pool (min)	20	200

[a] Represents total concentration of dispensable amino acids in the free pool.

Adapted from Waterlow et al., *Protein Turnover in Mammalian Tissues and in the Whole Body,* Elsevier/North Holland, New York, 1978.

and the movement of amino acids into or out of the pool over time.[14,15] Estimates of free pool size and flux are presented in Table 2. Note that the amounts of amino acids moving through the free pool each day are many times the actual free pool size. In the rat, amino acids in the free pool are replaced on the order of 50 times per day, while in the human, the total free pool is replaced approximately 6 times each day.

Flux rates presented in Table 2 represent averages for all amino acids. Significant differences exist among individual amino acids. For example lysine, which has a relatively large and stable free pool, has a half-life within the free pool of approximately 10 hr in the human, while leucine, which is much more metabolically active, has a half-life of 45 min.[15] These differences are important to consider when selecting an amino acid to represent the total free pool or as a metabolic tracer.[14,15]

C. AMINO ACID METABOLISM DURING AND AFTER EXERCISE

During endurance exercise, changes in protein turnover produce net protein breakdown with release of amino acids into the free pools. The metabolic roles and importance of these amino acids released during exercise remain uncertain, but understanding of the pathways is expanding rapidly. It is clear that the principal amino acids involved are the BCAA, alanine, and glutamine and that there are extensive organ-to-organ interactions.

The dominant features of this interorgan exchange are BCAA movement from the liver to skeletal muscles, with the return of alanine to the liver and glutamine to the gut (Figure 1). Movement of these amino acids among tissues serves to provide substrates for gluconeogenesis, assist in the elimination of nitrogen wastes, maintain glutamine levels, provide substrates for the purine nucleotide cycle, and maintain amino acid precursors for protein synthesis. Recent evidence from our laboratory,[10] which will be reviewed here, suggests that this interorgan exchange of amino acids is also related to the regulation of skeletal muscle protein synthesis.

Felig et al.[16] provided early evidence about amino acid movement among tissues. By examining arterial-venous differences in substrate concentrations across tissues, they observed that skeletal muscle had net BCAA uptake with alanine released in amounts exceeding its content in muscle proteins. The alanine released from skeletal muscle was removed by the liver. On the basis of these observations, these investigators proposed the existence of a glucose-alanine cycle for maintaining blood glucose levels and for shuttling nitrogen and gluconeogenic substrates from muscle to liver (Figure 1).

Extending these studies to exercise conditions, Felig[17] found no net amino acid uptake by muscle during short-term exercise. Felig concluded that the source of nitrogen for alanine synthesis appears to be amino acids endogenous to the working muscle. During prolonged exercise, however, amino acid movement between the splanchnic bed (liver and gut) and skeletal muscle is pronounced. Ahlborg et al.[18] examined arterial-venous differences across the splanchnic bed and across the leg in 6 untrained adult males during 4 hr of cycling exercise

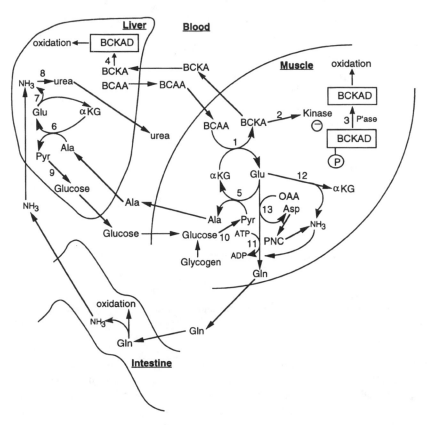

FIGURE 1 A summary of interorgan amino transport during exercise. The liver releases branched-chain amino acids (BCAA). The BCAA are imported by muscle where branched-chain aminotransferase (BCAAT; 1) catalyzes the transfer of the α-amino nitrogen from the BCAA to α-ketoglutarate (αKG) forming a branched-chain keto acid (BCKA) and glutamate (Glu). The BCKA inhibits the kinase (2) associated branched-chain amino acid dehydrogenase (BCKAD). This inhibition, coupled with the activity of a phosphatase (P'ase; 3), favor the dephosphorylated or active form of BCKAD. BCKA not oxidized in muscle are released and subsequently removed by the liver. Like muscle, liver BCKAD is dephosphorylated (4) which permits BCKA oxidation.

In muscle, the α-amino nitrogen of Glu is transferred to pyruvate (Pyr; when sufficient Pyr concentrations are present) to yield alanine (Ala) in a step catalyzed by alanine aminotransferase (AAT; 5). The Ala is released from muscle and extracted by the liver where the AAT reaction is reversed regenerating Glu and Pyr (6). Glu is deaminated via glutamate dehydrogenase (GDH; 7) to yield ammonia (NH_3) which is converted to urea in the urea cycle (8). Pyr is shuttled through gluconeogenesis (9) to form glucose which is released and subsequently transported into muscle. In muscle, glycolysis regenerates Pyr (10). This cycling of Ala and glucose between muscle and liver is referred to as the glucose-alanine cycle.

When muscle Pyr levels are low, nitrogen is removed from muscle via glutamine (Gln). Gln is formed from Glu and NH_3 in an ATP-dependent step catalyzed by glutamine synthetase (11). Potential NH_3 sources include the purine nucleotide cycle (PNC) and the GDH reaction (12). PNC cycle activity is dependent upon a continual supply of aspartate (Asp) which is formed from glutamate transamination with oxaloacetate (OAA) catalyzed by aspartate aminotransferase (13). Gln formed in muscle is released and transported primarily to the intestine where it is metabolized for energy. The NH_3 formed in Gln metabolism is released and transported to the liver where it can be detoxified in the urea cycle.

at 30% $\dot{V}O_2$ max. These investigators observed a significant increase in amino acid flux, including a fourfold increase in BCAA released from the splanchnic area and a corresponding increase in the uptake by exercising muscles. In return, muscles released alanine, which was removed by the liver for gluconeogenesis. These data demonstrate a change in amino acid flux during endurance exercise with BCAA movement from visceral tissues to skeletal muscles and a return of alanine as a precursor for hepatic glucose synthesis. After 3–4 hr of exercise, up to 60% of the glucose released from liver is derived from alanine.[19]

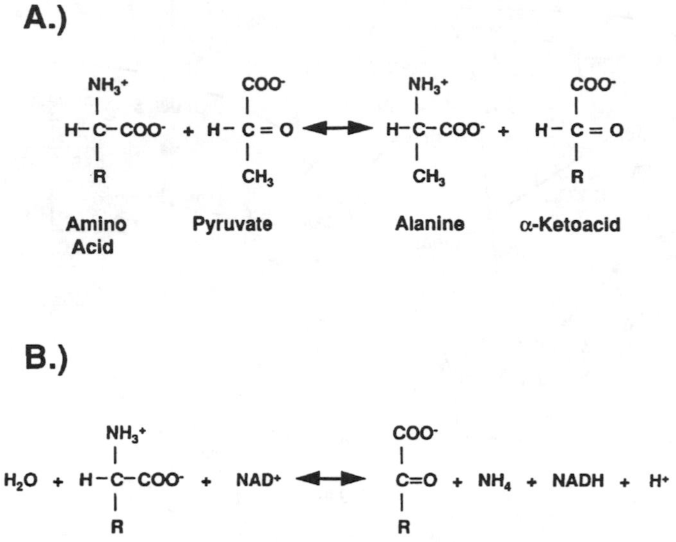

A.)

B.)

FIGURE 2 A.) Transamination of an amino acid into pyruvate, a reversible reaction catalyzed by an aminotransferase, and B.) oxidative deamination of an amino acid, a reversible reaction catalyzed by a deaminase.

Liver is the primary site for degradation of most amino acids. Hepatic tissue contains high concentrations of aminotransferases and deaminases which initiate amino acid degradation by removal of the α-amino group (Figure 2). However, the liver possesses very low branched-chain amino acid transferase (BCAAT) activity which results in BCAA release into the circulation (Figure 1).[20,21] Extrahepatic tissues, including kidney and skeletal muscle, contain BCAAT and are responsible for initiating the degradative pathway. Among these tissues, skeletal muscle appears to be the predominate tissue for BCAA degradation.[21-23]

BCAA catabolism is initiated by the reversible transamination of a BCAA to its corresponding α-keto acid with transfer of the α-amino group to α-ketoglutarate, forming glutamate (Figure 1). This step appears to be nearly at equilibrium with little physiological control. The second and rate-limiting step is decarboxylation of the branched-chain keto acid by branched-chain keto acid dehydrogenase (BCKAD). BCKAD activity is highly regulated by phosphorylation and dephosphorylation to the inactive and active forms, respectively. This step is stimulated by increases in the concentration of the leucine keto acid (α-ketoisocaproate). During periods of increased energy needs, such as starvation, trauma, and exercise, increased BCAA concentrations stimulate BCKAD, and the BCAA are oxidized for energy within skeletal muscle (Figure 3). In fact, recent evidence indicates that after only 5 min of cycling exercise at 70% $\dot{V}O_2$ max, the dephosphorylated (active) form of BCKAD is significantly increased.[24] During absorptive periods, when muscles use glucose as a primary fuel, muscle transaminates the BCAA and releases the keto acids into circulation for complete oxidation predominantly by the liver.[21,22]

While glutamate is formed *de novo* in skeletal muscle, there is no net release. Glutamate serves as an important intermediate in nitrogen metabolism. The amino nitrogen of glutamate can be transferred to pyruvate or oxaloacetate to form alanine and aspartate, respectively (Figure 1).[3,20] Alanine is released by the muscle for transport to the liver whereas aspartate is an important component of the purine nucleotide cycle within muscle (Figure 1). The purine nucleotide cycle serves to maintain muscle energy levels (regenerates the ATP pool) and produce free ammonia (NH_3). Ammonia may also be generated by glutamate deamination catalyzed by glutamate dehydrogenase (GDH; Figure 1). Earlier reports suggested that muscle GDH activity is very low or negligible.[25,26] However, recent evidence indicates that human

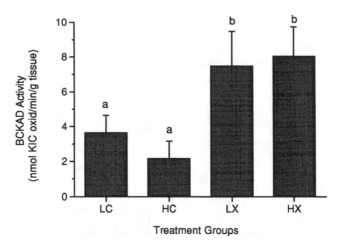

FIGURE 3 Exercise and dietary protein effects on BCKAD activity in skeletal muscle. Activities represent the amount of the BCKAD enzyme that is in the active form within the muscle. Activity was determined from *in vitro* oxidation of 2-keto-[1-^{14}C]-isocaproate with collection of $^{14}CO_2$. Abbreviations: LC, low-protein control; LX, low-protein exercised; HC, high-protein control; HX, high-protein exercised; KIC, alpha-keto isocaproate. Letters above bars indicate statistical significance at P <0.05. (Olken and Layman, unpublished data.)

glutamate dehydrogenase activity is quite high and sufficient to account for a significant portion of the increased ammonia flux that occurs during high-intensity exercise.[27,28]

The ammonia produced via the purine nucleotide cycle or GDH can combine with glutamate in an ATP-dependent reaction catalyzed by glutamine synthetase to form glutamine (Figure 1). Glutamine is ultimately released from muscle, with the majority being used by the gut as a primary energy source. Together, alanine and glutamine represent 60–80% of the amino acids released from skeletal muscle while they account for only 18% of the amino acids in muscle protein.[20,21]

Factors controlling alanine and glutamine formation in skeletal muscle during and after exercise have been studied extensively. Alanine aminotransferase (AAT) catalyzes the *de novo* synthesis of alanine in skeletal muscle via a reversible transamination reaction involving the transfer of the glutamate α-amino group to pyruvate yielding α-ketoglutarate and alanine. AAT functions at or near equilibrium such that factors altering glutamate and pyruvate concentrations will directly affect alanine production.[29] For example, transamination of aspartate or BCAAs increases the glutamate/α-ketoglutarate ratio which favors net alanine synthesis.[30] Similarly, an increase in muscle pyruvate concentration favors alanine formation.[29,30] Thus, in situations where pyruvate concentration is increased, alanine formation is favored, but when the muscle pyruvate pool is diminished both carbon and amino nitrogen are diverted to glutamine synthesis.[29]

Recent data from our laboratory illustrate this relationship between alanine and glutamine formation in skeletal muscle during and after exercise.[8] In a study with college-age men and women, we examined the effects of overnight fasting or pre-exercise meals on performance and amino acid metabolism. At 1-week intervals, 12 subjects performed 4 exercise/meal trials consisting of a fasting trial and 3 pre-exercise meals. For each of the 4 trials, subjects cycled for 90 min at 60% $\dot{V}O_2$ max either 90 min after consuming meals consisting of various cereal grains or at the same time for the fasting trial. Fasting trials were associated with lower carbohydrate oxidation rates and a greater reliance on fat as a fuel compared to the pre-exercise meal trials. Previous researchers have demonstrated that BCAA oxidation increases when carbohydrate oxidation is attenuated during exercise.[31,32] Thus, the fasted subjects in our study likely had an increased need to remove nitrogen from muscle compared to the fed subjects. With less available pyruvate from lower carbohydrate oxidation rates in the fasting

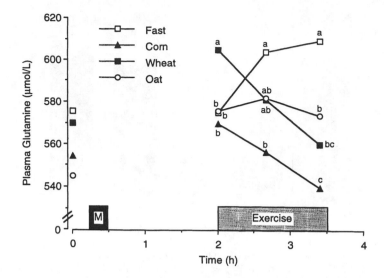

FIGURE 4 Plasma glutamine concentrations before subjects ingested either a corn, wheat, or oat cereal meal (M) and during 90 min of cycling exercise at 60% $\dot{V}O_2 \text{max}$. Values represent the mean of 12 subjects. Mean glutamine values during exercise increased in the fasting trial and decreased in the corn and wheat trials (P <0.05). Group means with the same letters at the same times are not significantly different. (Adapted from Paul, G. L. et al., *J. Nutr.,* 126, 1372, 1996.)

trials, glutamine formation increased. Conversely, glutamine concentration decreased during the fed trials (Figure 4).

In a second study, we utilized rats to examine the plasma glutamine/alanine relationship during recovery after 2 hr of exhaustive treadmill exercise.[10] Food was withheld from male rats 5 hr prior to exercise. Immediately after exercise, animals were fed via stomach tube either a nutritionally complete meal (M) or an isocaloric carbohydrate meal (CHO) corresponding to 15% of their daily energy intake or were food restricted (R). No difference existed in plasma insulin concentrations between M and CHO, but values were 3-fold higher than R. Hyperinsulinemia is known to stimulate skeletal muscle BCAA uptake and consequently lower plasma BCAA levels.[33] Accordingly, plasma BCAA concentrations were lower in CHO- and M-fed animals than R.

Enhanced plasma BCAA uptake by skeletal muscle increases the muscle free BCAA pool. Since the BCAAT reaction is essentially at equilibrium, increasing the muscle free BCAA pool elevates concentrations of the products, α-keto acids and glutamate.[21] To help discern the fate of muscle glutamate in the exercised animals, we measured plasma concentrations of alanine and glutamine. Plasma alanine concentrations were 25 and 100% greater in CHO and M, respectively, compared to R while plasma glutamine was 35 and 60% greater in R than M and CHO, respectively. These data suggest that BCAA flux through BCAAT was lower in R than CHO. BCAAT activity was likely highest in the M group since exogenous and endogenous BCAA were available to the muscles. These findings are in agreement with our earlier work examining BCAA oxidation in muscles.[4] Alanine synthesis, via pyruvate transamination with glutamate, was favored after CHO or M ingestion compared to R.

The muscle pyruvate pool in the R group was likely compromised. Such a condition would favor glutamine formation and release by muscle. A greater flux through BCAAT after M ingestion would explain the higher plasma alanine and glutamine concentrations compared to CHO, assuming that plasma alanine and glutamine removal was similar for the two groups. Alanine and glutamine absorption after the M feeding undoubtedly accounted for some of the difference between CHO and M, but absorption alone could not account for the large discrepancy. In addition to the relationship of alanine and glutamine, we also found inverse correlations between plasma alanine and leucine concentrations and plasma insulin and glutamine concentrations. These findings support the early hypothesis of Felig's group that plasma alanine appearance (muscle release) was related to plasma leucine disappearance (muscle uptake) and that plasma glutamine appearance was associated with non-fed conditions.[16]

Our results are consistent with the reasoning that the fate of muscle-free glutamate depends on pyruvate availability. If pyruvate is available, alanine formation and release is favored. Under conditions when the pyruvate supply is compromised such as fasting, nitrogen removal from muscle will proceed predominantly through glutamine.

The capacity of skeletal muscle for net amino acid degradation is limited, with the exception of the BCAA, aspartate, asparagine, and glutamate.[34] As mentioned above, BCKAD activity, the rate-limiting step in muscle BCAA oxidation, is increased during exercise.[4,24,35,36] This finding is consistent with direct evidence demonstrating increased ^{13}C-leucine oxidation rates during exercise.[37-40]

Carbohydrate intake before and during exercise appears to influence plasma BCAA changes. MacLean et al.[41] had subjects consume low-, moderate-, or high-carbohydrate diets for three days before cycling to exhaustion. When subjects consumed the low-carbohydrate diet, BCAA concentrations dropped 15–25% during exercise compared to the other groups. The moderate- and high-carbohydrate groups did not differ. In a separate study, volunteers that exercised to exhaustion with low pre-exercise glycogen stores experienced a 20–30% decrease in plasma BCAA concentrations whereas glycogen-loaded subjects were unaffected.[36] In addition, the authors noted that BCKAD activity increased 3.6-fold in the glycogen-depleted subjects. These data corroborate earlier reports that subjects with depleted glycogen stores at the start of exercise derive a greater percentage of their fuel requirement for exercise from amino acids compared to glycogen-loaded subjects.[31,42]

Plasma BCAA concentrations also decrease when carbohydrate is consumed during exercise. Davis et al.[43] had trained cyclists consume either a water placebo or 6 or 12% carbohydrate beverages while cycling to exhaustion. During the water placebo trial, BCAA did not change. However, BCAA decreased 15 and 25% during the 6 and 12% trials, respectively. Compared to the water placebo, plasma insulin concentrations increased when the 6 and 12% carbohydrate beverages were ingested leading the authors to conclude that insulin stimulated skeletal muscle BCAA uptake. Blomstrand et al.[44] observed nearly a 30% decrease in BCAA in subjects consuming a 5% carbohydrate beverage during a 30 km cross-country race, and Rennie et al.[32] reported a similar decrease in subjects consuming a glucose syrup every 15 min for 2 hr during treadmill exercise.

Exercise duration can also affect plasma BCAA responses. Short-duration endurance exercise (less than 45 min) does not appear to alter BCAA levels regardless of intensity,[45] whereas prolonged exercise (greater than 3 hr) apparently decreases plasma BCAA concentrations. After 3.75 hr of treadmill walking, Rennie et al.[37] found that plasma BCAA concentrations decline approximately 20%. Plasma BCAA concentrations are depressed 15–30% by 90 min bouts of running and cycling,[46] whereas ultraendurance activities such as a 100 km run or a 70 km cross-country ski race abate plasma BCAA levels 30–45%.[47,48]

Interpreting how prolonged exercise affects plasma BCAA concentrations is difficult because subjects in studies by Rennie et al.[37] and Refsum et al.[48] ingested carbohydrate throughout exercise. Though not reported, it is highly probable that carbohydrate was ingested by subjects during the 100 km run since carbohydrate foods and beverages are commonly consumed in these events.[49] Thus, insulin-stimulated BCAA uptake during exercise could have occurred as reported by Davis et al.[43]

BCAA movement from splanchnic tissue to muscle with the return of alanine to the liver and glutamine to the gut typifies the extensive interorgan amino acid exchanges that occur during exercise. The details of the organ-to-organ exchanges are summarized in the legend for Figure 1. The BCAA metabolized by muscle during exercise originate mostly from the plasma BCAA pool as we and others have reported significant plasma BCAA losses during exercise.[8,37,46-48] As discussed below, such losses have been implicated in causing fatigue during prolonged exercise and suggest a need for increased amino acid consumption during intensive exercise training.

D. BRANCHED-CHAIN AMINO ACIDS AND CENTRAL FATIGUE

Mood, performance, and the sense of well-being are all associated with levels of substances in the brain called neurotransmitters. While this research area remains to be elucidated, it is clear that neurotransmitters are important to brain function and can affect behavior and mood. One of the most studied of the neurotransmitters is serotonin.

A decrease in plasma BCAA concentrations during exercise may negatively affect exercise performance via changes in serotonin. Serotonin is synthesized in the brain from the amino acid tryptophan. The rate-limiting step in serotonin synthesis is brain uptake of plasma tryptophan since the brain enzymes involved in serotonin synthesis have a high capacity and do not approach saturation with substrate.[50,51] Furthermore, the rate constant of the committed step in serotonin synthesis, tryptophan hydroxylase, is similar to or above tissue tryptophan concentration.[52] Since tryptophan competes with BCAA and the other large-neutral amino acids phenylalanine, tyrosine, and methionine for brain uptake[53] (Figure 5), declining plasma BCAA concentrations during exercise would enhance brain tryptophan uptake. Hence, brain serotonin levels would increase, and in turn, compromise exercise performance via a sedative effect on the central nervous system. This is commonly referred to as the central fatigue hypothesis.[54]

Plasma tryptophan is found either circulating freely or bound to albumin.[55] The free form constitutes only 15–20% of total plasma tryptophan but can increase markedly during prolonged exercise as plasma free fatty acid (FFA) concentrations rise.[43,56] Plasma FFA elevations increase plasma free tryptophan levels by displacing the bound form of tryptophan from albumin.[56] In fact, increases in plasma free tryptophan directly correlate to plasma FFA increases during prolonged exercise.[43] This FFA effect during exercise may be important because free tryptophan is more available for transport into the brain than the bound form.[55]

Although the central fatigue hypothesis is physiologically sound, researchers have failed to link changes in plasma BCAA, tryptophan, or the ratio of tryptophan to the sum of the other large-neutral amino acids (trp:LNAA) with effects on exercise performance. We failed to observe any performance differences during a 6.4 km time trial that followed the 90 min of cycling exercise at 60% $\dot{V}O_2$ max described earlier,[8] even though there were significant trp:LNAA ratio differences among the oat, corn, wheat, and fasting groups at the start of the performance ride.[9] We concluded that although statistically significant, our trp:LNAA ratio differences were insufficient to impact physical performance.

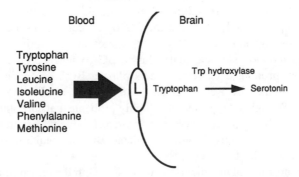

FIGURE 5 Competition for uptake of the large-neutral amino acids by the L-transport system (L) at the blood-brain barrier. A decrease of the other large-neutral amino acids relative to tryptophan favors brain tryptophan uptake. Tryptophan is readily converted to serotonin within the brain in a reaction catalyzed by tryptophan (Trp) hydroxylase.

Functionally significant trp:LNAA ratio differences were likely generated in the recent study by van Hall and others.[57] To induce large plasma BCAA and tryptophan concentration changes, subjects ingested a 6% carbohydrate beverage supplemented with tryptophan or a low or high dose of BCAA during a cycling ride to exhaustion at 70% $\dot{V}O_2$ max. Plasma amino acid changes associated with the high BCAA trial were estimated to reduce brain tryptophan uptake at exhaustion by 8–12% whereas tryptophan supplementation was estimated to increase tryptophan uptake 7- to 20-fold. Despite large plasma BCAA and tryptophan changes, no treatment differences were detected for the ride time to exhaustion. The authors suggested that serotoninergic activity during prolonged exhaustive exercise is unaffected by alterations in tryptophan supply or that manipulation of serotoninergic activity does not contribute to fatigue.

In a similar study, Blomstrand et al.[58] had glycogen-depleted subjects consume a 6% carbohydrate solution alone or supplemented with BCAA, or a water placebo during an exhaustive ride at 75% $\dot{V}O_2$ max. Ride time to exhaustion was improved during both carbohydrate trials compared to the water placebo. Although plasma BCAA concentrations increased 120% during the BCAA supplemented trials, no difference existed between the carbohydrate-containing beverages. BCAA infusion into glycogen-depleted subjects also does not appear to improve exercise performance.[59]

Blomstrand et al.[44] did report physical performance improvements when BCAAs were supplemented during a 42.2 km marathon competition. Compared to placebo ingestion, ingestion of the BCAA solution increased plasma BCAA concentrations by 140%. The authors suggested that this maintained a more favorable trp:LNAA ratio although ratio values were not reported. However, marathon times were not statistically different between placebo and BCAA groups until run times were subdivided into faster runners (less than 3.05 hr) and slower runners (3.05–3.30 hr). The rationale for selecting these cutoffs was not provided. In the same paper, subjects competing in a 30 km cross-country race, who also received BCAA supplementation during exercise, did not improve performance times. Hence, BCAA supplementation during either event did not appear to influence exercise performance.

Although physical performance may not be affected by plasma BCAA or tryptophan changes during exercise, such changes can influence post-exercise measurements of mood and cognitive performance. Our laboratory[8,9] measured plasma tryptophan and BCAA concentrations 30 and 60 min after subjects cycled 90 min then completed a 6.4 km performance ride. Plasma BCAA concentrations declined to below pre-meal and pre-exercise levels in all groups indicating a net BCAA loss from plasma.[8] The plasma trp:LNAA ratio was significantly higher during recovery in the fasting trial compared to the trials when a pre-exercise meal was ingested (Figure 6).[9] Perceptions of fatigue were also greater in the fasting trial compared to the fed trials, although no treatment effects were observed for the results of several cognitive tests.[9]

Other researchers have shown cognitive performance improvements during exercise recovery when subjects ingested BCAAs during exercise. Plasma trp:LNAA ratios were not reported in a study by Hassmén et al.,[60] but such supplementation is known to attenuate exercise-induced trp:LNAA ratio increases by elevating plasma BCAA concentrations. The authors evaluated performance on several cognitive tasks before and within the 1 hr after a 30-km cross-country run. During the run, subjects consumed either a mixture of BCAAs in a 5% carbohydrate solution or a placebo drink containing only the carbohydrates. When subjects consumed the BCAA during exercise, performance significantly improved on the more difficult tasks and was maintained on others. Scores on the latter tasks declined when the placebo was ingested. Interestingly, fatigue perception also tended to be higher when the placebo was ingested. These studies demonstrate that plasma tryptophan and LNAA changes during and after exercise are likely to have a greater influence on mood and mental acuity than physical performance.

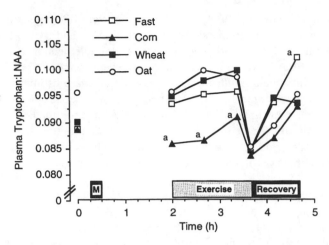

FIGURE 6 Plasma tryptophan:large-neutral amino acid (LNAA) ratio responses before and after subjects ingested either a corn, wheat, or oat cereal meal (M), and during cycling exercise and recovery. Values represent the mean of 12 subjects. a = significantly different from all corresponding time values (p <0.05). Increased perceptions of fatigue corresponded to the large increase in the ratio during the recovery period in the fasting trial compared to the fed trials. (From Paul, G. L. et al., *Am. J. Clin. Nutr.*, 64, 778, 1996. With permission from the American Institute of Nutrition.)

In summary, as carbohydrate stores become limited during exercise, plasma BCAA concentrations decline. This likely results from increased muscle BCAA uptake and oxidation associated with increased BCKAD activity. Carbohydrate ingested during exercise also lowers plasma BCAA concentrations, possibly by stimulating muscle BCAA uptake via modest increases in plasma insulin concentration. The decline in plasma BCAA concentrations during exercise (excluding ultra-endurance events) is approximately 20–30% irrespective of carbohydrate intake before or during exercise. This decline continues to occur during the first hour of recovery. Such declines in plasma BCAA are hypothesized to play a role in fatigue by favoring brain uptake of tryptophan, the precursor for serotonin synthesis. Although research in humans has failed to show that plasma trp:LNAA ratio changes alter exercise performance, such changes do affect measurements of cognitive reasoning and fatigue perception during the initial hour of recovery.

II. PROTEIN TURNOVER ASSOCIATED WITH EXERCISE

Muscle protein mass is determined by the relationship between the processes of protein synthesis and degradation. During periods of growth or protein accretion, protein synthesis rates exceed protein degradation rates. Growth thus results in a net accumulation of protein or positive balance of protein turnover. When rates of protein synthesis and degradation are equal, the period is defined as maintenance or net balance. Most of the research addressing changes in amino acid metabolism during exercise have examined the effects of endurance exercise and have focused on the use of amino acids as fuels. Few studies have examined changes in protein turnover during resistance exercise designed to produce muscle hypertrophy.

Studies examining the molecular basis for muscle hypertrophy have relied on animal models and used surgical procedures, weights, or chronic electrically stimulated contractions to produce chronic resistance or stretch on specific muscles.[61-65] Muscle hypertrophy appears to require full extension of the muscle and resistance, while high intensity levels and extended exercise durations do not produce hypertrophy. These procedures rapidly increase muscle weight and protein content and correspondingly increase muscle RNA content and protein synthesis rates. At the molecular level, these experimental models indicate that skeletal muscle hypertrophy is dependent upon stimulating transcription to increase muscle protein synthesis. The regulatory controls and limits of this response remain unknown.

Physical activity and exercise training are generally assumed to result in maintenance or enlargement of skeletal muscles; however, there is also general consensus that during endurance exercise protein synthesis is suppressed.[37,40,66-68] The magnitude of the depression in protein synthesis appears to be proportional to the duration and intensity of the activity.

While protein synthesis is suppressed during exercise, the effects of exercise on protein degradation are less clear. Reports indicate that protein degradation is increased,[37,69] decreased,[70] or unchanged.[40,68] These divergent responses are likely due to the different experimental protocols employed by the investigators. It is our belief that acute protein turnover changes, such as those observed during exercise and early recovery, are regulated more by changes in protein synthesis than degradation. Therefore, the following section will briefly discuss the various proteolytic pathways but will primarily focus on the effects of exercise on protein synthesis. Several review articles are available for readers interested in more detailed discussions about protein degradation during exercise.[5,19,71,72]

Protein breakdown occurs through four distinct pathways: (a) ATP-dependent, (b) ATP-independent, (c) calcium-dependent, and (d) lysosomal. The ATP-dependent pathway may or may not require protein conjugation with ubiquitin, a step which marks the protein for degradation through a pathway involving two large proteases. Although the ATP-dependent pathway is well defined, the proteases associated with the ATP-independent pathway are unknown. The calcium-dependent pathway involves the proteases calpains I and II whereas a wide array of cathepsins comprise the lysosomal pathway.

The calcium-dependent and lysosomal pathways are involved in increasing protein degradation rates after exercise. In muscles from exercised rats, 1 hr of exhaustive treadmill running nearly doubles calpain-mediated degradation rates,[73] whereas 1 hr of mild intensity swimming elevates cathepsin D activity.[74] An increase in calcium-dependent protease activity did not occur in the latter study,[74] suggesting that proteolytic pathway activities may be related to exercise mode, exercise intensity, or both. The roles of the ATP-independent and ATP-dependent pathways during exercise are unknown although the latter is upregulated after 1 d of food deprivation.[75] The mechanism of this upregulation involves enhanced gene expression of several pathway components including ubiquitin and subunits of the protease.[75,76] Although the ATP-dependent pathway is responsible for most of the accelerated proteolysis in early fasting, its contribution to the acute degradative responses associated with exercise is likely minimal since increased pathway activity is conferred at the transcriptional level.

One of the first reports of the influence of exercise on protein synthesis was by Dohm et al.,[74] examining protein synthesis in perfused rat muscles after exercise. These investigators noted that 1 hr of mild exercise produced by swimming decreased protein synthesis by 17%. A more strenuous 1 hr bout of treadmill exercise (28 m/min) decreased protein synthesis by 30%, whereas protein synthesis declined by 70% after an exhaustive 2–5 hr run. These results suggest that the extent of exercise-induced depression in muscle protein synthesis is dependent upon exercise intensity and duration. In support of this conclusion, rats exercising only 40 min at 21.5 m/min did not experience decreased muscle protein synthesis rates.[77]

Dohm et al.[69] also examined the effects of exhaustive running on protein degradation. They ran rats at 28 m/min for 4 hr and measured the urinary excretion of urea and 3-methylhistidine. Urea excretion increased by 31% during the first 12 hr after the exhaustive exercise bout. Urinary 3-methylhistidine, which is an indicator of muscle protein breakdown, also increased after exercise. However, the 3-methylhistidine increase did not occur until 12–36 hr after exercise. The studies by Dohm's group indicate that exhaustive exercise produces a catabolic condition in skeletal muscle by suppressing protein synthesis rates and stimulating protein degradation.[67,69,74]

Prolonged exercise also produces a catabolic state in humans. Rennie and others had 6 subjects complete 3.75 hr of treadmill exercise at 50% $\dot{V}O_2$ max and measured rates of protein synthesis and degradation.[37] Protein synthesis rates during exercise decreased 14% while degradation rates increased 54%. This study is also important because it is one of the few studies to make measurements during recovery after exercise. These investigators found that after exercise, synthesis rates increased 22% above the initial resting levels while protein degradation returned to pre-exercise levels. Similarly, Carraro and colleagues showed that 4-hr protein synthesis recovery values were elevated 22% compared to nonexercise conditions.[78] These investigators also found that production of some acute-phase proteins occurs in the liver during the early hours of recovery.[79] Synthesis of these proteins may provide a transient pool for other amino acids released by protein breakdown during exercise. In addition, skeletal muscle protein synthesis rates increase during the 24-hr following weight-lifting exercise.[80] Together, protein turnover changes after exercise suggest that recovery from both endurance and strength exercise is driven by increases in protein synthesis.

In vitro animal studies demonstrate that the decline in protein synthesis following exercise is independent of previous exercise training. Muscle incorporation rates of radio-labeled phenylalanine were measured in trained and untrained rats after a 2-hr swim. When values were compared to nonexercised rats, protein synthesis rates decreased approximately 30% irrespective of the trained state.[81,82]

The choice of metabolic tracer used to quantitate protein synthesis and degradation rates can influence the results and interpretations. Using a constant infusion of labeled leucine and lysine, Wolfe et al.[40,68] found decreases in protein synthesis of 48 and 17%, respectively, during 105 min of cycling exercise at 30% $\dot{V}O_2$ max. While both amino acids demonstrated that exercise inhibited protein synthesis, the magnitude of the response was significantly different depending on the amino acid tracer selected. These findings also suggest that while amino acid requirements for exercise appear to increase, the magnitude of the increase may be specific for each amino acid with the potential for unique effects on the BCAA.

While the acute effect of exercise on protein turnover is catabolic, the long-term effects of routine exercise do not lead to muscle atrophy. Routine exercise produces maintenance or hypertrophy of muscle mass. Only a few studies have looked at post-exercise recovery of protein turnover. Reports by Rennie et al.[37] and Devlin et al.[83] suggest that recovery occurs through stimulation of protein synthesis. We have also reported that within 4–8 hr following 2 hr of treadmill exercise at 26 m/min, protein synthesis rates in male rats recover to nonexercise control levels (Figure 7).[4]

A.   EFFECT OF FOOD INTAKE ON SHORT-TERM CHANGES IN PROTEIN SYNTHESIS

In our study,[4] muscle protein synthesis rates were depressed 26–30% 1 hr after exercise. We next examined if feeding the animals a 10 kcal (42 kJ) meal (approximately 15% of daily energy intake) of either a complete nutritional supplement or carbohydrate immediately after exercise could abate the suppressed protein synthesis rates observed 1 hr after exercise.[10] Feeding the carbohydrate meal after exercise attenuated the fall in protein synthesis, but rates were still 10% lower than nonexercised control animals. When animals were fed the complete nutritional supplement, protein synthesis rates were significantly greater than carbohydrate-fed animals and 8% greater than nonexercised control animals. Plasma insulin concentrations did not differ between feeding regimens and were 3-fold higher than controls. Correlation analyses revealed that protein synthesis rates were inversely related to plasma leucine concentration and directly related with plasma alanine concentration. These results indicate that an elevated flux through BCAAT is associated with minimizing the perturbations in protein synthesis induced by exercise. From a practical standpoint, these data suggest that feeding a nutritionally complete meal after exercise is more efficacious than feeding carbohydrate alone

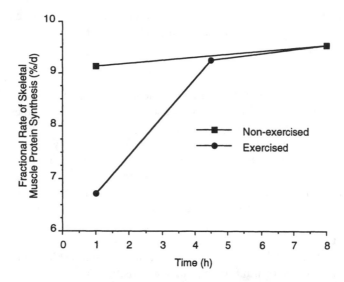

FIGURE 7 *In vivo* protein synthesis was determined in rats by constant infusion of ^{3}H-L-leucine after a 2-h exhaustive run on a motor-driven treadmill at 26 m/min. Control animals did not exercise. All animals were restricted from food for 20 hr prior to the experiment. Animals were killed at three time points during recovery and the fractional synthesis rate was determined for the gastrocnemius muscle. The exercise value at 1 hr is significantly different from all other (P <0.05). Pooled SEM is ±0.2%/d, N = 4. (Paul and Layman, unpublished data.)

for abating the exercise-induced decrease in muscle protein synthesis present during the early recovery hours.

Our animal data also demonstrate that increasing plasma insulin concentrations alone does not restore skeletal muscle protein synthesis rates after exercise; a supply of adequate amino acids is also required. This finding supports the recent work of Yoshizawa et al.[84] who induced a catabolic state in mice by withholding food for 18 hr. Muscle protein synthesis was stimulated after 1 hr by refeeding a nutritionally complete meal containing protein but not when protein was removed. As in our study, plasma insulin concentrations did not differ between meal conditions. When the insulin response to the complete meal was blocked with insulin anti-serum, the stimulatory effect on muscle protein synthesis was lost. The results of the above studies indicate that elevations in both plasma insulin and amino acids are essential for stimulating muscle protein synthesis during catabolic states, a conclusion supporting earlier data.[85]

B. MECHANISMS AND CONTROLS OF PROTEIN SYNTHESIS

Controls of muscle protein synthesis during and after exercise remain unknown. This section will discuss possible mechanisms involved in suppressing protein synthesis which helps create the catabolic state observed during endurance exercise.

As mentioned previously, high-intensity, exhaustive exercise bouts transiently decreases muscle protein synthesis rates. This effect is controlled presumably at the translational level of protein synthesis. Transcription is depressed, but RNA concentrations are unchanged during the relatively brief period of the exercise bout.

Translation of mRNA into protein is one of the most complex processes in biology and is a major consumer of energy in the cell. Translation can be divided into three phases: initiation, which implies the successful formation of the 80S ribosomal initiation complex; elongation, during which the mRNA is translated into protein; and termination, signified by the release of the completed protein from the ribosome. Potential regulatory controls of translation include (1) amino acid availability, (2) the energy state of the cell, (3) initiation factors, and (4) endocrine factors. Of these potential controls, the initiation factors and endocrine factors are of particular interest to us and will therefore be the primary focus of this section.

1. Amino Acid Availability

Exercise produces changes in plasma and tissue amino acid concentrations which could cause individual amino acids to be limiting as substrates for protein synthesis. The BCAA, alanine, and glutamine are the primary amino acids affected by exercise. As discussed earlier, levels of these amino acids in plasma during exercise depend heavily on the nutritional state of the individual. While plasma amino acid concentrations change during exercise, availability of amino acid substrates for muscle protein synthesis appears to be an unlikely level of control for several reasons. First, muscle contraction increases skeletal muscle amino acid uptake.[86] Second, exercise produces a temporary decrease and increase in muscle protein synthesis and degradation, respectively.[19,71,72] Taken together, these conditions assure a constant supply of amino acid precursors for protein synthesis. Additionally, the rate constant for tRNA synthetase is well below skeletal muscle amino acid concentrations which indicates that tRNA charging is not a likely factor limiting protein synthesis.[87]

2. Energy State of the Cell

Several researchers[12,70,88] have suggested that the energy state of the cell is the primary factor regulating protein synthesis. Decreases in the adenine nucleotide pool have been reported after *in vivo* muscle contraction.[70,88] Moreover, researchers have shown a direct relationship between decreases in muscle protein synthesis and muscle ATP concentrations.[12,70] Energy-requiring steps in translation include tRNA charging, dephosphorylation of eukaryotic initiation factor-2 (eIF-2), and subsequent formation of the ternary initiation complex, eIF-4F binding to mRNA, scanning of the mRNA for the correct starting site, and elongation of the growing peptide.

3. Initiation Factors

The majority of translational control of protein synthesis lies in the initiation phase, a complex sequence of steps involving at least 12 known eIFs.[89,90] A summary of the key steps and eIFs involved in the initiation phase of translation is illustrated in Figure 8.

Kinetic studies of translation indicate that there are two key regulatory steps in the initiation process.[91] The first regulation site in the initiation of protein synthesis is formation of the ternary initiation complex which occurs only if the initiation factor eIF-2 is bound with GTP. Consequently, after one round of initiation, eIF-2 is released bound to GDP. This GDP must be exchanged for GTP before eIF-2 can bind met-tRNA and participate in another round of initiation.[92] The guanine nucleotide exchange factor, eIF-2B, catalyzes this reaction, and regulates formation of the ternary initiation complex.[93]

eIF-2B activity can be modulated several ways, but by far the best studied mechanism is inhibition via phosphorylation of the α-subunit of eIF-2.[94] When phosphorylated, the affinity of the eIF-2 · GDP complex for eIF-2B is more than 100-fold greater than when unphosphorylated.[90] As a result, free eIF-2B becomes sequestered into an inactive complex, inhibiting the GDP exchange for GTP and subsequent initiation. Although eIF-2 phosphorylation changes have clearly been shown in liver, studies attempting to show this mechanism in skeletal muscle have not been successful.[90]

Another mechanism of altered eIF-2B activity less defined but suggested to occur in skeletal muscle involves phosphorylation of the ε-subunit of eIF-2B.[93,95] Three different protein kinases alter the activity of eIF-2B *in vitro*; however, it is inconclusive as to whether eIF-2B phosphorylation stimulates or inhibits its activity *in vivo*.[93,95,96]

The second key regulation step in the initiation of protein synthesis is recognition and unfolding of the mRNA to allow formation of the 48S pre-initiation complex.[91] This step

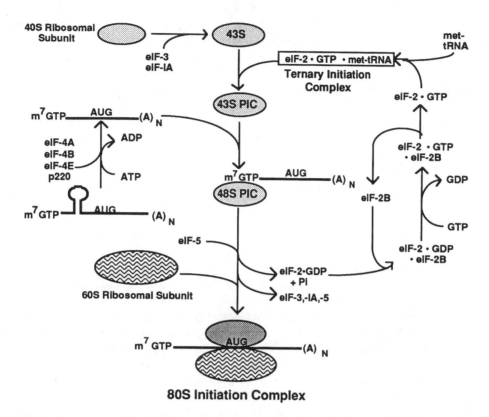

80S Initiation Complex

FIGURE 8 A summary of the initiation phase of translation. The initial steps of initiation involve the formation of a 43S ribosomal complex (40S ribosome + eukaryotic initiation factors [eIFs] 3 and IA) and a Ternary Initiation Complex (TIC; eIF-2 + GTP + met-tRNA). The TIC then binds the 43S ribosomal complex, resulting in a 43S Pre-Initiation Complex (PIC). Selected mRNA attachment to the 43S PIC forms the 48S PIC (m7GTP refers to the methylated GTP residue that "caps" the 5' terminus of eukaryotic mRNA). This step involves several other eIFs, namely eIF-4A, -4B, -4E and -4γ (p220). One of the functions of the eIFs at this step is to facilitate unwinding of secondary structures in the mRNA that are typically found between the 5' terminus and the translation start site (the AUG codon which codes for the methionine moiety of the TIC). Once the 43S PIC is properly positioned at the AUG codon, eIF-5 mediates hydrolysis of eIF-2-bound-GTP. This step releases all eIFs bound to the 48S PIC which allows for binding of the 60S ribosomal subunit to complete the formation of an active 80S ribosome. The newly formed 80S initiation complex then proceeds with the elongation phase of protein synthesis.

involves the group four eukaryotic initiation factors, namely: eIF-4A, eIF-4B, eIF-4E, and eIF-4γ (p220). Collectively, eIF-4A, eIF-4E, and p220 are referred to as eIF-4F. The group four eIF's facilitate initiation by binding to the mRNA and altering its structure. This allows for efficient movement of the ribosome along the mRNA to the start site for the elongation phase of protein synthesis.[89,91]

As with formation of the ternary initiation complex, phosphorylation plays a key role in formation of the 48S pre-initiation complex. One of the most studied factors in this regard is eIF-4E. eIF-4E is rapidly phosphorylated in response to hormones and growth factors,[97,98] resulting in a 3- to 4-fold increased affinity for mRNA binding than the nonphosphorylated form.[99] Increasing the phosphorylated form of eIF-4E is associated with enhanced eIF-4F activity and subsequently, increased protein synthesis rates. Another mechanism regulating eIF-4E activity involves a specific binding protein, termed 4E-BP1 (eIF-4E binding protein-1), or PHAS-I.[97,100] Nonphosphorylated 4E-BP1 specifically interacts with eIF-4E to inhibit mRNA binding and decrease translation rates.[100,101] Conversely, the interaction between eIF-4E and 4E-BP1 is diminished upon 4E-BP1 phosphorylation, allowing eIF-4E to bind mRNA and enhance translation rates.[101,102]

In summary, protein synthesis during exercise and recovery is thought to be regulated mostly at the level of translation efficiency, for this type of regulation allows the cell to alter protein synthesis rates rapidly and to reverse any alteration equally as rapidly. Short-term changes in translation rates are highly regulated by the activity of the eIFs, and phosphorylation/dephosphorylation appears to be the most prevalent control mechanism. The two key steps in the initiation process, namely the formation of the ternary initiation complex and the binding of the mRNA to the 43S pre-initiation complex, are potential sites where exercise-induced changes in protein synthesis may occur.

4.   Endocrine Factors

Endurance exercise also alters hormones and growth factors implicated in the regulation of muscle protein synthesis including insulin, growth hormone (GH), and insulin-like growth factor-I (IGF-I). Insulin appears to regulate both the initiation and elongation phases of translation,[103] but very little data exists directly addressing the role of insulin with respect to the regulation of protein synthesis rates during and following exercise. Insulin secretion is suppressed at the onset of exercise and remains blunted throughout, even when blood glucose levels rise. This has led some authors[104] to classify aerobic exercise as an insulin-deficient state.

The role insulin plays in regulating muscle protein synthesis rates after exercise is unclear. Balon et al.[105] failed to observe increases in protein synthesis or decreases in protein degradation in perfused rat muscles after high or moderate intensity exercise even though glucose and amino acid transport were stimulated. Thus, instead of directly stimulating the biosynthetic process, insulin might play a permissive role by facilitating or inducing the protein synthetic machinery.

Circulating GH levels are transiently increased by exercise.[106] This effect appears to be dependent on the intensity of exercise, as anaerobic forms of exercise are associated with higher GH release than aerobic forms.[107] GH has been shown by our laboratory (unpublished data) and others to promote protein anabolism by repartitioning available energy toward lean body mass and away from fat deposition.[108] Because exercise increases GH concentrations and the effects of exercise on body composition are similar to that of GH administration, it follows that GH may play a functional role in regulating muscle protein synthesis rates after exercise. However, the combination of exogenous GH treatment and exercise does not show additive or even significant increases in either muscle mass or muscle protein synthesis rates. Both Deyssig et al.[109] and Yarasheski et al.[110] failed to demonstrate further increases in muscle strength, size, or protein synthesis rates in young men by combining GH therapy with resistance exercise. Additionally, Yeh et al.[111] observed that administration of exogenous GH did not potentiate the effect of treadmill exercise on lean body mass in rats and Cooper et al.[112] found that endogenous GH did not play a role in increasing $\dot{V}O_2$ max, treadmill running time, or muscle succinate dehydrogenase activity (an indicator of aerobic conditioning) in rats during 4 wk of training. Thus, the marked improvement seen in cardiorespiratory function with exercise training is independent of GH. Despite the work done in this field, it remains unclear why circulating GH levels increase during exercise.

Many of GH's actions are mediated by insulin-like growth factor-I (IGF-I). IGF-I is synthesized in most tissues, including skeletal muscle, and it can act locally within the tissue or be released from the liver in response to circulating GH.[113] In addition, significant numbers of IGF-I receptors are detected in skeletal muscle.[114] The biological activity of IGF-I in serum and other extracellular fluids is modulated by at least six different highly specific insulin-like growth factor binding proteins (IGFBPs; IGFBP-1,-2,-3,-4,-5,-6). IGFBPs in extracellular fluids act to increase the half-life of IGF-I and/or block IGF activity whereas IGFBPs on the cell surface may enhance IGF-I activity.[115]

IGF-I is a potent stimulator of cell growth and differentiation in skeletal muscle.[113] Locally produced IGF-I may also be an important modulator of muscle protein synthesis, since synthesis rates after starvation/refeeding are proportional to changes in skeletal muscle IGF-I mRNA expression.[116] In addition, IGF-I stimulates protein synthesis by increasing the phosphorylation of 4E-BP1.[101] These findings suggest that IGF-I produced within muscle is involved in regulating protein synthesis at the level of translation initiation.

Serum IGF-I responses to exercise do not necessarily predict skeletal muscle IGF-I responses. Our laboratory[117] and others[118] have found no significant changes in serum IGF-I levels either with an acute bout of exercise or with endurance training. However, skeletal muscle IGF-I gene expression is enhanced in response to increased muscle load or exercise, even in the absence of GH.[119,120] These findings further support a role for muscle-derived IGF-I in regulating protein synthesis. Moreover, our laboratory and others have found that exercise increases circulating IGFBP-1 levels and strongly induces IGFBP-1 gene expression.[117,118,121] This finding may be important for IGF-I bioactivity in skeletal muscle since IGFBP-1 can potentially bring IGF-I to the muscle to exert its anabolic effects.

Exercise is associated with acute changes in serum insulin and GH concentrations. Insulin secretion is suppressed at the onset and throughout exercise whereas GH secretion is enhanced proportionately to the exercise intensity. Neither insulin nor GH appear to directly regulate muscle protein synthesis. However, insulin may facilitate the activity of other factors known to influence muscle protein synthesis rates including the eIF's whereas GH may exert its anabolic effect via IGF-I. Although no apparent association exists between serum IGF-I levels and rates of muscle protein synthesis, recent studies indicate that IGF-I produced within muscle in response to exercise may modulate muscle protein synthesis rates during recovery.

III. PHYSICAL ACTIVITY AND PROTEIN REQUIREMENTS

Exercise-induced changes in amino acid metabolism suggest an increased need for dietary amino acids (i.e., an increased protein requirement). During exercise, these changes include depression of muscle and whole body protein synthesis rates and apparent elevations in protein degradation.[5,12,71] Decreased protein synthesis and elevated degradation increases free amino acid availability for oxidation to energy and also for increased synthesis of stress-induced proteins.[79] In total, these changes lead to a net increase in amino acid use.

During recovery after exercise, muscle protein synthesis recovers to pre-exercise or nonexercised levels allowing the muscles to shift to an anabolic state for recovery. If the anabolic period leads to increased muscle mass, some increase in dietary protein is also required to support this growth.

The current Recommended Dietary Allowance (RDA) for protein (0.8 g/kg/d) is based on data derived primarily from sedentary subjects.[7] Because the RDA already contains a safety margin of 0.35 g/kg/d to assure adequate protein intake, no increment is added for work or training.[7] Recently, collective evidence from research techniques utilizing urea production, 3-methylhistidine excretion, and labeled amino acid isotopes indicates that both strength and endurance exercise increase amino acid utilization. Furthermore, results of nitrogen balance studies clearly show that the protein requirements of strength and endurance athletes exceed the current RDA. The following sections will review studies that demonstrate an increased protein need for those who regularly train. Furthermore, studies examining the effect of increased protein consumption on exercise performance and changes in body composition will be discussed.

A. EVIDENCE FOR INCREASED PROTEIN UTILIZATION DURING ENDURANCE AND STRENGTH EXERCISE

1. Urea Production

The major end products of amino acid degradation are carbon dioxide and urea. Urea is formed in the liver via the urea cycle and is the major route of nitrogen removal from the body (Figure 1). After formation, urea is released into the blood and is removed by the kidney and sweat glands.[122] Because urea formation is linked with amino acid degradation, increases in blood, urine, or sweat urea indicate an increase in protein breakdown.[123]

In general, serum and sweat urea increase during exercise while urinary urea decreases, changes that could result from hemoconcentration, an increased breakdown of amino acids and/or a decrease in urea clearance by the kidney. For example, Cerny[124] studied subjects cycling at 60–65% $\dot{V}O_2$ max for 2 hr. Both sweat and serum urea concentrations increased by 20% during exercise whereas urinary urea decreased by 50%. It was concluded that amino acids from protein degradation were available for conversion into urea during the 2-hr cycling session.

Rennie et al.[37] noted increased plasma urea and decreased urinary urea production during 3.75 hr of cycling at 50% $\dot{V}O_2$ max. Throughout the 24-hr recovery period, plasma urea concentration remained elevated. When renal clearance resumed normal rates 5 hr after exercise, urinary urea excretion showed marked increases that also lasted throughout recovery. From the urea data, the authors calculated that protein supplied 4–8% of the energy required for the exercise session.

Obtaining an accurate measurement of urea excreted in sweat is an important consideration if urea production is chosen to monitor protein and amino acid degradation during exercise. During 90 min of cycling at 45% $\dot{V}O_2$ max, Calles-Escandon et al.[125] showed that 30% of the total urea excretion was in the form of sweat losses. Lemon and Mullin[31] noted 154- and 66-fold increases in sweat urea nitrogen during 1 hr of cycling at 60% $\dot{V}O_2$ max in glycogen-depleted and glycogen-loaded subjects, respectively.

Urea production during exercise is apparently dependent upon exercise intensity. Subjects performing treadmill exercise at 41, 55, and 67% $\dot{V}O_2$ max had higher sweat urea and urine urea nitrogen levels immediately after exercise and after 3 d, respectively, only after the 55 and 67% $\dot{V}O_2$ max trials.[126] The researchers concluded that a protein utilization threshold exists somewhere between 41 and 55% $\dot{V}O_2$ max and that protein is utilized during the recovery period following exercise as well as during exercise.

The results of Calles-Escandon et al.[125] and Wolfe et al.[40] suggest that the lower limit of a "protein utilization threshold" may be around 45% $\dot{V}O_2$ max. In the former study,[125] urine and sweat urea losses during 90 min of cycling at 45% $\dot{V}O_2$ max increased 100%, whereas urea production was unaffected by 105 min of cycling at 30% $\dot{V}O_2$ max in the latter study.[40]

The use of protein as an energy source during exercise is also dependent on muscle glycogen levels. Using glycogen-loading techniques, Lemon and Mullin[31] demonstrated that protein accounted for 4.4% of the energy required to complete 1 hr of cycling at 60% $\dot{V}O_2$ max in glycogen-loaded subjects compared to 10.4% in glycogen-depleted subjects. Others also found that carbohydrate-depleted subjects utilize protein as an energy source more than carbohydrate-loaded subjects.[127]

2. 3-Methylhistidine Excretion

3-Methylhistidine (3-MH) is an amino acid formed by the methylation of specific histidine residues in the muscle contractile proteins.[128] Since it is not reutilized by the body and is excreted quantitatively in the urine, 3-MH excretion is assumed to be an index of contractile protein degradation.[128]

Urinary 3-MH is usually expressed as a ratio to urinary creatinine. It is known that urinary creatinine excretion is related to kidney function[129] and kidney function decreases during exercise.[130] Thus, expressing 3-MH as a ratio to creatinine helps account for possible changes in renal function that may occur during exercise. Moreover, since both 3-MH and creatinine are directly related to lean body mass,[131] using their ratio normalizes data for lean body mass differences among subjects.

3-MH excretion has been studied in response to isolated bouts of endurance or weightlifting exercise as well as repeated daily bouts of endurance or weightlifting exercise. For a plenary review of the findings, see the recent article by Hickson and Wolinsky.[132]

In general, 3-MH excretion changes minimally 24–72 hr after an isolated bout of endurance or weightlifting exercise. Trained and untrained subjects did not experience an increase from prerace values for 24 hr 3-MH excretion after a 10 km run.[133] Similarly, 3.75 hr of treadmill running at 50% $\dot{V}O_2$ max did not affect 24 hr 3-MH excretion.[31] Additionally, in separate 7-d periods, subjects performing single 60-min bouts of concentric or eccentric cycling exercise at 70 and 40% $\dot{V}O_2$ max, respectively, exhibited no change in 3-MH excretion over the 72 hr period following exercise.[134]

Hickson and others[135] reported that 3 sets of 3 exercises incorporating upper or lower body weightlifting exercises performed 4 d apart did not affect 3-MH excretion during the subsequent 24 hr. The workouts lasted approximately 35 min, and the exercises were performed at 75–80% 1RM (repetition maximum, or the amount of weight that can be lifted correctly one time). Similar results were found when a group of subjects who performed intensive weightlifting exercise were compared to a nonexercise control group.[136] The above results suggest that isolated bouts of either endurance or resistance exercise do not increase degradation of the muscle contractile proteins.

Results of studies examining the effect of repeated daily bouts of endurance exercise on 3-MH excretion are equivocal. Dohm et al.[137] reported that an 18.5 km (2 hr) run repeated daily for 1 wk significantly elevated 3-MH excretion (and 3-MH:creatinine ratios) on days 5 through 7 of exercise and on the first recovery day. Radha and Bessman[138] concluded that endurance exercise decreases 3-MH excretion. Subjects exercised on a treadmill 1 hr daily for 2 wk at 70% $\dot{V}O_2$ max. The average amount of 3-MH excreted daily for the 2-wk period was less than the average daily 3-MH excretion during a 1-wk control period. However, as creatinine excretion also fell during the exercise period, the 3-MH:creatinine ratio was not different between experimental conditions. These studies[137,138] should be interpreted with caution as differences in experimental protocols may have influenced the results. Several subjects in the study by Dohm et al.[137] did not refrain from consuming meat during the experimental period whereas meat-free diets were consumed by subjects in the Radha and Bessman study.[138] Since 3-MH and creatinine are found in muscle, meat-free diets should be consumed throughout the experimental period to eliminate exogenous 3-MH and creatinine contributions.[128] Also, differences in the exercise duration, intensity, or both could have affected the findings. Hence, direct comparisons of studies with different protocols may not be possible.

Repeated daily bouts of weightlifting exercise tend to increase 3-MH excretion. Hickson and Hinkelmann[139] conducted a 28 d study in which subjects were divided into an exercise or nonexercise control group. The exercise group performed 3 sets of 6 different weightlifting exercises 6 d/wk. During the final 14 d of training, 3-MH excretion tended to increase leading the authors to conclude that their weightlifting program was associated with increased skeletal muscle protein breakdown. A similar conclusion was reached by Pivarnik and others[140] and Frontera et al.[141] after 3-MH and 3-MH:creatinine ratios were elevated in 11 subjects during eleven consecutive days of resistance training and in older men (60–72 y) training the knee extensors and knee flexors at 80% 1 RM 3 times per week for 12 wk, respectively.

Data from studies examining 3-MH changes in response to isolated bouts and chronic weightlifting exercise help to illustrate the importance of a regular training program for gaining muscle mass. Since muscle growth is associated with higher rates of protein turnover (degradation and synthesis), it makes sense that an isolated bout of resistance exercise does not elevate 3-MH excretion and hence, muscle protein turnover. Practical experience tells us that adding muscle mass by lifting weights sporadically is not possible. Only when a regular training program is followed do gains in muscle mass occur. Obviously, if muscle protein degradation is elevated during a resistance training program, skeletal muscle protein synthesis rates must increase in order to support skeletal muscle repair, growth, and function. Indeed, recent evidence shows that weightlifting exercise increases skeletal muscle protein synthesis during the 24 hr period following exercise.[80]

3.   Metabolic Tracers

Stable isotopes, such as ^{13}C-leucine or ^{15}N-glycine, or radioactive isotopes, including ^{14}C-leucine, are used in humans to study amino acid oxidation during both endurance and resistance exercise. Additionally, stable amino acid isotopes can be used to determine protein requirements and estimate rates of whole body protein synthesis and degradation.

It is clear that endurance exercise elicits a rise in leucine oxidation. Elevated leucine oxidation rates occur at intensities as low as 25–30% $\dot{V}O_2$ max [39,40,68] and increase linearly with exercise intensity up to approximately 90% $\dot{V}O_2$ max.[39] However, it is unwarranted to draw the conclusion that human protein needs are elevated solely because the oxidation of leucine or any other single amino acid increases during endurance exercise. It may be that specific individual amino acid needs may increase with exercise. For example, Wolfe et al.[68] compared leucine and lysine metabolism during 105 min of cycling exercise at 30% $\dot{V}O_2$ max to determine if leucine metabolism was representative of the other essential amino acids. The authors found that the increase in lysine oxidation during exercise was small compared to the increase in leucine oxidation. It was concluded that leucine metabolism does not represent metabolism of the other essential amino acids during exercise.

Contrary to endurance exercise, weightlifting exercise does not increase leucine oxidation. Tarnopolsky and others[142] continuously infused leucine during a 1-hr resistance exercise session consisting of 9 separate exercises, each performed for 3 sets of 10 repetitions at 70% 1 RM. Leucine oxidation did not increase during exercise or the initial 2 hr of recovery, leading the authors to conclude that amino acids contribute little to the energy demands of resistance exercise.

Measurements of urea production, 3-MH excretion, and leucine oxidation have provided invaluable information about protein/amino acid metabolism in response to endurance and resistance exercise. However, these techniques have yielded very little information concerning recommended dietary protein intakes. Instead, recommended protein intakes for both endurance and strength athletes have come from experiments examining nitrogen balance.

B.   USE OF NITROGEN BALANCE TO DETERMINE PROTEIN REQUIREMENTS

Nitrogen balance occurs when the total nitrogen excreted in the urine, feces, and sweat is equal to the total nitrogen ingested (i.e., net nitrogen retention). Positive nitrogen balance occurs when total nitrogen excretion is less than total nitrogen consumption. For growth to occur (e.g., addition of muscle mass), positive nitrogen balance must exist.

Altering either daily protein intake or daily energy intake affects nitrogen balance. Gontzea et al.[143] and Iyengar and Rao[144] found that when subjects maintained a constant daily caloric intake, nitrogen balance was sensitive to changes in protein intake. Nitrogen balance is also altered if daily energy intake is changed while protein ingestion is kept constant.[145] Thus, a variable energy intake is one limitation to nitrogen balance studies. Other limitations include problems in accurately measuring all nitrogen intake and excretion and variable accommodation periods for adapting to new protein intakes.[146] Nonetheless, the wealth of data from nitrogen balance studies indicating that protein requirements increase in physically active individuals is convincing.

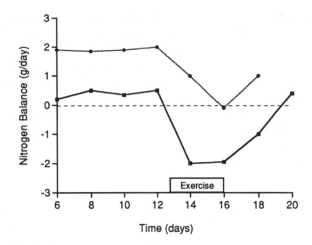

FIGURE 9 Nitrogen balance in subjects participating in several bicycle ergometer exercise sessions over a 4-d period (days 13–16 on graph). Subjects consumed 1.0 g/kg/d of protein (solid line) or 1.5 g/kg/d of protein (dotted line) for 12 d before and 4 d after the exercise period. (From Gontzea, I. et al., *Nutr. Rep. Int.*, 10, 35, 1974. With permission from Butterworths Publishers.)

1. Endurance Athletes

Gontzea and colleagues conducted two classic studies[143,147] on the effect of endurance exercise on nitrogen balance. In one study[143] (Figure 9), 30 subjects consumed a diet supplying 1.0 g/kg/d of protein along with an adequate energy supply to maintain nitrogen balance. After an equilibration period, subjects began a 4-d exercise program consisting of six 20-min bouts of cycling exercise at a workload ranging from 65–150 W. Each bout was separated by a 30-min rest period. During the 4 d of exercise, 29 of the 30 subjects experienced negative nitrogen balance leading the authors to conclude that 1.0 g/kg/d of protein does not cover the increased nitrogen consumption that occurs during periods of increased muscular exertion.

A second study from Gontzea's group[147] investigated the effect of exercise training on nitrogen balance (Figure 10). Twelve subjects repeated the dietary and exercise regimen employed in the earlier study[143] for 3 wk. Exercise intensity and duration were kept constant throughout the study. During the first 4 d, nitrogen balance became negative in all subjects

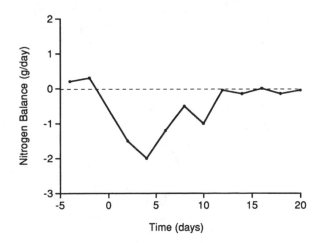

FIGURE 10 Nitrogen balance in subjects participating in a 20-d endurance exercise program. Subjects consumed 1.0 g/kg/d of protein for 32 d; the exercise program began after a 12-d control period (day +1 on the graph). (From Gontzea, I. et al., *Nutr. Rep. Int.*, 11, 231, 1975. With permission from Butterworths Publishers.)

confirming the earlier findings. However, by the end of the 3-wk period, nitrogen balance values were similar to the control period. Although the subjects required 18% less energy to complete the exercise task after 3 wk of training, their average nitrogen loss decreased by 90%. It was concluded that repeated bouts of exercise result in an adaptation which allows the body to conserve both energy and nitrogen. Similar adaptations occur during exercise training when only 0.57 g/kg/d of protein are ingested.[145]

Although the adaptation of sparing body nitrogen in response to protein deficiency lessens the magnitude of negative nitrogen balance, for most athletes the adaptation is insufficient to restore balance. Thus, to achieve nitrogen balance, daily protein intake, energy intake, or both must be increased.

Several nitrogen balance studies have been conducted to elucidate the protein needs of endurance and strength athletes. In general, protein requirements are calculated from a regression line generated by feeding exercising subjects various levels of protein both above and below the RDA (Figure 11). For example, Meredith and others[148] calculated that endurance athletes undertaking their normal daily training schedules required 0.94 g/kg/d dietary protein to maintain nitrogen balance. Nitrogen balance was calculated over the final 5 d of 3 separate 10-d periods during which subjects consumed diets containing either 0.6, 0.9, or 1.2 g/kg/d of protein. Tarnopolsky et al.[149] calculated that 1.37 g/kg/d dietary protein was required for endurance athletes to maintain nitrogen balance compared to 0.73 g/kg/d for sedentary controls. In this study, subjects consumed either 1.7 or 2.65 g/kg/d dietary protein. This requirement is similar to the 1.2–1.5 g protein/kg/d value reported by Friedman and Lemon.[150] These researchers found that nitrogen balance was negative when well-trained subjects consumed 0.89 g/kg/d protein but positive when 1.49 g/kg/d protein was ingested.

Based on nitrogen balance data, endurance athletes require a protein intake of 1.0–1.4 g/kg/d to maintain nitrogen balance. Interestingly, protein contributed only 6–10% to the total energy intake in the above studies. Thus, although the current RDA for protein is likely too low to cover the needs of endurance athletes during normal training, nitrogen balance will

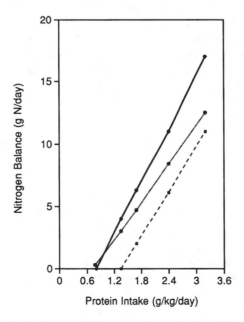

FIGURE 11 Predicted protein intakes to achieve zero nitrogen balance based on extrapolated data for endurance athletes (dashed line), bodybuilders (solid line), and sedentary individuals (dotted line). (From Tarnopolsky, M. A. et al., *J. Appl. Physiol.*, 64, 187, 1988. With permission from the American Physiological Society.)

be attained for most endurance athletes if a calorie-sufficient diet containing at least 10% of the calories as protein is consumed.

2. Strength Athletes

Weight training also leads to a daily protein requirement in excess of the current RDA. Laritcheva and others[151] concluded that nitrogen balance in weightlifters was affected by training intensity. During periods of preparation for international level contests, 2.2–2.6 g/kg/d of protein was needed to maintain nitrogen balance whereas a protein intake of 2.0 g/kg/d maintained a positive nitrogen balance during periods of less intense training. These findings support the earlier work of Celejowa and Homa[152] who found that 2.0–2.2 g/kg/d dietary protein was sufficient to maintain nitrogen balance during periods of moderate intensity strength training.

The protein requirement values required to maintain nitrogen balance in the above studies constituted intakes of 14–18% of total daily energy. In contrast, Tarnopolsky et al.[149] calculated that bodybuilders could maintain nitrogen balance while consuming 0.82 g/kg/d of protein (5% of total daily energy) and training at least 10 hr/wk, 1.5–2 hr/d. When the bodybuilders were fed their normal level of protein (2.77 g/kg/d or 18% of total daily energy), they produced a positive nitrogen balance of 13.4 g nitrogen/d compared to 1.06 g nitrogen/d during the experimental condition. However, Millward et al.[153] calculate that such a large positive nitrogen balance is equivalent to an impossibly large gain of more than 500 g lean tissue/d. Thus, the large positive balance reported by Tarnopolsky et al.[149] may have resulted from a lack of adaptation to the new intake.

In a latter study, Tarnopolsky and others[154] fed sedentary subjects and strength athletes diets containing 0.86, 1.4, or 2.4 g/kg/d of protein. The strength athletes maintained their normal training schedule during a 10-d adaptation period but performed a set exercise routine during the 3-d nitrogen balance period. Nitrogen balance data indicated that the protein requirement was 1.76 g/kg/d for strength athletes and 0.89 g/kg/d for the sedentary individuals. The latter value is very close to the current RDA for protein of 0.8 g/kg/d increasing the reliability of the calculated value for strength athletes.

The discrepancy between the nitrogen balance data of the two studies by Tarnopolsky and others[149,154] was attributed to an adaptation of nitrogen balance to the stress of training. Subjects in the initial study[149] were elite bodybuilders who had trained for 3 yr whereas subjects in the 1992 study[154] had less than 1 yr weight training experience. Interestingly, Lemon et al.[155] found that novice bodybuilders actively increasing muscle mass with a weightlifting program required 1.7 g/kg/d based nitrogen balance data from protein intakes of 2.67 and 0.99 g/kg/d. However, protein intake was significantly reduced from 1.35 g/kg/d during the 1-month adaptation period to 0.99 g/kg/d during the 3-d nitrogen balance period. As mentioned earlier, reduction in protein intake on energy-sufficient diets lower nitrogen balance values.[143,144] It is thus difficult to resolve the contribution of the decrease in protein consumption to the negative nitrogen balance observed on the lower protein intake. An underestimation of the nitrogen balance value at the lower protein intake would overestimate the protein requirement to achieve zero nitrogen balance.

It seems paradoxical that protein requirements would decrease in experienced weightlifters compared to novice weightlifters. The more experienced athletes would likely perform work with a greater intensity and volume because they are bigger and stronger. However, data from endurance athletes supports the notion that exercise improves the efficiency of the body for utilizing nitrogen.[147] A longitudinal study following the protein requirement of untrained subjects as they progress through a training program would be required to definitively answer this question.

The latter study by Tarnopolsky et al.[154] differs from other nitrogen balance studies because leucine oxidation and whole body protein synthesis were also measured. Since

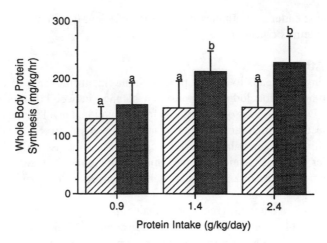

FIGURE 12 Whole body protein synthesis ± SD in strength athletes (solid bars) and sedentary controls (hacked bars) at three levels of protein intake. Bars with different letters indicate groups are different at P <0.05. (From Tarnopolsky, M. A. et al., *J. Appl. Physiol.,* 73, 1986, 1992. With permission from the American Physiological Society.)

proteins/amino acids have no storage form in the body, amino acids are oxidized as supply exceeds need.[156] Thus, the protein intake at which amino acid oxidation rapidly increases and/or the intake at which whole body protein synthesis plateaus may represent the most meaningful measure of protein intake.[156] In the strength athletes, whole body protein synthesis was greater when 1.4 g of protein/kg/d was consumed than 0.86 (Figure 12), but leucine oxidation was unchanged. Whole body protein synthesis failed to respond further when these subjects consumed 2.4 g of protein/kg/d; however, leucine oxidation was elevated indicating that the higher protein intake was too much. Changing the protein intake of sedentary subjects from 0.86–1.4 g/kg/d increased leucine oxidation without affecting whole body protein synthesis rates. Measurements of both whole body protein synthesis and leucine oxidation predicted that the protein requirements would be 1.41 and 0.90 g/kg/d for the strength athletes and sedentary controls, respectively, agreeing fairly closely with the nitrogen balance values.[154]

The experiments on strength athletes clearly indicate that the current RDA for protein of 0.8 g/kg/d is inadequate. Taken together, measurements of protein synthesis, leucine oxidation, and nitrogen balance indicate that strength/power athletes would benefit from protein intakes of 1.4–1.8 g/kg/d but that intakes exceeding 2.0 g/kg/d are unnecessary. Interestingly, such a protein intake is easily attainable if 15% of total energy intake is consumed as protein. For a 3200 kcal/d diet, this would represent 480 kcal/d from protein (3200 × 0.15). Since protein has an energy equivalence of 4 kcal per gram, 480 kcal/d would represent 120 g/d of protein (450 ÷ 4). An 80 kg (176 lbs) athlete consuming this diet would thus have a protein intake of 1.5 g/kg/d (120 ÷ 80).

Although both endurance and strength trained athletes can benefit from consuming protein in excess of the current RDA, the cause of the increased protein need differs between the two types of athlete. Examination of the amino acid utilization and protein turnover studies with endurance and strength trained subjects sheds light on why these differences occur. Following endurance exercise bouts exceeding 40% $\dot{V}O_2$ max, urea excretion is increased,[40,125,126] 3-MH excretion is typically unchanged,[138] and muscle protein synthesis is depressed.[37,40,66-68] These findings indicate that amino acids are oxidized for energy by endurance athletes and that the amino acids are coming from sources other than the muscle contractile proteins. Such sources likely include the liver and muscle free amino acid pool since depressed rates of muscle protein synthesis would make additional amino acids available for oxidation. In strength trained athletes, urea excretion and leucine oxidation increase at protein intakes exceeding 2.0 g/kg/d.[149,154] Moreover, amino acids are not used to any extent as an energy source during weightlifting exercise;[142] however, 3-MH excretion[139-141] and muscle protein synthesis rates increase.[80] Thus, protein turnover is elevated in strength athletes, and additional protein is required to supply the building blocks to support enhanced protein synthesis rates. However, protein/amino acids consumed in excess of need (i.e., 1.4–1.8 g/kg/d) will be oxidized.

C. EFFECTS OF PROTEIN INTAKE ON EXERCISE PERFORMANCE

The bottom line for any serious athlete is performance, and many athletes believe that optimal performance can only be achieved by consuming a high-protein diet.[157] Improvements in exercise performance can be defined in many ways. For endurance athletes, it may represent a decrease in the time required to complete an activity or the amount of time that a particular activity can be maintained (i.e., running or cycling to exhaustion). For strength athletes, obviously an increase in muscular strength would constitute enhanced performance whereas bodybuilders might be more concerned with increasing lean body mass. The vast majority of studies examining dietary effects on endurance exercise performance have focused on carbohydrate supplementation (see Chapters 3 and 22). Therefore, this review will be limited to the effect of protein supplementation on gains in muscular strength and/or changes in muscle mass.

One of the earliest studies examining the effect of protein supplementation on exercise performance was conducted on members of the U.S. military. Rasch et al.[158] supplemented the normal diet of one group with 0.7 g of protein/kg/d while a second group received a placebo. No differences were found between the improvements each group made in their physical fitness test scores measured by pull-ups, squat thrusts, standing broad jump, and bent knee sit-ups. The authors concluded that ingesting protein supplements did not enhance physical performance.

More recently, Tarnopolsky et al.[154] observed no difference in muscular strength when subjects consumed diets containing 0.86, 1.4, or 2.4 g/kg/d of protein. These results are not surprising since each diet was followed for only 13 d. It is unknown whether adherence to the higher protein diets would have elicited greater strength gains. However, previously untrained subjects consuming 1.35 or 2.62 g/kg/d of protein for 30 d also did not exhibit differences in muscular strength.[155] Moreover, no differences were found in lean body mass, muscle cross-sectional area, or muscle density. The authors speculated that increasing the duration of the study may have produced differences, a contention supported by the earlier findings of Consolazio and others.[159] In this study, 2 groups of men consumed diets containing 1.4 or 2.8 g/kg/d of protein while undergoing a 40-d physical conditioning program. The conditioning program incorporated aerobic exercise as well as calisthenics, isometric exercises, and other sporting activities. At the end of the experimental period, both groups showed a significant decrease in body fat with a subsequent increase in lean body mass; however, the increase was only significant for the group consuming 2.8 g/kg/d of protein.

Other researchers have shown greater increases in muscle mass on high-protein diets after only a month of resistance training. In elderly men, supplementing the normal diet with 23 g of protein per day for 4 wk improved thigh muscle gains compared to a nonsupplemented group.[160] In young males (average age 24 y), Fern et al.[161] observed greater body mass gains (2.8 vs. 1.5 kg) after 4 wk of weight training on a diet containing 3.3 vs. 1.3 g/kg/d of protein (Figure 13). However, infusions of ^{15}N-glycine revealed amino acid oxidation increased 160% in the high-protein group, indicating that 3.3 g/kg/d of protein exceeded the requirement.

It appears that protein intakes above 2.0 g/kg/d do not improve measurements of strength compared to lower intake levels. Furthermore, reports of enhanced lean body mass gains at protein intakes above 2.0 g/kg/d are equivocal. However, amino acid tracer studies indicate that such protein intakes are too high as amino acid oxidation rates substantially increase.

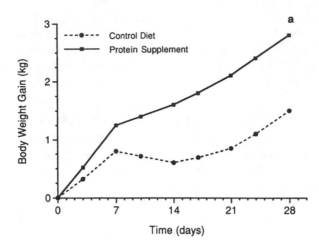

FIGURE 13   Body weight gain in subjects consuming either 1.3 g/kg/d of protein (dashed line) vs. 3.3 g/kg/d of protein (solid line) during 4 wk of strength training. a = significantly different from 1.3 g/kg/d group at P <0.005. (Adapted from Fern, E. B. et al., *Experentia*, 14, 168, 1991.)

Thus, studies examining strength performance and lean body mass gains are consistent with our earlier recommendation that strength athletes consume 1.4–1.8 g/kg/d of protein.

IV. SUMMARY AND CONCLUSIONS

Exercise produces diverse and dramatic changes in amino acid metabolism. Exercise alters movement of amino acids among tissues and changes amino acid oxidation rates and incorporation rates of amino acids into new proteins. During endurance exercise, these changes support increasing the use of amino acids (specifically the BCAA) as energy substrates for skeletal muscle and for the generation of alanine as a gluconeogenic substrate to maintain blood glucose. After exercise, the flux of amino acids is targeted on stimulating recovery of muscle protein synthesis.

Early investigations of changes in amino acid metabolism during exercise demonstrated movement of BCAA from the visceral tissues out to peripheral skeletal muscles with corresponding movement of nitrogen from muscle to the liver via alanine.[16-18,20] More recent work, including research in our laboratory,[10,21] has shown that BCAA are uniquely metabolized by skeletal muscle and appear to be an important energy substrate for exercising muscle. Muscle BCAA oxidation is regulated via substrate concentration and the energy state of the cell which controls the phosphorylation state of the rate limiting enzyme in the catabolic pathway.[21] BCAA catabolism in skeletal muscle is related to alanine or glutamine production for transport of amino nitrogen to the liver and kidney.[10]

Intense exercise produces short-term catabolic effects on protein turnover. Our research has shown that exhaustive exercise will depress muscle protein synthesis during exercise and the first few hours of recovery.[4,10] Recent findings in our laboratory show that post-exercise nutrition has a significant impact on the recovery rate.[10] Without food intake, recovery occurred slowly over a 4–8 hr period. With post-exercise carbohydrate feedings, recovery was accelerated by 60% 1 hr after exercise, and with a complete meal of amino acids, carbohydrates, and lipids, the rate of protein synthesis fully recovered and was actually above nonexercised control levels 1 hr after exercise. These data suggest the importance of post-exercise nutrition to support recovery from endurance exercise.

Amino acid flux during recovery emphasizes the importance of BCAA, insulin, and alanine. With the post-exercise feedings, there is an indirect relationship between leucine oxidation and alanine production and a direct relationship between alanine production and the rate of muscle protein synthesis.[10] These relationships are dependent on insulin availability. For rapid recovery of muscle protein synthesis, BCAA and glucose appear to be essential components of a post-exercise recovery meal.

The short-term changes in muscle protein synthesis suggest a regulatory mechanism at the level of translation. Our data indicate that RNA levels are constant and that the response time is likely associated with initiation factors.[4] Current research is exploring the roles of two initiation factors, eIF-2B and eIF-4E, in the control of short-term responses of muscle protein synthesis.

These changes in amino acid and protein metabolism associated with exercise lead to short-term changes in amino acid use for energy and longer-term changes in muscle mass. For individuals engaged in routine, intense exercise, these changes appear to increase the need for dietary protein. We suggest a protein intake of 1.4–1.8 g/kg/d for strength athletes and 1.2–1.4 g/kg/d for endurance athletes compared to the RDA of 0.8 g/kg/d. These requirements are viewed as adequate to support the needs for tissue building and replacement as well as increased amino acid use for energy.

REFERENCES

1. Goodman, M. N., Influence of aerobic exercise on fuel utilization by skeletal muscle, in *Nutrition and Aerobic Exercise*, Layman, D. K., Ed., ACS Symp. Ser. 294, American Chemical Society, Washington, D.C., 1986, 27.
2. Goodman, M. N., Amino acid and protein metabolism, in *Exercise, Nutrition, and Energy Metabolism*, Horton, E. S. and Terjung, R. L., Eds., Macmillan Publishing Co., New York, 1988, 89.
3. Hood, D. A. and Terjung, R. L., Amino acid metabolism during exercise and following endurance training, *Sports Med.,* 9, 23, 1990.
4. Layman, D. K., Paul, G. L., and Olken, M. H., Amino acid metabolism during exercise, in *Nutrition in Exercise and Sport,* Wolinsky, I. and Hickson, J. F., Eds., CRC Press, Boca Raton, FL, 1994, 123.
5. Paul, G. L., Dietary protein requirements of physically active individuals, *Sports Med.,* 8, 154, 1989.
6. Lemon, P. W. R., Do athletes need more dietary protein and amino acids?, *Int. J. Sports Med.,* 5, S39, 1995.
7. National Academy of Sciences National Research Council, *Recommended Dietary Allowances,* 10th ed., National Academy Press, Washington, D.C., 1989, 52.
8. Paul, G. L., Rokusek, J. T., Dykstra, G. L., Boileau, R. A., and Layman, D. K., Oat, wheat or corn ingestion cereal ingestion before exercise alters metabolism in humans, *J. Nutr.,* 126, 1372, 1996.
9. Paul, G. L., Rokusek, J. T., Dykstra, G. L., Boileau, R. A., and Layman, D. K., Pre-exercise meal composition alters plasma large-neutral amino acid responses during exercise and recovery, *Am. J. Clin. Nutr.,* 64, 778, 1996.
10. Paul, G. L. and Layman, D. K., Post-exercise feedings stimulate skeletal muscle protein synthesis and alter plasma amino acids, *FASEB J.,* 9, A746, 1995.
11. Meister, A., *Biochemistry of the Amino Acids,* Academic Press, New York, 1965.
12. Morgan, H. E., Earl, D. C. N., Broadus, A., Wolpert, E. B., Giger, K. E., and Jefferson, L. S., Regulation of protein synthesis in heart muscle. I. Effect of amino acid levels on protein synthesis, *J. Biol. Chem.,* 246, 2152, 1971.
13. Christensen, H. N., Role of amino acid transport and counter transport in nutrition and metabolism, *Physiol. Rev.,* 70, 43, 1990.
14. Waterlow, J. C., Garlick, P. J., and Millward, D. J., *Protein Turnover in Mammalian Tissues and in the Whole Body,* Elsevier/North Holland, New York, 1978.
15. Wolfe, R. R., in *Tracers in Metabolic Research,* Alan R. Liss, New York, 1984, 151.
16. Felig, P., Pozefsky, T., Marliss, E., and Cahill, G. F., Jr., Alanine: key role in gluconeogenesis, *Science,* 167, 1003, 1970.
17. Felig, P., Amino acid metabolism in exercise, *Ann. N.Y. Acad. Sci.* , 301, 56, 1977.
18. Ahlborg, G., Felig, P., Hagenfeldt, L., Hendler, R., and Wahren, J., Substrate turnover during prolonged exercise in man, *J. Clin. Invest.,* 53, 1080, 1974.
19. Dohm, G. L., Kasperek, G. J., Tapscott, E. B., and Barakat, H. A., Protein metabolism during endurance exercise, *Fed. Proc.,* 44, 348, 1985.
20. Ruderman, N. M., Muscle amino acid metabolism and gluconeogenesis, *Ann. Rev. Med.,* 26, 245, 1975.
21. Harper, A. E., Miller, R. H., and Block, K. P., Branched-chain amino acid metabolism, *Ann. Rev. Nutr.,* 4, 409, 1984.

22. Adibi, S. A., Metabolism of branched-chain amino acids in altered nutrition, *Metabolism,* 25, 1287, 1976.

23. Hutson, S. M., Cree, T. C., and Harper, A. E., Regulation of leucine and alpha-ketoisocaproate metabolism in skeletal muscle, *J. Biol. Chem.*, 253, 8126, 1978.

24. Rush, J. W. E., MacLean, D. A., Hultman, E., and Graham, T. E., Exercise caused branched-chain oxoacid dehydrogenase dephosphorylation but not AMP deaminase binding, *J. Appl. Physiol.,* 78, 2193, 1995.

25. Katz, A., Broberg, S., Sahlin, K., and Wahren, J., Muscle ammonia and amino acid metabolism during dynamic exercise in man, *Clin. Physiol. (Oxf.),* 6, 365, 1986.

26. Broberg, S. and Sahlin, K., Adenine nucleotide degradation in human skeletal muscle during prolonged exercise, *J. Appl. Physiol.,* 67, 116, 1989.

27. Wibom, R. and Hultman, E., ATP production rate in mitochondria isolated from microsamples of human muscle, *Am. J. Physiol.,* 259, E204, 1990.

28. Graham, T. E. and MacLean, D. A., Ammonia and amino acid metabolism in human skeletal muscle during exercise, *Can. J. Physiol. Pharmacol.,* 70, 132, 1992.

29. Garber, A. J., Karl, I. E., and Kipnis, D. M., Alanine and glutamine synthesis and release from skeletal muscle. II. The precursor role of amino acids in alanine and glutamine synthesis, *J. Biol. Chem.,* 254, 836, 1976.

30. Pardridge, W. M. and Davidson, M. B., Alanine metabolism in skeletal muscle in tissue culture, *Biochim. Biophys. Acta,* 585, 34, 1979.

31. Lemon, P. and Mullin, J. P., Effect of initial muscle glycogen levels on protein catabolism during exercise, *J. Appl. Physiol.,* 48, 624, 1980.

32. Rennie, M. J., Halliday, D., Davies, C. T. M., Edwards, R. G. T., Krywawych, S., Millward, D. J., and Matthews, D. E., Exercise induced increase in leucine oxidation in man and the effect of glucose, in *Metabolism and Clinical Implication of the Branched Chain Amino and Keto Acids,* Walser, M. and Williamson, J. R., Eds., Elsevier-North Holland, New York, 1981, 361.

33. Fernstrom, J. D. and Wurtman, R. J., Brain serotonin content: physiological regulation by plasma neutral amino acids, *Science,* 178, 414, 1972.

34. Goldberg, A. L. and Chang, T. W., Regulation and significance of amino acid metabolism in skeletal muscle, *Fed. Proc.,* 37, 2301, 1978.

35. Kasperek, G. J., Regulation of branched-chain 2-oxo acid dehydrogenase during exercise, *Am. J. Physiol.,* 256, E186, 1989.

36. Wagenmakers, A. J. M., Beckers, E. J., Brouns, F., Kuipers, H., Soeters, P. B., Van Der Vusse, G. J., and Saris, W. H. M., Carbohydrate supplementation, glycogen depletion, and amino acid metabolism during exercise, *Am. J. Physiol.,* 260, E883, 1991.

37. Rennie, M. J., Edwards, R. H. T., Krywawych, S., Davies, C. T. M., Halliday, D., Waterlow, J. C., and Millward, D. J., Effect of exercise on protein turnover in man, *Clin. Sci.,* 61, 627, 1981.

38. Hagg, S. A., Morse, E. L., and Adibi, S. A., Effects of exercise on rates of oxidation, turnover and plasma clearance of leucine in human subjects, *Am. J. Physiol.,* 242, E407, 1982.

39. Millward, D. J., Davies, C. T. M., Halliday, D., Wolman, S., Matthews, D., and Rennie, M. J., Effect of exercise on protein metabolism in humans as explored with stable isotopes, *Fed. Proc.,* 41, 2686, 1982.

40. Wolfe, R. R., Goodenough, R. D., Wolfe, M. H., Royle, G. T., and Nadel, E. R., Isotopic analysis of leucine and urea metabolism in exercising humans *J. Appl. Physiol.,* 52, 458, 1982.

41. MacLean, D. A., Spriet, L. L., and Graham, T. E., Plasma amino acid and ammonia responses to altered dietary intakes prior to prolonged exercise in humans, *Can. J. Physiol. Pharmacol.,* 70, 420, 1991.

42. Konopka, B. and Haymes, E., Effect of acute exercise on protein metabolism in women, *Med. Sci. Sports. Exer.,* 14, A112, 1982.

43. Davis, J. M., Bailey, S. P., Woods, J. A., Galiano, F. J., Hamilton, M. T., and Bartoli, W. P., Carbohydrate feedings delay alterations in plasma amino acids potentially involved in central fatigue, *Eur. J. Appl. Physiol.,* 65, 513, 1992.

44. Blomstrand, E., Hassmén, P., Ekblom, B., and Newsholme, E. A., Administration of branched-chain amino acids during sustained exercise — effects on performance and on plasma concentration of some amino acids, *Eur. J. Appl. Physiol.,* 63, 83, 1991.

45. Felig, P. and Wahren, J., Amino acid metabolism in exercising man, *J. Clin. Invest.,* 50, 2703, 1971.

46. Bazzarre, T. L., Murdoch, S. D., Wu, S. L., Herr, D. G., and Snider, I. P., Plasma amino acid responses of trained athletes to two successive exhaustion trials with and without interim carbohydrate feeding, *J. Am. Coll. Nutr.,* 11, 501, 1992.

47. Decombaz, J., Reinhardt, P., Anantharaman, K., Glutz, G., and Poortmans, J. R., Biochemical changes in a 100 km run: free amino acids, urea, and creatinine, *Eur. J. Appl. Physiol.,* 41, 61, 1979.

48. Refsum, H. E., Gjessing, L. R., and Stromme, S. B., Changes in plasma amino acid distribution and urine amino acids excretion during prolonged heavy exercise, *Scand. J. Clin. Invest.,* 39, 407, 1979.

49. Kaminsky, L. A. and Paul, G. L., Fluid intake during an ultramarathon running race: relationship to plasma volume and serum sodium and potassium, *J. Sports Med. Phys. Fitness,* 31, 417, 1991.

50. Bender, D. A., Uptake of tryptophan into the brain: dietary influences on serotoninergic function, *Biblthca. Nutr. Dieta.,* 38, 82, 1986.

51. Lovenberg, W. M., Biochemical regulation of brain function, *Nutr. Rev.,* 44, 6, 1986.

52. Pardridge, W. M., Blood-brain barrier transport of nutrients, *Nutr. Rev.,* 44, 15, 1986.

53. Pardridge, W. M., Regulation of amino acid availability to the brain, in *Nutrition and the Brain,* Wurtman, R. J. and Wurtman, J. J., Eds., Raven Press, New York, 1977, 141.

54. Newsholme, E. A., Acworth, I. N., and Blomstrand, E., Amino acids, brain neurotransmitters and a functional link between muscle and brain that is important in sustained exercise, in *Advances in Myochemistry,* Benzi, G., Ed., John Libby Eurotext Ltd., London, 1987, 127.

55. Wurtman, R. J., Hefti, F., and Melamed, E., Precursor control of neurotransmitter synthesis, *Pharmacol. Rev.,* 32, 315, 1981.

56. Scheider, W., The rate of access to the organic ligan binding region of serum albumin is entropy controlled, *Proc. Nat. Acad. Sci.,* 76, 2283, 1979.

57. van Hall, G., Raaymakers, J. S. H., Saris, W. H. M., and Wagenmakers, A. J. M., Ingestion of branched-chain amino acids and tryptophan during sustained exercise in man: failure to affect performance, *J. Physiol.,* 486, 789, 1995.

58. Blomstrand, E., Andersson, S., Hassmén, P., Ekblom, B., and Newsholme, E. A., Effect of branched-chain amino acid and carbohydrate supplementation on the exercise-induced change in plasma and muscle concentration of amino acids in human subjects, *Acta Physiol. Scand.,* 153, 87, 1995.

59. Varnier, M., Sarto, P., Martines, D., Lora, L., Carmignoto, F., Leese, G. P., and Naccarato, R., Effect of infusing branched-chain amino acid during incremental exercise with reduced muscle glycogen content, *Eur. J. Appl. Physiol.,* 69, 26, 1994.

60. Hassmén, P., Blomstrand, E., Ekblom, B., and Newsholme, E. A., Branched-chain amino acid supplementation during 30-km competitive run: mood and cognitive performance, *Nutrition,* 10, 405, 1994.

61. Goldberg, A. L., Work-induced growth of skeletal muscle in normal and hypophysectomized rats, *Am. J. Physiol.,* 213, 1193, 1967.

62. Goldberg, A. L., Biochemical events during hypertrophy of skeletal muscle, in *Cardiac Hypertrophy,* Alpert, N. R., Ed., Academic Press, New York, 1971, 301.

63. Goldspink, D. F., The influence of passive stretch on the growth and protein turnover of the denervated extensor digitorum longus muscle, *Biochem. J.,* 174, 595, 1978.

64. Laurent, G. J., Sparrow, M. P., and Millward, D. J., Muscle protein turnover in the adult fowl. II. Changes in rates of protein synthesis and breakdown during hypertrophy of the anterior and posterior latissimus dorsi muscle, *Biochem. J.,* 176, 407, 1978.

65. Wong, T. S. and Booth, F. W., Protein metabolism in rat tibialis anterior muscle after stimulated chronic eccentric exercise, *J. Appl. Physiol.,* 69, 1718, 1990.

66. Dohm, G. L., Hecker, A. L., Brown, W. E., Klain, G. J., Puente, F. R., Askew, E. W., and Beecher, G. R., Adaptation of protein metabolism to endurance training, *Biochem. J.,* 164, 705, 1977.

67. Dohm, G. L., Tapscott, E. B., Barakat, H. A., and Kasperek, G. J., Measurement of in vivo protein synthesis in rats during an exercise bout, *Biochem. Med.,* 27, 367, 1982.

68. Wolfe, R. R., Wolfe, M. H., Nadel, E. R., and Shaw, J. H. F., Isotopic determination of amino acid-urea interactions in exercise in humans, *J. Appl. Physiol.,* 56, 221, 1984.

69. Dohm, G. L., Williams, R. T., Kasperek, G. J., and van Rij, A. M., Increased excretion of urea and N$^\tau$-methylhistidine by rats and humans after a bout of exercise, *J. Appl. Physiol.,* 52, 27, 1982.

70. Bylund-Fellenius, A., Ojamaa, K. M., Flaim, K. E., Li, J. B., Wassner, S. J., and Jefferson, L. S., Protein synthesis versus energy state in contracting muscles of perfused rat hindlimb, *Am. J. Physiol.,* 246, E297, 1984.

71. Lemon, P. W. R. and Nagle, J. P., Effects of exercise on protein and amino acid metabolism, *Med. Sci. Sports Exer.,* 13, 141, 1981.

72. Booth, F. W. and Watson, P. A., Control of adaptations in protein levels in response to exercise, *Fed. Proc.,* 44, 2293, 1985.

73. Belcastro, A. N., Skeletal muscle calcium-activated neutral protease (calpain) with exercise, *J. Appl. Physiol.,* 74, 1381, 1993.

74. Dohm, G. L., Kasperek, G. J., Tapscott, E. B., and Beecher, G. R., Effect of exercise on synthesis and degradation of muscle protein, *Biochem. J.,* 188, 255, 1980.

75. Kettelhut, I. C., Pepato, M. T., Migliorini, R. H., Medina, R., and Goldberg, A. L., Regulation of different proteolytic pathways in skeletal muscle in fasting and diabetes mellitus, *Brazilian J. Med. Biol. Res.,* 27, 981, 1994.

76. Medina, R., Win, S. S., Hass, A., and Goldberg, A. L., Activation of the ubiquitin-ATP-dependent proteolytic system in skeletal muscle during fasting and denervation atrophy, *Biomed. Biochim. Acta,* 50, 347, 1991.

77. Bates, P. C., Millward, D. J., and Rennie, M. J., Re-examination of the effect of exercise on muscle protein synthesis in the rat, *J. Physiol.,* 315, 20P, 1981.

78. Carraro, F., Stuart, C. A., Hartl, W. H., Rosenblatt, J., and Wolfe, R. R., Effect of exercise and recovery on muscle protein synthesis in human subjects, *Am. J. Physiol.,* 259, E470, 1990.

79. Carraro, F., Hartt, W. H., Stuart, C. A., Layman, D. K., Jahoor, F., and Wolfe, R. R., Whole body and plasma protein synthesis in exercise and recovery in human subjects, *Am. J. Physiol.,* 258, D821, 1990.

80. Chesley, A., MacDougall, J. D., Tarnopolsky, M. A., Atkinson, S. A., and Smith, K., Changes in human muscle protein synthesis after resistance exercise, *J. Appl. Physiol.,* 73, 1383, 1992.

81. Davis, T. A. and Karl, I. E., Response of muscle protein turnover to insulin after acute exercise and training, *Biochem. J.,* 240, 651, 1986.

82. Davis, T. A., Klahr, S., and Karl, I. E., Insulin-stimulated protein metabolism in chronic azotemia and exercise, *Am. J. Physiol.,* 253, 164, 1987.

83. Devlin, J. T., Brodsky, I., Scrimgeour, A., Fuller, S., and Bier, D. M., Amino acid metabolism after intense exercise, *Am. J. Physiol.,* 258, E249, 1990.

84. Yoshizawa, F., Endo, M., Ide, H., Yagasaki, K., and Funabiki, R., Translational regulation of protein synthesis in the liver and skeletal muscle of mice in response to refeeding, *Nutr. Biochem.,* 6, 130, 1995.

85. Preedy, V. R. and Garlick, P. J., The response of muscle protein synthesis to nutrient intake in postabsorptive rats: the role of insulin and amino acids, *Biosci. Rep.,* 6, 177, 1986.

86. Goldberg, A. L., Jablecki, C., and Li, J. B., Effects of use and disuse on amino acid transport and protein turnover in muscle, *Ann. N.Y. Acad. Sci.,* 228, 190, 1974.

87. Tischler, M. E., Desautels, M., and Goldberg, A. L., Does leucine, leucyl-tRNA, or some metabolite of leucine regulate protein synthesis and degradation in skeletal and cardiac muscle, *J. Biol. Chem.,* 257, 1613, 1982.

88. Pain, V. M. and Manchester, K. L., The influence of electrical stimulation *in vitro* on protein synthesis and other metabolic parameters of rat extensor digitorum longus muscle, *Biochem. J.,* 118, 209, 1970.

89. Hershey, J. W. B., Translational control in mammalian cells, *Ann. Rev. Biochem.,* 60, 717, 1991.

90. Kimball, S. R. and Jefferson, L. S., Mechanisms of translational control in liver and skeletal muscle, *Biochimie,* 76, 729, 1994.

91. Morley, S., Signal transduction mechanisms in the regulation of protein synthesis, *Molec. Biol. Rep.,* 19, 221, 1994.

92. Singh, L. P., Aroor, A. R., and Wahba, A. J., Translational control of eukaryotic gene expression: role of the guanine nucleotide exchange factor and chain initiation factor-2, *Enzyme Protein,* 48, 61, 1994.

93. Price, N. and Proud, C., The guanine nucleotide-exchange factor, eIF-2B, *Biochimie,* 76, 748, 1994.

94. Clemens, M. J., Regulation of eukaryotic protein synthesis by protein kinases that phosphorylate initiation factor eIF-2, *Molec. Biol. Rep.,* 19, 201, 1994.

95. Welsh, G. I. and Proud, C. G., Glycogen synthase kinase-3 is rapidly inactivated in response to insulin and phosphorylates eukaryotic initiation factor eIF-2B, *Biochem. J.,* 294, 625, 1993.

96. Gilligan, M., Welsh, G. I., Flynn, A., Bujalska, I., Diggle, T. A., Denton, R. M., Proud, C., and Docherty, K., Glucose stimulates the activity of the guanine nucleotide-exchange factor eIF-2B in isolated rat islets of langerhans, *J. Biol. Chem.,* 271, 2121, 1996.

97. Hu, C., Pang, S., Kong, X., Velleca, M., and Lawrence, J., Jr., Molecular cloning and tissue distribution of PHAS-I, an intracellular target for insulin and growth factors, *Proc. Natl. Acad. Sci.,* 91, 3730, 1994.

98. Lin, T., Kong, X., Saltiel, A. R., Blackshear, P. J., and Lawrence, J. C., Jr., Control of PHAS-I by insulin in 3T3-L1 adipocytes, *J. Biol. Chem.,* 270, 18531, 1995.

99. Minich, W. B., Balasta, L., Goss, D. J., and Rhoads, R. E., Chromatographic resolution of *in vivo* phosphorylated and nonphosphorylated eukaryotic translation initiation factor eIF-4E: increased cap affinity of the phosphorylated form, *Proc. Natl. Acad. Sci.,* 91, 7668, 1994.

100. Haghighat, A., Mader, S., Pause, A., and Sonenberg, N., Repression of cap-dependent translation by 4E-binding protein-1: competition with p220 for binding to eukaryotic initiation factor-4E, *EMBO J.,* 14, 5701, 1995.

101. Graves, L. M., Bornfeld, K. E., Argast, G. M., Krebs, E. G., Kong, X., Lin, T. A., and Lawrence, J., Jr., cAMP- and rapamycin-sensitive regulation of the association of eukaryotic initiation factor 4E and the translational regulator PHAS-I in aortic smooth muscle cells, *Proc. Natl. Acad. Sci.,* 92, 7222, 1995.

102. Beretta, L., Gingras, A. C., Svitkin, Y. V., Hall, M. N., and Sonenberg, N., Rapamycin blocks the phosphorylation of 4E-BP1 and inhibits cap-dependent initiation of translation, *EMBO J.,* 15, 658, 1996.

103. Kimball, S. R., Vary T. C., and Jefferson, L. S., Regulation of protein synthesis by insulin, *Ann. Rev. Physiol.,* 56, 321, 1994.

104. Brooks, G. A., Fahey, T. D., and White, T. P., *Exercise Physiology: Human Bioenergetics and Its Applications,* 2nd ed., Mayfield Publishing Company, Mountain View, CA, 1996, 152.

105. Balon, T. W., Zorzano, A., Treadway, J. L., Goodman, N. M., and Ruderman, N. B., Effect of insulin on protein synthesis and degradation in skeletal muscle after exercise, *Am. J. Physiol.,* 258, E92, 1990.

106. Hartman, M. L., Veldhuis, J. D., and Thorner, M. O., Normal control of growth hormone secretion, *Hormone Res.,* 40, 37, 1993.

107. Weltman, A., Weltman, J. Y., Schurrer, R., Evans, W. S., Veldhuis, J. D., and Rogol, A. D., Endurance training amplifies the pulsatile release of growth hormone: effects of training intensity., *J. Appl. Physiol.*, 74, 410, 1993.

108. Zhao, X., Unterman, T. G., and Donovan, S. M., Human growth hormone but not human insulin-like growth factor-I enhances recovery from neonatal malnutrition in rats, *J. Nutr.*, 125, 1316, 1995.

109. Deyssig, R., Frisch, H., Blum, W. F., and Waldhor, T., Effect of growth hormone treatment on hormonal parameters, body composition and strength in athletes, *Acta Endocrinol.*, 128, 313, 1993.

110. Yarasheski, K. E., Zachwieja, J. J., Angelopulos, T. J., and Bier, D. M., Short-term growth hormone treatment does not increase muscle protein synthesis in experienced weight lifters, *J. Appl. Physiol.*, 74, 3073, 1993.

111. Yeh, J. K., Aloia, J. F., Chen, M., and Sprintz, S., Effect of growth hormone administration and treadmill exercise on the body composition of rats, *J. Appl. Physiol.*, 77, 23, 1994.

112. Cooper, D. M., Moromisato, D., Zanconato, S., Moromisato, M., Jensen, S., and Brasel, J. A., Effect of growth hormone suppression on exercise training and growth responses in young rats, *Pediatric Res.*, 35, 223, 1994.

113. Jones, J. I. and Clemmons, D. R., Insulin-like growth factors and their binding proteins: biological actions, *Endocrine Rev.*, 16, 3, 1995.

114. Livingston, N., Pollare, T., Lithell, H., and Arner, P., Characterization of insulin-like growth factor I receptor in skeletal muscles of normal and insulin resistant subjects, *Diabetologia*, 31, 871, 1988.

115. Bach, B. A. and Rechler, M. M., Insulin-like growth factor binding proteins, *Diabetes Rev.*, 3, 38, 1995.

116. Svanberg, E., Zachrisson, H., Ohlsson, C., Iresjö, B. M., and Lundholm, K. G., Role of insulin and IGF-I in activation of muscle protein synthesis after oral feeding, *Am. J. Physiol.*, 270, E614, 1996.

117. Gautsch, T. A., Kandl, S. M., Crabtree, S. L., Donovan, S. M., and Layman, D. K., Exercise stimulates hepatic insulin-like growth factor binding protein-1 (IGFBP-1) mRNA expression in rats, *FASEB J.*, 10, A206, 1996.

118. Koistinen, H., Koistinen, R., Selenius, L., Ylikorkala, O., and Seppälä, M., Effect of marathon run on serum IGF-I and IGF-binding protein 1 and 3 levels, *J. Appl. Physiol.*, 80, 760, 1996.

119. DeVol, D. L., Rotwein, P., Sadow, J. L., Novakofski, J., and Bechtel, P. J., Activation of insulin-like growth factor gene expression during work-induced skeletal muscle growth, *Am. J. Physiol.*, 259, E89, 1990.

120. Zanconato, S., Moromisato, D. Y., Moromisato, M. Y., Woods, J., Brasel, J. A., Leroith, D., Roberts, C. T., Jr., and Cooper, D., Effect of training and growth hormone suppression on insulin-like growth factor I mRNA in young rats, *J. Appl. Physiol.*, 76, 2204, 1994.

121. Hopkins, N. J., Jakeman, S., Cwyfan Hughes, S., and Holly, J. M. P., Changes in circulating insulin-like growth factor binding protein-1 (IGFBP-1) during prolonged exercise: effect of carbohydrate feeding, *J. Clin. Endo. Metab.*, 79, 1887, 1994.

122. Lemon, P. and Nagle, F., Effects of exercise on protein and amino acid metabolism, *Med. Sci. Sports Exer.*, 13, 141, 1981.

123. Haralambie, G. and Berg, A., Serum urea and amino nitrogen changes with exercise duration, *Eur. J. Appl. Physiol.*, 36, 39, 1976.

124. Cerny, F., Protein metabolism during two hour ergometer exercise, in *Metabolic Adaptations to Prolonged Physical Exercise*, Howald, H. and Poortmans, J. R., Eds., Birkhaser, Basel, Switzerland, 1975, 441.

125. Calles-Escandon, J., Cunningham, J. J., Snyder, P., Jacob, R., Huszar, G., Loke, J., and Felig, P., Influence of exercise on urea, creatinine, and 3-methylhistidine excretion in normal human subjects, *Am. J. Physiol.*, 246, E334, 1984.

126. Lemon, P., Dolny, D. G., and Yarasheski, K. E., Effect of intensity on protein utilization during prolonged exercise, *Med. Sci. Sports Exer.*, 16, A151, 1984.

127. Konopka, B. and Haymes, E., Effect of sweat collection methods on protein contribution, *Med. Sci. Sports Exer.*, 15, A99, 1983.

128. Munro, H. N. and Young, V. R., Urinary excretion of N^τ-methylhistidine (3-methylhistidine): a tool to study metabolic responses in relation to nutrient and hormonal status in health and disease of man, *Am. J. Clin. Nutr.*, 31, 1608, 1978.

129. Schroeder, L., Renal disease: nephrolithiasis, in *Nutrition in Health and Disease*, Anderson, L., Dibble, M., Turkki, P., Mitchell, H., and Rynbergen, H., Eds., J.B. Lippincott, Philadelphia, 1982, 537.

130. Refsum, H. E. and Stromme, S. B., Urea and creatinine production and excretion in urine during and after prolonged heavy exercise, *Scand. J. Clin. Lab. Invest.*, 33, 247, 1974.

131. Mendez, J., Lukaski, H. C., and Buskirk, E. R., Fat-free mass as a function of maximal oxygen consumption and 24-hour urinary creatinine and 3-methylhistidine excretion, *Am. J. Clin. Nutr.*, 39, 710, 1984.

132. Hickson, J. F. and Wolinsky, I., Research directions in protein nutrition for athletes, in *Nutrition in Exercise and Sport*, Wolinsky, I. and Hickson, J. F., Eds., CRC Press, Boca Raton, FL, 1994, 85.

133. Popp, R. L. and Farrar, R. P., Urinary 3-methylhistidine after acute exercise in highly vs moderately trained distance runners, *Med. Sci. Sports Exer.*, 16, 164A, 1984.

134. Plante, P. D. and Houston, M. E., Effects of concentric and eccentric exercise on protein catabolism in man, *Int. J. Sports Med.,* 5, 174, 1984.

135. Hickson, J. F., Wolinsky, I., Rodriguez, G. P., Pivarnik, J. M., Kent, M. C., and Shier, N. W., Failure of weight training to affect urinary indices of protein metabolism in men, *Med. Sci. Sports Exer.,* 18, 563, 1986.

136. Horswill, C. A., Layman, D. K., Boileau, R. A., Williams, B. T., and Massey, B. H., Excretion of 3-methylhistidine and hydroxyproline following acute weight-training exercise, *Int. J. Sports Med.,* 9, 245, 1988.

137. Dohm, G. L., Israel, R. G., Breedlove, R. L., Williams, R. T., and Askew, E. W., Biphasic changes in 3-methylhistidine excretion in humans after exercise, *Am. J. Physiol.,* 248, E588, 1985.

138. Radha, E. and Bessman, S. P., Effect of exercise on protein degradation: 3-methylhistidine and creatinine excretion, *Biochem. Med.,* 29, 96, 1983.

139. Hickson, J. F. and Hinkelmann, K., Exercise and protein intake effects on urinary 3-methylhistidine excretion, *Am. J. Clin. Nutr.,* 41, 246, 1985.

140. Pivarnik, J. M., Hickson, J. F., and Wolinsky, I., Urinary 3-methylhistidine excretion increases with repeated weight training exercise, *Med. Sci. Sports Exer.,* 21, 283, 1989.

141. Frontera, W. R., Meredith, C. N., O'Reilly, K. P., Knuttgen, J. G., and Evans, W. J., Strength conditioning in older men: skeletal muscle hypertrophy and improved function, *J. Appl. Physiol.,* 64, 1038, 1988.

142. Tarnopolsky, M. A., Atkinson, S. A., MacDougall, J. D., Senor, B. B., Lemon, P. W. R., and Schwarcz, H., Whole body leucine metabolism during and after resistance exercise in fed humans, *Med. Sci. Sports Exer.,* 23, 326, 1991.

143. Gontzea, I., Sutzescu, P., and Dumitrache, S., The influence of muscular activity on nitrogen balance and the need of man for proteins, *Nutr. Rep. Int.,* 10, 35, 1974.

144. Iyengar, A. and Rao, B. S. N., Effect of varying energy and protein intake on nitrogen balance in adults engaged in heavy manual labour, *Brit. J. Nutr.,* 41, 19, 1979.

145. Goranzon, H. and Forsum, E., Effect of reduced energy intake versus increased physical activity on the outcome of nitrogen balance experiments in man, *Am. J. Clin. Nutr.,* 41, 919, 1985.

146. Fuller, M. F. and Garlick, P. J., Human amino acid requirements: can the controversy be resolved?, *Annu. Rev. Nutr.,* 14, 217, 1994.

147. Gontzea, I., Sutzescu, P., and Dumitrache, S., The influence of adaptation to physical effort on nitrogen balance in man, *Nutr. Rep. Int.,* 11, 231, 1975.

148. Meredith, C. N., Zackin, M. J., Frontera, W. R., and Evans, W. J., Dietary protein requirements and protein metabolism in endurance-trained men, *J. Appl. Physiol.,* 66, 2850, 1989.

149. Tarnopolsky, M. A., MacDougall, J. D., and Atkinson, S. A., Influence of protein intake and training status on nitrogen balance and lean body mass, *J. Appl. Physiol.,* 64, 187, 1988.

150. Friedman, J. E. and Lemon, P. W. R., Effect of chronic endurance exercise on the retention of dietary protein, *Int. J. Sports Med.,* 10, 118, 1989.

151. Laritcheva, K. A., Yalovaya, N. I., Shubin, V. I., and Smirnov, P. V., Study of energy expenditure and protein needs of top weightlifters, in *Nutrition, Physical Fitness, and Health,* Parizkova, J. and Rogozkin, V. A., Eds., University Park Press, Baltimore, 1978, 144.

152. Celejowa, I. and Homa, M., Food intake, nitrogen, and energy balance in Polish weight lifters during a training camp, *Nutr. Met.,* 12, 259, 1970.

153. Millward, D. J., Bowtell, J. L., Pacy, P., and Rennie, M. J., Physical activity, protein metabolism and protein requirements, *Proc. Nutr. Soc.,* 53, 223, 1994.

154. Tarnopolsky, M. A., Atkinson, S. A., MacDougall, J. D., Chesley, A., Phillips, S., and Schwarcz, H. P., Evaluation of protein requirements for trained strength athletes, *J. Appl. Physiol.,* 73, 1986, 1992.

155. Lemon, P. W. R., Tarnopolsky, M. A., MacDougall, J. D., and Atkinson, S. A., Protein requirements and muscle mass/strength changes during intensive training in novice bodybuilders, *J. Appl. Physiol.,* 73, 767, 1992.

156. Young, V. R., Bier, D. M., and Pellet, P. L., A theoretical basis for increasing current estimates of the amino acid requirements in adult man with experimental support, *Am. J. Clin. Nutr.,* 50, 80, 1989.

157. Grandjean, A. C., Current nutritional beliefs and practices in athletes for weight/strength gains, in *Muscle Development: Nutritional Alternatives to Anabolic Steroids,* Garrett, W. E. and Malone, T. R., Eds., Ross Laboratories, Columbus, Ohio, 1988, 56.

158. Rasch, P. J., Hamby, J. W., and Burns, J. H., Protein dietary supplementation and physical performance, *Med. Sci. Sports Exer.,* 1, 195, 1969.

159. Consolazio, C. F., Johnson, H. L., Nelson, R. A., Dramise, J. G., and Skala, J. H., Protein metabolism during intensive physical training in the young adult, *Am. J. Clin. Nutr.,* 28, 29, 1975.

160. Frontera, W. R., Meredith, C. N., and Evans, W. J., Dietary effects on muscle strength gain and hypertrophy during heavy resistance training in older men, *Can. J. Sport Sci.,* 13, 13P, 1988.

161. Fern, E. B., Bileinski, R. N., and Schutz, Y., Effects of exaggerated amino acid and protein supply in man, *Experientia,* 47, 168, 1991.

Chapter 6

OVERVIEW OF HUMAN ENERGY TRANSFER AND NUTRITION

Catherine G. Ratzin Jackson

CONTENTS

I. HUMAN ENERGY TRANSFER

A. ENERGY CYCLE

The human organism captures and converts potential chemical energy from food macronutrients into usable chemical energy forms in a way similar to most living cells on earth. Carbon dioxide, a byproduct of animal energy metabolism, is cycled through the plant kingdom while oxygen, a byproduct of plant energy metabolism, is cycled through the animal kingdom; both processes use the byproducts of the other to transfer energy to useful forms. The particular way in which the human interconverts energy forms through the different pathways which phosphorylate adenosine 5'-diphosphate (ADP) to form 5'-adenosine triphosphate (ATP), the universal carrier of energy, are the objects of much study. The general principles have been elucidated in the past,[1] but much remains to be discovered.

B. ATP

Many sources are available for review which outline human energy metabolism.[2-7] All include a discussion of how substrates for utilization derived from food macronutrients (fats, carbohydrates, protein) are used in phosphorylating adenosine nucleotides to form the ATP molecule. ATP is the most important energy carrier molecule in the cell that directly supplies chemical energy to the cellular machinery which can be converted into cell work. All other energy reservoirs or cycles must first transfer their energy to forms of ATP with one or more phosphate groups which have been removed before use by the cell. This transfer of energy is often the limiting factor in physical activity.

As the ATP molecule releases its phosphate groups, energy is released to perform biological work. In terms of physical performance, it is the work of mechanical contraction of the muscles which is of greatest interest. The phosphate groups liberated from ATP to produce energy must be replaced to allow continuous energy transfer. The process where a phosphate is attached to ADP to form ATP is of greatest importance in understanding human energy metabolism (Figure 1).

C. HIGH ENERGY PHOSPHAGENS

The phosphagen system is named for the two high energy phosphate compounds, ATP and phosphocreatine (PCr), which enter into coupled energy transfer reactions. At rest the body is primarily in aerobic metabolism since most of the needs of the cell for oxygen can be met by blood flow related to a matched delivery of the cardiovascular system. During this time the phosphagen system functions continuously, particularly at the initiation of any movement, but it is not overly stressed. When an activity is begun, however, this balance cannot be maintained and the phosphagen system and all of its stores of phosphate are immediately mobilized. The higher the intensity the more rapidly this store will become depleted. In high intensity work, oxygen is difficult to deliver quickly and replenishment of the depleted phosphate groups from adenosine nucleotides must wait for the relatively slow mechanisms of the cardiovascular system to function. Under these circumstances approximately 80% of the ATP required for a 30 s activity may come from ATP derived anaerobically.[8]

During exercise or activity of any type the immediate source of ATP is that which is already stored and is coupled for acquisition of the phosphate group with PCr. As the phosphate groups are removed from ATP, ADP, adenosine 5′-monophosphate (AMP), and adenosine may remain in varying ratios or proportions. This particular system can provide energy only for brief periods of intense activity such as golf or tennis swings, sprints, or jumps. Under these circumstances the phosphate groups needed to replenish the adenosine forms are easily supplied in the exercise recovery period. While phosphocreatine is the immediate source of the phosphates and energy used to restore ADP to ATP, this coupled reaction with ATP cannot replete the system effectively until exercise or activity is terminated. During activity other sources of phosphate must be used. However, the hydrolysis of ATP is facilitated by increased activity of the ATPases found in muscle.

All humans seem to possess approximately the same ratio of PCr to ATP, which is 5 to 1, respectively, and is related to muscle mass. While highly intense activity such as sprinting can deplete phosphate groups within 10 s, a lower intensity activity can allow one to use this system for up to 3 min. The ATP is located in specific areas of muscle and tends to increase proportionally when the amount of muscle is increased. It appears that a ratio of ATP to muscle mass is established so that as muscle mass increases so does the amount of ATP. Enhancement of this ATP store over and above this established ratio is currently controversial.

Early theories of functioning of the phosphagen system suggested that PCr was the exclusive substrate for ATP resynthesis in intense activity.[9,10] It was widely accepted that glycolysis was the next immediate source of phosphates for energy and that one went through the energy delivery systems in ordered sequence. Experimental evidence shows that depletion

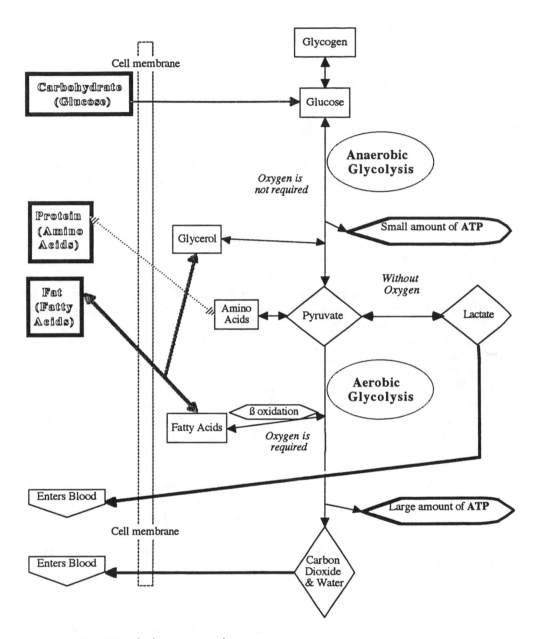

FIGURE 1   Interaction of substrates to produce energy.

of PCr is not necessary for mobilization of glycolysis and that PCr degradation and anaerobic glycolysis are simultaneously activated.[11-13] Reliable, noninvasive methods for estimating the amount of ATP which can be derived from this system are not yet developed. Work continues in developing a good match between direct and indirect measurements of aerobic and anaerobic contributions to intense activity.[14]

There is currently much interest in creatine supplementation to enhance muscle stores of total creatine and PCr. Skeletal muscle derives its supply from ingested dietary sources synthesized in the liver which enter the bloodstream. Biopsy studies have shown small increases of muscle PCr and total creatine with supplementation but ATP stores were unaffected.[15] Creatine supplementation may, however, delay fatigue and improve muscle performance in highly intense work.[16,17] It is widely accepted that there is little that can be done to effectively enhance access to the ATP of this system by sprint training.[18] There do not appear to be nutritional or exercise training practices which will allow higher amounts of ATP to be stored in muscle over and above established ratios of ATP to muscle mass.

D. GLYCOGENOLYSIS AND GLYCOLYSIS

Exercise may be of a duration or intensity beyond the capability of the phosphagen system to supply the immediate ATP need. At this point glucose or glycogen (which degrades to glucose) are mobilized for phosphate replacement producing both energy and lactate. Lactate is continuously formed in the cell to a certain degree and is easily transported to the blood stream due to its high permeability through the cell membrane. Baseline amounts of lactate have been established for normal individuals at rest such that the lack thereof is a clear sign of neuromuscular disease. When activity ensues, if intensity is not high, lactate in the system is rapidly cleared by other tissues and organs of the body, including muscle, which keep blood levels minimal. At other times, with high intensity and duration, lactate accumulation will be high enough to terminate activity by interfering with muscular contraction. It has long been accepted that this system can predominate in activities lasting from 1 to 3 min.

The first stages of glucose degradation are always anaerobic (without oxygen) and thus the designation is anaerobic glycolysis. Anaerobic glycolysis progresses to the formation of energy rich pyruvate. If oxygen delivery cannot be or is not increased sufficiently, the process remains anaerobic and pyruvate is converted to lactate. If this conversion of pyruvate to lactate occurs, anaerobic glycolysis results in very little energy transfer to produce ATP because the majority of the potential energy is left in the lactate. However, since this process is so rapid, the small amounts of ATP produced absolutely can supply a considerable amount of rephosphorylation of ATP due to the speed of the reaction. Lactate is thought to quickly cross the cell membrane into the blood where it can be cleared or taken out of the blood for use to create ATP elsewhere than the active muscle. Much of this lactate is used by other cells in the body to form ATP for their own use. However, the rate of clearance can be exceeded by the rate of production with the result that high levels of blood lactate accumulate. Under these circumstances exercise cannot continue for long periods because muscular contraction will soon be hindered.

Should activity continue to the point of greater activation of the aerobic system, many more ATPs can be formed by utilization of the phosphorylating system found at the inner mitochondrial membrane. The number of ATPs generated is much higher and produces much more energy transfer so that duration of activity is sustained.

In activities where one remains in anaerobic glycolysis, glycogen may not be completely degraded aerobically to water, an end product of aerobic metabolism. The precursors of glycogen thus formed may reassemble the glycogen molecule. This eliminates the need for high levels of additional carbohydrate in the diet immediately after activities of this type, a recommendation which is appropriately made for endurance activities.[19] The types of activity utilizing anaerobic glycolysis would include bodybuilding, weightlifting, and resistance exercises. A more fundamental concern in activities of this type would be that glycogen or carbohydrate loading, if done immediately before a bout of intense exercise, might make the muscle feel tight due to the compensatory storage of water with the glycogen. As water is not compressible, an injury may be the result.

Exclusively fueling this system is either glycogen stored in muscle or glucose brought into the cell and the subsequent degradation of glucose for energy. It is known that carbohydrate stores in muscle (glycogen) can be enhanced by dietary practices that favor a high carbohydrate diet (carbohydrate loading) which will in turn affect the length of performance.[20] However, not all activities benefit from this practice. The greatest benefit is derived when the activity is categorized as aerobic.

E. AEROBIC METABOLISM

If oxygen delivery can be increased through the enhanced functioning of the cardiovascular system, then substrates formed in glycolysis proceed to the aerobic system for oxidative phosphorylation which results in much more ATP production. The pyruvate formed during anaerobic glycolysis is then degraded to water and carbon dioxide when oxygen delivery increases, rather than converting to lactate and either being exported from the cell or accumulating in the blood. This produces approximately 18 times more ATP than would have been produced through anaerobic glycolysis. Additionally, the aerobic process will more efficiently clear the lactate previously produced and concurrently formed.

At the end of aerobic glycolysis, the glycogen or glucose is degraded to water and carbon dioxide and is thus not recoverable in a reversible reaction to glucose within the cell. Few precursors will remain and glycogen cannot be reformed except through intake of carbohydrate (glucose) in the diet. This scenario describes the endurance exerciser who participates in activities such as rhythmic aerobics, running, and other prolonged exercises. Carbohydrate or glycogen loading may be considered in these activities with the best practice being the conversion of the diet permanently to higher carbohydrate intake. A specificity of diet with respect to carbohydrate intake is suggested, based upon the metabolic pathway stressed in the activity; the need for carbohydrate is greater for the endurance exerciser than for the strength exerciser. This is an important concept for exercisers to understand if they are to use nutrition effectively to enhance performance of their activity.

If the exercise duration allows the aerobic system to predominate, ATP is formed in great quantities at the inner mitochondrial membrane. This system does not rely heavily on carbohydrate. While the carbohydrate contribution to energy production may diminish, aerobic metabolism cannot continue without some carbohydrate contribution. During aerobic metabolism the cell can now degrade other substrates effectively, the main one being fat (fatty acids). It is the hydrogens of the fat which can be used for ATP production; since fat contains great amounts of hydrogen concomitantly great amounts of ATP can be produced. Protein (amino acids) can also be used for ATP production and this occurs to a greater extent in the aerobic exerciser than in the anaerobic exerciser. By far the greatest amount of ATP can be produced from the degradation of fat (Figure 2). The difficulty usually encountered is that aerobic metabolism must first be overloaded and then stressed over long periods of time to produce enhanced levels of the enzymes necessary to use this pathway to a high degree at the cellular level.

Aerobic metabolism requires that oxygen be delivered in greater quantities than were previously necessary thus requiring a complex series of reactions in the body to match cardiac output and capillary blood flow to the needs of the cell. In terms of cellular metabolism the aerobic pathway is slow to become initiated and predominate during activity and is probably not used to a great degree until at least 5 min of continuous activity have elapsed. While the general principles of these energy transitions have been known for some time they are still not completely understood. Commonly misunderstood is the fact that energy production is not a question of the three "systems" taking turns serially or being able to "skip" systems. Rather it is a fact that all systems function at all times, and while one predominates, the others participate in greater or lesser degrees. The interaction of the three systems of energy delivery in the first 2 min of exercise is complex and not completely understood (Figure 3). In long duration activity the general patterns are somewhat clearer (Figure 4). Thus, it is important for exercisers to understand which energy system or systems predominate in their activity and to follow the specific dietary practices to enhance performance recommended by sport nutritionists.

F. SUBSTRATES: FAT, CARBOHYDRATE, AND PROTEIN

The three dietary sources of energy substrates are fat, carbohydrate, and protein. At rest and during normal daily activities, fats are the primary energy source, providing 80–90% of

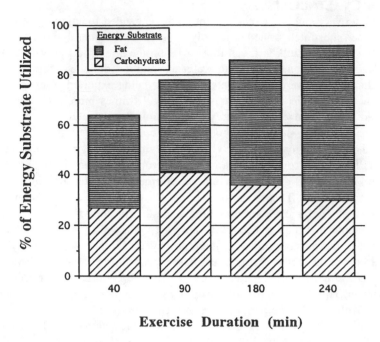

FIGURE 2 Interaction of carbohydrate and fat utilization during long duration exercise. Adapted from McArdle, W. D., Katch, F. I., and Katch, V. L., *Exercise Physiology: Energy, Nutrition, and Human Performance,* 3rd ed., Lea and Febiger, Philadelphia, 1991, p. 28.

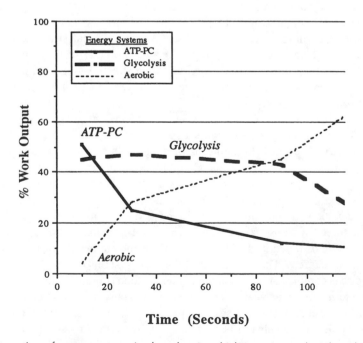

FIGURE 3 Interaction of energy systems in short-duration, high-intensity work. Adapted from McArdle, W. D., Katch, F. I., and Katch, V. L., *Exercise Physiology: Energy, Nutrition, and Human Performance,* 3rd ed., Lea and Febiger, Philadelphia, 1991, p. 206.

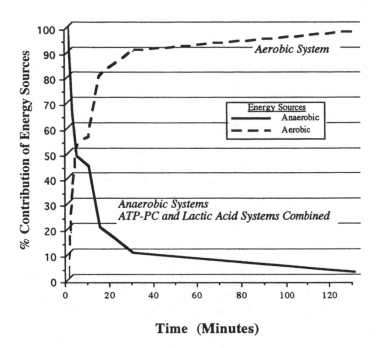

Time (Minutes)

FIGURE 4   Primary energy sources for long duration activity. Adapted from Fox, E. L., Bowers, R. W., and Foss, M. L., *The Physiological Basis for Exercise and Sports,* 5th ed., Brown and Benchmark, Dubuque, IA, 1989, p. 37.

the energy while carbohydrates and protein may provide 5–18% and 2–5%, respectively.[5] During exercise the proportion of each contribution will change.

Highly intense, anaerobic activities that stress the phosphagen system and begin to immediately mobilize the glycolytic system may not directly use any of the three substrates at the initiation of the activity. Post activity, the phosphagen system can be quickly restored. Anaerobic glycolysis does degrade some muscle glycogen which is used to generate additional ATP to sustain the intense, anaerobic activities. Post exercise the muscle glycogen must be restored, much of it from glycogen precursors remaining in the cell.

Whenever glycogen is degraded to water through aerobic glycolysis it must be replaced through carbohydrate in the diet. All ingested carbohydrates degrade in the digestive system predominantly to glucose with lesser contributions from galactose (milk sugar) and fructose (fruit sugar). The majority of galactose and fructose are converted to glucose in the cells lining the small intestine and most of the remainder is converted in the liver. Glucose is absorbed into the blood and transported to the body tissues for use or storage in the liver and muscles as glycogen.[21] Glycogen is composed of chains of individual glucose molecules which are linked together within the cells; glucose must be brought into the cell and then strung together as glycogen. The process of storage or replacement of glycogen is not rapid and can take up to 2 d to complete.[22]

Excessive depletion through exercise or diet may lead to insufficient carbohydrate available to provide glucose to regenerate muscle glycogen. If glucose supplies are low, the muscle glycogen cannot be restored.[23] The glucose available in the blood will be spared for use by the brain and the muscle will be left deficient in carbohydrate energy supply. If glucose levels fall below the levels necessary for proper brain function, other sources of glucose will be used. Protein can be degraded to its amino acids which can then be converted to pyruvate in the liver.[5] Two pyruvate molecules can be combined to form one glucose molecule which can then enter the blood. The primary source of protein for this process is muscle tissue; thus, glucose may be generated at the expense of muscle. This reaction may occur when the body is in starvation, when the individual consumes low levels of calories, or when the individual is under various forms of stress.

Fats, composed of glycerol and three fatty acids, can be used to provide glucose. The glycerol can be converted to glucose while the fatty acids cannot. The fatty acids must be degraded aerobically or they become ketones.[21] Ketones in the blood are toxic in large quantities; therefore, depending upon fat for the generation of glucose is not desirable. The alternative use of protein and fat rather than carbohydrate for glucose or glycogen restoration has negative implications. It becomes clear that an adequate amount of carbohydrate needs to be ingested for successful participation in any activity.

When aerobic glycolysis becomes the principle pathway of energy production the situation changes. Muscle glycogen is the initial source of glucose for aerobic energy; however, the duration of the activity may outlast the supplies stored within the muscle cell and other substrates, fats and protein, must be used.

During low intensity aerobic activities, fats are the preferred substrate for utilization (Figure 5). Fat is stored within the muscle cells and fat storage cells (adipocytes) as triglycerides; they also circulate in the blood as fatty acids. Triglycerides in adipocytes are easily liberated to the circulation for muscle use. The glycerol portion of a triglyceride can enter the glycolysis pathway in anaerobic metabolism and eventually become pyruvate to be used in aerobic glycolysis. The fatty acid portion of a triglyceride can undergo a process of β-oxidation which converts them to a compound that can be used in aerobic glycolysis to produce energy. Fatty acid use in aerobic metabolism results in far greater ATP production than that of carbohydrates. However, even when fats are the predominant energy source, carbohydrates must still be available. Carbohydrates are necessary to continuously prime the breakdown of fatty acids. Therefore, fats are never an exclusive energy source. Even when an overabundance of fat is available, if there are very low levels of carbohyrate to prime their breakdown, aerobic degradation of fat will stop. Other inhibitors of fat utilization

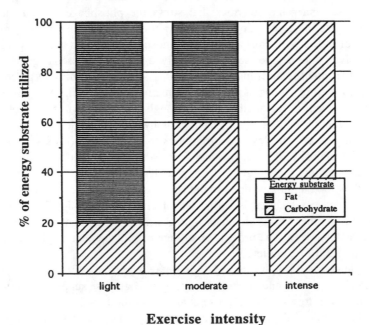

FIGURE 5 Interaction of carbohydrate and fat utilization during different intensities of exercise. Adapted from Sharkey, B. J., *Coaches Guide to Sport Physiology,* Human Kinetics Publishers, Champaign, IL, 1986, p. 84.

are high insulin levels, such as those found after a large intake of simple sugars, and high lactate levels.[24]

Proteins can be converted to pyruvate and can be used for energy production during aerobic activities. There is some disagreement among researchers as the level of contribution to energy delivery can be provided by protein which have ranged from 5% to 15% of the total energy during aerobic activity. Greater amounts of protein may be used as the duration of exercise increases.[25] It is generally agreed that the amount of ATP provided by protein is relatively small compared to fat and carbohydrate.

It has been established that all fat, carbohydrate, and protein can be utilized for energy production during physical activity. It is possible, and not uncommon, for the supply of energy substrates to outweigh the demand particularly through dietary excess. Protein is utilized for cellular structure, enzymes (the molecules that govern the breakdown and buildup of other chemicals), hormones (chemical messengers), blood borne carriers, and energy. Excess protein is not stored at any site in the body but may be converted to fat and stored in the adipocytes.

Carbohydrates are utilized for cellular structure, hormones, and energy. Excess carbohydrate is stored in muscle and liver as glycogen. These limited stores can be increased by a combination of a high carbohydrate diet and regular, activity-induced, depletion. When the glycogen storage capacity is exceeded, it is possible to convert carbohydrate to fat for storage in the adipocytes.

Fats are utilized for cellular structure, hormones, blood borne carriers, insulation, organ protection, and energy. Fats are the highest energy source available and the most easily stored. Fats are not usually converted to either protein or carbohydrate for storage. Fat storage occurs within muscle cells, for use during aerobic activity, and within adipocytes. Excess fat can also be found circulating in the blood and lining the walls of blood vessels. High levels of fat within the circulatory system are highly correlated with cardiovascular disease. It is clear that an excess of any one energy source may potentially result in an increase in fat storage.

G. POWER

While the above discussion focused on energy transitions which can be viewed as a complex series of interactions, there is another concept which must be considered. Because the work produced by muscle is the product of force times distance, the power generated by muscle is determined by work divided by time. Thus, more power is generated as the duration of work is shortened; nutritional practices should support this concept. Calculation of energy expenditure and energy intake, sometimes called "calories" or "joules," needed for optimal nutrition for sport and activity depend on these measurements. Walking, a simple activity, may place different demands upon the ability to deliver oxygen, and the energy intake and expenditure may not be the same under all conditions. As the speed of walking is increased and the time to cover a particular distance is shortened, the activity generates more power.[26] This results in an increased need for oxygen and energy production. All activity can be characterized by its frequency, intensity, and duration; understanding these relationships is fundamental to understanding the specificity of diet related to a particular activity. The influence of intensity of exercise on the substrate used to produce energy is great (Figure 4). Low intensity activities will rely more upon fat for the generation of energy while carbohydrate is utilized as power and intensity increases. There is also a relationship between duration of activity and substrate utilization (Figure 2). It becomes clear that if the desire is to diminish fat stores in the body, low intensity and long duration activities characterized as aerobic should be chosen. Conversely, if hypertrophy of muscle is desired, activities should be chosen which generate more power. Observations made of cellular effects of these two types of conditioning preclude, however, being able to mix the two types of activities and get maximum cellular benefit from both. Evidence has been presented which shows that, at the cellular level, the two types of activities may not produce desired results. While endurance training followed by strength training may not diminish either endurance or strength benefits at the cellular level the converse may not be true. It has been shown that endurance training in previously strength trained muscle may diminish the size of muscle fibers thereby suggesting that aerobic conditioning should be undertaken cautiously in athletes who wish to develop strength and hypertrophy in muscle.[27]

II. RELATIONSHIP OF SPECIFIC CELLS TO METABOLISM

A. MUSCLE FIBERS

There is a direct relationship between nutritional practices aimed at modifying energy production and specific characteristics of human muscle. Normal, nondiseased, human muscle has a mosaic of fiber types which can be viewed as possessing properties along a spectrum of capacities from highly aerobic to highly anaerobic.[28] Due to the difficulty of characterizing subsets of fiber types which may number up to nine identifiable groups, simpler groupings are usually chosen that describe three major groups of fibers identified histochemically as types I, IIa, and IIb. Physiological, anatomical, and biochemical properties can also be described and quantified. The fibers identified and studied with one property do not necessarily correlate with the other systems of classification, i.e., not all fibers identified histochemically as type I will show the same aerobic characteristics when identified physiologically.[29]

Type I [slow twitch (ST), slow twitch oxidative (SO), red, dark] fibers are those that have high capabilities for aerobic energy production. These fibers are stressed in endurance activities such as running, cycling, and swimming. All of the biochemical characteristics that support aerobic metabolism are at high levels in these fibers. There are elevated amounts of carbohydrate (glycogen, glucose) and fat (neutral lipids, triglycerides), the substrates for aerobic energy production. Aerobic conditioning enhances the ability of type I fibers to use energy substrates by increasing the amount and activity of the enzymes in the pathways for substrate utilization. It has been reported that individuals participating for long periods of time in endurance activities such as marathons have higher than expected percentages of type I fibers.[30] Whether these greater percentages of type I fibers are genetically inherited or are converted with prolonged aerobic training remains an open question. The type I fiber however does not have the capability to hypertrophy to a great degree, even if it is overloaded, perhaps due to the need to get oxygen to the center of the fiber.[30] The increase in cross-sectional area may reach a limit for efficient transport and diffusion of oxygen from the capillary to the center of the fiber. Thus the individuals who participate in and continually train using endurance activities stress the Type I fiber and will find that the muscles used will not enlarge greatly and that body fat stores tend to diminish. There is also a need to keep glycogen stores high through dietary ingestion of carbohydrate. Although it has long been accepted that muscle glycogen stores are the most important factor in successful endurance performance, the adaptations to fat metabolism have been investigated with conflicting results.[31,32]

Type II fibers (fast twitch, white, light) have two major subgroups, fast-twitch-oxidative-glycolytic (IIa, FTa, FOG) and fast-twitch-glycolytic (IIb, FTb, FG). Overall these fibers have high capabilities for producing energy anaerobically; however, the IIa also has a great ability for aerobic energy production, and therefore, is sometimes called "super fiber" in terms of performance. The IIa fiber, while fast twitch, can provide aerobic metabolism and can also hypertrophy the greatest of the type II subgroups. Type II fibers are stressed in resistance and power activities such as weightlifting and bodybuilding. All of the biochemical properties that support anaerobic metabolism are found in high levels in these fibers. Consequently, high amounts of glycogen are found particularly in the IIa fiber.[33] Conditioning enhances the ability of this fiber type to use energy substrates by increasing the amount and activity of enzymes which allow their use. It has not, however, been shown that individuals who participate in resistance activities over long periods of time have greater percentages of these fibers than are found in the general population of individuals who do not train or condition to a high degree.[34] Transitions between the percentages of IIa and the IIb fiber types with exercise along with significant and dramatic changes in their size have been shown, thereby either enhancing the aerobic (IIa) or the anaerobic (IIb) capacity of the muscle as a whole.[30] The type II fiber will significantly hypertrophy with use and is responsible for the great increase in muscle mass seen in strength conditioning and bodybuilding. There is also an effect of the speed of movement used to stress the fiber, as slower movements show more rapid increases in power[35] thereby increasing tension and hypertrophy to a greater degree than fast movements. It has been suggested that muscle fibers can split and increase their numbers (hyperplasia); however, this has not been conclusively proved in humans and there is evidence to both prove and disprove this theory.[36] The individuals who stress the use of these fibers will find that their muscles will enlarge and that they have a need for carbohydrate in their diet in order to produce energy through anaerobic glycolysis. There is also evidence that the amount of fat in the diet may directly affect testosterone production, which is known in turn to affect increases in muscle mass. Adequate fat in the diet may facilitate testosterone production while low fat diets are associated with clinically recognized decreases in production.[37]

B.   ADIPOCYTES

The greatest reserve of energy in the body is found in the adipocytes, whose only function is to store fat or triglyceride. They are found in superficial stores directly beneath the skin and in deep areas surrounding organs. The latter type of depot is termed essential fat. Adipocytes are known to significantly increase in number or show hyperplasia during the last 3 months of fetal development, the first year of life, and the prepubertal adolescent growth spurt.[38] An increase in number in pregnancy has been postulated, but this has not yet been proved. These are the only known times when the cells increase in number in an individual who is not morbidly obese.

The adipocytes are known to fill with a particular amount of lipid, triglyceride, which is under control of the brain. It is believed that a normal person increases fat stores by increasing the amount of triglyceride in each cell, rather than by increasing the fat cell number. Fat loss probably occurs by a decrease in the stores in each cell, rather than by the death of fat cells. The amount of filling has been shown to be approximately the same for all adipocytes in the body, thereby suggesting that one cannot "spot reduce" a particular area without reducing stores in the entire body first.[38] Obese individuals have been shown to have greater numbers of adipocytes which have greater lipid volumes than nonobese individuals. It is therefore postulated that hyperplasia may also be induced when the existing adipocytes can no longer accommodate filling.[39]

Not all human adipocytes throughout the body are of equal size and the metabolic characteristics of adipose tissue may vary in different locations.[40] Although the percent filling may be similar, the adipocytes themselves tend to be larger in the gluteo-femoral (buttocks) and femoral (thigh) region than in the abdominal region of young women as compared to young men.[41] These differences are not seen in middle-aged females and males. Gender hormones may influence the regional influx of triglyceride in and out of the cells in these regions. It is clear that the way the body stores fat is complex and is related to both the number, size, and filling of adipocytes.

Athletes of all types comprise a large portion of the millions of individuals who wish to modify, enhance, or diminish the fat stores in the body. Large groups of individuals use the thousands of diets and hundreds of weight loss programs available to them. Considering the fact that there are thousands of published diets, it cannot help but be noticed that if one of them worked successfully there would be no need for the others. It is seldom noted that caloric restriction must be coupled with exercise as the two practices are synergistic. Sound, scientifically based advice on proper and improper weight loss programs can be found in the position stand of the American College of Sports Medicine.[42] It is further recommended that manipulation of body fat stores not be done unless necessary and percentage body fat has been assessed by someone trained in the appropriate methods and how to interpret the results.

Body fat stores are assessed by many methods[43] with hydrostatic weighing considered the "gold standard" and skinfold caliper measurements considered the most practical. Considerable misinterpretation of results can be found in the popular literature. The assessment of body composition where the percentage of body fat is determined is most appropriately used as a tool to monitor progress rather than as an absolute number or criteria for performance. There is heightened awareness of these measurements in the general population but little understanding of what the percentages mean or how to apply the knowledge. The percentage body fat range for adult males is 10–25% for optimal health, 12–20% for optimal fitness, and more than 25% is considered obese.[44] The percentage body fat range for adult females is 18–33% for optimal health, 16–25% for ideal fitness, and more than 35% is considered obese.[44] Fitness requires not only keeping the range of body fat within acceptable limits but includes proper nutrition and the appropriate combination of activities known to produce "total fitness."[45] With the release of the first Surgeon General's report on physical activity and health,[46] it is clear that activity should be included along with sound nutritional practices to enhance the quality of life.

III. PRACTICAL APPLICATIONS OF UNDERSTANDING DAILY ENERGY BALANCE

The most accurate method of measuring energy expenditure is direct calorimetry where the subject is placed into an enclosed container and dissipated heat is measured directly. This is not practical under most circumstances, and the enclosures or rooms which are necessary to collect these data for exercise are extremely expensive and not available to most exercise physiologists. The method which is more practical is that of indirect calorimetry where products of biological oxidation, carbon dioxide, and oxygen are measured for certain periods of time using the gases expired through the airways during exercise compared to their amounts in ambient air. One liter of oxygen equates to use of 4.8 kcal (20.2 kJ).

In order to assess daily needs for energy (kcals) it is important to know the needs of the body for basal metabolism, the minimal rate of energy expenditure necessary for life.[47] An accurate measurement requires standardizing rest conditions (8 hr rest) and assuring that the subject is post absorptive (12–18 hr) and quiet during measurement.[48] Practically, 3–4 hr post absorption differs little from the more rigorous data collection for normal individuals for whom weight loss or weight gain programs are not being recommended. Results show differences in males and females (Table 10). While males on average are heavier and taller than females they tend to have almost one-third the body fat. Male lean body mass therefore is higher. Since this difference is made up of more muscle mass which is more metabolically

TABLE 1 **Profile of Physical and Metabolic Characteristics in Females and Males**

	Females	Males
Number of Subjects	25	24
Height (cm)	165	176
	(156–179)	(168–190)
Weight (kg)	58.2	68.5
	(42.4–70.5)	(53.1–80.3)
Body Fat (%)	25.6	10.7
	(18.4–34.8)	(4.5–26.0)
Lean Body Mass (LBM)	43.1	61.1
	(37.8–55.3)	(44.8–74.6)
Resting Oxygen Consumption		
ml/min	186	258
	(148–225)	(188–326)
ml/min/m²	115	141
ml/min/kg LBM	4.31	4.22
ml/min/kg Body Weight	3.20	3.77
J/min/kg Body Weight	67.2	79.2

Adapted from Bassett, D. R. and Nagle, F. J., in *Nutrition in Exercise and Sport*, 2nd ed., CRC Press, Boca Raton, FL, 1993; and Food and Nutrition Board, *Recommended Dietary Allowance*, 10th ed., National Academy Press, Washington, D.C., 1989.

active than adipose tissue, males have higher resting oxygen consumptions in all ways in which this is calculated. It is generally accepted that an average resting oxygen consumption (VO_2) is 3.5 ml/kg · min⁻¹ (1 MET or metabolic equivalent). It is important to note that in reality males have higher resting oxygen consumptions than females. As both genders age, the differences become more pronounced. It is more desirable to actually measure resting oxygen consumptions than to use the MET estimate when accurately assessing energy needs for weight loss or weight gain recommendations. In estimation there is a loss of precision which might render dietary recommendations unsuccessful.

While it is extremely important to understand the metabolic energy sources of activity for training and conditioning so that time is not wasted focusing on the wrong energy delivery system, it is also important to understand the overall energy needs of the body. An approximation of daily energy needs can be calculated[49] (Table 2). This is based on the assumption that there are no additional needs created by exercise or other increase in daily activity.[50] If additional activity is done, this amount of energy intake needs to be estimated and added to the daily requirement[51,52] (Table 3). It is suggested that for adaptation to take place for endurance activities the activity should expend approximately 300 kcals[53] (intensity) per minimally a 20 min (duration) exercise session done at least 3–4 d/wk (frequency). Examples of 300 kcal activities are provided in Table 4. The calculations for energy expenditure for muscular strength and muscular endurance activities[54] are found in Table 5. An extensive list providing energy expenditures for household, occupational, recreational, and sports activities can be found elsewhere.[54] Regardless of how precise one tries to calculate energy expenditure and energy need, it does remain that in many individuals the energy equation which states that energy in is equal to energy out is simply not true. The body in many cases remains the proverbial scientific "black box" and not yet all is understood with respect to controlling all the variables. When steady state is perturbed, lean body mass may be modified upward by

TABLE 2 A Method to Estimate Daily Energy Intake for Light to Moderate Activity

Age Category by Gender	kcal/kg	kcal/lb
Males		
11–14	55	25
15–18	45	20.5
19–24	40	18.2
25–50	37	16.8
51+	30	13.6
Females		
11–14	47	21.4
15–18	40	18.2
19–24	38	17.3
25–50	36	16.4
50+	30	13.6

Calculation: Determine your weight in either kg or lb. Then find your age category by gender and estimated kcal/kg or kcal/lb. Multiply both numbers to determine approximate daily energy intake.

Example: A 22-year-old female who weights 100 lb would multiply 100 × 17.3 kcal/lb = 1730 kcal/d. Additional activity should be added to this number.

Adapted from Ratzin, R. A., in *Nutriton for the Recreational Athlete,* CRC Press, Boca Raton, FL, 1995, chap. 6; and Ruud, J. S. and Wolinsky, I., in *Nutrition for the Recreational Athlete,* CRC Press, Boca Raton, FL, 1995, chap. 4.

overfeeding, obesity, pregnancy, and, in females, puberty. Lean body mass can be modified downward by such effects as androgens, underfeeding, anorexia, malnutrition, zero gravity, bed rest, aging, and, in males, puberty. Exercise in and of itself is actually a very minor affector of total body fat.[55]

IV. SUMMARY

Individuals who exercise should understand the energy transfer systems within the body and should choose modes of conditioning and training complementary to each other. The high energy phosphagens are utilized during the immediate activity period and transition to glycolysis and aerobic metabolism if exercise becomes more prolonged. While the phosphagen system is not appreciably modified by nutritional practices, glycolysis benefits from high carbohydrate intake. The aerobic system is enhanced by training and can use fats,

TABLE 3　Comparison of Kilocalories per Hour and per Minute Used by Two Different Weight Individuals

Activity	Weight 125 lbs Hour	125 lbs Min	205 lbs Hour	205 lbs Min
Archery	268 kcals	4.47 kcals	420 kcals	7.00 kcals
Baseball — infield or outfield	234	3.90	382	6.37
— pitching	299	4.98	488	8.13
Basketball — moderate	352	5.87	575	9.58
— vigorous	495	8.25	807	13.34
Bicycling — on level, 5.5 mph	251	4.18	409	6.81
— on level, 13.0 mph	537	8.95	877	14.62
Canoeing — 4 mph	352	5.87	565	9.42
Dancing — moderate	209	3.48	341	5.68
— vigorous	284	4.73	464	7.73
Fencing — moderate	251	4.18	409	6.81
— vigorous	513	8.55	837	13.95
Football	416	6.93	678	11.30
Golf — twosome	271	4.51	443	4.52
— foursome	203	3.38	332	5.53
Handball or hardball — vigorous	488	8.13	797	13.28
Horseback riding — walk	165	2.75	270	4.5
— trot	338	5.63	551	9.18
Motorcycling	182	3.03	297	4.95
Mountain Climbing	503	8.38	820	13.67
Rowing — pleasure	251	4.18	409	6.81
— rowing machine or sculling (20/min)	684	11.40	1116	18.6
Running — 5.5 mph	537	8.95	887	14.78
— 7.0 mph	669	11.15	1141	19.02
— 9.0 mph	777	12.95	1269	21.15
— 9.0 mph, 2.5% grade	907	15.12	1480	24.67
— 9.0 mph, 4% grade	959	15.98	1564	26.00
— 12.0 mph	984	16.40	1606	26.77
— in place, 140 counts/min	1222	20.37	1993	33.22
Skating — moderate	285		465	
— vigorous	513		837	
Skiing — downhill	483		789	
— level, 5.0 mph	586		956	
Soccer	447		730	
Squash	520		849	
Swimming — backstroke — 20 yds/min	194		316	
— 40 yds/min	418		682	
— breaststroke — 20 yds/min	241		392	
— 40 yds/min	482		786	
— butterfly	586		956	
— crawl — 20 yds/min	241		392	
— 50 yds/min	532		869	
— sidestroke	418		682	
Tennis — moderate	347		565	
— vigorous	488		797	
Volleyball — moderate	285		465	
— vigorous	489		797	

TABLE 3 **Comparison of Kilocalories per Hour and per Minute Used by Two Different Weight Individuals** *(continued)*

	Weight			
	125 lbs		205 lbs	
Activity	Hour	Min	Hour	Min
Walking — 2.0 mph	176		286	
— 110–120 paces/min	260		425	
— 4.5 mph	331		540	
— downstairs	333		544	
— upstairs	869		1417	
Water Skiing	391		638	
Wrestling, Judo, or Karate	643		1049	

Note: (1) Calculations for one minute of activity can be multiplied by the minutes of the activity if it lasts less than 1 hr (i.e., 20 min of wrestling for a 125 lb wrestler = 10.7 kcal/min × 20 min = 214 kcal per 20 min).

(2) Calculations can also be done for different body weights by dividing either weight column by the total body weight to find the calories for each pound. This number can be multiplied by the weight of the individual to find kilocalories per hour or minute (i.e., a 100 lb wrestler: 643 kcal per 125 lbs/hr/125 lbs = 5.1 kcal/lb/hr. 5.1 kcal/lb/hr × 100 lb = 510 kcal/hr).

The above data can also be completely personalized by first calculating an individual number of kilocalories per hour for a specific body weight [(2) above], and then multiplying by the number of minutes of activity.

Adapted from *Nutrition for Sport Success,* Swanson Center for Nutrition, Inc., 1984, p. 6; and Snyder, A. C., Welsh, R. S., and Hanisch, R. J., in *Nutrition for the Recreational Athlete,* CRC Press, Boca Raton, FL, 1995, chap. 5.

carbohydrates, and protein for ATP production. All systems benefit from exercise. Nutritional practices can be chosen to enhance performance from all systems.

Power activities require that exercise is done in short periods of time, and attention should be paid to the differences between muscular strength and muscular endurance activities as they may not enhance each other. The different types of muscle fibers should be understood with the intent of enhancing the specific fiber type used in activity for more effective use of time in training.

Adipocytes are the greatest energy reserve in the body, and much remains to be discovered as to their functioning. When there is a desire to modify fat stores in the body the individual should become educated in appropriate uses of body fat assessment and what the norms are for their age, gender, and activity status.

Assessing daily energy expenditure is difficult but can help in understanding nutritional needs of exercisers. Nutritional practices should be incorporated which support the activity choices. However, regardless of the choice, health should be a major concern. We now know that lower levels of activity than previously thought are sufficient to diminish the risk of disease.[56] A better understanding of metabolism and the nutritional practices which support the activity choices made will help to improve the quality of life for individuals who exercise.

TABLE 4 **Time Required to Expend 300 kcal and kcal per Minute for Different Aerobic Endurance Activities for Three Body Weights**

Activities	Minutes for 300 kcal Expenditure					
	Body Weights					
	59 kg	(kcal/min)	68 kg	(kcal/min)	77 kg	(kcal/min)
Aerobic dancing						
Medium intensity	49	6.12	43	6.98	38	7.90
High intensity	38	7.90	33	9.09	29	10.35
Cycling						
Leisure, 5.5 mph	79	3.80	69	4.35	61	4.92
Leisure, 9.4 mph	51	5.88	44	6.82	39	7.69
Racing	30	10.00	26	11.54	23	13.04
In-line skating	32	9.38	27	11.11	24	12.50
Jumping rope						
70/min	31	9.68	27	11.11	24	12.50
125/min	29	10.34	25	12.00	22	13.64
145/min	26	11.54	22	13.64	20	15.00
Rowing	55	5.46	47	6.38	42	7.14
Running, horizontal						
11.5 mi	38	7.90	33	9.09	29	10.35
9.0 min/mile	26	11.54	23	13.04	20	15.00
8.0 min/mile	24	12.50	21	14.29	19	15.79
7.0 min/mile	22	13.64	19	15.79	17	17.65
6.0 min/mile	20	15.00	17	17.65	15	20.00
5.5 min/mile	18	16.67	15	20.00	13	23.07
Nordic skiing, hard snow						
Level, moderate speed	43	6.98	37	8.11	33	9.09
Level, walking speed	36	8.33	31	9.68	27	11.11
Uphill, maximum speed	19	15.79	16	18.75	14	21.43
Swimming, freestyle						
20 yd/min	73	4.11	63	4.76	55	5.46
25 yd/min	58	5.17	50	6.00	44	6.82
35 yd/min	47	6.38	41	7.32	36	8.33
50 yd/min	33	9.09	28	10.71	25	12.00
treading, fast	30	10.00	26	11.54	23	13.04
treading, normal	82	3.66	71	4.23	63	4.76
Walking, normal pace						
asphalt road	63	4.75	55	5.46	49	6.12
fields and hills	62	4.84	54	5.56	47	6.38

From McArdle, W. D., Katch, F. I., and Katch, Y. L., *Exercise Physiology: Energy, Nutrition, and Human Performance,* 4th ed., Williams & Wilkins, Baltimore, 1996, pp. 769–781. With permission.

TABLE 5 **Kilocalories per Minute Used by Three Different Weight Individuals during Resistance Training**

Activities	59 kg	68 kg	77 kg
Free Weights	5.0	5.8	6.6
Hydra-Fitness	7.8	9.0	10.2
Nautilus	5.5	6.3	7.1
Universal	6.9	7.9	8.9

Adapted from McArdle, W. D., Katch, F. I., and Katch, V. L., *Exercise Physiology: Energy, Nutrition, and Human Performance,* 3rd ed., Lea Febiger, Philadelphia, 1991, chaps. 1, 6, 11.

REFERENCES

1. Gollnick, P. D., Free fatty acid turnover and the availability of substrates as a limiting factor in prolonged exercise, in *The Marathon: Physiological Medical, Epidemiological, and Psychological Studies,* Milvey, P., Ed., The New York Academy of Sciences, New York, 1977, 64.
2. Fox, E. L., Bowers, R. W., and Foss, M. L., *The Physiological Basis for Exercise and Sport,* 5th ed., Brown and Benchmark, Dubuque, IA, 1989, chap. 2.
3. Hargreaves, M., Ed., *Exercise Metabolism,* Human Kinetics,Champaign, IL, 1995.
4. Lamb, D. R. and Gisolfi, C. V., Eds., *Perspectives in Exercise Science and Sports Medicine: Volume 5, Energy Metabolism in Exercise and Sport,* Cooper Publishing Group, Carmel, IN, 1992,
5. McArdle, W. D., Katch, F. I., and Katch, V. L., *Exercise Physiology: Energy, Nutrition, and Human Performance,* 3rd ed., Lea and Febiger, Philadelphia, 1991, chaps. 1, 6, 11.
6. Williams, M. H., *Nutrition for Fitness and Sport,* 3rd ed., William C. Brown Publishers, Dubuque, IA, 1992.
7. Wolinsky, I. and Hickson, J. F., *Nutrition in Exercise and Sport,* 2nd ed., CRC Press, Boca Raton, FL, 1993.
8. Spriet, L. L., Anaerobic metabolism during high-intensity exercise, in *Exercise Metabolism,* Hargreaves, M., Ed., Human Kinetics, Champaign, IL, 1995, 1–36.
9. Margaria, R., Cerretelli, P., and Mangili, E., Balance and kinetics of anaerobic energy release during strenuous exercise in man, *J. Appl. Physiol.,* 19, 623, 1964.
10. Margaria, R., Oliva, D., Di Prampero, P. E., and Cerretelli, P., Energy utilization in intermittent exercise of supramaximal intensity, *Eur. J. Appl. Physiol.,* 26, 752, 1969.
11. Boobis, L. H., Williams, C., and Wooton, S. A., Human muscle metabolism during brief maximal exercise, *J. Physiol. Lond.,* 338, 21P, 1982, Abstract.
12. Jones, N. L., McCartney, N., Graham, T., Spriet, L. L., Kowalchuk, J. M., Heigenhayuser, G. J. F., and Sutton, J. R., Muscle performance and metabolism in maximal isokinetic cycling at slow and fast speeds, *J. Appl. Physiol.,* 59, 132, 1985.
13. Saltin, B., Gollnick, P. D., Eriksson, B.-O., and Piehl, K., Metabolic and circulatory adjustments at onset of maximal work, in *Onset of Exercise,* Gilbert, A. and Guille, P., Eds., University of Toulouse Press, Toulouse, France, 1971, 63–76.
14. Bangsbo, J., Gollnick, P. D., Graham, T. E., Juel, C., Kiens, B., Mizuno, M., and Saltin, B., Anaerobic energy production and O_2 deficit-debt relationship during exhaustive exercise in humans, *J. Physiol. Lond.,* 42, 539, 1990.
15. Harris, R. C., Soderlund, K., and Hultman, E., Elevation of creatine in resting and exercised muscle of normal subjects by creatine supplementation, *Clin. Sci.,* 83, 367, 1992.
16. Greenhaff, P. L., Casey, A., Short, A. H., Soderlund, K., and Hultman, E., Influence of oral creatine supplementation of muscle torque during repeated bouts of maximal voluntary exercise in man, *Clin. Sci.,* 84, 565, 1993.
17. Harris R. C., Viru, M., Greenhaff, P. L., and Hultman, E., The effect of oral creatine supplementation on running performance during maximal short-term exercise in man, *J. Physiol.,* 467, 74P, 1993, Abstract.
18. Nevill, M. S., Boobis, L. H., Brooks, S., and Williams, C., Effect of training on muscle metabolism during treadmill sprinting, *J. Appl. Physiol.,* 67, 2376, 1989.
19. Hermansen, L. and Vaage, O., Lactate disappearance and glycogen synthesis in human muscle after maximal exercise, *Am. J. Physiol.,* 233, E422, 1977.
20. Bergstrom, J., Hermansen, L., Hultman, E., and Saltin, B., Diet, muscle glycogen and physical performance, *Acta Physiol. Scand.,* 71, 140, 1967.
21. Guyton, A. C., *Textbook of Medical Physiology,* 8th ed., W. B. Saunders Co., Philadelphia, 1991, chaps. 67, 68.
22. Piehl, K., Time course for refilling of glycogen stores in human muscle fibers following exercise-induced glycogen depletion, *Acta Physiol. Scand.,* 90, 297, 1974.
23. Hultman, E. and Bergstrom, J., Muscle glycogen synthesis in relation to diet studied in normal subjects, *Acta Med. Scand.,* 182, 109, 1967.
24. Sharkey, B. J., *Coaches Guide to Sport Physiology,* Human Kinetics Publishers, Champaign, IL., 1986, chap. 5.
25. Steinberg, D., Metabolism, in *Best and Taylor's Physiological Basis of Medical Practice*, West, J. B., Ed., Williams and Wilkins, Philadelphia, 1990, 728.
26. Powers, S. K. and Howley, E. T., *Exercise Physiology: Theory and Application of Fitness and Performance*, 2nd ed., Brown and Benchmark, Dubuque, IA, 1994, chap. 4.
27. Hagerman, F. C., Energy metabolism and fuel utilization, *Med. Sci. Sports Exer.,* 24, S309, 1992.
28. Jackson, C. G. R., Dickinson, A. L., and Ringel, S. P., Skeletal muscle fiber area alterations in two opposing modes of resistance-exercise training in the same individual, *Eur. J. Appl. Physiol.,* 61, 37, 1990.
29. Romanul, F. C. A., Streter, F. A., Salmons, S., and Gergely, J., The effects of a changed pattern of activity on histochemical characteristics of muscle fibres, in *Exploratory Concepts in Muscular Dystrophy II,* Milhorat, E. A. T., Ed., Excerpta Medica, Amsterdam, 1974.
30. Dubowitz, V., *Muscle Biopsy, A Practical Approach,* 2nd ed., Bailliere Tindall, Philadelphia, 1988.

31. Costill, D., Daniels, J., Evans, W., Fink, W., Krahenbuhl, G., and Saltin, B., Skeletal muscle enzymes and fiber composition in male and female track athletes, *J. Appl. Physiol.,* 40, 149, 1976.
32. Hagenfeldt, L., Turnover of individual free fatty acids in man, *Fed. Proc.,* 34, 2236, 1975.
33. Jackson, C. G. R., Dickinson, A. W., Ringel S. P., and Barden, M. T., Histochemical profile of muscular cellular alterations following two modes of training in the same individual, unpublished data, 1994.
34. Jackson, C. G. R. and Dickinson, A. L., Adaptations of skeletal muscle to strength or endurance training, in *Advances in Sports Medicine and Fitness,* 1, Grana, W. A., Lombardo, J. A., Sharkey, B. J., and Stone, J. A., Eds., Year Book Medical Publishers, Chicago, 1988, 45.
35. Coyle, E. F., Costill, D. L., and Lesmes, G. R., Leg extension power and muscle fiber composition, *Med. Sci. Sports,* 11, 12, 1979.
36. Gollnick, P. D., Timson, B. F., Moore, R. L., and Riedy, M., Muscular enlargement and number of fibers in skeletal muscles of rats, *J. Appl. Physiol.,* 50, 936, 1981.
37. Ratzin, R. A., Effect of aerobic conditioning on resting serum testosterone levels and muscle fiber types in vegetarian and nonvegetarian sedentary males, Dissertation, University of Northern Colorado, Greeley, CO, 1990.
38. Katch F. I. and McArdle, W. D., *Nutrition, Weight Control, and Exercise,* Lea and Febiger, Philadelphia, 1988, chap. 6.
39. Hirsch, J. and Knittle, J. L., Cellularity of obese and nonobese human adipose tissue, *Fed. Proc.,* 29, 1516, 1970.
40. Rebuffe-Scrive, M., Adipose tissue metabolism and fat distribution, in *Human Body Composition and Fat Distribution,* Norgan, N. G., Ed., Euro-Nut, Wageningen, Holland, 1985, 212.
41. Sjostrom, L., Smith, U., Krotkiewski, M., and Bjorntorp, P., Cellularity in different regions of adipose tissue in young men and women, *Metabolism,* 21, 1143, 1972.
42. *Proper and Improper Weight Loss Programs,* American College of Sports Medicine Position Stand, P. O. Box 1440, Indianapolis, IN, 46206-1440.
43. Lohman T. G., Roche, A. F., and Martorell, R., *Anthropometric Standardization Reference Manual,* Human Kinetics Books, Champaign, 1988.
44. Lohman, T. G., ACSM Tutorial: Body Composition Assessment, presented at American College of Sports Medicine Annual Meeting, Baltimore, 1989.
45. *The Recommended Quantity and Quality of Exercise for Developing and Maintaining Cardiorespiratory and Muscular Fitness in Healthy Adults,* American College of Sports Medicine Position Stand, P. O. Box 1440, Indianapolis, IN, 46206-1440.
46. *1996 Surgeon General's Report on Physical Activity and Health,* Superintendent of Documents, P. O. Box 371954, Pittsburgh, PA, 15250-7954.
47. Durnin, J. V G. A. and Passmore, R., Eds., *Energy Work, and Leisure,* Heinemann, London, 1967.
48. Bassett, D. R. and Nagle, F. J., Energy metabolism in exercise and training, in *Nutrition in Exercise and Sport,* 2nd ed., Wolinsky, I. and Hickson, J. F., Eds., CRC Press, Boca Raton, FL, 1993.
49. Food and Nutrition Board, *Recommended Dietary Allowance,* 10th ed., National Academy Press, Washington, D.C., 1989.
50. Ratzin, R. A., Nutritional concerns for the vegetarian recreational athlete, in *Nutrition for the Recreational Athlete,* Jackson, C. G. R., Ed., CRC Press, Boca Raton, FL, 1995, chap. 6.
51. Ruud, J. S. and Wolinsky, I., Nutritional concerns of recreational strength athletes, in *Nutrition for the Recreational Athlete,* Jackson, C. G. R., Ed., CRC Press, Boca Raton, FL, 1995, chap. 4.
52. *Nutrition for Sport Success,* Swanson Center for Nutrition, Inc., 1984, p. 6.
53. Snyder, A. C., Welsh, R. S., and Hanisch, R. J., Nutritional concerns of recreational athletes who cross-train, in *Nutrition for the Recreational Athlete,* Jackson, C. G. R., Ed., CRC Press, Boca Raton, FL, 1995, chap. 5.
54. McArdle, W. D., Katch, F. I., and Katch, V. L., *Exercise Physiology: Energy, Nutrition, and Human Performance,* 4th ed., Williams & Wilkins, Baltimore, 1996, pp. 769–781.
55. Forbes, G. B., Body composition as affected by physical activity and nutrition, *Fed. Proc.,* 44, 343, 1985.
56. *Physical Activity, Physical Fitness, and Hypertension,* American College of Sports Medicine Position Stand, P. O. Box 1440, Indianapolis, IN, 46206-1440.

Chapter 7

EXERCISE AND THE B VITAMINS

_____ Priscilla M. Clarkson

CONTENTS

0-8493-8560-1/97/$0.00+$.50
© 1998 by CRC Press LLC

I. INTRODUCTION

Americans spend more than $1.5 billion annually on vitamin and other nutritional supplements.[1] A four month investigation by *Money* magazine showed that 35% of the dollars paid annually for supplements were spent for products with no scientifically proven health value. Beyond health claims that entice the general consumer, many supplements are marketed specifically to athletes or would-be athletes to enhance training and performance. The B vitamins, separately or combined with other products such as protein powders, are touted to provide performance boosts because of their physiological role in energy and red blood production.

Thiamin (vitamin B_1), riboflavin (vitamin B_2), niacin (vitamin B_3), pyridoxine (vitamin B_6), cobalamine (vitamin B_{12}), folic acid, pantothenic acid, and biotin comprise the B vitamins. Because there is little research on the latter two with regard to exercise and sport, they will not be discussed in this chapter. The B vitamins are essential organic nutrients that are water soluble. Unlike fat soluble vitamins that are stored in body fat, B vitamins generally cannot be stored in the body; although, tissue levels can become saturated to provide temporary storage when dietary intake is low. Excess ingestion of most water soluble vitamins will be excreted into the urine when the plasma levels exceed the renal threshold. Thus, these vitamins must be ingested in small amounts on a regular basis. Thiamin, riboflavin, niacin, and vitamin B_6 are all involved in energy-producing reactions in cells, while vitamin B_{12} and folic acid function in the production of red blood cells.

This chapter will evaluate whether athletes and those who exercise regularly require additional B vitamins for health and whether these supplements will improve performance. Before discussing the specific vitamins, measurement of dietary intake and status will be addressed.

II. ASSESSMENT OF STATUS

Nutritional status of a micronutrient must involve both assessment of dietary intake and biochemical measurements. The most accurate way to assess dietary intake is to biochemically analyze duplicate meals. This is costly and often impractical for assessing dietary intake in populations. More commonly, diet records, diet histories, and food frequency questionnaires are examined. However, these techniques are fraught with problems.[2] Several factors contribute to measurement errors of nutrient intake, and these are:

1. respondent biases,
2. interviewer biases,
3. respondent memory lapses,
4. incorrect estimation of portion sizes,
5. tendency to overestimate low intake and underestimate high intakes,
6. supplement use is not always taken into account,
7. coding and computation errors, and
8. errors associated with computer programs and associated data bases.[3,4]

Diet surveys tend to underestimate dietary intake.[3,5,6] For these reasons, deviations of 25% or less from the Recommended Dietary Allowance[7] (RDA) are not considered significant.

Assessing the absorption of a vitamin is important to accurately determine status, but this is a time consuming process and rarely done in studies of athletes. The most common means to assess vitamin status is from blood sampling, which provides a fairly accurate assessment of status. Because of the ease of acquiring blood samples, assessments can be made rapidly and multiple samples can be obtained. In some cases, the blood concentrations of a given vitamin are assessed, while for other vitamins, the enzyme activity for which the vitamin serves as a cofactor is assessed. Microbiological assays have been used where aliquots of diluted serum are added to the assay media that contains all the nutrients except one required for growth of a particular microbe. The growth rate would be proportional to the amount of the vitamin in the serum. High performance liquid chromatography (HPLC) analyses have been developed to accurately measure vitamin levels in serum, but these require a large sample volume. Analysis of vitamin concentrations or end products of reactions in urine samples is a less accurate measure of status and may reflect only recent ingestion of the vitamin, such as in the case of vitamin B_6. It should be noted that more than one measure of status for any vitamin is desirable.

For each of the B vitamins, the dietary source, RDA, and function will be addressed. This will be followed by a description of the dietary intake of athletes, status of athletes, changes due to exercise, and effects of supplementation.

III. THIAMIN

The richest dietary sources of thiamin are whole grains, pork, legumes, followed by other meats, fish, green vegetables, fruit, and milk.[3] Because of the availability of a wide variety of foods in western countries, thiamin deficiency is rare. The RDA for thiamin for adults is 0.5 mg/1000 kcal (0.5 mg/4184 kJ).[7] For those who consume less than 2000 kcal (8368 kJ) per day, the minimum intake of thiamin should be 1.0 mg/day.

Thiamin has no storage area in the body, rather it is bound to enzymes within tissues. Specifically it functions as a component of the coenzyme thiamin pyrophosphate (TPP).[8,9] TPP serves as a coenzyme for two major types of reactions: (1) for the action of transketolase in the pentose phosphate pathway and (2) for the oxidative decarboxylation of alpha-keto acids to carboxylics.[10] TPP acts as a coenzyme in the conversion of pyruvate to acetyl coenzyme A (CoA) and alpha-ketoglutarate to succinyl CoA, as well as the decarboxylation of branched chain amino acids. Because of thiamin's important role in carbohydrate metabolism, it has been targeted as an ergogenic aid that will increase endurance, delay fatigue, and enhance performance.[11]

A. DIETARY INTAKE AND STATUS

Diet records of athletes show that most athletes have adequate intake of thiamin.[12-26] This is likely due to the fact that thiamin intake is related to energy intake, and athletes tend to have a high energy intake to match their energy expenditure. Athletes who do not ingest sufficient energy or who obtain a high percentage of energy from low nutrient-density food (e.g., candy, sodas, diet sodas) may not ingest sufficient amounts of thiamin. Some adolescent gymnasts,[27] adolescent ballet dancers,[28] and college wrestlers[29,30] had thiamin intakes less than two-thirds the RDA. This is not surprising because these athletes typically restrict energy intake to maintain low body weights.

The most reliable technique to assess status is to determine the activity of a thiamin dependent enzyme in erythrocytes that is sensitive to thiamin depletion.[3] After a blood sample is obtained, the activity of transketolase is assessed in the erythrocytes. Next, TPP is added to the reaction. An increase in the activity of the enzyme will indicate a deficiency in thiamin. Thus, percent stimulation of TPP expressed as an activity coefficient provides an assessment of thiamin status. A value close to 1.0 indicates adequate status and a value of more than 1.25 indicates a high risk of deficiency.[8]

Thiamin status of athletes appears to be adequate,[18,21,25,26,31-34] and this most probably reflects adequate thiamin intake. Status has not been assessed for those athletes, who by not ingesting sufficient calories, may be at risk of lowered thiamin status.

B. EFFECTS OF EXERCISE

For elite athletes who do not ingest sufficient thiamin, it is possible that a thiamin deficiency can adversely affect performance. Steel[35] found that a group of Olympian athletes with high thiamin ingestion (based on data from questionnaires) had greater representation among the medal winners and finalists compared to a group with low (sub-optimal) thiamin ingestion. However, Wood et al.[36] found that an induced thiamin deficiency (500 µg thiamin for 4–5 weeks) did not affect cycle endurance performance or nerve conduction velocity. Deficiency was documented by low thiamin excretion, decreased erythrocyte transketolase activity, and elevation of the TPP test.

Early studies showed that thiamin supplementation in those with adequate status did not enhance performance.[37,38] Keys et al.[38] examined average thiamin intakes of 0.63, 0.53, 0.33, and 0.23 mg/1000 kcal (0.23 mg/4184 kJ) (based on analysis of all food ingested) for 10–12 weeks. No differences were found in cardiovascular parameters during a treadmill test or in measures of muscle strength. Thus, evidence that thiamin supplementation will enhance performance is equivocal.

IV. RIBOFLAVIN

Dairy products are the richest source of riboflavin, but riboflavin is also found in meat, cereals, and vegetables.[10] Riboflavin deficiency is rare in western countries. In the co-enzyme forms of FMN (flavin mononucleotide) and FAD (flavin adenine dinucleotide), riboflavin is involved in oxidative energy metabolism. The flavins have the ability to accept a pair of hydrogen atoms in mitochondrial metabolic processes and transport them to the electron transport system to be used in the formation of ATP. Flavins are also involved in a wide variety of reactions where electron transfer is necessary.[10] The RDA is 0.6 mg/1000 kcal (0.6 mg/4184 kJ) with a minimum intake of 1.2 mg for those who have an energy intake under 2000 kcal (8368 kJ).[7]

A. DIETARY INTAKE AND STATUS

Studies that have assessed dietary intake of athletes have found that most adult and adolescent athletes have an adequate or greater than adequate intake of riboflavin.[12,14-28] A recent study reported that riboflavin intake was significantly higher during the midluteal phase of the menstrual cycle;[39] the reason for this is not known.

One enzyme for which riboflavin serves as a co-factor (FAD) is glutathione reductase (GR). GR is found in erythrocytes (EGR), and measurement of stimulated EGR activity provides a reliable assessment of riboflavin status. When the body's riboflavin levels are low, EGR loses its saturation with FAD and its activity drops.[10,40] The assessment of EGR activity is performed with and without the addition of FAD to the sample. If the addition of FAD produces a marked increase in enzyme activity, riboflavin status is considered inadequate. Generally, an activity coefficient (EGRAC) less than 1.2 represents acceptable status and values greater than 1.4 indicate deficiency.

Biochemical deficiencies of riboflavin are rare in athletes.[21,25,34,41-43] Guilland et al.[26] reported that only 4% of male college athletes showed a biochemical deficiency based on EGR activation. In contrast, Haralambie[44] found evidence of inadequate riboflavin status in 8 out of 18 athletes also based on EGR activation. Inadequate status (EGR test) was found for young male and female Austrian athletes in boarding school for competitive sports.[32]

Rokitzki et al.[45] have recently criticized the use of only one assessment of riboflavin status, suggesting that riboflavin status based solely on enzyme activation can be misleading. When they examined a group of athletes using several tests, the enzyme activation test showed that athletes were well below the reference value, indicating adequate status. However, using a microbiological determination, it was found that 22% of the athletes did not attain the reference levels for nonathletes and, thus, had inadequate status.

Keith and Alt[41] found that 13 female athletes (track, tennis, and triathletes) had adequate riboflavin intake and riboflavin status based on EGRAC, however there was a trend for urinary riboflavin values/creatinine to be lower for the athletes compared with the sedentary group. While the latter change is sometimes indicative of decreased riboflavin status, it may also suggest greater retention or utilization of riboflavin by the trained athletes.[41]

B. EFFECTS OF EXERCISE

The beginning of an exercise program in previously sedentary men and women has been found to decrease riboflavin status.[46,47] These data may have important implications for older individuals who may not ingest sufficient amounts of riboflavin and begin an exercise program. Winters et al.[48] found that individuals between the ages of 50–67 years who started an exercise program showed a decreased riboflavin status after 4 weeks, as indicated by an increase in EGRAC and a decrease in riboflavin excretion. A small decrease in riboflavin status was also found for healthy obese subjects who were placed on a diet and exercise program.[49] In contrast, a mild intensity walking program did not affect riboflavin status in a group of pregnant women who were taking vitamin/mineral supplements.[50]

Subotičanec et al.[51] found that when Croatian children, 12–14 years of age, were placed on riboflavin supplements (2 mg/day) for 2 months, there was an increase in VO_2 max for only the boys who were initially deficient in riboflavin. An early study of riboflavin restriction showed that ingestion of riboflavin of 0.99 mg/day (0.31 mg/1000 kcal (0.31 mg/4184 kJ)) for 84–152 days did not affect aerobic or anaerobic performance.[52] Supplemental riboflavin has been found to have no effect on physical performance or aerobic capacity in subjects with adequate status.[42,51] In the Winters et al.[48] study mentioned above, subjects who had increased riboflavin intakes (0.9 μg/kcal (0.9 μg/4.184kJ)) did not show improvement in VO_2 max. Most studies showed that riboflavin status did not affect performance.

Heat exposure (49°C and 30% relative humidity) of 10 hours per day for 6 days resulted in an increased excretion of riboflavin that could indicate a lower requirement for riboflavin during heat stress.[53] However, this may also indicate that heat stress produces a malfunction in riboflavin usage that could result in lowered riboflavin status. A study of rats showed that high doses of riboflavin reduced the fall in body temperature during swimming.[54] Because of these preliminary findings, further studies of riboflavin status and thermoregulation are warranted.

Haralambie[44] found that muscle irritability assessed by electrical stimulation was decreased 70 min after ingestion of 10 mg of riboflavin. In other words, the current intensity necessary to elicit threshold excitation was higher after riboflavin ingestion. Haralambie[44] suggested that low riboflavin status may explain muscle hyperexcitability noted in some athletes. No studies have followed up on the effects of acute riboflavin ingestion on muscle activation.

V. NIACIN

Niacin is a general term to describe two compounds that act as vitamins, nicotinic acid and nicotinamide.[10,55] Nicotinamide serves as a precursor to pyridine nucleotides nicotinamide adenine dinucleotide (NAD) and nicotinamide adenine dinucleotide phosphate (NADP). These coenzymes function in energy metabolism by serving as proton and electron carriers.[3] NAD functions as an electron carrier in metabolic processes and functions as a coenzyme in many oxidative reactions. NADP serves as a hydrogen donor in reductive biosynthesis and is involved in the pentose phosphate pathways. Because nicotinic acid can increase flushing due to a release of histamine, many bodybuilders use niacin supplements to enlarge surface blood vessels prior to competition. Nicotinic acid has been found to be part of the glucose tolerance factor, but its role in this factor is unknown.[55]

A.   DIETARY INTAKE AND STATUS

The RDA for niacin is 19 mg/day for adult males and 15 mg/day for adult females (1 mg of niacin is equivalent to 60 mg of dietary tryptophan).[7] The requirement for niacin is usually linked to energy intake such that 6.6 niacin equivalents (NE)/1000 kcal (6.6 NE/4184 kJ) and a minimum of 13 NE for intakes of 2000 kcal (8368 kJ) or below are recommended. Cereals, legumes, and lean meat are sources of niacin. Niacin deficiency in industrialized countries is rare because of the fortification of foods (e.g., flour) with niacin.

Niacin consumption by adult athletes, dancers, and adolescent swimmers has been shown to be adequate.[2,13-23,56] However, 7.6% of adolescent ballet dancers and 11% of adolescent gymnasts consumed less than two-thirds of the RDA.[27,28] Ersoy[24] reported that the mean intake of niacin for 11-year-old gymnasts in Turkey was only 8.5 mg. These low intakes reflected inadequate energy intake.

There is no functional biochemical test for niacin status.[3,8,10] The most widely used method to assess status is the ratio of urinary excretion of N'-methylnicotinamide (NMN) and N'-methyl-2-pyridone-5-carboxylamide (2-pyridone) that are end products of niacin metabolism. A ratio lower than 1.0 would indicate deficiency. Another method that may not be as accurate is to assess NMN excretion expressed as mmol/mol of creatinine.

No biochemical deficiencies determined from blood samples were found for professional ballet dancers, highly trained male athletes, or ultramarathoners.[21,25,31] However, blood levels are not considered a sensitive test, yet no other data are available for athletes.

B.   EFFECTS OF EXERCISE

Several studies have reported no effect on performance after ingestion of niacin or nicotinic acid,[57-59] while other studies showed a decrement in performance.[60,61] Bergstrom et al.[57] found that muscle glycogen content was lower and arterial free fatty acid (FFA) levels were lower 90 min after the onset of exercise in subjects who had received niacin supplements (1.0 g intravenously and 0.6 g perorally) compared with control subjects. In a resting condition, Carlson and Oro[62] had three subjects ingest 200 mg nicotinic acid with an additional 100 mg 1 and 2 hours later. FFA were lowered immediately after the first dose. A dramatic increase in plasma FFA levels occurred after the second dose for two subjects and after the third dose for the third subject. The relationship of nicotinic acid, fatty acid release, and their effects on performance is not well understood.

Both acute and chronic effects of nicotinic acid on performance have been studied. Heath et al.[63] had subjects ingest 1 g of nicotinic acid 1 hour prior to a submaximal run. Subjects then ingested 3 g of nicotinic acid/day for 21 days. Compared to a control condition, the acute 1 g of nicotinic acid resulted in a lowering of FFA and an increase in the respiratory exchange ratio (RER). However, the effect on RER was blunted after 11 days and 21 days when the exercise was repeated. At 21 days the effect on FFA was also reduced. These results suggest an adaptation to the nicotinic acid ingestion.

Murray et al.[64] examined whether ingestion of nicotinic acid (280 mg/l) along with a carbohydrate-electrolyte drink would enhance performance. The average ingestion of nicotinic acid was about 330 mg for females and 521 mg for males. It was speculated that the combination of nicotinic acid and glucose would reduce FFAs and increase reliance on muscle glycogen and exogenous glucose. The exogenous glucose would theoretically prevent an adverse reduction in muscle glycogen. The nicotinic acid ingestion did blunt the FFA increase. However, there was no difference in performance time in the group who ingested the carbohydrate-electrolyte drink and nicotinic acid compared to placebo/control groups.

Due to the role of niacin in vasodilation, ingestion can increase skin blood flow and lower core temperature. Stephenson and Kolka[65] have recently examined doses of 300–400 mg of niacin to increase radiative and convective heat flux and found that niacin ingestion effectively increased sensible heat flux during exercise. Murray et al.[64] found that consumption of nicotinic acid did not affect rectal or skin temperatures during exercise at a temperature of 28°C, 56% relative humidity. The role of nicotinic acid in thermoregulation warrants further study.

VI. VITAMIN B$_6$

Vitamin B$_6$, pyridoxine, is commonly found in foods and deficiencies are rare.[8,10,66] Meat, fish, poultry, yeast, certain seeds, and bran are rich sources of vitamin B$_6$. After ingestion, most of the vitamin B$_6$ is carried to the liver where it is converted to pyridoxal 5'-phosphate (PLP), the active form of B$_6$. PLP is a coenzyme used in more than 60 metabolic processes, with many involved in amino acid metabolism. PLP is commonly associated with muscle glycogen phosphorylase, and it is thought that this enzyme may function as a storehouse for PLP. The RDA for vitamin B$_6$ is 2.0 mg/d for adult males and 1.6 mg/d for adult females.

A. DIETARY INTAKE AND STATUS

Adequate vitamin B$_6$ intakes have been reported for most male athletes.[20-23,31,67-71] Guilland et al.[25] found that two-thirds of male college athletes consumed only 69% of the RDA for vitamin B$_6$. Although several groups of female athletes were found to have adequate intakes of B$_6$,[22,72,73] other groups were found to have significantly low intakes.[20,23,27-29,67,74] Kaiseraure et al.[73] found that while eumenorrheic runners ingested adequate intakes of B$_6$ the amenorrheic subjects did not. Manore[75] points out that low vitamin B$_6$ ingestion can often be explained by low energy intake, especially in those athletes attempting to maintain low body weights, but low intakes may also be related to poor food choices.

Several biochemical markers exist to assess B$_6$ status but the two most frequently used are assessment of plasma PLP concentrations and erythrocyte aminotransferase activities (EAST).[3,8] Plasma PLP concentrations reflect tissue levels of vitamin B$_6$ in healthy persons. Other tests include the urinary excretion of B$_6$ degradation products (4-pyridoxic acid [4-PA]), tryptophan load test, kynurenine load test, and methionine load test. Urinary excretion provides information concerning recent dietary intake of vitamin B$_6$. To accurately assess status, it is recommended that at least two biochemical indices be used with one being the PLP test.

Few studies have assessed vitamin B$_6$ status of athletes. Three studies reported poor status in 35–60% of the athletes.[26,76,77] One of these studies used two tests for status (EAST and plasma PLP) and obtained values of 35% with poor status using EAST and only 17% using plasma PLP.[26] The other two studies only used the EAST test.[76,77] Blood samples of professional ballet dancers[25] and of 30 well-trained men[31] showed them to have adequate blood vitamin B$_6$ levels, yet this is not considered a sensitive index of status. Yates et al.[78] reported that an aerobic exercise program did not alter vitamin B$_6$ status (assessed by PLP and microbiological analysis of plasma total vitamin B$_6$) of pregnant women who were taking multivitamin/mineral supplement containing 10 mg vitamin B$_6$/d.

Using the EAST method, young male and female Austrian athletes had lower status than the reference value.[32] Raczyński[33] reported that 13% of Polish elite endurance athletes were at risk of B$_6$ deficiencies based on enzyme activation tests. Moreover, the risk was higher in athletes in pre-Olympic years and lowest in Olympic years. Rokitzki et al.[43] reported that of several groups of West German Athletes, more than 90% had inadequate status based on analysis of microbiological assays of blood, but based on enzyme activity, less than 5% had inadequate status. The authors criticized the latter test and suggested that several tests be used to obtain an accurate measure of status.

Coburn et al.[79] assessed vitamin B_6 levels in biopsies of the gastrocnemius muscle of 10 college age men who were placed on a diet low in vitamin B_6 for 6 weeks. While plasma PLP concentration decreased significantly, muscle levels showed no change. These data demonstrate that vitamin B_6 pools in skeletal muscle are resistant to depletion. This study also examined the effect of supplementing with vitamin B_6 for 6 weeks and found a small but nonsignificant increase in muscle B_6 levels. The authors concluded that skeletal muscle levels are constant and plasma levels are not a good indicator of tissue stores.

B. EFFECTS OF EXERCISE

Leklem and Shultz[80] reported that a 4500-meter run increased the blood levels of PLP in trained adolescent males. Also, other studies reported an increase in blood levels of PLP after endurance exercise.[81-83] This may be due to a release of PLP from muscle glycogen that has been transported in the blood to be used elsewhere as a co-factor for gluconeogenesis by the liver.[80,83] It has also been suggested that pyridoxal phosphate may be released from glycogen phosphorylase to provide glucose, via the glucose-alanine cycle, for muscle energy needs.[84] However, Crozier et al.[85] found that although exercise resulted in an increase in PLP in the plasma, the amount was unrelated to exercise intensity or duration. Moreover, the increase in PLP occurs within the first 5 min of exercise. Because of this rapid increase and lack of relationship to exercise intensity, Crozier et al.[85] suggest that the increase is more likely a concomitant event accompanying temporary protein shifts into the blood.

Although exercise results in an increase in vitamin B_6 in the urine, this does not suggest a need for vitamin B_6 supplementation. Rokitzki[86] found that after a marathon race only 1 mg of vitamin B_6 is lost, and they suggested that this could readily be replaced by a vitamin-rich diet. Moreover, another study found that 4-PA excretion in urine was significantly lower in trained athletes compared with controls,[87] which may indicate that the trained subjects could better conserve and store the vitamin. When N-acetyl-L-methionine (60 mg/kg) was given as a vitamin B_6 challenge, urinary excretion of 4-PA was increased in the trained subjects but decreased in the untrained. When dietary methionine is increased the demand for vitamin B_6 would be increased and thus the excretion of 4-PA would decrease, as happened in the untrained subjects. The authors suggest that the increased storage capacity in the trained athletes would allow for readily available vitamin B_6 necessary for the degradation of methionine and thus produce an increase in 4-PA excretion.

Despite the exercise-induced changes in vitamin B_6 levels, vitamin B_6 supplementation does not enhance performance in athletes. Lawrence et al.[88] examined swimming performance of trained swimmers who ingested 51 mg of pyridoxine hydrochloride or a placebo daily for 6 months. No significant difference was found between the groups in 100 yd (91.44 m) swimming times. Time-to-exhaustion was not altered in male cyclists who ingested 20 mg of vitamin B_6 per day.[89] Manore and Leklem[83] found that a combination of vitamin B_6 (2.4 mg/d) and a high carbohydrate diet (64% carbohydrate) for 1 week produced a decrease in FFA levels during endurance exercise. They recommended that athletes on high carbohydrate diets not supplement with vitamin B_6 above the RDA, as this may negatively affect substrate utilization and performance.

VII. FOLATE

Folate functions in the production of purines and pyrimidines (DNA synthesis).[8,10,90] In this role, folate is important for the production of rapidly proliferating cells such as erythrocytes. Folate is a term used for folic acid and related compounds that show folic acid activity. Fresh vegetables, especially uncooked leafy vegetables, are an important source of folate. Diets in western countries may not include sufficient vegetable intake, so that some folate deficiencies have been found. The RDA is set at 180 µg for adult females and 200 µg for adult males.[7] The 1989 RDAs are about 50% lower than those previously established.

Because of its role in DNA synthesis, a deficiency in folate produces abnormal cell replication in the hematopoietic system that is manifested by hypersegmented neutrophils, macrocytes in the peripheral blood, and megaloblasts in the bone marrow. Megaloblastic anemia can be the result of a folate deficiency or a vitamin B_{12} deficiency or both. Supplementing folate in the presence of vitamin B_{12} deficiency can correct megaloblastic anemia, but B_{12} deficiency will remain. Thus, folate supplementation can sometimes mask B_{12} deficiency.

A. DIETARY INTAKE AND STATUS

Several studies have found that a significant proportion of women athletes and adolescent ballet dancers and gymnasts did not consume two-thirds the RDA for folate.[25,27,28,72,91-93] In contrast, other studies have reported adequate intake of folate for both male and female athletes.[19-23] The studies concluding that some athletes consumed less than two-thirds the RDA were done before 1989 when the RDA was set at 400 µg/day. However, those studies that reported adequate intake were generally done after 1989 when the RDA was reduced to 200 ug/day. Unfortunately the latter studies did not assess intakes of those athletes most at risk, e.g. dancers, gymnasts.

Folate status is most commonly assessed by measurement of folate concentrations in the serum and red blood cells.[3] The latter is the better measure of long-term status.[8] Also, an increase in urinary excretion of formiminoglutamic acid (FIGLU) indicates low folate status because the enzyme that converts FIGLU to L-glutamate requires folate. However, reduced red blood cell folate and increased urinary excretion also could indicate vitamin B_{12} deficiency. If there is a vitamin B_{12} deficiency, the metabolism of folate intermediates is blocked.[8]

Few studies have assessed folate status of athletes. Singh et al.[21] found that ultramarathon runners had adequate blood levels and the mean value exceeded the normal range, reflecting the above normal intake of folate. Elmadfa[32] found that young male and female Austrian athletes had adequate status.

Despite possible folic acid deficiencies in athletes because of inadequate diets, no studies have assessed the relationship of folic acid status and exercise performance or the effect of folic acid supplementation on performance.

VIII. VITAMIN B_{12}

Vitamin B_{12} (cyanocobalamine) is only found in animal food products.[8,94] Deficiencies are rare but may occur in those who eat only foods derived from nonanimal sources. Vitamin B_{12} is required for normal red blood cell production because of its role in facilitating metabolism of folic acid. As mentioned earlier, deficiency in B_{12} or folate could result in megaloblastic anemia. Supplementing with B_{12} could correct the anemia, but the folate deficiency would remain. B_{12} is also important for nervous system function.

The RDA for adults is 2 µg/d.[7] It should be noted that the 1989 RDA for vitamin B_{12} is one-third to one-half lower than that established for the 1980 RDA. Because of cyanocobalamin's role in the formation and function of red blood cells, it is thought that vitamin B_{12} supplementation may enhance the oxygen carrying capacity of red blood cells and improve endurance performance.

A. DIETARY INTAKE AND STATUS

Those athletes who are on energy restricted diets may not be ingesting adequate amounts of vitamin B_{12}.[25,27,28,56,72] Strict vegetarian (vegan) athletes are not ingesting sufficient vitamin B_{12}, unless they consume soy products with B_{12}.[95] Vitamin B_{12} status is commonly assessed by serum or urine levels.[3] Based on analysis of blood samples, the limited data available suggest that athletes have adequate status. Normal B_{12} values were found for well-trained male endurance athletes[31] and young Austrian male and female athletes.[32]

Existing evidence suggests that vitamin B_{12} supplementation has no effect on performance.[96,97] Tin-May-Than et al.[97] injected nonanemic Burmese male subjects with 1 mg cyanocobalamin 3 times per week for 6 weeks and found that this did not improve aerobic exercise performance or measures of muscle strength and performance. Montoye et al.[96] had adolescent boys (age 12–17) consume 50 µg of vitamin B_{12} daily compared to a placebo group. No significant differences in time to run one-half mile or in the Harvard step-test score were found between the supplemented group or the placebo group after 7 weeks.

Studies have not fully examined whether the requirement for vitamin B_{12} is increased by exercise or training. The small percentage of athletes who do not ingest adequate amounts of vitamin B_{12} could easily improve their status through a proper diet or ingestion of small amounts of supplement. There are no data to suggest that vitamin B_{12} supplementation will enhance performance.

IX. VITAMIN B COMBINATIONS

A. DEFICIENCY AND PERFORMANCE

Van der beek et al.[98] had subjects restrict thiamin, riboflavin, or vitamin B_6, or combinations of these, for 11 weeks. Restriction was such that the diet contained no more than 55% of the Dutch RDA. Other vitamins were supplemented at twice the RDA level. The 11 week restriction had no effect on health, but status assessed through blood and enzymatic activation of these vitamins was lowered. Urinary levels also decreased. In concert with these changes, aerobic power, VO_2max, onset of blood lactate accumulation, and peak anaerobic power decreased when data were pooled over the 24 subjects. However, when subjects with just one or two vitamins restricted were analyzed, performance was not affected. Thus, the performance decrements could not be attributed to any one of these vitamins, but the combination. The authors suggested that the deficiencies in the three together negatively affect mitochondrial function. In another study van der Beek[99] reported that a combined restricted intake of thiamin, riboflavin, vitamin B_6, and vitamin C caused a decrease in VO_2max within a few weeks.

Powers et al.[100] examined the effect of a supplement containing iron, riboflavin, thiamin, and vitamin C in Gambian children (aged 11–14.5 years) who had subclinical vitamin deficiencies. The supplement improved the vitamin status of these children and improved their exercise capacity, relative to the placebo group. The effects of iron vs. the other vitamins with regard to performance improvement is not known.

When nonathletic adolescents at risk of B_6 and riboflavin deficiency (based on enzyme activation tests of blood samples) were given either 2 mg of riboflavin or 2 mg of pyridoxine per day for 2 months, improvement in status was found for the vitamin that they were taking.[51] While only the pyridoxine supplementation resulted in improved VO_2max, there was a positive correlation found between both pyridoxine and riboflavin status with VO_2max.

B. SUPPLEMENTATION AND PERFORMANCE

Singh et al.[101,102] had active men ingest a high potency multivitamin/mineral supplement that contained among other vitamins and minerals doses of the B vitamins in percentages many times higher than the RDA. The 12 weeks of supplementation did increase blood concentrations of thiamin, riboflavin, vitamins B_6, and B_{12} but did not affect VO_2 max, endurance capacity, or isokinetic strength tests. The authors concluded that vitamin supplementation had no effect on physically active men with normal biochemical measures of vitamin and mineral status and consuming an adequate diet.

Weight et al.[31] had 30 well-trained runners ingest a high potency multivitamin/mineral supplement for 3 months. Blood concentration of riboflavin and pyridoxine increased significantly but thiamin, nicotinic acid, cyanocobalamin, and folate did not. The supplement did not affect VO_2 max, peak running speed, or measures of lactate in the blood.[103] Barnett and Conlee[104] examined the effect of a marketed high potency vitamin/mineral supplement that also contained amino acids and an unsaturated fatty acid complex for 4 weeks and found no improvement in VO_2 max and no effect on other metabolic assessments. Consistent with these results, Telford et al.[105] found that a multivitamin/mineral supplement over 7–8 months had no effect on several measures of endurance and strength performance.

The effect of B complex supplementation on endurance capacity during a treadmill test was examined in physically active male college students.[106] The supplement contained 5 mg thiamin, 5 mg riboflavin, 25 mg niacin, 2 mg pyridoxine, 0.5 µg vitamin B_{12}, and 12.5 mg pantothenic acid. After 6 weeks of supplementation, there was no significant improvement in endurance capacity.

Bonke and Nickel[107] had one group of marksmen ingest a total of 90 mg thiamin, 60 mg B_6, and 120 µg B_{12} per day for 8 weeks and another group ingest 300 mg thiamin, 600 mg B_6, and 600 µg B_{12} per day for 8 weeks. Both groups improved firing accuracy. The authors speculated the elevated doses of the B vitamins may have a pharmacological effect by influencing receptor affinity for neurotransmitters. Along with the increased accuracy, a decrease in tremor was found.

In early studies, Keys and Henschel[108] had eight infantry men ingest 100 mg nicotinic acid amide, 5 mg of thiamine chloride, and 100 mg ascorbic acid daily for 4 weeks. Compared with the placebo, the supplementation did not result in greater improvement in physiological parameters during a 15 min submaximal marching treadmill test carrying a pack and rifle. In a follow-up study, Keys and Henschel[109] examined the effects of a supplement containing 5–17 mg thiamin, 10 mg riboflavin, 100 mg nicotinic acid, 10–100 mg vitamin B_6, 20 mg calcium pantothenate, and 100–200 mg ascorbic acid for 4–6 weeks. Twenty-six soldiers performed a strenuous treadmill run before and after supplementation. No beneficial effects on performance were found.

Colgan et al.[110] examined the effect of supplementation of hematopoietic nutrients for 12 weeks on nutritional status and performance in male and female endurance runners. The supplement contained 48 mg iron, 60 mg zinc, 2.4 mg folate, 150 mg pyridoxine, 500 mg ascorbic acid, and 100 µg cyanocobalamin. Status of the micronutrients improved, and there was an increase in VO_2max and time to exhaustion on a cycle ergometer. These authors suggested that micronutrients have many interactions with one another, so that supplementation with any one or two micronutrients may not be effective in improving performance. However, when a group of micronutrients that contribute to the same function (e.g., the production of red blood cells) are supplemented together, performance was enhanced. It should be noted that this study used higher levels of all constituents than in previous studies that showed no effect on performance.[103]

C.   RELATIONSHIP TO HEAT STRESS

Because these water soluble vitamins may be lost via sweating, Early and Carlson[111] suggested that vitamin B complex supplementation may enhance exercise in the heat. Henschel et al.[112] examined the effects of a supplement containing 200 mg ascorbic acid or 0.5 mg thiamin, 10 mg riboflavin, and 100 mg nicotinamide ingested for 3 days prior to exposure to heat for 2–4 days. During the heat exposure, the temperature was 110–120°F (43.3–48.9°C) in the day and 85–90°F (29.4–32.2°C) at night. The vitamin supplementation had no effect on sweat composition, water balance, strength tests, or exercise performance and recovery. Thus, the vitamin supplementation did not affect the rate and degree of acclimatization, the incidence of heat exhaustion, and the ability to perform work in the hot environment.[113]

Early and Carlson[111] studied the effect of one dose of a vitamin B supplement, containing 100 mg thiamin, 8 mg riboflavin, 100 mg niacinamide, 5 mg pyridoxine, 25 mg cobalamin, and 30 mg pantothenic acid in high school males. The supplement or a placebo was ingested 30 min before running ten 50-yd. (45.7 m) dashes during hot weather. The group who received the supplement showed less fatigue (drop off in running time) over the trials. These authors suggested that the amount of supplement and the combination of ingredients may be important for a supplement to be effective. They stated that the lower dosages of vitamins used in previous studies may not have been adequate to fulfill the additional vitamin requirement because of loss in sweat and heightened metabolic activity with exercise in the heat.

X. SUPPLEMENT USE

From the information available, there is no reason for athletes to supplement with any one B vitamin. Those who are at risk for a vitamin B deficiency are generally those athletes who are attempting to maintain low body weights and are on energy restricted diets. Adequate energy intake with good food choices should provide sufficient vitamin B intake for athletes. Some athletes ingest multivitamin mineral supplements containing 100% or less of the RDA as an insurance policy. There appears to be no harm in doing this, but neither may there be a benefit.

Thiamin and riboflavin appear harmless as supplements.[9,10,40] Under a physician's care, nicotinic acid in large doses of about 3 g/d have proven useful in lowering total cholesterol. However, side effects such as flushing, injury to the liver, skin conditions, and elevated blood glucose have been found with these large doses. In the niacinamide form, high doses are not harmful.[10,55]

Vitamin B_6 can have toxic effects in large doses (2–6 g pyridoxine/d) causing sensory and peripheral neuropathy.[10,66] Excessive levels of folate have been associated with insomnia, malaise, irritability, and gastrointestinal problems.[10,90] In the absence of folate deficiency, vitamin B_{12} supplements appear harmless, and physicians have sometimes used vitamin B_{12} as a placebo.[10,94]

In their review of supplement use among athletes, Sobal and Marquart[114] reported that multivitamins were the most frequently used type of supplement, and this was followed by vitamin C, iron, vitamin B complex, vitamin E, calcium, and vitamin A, in that order. Copeland and Fricker[115] reported that vitamin B complex vitamins were used by 626 out of 4064 athletes in a 1983 Australian Sports Medicine Federation Survey. In a group of 347 marathon runners at the 1987 Los Angeles marathon, only 6.9% of the runners reported taking vitamin B supplements although 21.9 % took multivitamin supplements.[116] The prevalence was slightly higher for the males and highest for the 35–45-year-olds. An interesting finding in a study by Bazzarre et al.[67] was that athletes who used supplements had greater dietary intake of B vitamins (excluding supplements) compared to nonusers.

XI. SUMMARY

Recent National Health and Nutrition Examination Survey (NHANES) data showed that for the 1988–91 survey year, most adults in the general population were ingesting amounts of thiamin, riboflavin, niacin, folate, and B_{12} sufficient to meet the RDA.[117] B_6 ingestion was adequate for men but slightly low for women, equaling 1.5 mg for 20–39-year-olds and 1.43 mg for 40–49-year-olds (compared to the RDA of 1.6 mg).

Because of high energy intakes to match the energy demands of exercise, most athletes are ingesting amounts of the B vitamins consistent with the RDA. However, athletes on energy restricted diets to maintain low body weights, such as gymnasts, dancers, and wrestlers, or athletes who are not ingesting a wide variety of foods, may not be meeting the RDA amounts. Niekamp and Baer[23] found that 11 of 12 collegiate cross country runners had adequate micronutrients due to high energy consumption and ingestion of a variety of foods. However, one runner who consumed a high energy diet consisting of only a few foods (most were of simple sugars) had low intake of thiamin, riboflavin, niacin, B_6, and folate.[23] Vegan athletes may not ingest sufficient amounts of B_{12} which is found in animal products.[95] Some athletes are not ingesting sufficient amounts of B_6 and possibly folate.[23,25,27-29,67,72,74,91-93]

In concert with findings that most athletes are consuming adequate amounts of these micronutrients are the findings that most athletes have adequate status. Riboflavin status may be impaired at the beginning of an exercise program, but an adequate diet should account for this.[46,47] Some athletes have compromised B_6 status.[26,32,33,43,76,77] However, controversy exists on whether measures of status have been accurate. Thus, additional data are needed to accurately determine vitamin status of athletes, particularly B_{12} and folate.

A couple of studies have indicated that nicotinic acid and riboflavin could be related to heat stress. Riboflavin excretion is exacerbated by exercise in the heat.[53] Nicotinic acid may be involved in thermoregulation.[65] Further studies are recommended to examine the role of these micronutrients in heat stress.

Deficiencies of the B vitamins can result in performance decrements.[98,99] Furthermore, those with compromised status, when given supplements, show improvement in performance. From the van der Beek study,[98,99] it is interesting to note that performance decrements occurred yet there was no noticeable effect on health. Thus, athletes who are not ingesting sufficient quantities of B complex vitamins may not realize that performance is deteriorating because they appear healthy. These athletes may benefit from a multivitamin/mineral supplement.

Generally, supplementation of moderate doses of B vitamins in athletes with adequate status does not result in improved performance.[101-105] However, one study showed that high doses of vitamin B complex were effective in improving marksmanship.[107] Also, when high doses of B_{12} and folate are supplemented along with other hematopoietic nutrients (zinc and iron), an increase in endurance was found.[110] While these two latter studies are provocative, further research is needed to fully document performance benefits. At this time, supplementation with B vitamins to improve athletic performance is unwarranted.

ACKNOWLEDGMENT

I would like to thank Drs. Melinda Manore, Stella Volpe, and Robert Murray for their expert review of this manuscript.

REFERENCES

1. Rock, A., Vitamin hype: why we're wasting $1 of every $3 we spend, *Money*, 82, September, 1995.
2. Pao, E. M. and Cypel, Y .S., Estimation of dietary intake, in *Present Knowledge in Nutrition*, 6th ed., Brown, M. L., Ed., International Life Sciences Institute, Washington, D.C., 1990, 399.
3. Gibson, R. S., *Principles of Nutritional Assessment,* Oxford University Press, New York, 1993, 37.
4. Garry, P. J. and Koehler, K. M., Problems in interpretation of dietary and biochemical data from population studies, in *Present Knowledge in Nutrition*, Brown, M. L., Ed., International Life Sciences Institute, Washington, D.C., 1990, 407.

5. Kaskoun, M. C., Johnson, R. K., and. Goran, M. I., Comparison of energy intake by semiquantitative food-frequency questionnaire with total energy expenditure by the doubly labeled water method in young children, *Am. J. Clin. Nutr.*, 60, 43, 1994.

6. Schoeller, D. A., How accurate is self-reported dietary energy intake?, *Nutr. Rev.*, 48, 373, 1990.

7. Food and Nutrition Board, National Research Council, *Recommended Dietary Allowances*, 10th ed., National Academy Press, Washington, D.C., 1989.

8. Bates, C. J., Thurnham, D. I., Bingham, S. A., Margetts, B. M., and Nelson, M., Biochemical markers of nutrient intake, in *Design Concepts in Nutritional Epidemiology*, Margetts, B. M. and Nelson, M., Eds., Oxford University Press, New York, 1991, 192.

9. Brown, M. L., Thiamin, in *Present Knowledge in Nutrition*, 6th ed., Brown, M. L., Ed., International Life Sciences Institute, Washington, D.C., 1990, 141.

10. Hunt, S. M. and Groff, J. L., *Advanced Nutrition and Human Metabolism*, West Publishing Company, St Paul, 1990.

11. Aronson, V., Vitamins and minerals as ergogenic aids, *Phys. Sportsmed.*, 14 (3), 209, 1986.

12. Ellsworth, N. M., Hewitt, B. F., and Haskell, W. L., Nutrient intake of elite male and female Nordic skiers, *Phys. Sportsmed.*, 13 (2), 78, 1985.

13. Adams, M. M., Porcello, L. P., and Vivian, V. M., Effect of a supplement on dietary intakes of female collegiate swimmers, *Phys. Sportsmed.*, 10 (7), 122, 1982.

14. Berning, J., Swimmers' nutrition, knowledge and practice, *Sports Nutr. News*, 4, 1, 1986.

15. Berning, J. R., Troup, J. P., VanHandel, P. J., Daniels, J., and Daniels, N., The nutritional habits of young adolescent swimmers, *Internat. J. Sport Nutr.*, 1, 20, 1991.

16. Burke, L. M. and Read, R. S. D., Diet patterns of elite Australian male triathletes, *Phys. Sportsmed.*, 15 (2), 140, 1987.

17. Peters, A. J., Dressendorfer, R. H., Rimar, J., and Keen, C. L.. Diet of endurance runners competing in a 20-day road race, *Phys. Sportsmed.*, 14 (7), 63, 1986.

18. Fogelholm, G. M., Himberg, J., Alopaeus, K., Grefm C., Laakso, J. T., Lehto, J. J., and Mussalo-Rauhamaa, H., Dietary and biochemical indices of nutritional status in male athletes and controls, *J. Am. Coll. Nutr.*, 11, 181, 1992.

19. Nutter, J., Seasonal changes in female athletes' diets, *Internat. J. Sport Nutr.*, 1, 395, 1991.

20. Faber, M. and Benadé, A. J. S., Mineral and vitamin intake in field athletes (discus-, hammer-, javelin-throwers and shotputters), *Internat. J. Sports Med.*, 12, 324, 1991.

21. Singh, A., Evans, P., Gallagher, K. L., and Deuster, P. A., Dietary intakes and biochemical profiles of nutritional status of ultramarathoners, *Med. Sci. Sports Exer.*, 25, 328, 1993.

22. Nieman, D. C., Butler, J. V., Pollett, L. M., Dietrich, S. J., and Lutz, R. D., Nutrient intake of marathon runners, *J. Am. Diet. Assoc.*, 89, 1273, 1989.

23. Niekamp, R. A. and Baer, J. T., In-season dietary adequacy of trained male cross-country runners, *Internat. J. Sport Nutr.*, 5, 45, 1995.

24. Ersoy, G., Dietary status and anthropometric assessment of child gymnasts, *J. Sports Med. Phys. Fit.*, 31, 577, 1991.

25. Cohen, J. L., Potosnak, L., Frank, O., and Baker, H., A nutritional and hematological assessment of elite ballet dancers, *Phys. Sportsmed.*, 13 (5), 43, 1985.

26. Guilland, J., Penaranda, T., Gallet, C., Boggio, V., Fuchs, F., and Klepping, J., Vitamin status of young athletes including the effects of supplementation, *Med. Sci. Sports Exer.*, 21, 441, 1989.

27. Loosli, A. R., Benson, J., Gillien, D. M., and Bourdet, K., Nutrition habits and knowledge in competitive adolescent female gymnasts, *Phys. Sportsmed.*, 14(8), 118, 1986.

28. Benson, J., Gillien, D. M., Bourdet, K., and Loosli, A. R., Inadequate nutrition and chronic calorie restriction in adolescent ballerinas, *Phys. Sportsmed.*, 13 (10), 79, 1985.

29. Steen, S. N. and McKinney, S., Nutritional assessment of college wrestlers, *Phys. Sportsmed.*, 14 (11), 101, 1986.

30. Short, S. H. and Short, W. R., Four-year study of university athletes' dietary intake, *J. Am. Diet. Assoc.*, 82, 632, 1983.

31. Weight, L. M., Noakes, T. D., Labadarios, D., Graves, J., Jacobs, P., and Berman, P. A., Vitamin and mineral status of trained athletes including the effects of supplementation, *Am. J. Clin. Nutr.*, 47, 186, 1988.

32. Elmadfa, I. and Rupp, B., Nutritional status of young athletes, in *New Aspects of Nutritional Status*, No. 51, Somogyi, J. C., Elmadfa, I., and Walter, P., Eds., Karger, Basel, 1994, 163.

33. Raczyński, G. and Szczepańska, B., Longitudinal studies on vitamin B_1 and B_6 status in Polish elite athletes, *Biol. Sport*, 10, 189, 1993.

34. Rokitzki, L., Berg, A., and Keul, J., Blood and serum status of water- and fat-soluble vitamins in athletes and non-athletes, *Internat. J. Vit. Nutr. Res.*, 30, 192, 1989.

35. Steel, J. E., A nutritional study of Australian Olympic athletes, *Med. J. Aust.*, 2, 119, 1970.

36. Wood, B., Gijsbers, A., Goode, A., Davis, S., Mulholland, J., and Breen, K., A study of partial thiamin restriction in human volunteers, *Am. J. Clin. Nutr.*, 33, 848, 1980.

37. Karpovich, P. V. and Millman, N., Vitamin B_1 and endurance, *New Engl. J. Med.*, 226, 881, 1942.
38. Keys, A., Henschel, A. F., Mickelsen, O., and Brozek, J. M., The performance of normal young men on controlled thiamine intakes, *J. Nutr.*, 26, 399, 1943.
39. Martini, M. C., Lampe, J.W., Slavin, J. L., and Kurzer, M. S., Effect of the menstrual cycle on energy and nutrient intake, *Am. J. Clin. Nutr.*, 60, 895, 1994.
40. McCormick, D. B., Riboflavin, in *Present Knowledge in Nutrition*, 6th ed., Brown, M. L., Ed., International Life Sciences Institute, Washington, D.C., 1990, 1146.
41. Keith, R. E. and Alt, L. A., Riboflavin status of female athletes consuming normal diets, *Nutr. Res.*, 11, 727, 1991.
42. Tremblay, A., Boilard, B., Breton, M. F., Bessette, H., and Roberge, A. G., The effects of riboflavin supplementation on the nutritional status and performance of elite swimmers, *Nutr. Res.*, 4, 201, 1984.
43. Rokitzki, L., Sagredos, A. N., Reuß, F., Cufi, D., and Keul, J., Assessment of vitamin B_6 status of strength and speedpower athletes, *J. Am. Coll. Nutr.*, 13, 87, 1994.
44. Haralambie, G., Vitamin B_2 status in athletes and the influence of riboflavin administration on neuromuscular irritability, *Nutr. Metab.*, 20, 1, 1976.
45. Rokitzki, L., Sagredos, A., Keck, E., Sauer, B., and Keul, J., Assessment of vitamin B_2 status in performance athletes of various types of sports, *J. Nutr. Sci.Vit.*, 40, 11, 1994.
46. Belko, A. Z., Obarzanek, E., Kalwarf, H. J., Rotter, M. A., Bogusz, S., Miller, D., Haas, J. D., and Roe, D. A., Effects of exercise on riboflavin requirements of young women, *Am. J. Clin. Nutr.*, 37, 509, 1983.
47. Soares, M. J., Satyanarayana, K., Bamji, M. S., Jacob, C. M., Ramana, Y. V., and Rao, S. S., The effect of exercise on the riboflavin status of adult men, *Br. J. Nutr.*, 69, 541, 1993.
48. Winters, L. R., Yoon, J. S., Kalwarf, H. J., Davies, J. C., Berkowitz, M. G., Haas, J., and Roe, D. A., Riboflavin requirements and exercise adaptation in older women, *Am. J. Clin. Nutr.*, 56, 526, 1992.
49. Van Dale, D., Schrijver, J., and Saris, W. H. M., Changes in vitamin status in plasma during dieting and exercise, *Internat. J. Vit. Nutr. Res.*, 60, 67, 1990.
50. Lewis, R. D., Yates, C. Y., and Driskell, J. A., Riboflavin and thiamin status and birth outcome as a function of maternal aerobic exercise, *Am. J. Clin. Nutr.*, 48,110, 1988.
51. Subotičanec, K., Stavljenić, A., Schalch, W., and Buzina, R., Effects of pyridoxine and riboflavin supplementation on physical fitness in young adolescents, *Internat. J. Vit. Nutr. Res.*, 60, 81, 1990.
52. Keys, A., Henschel, A. F., Mickelsen, O., Brozek, J. M., and Crawford, J. H., Physiological and biochemical functions in normal young men on a diet restricted in riboflavin, *J. Nutr.*, 27, 165, 1944.
53. Tucker, R. G., Mickelsen, O., and Keys, A., The influence of sleep, work, diuresis, heat, acute starvation, thiamine intake and bed rest on human riboflavin excretion, *J. Nutr.*, 72, 251, 1960.
54. Di Macco, G., Vitamin e affaticamento (ricerche sperimentali), *Medna Sport*, 4, 271, 1964, as cited in Ref. 44.
55. Jacob, R. A. and Swendseid, M. E., Niacin, in *Present Knowledge in Nutrition*, 6th ed., Brown, M. L., Ed., International Life Sciences Institute,Washington, D. C., 1990, 163.
56. Walberg-Rankin, J., A review of nutritional practices and needs of bodybuilders, *J. Str. Cond. Res.*, 9, 116, 1995.
57. Bergstrom, J., Hultman, E., Jorfeldt, L., Pernow, B., and Wahren, J., Effect of nicotinic acid on physical working capacity and on metabolism of muscle glycogen in man, *J. Appl. Physiol.*, 26, 170, 1969.
58. Norris, B., Schade, D. S., and Eaton, R. P., Effects of altered free fatty acid mobilization on the metabolic response to exercise, *J. Clin. Endocrin. Metab.*, 46, 254, 1978.
59. Hilsedager, D. and Karpovich, P. V., Ergogenic effect of glycine and niacin separately and in combination, *Res. Q. Am. Assoc. Health Phys. Educ. Recreat.*, 35, 389,1964.
60. Galbo, H., Holst, J. J., Christensen, N. J., and Hilsted, J., The effect of nicotinic acid and propranolol on glucagon and plasma catecholamine response to prolonged exercise in man, *Diabetologia*, 11, 343, 1975.
61. Pernow, B. and Saltin, B., Availability of substrates and capacity for prolonged heavy exercise in man, *J. Appl. Physiol.*, 31, 416, 1971.
62. Carlson, L. A. and Oro, L., The effect of nicotinic acid on the plasma free fatty acids, *Acta Med. Scand.,*172, 641, 1962.
63. Heath, E. M., Wilcox, A. R., and Quinn, C. M., Effects of nicotinic acid on respiratory exchange ratio and substrate levels during exercise, *Med. Sci. Sports Exer.*, 25, 1018, 1993.
64. Murray, R., Bartoli, W. P., Eddy, D. E., and Horn, M. K., Physiological and performance responses to nicotinic-acid ingestion during exercise, *Med. Sci. Sports Exer.*, 27, 1057, 1995.
65. Stephenson, L. A. and Kolka, M. A., Increased skin blood flow and enhanced sensible heat loss in humans after nicotinic acid ingestion, *J. Therm. Biol.*, 20, 409, 1995.
66. Merrill, A. H. and Burnham, F. S., Vitamin B-6, in *Present Knowledge in Nutrition*, 6th ed., Brown, M. L., Ed., International Life Sciences Institute, Washington, D. C., 1990, 155.
67. Bazzarre, T. L., Scarpino, A., Sigmon, R., Marquart, L. F., Wu, S. L., and Izurieta, M., Vitamin-mineral supplement use and nutritional status of athletes, *J. Am. Coll. Nutr.*, 12, 162, 1993.
68. Hickson, J. F., Schrader, J., Pivarnik, J. M., and Stockton, J. E., Nutritional intake from food sources of soccer athletes during two stages of training, *Nutr. Rep. Internat.*, 34, 85, 1986.

69. Jensen, C. D., Zaltas, E. S., and Whittam, J. H., Dietary intakes of male endurance cyclists during training and racing, *J. Am. Diet. Assoc.*, 92, 986, 1992.

70. Saris, W. H. M., van Erp-Baart, M. A., Brouns, F., Westerterp, K. R., and ten Hoor, F., Study on food intake and energy expenditure during extreme sustained exercise, the Tour de France, *Internat. J. Sports Med.*, 10, S26, 1989.

71. Worme, J. D., Doubt, T. J., Singh, A., Ryan, C. J., Moses, F. M., and Deuster, P. A., Dietary patterns, gastrointestinal complaints, and nutrition knowledge of recreational triathletes, *Am. J. Clin. Nutr.*, 51, 690, 1990.

72. Welch, P. K., Zager, K. A., Endres, J., and Poon, S. W., Nutrition education, body composition, and dietary intake of female college athletes, *Phys. Sportsmed.*, 15 (1), 63, 1987.

73. Kaiserauer, S., Snyder, A. C., Sleeper, M. and Zierath, J., Nutritional, physiological, and menstrual status of distance runners. *Med. Sci. Sports Exer.*, 21, 120, 1989.

74. Keith, R. E., O'Keeffe, K. A., Alt, L. A., and Young, K. L., Dietary status of trained female cyclists, *J. Am. Diet. Assoc.*, 89, 1620, 1989.

75. Manore, M. M., Vitamin B_6 and exercise, *Internat. J. Sport Nutr.*, 4, 889, 1994.

76. Fogelholm, M., Ruokonen, I., Laakso, J. T., Vuorimaa, T., and Himberg, J., Lack of association between indices of vitamin B_1, B_2, and B_6 status and exercise-induced blood lactate in young adults, *Internat. J. Sport Nutr.*, 3, 165, 1993.

77. Telford, R. D., Catchpole, E. A., Deakin, V., McLey, A. C., and Plank, A. W., The effect of 7 to 8 months of vitamin/mineral supplementation on the vitamin and mineral status of athletes, *Internat. J. Sport Nutr.*, 2, 123, 1992.

78. Yates, C. Y., Boylan, L. M., Lewis, R. D., and Driskell, J. A., Maternal aerobic exercise and vitamin B-6 status, *Am. J. Clin. Nutr.*, 48, 117, 1988.

79. Coburn, S. P., Ziegler, P. J., Costill, D. L., Mahuren, J. D., Fink, W. J., Schaltenbrand, W. E., Pauly, T. A., Pearson, D. R., Conn, P. S., and Guilarte, T. R., Responses of vitamin B-6 content of muscle to changes in vitamin B-6 intake in men, *Am. J. Clin. Nutr.*, 53, 1436, 1991.

80. Leklem, J. E. and Shultz, T. D., Increased plasma pyridoxal 5′-phosphate and vitamin B_6 in male adolescents after a 4500-meter run, *Am. J. Clin. Nutr.*, 38, 541, 1983.

81. Hatcher, L. F., Leklem, J. E., and Campbell, D. E., Altered vitamin B_6 metabolism during exercise in man, effect of carbohydrate modified diets and vitamin B_6 supplements, *Med. Sci. Sports Exer.*, 14, 112A, 1982.

82. Hofmann, A., Reynolds, R. D., Smoak, B. L., Vallanueva, V. G., and Deuster, P. A., Plasma pyridoxal and pyridoxal 5′-phosphate concentration in response to ingestion of water of glucose polymer during a 2-h run, *Am. J. Clin. Nutr.*, 53, 84, 1991.

83. Manore, M. M. and Leklem, J. E., Effect of carbohydrate and vitamin B_6 on fuel substrates during exercise in women, *Med. Sci. Sports Exer.*, 20, 233, 1988.

84. Belko, A. Z., Vitamins and exercise — an update, *Med. Sci. Sports Exer.*, 19, S191, 1987.

85. Crozier, P. G., Cordain, L., and Sampson, D. A., Exercise-induced changes in plasma vitamin B-6 concentrations do not vary with exercise intensity, *Am. J. Clin. Nutr.*, 60, 552, 1994.

86. Rokitzki, L., Sagredos, A. N., Reuß, F., Büchner, M., and Keul, J., Acute changes in vitamin B_6 status in endurance athletes before and after a marathon, *Internat. J. Sport Nutr.*, 4, 154, 1994.

87. Dreon, D. M. and Butterfield, G. E., Vitamin B_6 utilization in active and inactive young men, *Am. J. Clin. Nutr.*, 43, 816, 1986.

88. Lawrence, J. D., Smith, J. L., Bower, R. C., and Riehl, W. P., The effect of alpha-tocopherol (vitamin E) and pyridoxine HCL (vitamin B_6) on the swimming endurance of trained swimmers, *J. Am. Coll. Health Assoc.*, 23, 219, 1975.

89. Virk, R., Dunton, V., and Leklemm J., The effect of vitamin B_6 supplementation on fuel utilization during exhaustive exercise, *FASEB*, 6, A1374, 1992.

90. Krumdieck, C. L., Folic acid, in *Present Knowledge in Nutrition*, 6th ed., Brown, M. L., Ed., International Life Sciences Institute, Washington, D. C., 1990, 179.

91. Lamar-Hildebrand, N., Saldanha, L., and Endres, J., Dietary and exercise practices of college-aged female body builders, *J. Am. Diet. Assoc.*, 89, 1308, 1989.

92. Calabrese, L. H., Kirkendall, D. T., Floyd, M., Rapoport, S., Williams, G. W., Weiker, G. G., and Bergfeld, J. A., Menstrual abnormalities, nutritional patterns, and body composition in female classical ballet dancers, *Phys. Sportsmed.*, 11 (2), 86, 1983.

93. Bazzarre, T. L., Marquart, L. F., Izurieta, M., and Jones, A., Incidence of poor nutritional status among triathletes, endurance athletes and control subjects, *Med. Sci. Sports Exer.*, 18, S90, 1986.

94. Herbert, V., Vitamin B-12, in *Present Knowledge in Nutrition*, 6th ed., Brown, M. L., Ed., International Life Sciences Institute,Washington, D. C., 1990, 170.

95. Janelle, K. C. and Barr, S. I., Nutrient intakes and eating behavior of vegetarian and nonvegetarian women, *J. Am. Diet. Assoc.*, 95, 180, 1995.

96. Montoye, H. J., Spata, P. J., Pinckney, V., and Barron, L., Effect of vitamin B_{12} supplementation on physical fitness and growth of young boys, *J. Appl. Physiol.*, 7, 589, 1955.

97. Tin-May-Than, Ma-Win-May, Khin-Sann-Aung, and Mya-Tu, M., The effect of vitamin B_{12} on physical performance capacity, *Br. J. Nutr.,* 40, 269, 1978.

98. van der Beek, E. J., van Dokkum, W., Wedel, M., Schrijver, J., and van den Berg, H., Thiamin, riboflavin and vitamin B_6: Impact of restricted intake on physical performance in man, *J. Amer. Coll. Nutr.*, 13, 629, 1994.

99. van der beek, E. J., van Dokkum, W., Schrijver, J., Wedel, M., Gailland, A. W. K., Wesstra, A., van de Weerd, H., and Hermus, R. J. J., Thiamin, riboflavin, and vitamins B_6 and C, Impact of combined restricted intake on function performance in man, *Am. J. Clin. Nutr.,* 48, 1451, 1988.

100. Powers, H. J., Bates, C. J., Lamb, W. H., Singh, J., Gelman, W., and Webb, E., Effects of a multivitamin and iron supplement on running performance in Gambian children, *Hum. Nutr. Clin. Nutr.,* 39C, 427, 1985.

101. Singh, A., Moses, F. M., and Deuster, P. A., Chronic multivitamin-mineral supplementation does not enhance physical performance, *Med. Sci. Sports Exer.,* 24, 726, 1992.

102. Singh, A., Moses, F. M., and Deuster, P. A., Vitamin and mineral status in physically active men, effects of a high potency supplement, *Am. J. Clin. Nutr.*, 55, 1, 1992.

103. Weight, L. M., Myburgh, K. H., and Noakes, T. D., Vitamin and mineral supplementation, effect on the running performance of trained athletes, *Am. J. Clin. Nutr.,* 47, 192, 1988.

104. Barnett, D. W. and Conlee, R. K., The effects of a commercial dietary supplement on human performance, *Am. J. Clin. Nutr.,* 40, 586, 1984.

105. Telford, R. D., Catchpole, E. A., Deakin, V., Hahn, A. G., and Plank, A. W., The effect of 7 to 8 months of vitamin/mineral supplementation on athletic performance, *Internat. J. Sport Nutr.*, 2, 135, 1992.

106. Read, M. H. and McGuffin, S. L., The effect of B-complex supplementation on endurance performance, *J. Sports Med.,* 23, 178, 1983.

107. Bonke, D. and Nickel, B., Improvement of fine motoic movement control by elevated dosages of vitamin B_1, B_6, and B_{12} in target shooting, *Internat. J. Vit. Nutr. Res.,* 30, 198, 1989.

108. Keys, A. and Henschel, A. F., High vitamin supplementation (B_1, nicotinic acid and C) and the response to intensive exercise in U. S. Army infantrymen, *Am. J. Physiol.,* 133, 350, 1941.

109. Keys, A. and Henschel, A. F., Vitamin supplementation of U. S. Army rations in relation to fatigue and the ability to do muscular work, *J. Nutr.,* 23, 259, 1942.

110. Colgan, M., Fiedler, S., and Colgan, L. A., Micronutrient status of endurance athletes affect hematology and performance, *J. Appl.Nutr.,* 43, 16, 1991.

111. Early, R. G. and Carlson, B. R., Water-soluble vitamin therapy in the delay of fatigue from physical activity in hot climatic conditions, *Int. Z. Angew. Physiol.,* 27, 43, 1969.

112. Henschel, A., Taylor, H. L., Mickelsen, O., Brozek, J. M., and Keys, A., The effect of high vitamin C and B intake on the ability of man to work in hot environments, *Fed. Proc.,* 3, 18, 1944.

113. Mayer, J. and Bullen, B., Nutrition and athletic performance, *Physiol. Rev.,* 40, 369, 1960.

114. Sobal, J. and Marquart, L. F., Vitamin/mineral supplement use among athletes, A review of the literature, *Internat. J. Sport Nutr.*, 4, 320, 1994.

115. Copeland, I. and Fricker, P. A., Vitamins in sport, who is at risk?, *Clin. J. Sport Med.,* 4, 151, 1994.

116. Nieman, D. C., Gates, J. R., Butler, J. V., Pollett, L. M., Dietrich, S. J., and Lutz, R. D., Supplementation patterns in marathon runners, *J. Am. Diet. Assoc.,* 89, 1615, 1989.

117. Alaimo, K., McDowell, M. A., Briefel, R. R., Bischoff, A. M., Caughman, C. R., Loria, C. M., and Johnson, C. L., Dietary intake of vitamins, minerals, and fiber of person ages 2 months and over in the United States: third national health and nutrition examination survey, Phase 1, 1988–1991. Advance data from vital and health statistics: No. 258. Hyattsville, MD: National Center for Health Statistics, 1994. [Department of Health and Human Services publication, Public Health Service 95-1250 (11/94)]

Chapter 8

TRACE MINERALS AND EXERCISE

_____ Emily M. Haymes

CONTENTS

I. INTRODUCTION

Trace minerals are defined as those minerals essential for life found in the body in quantities less than 5 g. Although there is some disagreement about the need for some of the trace minerals, the following minerals are considered to be essential: iron, iodine, zinc, copper, chromium, selenium, manganese, cobalt, silicon, nickel, molybdenum, vanadium, and arsenic. Very little information is available relative to exercise for most of the trace minerals. On the other hand, the role of iron in exercise has been thoroughly investigated. Recent research has

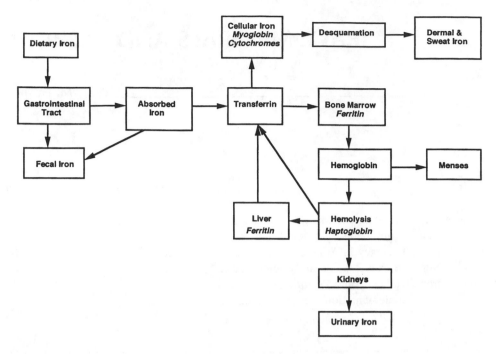

FIGURE 1   Metabolism of iron in the human body including pathways for excretion.

focused on zinc, copper, and chromium metabolism during exercise. The following discussion will be limited to those trace minerals that have been studied in exercising individuals.

II.   IRON

Iron is the trace mineral found in the body in greatest amounts. Distribution of iron in the body and avenues of excretion are illustrated in Figure 1. Because two-thirds of the iron is found in hemoglobin, its presence or absence greatly affects oxygen transport in the blood. Small amounts of iron are found in the muscles as myoglobin and iron containing enzymes in the mitochondria including the cytochromes. Iron is stored primarily in the bone marrow as ferritin and hemosiderin. The average man will store about 1000 mg of iron, but the average woman will only have about 300 mg of stored iron.

A.   IRON REQUIREMENTS AND DEFICIENCY

Iron is lost from the body through desquamation of cells from the skin, through the gastrointestinal tract and through the urinary tract (see Figure 1). Daily iron loss by adult men is 1.0 mg and by adult women who are not menstruating is 0.8 mg.[1] Women who are menstruating lose additional iron through the menses which average 0.6 mg/day and increases the requirement to 1.4 mg/day. Iron loss through the menses will exceed 1.4 mg/day in about 10% of adult women and increase the requirement to more than 2.2 mg/day.[2] During pregnancy women need additional iron for expanding their red cell volume (450 mg), for the fetus (290 mg), and for the placenta (25 mg). Because cessation of the menses saves about 270 mg of iron, pregnant women will need an additional 500 mg or 2 mg/day during pregnancy.[3]

Adolescents require more iron (0.2 mg/day) during the adolescent growth spurt (ages 11–18 years) to support the growth and expand blood volume in addition to replacing iron losses. Once menarche occurs, girls will need even more iron to replace blood lost through the menses. Adolescent girls (ages 12–16 years) require approximately 1.7 mg/day.[4]

Based on an average iron absorption of 10%, the recommended dietary allowance (RDA) for iron is 10 mg/day for men aged 19 and older and women after menopause.[5] The RDA for boys 11–18 years is 12 mg/day while the RDA for girls 11–18 years and nonpregnant women ages 19 to menopause is 15 mg/day. During pregnancy, a supplement providing 30–60 mg iron/day is recommended in addition to the normal recommendation for nonpregnant women.

The amount of iron absorbed from food varies considerably and averages about 10% under normal circumstances. Iron absorption is increased when iron stores are depleted and may exceed 20% in iron deficient persons. Two forms of food iron, heme and nonheme iron, are absorbed through the walls of the small intestine by different mechanisms. About 40% of the iron found in meat, fish, and poultry is heme iron. Heme iron is more easily absorbed (about 23%) and is not affected by other foods in a meal. Nonheme iron is the form found in vegetables and grains and makes up the remaining 60% of the iron in meat, fish, and poultry. Absorption of nonheme iron varies from 3–8% depending on the presence of enhancing and inhibiting factors in the meal and the amount of iron stored in the body.[6] The presence of meat, fish, and poultry in a meal enhances the absorption of nonheme iron. Ascorbic acid (vitamin C) also increases nonheme iron absorption. Tannic acid (found in tea), phytic acid (found in whole grains), and bran are inhibitors of nonheme iron absorption. Large quantities of calcium, phosphate, and zinc, as might be found in a mineral supplement, will interact and inhibit absorption of nonheme iron.[3]

If a person consumes and absorbs less iron than (s)he loses, the negative iron balance will eventually drain the iron stores of the body. There are three stages of iron deficiency: iron depletion, iron deficient erythropoiesis, and iron deficiency anemia. The first stage, iron depletion, develops as the body's stores are depleted. Depletion of the bone marrow iron stores can be detected by the absence of or only traces of iron in a bone marrow biopsy. Plasma ferritin concentration is closely correlated with the amount of iron stored and is a more practical method of detecting iron depletion. Plasma ferritin concentrations of 12 µg/l or less are an indication that iron stores are depleted.[7]

As iron stores are depleted, iron absorption increases. Depletion of iron stores reduces the amount of iron available for hemoglobin formation. Because less hemoglobin is formed, protoporphyrin used to form heme is released into the blood. This is known as a free erythrocyte protoporphyrin (FEP). Transferrin, a plasma protein that transports iron in the blood, is produced in greater quantities. If the total quantity of iron in the blood does not increase proportionately, the saturation of transferrin with iron decreases. When the FEP concentration exceeds 100 µg/dl RBC and the transferrin saturation falls below 16%, the second stage of iron deficient erythropoiesis has developed. Recent evidence suggests increases in serum transferrin receptors may be a more sensitive indicator of tissue iron deficiency than FEP.[8]

Hemoglobin concentration remains within the normal range until the third stage develops. Anemia is defined as a hemoglobin concentration of less than 12 g/dl for women, less than 13 g/dl for men, and less than 11 g/dl during pregnancy.[3] Iron deficiency anemia is characterized not only by low hemoglobin and ferritin concentrations, low transferrin saturation, and elevated FEP concentrations, but also by erythrocytes that are microcytic (smaller than normal) and hypochromic (low in iron).

Iron deficient erythropoiesis in the U.S. population is most common in adolescent girls aged 15–19 years (14%), adolescent boys aged 11–14 years (12%), and nonpregnant women aged 20–44 years (9.6%).[9] Another study reported that low ferritin concentrations indicative of iron depletion were found in more than 20% of the adolescent girls aged 12–18 years and

TABLE 1   Prevalence of Iron Deficiency Among Athletes

Study	Sport	Gender	Low[a] Ferritin	Iron[b] Deficiency	Anemia[c]
Balaban[12]	Runners	Women	25%	—	5.4%
		Men	8%	—	5.7%
Colt[14]	Runners	Women	28%	—	0
		Men	3.5%	—	1.2%
Deuster[16]	Runners	Women	35%	—	—
Haymes[17]	Runners	Women	30%	9%	0
Pate[19]	Runners	Women	20%	—	2.8%
Robertson[20]	Runners	Men	8%	8%	—
Nickerson[18]	Runners	Girls	—	34%	5.7%
		Boys	—	8%	—
Clement[23]	Skiers	Women	21%	—	7%
		Men	13%	—	0
Haymes[24]	Skiers	Women	20%	20%	0
		Men	11%	0	0
Rowland[27]	Swimmers	Girls	47%	—	0
		Boys	0	—	6.7%
Risser[26]	Variety	Women	31%	18%	7%
Willows[28]	Variety	Girls	11%	—	—
		Boys	5%	—	—
Brown[13]	Track	Girls	44%	—	12.5%
U.S. Population[9-11]		Girls	24.5%	14.2%	5.9%
		Women	21.1%	9.6%	5.8%
		Boys	11.9%	0.1%	2.6%
		Men	1.7%	0.6%	2.9%

[a]   Ferritin <12 ug/l.
[b]   Ferritin <12 ug/l and transferrin saturation <16%.
[c]   Hemoglobin <12 g/dl for women and <13 g/dl for men.

women aged 18–45 years and 10% of the adolescent boys aged 12–18 years.[10] Iron deficiency anemia was found in approximately 6% of the women and adolescent girls.[11]

B.   IRON DEFICIENCY IN ATHLETES

Low ferritin concentrations and depleted bone marrow iron stores have been found in both men and women runners.[12-21] Poor iron status has also been observed in women athletes competing in other sports including field hockey, cross country skiing, crew, basketball, and softball (Table 1).[22-29] The questions are: (1) is the proportion of athletes who are iron depleted greater than that found in the general population and (2) do low ferritin concentrations mean that the iron stores are depleted?

In the case of men distance runners the answer to the first question is probably yes. Low plasma ferritin in men is very rare in the normal population. Because many of the studies of women runners have not used a plasma ferritin <12 μg/l as a criteria for iron depletion, it is more difficult to compare the incidence of iron depletion in runners with the normal population. Several recent studies reported no significant differences in plasma ferritin between women distance runners and control groups matched for age.[12,17,19] However, the prevalence of subnormal ferritin concentrations is significantly greater in women athletes than nonathletes.[30] Some of the variation in ferritin concentration among studies could be due to recent strenuous exercise. Lampe and colleagues[31] observed significantly increased serum ferritin concentrations for 3 days following a marathon. Transferrin saturation has been observed to increase during heavy training and decrease during periods of relative rest.[32] Elevation of either ferritin or transferrin saturation by intense exercise bouts could mask iron depletion and iron deficient erythropoiesis in an athlete. Plasma ferritin is also increased by infection and inflammation which would mask depleted iron stores. Immediately following prolonged exercise (e.g., triathlon) serum iron was significantly decreased but plasma ferritin was elevated for 48 hours after the race.[33] Taylor and colleagues suggested changes in ferritin and iron were likely due to an acute phase response to inflammation.[33] Moore and others observed a significant decrease in serum iron after 2 weeks of intense military training which is also a part of the acute phase response.[34]

Under normal circumstances low ferritin concentrations and reduced bone marrow iron are adequate evidence of iron depletion. Eichner[35] has suggested that low plasma ferritin in athletes is due to an expanded plasma volume. However, this explanation does not appear to be valid in the case of elite male distance runners who were found to have a mean serum ferritin of 32 μg/l.[36] Because the median serum ferritin for adult males is 94 μg/l,[10] this would require a threefold expansion of the plasma volume which is highly unlikely. An expanded plasma volume has been observed in some distance runners, but the 15% difference in plasma volume could not explain the 78% reduction in serum ferritin.[37] Magnusson and colleagues found that all of the runners with low serum ferritin had at least traces of hemosiderin in their bone marrow and normal FEP concentrations and concluded that none was truly iron deficient.[37]

Several studies have examined whether iron status changes during training. Significant reductions in ferritin have been observed in some studies[22,38-41] but not in others.[24,31,34,42] Transient reductions in hemoglobin concentration have been observed at the beginning of training that may be due to red blood cell destruction and/or an expansion of plasma volume. Hemoglobin is restored to normal concentrations after a few weeks of training accompanied by significant increases in FEP and transferrin.[43] Increases in FEP would be expected if inadequate iron was available to support hemoglobin formation while increases in transferrin occur when iron stores are depleted. The restoration of hemoglobin during training puts an added strain on the iron stores.

Many athletes have hemoglobin concentrations that are in the lower part of the normal range.[44-46] However, the incidence of iron deficiency anemia is relatively low and appears to be no more prevalent than in the normal population. Low hemoglobin concentration in some athletes may be due to plasma volume expansion.[47,48] Pate[49] has described low hemoglobin concentration as suboptimal and suggests it may be detrimental to performance. Because most of the oxygen transported in the blood is bound to hemoglobin, a reduction in hemoglobin concentration necessitates an increase in cardiac output to maintain oxygen delivery to the tissues.[50] On the other hand, increased plasma volume could be beneficial because of decreased resistance to blood flow, improved sweating, and a larger stroke volume.[35,48] Red cell mass may also increase during training, however, the results of studies are equivocal.[44,48,51,52]

Reduced hemoglobin concentration in athletes may be due to increased red blood cell destruction. Evidence of red cell destruction includes reduced haptoglobin concentration, increased plasma hemoglobin concentration, and the presence of hemoglobin in the urine (hemoglobinuria). When red blood cells are destroyed in the blood vessels (intravascular hemolysis), the hemoglobin is released and picked up by haptoglobin (Figure 2). The haptoglobin is then removed from the blood as it passes through the liver, and the haptoglobin concentration decreases. If more hemoglobin is released than can be bound to haptoglobin, the hemoglobin concentration in the plasma rises. Excess plasma hemoglobin will be removed in the kidneys and excreted in the urine. Several studies have reported evidence of intravascular hemolysis in runners and swimmers,[53-58] however, other studies did not find any evidence of hemolysis.[44,59] If anemia is due to intravascular hemolysis, the red cell volume will be increased (macrocytic) rather than decreased (microcytic). Magnusson and colleagues[55] suggested that heme iron removed from haptoglobin by hepatocytes may be stored in the liver. Plasma ferritin reflects iron storage in the bone marrow. Even though plasma ferritin was low, hemoglobin synthesis would not be impaired because iron could be transported from the liver to the bone marrow by transferrin. Robertson and others[20] found elevated transferrin in male runners who ran 80 km or more weekly which they suggested

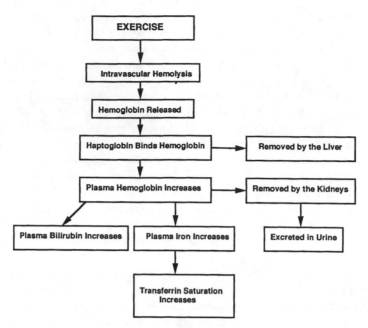

FIGURE 2   Exercise-induced, intravascular hemolysis and the fate of heme iron.

might "reflect increased movement of iron from the reticuloendothelial system to the erythroid bone marrow."

C.   NEGATIVE IRON BALANCE IN ATHLETES

The most likely causes of iron depletion in women athletes are:

1. inadequate iron intake,
2. reduced iron absorption due to diets with low bioavailability,
3. excessive iron loss through the menses,
4. excessive iron loss through sweating,
5. gastrointestinal blood loss, and
6. excretion of iron in the urine.

One of the most likely causes of iron depletion among women is low iron intake. Approximately 50% of all women and girls over the age of 11 years in the United States consume less than 10 mg of iron/day. Low iron intake may also contribute to iron depletion in adolescent boys and children. About 50% of all children under the age of 11 years have less than adequate iron intakes. Average dietary iron intake is 6 mg/1000 kcal.

Women runners typically consume 2000–2500 kcal/day (8372–10,465 kJ/day) or about 12–15 mg iron/day.[17,60-62] If they lose 1.5 mg iron daily through desquamation and the menses, assuming that 10% of the iron is absorbed would result in negative iron balance for some of these women (1.2 mg – 1.5 mg = –0.3 mg). Many women runners consume diets low in meat and high in fiber which reduces iron bioavailability to less than 10%.[17,60-62] Women runners with a bioavailable iron intake of 0.9 mg/day are more likely to be in negative iron balance than women with a bioavailable iron intake of 1.5 mg/day.

Iron loss through the menses averages 0.6 mg/day.[4] Approximately 25% of menstruating women lose 0.9 mg iron or more through the menses.[4] These women would be more likely to be in negative iron balance and become iron deficient.[2] Many of the women athletes who are iron depleted may have greater blood losses through the menses. Some women athletes

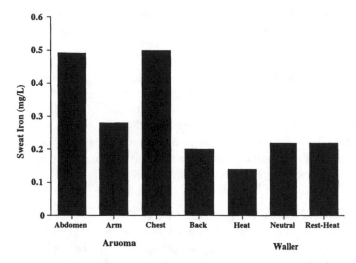

FIGURE 3 Sweat iron concentration during exercise measured at various sites by Aruoma[67] and from the arm in different environments by Waller.[68]

are amenorrheic (three or fewer menses per year) and lose very little iron through the menses. Deuster and colleagues[63] found no significant difference in serum ferritin concentrations of eumenorrheic and amenorrheic women distance runners. However, a greater percentage of the amenorrheic runners (46%) were iron depleted than eumenorrheic runners (31%). Perry and colleagues[64] found amenorrheic and eumenorrheic runners with disordered eating habits were more likely to have low transferrin saturations.

Excretion of iron through sweating is a potential cause of negative iron balance in both women and men. Sweat iron concentrations of 0.13–0.50 mg/l have been reported for men and women during exercise.[65-68] Higher sweat iron concentration have been reported for men and women resting in hot environments (0.17–1.6 mg/l).[69-71] Waller and Haymes[68] found lower sweat iron concentations during exercise in the heat than during rest in the heat or exercise in a neutral environment (Figure 3). Athletes training in hot environments may lose 1–2 l of sweat/hour. An athlete sweating at a rate of 1 l/hour for several hours of training could lose a substantial amount of iron. However, part of the iron excreted in the sweat may come from desquamated skin cells that are normally lost each day. Mean iron uptake by the skin is 0.24 mg/day, but it varies directly with the percent transferrin saturation.[72] Iron deficient athletes are likely to have low cell-rich sweat iron losses. Recent evidence suggests that the amount of iron excreted in the sweat may be overestimated if only the first sweat excreted is sampled.[73] Subsequent sweat samples were found to have a much lower iron concentration.[73] Sweat iron concentration during exercise has also been found to decrease over time.[68] This is consistent with the theory that the initial sweat is contaminated with iron from cellular debris and the environment.

Distance runners may lose some iron through gastrointestinal bleeding. The incidence of gastrointestinal bleeding reported among runners ranges from 8 to 85%.[74-79] Both qualitative and quantitative techniques have been used to detect blood in the feces. When a quantitative method, HemoQuant, was used, the average amounts of hemoglobin lost in races ranging from 10 km through a marathon were 1.5 mg/g and 2.25 mg/g of stool, respectively.[77,78] This would be about 1.0 –1.5 mg iron/day or about twice the normal rate of iron loss through the feces. Presence of blood in the feces was more frequent when running at faster speeds in one study[76] but not in two others.[79,80] Bleeding into the gastrointestinal tract may be due to vasoconstriction of splanchnic vessels during heavy exercise.[78] In an ultramarathon race, symptoms of lower gastrointestinal tract distress were significantly related to the presence of fecal blood.[79] Use of aspirin or nonsteroidal antiinflammatory drugs by exercising persons may increase bleeding and the amount of iron lost through the gastrointestinal tract,[77] however, two recent studies reported that runners with gastrointestinal bleeding were not more likely to use nonsteroidal anti-inflammatory drugs.[79,80]

The amount of iron lost in the urine of runners was 0.18 mg/day or about twice the normal rate of 0.1 mg/day.[37] Possible sources of this iron are hemosiderin, transferrin, hemoglobin, and red blood cells. Following distance runs increased red cell counts were found in the urine of most runners.[81] Transferrin has also been found in the urine of distance runners.[82] Evidence of hematuria has been observed in 17–18% of runners following marathon runs.[83,84] One possible cause of hematuria is trauma to the bladder wall during running.[85] Because the amount of iron found in the urine is relatively small, it is unlikely that this is a major source of iron loss in most exercising individuals.

D. IRON DEFICIENCY AND PERFORMANCE

There is ample evidence that iron deficiency anemia has a significant negative effect on physical work capacity and maximal oxygen uptake.[86-88] When hemoglobin concentration is low, the amount of oxygen transported by the blood is reduced. During maximal exercise cardiac output cannot increase to compensate for the lower oxygen transport. The question is, does iron deficiency without anemia have a negative effect on physical performance?

Theoretically iron depletion could have an adverse effect on the amounts of myoglobin, cytochromes, and iron containing enzymes in muscle. Animal studies in which rats with iron deficiency anemia were transfused to restore hemoglobin concentration still had reduced endurance capacities in comparison to nonanemic rats.[89-91] Iron deficient rats have significantly lower concentrations of cytochromes c, b, and a, and the activities of cytochrome oxidase, pyruvate-malate oxidase, succinate dehydrogenase, and NADH dehydrogenase are significantly lower than in skeletal muscle of normal rats.[92,93] Iron repletion restores maximal oxygen uptake and hemoglobin concentration faster than muscle enzyme activity and endurance which follow similar patterns.[92]

Men and women who are iron deficient but have hemoglobin concentrations that are borderline for anemia (approximately 12 g/dl) have significantly lower heart rates during exercise after only 2 days of iron therapy.[94] Iron deficient adults also have higher blood lactate concentrations following maximal exercise than subjects with normal hemoglobin concentrations.[29,94] Celsing and associates[86] attempted to simulate the animal studies with men by doing repeated phlebotomies to deplete the iron stores over a 9 week period. Following transfusion that restored normal hemoglobin levels, maximal oxygen uptake, endurance time, and blood lactate returned to prephlebotomy levels. Because no significant impairment in muscle enzyme activity was observed during this study, the length of the iron deficiency period may have been too short to deplete the tissue iron.

E. IRON SUPPLEMENTATION

Because many women are iron depleted or iron deficient, there has been much interest in the use of iron supplements. It is well established that iron therapy is beneficial in increasing iron concentration and physical work capacity and reducing exercise heart rate and lactate in persons with iron deficiency anemia.[95,96] The question is whether iron supplements would be beneficial to athletes or physically active persons who are not anemic.

Several studies have examined changes in hematologic status of athletes taking iron supplements during training. The results of these studies are summarized in Table 2. Most of the studies that did not observe any significant changes in hemoglobin or iron status used low dosages of iron (18 mg/day) and athletes who were not iron deficient.[24,97,98] When supplements containing larger dosages of iron (50 mg/day or more) have been given to iron deficient athletes, significant improvements in iron status have been observed.[29,99-108] Use of

TABLE 2   Iron Supplementation during Training

Study	Sport	Amount of Iron	Increased Hemoglobin	Increased Ferritin
Cooter[97]	Basketball	18 mg	No	—
Haymes[24]	Cross-Country Skiing	18 mg	No	No
Pate[98]	Variety	50 mg	No	—
Matter[99]	Running	50 mg	No	Yes
Nickerson[100]	Running	60 mg	Yes	Yes
Hunding[46]	Running	60 mg	Yes	—
Yoshida[106]	Running	60 mg	No	Yes
Lamanca[101]	Endurance	100 mg	Yes	Yes
Newhouse[102]	Running	100 mg	No	Yes
Klingshirn[108]	Running	100 mg	No	Yes
Fogelholm[107]	Variety	100 mg	No	Yes
Clement[103]	Running	100 mg	No	Yes
	Running	200 mg	Yes	Yes
Plowman[104]	Running	234 mg	Yes	—
Schoene[29]	Variety	270 mg	Yes	Yes
Rowland[105]	Running	300 mg	No	Yes

iron supplements may also be beneficial in preventing iron depletion from developing in some girl and women athletes during prolonged endurance training.[24,39,41,109]

Most studies of iron supplementation have not found improved exercise performance in nonanemic iron deficient women athletes.[29,99,101,102,107,108,110] Only one study found that adolescent girl runners improved in endurance after 4 weeks of iron supplementation.[105] Competitive women runners could also run 3000 m faster after 8 weeks of iron supplementation.[106] However, use of iron supplements by women athletes has been found to reduce blood lactate concentrations following heavy exercise[29,101] and to increase the running velocity at which the onset of blood lactate accumulation (OBLA) occurred.[106] Reduction in blood lactate could be due to an improvement in aerobic metabolism in the muscles.

F.   IRON TOXICITY

Use of iron supplements with dosages of 75 mg or more indiscriminantly by athletes is not advised because of the possibility of iron toxicity. Intake of large iron dosages may interfere with the absorption of zinc.[3] Some individuals have a genetic disorder called hemochromatosis that causes them to absorb and store large amounts of iron which can damage the liver. For these reasons it is preferable to screen athletes for iron deficiency at the annual physical examination. Those athletes who are diagnosed as iron depleted should be given iron supplements. Some girls and women may choose to take a low dosage iron supplement (15 mg/day) to ensure an adequate daily iron intake.

Iron is a transition metal that can serve as a catalyst for lipid peroxidation if it is unbound. Transferrin acts as an antioxidant because it binds unbound iron. Aruoma and colleagues[111] found untreated hemochromatosis patients have significant amounts of unbound iron in the plasma. Following phlebotomy treatments, unbound iron decreased significantly in direct proportion to the decline in plasma ferritin. Elevated iron stores in males have been linked to increased risk of cancer[112] and myocardial infarction.[113] Although Magnusson and colleagues[114] did not find that ferritin was a significant risk factor for myocardial infarction, they did find that men and women with low transferrin levels were at increased risk. It has been suggested that high levels of physical activity are beneficial in lowering the risk of coronary heart disease because they reduce body iron stores. Lakka and colleagues[115] found middle-aged men who exercised more than 3 times/week had 20% lower serum ferritin levels than men who exercised less than once per week. Further research is needed on iron stores, physical activity, and the incidence of chronic diseases.

III. ZINC

Another essential mineral in many metabolic pathways is zinc. Zinc is a part of many enzymes including lactate dehydrogenase, carbonic anhydrase, alkaline phosphatase, alcohol dehydrogenase, and superoxide dismutase. Approximately 2 g of zinc is stored in the body primarily in the muscles and bones. Bone zinc is not mobilized during negative zinc balance, however, muscle catabolism is accompanied by the release of zinc into the plasma.[116] Zinc in blood is found primarily in erythrocytes with much smaller amounts found in plasma. It is thought that plasma zinc is a part of the exchangeable zinc pool which can be mobilized during stress and is useful as an index of zinc deficiency.[117] Zinc deficiency results in growth retardation, delayed sexual maturation, anorexia, loss of taste acuity, depressed immune responses, and impaired wound healing.

A. ZINC INTAKE

Foods which contribute the greatest amount of zinc to the diet are meats, seafood, and poultry. Plants containing phytate and dietary fiber are not good sources because they inhibit zinc absorption. The RDA for zinc is 15 mg/day for men and 12 mg/day for women.[5] Mean dietary zinc density is 5 mg/1000 kcal with the average woman consuming 10 mg/day and the average man consuming 16 mg/day.[118,119] Some female athletes have zinc intakes which are below the RDA.[16,120,121] For example, Deuster and colleagues[16] found that more than 40% of the elite women marathon runners they studied consumed less than 10 mg/day. Mean zinc intake for several athletic groups is reported in Table 3.

B ZINC DEPLETION IN ATHLETES

Several studies have reported that plasma zinc concentration is below the normal range (80–130 µg/dl) in many athletes. Dressendorfer and Sockolov[122] found that 23% of the male

TABLE 3   Mean Food Zinc and Copper Intakes of Athletes

Study	Sport	Sex	Zinc mg/day	Copper mg/day
Deuster[137]	Runners	Women	10.3	—
	Untrained	Women	10.0	—
Singh[124]	Marathon	Women	13.1	2.1
	Untrained	Women	9.9	1.5
Lukaski[150]	Swimmers	Women	10.4	1.3
	Control	Women	9.8	1.2
	Swimmers	Men	15.6	1.6
	Control	Men	15.2	1.8
Hackman[154]	Runners	Men	7.4	—
	Untrained	Men	5.7	—
Singh[129]	Ultramarathon	Both	14.3	1.8
Fogelholm[128]	Endurance	Men	17.7	—
	Controls	Men	14.1	—
Fogelholm[126]	Variety	Men	16.6–17.9	—
	Control	Men	14.2–14.9	—
Fogelholm[127]	Skiers	Women	15.8	—
	Control	Women	10.5	—
	Skiers	Men	21.9	—
	Control	Men	14.1	—
Benson[120]	Dancers	Girls	7.6	—
U.S. Population[119]		Girls	10.1	0.8
		Boys	15.8	1.2
		Women	9.7	0.9
		Men	16.4	1.2

runners they examined had less than 65 µg zinc/dl serum. The runners had significantly lower serum zinc concentrations than a group of nonrunning men. Haralambie[123] also found 23% of the men and 43% of the women athletes examined had serum zinc below the normal range. Women marathon runners have plasma zinc concentrations that are near the lower limit of the normal range, and 22% were below the normal range.[16,124] Other studies have found no significant difference in plasma zinc between male and female athletes and nonathletes with all groups within the normal range.[125-130]

There are several possible reasons for low plasma zinc concentrations in athletes including low dietary zinc intake, excessive zinc loss during exercise, expansion of the plasma volume during training which dilutes the zinc concentration, and redistribution of plasma zinc to other tissues. Although some athletes have low zinc intakes, Deuster and colleagues[16] found a low correlation between zinc intake and plasma zinc. They did find, however, that zinc intake was significantly correlated with erythrocyte zinc (r = 0.35). Plasma zinc concentration declines when dietary zinc is restricted to less than 4 mg/day.[117] Therefore, low zinc intake could be a contributing factor in zinc depletion for some athletes.

Zinc is excreted in the urine, sweat, and feces. Normal loss through the skin for sedentary men has been estimated to be 0.76 mg/day.[131] Zinc concentration of the sweat has been reported to be as high as 1.15 mg/liter of sweat.[132] Men and women exposed to a hot environment for 1 week have significantly decreased serum zinc concentrations.[133] It is quite possible that individuals who exercise or are exposed to heat lose more zinc through the sweat than estimated for sedentary individuals. Results of two studies that examined sweat zinc during exercise are presented in Figure 4.[67,134] Increased excretion of zinc through the urine has also been observed following exercise.[135,136] Highly trained women runners excreted more zinc in the urine than untrained women.[137] Although the combination of increased zinc excretion and low zinc intake could be responsible for the low plasma zinc concentration observed in many athletes, elevated zinc intake appears to enhance urinary zinc loss. Male runners consuming a zinc supplement (50 mg/d) had significantly greater urinary zinc losses following a 2 hour run compared to placebo trials.[138]

Expansion of the plasma volume during training could also dilute the plasma zinc concentration. About 75% of the plasma zinc is bound to albumin and the remainder is bound to alpha-macroglobulin. During training, the concentration of alpha-macroglobulin increases and the relative decrease in albumin is much less than the increase in plasma volume.[123] It would seem less likely that plasma volume expansion was the cause of the low plasma zinc concentrations, although it may be a contributing factor. Simpson and Hoffman-Goetz[139]

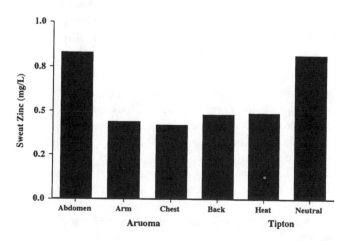

FIGURE 4 Sweat zinc concentration during exercise measured at various sites by Aruoma[67] and from the arm in different environments by Tipton.[134]

found that correcting serum zinc for plasma volume changes eliminated the significant decrease observed 2 hours following high intensity exercise but did not affect the significant reduction in serum zinc observed 24 hours after a 2-hour, moderate-intensity exercise bout.

There is also evidence that zinc may be redistributed within the body during and following exercise. Some studies have reported an increase in plasma zinc concentration immediately following short, intense exercise bouts[117,136,140-143] while other studies reported no increase after distance runs but significant decreases 2–24 hours post exercise.[135,136,138] The increase in plasma zinc immediately following intense exercise bouts is reduced following endurance training.[141] It has been suggested that increased plasma zinc could be due to muscle catabolism during exercise, however, Nosaka and Clarkson[144] found no changes in plasma zinc following eccentric exercise that resulted in muscle soreness and elevated plasma creatine kinase activity. On the other hand, decreased erythrocyte zinc concentration is seen after exercise accompanied by a decrease in carbonic anhydrase I concentration in the erythrocyte.[140] Both plasma and erythrocyte zinc returned to normal 30 min post exercise. The increase in plasma zinc is probably due to a shift from the erythrocyte.

Stresses, including exercise, stimulate the uptake of zinc by the liver and synthesis of metallothionen and are accompanied by a reduction in plasma zinc.[145] Stress stimulates an acute phase response which is associated with significant decreases in both plasma zinc and iron. U.S. Navy SEAL trainees undergoing physical and psychological stresses of Hell Week (5 days) had significantly lower plasma zinc concentrations but no increase in urinary zinc loss.[146] The results are consistent with zinc removal by other tissues. Plasma zinc also decreased in soldiers during field exercises lasting 34 days, however, urinary zinc loss increased.[147] Because the soldiers lost weight during the field exercises, Miyamura and colleagues[147] suggested that muscle catabolism may have been responsible for increasing zinc excretion.

Low plasma zinc during training may be due to a redistribution of zinc to the erythrocyte or liver. Elite women marathon runners have significantly higher erythrocyte zinc and slightly lower plasma zinc concentrations than untrained women.[124] Male endurance athletes also have significantly higher erythrocyte zinc than nonathletes.[128] Ten weeks of running training increased erythrocyte zinc concentration, specifically carbonic anhydrase I-derived zinc, and reduced albumin-bound plasma zinc.[141] No significant changes in alpha-macroglobulin-bound plasma zinc occurred with training. Erythrocyte zinc also increased in female college students after 24 weeks of a fitness training program.[148] Plasma zinc decreased significantly after 5 months of middle-distance running training and remained low over the remainder of the 9 month training season.[149] On the other hand, no changes in plasma zinc were observed over 12 weeks of training or a 6 month competitive swimming season.[150,151] However, Dolev[151] did find a significant increase in mononuclear cell zinc content following 12 weeks of training.

C. ZINC SUPPLEMENTATION

Zinc supplements are used by some athletes to improve their zinc status. Singh et al. found 21% of the elite marathon runners they studied took zinc supplements.[124] Because zinc is a part of lactate dehydrogenase, a zinc deficiency could potentially affect anaerobic muscle performance. Some evidence has been reported that zinc supplements increase muscle endurance in rats[152] and humans.[153] Krotkiewski and colleagues[153] used a large zinc supplement (135 mg/day) and found that isometric endurance but not isokinetic endurance was increased. Lukaski and colleagues[125] found no relationship between VO_2max and either plasma or erythrocyte zinc of trained athletes. In a subsequent study, neither a low zinc intake (3.6 mg/day) for 120 days nor a diet supplemented with zinc (33.6 mg/day) for 30 days significantly changed VO_2max.[117]

Zinc supplements should be used with caution. Copper absorption is inhibited by zinc supplements containing 50 mg.[154] Larger zinc supplements (160 mg/day) reduce high-density lipoprotein (HDL) cholesterol concentration.[155] Because HDL is beneficial in removing cholesterol, they are antiatherogenic. A lower HDL cholesterol suggests that large zinc supplements may be atherogenic. There is evidence that zinc supplements may reverse the positive effect of exercise in increasing HDL-cholesterol.[156] Zinc supplements containing less than 30 mg do not appear to affect HDL-cholesterol.[157] Elevated zinc intake also appears to suppress immunity. Although zinc supplements (50 mg/d) reduced the formation of superoxide anions by polymorphonuclear lymphocytes, T cell (lymphocyte) activity was depressed post exercise.[138] Supplementing the diet with more than 15 mg of zinc/day is not recommended.

IV. COPPER

Copper is another trace mineral that has attracted the attention of exercise physiologists because it is part of cytochrome oxidase, the final step in the electron transport system. Another copper containing protein, ceruloplasmin, functions as a ferrioxidase oxidizing iron from Fe (II) to Fe (III) for incorporation into ferritin and transferrin. Copper is also part of superoxide dismutase, a free radical scavenger that protects tissues from peroxidation.

A. COPPER INTAKE

There is no RDA for copper, however, the recommended safe and adequate copper intake is 1.5–3.0 mg/day.[5] The best sources of copper are shellfish, organ meats, legumes, and nuts. Copper bioavailability is reduced by zinc intakes that are 1.5 RDA or more and by diets that are high in fructose.[5] One recent study reported that men consumed about about one-half the recommended amount (1.2 mg/day) and women consumed even less (0.9 mg/day).[119] Women and men athletes appear to consume slightly more copper than the average adult (Table 3).

B. COPPER STATUS AND EXERCISE

Copper is found in the blood in both the plasma and erythrocytes. Normal plasma copper concentration ranges from 11 to 22 µmol/l. Copper in the plasma includes that bound to ceruloplasmin, a protein important in iron metabolism, and that carried by albumin. Erythrocyte copper includes that bound to superoxide dismutase (SOD). Although plasma copper is frequently used as an indicator of copper status, the erythrocyte SOD may be a better indication of copper status.[5]

Several studies have examined plasma copper in athletes and reported mixed results. Lukaski and colleagues[125] and Haralambie[158] reported significantly higher plasma copper in male athletes compared to controls. Resina and colleagues[159] found significantly lower plasma copper in distance runners than controls but no difference in plasma copper between professional soccer players and controls.[160] Female athletes have higher serum copper concentrations than males.[130,143] Decreases in plasma copper and ceruloplasmin were observed after several months of competitive swim training in one study.[161] In another study no significant change in plasma copper or ceruloplasmin concentration was found in women or men swimmers over a 6 month competitive swimming season.[150] However, erythrocyte SOD activity increased during swim training.[150] SOD contains both copper and zinc, but the activity of this enzyme depends on copper. SOD is an important enzyme that protects tissues from free radicals by converting superoxide anions to peroxides.

Plasma copper and ceruloplasmin concentrations have been found to increase during prolonged exercise,[142,158,162,163] decrease,[143] or remain relatively constant (Figure 5).[135] Ohla and colleagues[162] also found significant increases in plasma copper during graded exercise that were greater for trained than untrained subjects. Haralambie[158] observed a decrease in plasma copper but not ceruloplasmin during the early minutes of exercise and suggested that

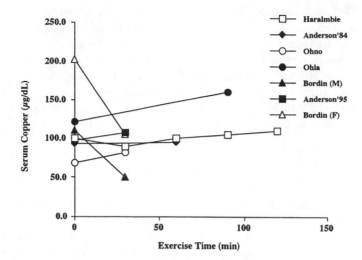

FIGURE 5 Changes in serum copper during exercise. Data from Anderson et al.,[135] Haralambie,[158] Ohla et al.,[162] Ohno et al.,[163] Anderson et al.,[142] and Bordin.[143]

copper might be mobilized from the ceruloplasmin. Plasma copper was inversely correlated with the catecholamines dopamine, norepinephrine, and epinephrine after 30 min of recovery from exercise but not immediately following exercise.[163]

Excessive loss of copper through sweating could be responsible for the lower plasma copper observed in some studies. Prolonged heat exposure led to a reduction in plasma copper but not ceruloplasmin.[133] Sweat copper concentration in resting men is approximately 0.11 mg/l and sedentary men lose 0.41 mg/day through the skin.[131] The copper content of the sweat during exercise varied according to the site[67] and was higher during exercise in a thermoneutral environment than in a hot environment.[164] Although heavy sweating during exercise could lead to excessive loss of copper, the increased caloric intake of exercising individuals may prevent a negative copper balance from occurring.

V. CHROMIUM

Chromium is of interest because it enhances glucose tolerance and affects lipid metabolism. Increased chromium concentration may decrease the amount of insulin needed for glucose uptake by the tissues.[165] Noninsulin-dependent diabetics had lower fasting blood glucose concentrations after 6 weeks of chromium supplementation.[166] Supplementing the diet with chromium picolinate has been found to decrease total and LDL-cholesterol and increase HDL-cholesterol.[166]

A. CHROMIUM AND THE DIET

Although there is no RDA for chromium, the recommended intake is 50–200 µg/day. The amount of chromium in the U.S. diet is quite small (5–150 µg/day) probably due to the highly refined nature of many foods consumed. The best sources of chromium in the diet are meats, whole grains, brewer's yeast, nuts, cheese, and molasses.[165]

Foods that are high in simple sugars, especially glucose, stimulate an increased insulin response.[167] Among subjects with the greatest insulin responses, >718 pmol/l, there was no relationship between the insulin response and chromium excretion in the urine.[167] However, in subjects with smaller insulin responses to carbohydrates, increases in chromium excretion were related to the increase in insulin.[167]

B. EXERCISE AND CHROMIUM

Recent studies have examined the effects of exercise on serum and urine chromium concentrations. Increases in serum chromium, glucose, and insulin have been observed immediately after a run, but 2 hours after the run only chromium was still elevated.[168] Urinary chromium excretion was doubled following exercise which suggests that physically active people may have a greater need for chromium.[135] The amount of chromium excreted in response to exercise appears to be related to the individual's fitness level. Trained runners had lower basal urinary chromium losses and greater increases in urinary chromium in response to exercise than untrained men.[169] Anderson and colleagues[169] suggested that lower basal urinary chromium in trained subjects may be due to excessive chromium losses during training leading to chromium depletion. Studies of chromium losses during training are needed to test this hypothesis.

Dietary intake prior to exercise affects the amount of chromium excreted during exercise. Carbohydrate loading for 3 days prior to exercise resulted in significantly lower urinary chromium excretion following exercise compared to a normal mixed diet.[170] Serum cortisol concentrations were also significantly lower post-exercise following carbohydrate loading and there was a significant positive correlation between serum cortisol and urinary chromium. Because serum cortisol is considered a valid indicator of stress, the reduction in urinary chromium following carbohydrate loading could be due to a reduction in stress.[170]

Chromium picolinate is included in ergogenic products that are being advertised as beneficial to athletes. Most of the research support for these claims has come from two studies by Evans.[166] In the first study, students enrolled in a weight training class were given chromium picolinate (200 µg Cr) for 40 days. Subjects receiving chromium significantly increased their lean body mass while those receiving a placebo had only a slight increase in lean body mass. The second study involved football players who were given the same chromium picolinate supplement for 6 weeks during a weight-training program. Football players receiving chromium had greater increases in lean body mass than those receiving the placebo. Evans[166] suggested that additional chromium was needed for insulin to regulate fat utilization and muscle development. Hasten and colleagues[171] attempted to replicate Evans' study on weight lifting. Both men and women students enrolled in a 12 week weight lifting program were given either chromium picolinate (200 µg Cr) or a placebo. Significantly greater increases in lean body mass were observed only in the women on the chromium supplement. No significant differences in muscle strength gains were observed between the treatments. Evans and Pounchnik[172] supplemented the diets of males and females enrolled in an aerobics class with 400 and 200 µg chromium, respectively, for 12 weeks. Half the subjects received chromium tripicolinate, and the other half received chromium dinicotinate. Significant increases in lean body mass were found only in the subjects receiving chromium tripicolinate. However, no placebo or control group was included in the study.

Two recent studies have failed to replicate the significant increases in lean body mass and decreases in body fat following chromium picolinate supplementation.[173,174] Clancy et al.[173] found no significant effect of 200 µg chromium on lean body mass, body fat, or strength in football players following 9 weeks of supplementation. Hallmark and colleagues[174] also failed to find any significant effects of chromium supplementation (200 µg) in males participating in strength training for 12 weeks on lean body mass, body fat, or strength. Changes in lean body mass in both studies were measured using hydrostatic weighing. Urinary chromium excretion was significantly greater in the supplemented subjects in both studies. Clarkson[175] concluded from her review of the research on chromium that further well-controlled studies are required before recommending chromium supplements as an aid to increasing muscle mass.

VI. SUMMARY

Iron is the trace mineral that has been studied most extensively with respect to exercise. Iron depletion is relatively common among women athletes, but the prevalence among athletes does not appear to be greater than among age-matched peers in the U.S. population. Possible causes of iron depletion in women athletes include inadequate intake of iron and iron loss through the menses, sweat, and gastrointestinal bleeding. Iron deficiency anemia reduces physical work capacity and endurance.[86-88] The effects of iron depletion without anemia on performance are more variable. Iron supplements (50 mg/day or more) are effective in increasing plasma ferritin of iron depleted athletes but should be used cautiously and only after iron depletion has been verified.

Low serum zinc concentrations in athletes have been reported in several studies.[122-124] Elevated zinc excretion through the urine and sweat coupled with a low zinc intake is a possible cause of hypozincemia. Zinc is redistributed among the tissues during exercise, and low plasma zinc during training may be due to increased uptake by the liver and skeletal muscles. Zinc supplements in excess of the RDA are not recommended because of its inhibition of copper absorption,[154] immune function,[138] and HDL-cholesterol.[155]

Plasma copper and ceruloplasmin increase during prolonged exercise[158,162] but decrease[161] or do not change with training.[150] The copper containing enzyme SOD increases with training.[150] Excretion of copper in sweat is a possible cause of lower plasma copper. Chromium excretion in the urine following exercise is greater than at rest[135] and is higher when the carbohydrate content of the diet is low.[170] The effects of chromium supplements on lean body mass has produced mixed results and requires further research.

REFERENCES

1. Hallberg, L., Iron, in *Nutrition Reviews' Present Knowledge in Nutrition*, 5th ed., The Nutrition Foundation, Washington, D.C., 1984, chap. 32.
2. Hallberg, L., Hogdahl, A.M., Nilsson, L, and Rybo, G., Menstrual blood loss and iron deficiency, *Acta Med. Scand.*, 180, 639, 1966.
3. Herbert, V., Recommended dietary intakes (RDI) of iron in humans, *Am. J. Clin. Nutr.*, 45, 679, 1987.
4. Hallberg, L. and Rossander-Hulten, L., Iron requirements in menstruating women, *Am. J. Clin. Nutr.*, 54, 1047, 1991.
5. Food and Nutrition Board, National Research Council, *Recommended Dietary Allowances*, 10th ed., National Academy Press, Washington, D.C., 1989.
6. Monsen, E.R., Hallberg, L., Layrisse, M., Hegsted, D.M., Cook, J.D., Mertz, W., and Finch, C.A., Estimation of available dietary iron, *Am. J. Clin. Nutr.*, 31, 134, 1978.
7. Cook, J.D. and Finch, C.A., Assessing iron status of a population, *Am. J. Clin. Nutr.*, 32, 2115, 1979.
8. Skikne, B.S., Flowers, C.H., and Cook, J.D., Serum transferrin receptor: a quantitative measure of tissue iron deficiency, *Blood*, 75, 1870, 1990.
9. Expert Scientific Working Group, Summary of a report on assessment of the iron nutritional status of the United States population, *Am. J. Clin. Nutr.*, 42, 1318, 1985.
10. Cook, J.D., Finch, C.A., and Smith, N.J., Evaluation of the iron status of a population, *Blood*, 48, 449, 1976.
11. Dallman, P., Yip, R., and Johnson, C., Prevalence and causes of anemia in the United States, 1976 to 1980, *Am. J. Clin. Nutr.*, 39, 437, 1984.
12. Balaban, E.P., Cox, J.V., Snell, P., Vaughan, R.H., and Frenkel, E.P., The frequency of anemia and iron deficiency in the runner, *Med. Sci. Sports Exer.*, 21, 643, 1989.
13. Brown, R.T., McIntosh, S.M., Seabolt, V.R., and Daniel, W.A., Iron status of adolescent female athletes, *J. Adolesc. Health Care*, 6, 349, 1985.
14. Colt, E. and Heyman, B., Low ferritin in runners, *J. Sports Med. Phys. Fitness*, 24, 13, 1989.
15. Ehn, L., Carlmark, B., and Hoglund, S., Iron status in athletes involved in intense physical activity, *Med. Sci. Sports Exer.*, 12, 61, 1980.
16. Deuster, P.A., Dyle, S.B., Moser, P.B., Vigersky, R.A., Singh, A., and Schoomaker, E.B., Nutritional survey of highly trained women runners, *Am. J. Clin. Nutr.*, 45, 954, 1986.
17. Haymes, E.M. and Spillman, D.M., Iron status of women distance runners, *Int. J. Sports Med.*, 10, 430, 1989.

18. Nickerson, H.J., Holubets, M.C., Weller, B.R., Haas, R.G., Schwartz, S., and Ellefson, M.E., Causes of iron deficiency in adolescent athletes, *J. Pediatr.*, 114, 657, 1989.

19. Pate, R.R., Dover, V., Goodyear, L., Jun-Zong, P., and Lambert, M. Iron storage in female distance runners, in *Sport, Health, and Nutrition*, Katch, F.I., Ed., Human Kinetics, Champaign, IL, 1986, chap. 9.

20. Robertson, J.D., Maughan, R.J., Milne, A.C., and Davidson, R.J.L., Hematological status of male runners in relation to the extent of physical training, *Int. J. Sport Nutr.*, 2, 366, 1992.

21. Wishnitzer, R., Vorst, E., and Berrebi, A., Bone marrow iron depression in competitive distance runners, *Int. J. Sports Med.*, 4, 27, 1983.

22. Diehl, D.M., Lohman, T.G., Smith, S.C., and Kertzer, R., Effects of physical training and competition on the iron status of female field hockey players, *Int. J. Sports Med.*, 7, 264, 1986.

23. Clement, D.B., Lloyd-Smith, D.R., MacIntyre, J.G., Matheson, G.O., Brock, R., and DuPont, M., Iron status in winter Olympic sports, *J. Sports Sci.*, 5, 261, 1987.

24. Haymes, E.M., Puhl, J.L., and Temples, T.E., Training for cross-country skiing and iron status, *Med. Sci. Sports Exer.*, 18, 162, 1986.

25. Parr, R.B., Bachman, L.A., and Moss, R.A., Iron deficiency in female athletes, *Phys. Sportsmed.*, 12 (4), 81, 1984.

26. Risser, W.L., Lee, E.J., Poindexter, H.B.W., West, M.S., Pivarnik, J.M., Risser, J.M.H., and Hickson, J.F., Iron deficiency in female athletes: its prevalence and impact on performance, *Med. Sci. Sports Exer.*, 20, 116, 1988.

27. Rowland, T.W. and Kelleher, J.F., Iron deficiency in athletes: insights from high school swimmers, *Am. J. Dis. Child.*, 142, 197, 1989.

28. Willows, N.D., Grimston, S.K., Smith, D.I., and Hanby, D.A., Iron and hematological status among adolescent athletes tracked through puberty, *Pediat. Exer. Sci.*, 7, 253, 1995.

29. Schoene, R.B., Escourrou, P., Robertson, H.T., Nilson, K.L., Parsons, J.R., and Smith, N.J., Iron repletion decreases maximal exercise lactate concentrations in female athletes with minimal iron-deficiency anemia, *J. Lab. Clin. Med.*, 102, 306, 1983.

30. Fogelholm, M., Indicators of vitamin and mineral status in athlete's blood: a review, *Int. J. Sport Nutr.*, 5, 267, 1995.

31. Lampe, J.W., Slavin, J.L., and Apple, F.S., Poor iron status of women runners training for a marathon, *Int. J. Sports Med.*, 7, 111, 1986.

32. Banister, E.W. and Hamilton, C.L., Variations in iron status with fatigue modelled from training in female distance runners, *Eur. J. Appl. Physiol.*, 54, 16, 1985.

33. Taylor, C., Rogers, G., Goodman, C., Baynes, R.D., Bothwell, T.H., Bexwoda, W.R., Kramer, F., and Hattingh, J., Hematologic, iron-related, and acute-phase protein responses to sustained strenuous exercise, *J. Appl. Physiol.*, 62, 464, 1987.

34. Moore, R.J., Friedl, K.E., Tulley, R.T., and Askew, E.W., Maintenance of iron status in healthy men during an extended period of stress and physical activity, *Am. J. Clin. Nutr.*, 58, 923, 1993.

35. Eichner, E.R., The anemias of athletes, *Phys. Sportsmed.*, 14, 122, 1986.

36. Martin, D., Vroom, D.H., May, D.F., and Pilbeam, S.P., Physiological changes in elite male distance runners training for Olympic competition, *Phys. Sportsmed.*, 14 (1), 152, 1986.

37. Magnusson, B., Hallberg, L., Rossander, L., and Swolin, B., Iron metabolism and "sports anemia." I. A study of several iron parameters in elite runners with differences in iron status, *Acta Med. Scand.*, 216, 149, 1984.

38. Blum, S.M., Sherman, A.R., and Boileau, R.A., The effects of fitness-type exercise on iron status in adult women, *Am. J. Clin. Nutr.*, 43, 456, 1986.

39. Nickerson, H.J., Holubets, M., Tripp, A.D., and Pierce, W.E., Decreased iron stores in high school female runners, *Am. J. Dis. Child.*, 139, 1115, 1985.

40. Roberts, D. and Smith, D., Serum ferritin values in elite speed and synchronized swimmers and speed skaters, *J. Lab. Clin. Med.*, 116, 661, 1990.

41. Lyle, R.M., Weaver, C.M., Sedlock, D.A., Rajaram, S., Martin, B., and Melby, C.L., Iron status in exercising women; the effects of oral iron therapy vs increased consumption of muscle foods, *Am. J. Clin. Nutr.*, 56, 1049, 1992.

42. Pratt, C.A., Woo, V., and Chrisley, B., The effects of exercise on iron status and aerobic capacity in moderately exercising adult women, *Nutr. Res.*, 16, 23, 1996.

43. Frederickson, L.A., Puhl, J.L., and Runyan, W.S., Effects of training on indices of iron status of young female cross-country runners, *Med. Sci. Sports Exer.*, 15, 271, 1983.

44. Brotherhood, J., Brozovic, B., and Pugh, L., Hematological status of middle and long distance runners, *Clin. Sci.*, 48, 135, 1975.

45. Clement, D.B., Asmundson, R.C., and Medhurst, C.W., Hemoglobin values: comparative survey of the 1976 Canadian Olympic team, *Can. Med. Assoc. J.*, 117, 614, 1977.

46. Hunding, A., Jordal, R., and Paulev, P.E., Runner's anemia and iron deficiency, *Acta Med. Scand.*, 209, 315, 1981.

47. Convertino, V.A., Brock, P.J., Kell, L.C., Bernauer, E.M., and Greenleaf, J.E., Exercise training-induced hypervolemia: role of plasma albunim, renin, and vasopressin, *J. Appl. Physiol.*, 48, 665, 1980.

48. Dill, D.B., Braithwaite, K., Adams, W.C., and Bernauer, E.M., Blood volume of middle-distance runners: effect of 2300-m altitude and comparison with non-athletes, *Med. Sci. Sport*, 6, 1, 1974.

49. Pate, R.R., Sports anemia: a review of the current research literature, *Phys. Sportsmed.*, 11 (2), 115, 1983.

50. Freedson, P.S., The influence of hemoglobin concentration on exercise cardiac output, *Int. J. Sports Med.*, 2, 81, 1981.

51. Glass, H.L., Edwards, R.H.T., DeGarreta, A.C., and Clark, J.C., ¹¹CO red cell labeling for blood volume and total hemoglobin in athletes: effect of training, *J. Appl. Physiol.*, 26, 131, 1969.

52. Holmgren, A., Mossfeldt, F., Sjostrand, T., and Strom, G., Effect of training on work capacity, total hemoglobin, blood volume, heart volume and pulse rate in recumbent and upright positions, *Acta Physiol. Scand.*, 50, 72, 1960.

53. Dufaux, B., Hoedegrath, A., Streitberger, I., Hollman, W., and Assmann, G., Serum ferritin, transferrin, haptoglobin, and iron in middle- and long-distance runners, elite rowers, and professional racing cyclists, *Int. J. Sports Med.*, 2, 43, 1981.

54. Weight, L.M., Byrnes, M.J., and Jacobs, P., Haemolytic effects of exercise, *Clin. Sci.*, 81, 147, 1991.

55. Magnusson, B., Hallberg, L., Rossander, L., and Swolin, B., Iron metabolism and "sports anemia." II. A hematological comparison of elite runners and control subjects, *Acta Med. Scand.*, 216, 156, 1984.

56. Miller, B.J., Pate, R.R., and Burgess, W., Foot impact force and intravascular hemolysis during distance running, *Int. J. Sports Med.*, 9, 56, 1988.

57. Puhl, J.L., Runyon, W.S., and Kruse, S.J., Erythrocyte changes during training in high school women cross-country runners, *Res. Quart. Exer. Sport*, 52, 484, 1981.

58. Selby, G.B. and Eichner, E.R., Endurance swimming, intravascular hemolysis, anemia, and iron depletion, *Am. J. Med.*, 81, 791, 1986.

59. Steenkamp, I., Fuller, C., Graves, J., Noakes, T.D., and Jacobs, P., Marathon running fails to influence RBC survival rates in iron-replete women, *Phys. Sportsmed.*, 14, 89, 1986.

60. Manore, M.M., Besenfelder, P.D., Wells, C.L., Carroll, S.S., and Hooker, S.P., Nutrient intakes and iron status in female long-distance runners during training, *J. Am. Diet. Assoc.*, 89, 257, 1989.

61. Snyder, A.C., Dvorak, L.L., and Roepke, J.B., Influence of dietary iron source on measures of iron status among female runners, *Med. Sci. Sports Exer.*, 21, 7, 1989.

62. Pate, R.R., Miller, B.J., Davis, J.M., Slentz, C.A., and Klingshirn, L.A., Iron status of female runners, *Int. J. Sport Nutr.*, 3, 222, 1993.

63. Deuster, P.A., Kyle, S.B., Moser, P.B., Vigersky, R.A., Singh, A., and Schoonmaker, E.B., Nutritional intakes and status of highly trained amenorrheic and eumenorrheic women runners, *Fert. Steril.*, 46, 636, 1986.

64. Perry, A.C., Crane, L.S., Applegate, B., Marquez-Sterling, S., Signorile, J.F., and Miller, P.C., Nutrient intake and psychological and physiological assessment in eumenorrheic and amenorrheic female athletes, *Int. J. Sport Nutr.*, 6, 3, 1996.

65. Paulev, P.E., Jordal, R., and Pedersen, N.S., Dermal excretion of iron in intensely training athletes, *Clin. Chim. Acta*, 127, 19, 1983.

66. Lamanca, J.J., Haymes, E.M., Daly, J.A., Moffatt, R.J., and Waller, M.F., Sweat iron loss of male and female runners during exercise, *Int. J. Sports Med.*, 9, 52, 1988.

67. Aruoma, O.I., Reilly, T., MacLaren, D., and Halliwell, B., Iron, copper and zinc concentrations in human sweat and plasma: the effects of exercise, *Clin. Chim. Acta*, 177, 81, 1988.

68. Waller, M.F. and Haymes, E.M., The effects of heat and exercise on sweat iron loss, *Med. Sci. Sports Exer.*, 28, 197, 1996.

69. Coltman, C.A. and Rowe, N.J., The iron content of sweat in normal adults, *Am. J. Clin. Nutr.*, 18, 270, 1966.

70. Hussein, R. and Patwardhan, V.N., Iron content of thermal sweat in iron-deficiency anemia, *Lancet*, 1, 1073, 1959.

71. Vellar, O.D., Studies on sweat losses of nutrients. I. Iron content of whole body sweat and its association with other sweat constituents, serum iron levels, hematological indices, body surface area, and sweat rate, *Scand. J. Clin. Lab. Invest.*, 21, 157, 1968..

72. Green, R., Charlton, R., Seftel, H., Bothwell, T.H., Mayet, F., Adams, B., Finch, C., and Layrisse, M., Body iron excretion in man: a collaborative study, *Am. J. Med.*, 45, 336, 1968.

73. Brune, M., Magnusson, B., Persson, H., and Hallberg, L., Iron losses in sweat, *Am. J. Clin. Nutr.*, 43, 438, 1986.

74. Porter, A.M.W., Do some marathon runners bleed into the gut?, *Br. Med. J.*, 287, 1427, 1983.

75. McCabe, M.E., Peura, D.A., Kadakia, S.C., Bocek, Z., and Johnson, L.F., Gastrointestinal blood loss associated with running a marathon, *Dig. Dis. Sci.*, 31, 1229, 1986.

76. McMahon, L.F., Ryan, M.J., Larson, D., and Fisher, R.L., Occult gastrointestinal blood loss in marathon runners, *Ann. Intern. Med.*, 100, 846, 1984.

77. Robertson, J.D., Maughan, R.J., and Davidson, R.J.L., Fecal blood loss in response to exercise, *Br. Med. J.*, 295, 303, 1987.

78. Stewart, J.G., Ahlquist, D.A., McGill, D.B., Ilstrup, D.M., and Schwartz, S., Gastrointestinal blood loss and anemia in runners, *Ann. Intern. Med.*, 100, 843, 1984.

79. Baska, R.S., Moses, F.M., Graeber, G., and Kearney, G., Gastrointestinal bleeding during an ultramarathon, *Dig. Dis. Sci.*, 35, 276, 1990.

80. Lampe, J.W., Slavin, J.L., and Apple, F.S., Iron status of active women and the effect of running a marathon on bowel function and gastrointestinal blood loss, *Int. J. Sports Med.*, 12, 173, 1991.

81. Fassett. R.G., Owen, J.E., Fairley, J., Birch, D.F., and Fairley, K.F., Urinary red-cell morphology during exercise, *Br. Med. J.*, 285, 1455, 1982.

82. Poortmans, J.R., Exercise and renal function, *Sports Med.*, 1, 125, 1984.

83. Boileau, M., Fuchs, E., Barry, J.M., and Hodges, C.V., Stress hematuria: athletic pseudonephritis in marathoners, *Urology*, 15, 471, 1980.

84. Siegal, A.J., Hennekens, C.H., Solomon, H.S., and Van Boekel, B., Exercise-related hematuria: findings in a group of marathon runners, *J. Am. Med. Assoc.*, 241, 391, 1979.

85. Blacklock, N.J., Bladder trauma in the long-distance runner, *Br. J. Urology*, 49, 129, 1977.

86. Celsing, F., Blomstrand, E., Werner, B., Pihlstedt, P., and Ekblom, B., Effects of iron deficiency on endurance and muscle enzyme activity in man, *Med. Sci. Sports Exer.*, 18, 156, 1986.

87. Edgerton, V.R., Ohira, Y., Hettiarachchi, J., Senewiratne, B., Gardner, G.W., and Barnard, R.J., Elevation of hemoglobin and work tolerance in iron deficient subjects, *J. Nutr. Sci. Vit.*, 27, 77, 1981.

88. Gardner, G.W., Edgerton, V.R., Senewiratne, B., Barnard, R.J., and Ohira, Y., Physical work capacity and metabolic stress in subjects with iron deficiency anemia, *Am. J. Clin. Nutr.*, 30, 910, 1977.

89. Davies, K.J.A., Donovan, C.M., Refino, C.J., Brooks, G.A., Packer, L., and Dallman, P.R., Distinguishing effects of anemia and muscle iron deficiency on exercise bioenergetics in the rat, *Am. J. Physiol.*, 246, E535, 1984.

90. Finch, C.A., Miller, L.R., Inamdar, A.R., Person, R., Seiler, K., and Mackler, B., Iron deficiency in the rat: physiological and biochemical studies of muscle dysfunction, *J. Clin. Invest.*, 58, 447, 1976.

91. Finch, C.A., Gollnick, P.D., Hlastala, M.P., Miller, L.R., Dillmann, E., and Mackler, B., Lactic acidosis as a result of iron deficiency, *J. Clin. Invest.*, 64, 129, 1979.

92. Davies, K.J.A., Maguire, J.J., Brooks, G.A., Dallman, P.R., and Packer, L., Muscle mitochondrial bioenergetics, oxygen supply, and work capacity during dietary iron deficiency and repletion, *Am. J. Physiol.*, 242, E418, 1982.

93. McLane, J.A., Fell, R.D., McKay, R.H., Winder, W.W., Brown, E.B., and Holloszy, J.O., Physiological and biochemical effects of iron deficiency on rat skeletal muscle, *Am. J. Physiol.*, 241, C47, 1981.

94. Ohira, Y., Edgerton, V.R., Gardner, G.W., Gunawardena, K.A., Senewiratne, B., and Ikawa, S., Work capacity after iron treatment as a function of hemoglobin and iron deficiency, *J. Nutr. Sci. Vit.*, 27, 87, 1981.

95. Gardner, G.W., Edgerton, V.R., Barnard, R.J., and Bernauer, E.M., Cardiorespiratory, hematological and physical performance responses of anemic subjects to iron treatment, *Am. J. Clin. Nutr.*, 28, 982, 1975.

96. Ohira, Y., Edgerton, V.R., Gardner, G.W., Senewiratne, B., Barnard, R.J., and Simpson, D.R., Work capacity, heart rate and blood lactate responses to iron treatment, *Br. J. Haematol.*, 41, 365, 1979.

97. Cooter, G.R. and Mowbray, K., Effects of iron supplementation and activity on serum iron depletion and hemoglobin levels in female athletes, *Res. Quart.*, 49, 114, 1978.

98. Pate, R.R., Maguire, M., and Van Wyk, J., Dietary supplementation in women athletes, *Phys. Sportsmed.*, 7 (9), 81, 1979.

99. Matter, M., Stittfall, T., Graves, J., Myburgh, K., Adams, B., Jacobs, P., and Noakes, T.D., The effect of iron and folate therapy on maximal exercise performance in female marathon runners with iron and folate deficiency, *Clin. Sci.*, 72, 415, 1987.

100. Nickerson, H.J. and Tripp, A.D., Iron deficiency in adolescent cross-country runners, *Phys. Sportsmed.*, 11, 60, 1983.

101. Lamanca, J.J. and Haymes, E.M., Effects of iron repletion on VO$_2$max, endurance, and blood lactate, *Med. Sci. Sports Exer.*, 25, 1386, 1993.

102. Newhouse, I.J., Clement, D.B., Taunton, J.E., and McKenzie, D.C., The effects of prelatent/latent iron deficiency on work capacity, *Med. Sci. Sports Exer.*, 21, 263, 1989.

103. Clement, D.B., Taunton, J.E., McKenzie, D.C., Sawchuk, L.L., and Wiley, J.P., High- and low-dosage iron-supplementation in iron-deficient, endurance trained females, in *Sport, Health, and Nutrition*, Katch, F.I., Ed., Human Kinetics, Champaign, IL, 1986, chap. 6.

104. Plowman, S.A. and McSwegin, P.C., The effects of iron supplementation on female cross-country runners, *J. Sports Med. Phys. Fitness*, 21, 407, 1981.

105. Rowland, T.W., Deisroth, M.B., Green, G.M., and Kelleher, J.F., The effect of iron therapy on exercise capacity of nonanemic iron-deficient adolescent runners, *Am. J. Dis. Child.*, 142, 165, 1988.

106. Yoshida, T., Udo, M., Chida, M., Ichioka, M., and Makiguchi, K., Dietary iron supplement during severe physical training in competitive distance runners, *Sports Training Med. Rehab.*, 1, 279–285, 1990.

107. Fogelholm, M., Jaakkola, L., and Lammpisjarvi, T., Effects of iron supplementation in female athletes with low serum ferritin concentration, *Int. J. Sports Med.*, 13, 158, 1992.

108. Klingshirn, L.A., Pate, R.R., Bourque, S.P., Davis, J.M., and Sargent, R.G., Effect of iron supplementation on endurance capacity in iron-depleted female runners, *Med. Sci. Sports Exer.*, 24, 819, 1992.

109. Rajaram, S., Weaver, C.M., Lyle, R.M., Sedlock, D.A., Martin, B., Templin, T.J., Beard, J.L., and Percival, S.S., Effects of long-term moderate exercise on iron status in young women, *Med. Sci. Sports Exer.*, 27, 1105, 1995.

110. Telford, R.D., Bunney, C.J., Catchpole, E.A., Catchpole, W.R., Deakin, V., Gray, B., Hahn, A.G., and Kerr, D.A., Plasma ferritin concentration and physical work capacity in athletes, *Int. J. Sport Nutr.*, 2, 335, 1992.

111. Aruoma, O.I., Bomford, A., Polson, R.J., and Halliwell, B., Nontransferrin-bound iron in plasma from hemochromatosis patients: effect of phlebotomy therapy, *Blood*, 72, 1416, 1988.

112. Stevens, R.G., Jones, D.Y., Micozzi, M.S., and Taylor, P.R., Body iron stores and the risk of cancer, *New Engl. J. Med.*, 319, 1047, 1988.

113. Salonen, J.T., Nyyssonen, K., Korpela, H., Tuomilehto, J., Seppanen, R., and Salonen, R., High stored iron levels are associated with excess risk of myocardial infarction in eastern Finnish men, *Circulation*, 86, 803, 1992.

114. Magnusson, M.K., Sigfusson, N., Sigvaldason, H., Johannesson, G.M., Magnusson, S., and Thorgeirsson, G., Low iron-binding capacity as a risk factor for myocardial infarction, *Circulation*, 89, 102, 1994.

115. Lakka, T.A., Nyyssonen, K., and Salonen, J.T., Higher levels of conditioning leisure time physical activity are associated with reduced levels of stored iron in Finnish men, *Am. J. Epidem.*, 140, 148, 1994.

116. Sandstead, H.H. and Evans, G.W., Zinc, in *Nutrition Reviews' Present Knowledge in Nutrition*, 5th ed., The Nutriton Foundation, Washington, D.C., 1984, chap. 33.

117. Lukaski, H.C., Bolonchuk, W.W., Klevay, L.M., Milne, D.B., and Sandstead, H.H., Changes in plasma zinc content after exercise in men fed a low-zinc diet, *Am. J. Physiol.*, 247, E88, 1984.

118. Patterson, K.Y., Holbrook, J.T., Bodner, J.E., Kelsay, J.L., Smith, J.C., and Veilon, C., Zinc, copper, and manganese intake and balance for adults consuming self-selected diets, *Am. J. Clin. Nutr.*, 40, 1397, 1984.

119. Pennington, J.A.T., Young, B.E., and Wilson, D.B., Nutritional elements in U.S. diets: results from the total diet study, 1982 to 1986, *J. Am. Diet. Assoc.*, 89, 659, 1989.

120. Benson, J., Gillien, D.M., Bourdet, K., and Loosli, A.R., Inadequate nutrition and chronic calorie restriction in adolescent ballerinas, *Phys. Sportsmed.*, 13 (10), 79, 1985.

121. Loosli, A.R., Benson, J., Gillien, D.M., and Bourdet, K., Nutrition habits and knowledge in competitive adolescent female gymnasts, *Phys. Sportsmed.*, 14(8), 118, 1986.

122. Dressendorfer, R.H. and Sockolov, R., Hypozincemia in runners, *Phys. Sportsmed.*, 8 (4), 97, 1980.

123. Haralambie, G., Serum zinc in athletes in training, *Int. J. Sports Med.*, 2, 135, 1981.

124. Singh, A., Deuster, P.A., and Moser, P.B., Zinc and copper status of women by physical activity and menstrual status, *J. Sports Med. Phys. Fitness*, 30, 29, 1990.

125. Lukaski, H.C., Bolonchuk, W.W., Klevay, L.M., Milne, D.B., and Sandstead, H.H., Maximum oxygen consumption as related to magnesium, copper, and zinc nutriture, *Am. J. Clin. Nutr.*, 37, 407, 1983.

126. Fogelholm, G.M., Himberg, J.-J., Alopaeus, K., Gref, C.-G., Laakso, J.T., Lehto, J.J., and Mussalo-Raukamaa, H., Dietary and biochemical indices of nutritional status in male athletes and controls, *J. Am. Coll. Nutr.*, 11, 181, 1992.

127. Fogelholm, M., Rehuven, S., Gref, C.-G., Laakso, J.T., Lehto, J., Ruokonen, I., and Himberg, J.J., Dietary intake and thiamin, iron, and zinc status in elite Nordic skiers during different training periods, *Int. J. Sport Nutr.*, 2, 351, 1992.

128. Fogelhom, M., Laakso, J., Lehto, J., and Ruokonen, I., Dietary intake and indicators of magnesium and zinc status in male athletes, *Nutr. Res.*, 11, 1111, 1991.

129. Singh, A., Evans, P., Gallagher, K.L., and Deuster, P.A., Dietary intakes and biochemical profiles of ultra-marathoners, *Med. Sci. Sports Exer.*, 25, 328, 1993.

130. Wang, W.-C., Heinonen, D., Mukela, P., and Nauto, V., Serum selenium, zinc and copper in Swedish and Finnish orienteers. A comparative study, *Analyst*, 120, 837, 1995.

131. Jacob, R.A., Sandstead, H.H., Munoz, J.M., Klevay, L.M., and Milne, D.B., Whole body surface loss of trace metals in normal males, *Am. J. Clin. Nutr.*, 34, 1379, 1981.

132. Prasad, A.S., Schulert, A.R., Sandstead, H.H., and Miale, A., Zinc, iron, and nitrogen content of sweat in normal and deficient subjects, *J. Lab. Clin. Med.*, 62, 84, 1963.

133. Uhari, M., Pakarinen, A., Hietala, J., Nurmi, T., and Kouvalainen, K., Serum iron, copper, zinc, ferritin, and ceruloplasmin after intense heat exposure, *Eur. J. Appl. Physiol.*, 51, 331, 1983.

134. Tipton, K., Green, N.R., Haymes, E.M., and Waller, M., Zinc loss from sweat of athletes exercising at high and neutral temperatures, *Int. J. Sport Nutr.*, 3, 261, 1993.

135. Anderson, R.A., Polansky, M.M., and Bryden, N.A., Strenuous running: acute effects on chromium, copper, zinc, and selected clinical variables in urine and serum of male runners, *Biol. Trace Elem. Res.*, 6, 327, 1984.

136. Van Rij, A.M., Hall, M.T., Dohm, G.L., Bray, J., and Pories, W.J., Changes in zinc metabolism following exercise in human subjects, *Biol. Trace Elem. Res.*, 10, 99, 1986.

137. Deuster, P.A., Day, B.A., Singh, A., Douglass, L., and Moser-Veillon, P.B., Zinc status of highly trained women runners and untrained women, *Am. J. Clin. Nutr.*, 49, 1295, 1989.

138. Singh, A., Failla, M.L., and Deuster, P.A., Exercise-induced changes in immune function: effects of zinc supplementation, *J. Appl. Physiol.*, 76, 2298, 1994.

139. Simpson, J.R. and Hoffman-Goetz, L., Exercise, serum zinc, and interleukin-1 concentrations in man: some methodological considerations, *Nutr. Res.*, 11, 309, 1991.

140. Ohno, H., Yamashita, K., Doi, R., Yamamura, K., Kondo, T., and Taniguchi, N., Exercise-induced changes in blood zinc and related proteins in humans, *J. Appl. Physiol.*, 58, 1453, 1985.

141. Ohno, H., Sato, Y., Ishikawa, M., Yahata, T., Gasa, S., Doi, R., Yamamura, K., and Taniguchi, N., Training effects on blood zinc levels in humans, *J. Sports Med. Phys. Fitness*, 30, 247, 1990.

142. Anderson, R.A., Bryden, N.A., Polansky, M.M., and Deuster, P.A., Acute exercise effects on urinary losses and serum concentrations of copper and zinc of moderately trained and untrained men consuming a controlled diet, *Analyst*, 120, 861, 1995.

143. Bordin, D., Sartorelli, L., Bonanni, G., Mastrogiacomo, I., and Scalco, E., High intensity physical exercise induced effects on plasma levels of copper and zinc, *Biol.Trace Elem. Res.*, 36, 129, 1993.

144. Nosaka, K. and Clarkson, P.M., Changes in plasma zinc following high force eccentric exercise, *Int. J. Sport Nutr.*, 2, 175, 1992.

145. Oh, S.H., Deagen, J.T., Whanger, P.D., and Weswig, P.H., Biological function of metallothionein. V. Its induction in rats by various stresses, *Am. J. Physiol.*, 234, E282, 1978.

146. Singh, A., Smoak, B.L., Patterson, K.Y., LeMay, L.G., Veillon, C., and Deuster, P.A., Biochemical indicies of selected trace minerals in men: effect of stress, *Am. J. Clin. Nutr.*, 53, 126, 1991.

147. Miyamura, J.B., McNutt, S.W., Lichton, I.J., and Wenkam, N.S., Altered zinc status of soldiers under field conditions, *J. Am. Diet. Assoc.*, 87, 595, 1987.

148. Fogelholm, M., Micronutrient status in females during a 24-week fitness-type exercise program, *Ann. Nutr. Metab.*, 36, 209, 1992.

149. Couzy, F., Lafarue, P., and Guezennec, C.Y., Zinc metabolism in the athlete: influence of training, nutrition and other factors, *Int. J. Sports Med.*, 11, 263, 1990.

150. Lukaski, H.C., Hoverson, B.S., Gallagher, S.K., and Bolonchuk, W.W., Physical training and copper, iron, and zinc status of swimmers, *Am. J. Clin. Nutr.*, 51, 1093, 1990.

151. Dolev, E., Burstein, R., Lubin, F., Wishnitzer, R., Chetrit, A., Skofi, M., and Deuster, P.A., Interpretation of zinc status in a strenuously exercising population, *J. Am. Diet. Assoc.*, 95, 482, 1995.

152. Richardson, J.H. and Drake, P.D., The effects of zinc on fatigue of striated muscle, *J. Sports Med. Phys. Fitness*, 19, 133, 1979.

153. Krotkiewski, M., Gudmundsson, M., Backstrom, P., and Mandroukas, K., Zinc and muscle strength and endurance, *Acta Physiol. Scand.*, 116, 309, 1982.

154. Hackman, R.M. and Keen, C.L., Changes in serum zinc and copper levels after zinc supplementation in running and nonrunning men, in *Sport, Health, and Nutrition,* Katch, F.I., Ed., Human Kinetics, Champaign, IL, 1986, chap. 8.

155. Hooper, P.L., Visconti, L., Garry, P.J., and Johnson, G.E., Zinc lowers high-density lipoprotein-cholesterol levels, *J. Am. Med. Assoc.*, 244, 1960, 1980.

156. Goodwin, J.S., Hunt, W.C., Hooper, P., and Garry, P.J., Relationship between zinc intake, physical activity, and blood levels of high-density lipoprotein cholesterol in a healthy elderly population, *Metabolism*, 34, 519, 1985.

157. Crouse, S.F., Hooper, P.L., Atterbom, H.A., and Papenfuss, R.L., Zinc ingestion and lipoprotein values in sedentary and endurance trained men, *J. Am. Med. Assoc.*, 252, 785, 1984.

158. Haralambie, G., Changes in electrolytes and trace elements during long-lasting exercise, in *Metabolic Adaptations to Prolonged Physical Exercise*, Howald, H. and Poortmans, J., Eds., Birkhauser Verlag, Basel, 1975, p. 340.

159. Resina, A., Fedi, S., Gatteschi, L., Rubenni, M.G., Giamberardino, M.A., Trabassi, E., and Imreh, F., Comparison of some serum copper parameters in trained runners and control subjects, *Int. J. Sports Med.*, 11, 58, 1990.

160. Resina, A., Gatteschi, L., Rubenni, M.G., Giamberardino, M.A., and Imreh, F., Comparison of some serum copper parameters in trained professional soccer players and control subjects, *J. Sports Med. Phys. Fitness,* 31, 413, 1991.

161. Dowdy, R.P. and Burt, J., Effect of intensive long-term training on copper and iron nutriture in man, *Fed. Proc.*, 39, 786, 1980.

162. Ohla, A.E., Klissouras, V., Sullivan, J.D., and Skoryna, S.C., Effect of exercise on concentration of elements in the serum, *J. Sports Med. Phys. Fitness*, 22, 414, 1982.

163. Ohno, H., Yahata, T., Hirata, F., Yamamura, K., Doi, R., Harada, M., and Taniguchi, N., Changes in dopamine-β-hydroxylase, and copper, and catecholamine concentrations in human plasma with physical exercise, *J. Sports Med. Phys. Fitness*, 24, 315, 1984.

164. Tipton, K., Green, N.R., Waller, M., and Haymes, E.M., Mineral losses from sweat in athletes exercising at two different temperatures, *FASEB J.*, 6, A768, 1991.

165. Pi-Sunyer, F.X. and Offenbacher, E.G., Chromium, in *Nutrition Review's Present Knowledge in Nutrition*, 5th ed., The Nutrition Foundation, Washington, D.C., 1984, chap. 40.

166. Evans, G.W., The effect of chromium picolinate on insulin controlled parameters in humans, *Int. J. Biosocial Med. Res.*, 11, 163, 1989.

167. Anderson, R.A., Bryden, N.A., Polansky, M.M., and Reiser, S., Urinary chromium excretion and insulinogenic properties of carbohydrates, *Am. J. Clin. Nutr.*, 51, 864, 1990.

168. Anderson, R.A., Polansky, M.M., Bryden, N.A., and Guttman, H.N., Strenuous exercise may increase dietary needs for chromium and zinc, in *Sport, Health, and Nutrition*, Katch, F.I., Ed., Human Kinetics, Champaign, IL, 1986, chap. 7.

169. Anderson, R.A., Bryden, N.A., Polansky, M.M., and Deuster, P.A., Exercise effects on chromium excretion of trained and untrained men consuming a constant diet, *J. Appl. Physiol.*, 64, 249, 1988.

170. Anderson, R.A., Bryden, N.A., Polansky, M.M., and Thorp, J.W., Effects of carbohydrate loading and underwater exercise on circulating cortisol, insulin and urinary losses of chromium and zinc, *Eur. J. Appl. Physiol.*, 63, 146, 1991.

171. Hasten, D.L., Rome, E.P., Franks, B.D., and Hegsted, M., Effects of chromium picolinate on beginning weight training students, *Int. J. Sport Nutr.*, 2, 343, 1992.

172. Evans, G.W. and Pounchnik, D.J., Composition and biological activity of chromium-pyridine carboxylate complexes, *J. Inorgan. Biochem.*, 49, 177, 1993.

173. Clancy, S.P., Clarkson, P.M., DeCheke, M.E., Nosaka, K., Freedson, P.S., Cunningham, J.J., and Valentine, B., Effects of chromium picolinate supplementation on body composition, strength, and urinary chromium loss in football players, *Int. J. Sport Nutr.*, 4, 142, 1994.

174. Hallmark, M.A., Reynolds, T.H., DeSouza, C.A., Dotson, C.O., Anderson, R.A., and Rogers, M.A., Effects of chromium and resistive training on muscle strength and body composition, *Med. Sci. Sports Exer.*, 28, 139, 1996.

175. Clarkson, P.M., Nutritional ergogenic aids: chromium, exercise, and muscle mass, *Int. J. Sport. Nutr.*, 1, 289, 1991.

Chapter 9

NUTRITION AND BONE IN PHYSICAL ACTIVITY AND SPORT

John J. B. Anderson
Mark Stender
Pamela Rondano
Lindsay Bishop
Amy B. Duckett

CONTENTS

0-8493-8560-1/97/$0.00+$.50
© 1998 by CRC Press LLC

I.   INTRODUCTION

The focus of this chapter is to provide an understanding of the impact of nutrition on the bone health of both male and female athletes. Bone health is examined in relation to the critical nutrients needed for bone development and maintenance, as well as in relation to the effect of physical activity on bone mass density. Emphasis is placed on female athletes because of the interactions among athletic activity, menstrual status, and diet.

II.   NUTRITIONAL NEEDS AND BONE HEALTH OF ATHLETES

Many nutrients are required for normal development and maintenance of the organic matrix and the mineral phases of dynamic bone tissues. Adequate energy and protein together support tissue growth and development. Though sufficient consumption of both is necessary for bone development and mineralization, micronutrients do not appear to be so critical to the development of bone length. For the athlete, maintenance of bone health is essential for performance. The nutrients critical for the support of mineralized bone tissue are reviewed in the next section, followed by an outline of the dietary recommendations for athletes.

A.   MACRONUTRIENTS AND ENERGY

Energy is extracted from chemical bonds of the hydrocarbon backbones of the macronutrients (carbohydrates, fats, and proteins) after metabolic degradation and entry into the citric acid cycle. Foods that supply the macronutrients also generally carry the micronutrients, therefore, adequate energy consumption from foods is critical for sufficient intakes of the micronutrients to support cellular and extracellular processes. If too little energy is consumed each day, micronutrient intakes will also be low, unless a multi-nutrient supplement is taken daily.

Athletes have special needs to maintain energy balance because of their high levels of energy expenditure in physical activities. Intakes that achieve the energy Recommended Dietary Allowance (RDA)[1] may not be adequate for athletes (see Chapter 2). Many athletes, particularly runners, eat a diet that may be deficient in total calories compared to their energy requirements.[2] Low energy intakes that contribute to negative energy balance adversely affect protein utilization and potentially compromise functional tissue protein, including skeletal muscle, for gluconeogenesis.

B. PROTEIN

Athletes need adequate intakes of protein not only for renewal of lean body mass and musculature, but also for energy that is derived from the organic structures of the amino acids. In general, athletes have slightly greater needs for protein compared with relatively sedentary individuals. An allowance of 1.0 g/kg body weight/day will meet the needs of practically all athletes, whereas 0.8 g/kg body weight/day is recommended for nonathletes.[1]

The protein requirements of athletes can be met from both animal and plant sources. Animal sources of protein include meat, fish, and poultry. Having a protein score equivalent to that of meat proteins, soy beans are considered a high-quality plant protein source.

Epidemiologic investigations show adverse effects of regular consumption of high protein diets in young adult women on bone mineral content (BMC) and bone mineral density (BMD).[3] One group has even hypothesized that high-protein diets contribute to hip fractures.[4] A review of a large series of studies of the effect of dietary protein on urinary calcium losses by Kerstetter and Allen[5] demonstrated that large amounts of animal protein increases urinary calcium losses. The calciuretic effect is both acute and, if dietary practices are persistent, also chronic. The absence of hypercalciuria after the consumption of soy protein suggests that the effect of animal protein is specific for amino acids that are plentiful in animal but not plant proteins. The mechanism for the protein-induced hypercalciuria has not been established, but several possibilities exist, including excess acid (H^+) production, stimulation of insulin and glucagon, and increased urinary sulfate excretion.

An important effect of high animal protein consumption is the generation of excess hydrogen ions (acid) and thereby extra work for the kidneys to remove these ions in order to defend against pH lowering. The urinary pH of meat-eating omnivores is significantly lower than the pH of strict vegetarians which are often in the alkaline range. Within reasonable limits of protein intake, however, the renal and other organ adjustments to the increased hydrogen ions are sufficient to minimize the losses of calcium in the urine of meat-eaters. This conclusion is not entirely based on hard data, but the studies of lactoovovegetarians suggest that the measurements of BMC and BMD of elderly lactoovovegetarians are not different from those of omnivorous women.[6,7] In these studies, dietary protein had a positive effect on bone mass.

Long-term experimental data of high-protein (animal) dietary patterns on bone measurements are lacking, but they are necessary to establish with reasonable certainty any adverse role of chronic intakes of animal proteins in the development of osteoporosis.

C. VITAMINS
1. Vitamin A and β-Carotene

Vitamin A, and possibly β-carotene, most likely plays an important role in the metabolism of bone cells, but little direct evidence exists for specific roles of retinol or retinoic acid. β-carotene is stored in fat cells located in bone marrow and in other fat depots in the body.

Adequate consumption of these two nutrients serves as a marker of a reasonably well-balanced diet, since fruits and vegetables provide practically all of the β-carotene and much of the vitamin A after intestinal digestion of β-carotene and other carotenoid molecules in plant foods.

Athletes with low circulating levels of vitamin A are probably at greater risk for musculoskeletal injuries and possibly fractures. Research evidence, however, to support this possibility is lacking.

2. Vitamin D

Although few investigations of vitamin D status of adolescents and young adults have been reported, published data suggest that even adolescents and young adults may have circulating levels of vitamin D metabolites that are indicative of deficiency, especially in the winter months. Therefore, if athletes receive little exposure to ultraviolet light and consume little vitamin D, they may become insufficient or frankly deficient.[8] Indoor athletes may need to pay more attention to the adequacy of their vitamin D status.

The primary reasons for deficits in vitamin D status are insufficient exposures to ultraviolet light for skin biosynthesis of the vitamin and limited intakes of vitamin D from foods, mainly fortified dairy products and fish. Supplementation of athletic individuals with vitamin D and calcium at RDA levels, at least in the winter and early spring months, may be a practical solution to the problem of vitamin D deficiency or insufficiency among female athletes living in northerly or southerly latitudes.

3. Vitamin K

A new role of vitamin K, in addition to its function in blood clotting, has recently been discovered. Vitamin K is required for the synthesis of a bone extracellular protein known as osteocalcin or bone GLA-protein. (The GLA signifies glutamic acid residues, which are abundant in these vitamin K-dependent proteins.) This protein has similar calcium-binding GLA groups as prothrombin. Osteocalcin is produced only by osteoblasts in bone tissues, and it may be involved in the initial step of mineralization of the collagen matrix of bone but not of collagen in other connective tissues of the body. Under conditions of vitamin K deficiency, osteocalcin is reduced in the number of gamma carboxylations of GLA residues. When intakes of vitamin K are adequate, this bone matrix protein is made in sufficient amounts. The synthesis of two additional bone matrix proteins also appears to be dependent on the availability of vitamin K from the diet.

Athletes may be low in vitamin K in both the diet and blood circulation. No reports, however, have been published specifically on the vitamin K status of athletes, nor have vitamin K replacement studies of athletes been conducted. Therefore, it is difficult to determine if athletes have undercarboxylation of their circulating osteocalcin, as has been shown for elderly subjects.[9] Vitamin K deficiency may also serve as a marker of a deficiency of vitamin D and therefore is linked to osteoporosis and fractures by complex mechanisms operating in osteoblasts. In a multicenter supplement study of elderly Japanese women with 1α-hydroxyvitamin D, bone mass was shown to be increased after 24 or 48 weeks of vitamin K therapy.[10] In fact, one study demonstrated that dialysis patients with a higher vitamin K status sustained fewer fractures than dialysis patients with low vitamin K status.[11] Thus, it appears that vitamin K nutriture remains important for bone health in athletes throughout life.

4. Vitamin E

Little information about the role of vitamin E in bone cells has been published, but clearly this antioxidant nutrient is needed to protect points of unsaturation in structural lipids in membranes of the envelope and internal organelles of bone cells, as in all other tissues of the body.

5. Vitamin C (Ascorbic Acid)

Vitamin C plays a critical role in the formation of the matrix proteins, namely collagen. Ascorbic acid may be one of the more critical micronutrients needed by athletes for musculoskeletal tissue repair and wound healing (see also iron and zinc below). For example, post-translational modification of the collagen molecule, i. e., hydroxylations of proline and lysine residues, requires vitamin C and iron for these enzymatic steps that lead to collagen maturation.

6. B Vitamins

A few B vitamins play important roles in bone tissue, especially in relation to their actions as enzyme activators in energy pathways in bone cells and in 1-carbon transfer steps relating to nucleic acid metabolism and cell division. Folate and vitamin B_{12} are especially essential for the recruitment and differentiation of new cells derived from bone marrow progenitor cells. Low folic acid intakes may have adverse effects on cholesterol metabolism and other aspects of cellular protection against free radicals.

Several other B vitamins, notably vitamin B_6, also play critical roles in the metabolism of bone tissue, especially in the activities of osteoblasts that produce the organic matrix and of osteoclasts that initiate bone resorption. Relatively little is known of the direct or indirect roles of these vitamins on bone cells, and the dietary amounts needed for optimal bone health are only estimated. Limited intakes of fruits and vegetables by the U.S. population in national food surveys suggest, however, that many athletes may have deficiencies of several B vitamins that have important roles in bone cell metabolism.

D. MINERALS
1. Calcium

Osteopenia is a common finding in amenorrheic athletes, and therefore adequate calcium intakes by female athletes is critical, especially for those athletes who are not producing estrogens and other sex hormones. Males also need adequate intakes of calcium, but they typically consume enough from dairy products alone. Dietary calcium intakes by females in the United States typically average considerably below the RDAs for calcium, starting at age 11 years. Unfortunately, this generally holds true for female athletes as well. The RDAs for females and males are 1200 mg of calcium per day from 11 through 24 years and 800 from age 25 years.[1] The National Institute of Health (NIH) Consensus Conference on Calcium in 1994 suggests that calcium intakes should be 1200–1500 mg/day for adolescents and young adults (11–24 years) and 1000 mg/day for adults 25–50 years.[12] Many nutritionists are not in agreement with the NIH recommendation of 1500 mg/day because it is practically impossible to obtain compliance with such a high requirement, even with supplementation. Furthermore, the scientific evidence of skeletal benefits in support of a daily recommendation of 1500 mg of calcium alone is not convincing. (Calcium plus vitamin D, however, may be more effective than calcium alone.) No harm, of course, would be anticipated from an intake of 1500 mg/day or even an intake as high as 2000, a value now considered the upper limit of safety. (No specific upper limit of safety of calcium consumption from foods and supplements has been published by federal agencies.) However, high-calcium dairy foods provide many other nutrients in addition to calcium that boost the nutritional status of individuals, whereas calcium supplements contain only calcium and an anion, such as carbonate or lactate.

Since approximately 90% of female BMC and BMD is accumulated by 16–18 years of age,[13,14] girls clearly must amass a large amount of their peak bone mass (PBM) during the period from the start of premenarche (roughly ages 9–11 in the United States and other affluent nations) to the end of their adolescent development. Males typically have a longer period for PBM accrual. This brief window of 6 years or so is a critical time for accruing an estimated 40–50% of the PBM, as assessed at age 30. (Calcium balance data also support this timing of PBM accrual at approximately age 30.[15]) Calcium intake in adequate amounts during this 6-year time-frame is clearly important. The few published scientific reports suggest that the premenarcheal skeleton may be more responsive to higher calcium intakes then the peri- or post-menarcheal bone tissue.[16] The BMC and BMD gains of postmenarcheal girls resulting from calcium supplements are surprisingly small.[16-18] Postmenarcheal girls definitely increase their values of BMC and BMD, but the same high level of calcium intake from supplements is much less effective after menarche than before menarche.[17,18] A prospective study of postpubertal girls from 13–17 years showed only small gains in BMC and BMD.[19] The hormones of development likely dominate the physiology of postmenarcheal growth during this time and, consequently, energy and the macronutrients drive skeletal development and mineralization much more so than the intake of calcium or any other micronutrient.[20]

Despite the understanding that osteoporosis is a calcium-deficiency disease, large amounts of dietary calcium alone do not consistently result in enhanced bone formation or increased BMC. Thus, the relative ineffectiveness of dietary or supplemental calcium plus diet or other nutrient combinations, such as the combined use of calcium and vitamin D, must be considered in an effort to maintain BMC *and* to prevent bone loss in amenorrheic female athletes. Further research on the role of these and other nutrient combinations in promoting bone health of athletes is needed.

Chronic calcium supplement studies of female athletes have not been conducted. Supplement studies of post-menopausal women employing both calcium and vitamin D, however, have been successful in preserving BMC and even in increasing it.

In addition to adequate calcium intakes by athletes, a number of reports have supported the benefit of regular physical activity in conjunction with RDA intake levels of dietary calcium in order to enhance bone mass and to prevent the development of low bone mass.[21] Athletic females may possibly have more efficient utilization of the calcium in their diets than non-athletic females, but this point has not been adequately supported yet by published research.[22,23]

In summary, adequate dietary calcium is required for both developing peak bone mass and for maintaining bone mass by athletes of both genders. Adequate vitamin D intake is also essential for enhancing the intestinal absorption of calcium from the diet. Optimal bone health depends, therefore, on these two important micronutrients, as well as others (See below).

2. Phosphorus

Phosphorus intakes practically always exceed those of calcium because nearly all foods contain plentiful amounts of phosphorus, but only a few contain calcium. Thus, phosphorus deficiency seldom occurs in adults and the elderly. Oftentimes, our diets provide too much phosphorus with respect to calcium. The absorbed phosphate ions promptly decrease the serum calcium concentration, which in turn stimulates parathyroid hormone (PTH) secretion and its elevation in blood. PTH enhances renal reabsorption of calcium by the kidneys; however, this action does not compensate for the loss of calcium in the GI secretions. The net result is a loss of calcium from the skeleton.

Most Americans consume an excess of phosphorus in relation to calcium, thus skewing the dietary calcium-to-phosphorus (Ca:P) ratio. Although RDAs do exist for phosphorus (and they are identical to those for calcium throughout the life cycle), average daily intakes invariably exceed the RDAs.[24] Furthermore, phosphorus in foods is readily removed during digestion and phosphate ions are rapidly absorbed, unlike calcium ions which are slowly absorbed.[25] Therefore, the most important characteristic of high dietary phosphorus consumption, including phosphate additives in many processed foods and cola drinks, is the typically low Ca:P ratio that results. Because so many American foods are processed with phosphates, women (and men) may potentially be placed at risk for the development of osteoporotic fractures because of the low Ca:P ratio of their diets.[24,26]

The consumption of foods which contain phosphate additives by many athletes in the U.S. population has been increasing in recent years.[27] This increment plus the behaviors of women who avoid or reduce the consumption of the recommended number (two or more) of servings of dairy products each day are considered to be important risk factors for low bone mass and subsequent osteoporotic fractures among female athletes. Males are much less likely to have fractures because of inadequate dietary intakes of calcium or excessive amounts of phosphorus.

3.   Magnesium

The literature on the association of magnesium and bone mass is extremely limited. Only one prospective human trial involving magnesium supplementation has been conducted, and the results from this Israeli study[28] are inconclusive. Clearly, the magnesium-calcium-bone triad needs greater investigation. Some researchers have suggested that high intakes of calcium from supplements may inhibit or otherwise interfere with magnesium absorption and thereby have an adverse effect on the function of magnesium in bone and other tissues. This idea has not yet been validated experimentally in humans. Athletes need to have intakes of magnesium that meet or exceed the RDA level.

The ratio of calcium to magnesium in typical American diets ranges between 3:1 and 4:1, but some investigators suggest that the optimal dietary ratio should be closer to 2:1. Further long-term studies are needed in this area.

4.   Sodium

High sodium intakes lead to increased urinary calcium losses. Persistent net losses of urinary calcium must ultimately be derived from the skeleton. Therefore, extended periods of high sodium intakes could contribute to low bone mass, osteoporosis, and fractures. Data obtained from postmenopausal women placed on a high sodium diet not only increase their urinary calcium/creatinine ratio but also their urinary ratio of hydroxyproline/creatinine.[29] The greatest effect of sodium on urinary calcium losses has been shown to occur when calcium intakes are low, the typical situation among elderly women and many adolescent females. Elevations in PTH and 1,25-dihydroxyvitamin D most likely accompany the sodium-induced renal losses of calcium, although this point is not yet settled. A moderate sodium intake would, nevertheless, seem to be a logical recommendation to delay or prevent bone loss, especially among low-calcium consuming adolescent and adult athletes.

Athletes lose significant amounts of sodium in sweat and excreta that must be replenished by dietary sources. Inadequate sodium consumption, however, is seldom a concern because of the widespread use of sodium-processing in American foods. If an athlete avoids high-sodium foods and does not practice discretionary use of table salt, the potential for deficiency is conceivable.

5.   Potassium

Potassium replacement is critical for health since it has essential roles within cells. Most foods provide adequate amounts of potassium, but fruits and vegetables are especially rich in this mineral. Athletes have an obligation to consume enough potassium to support their activities and, surprisingly, reported deficits of this nutrient have been very rare.

6.   Iron

Iron is essential for the enzymatic post-translational conversion of proline and lysine residues to hydroxyproline and hydroxylysine in newly formed collagen prior to secretion by osteoblasts into extracellular fluids of the nascent bone matrix. Vitamin C is also required in these same reaction steps (See above section). Non-heme iron absorption may be improved by Vitamin C or an acid diet but not by and alkaline or high fiber diet, both of which exist in vegetarian diets. Iron is also lost in sweat. Iron deficiency is common among male and female endurance athletes. Women runners especially, have been found to have marginal iron nutritional status because of low serum ferritin.[30] Athletes can be iron deficient, i.e., low serum ferritin and iron stores, without other laboratory evidence of anemia, i.e., normal red cell number and hematocrit. The reduced iron status can adversely influence athletic performance.

7.   Zinc

Like iron, zinc has important functions in bone cells and especially in tissue repair from injuries and in wound healing. Compared to untrained control women runners, highly trained women runners have significantly greater amounts of urinary zinc losses. This urinary loss of zinc suggests a higher rate of turnover of zinc in skeletal muscle[31] and possibly in the skeleton, a storehouse of the body's zinc. Further research is needed to establish whether endurance runners, male or female, are zinc deficient. Serum concentrations of zinc in female runners suggest that these athletes have marginal zinc status.[30]

8.   Fluoride

At reasonable intake levels (1 ppm or somewhat higher) fluoride ions consumed in drinking water, via dietary sources, or from consumer tooth-protective products can have positive effects on developing bone tissue (and tooth enamel) by increasing the surface hardness of the crystals in the mineral phase of the skeleton. On the other hand, too much fluoride can make the crystals more fracture-prone because of their strong chemical properties. A subsequent reduction in bone strength has been demonstrated in supplementation trials of osteoporotic patients.[32] Therefore, a narrow window exists in which fluoride ions can benefit mineralized tissues, i.e., bones and teeth. High consumption of fluoride also has adverse effects on gastrointestinal function in addition to increasing fracture rates and risk of fractures.[33] New slow-release preparations of fluoride, however, eliminate most of these problems, and these new drugs have been shown to increase bone mass of osteoporotic women, as shown by a recent report.[34]

9.   Other Trace Elements

Several trace elements, including iron, copper, manganese, and boron may have important roles in bone metabolism, either the mineral phase or in the activities of bone cells, such as in the formation of the matrix proteins like collagen. Human experimental evidence, however, is not sufficient to conclude that dietary deficits of these elements are critical to bone health. One report suggests that supplementation with combinations of zinc, copper, and magnesium, along with calcium (1000 mg/day), may improve spinal bone mass in postmenopausal women. In comparison, women who received the trace elements alone, calcium alone, or placebo lost spinal bone density over this 2-year trial.[35] Little data exist on the relationships of single trace elements alone and bone mass. Therefore, it presently is not possible to make dietary micronutrient recommendations with respect to optimizing bone mass.

E.   NON-NUTRIENTS: DIETARY FIBER AND OTHER COMPONENTS OF PLANT FOODS

The effect of dietary fiber on bone tissue is generally neutral. A few studies have shown significant negative effects of fiber on intestinal calcium absorption because of reduced bioavailability of calcium ions in the luminal milieu of the gut, but no long term study has found an adverse effect of high fiber diets on bone mass. One study of late adolescent girls (18–20 years) suggested that high fiber intakes led to later age of menarche, lower body weights, lower circulating estrogens, and lower bone densities at several sites.[36] However, dietary fiber intakes at the recommended levels of 20–30 g/day, which few Americans obtain, are not likely to have an adverse influence on bone mass during the later years of life since bone development and growth have long been completed. A high fiber intake may decrease the absorption of iron (see above under Iron).

Several other molecules found in plant foods have been suggested to influence calcium metabolism or bone tissue and, hence, bone mass. It appears that sufficient amounts of these molecules are ingested by some consumers to be of concern to toxicologists. These phyto-molecules include phytoestrogens, oxalates, molecules found in caffeine/tea, and many others. Except for oxalates, little knowledge exists about these 10,000 or more natural chemicals produced by diverse species of the plant kingdom. Oxalates in spinach and rhubarb have been shown to substantially reduce calcium absorption because of their chelation or tight binding of calcium ions within the gut lumen.[37] The effects of phytoestrogens on bone cells are presently being investigated in a number of laboratories. Phytoestrogens, such as genistein in soy and soy products, have weak agonistic effects on osteoblasts or related cells studied in tissue culture, and therefore they may help to retain bone mass, somewhat like estrogenic molecules do. Understandings of the mechanisms of phytoestrogens and other phytomolecules on bone tissue are just beginning to unfold.[38] This area of investigation is potentially enormous and largely uncharted.

F. SUMMARY

Nutrients considered critical for bone development and maintenance of bone tissue by athletes are calcium, phosphorus, and vitamin D. Vitamin K may also fall in this critical category, but more information is needed before this classification can be made. (Many other micronutrients are also essential to the healthy functioning of bone cells, but less is known about these other nutrients. For example, the roles of magnesium and zinc in bone tissue have not yet been resolved.) These nutrients need to be provided in optimal, but not excessive, amounts for bone health. Protein and energy are nutrient variables that are absolutely essential for optimal skeletal development but not for BMC per se. In addition, several other micron-utrients and a few non-nutrients may also be important and essential for bone, but deficiencies of these nutrients have not been shown to have major effects on bone. Finally, excessive intakes of a few specific nutrients also can have severe deleterious effects on bone tissue; these include phosphorus, protein, vitamin D, sodium, and fluoride. Little is known of the influences on bone of non-nutrient components derived from plant sources, but phytoestrogens, such as genistein, are receiving interest by researchers because of their potential for preventing bone loss. Dietary recommendations for bone health of athletes are listed in Table 1.

TABLE 1   Recommended Intakes of Nutrients for Adult Athletes in Relation to Bone Health

Nutrient Variable	Females (18 & Older)	Males (18 & Older)
Energy, kcal	2200 (RDA) +	2900 (RDA) +
Protein, g	50 (RDA) +	63 (RDA) +
Calcium, mg[a]	1200 (RDA) +	350 (RDA)
Magnesium, mg	280 (RDA) +	350 (RDA) +
Vitamin D, IU[b]	400 (RDA)	400 (RDA)
Vitamin K, μg	70 (RDA) +	65 (RDA) +

Note: RDA = Recommended Dietary Allowance.[1] + = Additional amounts.

[a]   Amenorrheic females need to consume at least this amount.
[b]   Vitamin D equivalents: 400 IU = 10 μg.

III. FOOD CONSUMPTION AND THE HEALTH OF ATHLETES

Nutrients are provided by the foods and beverages consumed in the diet. In order to obtain the essential nutrients and non-nutrients in amounts that support good health, including the optimal functioning of musculoskeletal tissues, athletes need to make wise selections of foods and beverages. This section focuses on the food guide pyramid, food labeling, and the nutritive value of the major beverages, nonalcoholic and alcoholic, consumed in the United States.

A. BASIC FOOD GUIDE/PYRAMID

The guidelines for nutrient intake presented by the Basic Food Guide/Pyramid (see Chapter 1) are critical for athletes. Typical nutrient deficiencies among athletes are found in the dairy group (inadequate calcium intakes), the protein group (inadequate heme iron intakes from meats and poultry), and the vegetable group (general inadequacy of micronutrients).

Calcium is not abundantly distributed in foods, but dairy products provide good amounts (200–400 mg) in each serving. For adolescents, 3–4 servings per day are required to meet the RDA of 1200 mg/day, whereas for adults 2–3 servings a day are sufficient to yield 800 mg, the current adult RDA. Other foods providing calcium in substantial amounts include dark greens (except for spinach whose calcium is not bioavailable),[37,39] small fishes with soft bones, and breads and other baked goods prepared with calcium propionate. In the typical adult American diet, roughly 60% of all calcium is derived from dairy products, about 25% from bakery products, approximately 10% from vegetables (dark greens) and fruits, and another 5% from miscellaneous foods. The food industry has voluntarily undertaken calcium fortification of new products in order to improve calcium intakes of females.[24] Calcium-fortified foods, such as breads and orange juices, are just beginning to have an impact on calcium intakes, but the extent of the benefit of calcium fortification of foods has not yet been assessed.

Iron is not widely distributed in foods; however, red meats (heme iron) and legumes (non-heme iron) are good sources. (Dried fruits also have fairly high amounts of non-heme iron.) In addition, the protein food group (meats) provides adequate amounts of zinc.

Dark, leafy, green and the red/orange/yellow vegetables provide many critical micronutrients in the diet, including some of the B vitamins (except vitamin B_{12} or cobalamin), vitamin C, β-carotene and related molecules, magnesium, and other minerals.

Athletes need to consume adequate numbers of servings in these three groups, as well as the recommended numbers in the other groups of the pyramid, in order to meet or exceed their age-specific RDAs for the critical nutrients, dietary fiber, and many important non-nutrients.

Lactose-intolerant athletes may wish to use lactase-treated milks or cultured dairy products, such as buttermilk. African-Americans are especially likely to be lactose intolerant. Many low-lactose products are now available in the markets, including regular milks and cultured milks. For example, buttermilk is a sour milk made typically from skim milk that has a culture of acid-producing bacteria added to it. These products have little or no lactose remaining after treatment, and they should be well tolerated by any athlete with milk intolerance (but not by those with a milk allergy).

B. VEGETARIAN FOOD GUIDE/PYRAMID

The nutrient needs of the vegetarian athlete are not different from the nonvegetarian athlete. Adequate energy and protein must be supplied by the diet to obtain the essential nutrients and non-nutrients from all of the food groups. The Vegetarian Food Guide/Pyramid outlines the suggested numbers of servings needed to meet the nutrient requirements of the vegetarian athlete. The female Vegetarian Pyramid appears in Chapter 17.

Protein (2–3 servings per day) is supplied by legumes, seeds, and soybeans; however, the remainder of the pyramid is identical to the basic food guide/pyramid (see Chapter 2). The vegetarian athlete must closely monitor iron, B_{12}, and zinc status. Since B_{12}, or cobalamin, is not provided by any plant food, supplementation at the level of the RDA may be necessary.

C. FOOD LABELING

The new food labeling information (Nutrition Facts panel) is based on a 2000 kcal (8400 kjoule) diet. Some labels also provide information on a 2500 kcal (10,500 kjoule) diet. The percent daily values (%DVs or PDVs) of major nutrients are useful in assessing the total intake of a nutrient or energy of an individual. For example, calcium intake from the foods and beverages in a day's intake can be totaled and compared to the age-specific RDA for calcium of a female athlete. This exercise can be done for other critical nutrients in order to assess the adequacy of an athlete's diet and her overall nutritional status.

D. SOFT DRINKS: COLAS, NON-COLAS, FRUIT DRINKS

Cola drinks typically contain phosphoric acid that provides approximately 60 mg of phosphorus per 12-oz. (355 ml) can. These drinks, however, provide no calcium, so that if they substitute for milk as a beverage, not only is phosphorus intake increased, but calcium consumption is avoided. This combination can exacerbate the Ca:P ratio, potentially contributing to elevations in serum parathyroid hormone and losses in bone mass.[40]

E. ALCOHOLIC BEVERAGES

Alcoholic beverages provide energy from the ethanol molecules and, in the case of most beers and some other beverages, additional calories from carbohydrates. Also alcohol acts as a mild diuretic that contributes to excessive water loss and to dehydration, both of which should be avoided by athletes. Athletes need to recognize these potentially adverse effects of even moderate alcohol consumption without adequate fluid (water) replacement.

F. PATTERNS OF MEALS AND SNACKS

Regular patterns of meal-eating are probably beneficial to performance in sports and other demanding forms of physical activity, such as ballet dancing. The reason is that nutrient balance and food variety are better achieved. Also, bowel movements tend to be more regular under such patterns (see also Chapter 2).

The typical food intakes of many athletic girls and young adult women supply calcium in amounts far below the RDA of 1200 mg/day, primarily because they do not choose dairy products as frequently as recommended (3–4 servings each day) to optimize PBM. The behaviors associated with the limited selection of dairy products are complex, but several reasons are given for the avoidance of dairy products. One, for example, is that milk and cheese are animal foods, and many young people have become vegans (strict) or partial vegetarians. Another is that dairy products are considered to be high in fat and, therefore, they are shunned by weight-conscious adolescents. A third is that milk is not considered preferable in comparison to cola or other nondairy drinks. Unfortunately, not enough young people understand the important contributions that low-fat dairy products make toward a healthy nutritional status with respect to calcium, protein, vitamin D, riboflavin, folic acid, vitamin B_{12} (cobalamin), and several other micronutrients.[41,42]

Premenarcheal female athletes clearly need the most calcium to support their robust gains in BMC, and then peri- and post-menarcheal females need sufficient amounts of calcium to support their continued skeletal accrual of calcium in the mineral phase of bone tissue. These groups of females should receive focused nutrition education in order to improve their overall nutritional consumption patterns. They must be certain to include calcium-rich foods in their diets each day. Some female athletes may become pregnant soon after their athletic competition ends. Thus, it is highly desirable for them to have good nutritional intakes well before conception to reduce the risk of poor pregnancy outcomes. Calcium, iron, and folic acid are in critical need during pregnancy.

So many low-fat or no-fat dairy products are available in the food markets today that females (and males) can readily make healthy food choices for the provision of optimal intakes of calcium and other essential micronutrients. Unfortunately too many young females either do not heed the nutritional knowledge they possess, or else they have not received adequate information about the nutrient composition of foods, especially calcium-rich foods. Nutrition education among young women is greatly deficient in the United States.

The role of nutrient supplements as part of the nutrient supply of athletes has not been well examined with experimentally sound study designs. It would seem highly advisable, however, for female athletes to take a one-a-day type multiple micronutrient supplement with a meal, such as the dinner meal after physical activities have concluded for the day. The amounts of each nutrient in these supplements should approximate the RDA (or USRDA used in drug labeling) of the specific nutrient. For example, the iron content should not exceed 18 mg per pill (100% of the USRDA, but slightly higher than 100% of the RDA of 15 mg/day) in the absence of documented deficiency (see case below for iron treatment of an individual with documented anemia).

Calcium supplementation, often coupled with vitamin D (400–800 IU/day), has become commonplace in the armamentarium of physicians to improve the calcium nutritional status of patients. Prior to recommending a daily dosage of 500 or 1000 mg of calcium, it would be wise to obtain either a 24-hour recall of total food and drink consumption or a quick-and-dirty calcium frequency questionnaire based on the commonly consumed calcium-rich foods.[43,44] Many choices of calcium supplements exist, but bioavailable calcium carbonate tablets, if tolerated, remain the most economical sources containing approximately 40% elemental calcium.

Other questions of importance are the ascertainment of "typical" pattern of eating and whether nutrient supplementation is already being used by the athlete. If a dietitian-nutritionist is available to administer the questionnaire of choice and to solicit other information about usual dietary practices of the patient, better assurance of optimal dosage of supplemental calcium can be attained. For example, a female athlete may often consume the same foods every day, thereby greatly reducing variety and increasing the chances of developing a deficiency of one or more micronutrients. Calcium-rich foods may not be purchased by female athletes because of their short storage time and the need to go to the market frequently. Athletes need to eat according to the Basic Food Guide/Pyramid (see Chapter 1) and to try to achieve more variety in their food choices.

G. SUMMARY

The wise selection of foods by athletes, both females and males, is necessary for obtaining not only all the essential nutrients in approximately the "right" amounts but also the non-nutrients whose roles in health are taking on increasing importance. The Basic Food Guide/Pyramid is the best tool available for guidance about the number of servings needed each day for the support of optimal health. For vegetarians, a modified food guide is available. Caution is given to athletes about excessive use of phosphorus-containing soft drinks and alcoholic beverages. Meal patterns for athletes need special attention.

IV. BONE CHANGES WITH EXERCISE

Exercise or mechanical stress is a critical factor in the development and maintenance of optimal bone density. In the normal physiologic state adult bone mass undergoes a continual process of resorption and formation to respond to various environmental stresses. A balance of several factors including menstrual status, body weight, diet, and genetics determines an individual's bone mineral density.

A. BONE STRUCTURES AND TURNOVER RATES

Bone is a dynamic tissue with a slow turnover. It is composed of two types of bone tissue, cancellous (trabecular) and cortical (compact). Individual bones are formed by a process called bone modeling, and each bone contains differing proportions of cancellous and cortical bone. For example, vertebral bones of the spinal column contain much higher amounts of cancellous bone tissue than other bones. Long bones, such as the femur, contain much more cancellous tissue at the ends, i.e., hips and knees, than in the shaft region. Cancellous bone typically is more metabolically active than cortical bone tissue and therefore it turns over faster than cortical tissue. For females, this fact takes on greater importance after menopause. With reduced estrogen levels, the higher rates of resorption of bone tissue, especially of vertebrae, hips, and wrists, results in the loss of bone mass and sets the stage for the development of osteoporosis.

Bone development in early life is referred to as modeling. After skeletal growth (height) is completed, approximately 16–18 years in females and 20–22 years in males, modeling ceases and remodeling becomes the sole process through which bones change. Modeling of the long bones of the limbs involves new cell formation at epiphyses, the subsequent formation of cartilage, and the final replacement by bone (mineralized) tissue. Even though some resorption of bone tissue must occur to increase the length of bones and to develop the shape needed for the supporting and movement functions of the body, modeling is dominated by the formation of bone.

Bone remodeling is the process through which bone is lost at any age, primarily after skeletal growth (height) has been completed. In this process, bone resorption by osteoclasts precedes bone formation by osteoblasts, but the net effect is a loss of bone mass because osteoblasts cannot form as much bone during each remodeling cycle as is removed by osteoclasts. The rates of bone remodeling vary in young adult women, but it is probably set at a higher level in athletes, especially those participating in weight-bearing sports.

B. PEAK BONE MASS AND OPTIMAL SKELETAL DEVELOPMENT

Adults must consume adequate amounts of calcium and other nutrients prior to the onset of puberty, and they must continue this consumption pattern until early adulthood in order to optimize peak bone mass (PBM) development. The calcium requirements for practically all females below 25 years of age can typically be met by intakes of approximately 1000 mg/day, but 1200 mg/day (the RDA) may be a safer value to use. Females beyond the mid-20s should consume at least 800 mg/day, the RDA. Males need to meet or exceed the same RDA values in order to achieve peak bone mass.

Bone consolidation continues after growth in height ceases. The gains in bone mass during the 20s are small compared to during prepuberty, but it is thought that the gains can be enhanced by healthy behaviors. Two important factors which contribute to optimal PBM development are adequate intakes of calcium from calcium-rich foods and regular physical exercise in weight-bearing activities. A positive interaction may exist between these two bone-promoting factors to improve bone mass even further. Athletes who restrict energy intake, i.e., dieting, may need to take calcium supplements.

Primary prevention of low bone mass (osteopenia) and subsequent osteoporotic fractures in both males and females can best be achieved by adopting healthy behaviors (calcium intake and physical activity) early in life, starting in the prepubertal years and continuing into adulthood. It is never too late to start.

C. MEASUREMENT OF BONE MASS AND DENSITY

Bone mineral density is currently measured via dual energy x-ray absorptiometry (DEXA) or quantitative computed tomography (QCT). Both techniques have a margin of error which often exceeds the observed changes in bone density.

DEXA is most commonly used to measure BMC and estimate BMD. X-rays of two different energies are used to correct for soft tissues surrounding bone at different sites of the skeleton. With DEXA instruments, total-body bone mass, hip mass, forearm mass, and vertebral mass measurements can be made. (Mass is measured as BMC.) Other machines, such as single-photon absorptiometry (SPA), have previously been used to measure forearm and calcaneus bone mass. Because this instrument requires the use of a radioactive source with a relatively short life, the long-lasting x-ray machines have become dominant in clinical and research use and SPA instruments are seldom employed today.

The reproducibility of these DEXA machines is of the order of 1–2% for each measurement site.

D. BENEFITS OF LOADING ACTIVITIES ON BONE MASS AND DENSITY

Upper body loading activities, including strength exercises and resistance training, have been demonstrated to improve both BMC and BMD of the vertebrae and hips, as well as to increase muscle strength, although research findings have not all been consistent. These loading activities must be continued on a regular basis (3 or 4 times a week for sufficient repetitions) in order to maintain the skeletal and muscle improvements.[45] Athletes who employ these types of activities along with their routine workouts of their specific sports and who consume healthy diets should be able to maintain high fitness levels and hopefully high performance levels, in addition to enhancing their bone measurements. Amenorrheic athletes, of course, will not obtain the same skeletal benefits of loading activities as eumenorrheic athletes because of the well established promotion and preservation of skeletal mass by estrogens (see above). What is not clear at this time is whether exercising eumenorrheic athletes (and male athletes) obtain an additional positive interactive benefit between dietary calcium and BMC as a result of optimal or near optimal levels of each variable. Further studies are needed to clarify these issues of nutrient-exercise interactions.

E. SUMMARY

The effects of exercise, especially intense competitive athletics, depend to a large extent on the specific type(s) of activity utilized in a given sport. For example, amenorrheic female endurance runners, but not necessarily athletes in all other sports who are amenorrheic, have greater reductions of bone mass and density in the upper body, especially the vertebrae, than in the lower extremities. Nevertheless, when bone loss of the proximal femur becomes so great, fractures can also occur at this site. High intakes of calcium may delay or even prevent the fractures in amenorrheic athletes, but experimental evidence has not yet been provided to substantiate this contention. Athletes who do power and strength exercises to improve their muscle strength generally have improved bone mass at the sites involved in the exercises and to a lesser extent at distal sites that are involved as struts (legs) for the support of the body. Therefore, repetitive exercises of sufficient demand generally contribute to improved bone measurements and improved microarchitecture of the skeleton because of the loading forces placed on the bone sites through muscle attachments and weight-bearing sites of the skeleton. The major exception to this generalization is amenorrheic female endurance athletes (or even possibly hypogonadal male endurance athletes) who lose bone tissue and continue to lose it at all skeletal sites, despite the minimal early and short-lived benefits at weight-bearing sites, without estrogen replacement therapy and/or possibly calcium supplementation. Further experimental research is needed to find ways to counter the loss of bone mass of amenorrheic runners and other female athletes who have similar major losses of bone tissue related to their athletic endeavors.

V. BONE HEALTH IN THE FEMALE ATHLETE

The bone health of the female athlete involves consideration of several factors in addition to adequate calcium intake. Eating habits and menstrual cycle irregularities directly impact the bone health of the female athlete.

A. ETIOLOGY OF ATHLETIC AMENORRHEA

In the general population the reported rates of amenorrhea are 2–5%.[46] In a review of six studies, the rates among athletes vary widely from 3.4 to 66%, with amenorrhea having the greatest prevalence in distance runners, ballet dancers, and gymnasts.[47] Several etiologic factors have been proposed to explain the amenorrheic state, including training intensity and volume, nutritional inadequacies, reproductive immaturity, psychological stress, and body composition changes. The perceived psychological stress from competition and training are difficult to isolate from other psychological stresses. However, amenorrheic runners have been reported to perceive more stress with their activity than eumenorrheic runners.[48] Interestingly, no difference was seen in depression, hypochondriasis, anxiety, or obsessive/compulsive tendencies. The multifactorial nature of the menstrual disturbances with exercise makes it difficult to assess the relative importance of each factor; however, training intensity and volume are likely to play a major contributing role. Studies have shown the incidence of amenorrhea to be dependent,[49,50] as well as independent,[51] on one or more of the mentioned factors.

B. PATHOPHYSIOLOGY OF ATHLETIC AMENORRHEA

Though the precise mechanism is unknown, exercise-associated amenorrhea is considered a form of hypothalamic amenorrhea. Neuroendocrinologic studies show various factors including corticotropin releasing hormone (CRH), cortisol, and beta-endorphin exert an inhibitory effect on the hypothalamic pituitary ovarian (H-P-O) axis and the hypothalamic gonadotropin-releasing hormone (GnRH) pulse generator resulting in decreased estrogen levels and disruption of regular menstrual cycling.

Exercise has been shown to acutely activate the hypothalamic pituitary adrenal (H-P-A) axis.[52] Loucks et al.[53] studied the H-P-A and H-P-O axes during the early follicular phase in eumenorrheic sedentary women, eumenorrheic athletes, and amenorrheic athletes. During the 24-hour analysis period, the three groups did not differ in adrenocorticotropic hormone (ACTH) pulse pattern or in cortisol pulse frequencies; however, both groups of athletes exhibited elevated serum cortisol levels in the morning, with the amenorrheic athletes maintaining their elevation of cortisol throughout the day and evening.

Exercise-related amenorrhea is associated with low levels of both estrogen and progesterone. In the acute setting, physical activity increases plasma concentrations of estradiol (E_2) and progesterone; however, levels return to normal within 2 hours of cessation of exercise.[54] Boyden et al.[55] found a significant decrease in the E_2 plasma concentration after 19 eumenorrheic women increased their running distance by 50 miles per week from baseline. Of the

TABLE 2   Prospective Studies of BMD of Female Athletes

| Study | Subjects | BMD | | Estrogen |
		Pre-	Post-	
Baer et al., 1993[73]	Runners	Lumbar: • No significant difference between Amenorrheics and Eumenorrheics	• No significant difference between Amenorrheics and Eumenorrheics	• Estradiol: Amenorrheics < Eumenorrheics

19 subjects 18 developed menstrual changes consisting mainly of oligomenorrhea but none developed amenorrhea. Interestingly, total body weight did not change but the subjects became leaner. A study comparing reproductive hormones of amenorrheic, oligomenorrheic, and eumenorrheic women runners and controls with daily blood sampling over a 21-day period showed significantly decreased E_2 and progesterone concentrations in oligomenorrheic and amenorrheic runners compared to controls and eumenorrheic runners.[56] In a large group (N = 205) of runners of varying activity levels, Hetland et al.[50] found that sex hormone disturbances were significantly related to training intensity. The elite runners had reductions of up to 25–44% of estradiol and progesterone, respectively, as compared to the normally active women who had little or no reduction in these hormones.

C.   BONE LOSS IN AMENORRHEIC AND OLIGOMENORRHEIC ATHLETES

Including the studies mentioned, the majority of studies on the relationship between athletic participation and estrogen hormonal status in female athletes have been cross-sectional in nature, rather than prospective, which is considered the gold standard. Well-designed prospective studies with the inclusion of appropriate control subjects are needed to provide a better understanding of how female athletes can better preserve and maximize their musculoskeletal tissues.

In this brief review of the literature, studies that measured BMD and either measured serum estrogens or evaluated menstrual status are highlighted. Table 2 provides data obtained in the one prospective study found in the literature search undertaken from 1990 until present.

Tables 3 and 4 include the research findings of studies that were cross-sectional in nature. Table 3 includes reports that provided information on both BMD and measured circulating estrogens and Table 4 reports on those publications that measured BMD but only evaluated menstrual status without determining estrogens in blood.

The mechanistic explanation of the loss of bone mass in amenorrheic and possibly oligomenorrheic athletes most probably relates to the reduction of serum estrogens. When females become hypoestrogenic, they begin to lose bone mass, as measured by DEXA. This loss likely results from the removal of the estrogenic inhibition on the action of PTH on osteoblasts in bone, especially those cells located on trabecular surfaces. Serum PTH concentrations do not have to be elevated for effective resorptive activity of PTH in bone tissues, especially cancellous tissue. Therefore, the loss of estrogen production by the ovaries can

TABLE 3   Cross-Sectional Studies, BMD, and Estrogen Measurements

Study	Subjects	BMD	Estrogen
Snead et al., 1992[56]	Runners	• Lumbar Spine: Amenorrheics and Oligomenorrheics < Eumenorrheics and Controls	• 17β-estradiol and Progesterone: Controls and Eumenorrheics > Oligomenorrheics and Amenorrheics
Hetland et al., 1993[50]	Running	• Lumbar: Amenorrheics < Eumenorrheics	• Estradiol and Progesterone: Runners had significantly lower baseline levels and fluctuations than normally active women

TABLE 4 Cross-Sectional Studies of BMD of Female Athletes

Study	Subjects	BMD
Young et al., 1994[82]	Dancers	• BMD was elevated at weight-bearing sites (femoral neck, Wards triangle, trochanter) • BMD deficits similar to those found in anorexics in non-weight bearing sites
Haenggi et al., 1994[71]	Non-athletes	• BMD is lower in amenorrheic women than in regularly menstruating, age-matched controls • Hormone-replacement therapy resulted in increased BMD
Myerson et al., 1992[75]	Runners	• Amenorrheics < Eumenorrheics, but not significantly different from Controls • Especially pronounced in the lumbar spine
Wolman et al., 1992[81]	Elite Athletes	• Amenorrheics < Eumenorrheics and OCA users
Snead et al., 1992[79]	Runners	• Lumbar Spine: Oligomenorrheics and Amenorrheics < Eumenorrheics • Proximal Femur: No significant difference
Rutherford, 1993[78]	Triathletes and Runners	• Lumbar Spine, Arm, Trunk, Total Spine: Amenorrheics < Eumenorrheics • Lumbar and Total Spine: Amenorrheics < Controls

result in significant losses of bone mass, and this loss can be very rapid in low calcium and vitamin D consumers.

D. MUSCULO-SKELETAL COMPLICATIONS AND FRACTURES

For female athletes with menstrual disorders, the significance of stress fractures as a sign of potential bone fragility should be strongly emphasized.

The heightened risk of osteoporosis and fractures in other states of estrogen and progesterone deficiency has been well documented.[57-59] Risk factors include menopause, young females with hyperprolactinoma, ovarian failure, or castration. Female athletes with exercise-associated menstrual irregularity have been shown to have an increased incidence of musculoskeletal injuries. In a retrospective study, Lloyd et al.[60] found that female distance runners who had stopped their running program because of injury were more likely to have had irregular or absent menses while running and were also less likely to have used exogenous estrogen in the form of oral contraceptives. The same study reviewed the medical histories of college female athletes and found the frequency of stress fractures in those with irregular menses to be almost four times greater than that of the normally menstruating athletes. In this study regular menses were defined as cycles occurring every 25–35 days or 10–13 cycles per year whereas irregular cycles were defined as any other cycle pattern, including amenorrhea. The frequency of soft tissue injuries was the same for both groups. Although this study did not measure serum values of sex hormones, it is likely that athletes clinically defined as hypoestrogenic, as manifested by irregular menses, were at increased risk of stress fractures but not of soft-tissue injuries.

The location of fractures in postmenopausal females is most commonly in trabecular bone, such as the hip, vertebra, and distal radius. These sites are in striking contrast to amenorrheic athletes, even those with very low trabecular BMD. Fractures in amenorrheic athletes are generally seen in weight-bearing cortical bones such as the tibia, femur, and metatarsal. The site of the fracture does depend on the type of activity. In a sport like rowing, the stress is primarily on the upper body, and it is more common to see stress fractures of the ribs or pars interarticularis. Research on a direct cause-effect relationship between stress fractures and low BMD is sparse. In a case-control study, 25 athletes (19 women) with stress fractures, matched for sex, age, weight, height, and exercise history with controls, had significantly lower BMD at the lumbar spine and proximal femur.[61] Most athletes in the study were runners, and not one of the stress fractures occurred in the spine. A subgroup of six athletes with stress fractures of the femoral neck, which is predominantly cortical bone, had significantly lower BMD at this site than did the matched controls. This same study found the following factors in addition to lower bone density that differentiated subjects with stress fractures from control subjects: lower dietary calcium intake, increased incidence of current menstrual irregularity, and a lower incidence of oral contraceptive use in the stress fracture group. Both groups had a similar history soft tissue injuries such as muscle tears, runner's knee, iliotibial band friction syndrome, and achilles tendonitis.

Clearly further studies are needed to fully delineate the interplay of etiologic factors, especially inadequate dietary intakes, contributing to stress fractures in female athletes.

E.   FEMALE ATHLETE TRIAD — DISORDERED EATING, AMENORRHEA, OSTEOPENIA

Numerous beneficial effects have been found in exercising female subjects, but evidence has mounted over the past 25 years demonstrating that high levels of exercise combined with other factors, such as inadequate nutrition and low body weight and fat, can contribute to menstrual disturbances.[49,62] These disturbances typically result in reductions in bone mass and bone mineral density, both of which may not be reversible.

The triad consists of three associated medical disorders: disordered eating, amenorrhea, and osteoporosis. The reported prevalence of disordered eating among female athletes is varied, as is the defined criteria; however, based on a number of studies, it has been reported in the 15–62% range.[63] In pursuit of improved performance and an ideal body image, athletes have commonly gone to dietary extremes to decrease body fat stores. This individual concern may be further exacerbated by coaches, trainers, or parents who define weight goals for the athletes. Society has also fostered the belief that thinness is associated with fitness and beauty. A questionnaire administered to 182 female college athletes revealed that 32% had at least one weight-control behavior defined as pathogenic.[64] These abnormal behaviors included binging more than twice a week, self-induced vomiting, and the use of laxatives, diet pills, or diuretics. The authors found that half of the athletes who believed they had a history of obesity also demonstrated a pathogenic weight-control behavior. Possible explanations for the prevalence of eating disorders among female athletes are summarized in Table 5.

Although many athletes with disordered eating do not meet the full criteria for anorexia nervosa or bulimia nervosa they typically remain at risk for serious hormonal, psychological, and skeletal problems. The criteria, as defined by the American Psychiatric Association's *Diagnostic and Statistical Manual of Mental Disorders* (DSM IV)[65] for anorexia nervosa and bulimia nervosa, are listed in Table 6.

The disordered eating may contribute to menstrual dysfunction, and in turn each of these is a known contributor to osteopenia. Multiple etiologic factors exist in athletic amenorrhea, but the most frequent associations found for amenorrheic athletes are high intensity exercise

TABLE 5   Possible Explanations for the Prevalence of Eating Disorders among Female Athletes

- competitive athletic atmosphere
- constant pressure to succeed
- heightened body awareness
- compulsiveness and perfectionism
- fluctuation of self-esteem with fluctuation of performance
- ability to block pain and hunger
- willingness to take unnecessary risks to win
- importance of aesthetics in sport or dance
- belief that body leanness optimizes performance
- lack of identity beyond the sport or dance

From American Psychiatric Association, *Diagnostic and Statistical Manual of Mental Disorders IV (edition 4)*, Washington, D.C., 1994.

TABLE 6   Diagnostic Criteria for Anorexia Nervosa and Bulimia Nervosa

Anorexia Nervosa

• Refusal to maintain body weight over a minimal normal weight for age and height, e.g., weight loss leading to maintenance of body weight 15% below that expected; or failure to make expected weight gain during period of growth, leading to body weight 15% below that expected.
• Intense fear of gaining weight or becoming fat, even though underweight.
• Disturbance in the way in which one's body weight, size, or shape is experienced; e.g., the person claims to "feel fat" even when emancipated or believes that one area of the body is "too fat" even when obviously underweight.
• In females, absence of at least three consecutive menstrual cycles when otherwise expected to occur (primary or secondary amenorrhea).

Bulimia Nervosa

• Recurrent episodes of binge eating (rapid consumption of a large amount of food in a discrete period of time).
• A feeling of lack of control over eating behavior during the eating binges.
• Regular practice of either self-induced vomitting, use of laxatives or diuretics, strict dieting or fasting, or vigorous exercise to prevent weight gain.
• A minimum of two binge eating episodes a week for at least three months. Persistent over concern with body shape and weight.

Adapted from American Psychiatric Association, *Diagnostic and Statistical Manual of Mental Disorders IV (edition 4)*, Washington, D.C., 1994.

and poor nutritional status. It has been shown that severe protein-calorie restriction can produce both hypercortisolism and amenorrhea.[66]

Osteoporosis can be defined as premature bone loss or inadequate bone formation, each resulting in low bone mass and a high risk of fractures. Combined with appropriate physiologic and nutritional conditions, regular exercise/mechanical stress is known to increase bone mineral density. In amenorrheic athletes, such as distance runners, estrogen and progesterone deficiencies, and most likely nutritional inadequacies, have been shown to overwhelm the trophic effects of exercise on bone and result in decreased bone mineral density and increased risk of stress fractures. Interestingly, studies of amenorrheic gymnasts have shown greater BMD measurements at most skeletal sites compared with nonexercising controls.[67] These differences among sport-specific athletes suggest that the type of activity may possibly serve as a critical factor in the risk of bone density loss during the amenorrheic state.

F.   TREATMENT OF FEMALES WITH ATHLETIC-RELATED INJURIES AND MENSTRUAL DISORDERS

The presentation of female athletes with overuse injuries is often a manifestation of multiple etiologic factors which should ideally be modified before a full return to activity. The scope of the presenting problem usually goes beyond that seen at the surface, and the physician should be alerted to uncover the presence of any other potential aspects of the female athlete triad. Just as the etiologic components of the female athlete triad are multi-dimensional, the solutions are multi-dimensional as well. Many athletes are not willing to discuss disordered eating particularly when they feel they have presented with a complaint such as a painful shin. It may take several visits before the athlete is willing to reveal any problematic dietary practices.

To appreciate the athlete's complete diagnoses one must evaluate the athletes training regimen, nutrition, dietary practices, menstrual status, medications, and in cases of exercise associated amenorrhea a complete physical exam and selected blood work. Fortunately with increased physician awareness of the female athlete triad, screening for risks factors in the preparticipation physical exams is the first step in primary prevention. In addition to modification of risk factors, the specific treatment for stress fractures varies somewhat according to site but in very general terms requires 4–8 weeks of rest from the offending activity and if weight bearing is painful the use of crutches. Furthermore an attempt should be made to modify any contributing biomechanical abnormalities such as overpronation. A look at the athlete's training regimen often reveals a recent change in terrain, a sudden increase in training volume or intensity, as well as exercising in old or worn footwear. More complicated treatment is usually necessary for certain anatomic sites such as the superior cortex of the femoral neck or the anterior tibia which generally require orthopedic consultation.

Disordered eating and macronutrient deficiencies may directly increase the risk of bone injury and also indirectly by contributing to menstrual disturbances. For many athletes the disordered eating is a way of life requiring experienced psychological counseling to promote healthy dietary habits. Studies of females with anorexia nervosa and secondary amenorrhea have been shown to have increased excretion and decreased absorption of calcium;[68] therefore, increased calcium intake alone is not likely sufficient to improve bone mineral density. In a study of amenorrheic, anorexic females, Bachrach et al.[69] illustrated the importance of weight gain. Weight gain had an independent effect on bone mineral accretion, and recovery of bone mineral density occurred before the resumption of menses.

In the presence of sports-induced menstrual disorders a reduction in activity level can help restore normal patterns; however, for the elite athlete with amenorrhea or oligomenorrhea a reduction in activity or an increase in weight are not welcomed options. Even in the absence of injury, evaluation and treatment of athletic amenorrhea, particularly in adolescents, is critical. The first step in treating athletic amenorrhea should involve educating the patient on the likely causes, risk factors, and potential complications. Often athletes will be more motivated to treat menstrual disturbances knowing the increased risk of injury and missing time from participation. Furthermore, as the most significant bone loss occurs early in the amenorrheic period, early treatment is a must.

For many female athletes, hormone replacement is a reasonable option as part of a larger management plan. The vast majority of research on the benefits of estrogen and progesterone treatment for maintaining or improving bone mineral density in the amenorrheic state has been with postmenopausal females. Research on the bone effects in females with athletic amenorrhea or oligomenorrhea is sparse. Specific doses of hormonal therapy for athletic amenorrhea to protect against bone loss is unknown. For postmenopausal females the protective dose of conjugated estrogens is 0.625 mg daily or 0.3 mg if combined with calcium supplementation.[70] These dosages can not be assumed to apply to athletes because of the numerous differences between postmenopausal females and amenorrheic athletes. Haenggi et al.[71] studied young females with hypothalamic amenorrhea (aged 18–45 years) excluding athletes and followed them for 12–24 months after the initiation of 0.03 mg ethinylestradiol and 0.15 mg desogrestrel daily for 21 days per month. Compared with pre-treatment BMD the post-treatment values revealed significant rises in BMD at the lumbar spine and Ward's triangle but no significant changes at the femoral neck, tibial diaphysis, and tibial epiphysis. With the exclusion of athletes from this study, the findings are difficult to apply to athletic amenorrhea.

It is commonly felt, however, that for athletes low dosage combined (estrogen plus progestin) oral contraceptives provide a sufficient dose of estrogen to maintain bone density as well as provide contraception. Some athletes are content at being amenorrheic, finding the resumption of menses an unwanted inconvenience and/or they are resistant to having hormonally induced regular menstrual bleeding. For these patients an option of both decreasing exercise intensity or duration and improving nutrition may be tried for up to 6 months, but generally thereafter hormonal therapy is strongly suggested if amenorrhea persists.

G. SUMMARY

Bone health in girls and young adult women relates to the continuous progression of the normal developmental sequence that precedes and follows the onset of menstruation or menarche. Females who are very athletic and have either delayed menarche and primary amenorrhea or secondary amenorrhea may compromise their bone health because of the low circulating levels of serum estrogens.

Athletes with symptomatic menstrual disturbances such as amenorrhea or oligomenorrhea have deficient hormone levels leading to adverse consequences on bone mass. As far as the asymptomatic individual is concerned, only one group of investigators[72] has found an associated bone loss with deficient hormone levels. A critical degree of alteration from normal menstrual function must exist for an adverse effect on BMC to occur.

VI. CASE STUDY OF A FEMALE DISTANCE RUNNER

An 18-year-old freshman distance runner presented to the sports medicine clinic during the middle of the fall cross country season complaining of pain in the mid-left thigh and right proximal as well as distal tibia. Pain was primarily aggravated with running and progressively worsening over the preceding 3 weeks. She had been self-medicating with over-the-counter, non-steroidal anti-inflammatories as she figured she could "run through" the pain. She also noted a recent general decrease in energy over the past month and complained of feeling lightheaded during intense interval training and a slowing of her usual race times.

Her past medical history was significant for iron deficiency anemia 2 years ago, left tibial stress fracture 1 year ago, and asthma which was well controlled with a low-dose inhaled steroid and bronchodilator.

Past gynecological history included menarche at age 13 and an irregular menstrual pattern ever since (a range of 5–10 menses per year). Periods of oligomenorrhea generally worsened during times of intense physical training. After development of the tibial stress fracture in high school she was started on an oral contraceptive pill; however, she stopped taking this after 3 months because of side effects relating to mood changes and dysphoria. She was unwilling to try another pill with a different side effect profile. During the 6 months prior to her current complaints she had three menstrual cycles which were roughly evenly spaced apart.

General dietary intake questioning provoked an easily observable degree of apprehension. discomfort, and suspicious pauses. Specific questions screening for abnormal/dysfunctional dietary practices such binging, purging, laxative or diuretic use were all abruptly denied. She also denied any fluctuations in weight over the past 18 months.

With her known history of oligomenorrhea and stress fracture she had been strongly encouraged at the start of the cross-country season to report any early signs of pain in the lower extremities associated with running and was encouraged to reconsider starting an oral contraceptive pill with a different side effect profile from the previous pill. She had been counseled about the long term risk of osteoporosis in addition to the importance of regular menstrual cycles and proper nutrition in the attainment of peak bone mass.

Physical exam revealed a well developed, white female, weight 125 pounds, height 65 inches, blood pressure 110/70, pulse 72, and a rather pale complexion. The left femur was tender to deep palpation at midshaft, and fulcrum test was positive. Her right tibia revealed tenderness focally to palpation at the proximal one-third as well as distal one-third of the medial cortex. The remainder of the physical, including gynecological exam, was otherwise unremarkable and unrevealing for any pathological causes of oligomenorrhea.

TABLE 7 Laboratory Analysis of Iron Status of Case

	Ferritin (μg/dl) (Normal 10–291)	Hb (g/dl) (Normal 10–16)	MCV (fl) (Normal 81–99)	Hct (Normal 37–47)
4 months prior presentation	—	12.1	—	—
At presentation	5.0	9.5	86.7	28.6
4 wks post initiation of ferrous sulfate	—	11.9	87.4	36.4
10 wks post initiation of ferrous sulfate	16	12.7	87.7	39.6

A. INVESTIGATION AND RESULTS

Laboratory analyses revealed the values relative to iron status shown in Table 7. Other data obtained included:

- Plain film radiographs of left femur and right tibia that were normal.
- Stool samples for occult blood loss that were negative.
- Total iron that was 21 μg/l (Normal 40–180 μg/l).
- Screening tests to rule out other pathologic causes of oligo/amenorrhea were within normal limits and included: pregnancy test, thyroid function tests, prolactin, luteinizing hormone (LH), and follicle stimulating hormone (FSH). Both LH and FSH were in the low–normal range.
- A Technecium-labeled bone scan revealed findings consistent with stress fractures at the left femur midshaft, right tibia proximal, and distal posteromedial cortex, as well as an old stress fracture at the distal left tibia posteromedial cortex.

B. DIAGNOSES

Four diagnoses were made for this 18-year-old female athlete:

- Multiple stress fractures.
- Iron deficiency anemia.
- Exercise-associated oligomenorrhea.
- Probable eating disorder.

C. MANAGEMENT

The management of this complicated case was as follows:

- Athlete was educated on the importance of healthy dietary habits including adequate caloric and nutrient intake particularly with regard to iron and calcium; as well she was counseled on the role of nutrition and regular cyclical menses in relation to the attainment and maintenance of peak bone mass and the prevention of future stress fractures.
- Training activity was decreased and changed to nonimpact-loading activities including swimming and easy cycling.
- Patient was not agreeable to trying another oral contraceptive pill with a different side-effect profile; however, she was agreeable to hormone replacement therapy consisting of conjugated estrogens 0.625 mg orally on days 1–25 and medroxyprogesterone acetate 5 mg on days 16–25 of each month.
- Ferrous sulfate 325 mg orally three times daily was administered initially. Later, this dose was given only two times and then once a week until iron parameters normalized.

• Subsequent DEXA BMD measurements revealed the following (values given as a percentage of BMD as compared to sex- and age-matched controls): left hip 100%, lumbar spine 89%, total body 92%. These BMD measures proved to be an excellent motivational tool for the athlete, as she was convinced that she truly did have significant medical and behavioral problems.

D. FOLLOW-UP

At one month the athlete showed good compliance with medication as manifested by the re-appearance of menses and with the red blood cell indices returning toward normal. Follow-up at 10 weeks revealed satisfactory healing (clinically) of the stress fractures. A slow gradual return to running was allowed, which was well tolerated.

In summary, this case required considerable consultation among sports medicine staff and other colleagues in the University of North Carolina Hospitals. She illustrates the great need for education among highly competitive athletes about diet and osteoporosis.

VII. CONCLUSIONS

Good nutrition is important for maintaining a high level of performance for all athletes. The role of nutrients in the development of low bone mass and fractures among female athletes is further complicated by the influences of other factors of the female athlete triad, namely amenorrhea and eating disorders. Low calcium consumption remains a nutritional problem among female athletes because so many of them avoid calcium-rich dairy products on the presumption that these foods are high in fat content. In addition to calcium, several other nutrient deficiencies (severe) or insufficiencies (less severe), especially of iron, have been found among female athletes who have poor food habits and who do not take advantage of sound nutritional advice. Vegetarian athletes, either partial or total, typically need nutrition counseling in order to assure adequate intakes of several micronutrients. Supplementation with micronutrients (vitamins and minerals) does not make a bad diet good, but it may help many athletes with marginal intakes of calcium, iron, zinc, magnesium, and one or more vitamins. Nutrition education should remain one of the important components of any successful athletic program for athletes, and sports medicine physicians and trainers should emphasize the benefits of a sound nutritional approach in the prevention of sports-related injuries and fractures.

While it is generally perceived that athletic participation, be it recreational or at the elite level, is part of a healthy lifestyle, this is unfortunately not always the case. In combination with nutritional inadequacies and the related reproductive hormone disturbances, very good evidence exists for alarming concern about the deleterious effects of heavy physical training on bone health. As illustrated in the case of the female cross-country runner, several factors, particularly a diet low in calcium, iron, and total calories along with the menstrual disturbances, are truly unhealthy for both the short term as it pertains to stress fractures and more significantly for the long-term consequences of osteoporosis with its related fractures and disability.

As important as it may be for health professionals to promote a lifestyle of regular physical activity, it is equally important to encourage sound nutritional habits. Primary prevention is the greatest tool to help reduce any unnecessary harm from sports participation, and it is best done in the pre- and early adolescent ages (involving the athlete, parents, coaches, and trainers), when bone mass development is so critical and when education may have the greatest preventive effect.

REFERENCES

1. *Recommended Dietary Allowances, 10th ed.*, Subcommittee on Dietary Allowances, Food and Nutrition Board, National Research Council, National Academy Press, Washington, D.C., 1989.
2. Horvath, P.J., Eagen, C.K., Leddy, J.J., and Pendergast, D.R., Effect of dietary fat level on performance and metabolism in trained male and female runners, *FASEB J.*, 10, A288, 1996.
3. Metz, J., Anderson, J.J.B., and Gallagher, P.N., Jr., Intakes of calcium, phosphorus, protein and level of physical activity are related to radial bone mass in young adult women, *Am. J. Clin. Nutr.*, 58, 537, 1993.
4. Abelow, B.J., Holford, T.R., and Insogna, K.L., Cross-cultural association between dietary animal protein and hip fracture: a hypothesis, *Calcf. Tissue Int.*, 150, 14, 1992.
5. Kerstetter, J.E. and Allen, L.H., Dietary protein increases urinary calcium, *J. Nutr.*, 120, 134, 1990.
6. Tylavsky, F.A. and Anderson, J.J.B., Dietary factors in bone health of elderly lactoovovegetarian and omnivorous women, *Am. J. Clin. Nutr.*, 48, 842, 1988.
7. Hunt, I.F., Murphy, M.J., Henderson, C., Clark, V.A., Jacobs, R.M., Johnston, P.K., and Coulson, A.H., Bone mineral content in postmenopausal women: comparison of omnivores and vegetarians, *Am. J. Clin. Nutr.*, 50, 517, 1989.
8. Lamberg-Allardt, M., Ala-Houhala, M., Ahola, M., Parvianained, M.T., Rasanen, L., and Visakorpi, J., Vitamin D status of children and adolescents in Finland, *Ann. Nutr. Metab.*, 30, 267, 1986.
9. Plantalech, L., Guillaumont, M., Leclercq, M., and Delmas, P.D., Impaired carboxylation of serum osteocalcin in elderly women, *J. Bone Min. Res.*, 6, 1211, 1991.
10. Orimo, H., Shiraki, M., Fujita, T., Inoue, T., and Kushida, K., Clinical evaluation of menatetrenone in the treatment of involutional osteoporosis, *J. Bone Miner. Res.*, 7(Suppl. 1), S122, 1992.
11. Kohlmeier, M., Saupe, J., and Shearer, M.J., Risk of bone fracture in hemodialysis patients is related to vitamin K status, *J. Bone Miner. Res.*, 10, 5361, 1995.
12. NIH Consensus Conference, *Optimal Calcium Intake*, Bethesda, MD, 1995. (Also see *J. Am. Med. Assoc.*, 272, 1942, 1994.)
13. Bonjour, J.P., Theintz, G., Buchs, B., Slosman, D., and Rizzoli, R., Critical years and stages of puberty for spinal and femoral bone mass accumulation during adolescence, *J. Clin. Endocrinol. Metab.*, 73, 555, 1991.
14. Theintz, G., Buchs, B., Rizzoli, R., and Bonjour, J.P., Longitudinal monitoring of bone mass accumulation in healthy adolescents: evidence for a marked reduction after 16 years of age at levels of lumbar spine and femoral neck in female subjects, *J. Clin. Endocrinol. Metab.*, 75, 1060, 1992.
15. Matkovic, V. and Heaney, R.P., Calcium balance during human growth: evidence for threshold behavior, *Am. J. Clin. Nutr.*, 55, 992, 1992.
16. Johnston, C.C., Jr., Miller, J.Z., Slemenda, C.W., Reister, T.K., Christian, J.C., and Peacock, M., Calcium supplementation and increases in bone mineral density in children, *New Engl. J. Med.*, 327, 82, 1992.
17. Matkovic, V., Fontana, D., Tomineac, C., Goel, P., and Chesnut, C.H., III, Factors that influence peak bone mass formation: a study of calcium balance and the inheritance of bone mass in adolescent females, *Am. J. Clin. Nutr.*, 52, 878, 1990.
18. Lloyd, T., Andon, M.B., Rollings, N., Martel, J.K., Landis, J.R., Demers, L.M., Eggli, D.F., Kielselhorst, K., and Kulin, H.E., Calcium supplementation and bone mineral density in adolescent girls, *J. Am. Med. Assoc.*, 270, 841, 1993.
19. Katzman, D.K., Bachrach, L., Carter, D.R., and Marcus, R., Clinical anthropometric correlates of bone mineral acquisition in healthy adolescent girls, *J. Clin. Endocrinol. Metab.*, 73, 1332, 1991.
20. Anderson, J.J.B., The role nutrition in the functioning of skeletal tissue, *Nutr. Rev.*, 50, 388, 1992.
21. Anderson, J.J.B. and Metz, J.A., Contributions of dietary calcium and physical activity to primary prevention of osteoporosis in females, *J. Am. Coll. Nutr.*, 12, 378, 1993.
22. Kanders, B., Dempster, D.W., and Lindsay, R., Interaction of calcium nutrition and physical activity on bone mass in young women, *J. Bone Miner. Res.*, 3, 145, 1988.
23. Halioua, L. and Anderson, J.J.B., Lifetime calcium intake and physical activity habits: independent and combined effects on the radial bone of health premenopausal Caucasian women, *Am. J. Clin. Nutr.*, 49, 534, 1989.
24. Anderson, J.J.B. and Barrett, C.J.H., Dietary phosphorus: the benefits and problems, *Nutr. Today*, 20, 29, 1994.
25. Anderson, J.J.B., Dietary calcium and bone mass through the lifecycle, *Nutr. Today*, 25, 9, 1990.
26. Calvo, M.S., Dietary phosphorus, calcium metabolism, and bone, *J. Nutr.*, 123, 1627, 1993.
27. Calvo, M.S. and Youngmee, K.P., Changing phosphorus content of the U.S. diet: potential for adverse effects on bone, *J. Nutr.*, 126, 1168S, 1996.
28. Stendig-Lindberg, G., Tepper, R., and Leichter, I., Trabecular bone density in a two year controlled trial of peroral mangnesium osteoporosis, *Magnesium Res.*, 6, 155, 1993.
29. Nordin, B.E.C. and Need, A.G., The effect of sodium on calcium requirement, in *Nutrition and Osteoporosis, vol. 9, Advances in Nutritional Research,* Draper, H.H., Ed., Plenum Press, New York, 1994, 209.
30. Deuster, P.A., Kyle, S.B., Moser, P.B., Vigersky, R.A., Singh, A., and Schoomaker, E.B., Nutritional survey of highly trained women runners, *Am. J. Clin. Nutr.*, 45, 954, 1986.

31. Deuster, P.A., Day, B.A., Singh, A., Douglas, L., and Moser-Veillon, P.B., Zinc status of highly trained women runners and untrained women, *Am. J. Clin. Nutr.*, 49, 1295, 1989.

32. Riggs, B.L., Hodgson, S.F., O'Fallon, W.M., Chao, E.Y.S., Wahner, H.W., Muhs, J.M., Cedel, S.L., and Melton, L.J., III, Effect of flouride treatment on the fracture rate in postmenopausal women with osteoporosis, *N. Engl. J. Med.*, 322, 802, 1990.

33. Klerekoper, M., Peterson, E., Phillips, D., Nelson, D., Tilley, B., and Parfitt, A.M., Continuous sodium flouride therapy does not reduce vertebral fracture rate in postmenopausal osteoporosis, *J. Bone Miner. Res.*, 4(Suppl. 1), S376, 1989.

34. Pak, C.Y.C., Sakhaee, K., Bell, N.H., Licata, N., and Johnston, C., Comparison of nonrandomized trials with slow-release sodium flouride with a randomized placebo-controlled trial on postmenopausal osteoporosis, *J. Bone Miner. Res.*, 11, 160, 1996.

35. Strause, L., Saltman, P., Smith, K.T., Bracker, M., and Andon, M.B., Spinal bone loss in postmenopausal women supplemented with calcium and trace minerals, *J. Nutr.*, 124, 1060, 1994.

36. Dhuper, S., Warren, M.P., Brooks-Gunn, J., and Fox, R., Effects of hormonal status on bone density in adolescent girls, *J. Clin. Endocrinol. Metab.*, 71, 1083, 1990.

37. Weaver, C.M., Martin, B.R., and Heaney, R.P., Calcium absorption from foods, in *Nutritional Aspects of Osteoporosis, Serono Symposium No. 85*, Burckhardt, P. and Heaney, R.P., Eds., Raven Press, New York, 1991, 133.

38. Anderson, J.J.B., Ambrose, W.W., and Garner, S.C., Orally dosed genistein from soy and prevention of cancellous bone loss in two ovariectomized rat models, *J. Nutr.*, 125, 799S, 1995.

39. Heaney, R.P. and Weaver, C.M., Calcium bioavailability from spinach, *Am. J. Clin. Nutr.*, 47, 707, 1988.

40. Wyshak, G. and Frisch, R.E., Carbonated beverages, dietary calcium, the dietary calcium-phosphorus ratio and bone fractures in boys and girls, *J. Adolesc. Health*, 15, 210, 1994.

41. Barger-Lux, M.J., Heaney, R.P., Packard, P.T., Lappe, J.M., and Recker, R.R., Nutritional correlates of low calcium intake, *Clin. Appl. Nutr.*, 2, 39, 1992.

42. Miller, G.D., Jarvis, J.K., and McBean, L.D., *Handbook of Dairy Foods and Nutrition*, CRC Press, Boca Raton, FL, 1995.

43. Musgrave, K.O., Giambalvo, L., Leclerc, H.L., Cook, R.A., and Rosen, C.J., Validation of quantitative food frequency questionnaire for calcium supplementation, *J. Am. Diet Assoc.*, 89, 1484, 1989.

44. Hertzler, A.H., Assessment of calcium intakes of adults and the elderly, Dept. of Nutrition and Foods, and Virginia Cooperative Extension, Virginia Polytechnical Institute and State University, Blacksburg, VA, 1993 (mimeograph).

45. Dalsky, G., Stocke, K., Ehsani, A., Slatopolsky, E., Lee, W., and Birge, S.J., Jr., Weight-bearing exercise training and lumbar bone mineral content in postmenopausaul women, *Ann. Int. Med.*, 108, 824, 1988.

46. Loucks, A.B. and Horvath, S.M., Athletic amenorrhea: a review, *Med. Sci. Sports Exer.*, 17, 45, 1985.

47. Otis, C.L., Exercise-associated amenorhea, *Clin. Sports Med.*, 11, 351, 1992.

48. Schwartz, B., Cumming, D.C., Riordan, E., Selye, M., Yen, S.S.C., and Rebar, R.W., Exercise-associated amenorrhea: a distinct entity?, *Am. J. Obstet. Gynecol.*, 141, 662, 1981.

49. Bullen, B.A., Skrinar, G. S., Beitins, I.Z., vonMering, G., Turnbull, B.A., and McArthur, J.W., Induction of menstrual disorders by strenuous exercise in untrained women, *N. Engl. J. Med.*, 312, 1349, 1985.

50. Hetland, M.L., Haarbo, J., and Christiansen, C., Running induces menstrual disturbances but bone mass is unaffected, except in emenorrheic women, *Am. J. Med.*, 95, 53, 1993.

51. Baker, E.R., Mathur, R.S., Kirk, R.F., and Williamson, H.O., Female runners and secondary amenorrhea: correlation with age, parity, mileage, and plasma hormonal and sex-hormone-binding globulin concentrations, *Fertility Sterility*, 36, 183, 1981.

52. Farrell, P.A., Gustafson, A.B., Gaarthwaite, T.L., Kalthoff, R.K., Cowley, A.W., Jr., and Morgan, W.P., Influence of endogenous opioids on the response of selected hormones to exercise in humans, *J. Appl. Physiol.*, 61, 1051, 1986.

53. Loucks, A.B., Mortola, J.F., Girton, L., and Yen, S.S.C., Alterations in the hypothalamic-pituitary-ovarian and hypothalamic-pituitary-adrenal axes in athletic women, *J. Clin. Endocrinol. Metab.*, 68, 402, 1989.

54. Bonen, A., Ling, W., MacIntyre, K., Neil, R., McGrail, J.C., and Belcastro, A.N., Effects of exercise on the serum concentrations of FSH, LH, progesterone and estradiol, *Eur. J. Appl. Physiol.*, 42, 15, 1979.

55. Boyden, T.W., Paramenter, R.W., Stanforth, P., Rotkis, T., and Wilmore, J.H., Sex steroids and endurance running in women, *Fertility Sterility*, 39, 629, 1983.

56. Snead, D.B., Weltman, A., Weltman, J.A., Evans, W.S., Veldhuis, J.D., Varma, M.M., Teates, C.D., Dowling, E.A., and Rogol, A.D., Reproductive hormones and bone mineral density in women runners, *J. Appl. Physiol.*, 72, 2149, 1992.

57. Osteoporosis: Consensus Conference, *J. Am. Med. Assoc.*, 252, 799, 1984.

58. Schlechte, J.A., Sherman, B., and Martin, R., Bone Density in amenorrheic women with and without hyperprolactinemia, *J. Clin. Endocrinol. Metab.*, 56, 1120, 1983.

59. Lindsay, R., Hart, D.M., Forrest, C., and Baird, C., Prevention of spinal osteoporosis in oophorectomized women, *Lancet*, 2, 1151, 1980.

60. Lloyd, T., Triantafyllou, S.J., Baker, E.R., Houts, P.S., Whiteside, J.A., Kalenak, A., and Stumpf, P.G., Women athletes with menstrual irregularity have increased musculoskeletal injuries, *Med. Sci. Sports Exer.*, 18, 374, 1986.

61. Myburgh, K.H., Hutchins, J., Fataar, A.B., Hough, S.F., and Noakes, T.S., Low bone density is an etiologic factor for stress fractures in athletes, *Ann. Int. Med.*, 113, 754, 1990.

62. Warren, M.P., The effects of exercise on pubertal progression and reproductive function in girls, *J. Clin Endocrinol. Metab.*, 51, 1150, 1980.

63. Barnett, N.P. and Wright, P., Psychological considerations for women in sports, *Clin. Sportsmed.*, 13, 297, 1994.

64. Rosen, L.W., McKeag, D.B., Hough, D.O., and Curley, V., Pathogenic weight-control behavior in female athletes, *Phys. Sportsmed.*, 14, 79, 1986.

65. American Psychiatric Association, *Diagonostic and Statistical Manual of Mental Disorders IV (edition 4)*, Washington, D.C., 1994.

66. Fichter, M.M. and Pirke, K.M., Effect of experimental and pathological weight loss upon the hypothalamo-pituitary-adrenal axis, *Psychoneuroendocrinology*, 11, 295, 1986.

67. Kirchner, E.M., Lewis, R.D., and O'Connor, P.J., Bone mineral density and dietary intake of female college gymnasts, *Med. Sci. Sports Exer.*, 27, 543, 1995.

68. Abrams, S.A., Silber, T.J., Esteban, N.V., Vieira, N.E., Stuff, J.E., Meyers, R., Majd, M., and Yergey, A.L., Mineral balance and bone turnover in adolescents with anorexia nervosa, *J. Pediatr.*, 123, 326, 1993.

69. Bachrach, L.K., Katzman, D.K., Litt, I.F., Guido, D., and Marcus, R., Recovery from osteopenia in adolescent girls with anorexia nervosa, *J. Clin. Endocrinol. Metab.*, 72, 602, 1991.

70. Ettinger, B., Genant, H.K., and Cann, C.E., Postmenopausal bone loss is prevented by treatment with low dosage estrogen with calcium, *Ann. Int. Med.*, 106, 40, 1987.

71. Haenggi, W., Casez, J.P., Birkhaeuser, M.H., Lippuner, K., and Jaeger, P., Bone mineral density in young women with long-standing amenorrhea: limited effect of hormone replacement therapy with ethinylestradiol and desogrestrel, *Osteoporosis Int.*, 4, 99, 1994.

72. Prior, J.C., Vigna, Y.M., Schechter, M.T., and Burgess, A.E., Spinal bone loss and ovulatory disturbances, *N. Engl. J. Med.*, 323, 1221, 1990.

73. Baer, J.T., Taper, L.J., Gwazdauskas, F.G., Walburg, J.L., Novascone, M., Ritchey, S.J., and Thye, F.W., Diet, hormonal, and metabolic factors affecting bone mineral density in adolescent amenorrheic and eumenorrheic female runners, *J. Sports Med. Phys. Fitness*, 32, 51, 1993.

74. Lindberg, J.S., Fears, W.B., Hunt, M.M., Powell, M.R., Boll, D., and Wade, C.E., Exercise-induced amenorrhea and bone density, *Ann. Intern. Med.*, 101, 647, 1984.

75. Myerson, M., Gutin, B., Warren, M.P., Wang, J., Lichtman, S., and Pierson, R.N., Total bone density in amenorrheic runners, *Obstet. Gynecol.*, 79, 973, 1992.

76. Nelson, M.E., Fischer, E.C., Catsos, P.D., Meredith, G.N., Turksoy, R.N., and Evans, W.J., Diet and bone status in amenorrheic runners, *Am. J. Clin. Nutr.*, 43, 910, 1986.

77. Robinson, T., Snow-Harter, C., Gillis, D., Taafe, R., Shaw, J., and Marcus, R., Bone mineral density and menstrual cycle status in competitive female runners and gymnasts, *Med. Sci. Sports Exer.*, 25, S49, 1993.

78. Rutherford, O.M., Spine and total body bone mineral density in amenorrheic endurance athletes, *J. Appl Physiol.*, 74, 2904, 1993.

79. Snead, D.B., Stubbs, C.C., Weltman, J.Y., Evans, W.S., Veldhuis, J.D., Rogol, A.D., Teates, C.D., and Weltman, A., Dietary patterns, eating behaviors, and bone mineral density in women runners, *Am. J. Clin. Nutr.*, 56, 705, 1992.

80. Snow-Harter, C.M., Bone health and prevention of osteoporosis in active and athletic women, *Clin. Sports Med.*, 13, 398, 1994.

81. Wolman, R.L., Clark, P., McNally, E., Harries, M.G., and Reeve, J., Dietary calcium as a statistical determinant of spinal trabecular bone density in amenorrheic and oestrogen-replete athletes, *Bone Miner.*, 17, 415, 1992.

82. Young, N., Formica, C., Szmukler, G., and Seeman, E., Bone density at weight-bearing and nonweight-bearing sites in ballet dancers: the effects of exercise, hypogonadism, and body weight, *J.Clin. Endocrinol. Metab.*, 78, 449, 1994.

83. American Psychiatric Association, *Diagnostic and Statistical Manual of Mental Disorders IV (edition 4)*, Washington, D.C., 1994.

Chapter 10

NUTRITIONAL ANTIOXIDANTS AND PHYSICAL ACTIVITY

_____ Mitchell M. Kanter

CONTENTS

I. INTRODUCTION

The processes of oxidant stress and subsequent free radical production and their pertinence to physical exercise have received much scrutiny in the past decade. Various lay publications, clinicians, and some scientists have gone so far as to intimate that free radicals are responsible for the apparent spate of pathologies that seem to have afflicted many elite-level distance athletes in recent years.

Although a number of epidemiological and cross-sectional studies are suggestive of a link between free radical production, ingestion of diets low in some antioxidants, and a number of disease processes,[1,2] there are no strong data (epidemiological or otherwise) that could even remotely link physical exercise to the early onset of diseases induced by free radicals. Nevertheless, there is a growing belief in some quarters that there is a "dark side" to physical exercise. This belief is buoyed, to an extent, by the fact that habitual physical exercise, which promotes a number of adaptations that should make an individual stronger and healthier (e.g., increased cardiac function, improved glucose tolerance, lower blood pressure in hypertensives), has still not been shown to be an effective means of improving mean or maximal lifespan in most organisms.

Although most species are endowed with a ubiquitous enzymatic antioxidant defense system, it has also been suggested that physical exercise may outstrip the body's endogenous defenses. If this is true, it is theoretically possible that exercise can serve to make an individual more susceptible to free radical-induced muscle damage, muscle soreness, and infection, among other things. Therefore, the use of ingestible antioxidants has been recommended as a means of providing additional protection against potential exercise-induced free radical damage.

A consensus of opinion regarding the role of physical activity in the initiation of free radical-mediated reactions, the damage that may be evoked by exercise-induced free radicals, and the possible efficacy of diets rich in antioxidants (or supplements) has not been firmly established. Nevertheless, there is a large and growing body of literature concerning these issues. After a brief presentation on free radical chemistry, this chapter will review the available literature on exercise-induced free radical generation and lipid peroxidation, as well as the known effects of various nutritional antioxidants, including vitamins C and E, and other antioxidant mixtures.

II.   FREE RADICALS AND LIPID PEROXIDATION: THEIR RELEVANCE TO PHYSICAL ACTIVITY

A free radical may be defined as a molecule with one or more unpaired electrons in an orbital.[3] The presence of unpaired electrons tends to make a molecular species highly reactive, and when these reactive molecules come in contact with other stable molecules they can set in motion a sequence of potentially damaging reactions. Among other things, free radical chain reactions can damage protein, lipid, and DNA structures.

Various studies have indicated that free radical production in biological systems may be increased secondary to an elevation in oxygen consumption.[4-6] It has been estimated that between 2–5% of the oxygen reduced via the mitochondrial electron transport chain is converted to hydrogen peroxide and free radicals.[7,8] In addition, increases in circulating catecholamine levels,[9] lactic acid production,[10] and core temperature,[11] as well as transient hypoxia and reoxygenation of tissues[12] have all been implicated as promoters of free radicals. Any or all of these phenomena may occur during or as a result of physical activity; therefore, exercise has been strongly implicated as a key initiator of free radicals.

Although proteins and DNA are generally the most prevalent targets of biological attack by free radicals, it is the damage that affects lipids, or lipid peroxidation, that has been the most well-researched biological phenomenon occurring as a result of free radical generation. Lipid peroxidation is the oxidative deterioration of polyunsaturated fats.[13] It involves the reaction of oxygen and polyunsaturated lipids to form lipid free radicals and hydroperoxide radicals, which in turn promote additional free radical reactions.[14] (*Note:* Lipid peroxidation is often thought of as a process that evokes negative biological consequences. It should be remembered, however, that it serves a role in a number of biosynthetic reactions and, as such, promotes numerous positive and necessary consequences as well.[3])

In light of the fact that cell membranes are composed to a large extent of polyunsaturated lipids and various protein structures, they are generally a key site of free radical attack.[15] Furthermore, the presence of iron (which serves as a potent catalyst in the generation of free radicals)[16] in mitochondrial membranes further increases the susceptibility of this organelle to free radical attack. The relevance of this phenomenon as it relates to physical exercise is clear if one remembers that the mitochondria are the key cellular sites of aerobic metabolism; the simultaneous presence of unsaturated lipids, oxygen, unpaired electrons, and iron in the mitochondrial membrane are what apparently makes this organelle particularly sensitive to free radical mediated damage.

III. ROLE OF SCAVENGER ENZYMES

It has become increasingly obvious that aerobic organisms are continually exposed to agents that promote oxidant stress, both endogenously (via respiration) and exogenously (via pollutants, drug, etc.). Millions of years ago as the atmosphere was transformed from an anaerobic environment to a largely aerobic environment, organisms were forced to evolve mechanisms not only for the utilization of oxygen but also for defense against its toxic by-products.[17] As a result, aerobic organisms possess several different mechanisms that provide protection against uncontrolled free radical reactions.[14] The enzymes superoxide dismutase, glutathione peroxidase, and catalase are part of this elaborate defense system that is present in mammalian cells. Along with support enzymes such as glutathione reductase and glucose-6-phosphate dehydrogenase,[18] these enzymes work in concert to detoxify free radicals produced as a result of daily living.

Numerous studies have demonstrated that habitual physical exercise serves to increase the activity of various antioxidant enzymes in a number of tissues,[19-25] suggesting greater protection. Nevertheless, some researchers have suggested that the increased generation of reactive oxygen species during physical exercise may outstrip the inherent protective capacity of our endogenous defense system,[26,27] thus providing a rationale for the use of exogenous antioxidant supplements by individuals who habitually perform strenuous physical exercise.

IV. ANTIOXIDANT NUTRIENTS

There are a number of nutritional components with purported antioxidant properties (for example, see Table 1). However, in recent years the major focus of nutritional research has been on the vitamins E and C and beta carotene (a vitamin A precursor). Of these nutrients, vitamin E is of particular importance because of its association with cell membranes.[28] Vitamin E is often used synonymously with the term alpha tocopherol. In fact, vitamin E is a generic term for all of the tocopherols and tocotrienols, of which there are eight naturally occurring vitamin E derivatives.[29] Alpha tocopherol has the highest biological availability of the vitamin E derivatives. Vitamin E acts as a cell membrane stabilizer;[28] it can scavenge a number of free radicals, including the damaging singlet oxygen radical.[30]

Principle food sources of vitamin E include vegetable oils, nuts, wheat germ, and seed oils. Fruits, vegetables, and meats contain small amounts of vitamin E. Vitamin E deficiency is extremely rare in healthy human subjects,[31] and most of our understanding of deficiency symptoms has been gleaned from animal studies.[32] In rats, vitamin E deficiency promotes a decline in endurance performance and a decline in mitochondrial respiratory control.[4]

It should be noted that foods high in carbohydrate tend to be low in vitamin E. Therefore, people who habitually ingest high carbohydrate, low fat diets may inadvertently be consuming marginal to low vitamin E diets, and those consuming high polyunsaturated fat diets may require greater-than-RDA intakes of vitamin E.[33-35]

At the other extreme, vitamin E toxicity is not widely reported in humans, and intakes as high as 200 times the recommended dietary allowance have been administered without apparent negative consequences.[36]

Vitamin C is an essential water soluble vitamin, and it is considered the most important antioxidant in the watery fluids outside the body cells.[37] A primary role of vitamin C is to aid in the regeneration of oxidized vitamin E. Vitamin C also quenches singlet oxygen and other water soluble radicals.[38]

TABLE 1   Key Nutrients that Display Direct or Indirect Antioxidant Properties

Vitamin E

Quenches singlet oxygen
Stabilizes superoxide anion
Stabilizes hydroxyl radical

Vitamin C

Quenches singlet oxygen
Stabilizes hydroxyl radical
Regenerates reduced vitamin E

Beta Carotene

Quenches singlet oxygen

Copper
Zinc

Component of cytosolic superoxide dismutase

Manganese

Component of mitochondrial superoxide dismutase

Selenium

Component of glutathione peroxidase

Iron

Component of catalase

Although vitamin C deficiency symptoms (such as scurvy) are well documented, the problem of vitamin C deficiency has largely been eradicated in Westernized countries because of the prevalence and availability of ascorbate-rich foods in most cultures. Good food sources of vitamin C include citrus fruits, cantaloupes, tomatoes, strawberries, green leafy vegetables, and cauliflower.

Because vitamin C activity in foods can be compromised by factors such as heat and light[37] and physiological demand for vitamin C can apparently be affected by environmental factors such as smog, cigarette smoke, etc.,[32] many scientists and nutritionists believe that present RDA levels for ascorbate are inadequate for most people.[39] However, chronic megadose ingestion of ascorbate supplements are not benign. Various studies have indicated an increase in renal stone formation,[40] gastrointestinal disturbances,[41] erythrocyte hemolysis,[42] and numerous other pathologies in patients who habitually ingested high doses of vitamin C. Vitamin C has also demonstrated prooxidant properties *in vitro*,[43] and it has been suggested that megadose vitamin C intakes can predispose some individuals to iron overload toxicity symptoms.[43]

Beta carotene is one of a group of compounds called carotenoids that are part of the red, orange, and yellow pigments found in many plants. Beta carotene is the most well-researched of the carotenoids, and it has been shown in *in vitro* studies to quench superoxide anions as well as singlet oxygen.[44,45] There are actually more than 650 natural carotenoids; many of these carotenoids, such as lutein, zeaxanthin, and lycopene, may have more potent antioxidant effects than beta carotene, although additional research regarding their antioxidant properties is necessary.

Additional compounds with purported antioxidant properties include ubiquinone, which also serves as a redox component in the electron transport chain; glutathione, which has been reported to scavenge hydroxyl radicals and singlet oxygen and to regenerate vitamin E;[46] and selenium, which functions primarily as a component of the glutathione peroxidase enzyme.

V.   ANTIOXIDANTS AND EXERCISE PERFORMANCE

In well-fed subjects, data regarding the potential ergogenic effects of antioxidant supplements suggest little or no benefit. Early studies done by Cureton[47] in the 1950s suggested that vitamin E (via wheat germ oil) could enhance physical performance. However, doubts have been raised regarding the results of these studies because of numerous methodological problems. More recent studies have failed to show an effect of either vitamin E[48-50] or vitamin C[51-53] supplementation on aerobic or anaerobic performance. An exception is a study by Simon-Schnass and Pabst,[54] who reported positive alterations in the anaerobic threshold in mountain climbers who consumed 400 mg vitamin E/day for 10 weeks at altitude. Few studies at sea level have reported as dramatic an effect.

When a vitamin deficiency exists (particularly vitamin E), however, numerous studies have demonstrated a decrement in physical performance, strongly suggesting that supplementation can be beneficial under these conditions. Davies et al.[4] and Gohil et al.[55] demonstrated decrements in running performance in rats maintained on a vitamin E-deficient diet. Vitamin E deficiency has also been reported to decrease oxidative phosphorylation in liver, increase red cell hemolysis, and decrease respiratory control in muscle.[56] Any of these perturbations would more than likely produce a decrement in physical performance as well.

A decrement in running performance was also reported by Packer et al.[57] in guinea pigs maintained on a vitamin C deficient diet. However, few additional studies have looked at the effects of vitamin C deficiency on physical performance in large measure because most animal species are capable of de novo ascorbate synthesis.

Selenium and glutathione deficiencies have also been studied in exercising subjects. Selenium deficiency reportedly increased lipid peroxidation in rat skeletal muscle mitochondria,[58] and Goldfarb and Sen[46] reported that glutathione-deficient rats could run only half as far as saline control animals.

VI.   LIPID PEROXIDATION, MUSCLE INJURY, AND OTHER SEQUELAE TO PHYSICAL ACTIVITY

If antioxidants are to exert a beneficial effect in exercising individuals, it is likely that the processes of tissue damage, lipid peroxidation, and/or immune function, rather than performance, would be affected in a positive manner. Although current data are far from conclusive, a number of studies tend to suggest that this is in fact the case.

A recent report by Hartmann et al.[59] indicated that short-term vitamin E supplementation (800 mg administered 12 and 2 h prior to exercise and 22 h after exercise) reduced DNA damage in peripheral white blood cells following exhaustive exercise. Following 2 weeks of supplementation with 1200 mg vitamin E/day, a diminution in DNA damage was noted as well.

These data support earlier studies by Sumida et al.[60] who reported a decrease in serum enzyme markers indicative of tissue damage in human subjects who consumed 300 mg vitamin E for 4 weeks and Cannon et al.[61] who demonstrated a more rapid decline in serum creatine kinase levels following exercise in subjects who ingested 800 mg vitamin E for 48 days. In addition, a recent report by Rokitzi et al.[62] indicated that subjects who ingested a mixture of 400 IU vitamin E and 200 mg vitamin C per day for 4.5 weeks prior to a marathon demonstrated a smaller post-race rise in serum CK levels than subjects who consumed a placebo.

In a critical review of the literature regarding the significance of vitamin E in physical activity, Kagan et al.[63] cite a number of animal trials that demonstrated that the requirement from vitamin E is elevated significantly with intense exercise. For example, Jackson et al.[64] noted that vitamin E supplementation (240 mg for 42–45 days) promoted less severe muscle damage in exercised rats and mice than did a control diet and that vitamin E deficient animals were more susceptible to tissue damage than their standard fed or supplemented counterparts.

However, it should be noted that contradictory studies do exist. Kanter and Eddy,[65] Warren et al.,[66] Robertson et al.,[67] and Helgheim et al.[68] have all reported no effects of vitamin E supplementation on serum enzyme changes post exercise.

Kanter and Eddy[65] and Warren et al.[66] used eccentric exercise in their studies. Furthermore, many of the aforementioned studies employed different vitamin dosing regimens and different intensities of physical activity. Any or all of these differences in research design may account for the variations in the data.

In recent years, numerous studies have suggested that antioxidant supplementation could suppress the exercise-induced rise in various lipid peroxide markers. In light of the fact that a relationship between markers of lipid peroxidation and tissue damage has been reported,[69,70] a diminution in exercise induced lipid peroxide markers could have acute and longer term physiological implications.

Typical of these studies is the report by Sumida et al.,[60] in which 4 weeks of vitamin E supplementation significantly decreased the serum level of TBARS (thiobarbituric acid reactive substances — a commonly used marker of lipid peroxide formation) in human subjects.

The results of Sumida et al.[60] support the earlier findings of Dillard et al.,[71] who reported a decrease in expired pentane levels (pentane is a marker of linoleic acid peroxidation) following exercise in subjects who ingested 1200 IU vitamin E daily for 2 weeks, and Kanter et al.,[72] who noted a decline in serum TBARS and expired pentane at rest and following exercise in subjects who ingested a mixture of vitamin E (800 IU/day), vitamin C (1000 mg/day), and beta carotene (30 mg/day) for 4 weeks.

Data from "alternative" human populations have suggested a benefit of vitamin E supplementation as well. In a series of studies, Meydani et al.[73,74] found that vitamin E supplements (800 IU/day for 48 days) diminished markers of lipid peroxidation in older subjects, and the aforementioned study by Simon-Schnass and Pabst[54] demonstrated lower breath pentane in vitamin E-supplemented mountain climbers who performed strenuous work at altitude.

Studies with animals have produced similar results. For example, Goldfarb and Sen[46] noted a decline in TBARS in skeletal muscle and blood of supplemented (250 IU vitamin E/day for 5 weeks) rats, and Brady et al.[75] reported similar findings in liver of rats swum to exhaustion following 4 weeks of supplementation. Kumar et al.[76] found that supplementation with vitamin E for 60 days significantly decreased the exercise-induced rise in cardiac malondialdehyde levels in rats exercised to exhaustion.

A number of studies involving vitamin C supplementation have also suggested enhanced protection in exercising subjects. Jakeman and Maxwell[77] demonstrated that vitamin C (400 mg/day for 21 days) promoted less low-frequency fatigue (indicative of exercise-induced muscle damage) than did vitamin E or a placebo. Recovery of maximal voluntary contraction during a 24 hour period post-exercise was also greater in vitamin C supplemented subjects. Kaminski and Boal[78] reported less calf muscle soreness in subjects who consumed 3 g vitamin C for 3 days prior to and 4 days after strenuous calf exercise.

Peters et al.[79] noted that runners who consumed 600 mg vitamin C for 3 weeks prior to a 42 km race reported fewer cases of upper respiratory tract infection than did runners who were not supplemented. On the other hand, a recent report by Nieman et al.[80] found no effect of vitamin C supplementation (1000 mg/day for 1 week) on various indices of immune function following a 2.5 hour run. The relatively short supplementation period in the Nieman study may have accounted in part for these apparently contradictory findings. Regardless, in none of these studies did the investigators measure markers of lipid peroxidation or oxidant stress. Therefore, it is impossible to ascertain if their observations are supportive of the link between exercise, vitamin C supplementation, and free radical generation.

Data to support the potential protective role of other individual antioxidant supplements in exercising subjects are scarce. Information does exist to support the need for selenium supplements, for example, in selenium-deficient animals who perform physical exercise.[58,81] However, well-fed animals who exercise apparently do not derive a benefit from selenium supplements. Similarly, research on well-fed, exercising human subjects does not support the need for coenzyme Q_{10} supplements,[82-84] and no studies to date have looked at the individual effects of beta carotene in physically active subjects. Studies in which subjects consumed beta carotene as part of a supplement containing other nutrients have suggested a possible beneficial effect in diminishing exercise-induced lipid peroxidation and tissue damage.[39,85]

VII. TO SUPPLEMENT OR NOT TO SUPPLEMENT?

Despite the growing interest of the scientific community on the relationship between physical activity, free radical generation, and lipid peroxidation, it is still impossible to state with certainty whether active people would benefit by consuming an antioxidant supplement. Despite the relatively large number of studies performed to date on a number of antioxidant nutrients (most notably vitamin E), the lack of uniformity in study design has made it difficult to compare results from study to study. Differences in exercise protocol, vitamin dosing regimens, and supplements employed, among other things, have compounded our inability to draw more definitive conclusions from the data. Coupled with the fact that various markers that are purported to measure free radical-mediated lipid peroxidation and tissue damage have been questioned for their reliability and specificity,[86,87] interpretation of results is often difficult as well.

Furthermore, it has long been assumed that dead or dying cells undergo lipid peroxidation more readily than normal cells,[88] leading some scientists to the question whether free radicals and lipid peroxides are actually produced in abundance during physical activity and subsequently contribute to tissue damage, or if they are primarily a product of exercise induced damage and its resultant enhancement in the immune response. Questions such as these are not trivial and need to be answered more fully if we are to be in a position to accurately predict the antioxidant needs of the active person or sportsman.

Nevertheless, trends in the available literature certainly suggest that antioxidant supplements can be beneficial for active people under certain conditions. In a recent article, Blumberg[89] suggested that whether an individual or a population should consider choosing a nutritional supplement is dependent on a number of key factors. These include: the probability that the intervention is efficacious; the probability that the scientific evidence is correct; the probability that increasing intake/status is toxic; the cost of the intervention; and the impact of delaying a potentially beneficial recommendation. Based on these criteria, it seems likely that physically active people will, at worst, be spending money unnecessarily if they choose to supplement and, at best, will derive a real benefit from supplementation.

This is not to imply that indiscriminate supplementation poses no risks. As stated earlier, chronic megadose intakes of vitamin C, for example, have been associated with iron-overload toxicity symptoms,[43] among other things, and the potential negative effects of long-term, high-dose intakes of supplements such as coenzyme Q_{10}, glutathione, etc. are largely unknown.

Recent data from a number of longitudinal population studies, most notable the National Health and Nutrition Examination Survey (NHANES) study,[90] strongly suggest that foods that tend to be high in traditional antioxidant nutrients (i.e., fruits, vegetables), tend to be low in the typical Western-style diet. In fact, the NHANES data indicate that more than 90% of the study participants consume less than recommended daily amounts of fruits and vegetables.

These data certainly lend credence to the notion that people in general, and active people in particular, might benefit by increasing their daily antioxidant intake.

Furthermore, it has been suggested that the amount of vitamin E supplied in the "normal" American diet is about two-thirds of the recommended daily value.[46] Coupled with the fact that the standard recommendation for physically active people is to eat a diet high in carbohydrate, low in total fat, and proportionally high in polyunsaturated fat (that is, a diet that tends to be low in vitamin E), the benefits of supplementation for active people cannot be discounted.

This chapter has focused primarily on the potential benefits of a small number of nutrients, notably vitamins C and E, for physically active people, largely because the majority of the available literature deals with these nutrients. It should be noted, however, that numerous other nutrients serve as a part of the body's antioxidant defense system, principally in conjunction with the various antioxidant enzymes. For example, copper and zinc are a part of the structure of cytosolic superoxide dismutase (SOD); manganese is part of mitochondrial SOD; selenium is necessary for glutathione peroxidase activity; and iron serves as a part of the structure of catalase. As mentioned previously, all of these enzymes play a role in the detoxification of free radicals, and numerous studies have demonstrated that the activity of these enzymes is affected by both acute and chronic physical exercise.[19-25] Therefore, the possibility that the requirements for any or all of these nutrients might be different in people who exercise habitually cannot be ruled out.

Finally, the question as to whether an individual should attempt to derive his or her nutrients via the diet or by supplementation merits some discussion. Although it is beyond the scope of this review to fully discuss the pros and cons of whole foods versus supplements, it should be pointed out that nutrients taken in isolation are not always adequately absorbed into the body. In our laboratory, we have attempted to administer vitamin E supplements in pill form with water to subjects prior to exercise, and we found that the vitamin was not absorbed for at least 4 hours after ingestion. When the pill was administered subsequent to a meal containing a nominal amount of fat, absorption was more rapid and complete (unpublished observation). This suggests that whole foods or combinations of foods and beverages consumed together can often promote greater absorption and, potentially, greater protection.

VIII.   SUMMARY

Numerous studies suggest that physical exercise can promote a rise in free radical production and subsequent lipid peroxidation via a number of mechanisms, including a rise in oxygen consumption, and elevations in circulating catecholamine levels, lactic acid production, and core body temperature.[4,5,9-11] It has further been suggested that strenuous or prolonged exercise may unduly tax the body's endogenous antioxidant defenses, necessitating the consumption of additional antioxidant nutrients.[26,27]

Research on a number of antioxidant nutrients, most notably vitamin E, suggest that this may be the case. Various studies have indicated that vitamin E can decrease blood and tissue markers purportedly indicative of lipid peroxidation and tissue damage.[4,54,55] It has also been demonstrated that subjects who consumed high levels of vitamin C prior to a marathon running event (42 km) suffered fewer incidences of upper respiratory tract infection following the race than their non-supplemented counterparts.[79] However, it should be noted that a number of studies that indicate no benefit of antioxidant nutrient consumption exist as well.

The contradictory data that presently exist may be the result of differences in dosing regimens, exercise protocols, subject populations, and/or a combination of these factors. A lack of sensitive and specific *in vivo* markers of lipid peroxidation, free radical generation, and tissue damage have also contributed to our relative lack of understanding regarding the potential of antioxidant nutrients for active people.

Based on the literature, it seems unlikely that moderate supplementation with vitamins C and E (approximately 400 mg of vitamin C/day; 400 IU of vitamin E/day) will cause harm and might serve as an "insurance policy" for physically active people. Future research with more sophisticated methodologies will undoubtedly shed more light on this issue.

REFERENCES

1. Halliwell, B., Oxidants and human disease: some new concepts, *FASEB J.,* 1, 358, 1987.
2. Kanter, M.M., Free radicals, exercise and antioxidant supplementation, *Intl. J. Sport Nutr.,* 4, 205, 1994.
3. Halliwell, B. and Chirico, S., Lipid peroxidation: its mechanism, measurement and significance, *Am. J. Clin. Nutr.,* 57(Suppl.), 715S, 1993.
4. Davies, K.J.A., Quintanilha, A.T., Brooks, G.A., and Packer, L., Free radicals and tissue damage produced by exercise, *Biochem. Biophys. Res. Comm.,* 107, 1198, 1982.
5. Jenkins, R.R., Free radical chemistry: relationship to exercise, *Sports Med.,* 5, 156, 1988.
6. Sjodin, B., Hellsten Westing, Y., and Apple, F.S., Biochemical mechanisms for oxygen free radical formation during exercise, *Sports Med.,* 10, 236, 1990.
7. Chance, B., Eleff, S., and Leigh, J.S., Jr., Noninvasive, nondestructive approaches to cell bioenergetics, *Proc. Natl. Acad. Sci. U.S.A.,* 77, 7430, 1980.
8. Loschen, S., Azzi, A., and Flohe, L., Mitochondrial H_2O_2 formation: relationship with energy conservation, *FEBS Lett.,* 33, 84, 1973.
9. Cohen, G. and Heikkila, R., The generation of hydrogen peroxide, superoxide and hydroxyl radical by 6-hydroxydopamine dialuric acid and related cytotoxic agents, *J. Biol. Chem.,* 249, 2447, 1974.
10. Demopoulos, H.B, Santomier, J.P., Seligman, M.L., and Pietronigro, D.D., Free radical pathology: Rationale and toxicology of antioxidants and other supplements in sports medicine and exercise science, in *Sport, Health and Nutrition,* Katch, F.I., Ed., Human Kinetics Publishers, Champaign, IL, 1986, 139.
11. Salo, D.C., Donovan, C.M, and Davies, K.J.A., HSP70 and other possible heat shock or oxidative stress proteins are induced in skeletal muscle, heart and liver during exericse, *Free Rad. Biol. Med.,* 11, 239, 1991.
12. Merry, P., Kidd, B.L., Claxson, A., and Blake, D.R., Synovitis of the joint is an example of reperfusion injury, in *Free Radicals, Metal Ions and Biopolymers,* Beaumont, P.C., Kidd, B.L., Claxson, A., and Blake, D.R., Eds., Richelieu Press, London, 1989, 199.
13. Tappel., A., Lipid peroxidation damage to cell components, *Fed. Proc.,* 32, 1870, 1973.
14. Bus, J.S. and Gibson, J.E., Lipid peroxidation and its role in toxicology, in *Reviews in Biochemical Toxicology, Vol. 1,* Bend, J.R, Hodgson, E., and Philpot, R.M., Eds., North-Holland, New York, 1979, 125.
15. Demopoulos, H.B., The basis of free radical pathology, *Fed. Proc.,* 32, 1859, 1973.
16. McCord, J.M. and Day, E.D., Jr., Superoxide dependent production of hydroxyl radical catalyzed by iron-EDTA complex, *FEBS Lett.,* 86, 139, 1978.
17. Fridovich, I., Superoxide dismutase in biology and medicine, in *Pathology of Oxygen,* Autor, A., Ed., Academic Press, New York, 1982, 1.
18. Vina, J., *Glutahione: Metabolism and Physiological Function,* Vina, J., Ed., CRC Press, Boca Raton, FL, 1993.
19. Alessio, H.M. and Goldfarb, A.H., Lipid peroxidation and scavenger enzymes during exercise: adaptive response to training, *J. Appl. Physiol.,* 64, 1333, 1988.
20. Hammeren, J., Powers, S., Lawler, J., Criswell, D., Lowenthal, D., and Pollock, M., Exercise training-induced alterations in skeletal muscle oxidative and antioxidant enzyme activity, *Int. J. Sports Med.,* 13, 412, 1993.
21. Higuchi, M., Cartier, L.J., Chen, M., and Holloszy, J.O., Superoxide dismutase and catalase in skeletal muscle: adaptive response to exercise, *J. Gerontol.,* 40, 281, 1985.
22. Jenkins, R.R., Friedland, R., and Howald, H., The relationship of oxygen uptake to superoxide dismutase and catalase activity in human muscle, *Int. J. Sports Med.,* 95, 11, 1984.
23. Ji, L.L. and Fu, R.G., Responses of glutathione system and antioxidant enzymes to exhaustive exercise and hydroperoxide, *J. Appl. Physiol.,* 72, 549, 1992.
24. Ji, L.L., Fu, R.G., and Mitchell, E.W., Glutathione and antioxidant enzymes in skeletal muscle: effects of fiber type and exercise intensity, *J. Appl. Physiol.,* 73, 1854, 1992.
25. Kanter, M.M., Hamlin, R.L., Unverferth, D.V., Davis, H.W., and Merola, A.J., Effect of exercise training on antioxidant enzymes and cardiotoxicity of doxorubicin, *J. Appl. Physiol.,* 59, 1298, 1985.
26. Ohno, H., Sato, Y., Yamashita, K., Doi, R., Arai, K., Kondo, T., and Taniguchi, N., The effect of brief physical exercise on free radical scavenging enzyme systems in human red blood cells, *Can J. Physiol. Pharmacol.,* 64, 1263, 1986.
27. Pincemail, J., Derby, C., Camus, G., Pirnay, F., Bouchez, R., and Massaux, L., Tocopherol mobilization during intensive exercise, *Arch. Int. Physiol. Biochem.,* 94, S43, 1986.
28. Bjorneboe, A., Bjorneboe, G.A., and Drevon, C.A., Absorption, transport and distribution of vitamin E, *J. Nutr.,* 120, 233, 1990.

29. Fritsma, G.A., Vitamin E and autoxidation, *Am. J. Med. Tech.*, 49, 453, 1983.
30. Fahrenholtz, S.R., Doleiden, F.H., Trozzolo, A.M., and Lamola, A.A., On the quenching of singlet oxygen by alpha-tocopherol, *Photochem. Photobiol.*, 20, 505, 1974.
31. Losowsky, M.S. and Leonard, P.J., Evidence of vitamin E deficiency in patients with malabsorption or alcoholism and the effects of therapy, *Gut*, 8, 539, 1967.
32. Zapsilas, C. and Anderle Beck, R., *Food Chemistry and Nutritional Biochemistry*, John Wiley and Sons, 1985, 273.
33. Buckingham, K.W., Effect of dietary polyunsaturated/saturated fatty acid ratio and dietary vitamin E on lipid peroxidation in the rat, *J. Nutr.*, 115, 1425, 1985.
34. Harris, P.L. and Embree, N.D., Quantitative consideration of the effect of polyunsaturated fatty acid content of the diet upon the requirements for vitamin E, *Am. J. Clin. Nutr.*, 13, 385, 1963.
35. Food and Nutrition Board, National Research Council, *Recommended Dietary Allowances*, 10th ed., National Academy Press, Washington, D.C., 1989.
36. Bendich, A. and Machlin, L.J., Safety of oral intake of vitamin E, *Am. J. Clin. Nutr.*, 48, 1088, 1988.
37. Bendich, A., Machlin, L.J., Scandurra, O., Burton, G.W., and Wayner, D.D.M., The antioxidant role of vitamin C, *Adv. Free Radical Biol. Med.*, 2, 419, 1986.
38. Frei, B., England, L., and Ames, B.N., Ascorbate is an outstanding antioxidant in human blood plasma, *Proc. Natl. Acad. Sci. U.S.A.*, 86, 6377, 1989.
39. Kanter, M.M., Free radicals and exercise: effects of nutritional antioxidant supplementation, in *Exercise and Sports Sciences Reviews*, Holloszy, J., Ed., 1995, 23.
40. Briggs, M.H., Garcia-Webb, P., and Davies, P., Urinary oxalate and vitamin C supplements, *Lancet*, 2, 201, 1973.
41. Coulehan, J.L., Kapner, L., Eberhard, S., Taylor, F.J., and Rogers, K.D., Vitamin C and upper respiratory illness in Navajo children: preliminary observations, *Ann. N.Y. Acad. Sci.*, 258, 513, 1974.
42. Mengel, C.E. and Greene, H.L., Ascorbic acid effects on erythrocyte, *Ann. Intern. Med.*, 84, 490, 1976.
43. Herbert, V., Does Mega-C do more good than harm, or more harm than good?, *Nutr. Today*, Jan/Feb, 28, 1993.
44. Bendich, A., Carotenoids and the immune response, *J. Nutr.*, 119, 112, 1989.
45. Isler, O., Ed., *Carotenoids*, Berkhauser Verlag, Basel, 1971.
46. Goldfarb, A.H. and Sen, C.K., Antioxidant supplementation and the control of oxygen toxicity during exercise, in *Exercise and Oxygen Toxicity*, Sen, C., Packer, L., and Hanninen, O., Eds., Elsevier Press, New York, 1994.
47. Cureton, T.K., Effect of wheat germ oil and vitamin E on normal human subjects in physical training programs, *Am. J. Physiol.*, 179, 628, 1954.
48. Sharman, I.M., Down, M.G., and Sen, R.N., The effects of vitamin E and training on physiological function and athletic performance in adolescent swimmers, *Br. J. Nutr.*, 6, 256, 1971.
49. Shephard, R.J., Campbell, R., Pimm, P., Stuart, D., and Wright, G.R., Vitamin E, exercise, and the recovery from physical activity, *Eur. J. Appl. Physiol.*, 33, 119, 1974.
50. Talbot, D. and Jamieson, J., An examination of the effect of vitamin E on the performance of highly trained swimmers, *Can. J. Appl. Sport Sci.*, 2, 67, 1977.
51. Bramich, K. and McNaughton, L., The effects of two levels of ascorbic acid on muscular endurance, muscular strength and on VO_2 max, *Int. Clin. Nutr. Rev.*, 7, 5, 1987.
52. Keith, R.E., Vitamins in sport and exercise, in *Nutrition in Exercise and Sport*, Hickson, J.E. and Wolinsky, I., Eds., CRC Press, Boca Raton, FL, 1989, 233.
53. Keren, G. and Epstein, Y., The effect of high dosage vitamin C intake on aerobic and anaerobic capacity, *J. Sports Med.*, 20, 145, 1980.
54. Simon-Schnass, I. and Pabst, H., Influence of vitamin E on physical performance, *Int. J. Vit. Nutr. Res.*, 58, 49, 1988.
55. Gohil, K., Packer, L., De Lumen, B., Brooks, G.A., and Terblanche, S.E., Vitamin E deficiency and vitamin C supplements: exercise and mitochondrial oxidation, *J. Appl. Physiol.*, 60, 1986, 1986.
56. Sen, C.K., Oxidants and antioxidants in exercise, *J. Appl. Physiol.*, 79, 675, 1995.
57. Packer, L., Gohil, K., DeLumen, B., and Terblanche, S.E., A comparative study on the effects of ascorbic acid deficiency and supplementation on endurance and mitochondrial oxidative capacities in various tissues of the guinea pig, *Comp. Biochem. Physiol.*, 83B, 235, 1986.
58. Ji, L.L., Stratman, F.W., and Lardy, H.A., Antioxidant enzyme systems in rat liver and skeletal muscle, *Arch. Biochem. Biophys.*, 263, 150, 1988.
59. Hartman, A., Nieb, A.M., Grunert-Fuchs, M., Poch, B., and Speit, G., Vitamin E prevents exercise-induced DNA damage, *Mutation Res.*, 346, 195, 1995.
60. Sumida, S., Tanaka, K., Kitao, H., and Nakadomo, F., Exercise-induced lipid peroxidation and leakage of enzymes before and after vitamin E supplementation, *Int. J. Biochem.*, 21, 835, 1989.
61. Cannon, J.G., Orencole, S.F., Fielding, R.A., Meydani, M., Meydani, S.N., Fiaterone, M.A., Blumberg, J.B., and Evans, W.J., Acute phase response to exercise: interaction of age and vitamin E on neutrophils and muscle enzyme release, *Am. J. Physiol.*, 259, R1214, 1990.

62. Rokitzi, L., Logemann, E., Sagredos, A.N., Murphy, M., Wetzel-Roth, W., and Keul, J., Lipid peroxidation and antioxidative vitamins under extreme endurance stress, *Acta Physiol. Scand.*, 154, 149, 1994b.

63. Kagan, V.E., Spirichev, V.B., Serbinova, E.A., Witt, E., Erin, A.N., and Packer, L., The significance of vitamin E and free radicals in physical exercise, in *Nutrition in Exercise and Sport, 2nd Edition*, Wolinsky, I. and Hickson, J., Jr., Eds., CRC Press, Boca Raton, FL, 1994, 185.

64. Jackson, M.J., Jones, D.A., and Edwards, R.H.T., Biology of vitamin E, in *Proceedings of a Ciba Foundation Symposium*, Porter, R. and Wheelan, J., Eds., Pitman Medical Ltd., London, 1983, 224.

65. Kanter, M.M. and Eddy, D.E., Effect of antioxidant supplementation on serum markers of lipid peroxidation and skeletal muscle damage following eccentric exercise, *Med. Sci. Sport Exer.*, 24, S17, 1992.

66. Warren, J.A., Jenkins, R.R., Packer, L., Witt, E.H., and Armstrong, R.B., Elevated muscle vitamin E does not attenuate eccentric exercise-induced muscle injury, *J. Appl. Physiol.*, 72, 2168, 1992.

67. Robertson, J.D., Crosbie, L., Maughan, R.J., Leiper, J.B., and Duthie, G.C., Influence of vitamin E supplementation on muscle damage following endurance exercise, *Int. J. Vit. Nutr. Res.*, 60,171, 1990.

68. Helgheim, I., Hetland, O., Nilsson, S., Ingjer, F., and Stromme, S.B., The effects of vitamin E on serum enzyme levels following heavy exercise, *Eur. J. Appl. Physiol.*, 40, 283, 1979.

69. Guaduel, Y., Menasche, P., and Duvelleroy, M., Enzyme release and mitochondrial activity in reoxygenated cardiac muscle: relationship with oxygen-induced lipid peroxidation, *Gen. Physiol. Biophys.*, 8, 327, 1989.

70. Kanter, M.M., Lesmes, G.R., Kaminsky, L.A., La Ham-Saeger, J., and Nequin, N.D., Serum creatine kinase and lactate dehydrogenase changes following an eighty kilometer race: relationship to lipid peroxidation, *Eur. J. Appl. Physiol.*, 57, 60, 1988.

71. Dillard, C.J., Litov, R.E., Savin, R.E., Dumelin, E.E., and Tappel, A.L., Effects of exercise, vitamin E, and ozone on pulmonary function and lipid peroxidation, *J. Appl. Physiol. Respirat. Environ. Exer. Physiol.*, 45, 927, 1978.

72. Kanter, M.M., Nolte, L.A., and Holloszy, J.O., Effects of an antioxidant vitamin mixture on lipid peroxidation at rest and postexercise, *J. Appl. Physiol.*, 74, 965, 1993.

73. Meydani, M., Protective role of dietary vitamin E on oxidative stress in aging, *Age*, 15, 89, 1992.

74. Meydani, M., Evans, W.J., Handelman, G., Biddle, L., Fielding, R.A., Meydani, S.N., Burrill, J., Fiatarone, M.A., Blumberg, J.B., and Cannon, J.G., Protective effect of vitamin E on exercise-induced oxidative damage in young and older adults, *Am. J. Physiol.*, 264, R992, 1993.

75. Brady, P.S., Brady, L.J., and Ullrey, D.E., Selenium, vitamin E and the response to swimming stress in the rat, *J. Nutr.*, 109, 1103, 1979.

76. Kumar, C.T., Reddy, V.K., Prasad, M., Thyagaraju, K., and Reddanna, P., Dietary supplementation of vitamin E protects heart tissue from exercise-induced oxidant stress, *Mol. Cell. Biochem.*, 111, 109, 1992.

77. Jakeman, P. and Maxwell, S., Effect of antioxidant vitamin supplementation on muscle function after eccentric exercise, *Eur. J. Appl. Physiol.*, 67, 426, 1993.

78. Kaminski, M. and Boal, R., An effect of ascorbic acid on delayed-onset muscle soreness, *Pain*, 50, 317, 1992.

79. Peters, E.M, Goetzsche, J.M., Grobbelaar, B., and Noakes, T.D., Vitamin C supplementation reduces the incidence of postrace symptoms of upper-respiratory-tract infection in ultramaration runners, *Am. J. Clin. Nutr.*, 57, 170, 1993.

80. Nieman, D.C., Nehlsen-Cannarella, S.L., Henson, D.A., Butterworth, D.E., Fagoaga, O.R., Warren, B.J., and Rainwater, M.K., Carbohydrate, ascorbic acid, and the immune response to running, *Int. J. Sports Med.*, (in press).

81. Ji, L.L., Stratman, F.W., and Lardy, H.A., Antioxidant enzyme response to selenium deficiency in rat myocardium, *J. Amer. Col. Nutr.*, 11, 79, 1992.

82. Shimomura, Y., Suzuki, M., Sugiyama, S., Hanaki, Y., and Ozawa, T., Protective effect of coenzyme Q-10 on exercise-induced muscular injury, *Biochem. Biophys. Res. Commun.*, 176, 349, 1991.

83. Snider, I.P., Bazzarre, T.L., Murdoch, S.D., and Goldfarb, A., Effects of Coenzyme Athletic Performance System as an ergogenic aid on endurance performance to exhaustion, *Int. J. Sports Nutr.*, 2, 272, 1992.

84. Zuliani, U., Bonetti, A., Campana, M., Cerioli, G., Solito, F., and Novarini, A., The influence of ubiquinone (CoQ10) on the metabolic response to work, *J. Sports Med. Phys. Fitness*, 29, 57, 1989.

85. Viguie, C.A., Packer, L., and Brooks, G.A., Antioxidant supplementation affects indices of muscle trauma and oxidant stress in human blood during exercise, *Med. Sci. Sport. Exer.*, 21, S16, 1989.

86. Halliwell, B. and Gutteridge, J.M.C., *Free Radicals in Biology and Medicine*, Clarendon Press, Oxford, 1985, 162.

87. Wong, S.H.Y., Knight, J.A., Hopfer, S.M., Zaharia, O., Leach, C.N., and Sunderman, F.W., Lipoperoxides in plasma as measured by liquid-chromatographic separation of malondialdehyde-thiobarbituric acid adduct, *Clin. Chem.*, 33, 214, 1987.

88. Gutteridge, J.M.C., Lipid Peroxidation: Some problems and concepts, in *Oxygen Radicals and Tissue Injury: Proceedings of an Upjohn Symposium*, Halliwell, B., Ed., FASEB, Bethesda, MD, 1988, 9.

89. Blumberg, J., Are antioxidants at an awkward age?, *J. Amer. Coll. Nutr.*, 13, 218, 1994.

90. Patterson, B.H., Block, G., Rosenberger, W.F., Pee, D., and Kahle, L.L., Fruit and vegetables in the American diet: data from the NHANES II survey, *Am. J. Pub. Health*, 80, 1443, 1990.

Chapter 11

WATER AND ELECTROLYTES DURING PHYSICAL ACTIVITY

_____ Leo C. Senay, Jr.

CONTENTS

0-8493-8560-1/97/$0.00+$.50
© 1998 by CRC Press LLC

I.   INTRODUCTION

When an individual begins to exercise, the increase in metabolic activity in skeletal muscle initiates a number of events in the body. To supply the oxygen demand of skeletal muscle, cardiac output increases and the increase in blood flow to skeletal muscle is accommodated by dilation of resistance blood vessels and an increase in open capillaries. The increase in area of fluid exchange across the capillary walls combines with the increase in production of osmotically active substances by the skeletal muscle to alter resting body fluid dynamics. Water, ions, and molecules rapidly move in and out of the vascular volume and the interstitial space (ISF). With exercise, body temperature increases and, in most instances, stimulates the heat dissipation mechanisms of the body. Cutaneous vasodilation will take place thus increasing heat exchange from the body to the environment. If heat transfer by radiation and convection is not adequate, sweating is then stimulated and heat is then lost by evaporation of water from the surface of the body. Sweat superimposes a new set of circumstances upon those already in place during exercise. Water loss leads to dehydration and, to maintain and replenish body fluid volumes, fluid replacement during and after exercise is necessary. This chapter will be concerned with the body fluid changes that take place during and after exercise. Particular attention will be paid to the mechanisms involved and strategies of rehydration.

Fluid and electrolyte research in recent years has more or less been focused on finding the ingested elixir that will both satisfy electrolyte needs and bring about improvements in performance.[1,2] Indeed the results of these studies can be seen in the present and past recommendations as to fluid intake during exercise by the American College of Sports Medicine.[3-5] Before we can review the findings dealing with water and electrolytes during activity, it is necessary to possess a common fund of information.

II.   BASIC CONSIDERATIONS

A.   PROPERTIES OF WATER

Water has several colligative properties that are used to the body's advantage. The first, and perhaps foremost, is the high specific heat of water. The specific heat of water equals 1 when 1 kg of water is heated 1°C between 15 and 16°C. The heat necessary to do this is defined as 1000 calories (4186 joules) or 1 kg cal. An average 70 kg male contains some 42 kg of water which is present to various degrees in all tissues.[6-8] Because of the presence of tissue protein, fat, etc. the specific heat of the body is 0.83.[9] Therefore, in order to raise the body temperature of a 70 kg man 1°C his heat content must increase 58 kg calories (242.8 Kjoules). If a similar quantity of liquid mercury were to have its temperature raised 1°C it would take only 2.3 kg cal (9.63 kJ) to do so. Thus, water is heat buffer in the human body. High specific heat combined with the fluidity of water also assists in the convective transfer of heat within the body from areas of heat production to areas of heat dissipation. The heat transport occurs with a minimal increase in blood temperature.

Water has a high heat of vaporization. To heat 1 kg of water from 20 to 100°C requires 80 kg calories(334 kilojoules) but to cause the water to boil, another 540 kg calories (2.26 megajoules) must be added. The connection to exercise physiology is the evaporation of sweat: for every gram of sweat evaporated (liquid to vapor) from the skin, the body loses 0.58 kg calories (2.43 kilojoules) of heat.[10]

The chemical reactions within the human body depend upon the solvent power of water. Without proper hydration, most of the chemical reactions within a cell will not occur or will not occur as efficiently. In addition to a role in cell metabolism as a solvent, the ionic environment of the body is owed to the ability of water to dissolve and thus allow transport of various electrolytes needed to maintain a proper internal environment.

B.   ELECTROLYTES AND BODY FUNCTION

The function of cells in the human body depend upon the maintenance of a proper electrolyte environment both in and outside the cell. Excitability of nerve, skeletal muscle, cardiac muscle, etc. all depend upon the ionic gradients that exist across the cell membrane.[11] Thus our ability to move is dependent upon the presence of electrolytes within the body water contents.

III.   BODY FLUID COMPARTMENTS

A.   METHODS OF DETERMINATION

Total body water in living humans can be determined by the use of agents which freely distribute throughout all fluid compartments in the body.[6,7] Certain small volumes are slow to equilibrate with the selected marker (see below). The markers of choice for total body water are tritiated water wherein the water molecules contain one radioactive hydrogen ion and, if radioactivity is to be avoided, deuteriated (heavy) water. The usual equilibration time of 3 hr after ingestion has yielded similar results for both types of tracer. For males and females in the age groups of 16–30 yr the average water content expressed as percent of body weight is 60 and 50%, respectively.[7,12] Extended to the entire population, 95% of males lie in the range of 49.6–68% while the range for females is 44.1–57.6%. The reason for the difference in water content between the sexes is because a greater proportion of the body weight of females is fat and adipocytes contain little water (usually assumed to be 10%).[6] As noted above, there are body compartments whose volumes are difficult to ascertain and whose contribution to measurement of total body water may be variable. These volumes are in dense connective tissue and cartilage which contain 7.5% of body water; bone contains a similar amount, but transcellular water, which is water present in secretions such as the cerebrospinal and intestinal fluids, etc.,[6,7] can be quite variable. If we consider a 70 kg man and a 55 kg woman, their respective total body water would be 42 and 27.5 kg. To divide body water into its two major components, extra and intracellular, the size of the extracellular volume (ECV) must be determined and subtracted from the total body water measurement. It is not presently possible to directly measure intracellular volume (ICV). The determination of ECV can be done using a number of inorganic and organic compounds. However, each substance that has been used measures a slightly different volume.[6,7] The distribution seems to vary with the size of the tracer employed. For example, inulin with a molecular weight of 5000 indicates an ECV of 12–14 l while radioactive sulphate (SO^4), measures a volume of 23 l in our 70 kg man. Using the inulin volume, the ECV will be considered to be 14 l. Thus intracellular volume would amount to 22 kg (see below). The reader will note that kilogram and liter have been used interchangeably, because at body temperature there is little error equating 1 kg with 1 l of water.

The ECV can in turn be divided into interstitial and intravascular volumes by measuring plasma volume. This can be done directly by dye dilution or radioiodinated albumin or indirectly through marking a small volume of erythrocytes with a radioactive marker and determining the dilution of this marker and estimating the total body hematocrit. The plasma volume (PV) of our 70 kg man has been estimated at slightly more than 3 l (7.5% of body water). ISF volume is then calculated to be 11 l.

In summary, the total body water of a 70 kg man is divided as follows: 15% in bone, GI tract, cerebrospinal fluid, and dense connective tissue; 53% within cells; and 33% in the

ECV. The latter volume consists of 7.5% of body water in the PV leaving about 25% of body water in the ISF. The partitioning of total body water in our 55 kg female can be done in a similar fashion.

B.   BODY COMPARTMENT FLUID EXCHANGES

Water readily traverses all cell membranes in the human body. The direction in which water moves is determined mainly by osmotic and hydrostatic gradients. From ISF to the cell interior, for example, the movement of water is determined by the activity of the ATPase Na-K pump. If the activity of the pump is decreased or prevented, sodium (Na) moves into the cell followed closely by water. The cell will then swell.

In exercise, the exchange between the two components of ECV are of greatest concern. In general, two opposing forces operate; one retains fluid within the vascular volume, the other moves fluid out of the vascular volume. Each of these forces is made up of a number of contributing factors. As first clearly noted by Starling,[13] the hydrostatic pressure within the capillaries is the prime reason for fluid exiting the capillary. The hydrostatic pressure brought to bear on a capillary wall is in turn a function of blood volume, cardiac output, and peripheral resistance. With exercise, the contracting muscles add to the forces causing fluid to move from the vascular system to the interstitial spaces by the production of osmotically active particles through aerobic and anaerobic metabolism.

The plasma proteins are the main cause of fluid retention in the capillaries. Since most osmotically active particles appear to move across capillary walls much more readily than protein molecules, it is these large molecules that exert an osmotic pressure (usually referred to as protein oncotic pressure) that counters the hydrostatic pressure noted above. Starling[13] was of the opinion that plasma proteins did not leave the vascular volume, and his opinion is still reflected today by various authors who imply that whatever protein is present in the interstitial space is minor when compared to that within the plasma.[6,8] However, the student of exercise should consider the following: only 40% of those proteins we consider plasma proteins are present at any one time within the vascular volume.[14] In humans, the total plasma protein concentration approximates 7 g/dl. The total amount of protein within the vascular bed in our 70 kg man is then some 210 g. Radioactive tracer studies note that the amount of protein referred to as plasma protein is some 500 g or more.[14] Where is the balance of the protein? It is in the interstitial space and lymph. Protein within the vascular volume does move across capillary walls either by moving through intercellular clefts or, more likely, through the process of pinocytosis.[15] Here, invaginations of capillary walls occur and these invaginations become small vacuoles whose content is that of the plasma in contact with the wall when the vacuole is formed. The vacuoles then move across the endothelial cell by a process resembling diffusion, and the contents of the vacuole are "dumped" into the interstitial space. There is little or no such traffic from interstitial space to the capillary lumen. That such traffic does indeed occur can be inferred by a simple experiment. If albumin is labeled with Evans Blue dye and the concentration of dyed albumin is followed for 24 hr, the dyed albumin disappears from the vascular volume at a rate equal to 3–5% of the labeled protein per hour.[16] Such a rate of disappearance far exceeds that of albumin clearance by the gastrointestinal tract. In addition, radioactive tracer studies have shown that there is a 24–36 hr turnover for the entire plasma albumin contents.[14] The exiting protein is replaced by that returning from the interstitial spaces via the lymphatic system. The amount of protein that is referred to as plasma protein in the ISF amounts to some 315 g in a volume of 11 l thus giving an average concentration of 2.9 g/dl of interstitial space. No one can clearly answer as to just where this protein is in interstitial space for the following reasons: Interstitial space contains hyaluronic acid, and in low concentrations (<1%), this substance causes watery fluids to gel. The hyaluronic gels have been shown to exclude albumin.[17] This exclusion is only partial, not total. However, if there exists water channels within interstitial space it would appear logical that the concentration of protein within these watery channels would be considerably higher than the average noted above. Which, of these concentrations of protein, that within the gel matrix or that within the watery channels, must we consider to be one of the forces moving water out of the capillaries? Later, we shall explore the role of the extravascular protein in the fluid volume shifts caused by exercise and by heat exposure.

Finally, the size of the ISF compartment appears to be determined by events in the vascular volume and within the cells. There is no process that is specific for solely increasing or decreasing the size of this compartment in a healthy individual. In general, the size of this compartment in a resting subject seems to be passively determined by the fibrous structures within the interstitial space, the gel matrix, and the rate at which protein is returned to the vascular volume via the lymph.[17] The ISF does have a potential to hold considerable quantity of fluid for its compliance (volume change per unit of pressure change) appears to be similar to the circulatory bed.[18] This potential is usually fulfilled when removal of protein and fluid from the space is inhibited or slowed. The most common example would be the swelling of the feet and ankles of airplane passengers during long journeys.

IV. IONIC CONTENTS OF BODY FLUID COMPARTMENTS

To appreciate the ion species and concentrations in the various fluid compartments, the total amount of these ions in the body should be known. For example, for an average male, the total amount of body sodium (Na) amounts to some 4150 milliequivalents.[7] About 40% of this is in bone and the rest mainly in the ECV. The quantity of Na that is of immediate interest is that which has been dubbed "readily exchangeable." A good way to visualize this concept is to remember that readily exchangeable means that it quickly equilibrates with a radioactive ion of the same species. The readily exchangeable Na totals 2900 meq and the extracellular concentration ranges between 138 and 145 meq/l of plasma. A more precise but less used concentration expression is per kilogram of water but this demands correction for the volume of plasma occupied by the large protein molecules.[19] When done, the concentration of Na is noted as ranging from 148 to 156 meq/kg of plasma water. Na and other extracellular ions can only be compared from subject to subject if the latter expressions are used but for some reason, exercise physiologists in general appear to prefer the clinical values based on per liter of plasma. Multiplying the Na concentration in the ECV by 14 (the ECV volume) reveals that of the readily exchangeable Na about 70% is in the ECV. The remaining exchangeable Na is found in bone, dense connective tissue, and cartilage. The contribution of the small quantity of intracellular sodium to this fraction is minimal.

Similar figures exist for the chief intracellular cation, potassium (K).[7] The total body K of our 70 kg man is 3700 meq, and the readily exchangeable portion amounts to 3400 meq. Of this total, 56–70 meq (4–5 meq/l) are in the ECV. Approximately 90% of the total body K is in the ICV (150 meq/l) with very little in bone (8%). Clearly, the cellular portion of K is mobile and rapidly equilibrates with an injected tracer.

For chloride (Cl), the main anion of extracellular space, total body amount is 2550 meq of which 2150 is readily exchangeable.[7] The total amount of Cl in the extracellular space amounts to some 1400–1450 meq in our 70 kg subject, with most of that residing in the ECV (4–5 meq/l), the remaining being distributed similarly to Na. As noted above, the distribution of ions, particularly Na and K across cell membranes, is maintained by a metabolic process utilizing a membrane-resident carrier complex that is also an enzyme that utilizes energy stored in the ATP molecule. Basically, Na moves down a concentration gradient into the cells where the [Na] ~10 meq/l while K, with an intracellular concentration of ~150 meq/l, diffuses out of the cell. The ATPase pump moves the Na out of the cell and at the same time moves K into the cell. Note that this movement takes place against a concentration gradient in both directions and therefore work must be done to move these ions. For every three Na ions pumped out of a cell, two K are moved in. In excitable tissue (nerve, muscle) the resulting ion distribution across the membrane is responsible for the resting membrane potential, and, once excited (an action potential) the distribution of ions is also critical to the development of an action potential.[11]

The difference in protein concentration between the intravascular volume and the ISF influences the distribution of the diffusible ions between these two compartments. Such a situation is usually described as a Gibbs-Donnan equilibrium wherein the presence of a nondiffusible ion on one side of a semi-permeable membrane (capillary wall for example) determines the distribution of diffusible ions on both sides of the membrane.[8] In the vascular volume, at arterial pH, the protein molecules (particularly albumin) bear negative charges since the protein is on the alkaline side of its iso-electric point. Therefore, the negative charges on the protein must be electrically neutralized by positive charges and, in mammals, the positive charge is present on the Na ion. Since more negative charges (protein) exist in capillaries than in the ISF in contact with the capillaries, there is a slightly greater amount of Na and a slightly lower amount of Cl within the vascular volume than in the interstitial space. Of what importance is this difference? Pure albumin at concentrations equal to that in plasma exerts an oncotic pressure of approximately 19 mmHg.[14] When the negative charges at body pH are joined with an equal number of Na ions, the measured oncotic pressure then rises from 25 to 28 mmHg. Thus the osmotic pressure of plasma is somewhat greater than that in the interstitial fluid. Any movement of protein or water from one of these extracellular compartments to another will influence this distribution.

V. THE EFFECT OF EXERCISE ON CONTENTS AND SIZE OF BODY FLUID COMPARTMENTS

In 1968, Oscai et al.[20] presented evidence that an individual going from being untrained to trained via daily bouts of rhythmic exercise (running) also enjoyed an increase in blood volume. Since then, there have been a number of confirmatory studies. The general finding is an increase in blood volume through an increase in both plasma and red cell volume. However, the increases in these two fractions are not uniform, for the plasma volume increases proportionately more than does the red cell volume.[21]

The mechanisms invoked by the stimulus of exercise to bring about the volume increase are still being studied and debated.[21,22] If an untrained individual exercises at a level that requires 50–75% of his/her maximum oxygen consumption (VO$_2$max) for at least 1 hr at a cool environmental temperature, blood samples taken before exercise begins and 24 hr post exercise will usually indicate an increase in plasma volume. Indeed, Senay (unpublished) found that 45 min of exercise at 40–50% of VO$_2$max served to increase blood volume when blood samples were taken the day after exercise. There appears to be an inverse relationship between intensity of exercise and time of exercise in order to bring about plasma volume expansion. The more intense the exercise, the shorter the performance time needed to increase plasma volume.[24,25] If the individual continues upon a daily bout of exercise, blood volume will increase and finally stabilize at levels some 5–20% greater than the original volume.[21] The increase in any one person depends upon a number of items: just how untrained was the individual to start with? For example Saltin et al.[23] first had subjects undergo prolonged bed rest, then trained them. In these subjects, the average increase in plasma volume was some 16%. It would seem reasonable to expect that the volume expansion could be linked to the VO$_2$max of the subject before training began. The intensity of the training may play a role in determining blood volume expansion. Whether or not the type of rhythmic exercise influences volume expansion doesn't seem to have been addressed: that is does exercise on a cycle ergometer lead to the same expansion as running? Little information exists on blood volume expansion in females, but considering paired studies of males and females wherein few differences were discerned, it is probable that females respond to exercise training as do males.[26,27] Age does not seem to be a factor, for elderly subjects have been shown to be capable of blood volume expansion with exercise training.[25]

What then are the physiologic processes that bring about the expansion of blood volume with repetitive exercise? Are events bringing about short-term expansion the same as that in place after weeks or months of training? Does this expansion extend to the entire extracellular volume? If blood samples are drawn from a subject before, during, and after each training bout, blood analysis supports the following general scenario. During the exercise, fluid is lost from the vascular volume. The amount that is lost depends on the position of the subject before exercise begins while the amount of plasma volume reduction may depend upon the type (cycle vs running) and intensity of exercise.[22,23] Simultaneously, the plasma concentration of certain hormones significantly increase. These include several that are directly concerned with fluid and electrolyte balance, i.e., aldosterone, (ALD), anti-diuretic hormone (ADH), and atrial natriuretic peptide (ANP).[28-30] Other hormones — epinephrine, norepinephrine, growth hormone — also increase but are not directly related to volume and electrolyte control. The increases in ALD and ADH were the basis of the first simplistic explanation of how plasma volume (and hence, blood volume) enlarged beginning with the first bout of exercise training. The reasoning was straightforward: the increase in ALD and ADH were responsible for water and salt retention after exercise ceased and thus, plasma volume expanded. ALD does indeed increase the kidney reabsorption of Na. However, Na is not confined to the plasma volume and difficulties with this explanation occurred when the subjects were weighed before each exercise session. Based upon the idea that ALD and ADH were responsible for Na and water retention, an increase in plasma volume of 5–10% had to reflect a similar increase in the entire extracellular volume, because both Na and water pass freely across capillary walls. If the extracellular volume expanded by 10% the subject would show a weight gain of some 1.4 kg (3.1 lb). If water and salt retention were the basis of continued expansion, then body weight should also continue to rise. The magnitude of weight gain is considerably less than this and therefore, for the short term plasma volume expansion another explanation must be sought.[31] During exercise, fluid leaves the vascular volume. The loss depends upon the position and rigor of the exercise.[32,33] The contraction of skeletal muscle produces osmotically active ions and molecules that cause water to move out of the vascular volume. In addition, lymph flow from the active muscle mass is increased, and if the exercise increases body temperature, lymph flow from the skin also increases because of the increase in skin blood flow necessary for body cooling (see below).[34] As noted above, considerable protein exists in the interstitial fluid and the increase in the movement of fluid through the ISF moves protein into the vascular volume via the lymph ducts.[35] Because of the exercise, the movement into the vascular volume exceeds the rate at which protein escapes from the vascular volume. The oncotic pressure exerted by this added protein causes water to be retained within the vascular volume. For each gram of protein returned to the vascular bed, 15 ml of water are also added to the blood volume.[36] An increase in total circulating plasma protein of 13–20 g can increase plasma volume by 200–300 ml. The water must come from interstitial space, because the subjects, for the most part, do not gain sufficient weight to account for an expansion of extracellular volume.[35] Calculations indicate that the movement of protein and water into the vascular volume causes an increase in the concentration of protein within the ISF. In order to re-establish the former ratio of protein concentration in and outside the vascular volume, approximately 1 kg of water and attendant salt should be added to the extracellular volume. Indeed, in well-controlled experiments this is what happens.[21,24,30] While this explanation is sound for the volume expansion early in exercise training (1 wk or so), certain other events must be added to explain volume expansion in the trained subject. Red cell production increases, but the red cell addition to the vascular volume is not in proportion to the expansion of the PV, thus the "anemia" of training.[23,37] The sensitivity of volume receptors decreases. If a person were to have his/her volume expanded with saline, the increase in volume would be excreted in 24 hr. As exercise training continues the volume receptors appear to adapt to the increase in volume.[38] The increase does not cause a matching increase in arterial blood pressure and therefore the increase in blood volume must be matched by an increase in the capacitance of the circulatory system. Certainly, ALD and ADH aid in the retention of salt and water such that volume expansion may occur. Additionally, protein synthesis probably increases but we do not possess evidence as to this event. Finally, what happens when a person ceases training? It has been found that one of the first events that occurs is a reduction in total circulating protein within the vascular volume and with this protein reduction, water no longer is held in the vascular volume and reduction in blood volume occurs.[39] Depending on the intensity and length of the training program, return to pre-training values for total circulating plasma protein and PV can take 3–4 wks. Therefore, in order to maintain an increased blood volume the person must continue to exercise. The continued influx of protein into the vascular volume supports the increase in PV. Continued exercise is also necessary in setting the sensitivity of the various body volume receptors.

Whether or not ISF volume is changed in training is an open question. Because of physical constraints and the function of the lymphatic system, it seems unlikely but this is only a guess.

Is it to the advantage of a person to attain and maintain an increase in blood volume? Suppose an untrained person has a blood volume of 5 l divided into 2.75 l of plasma and 2.25 l of red cells (a hematocrit of 0.45). The individual sits on a cycle ergometer and starts to work at 50% of his/her VO_2max. Serial blood samples usually reveal that with exercise the hematocrit increases because the amount of plasma decreases. It is not unusual for such a subject to lose 15% of his/her plasma volume with 30 min of cycle ergometer exercise.[40] The absolute loss in this case would be 413 ml of plasma leaving behind 2.34 l. Now the subject undergoes a vigorous training program and plasma volume expands some 15%; an increase of some 413 ml. If the subject now exercises as before (50% VO_2max) he/she will again lose 15% of his/her plasma volume (474 ml) but now the amount of plasma remaining in the vascular volume is 2.69 l. The increase in blood volume would have a positive effect upon cardiac output allowing better maintenance of muscle and skin circulation.

Rhythmic exercise training does influence the enzyme concentrations in skeletal muscle and may result in muscle hypertrophy, but there seems not to be any remarkable changes in intracellular volume of the lean body mass.[41] What usually does occur is a reduction in fat stores, and since fat contains little water, the amount of water in the body as percent of body weight increases.

VI.　INFLUENCE OF RHYTHMIC EXERCISE UPON BODY FLUID COMPONENTS

There are a number of studies concerned with changes in blood volume during exercise. Senay and Pivarnik[22] grouped such studies into four categories: short-term exercise (less than 30 min), intermediate-term exercise (from 30 min to several hours), distances of 42.2 km or longer, and exercise rates equal to and exceeding VO_2max. Here, the division will be based on whether sweating is sufficient to influence body fluid concentrations and dynamics. In the classification noted above, the first and last categories do not include significant sweating or fluid intake. Many of the intermediate studies have subjects exercising with and without fluid replacement while significant sweat loss occurs.

In discussing the effect of training upon plasma volume, it was noted that during the actual exercise plasma volume underwent a reduction due to the increase in forces causing water to move out of the vascular volume. This is particularly true of exercise done in the upright posture on a cycle ergometer.[33,40] The responses seem to be consistent in this form of exercise. However, in subjects walking on a treadmill the dynamics of plasma volume appeared to depend upon the individual subject, because the exercise was uniform, but the plasma volume changes were not.[33] Some subjects showed a volume reduction, others an increase, while others did not change from control values. This was a short-term study comparing progressively increasing cycle and treadmill exercise, several other differences were noted.[33]

In all forms of rhythmic exercise, the concentration of plasma K ([K]) increases. The amount of increase depends upon the number of contracting muscle fibers for the K appearing in the plasma is a by-product of muscle membrane action potentials. For each muscle fiber, each membrane action potential is accompanied by the loss of K from inside the muscle cell. While individual fiber loss is small, the combined effect of all active muscle fiber is sufficient to raise extracellular [K] 1–2 meq/l.

Nose et al.[42] reported data from a study where subjects exercised to exhaustion in a step wise manner. A curvilinear relationship was noted for plasma Na concentration ([Na]) and exercise intensity. The authors suggested that the increase in [Na] was related to the increase in blood lactate. What this study does illustrate well is the fact that the increase in osmotic gradient from contracting muscle to blood moves proportionately more water than ions out of the vascular volume.

Lundvall et al.[43] studied the transfer of fluid between blood and tissue during rhythmic exercise. They had 19 male subjects pedal a cycle ergometer for 6 min on three separate occasions. The exercise levels were light (300 kilopond m/min; 1 kilopond equals 9.8 Newtons), moderate (900 kpm/m), and heavy (1200–1500 kpm/m). Leg volumes were measured before and after exercise. The increase in leg volume was proportional to the work load. Since the legs contained the active muscle, the calculated change in leg volume was compared with the reduction in plasma volume. The increase in leg volume during heavy exercise averaged 1100 ml but the plasma volume revealed a net loss of only 600 ml. With heavy exercise, plasma osmolarity[7] increased some 22 mosm/kg of plasma water and the authors suggested that 500 ml of fluid had entered the vascular volume because of two events; an increased osmotic gradient from inactive tissue to blood and a decrease in capillary hydrostatic pressure. Later experiments on animals supported this hypothesis.[44] In summary, it is usual in short term exercise, where sweating does not influence body fluid dynamics, for fluid to leave the vascular volume. Evidence indicates that this fluid is hypotonic to plasma, because it apparently does not contain a full complement of plasma ions. Protein in small amounts also leaves the circulation but the remaining amount because of water loss from the circulation undergoes a relative increase in concentration. Combined with the plasma ions and with ions and molecules entering the blood volume there is a marked increase in plasma osmolarity (see above). This increase in osmolarity is not only due to the metabolic activity of skeletal muscle which is responsible for elevating [K] and [PO_4] but also the increases in glucose and lipid content of plasma because of the increased secretion of catecholamines and glucagon.[46,47] Clearly, there is a limit to the amount of fluid that leaves the vascular volume. Greenleaf et al.[45] indicate the upper limit of PV loss to be in the neighborhood of 20% of the resting PV. Several factors apparently limit PV loss. The first was noted above, i.e., the increase in plasma osmotic pressure. A second as shown by Sjogaard and Saltin[48] was that most of the water that left the vascular volume was present in the intercellular spaces of skeletal muscle. It was only with maximum exercise that water entered the skeletal muscle cells. The geometry of skeletal muscle cells does seem to impose structural limitations upon the amount of fluid that could enter. The amount of fluid in the interstitial spaces would be determined by the compliance of this space plus the rate of return to the vascular volume via the lymph ducts.

What happens when short-term intensive exercise ceases? In general there is a rapid return to control concentrations of ions.[49,50] If the exercise had been of sufficient intensity and length, protein content would be increased. Blood lactate levels rapidly fall as lactate is converted into glycogen in skeletal muscle and liver. Hormone levels, particularly ADH return to control levels as does ALD.[51,52] Some of these changes, such as the return of plasma volume and particularly the return of K into the skeletal muscle cells via the ATPase pump occur rapidly for blood samples taken at the end of exercise are quite different from those taken 5 min to an hour later.[42,52]

VII.   WATER AND ELECTROLYTE BALANCE DURING EXERCISE

When heat loss by convection and radiation is insufficient to prevent an elevation in body heat content, the increase in blood temperature flowing through the anterior hypothalamus stimulates the appropriate neurons in this area to initiate sweat gland activity. The secreted sweat spreads over the body surface from which it evaporates and in doing so removes heat from the skin surface. Usually, the circulation to the skin increases before active sweating occurs and thus there is an increase in the convective transfer of heat from contracting muscles to the surface of the body where heat exchange occurs. Heat exchange from the surface of the human body is a complex issue and for our purposes, our interest will be directed at sweat production.[53]

A.   INFLUENCE OF SWEATING ON BODY FLUID VOLUMES

If an individual sweats while exercising and does not ingest fluids, the amount and composition of sweat will determine to great extent what changes will occur within the fluid compartments of the body. The immediate source of water for the sweat glands is from the interstitial space though it can be shown that each gland appears to be served by capillaries. Sweat that rises to the skin surface is hypotonic to blood plasma and fluid in the interstitial spaces.[54,55] Therefore, osmotically active particles must be left behind in the cutaneous interstitial space. The osmotic gradient from blood to the cutaneous interstitial space increases and water must leave the vascular compartment. The osmotic pressure of blood then increases and fluid enters the blood from the extracutaneous cell volume. There has been a debate over how much each of the body fluid compartments eventually contributes to the volume of water lost via the eccrine sweat glands. Adolph and others reported that plasma volume lost water at a rate 2.5 times that of the rest of the body.[56,57] Plasma is 93% water while the total body water is 60% of body weight. The proportional water loss for plasma should mirror the ratio 93/65, and in a study by Senay,[57] the ratio was close to this and it certainly wasn't 2.5. If one looks at the water content of various tissues in the body, clearly the contribution of each tissue to satisfying osmotic gradients from the intracellular compartment to the interstitial fluid via the blood will vary as to the water content of the tissue.[6] Several studies addressed this issue and reported that during bouts of intermediate exercise (30 min to 2 hr) the largest contributor to water loss by sweating was, with one exception, found to be the extracellular compartment which was the source of about 55% of the lost water.[58-61] Plasma contributed 10% to the sweat loss while the intracellular volume contributes approximately 45%. If we assume that our 70 kg subject lost 3% of his body weight via sweating, the 2.1 kg loss would be partitioned into a 0.21 kg loss from plasma, a 1.16 kg ISF loss, and a reduction in ICF of 0.95 kg. However, it should be added that the distribution of water loss changes after exercise ceases. Nose et al.[61] dehydrated subjects some 2.3% of body water. Plasma volume was decreased 9.4% at the end of exercise. The plasma volume reduction was only 5% 30 min later, and at 60 min the reduction was at 5.6%. The authors identified the ISF as the source of the added water. The post-exercise equilibration of water can be ascribed to the decrease in hydrostatic pressure within the circulatory bed with the end of exercise. Thus, the reduction measured immediately at the end of exercise combines both hydrostatic and osmotic losses from the plasma volume. Astrand and Saltin[62] also saw a similar event at the end of a cross-country ski race. The reduction in hydrostatic pressure following exercise allows protein oncotic pressure to assert its influence as to water content of the vascular volume. The partial re-establishment of plasma volume probably plays a role in the treatment advocated by Noakes for long distance runners who collapse after finishing the race.[63]

B. SWEAT ELECTROLYTES AND FLUID COMPARTMENTS

There is considerable subject variation in sweat content. Indeed, variation is present in an individual. Based on the work of Robinson and others,[64,65] we know that the Na and Cl content of sweat depends upon the amount present in the diet. Placing a person on a low salt diet will reduce the amount of salt in the sweat. The amount of Na reabsorbed is influenced by the mineralocorticoid ALD. Reductions in Na intake stimulate an increase in secretion of ALD whose action in the collecting duct of the kidney tubule and in the sweat gland duct increases the reabsorption of Na and thus conserves body Na.[55]

Na is the principle cation in extracellular fluid, and the volume of the extracellular fluid depends upon an adequate quantity of the ion being present. One other property of Na should be noted and that is the contribution of Na and Cl to the osmotic pressure of extracellular fluid. Together, they are responsible for about 96% of extracellular osmolarity. It must be noted that Na (and other ions) play dual roles in the body; the first is as a specific ion species that take part in specific biologic processes and a nonspecific role in osmotic pressure. With these facts in mind, if we assign a [Na] of 140 meq/l to the extracellular volume of our 70 kg man, a total of 1960 meq of Na would be present in the extracellular volume. What happens if our subject loses 2 l of sweat with a Na concentration ([Na]) and [Cl] of 50 meq/l? The subject ingests water equal to sweat loss and assumes that all the water is absorbed (see below). If the water only entered the ECV, the volume would be the same 14 l, but the concentration of Na would be reduced to 133 meq/l. A similar reduction for Cl would also occur. With the reduction in ion concentration would also come a reduction in osmolarity of 5–6%. Such a decrease would result in a decrease in the secretion of ADH and cause an increase in free water clearance by the kidney until the body fluid osmolarity had returned to the pre-sweating level. If this happens, we now have a [Na] of 140 meq/l but an ECV of 13.3 l. As reported by Nose et al.[66] similar results are seen when subjects replace sweat loss with only water. However, in real life, only 51% of the ingested water was retained in the body because reduction in osmolarity reduced ADH production and increased free-water clearance by the kidney.

What would have happened had water not been ingested? If water and salt loss were confined to the ECV, the ECV would now be 12 l with a [Na] of 155 meq/l. Of course this does not occur because, as noted above, water will move according to osmotic gradients, and as noted by Lundvall, water will move from plasma and from the intracellular volume until equilibration occurs.[44] In addition to water movement, ADH secretion will increase causing the kidney to conserve water, and aldosterone levels will remain elevated also.[67] The events in "real life" show that blood volume is conserved at the expense of osmolarity. With dehydration, excretion of water and ions decreases and body fluid osmolarities increase. What results is a subject whose total body water has been reduced as above with about 55% of the loss coming from the ECV.[58-61] Thus the ECV has been reduced some 1.1 l and if [Na] returned to its original value of 140 meq/l, an additional 54 meq would have to be excreted. The usual result is that the excess ions are not excreted and body fluid osmolarity increases.

C. PHYSIOLOGIC CONSEQUENCES OF HYPOHYDRATION

When individuals engage in exercise and sweating is necessary for body cooling, such persons do not voluntarily ingest an amount of fluid equal to sweat loss.[68] Without encouragement or prompting, exercising and/or heat exposed subjects ingest volumes of fluid ranging from one-third to two-thirds of the volume lost in sweat. Until recent times, athletes engaged in such sports as distance running, football, soccer, and rugby were not encouraged to replace water lost in sweat.[63] Laboratory studies have shown that when inadequate water intake occurs, body fluid osmolarities increase, there is an increase in ionic concentrations, and the circulating blood volume decreases.

1. Blood Volume Reduction

With sweating, plasma volume is reduced with a consequent increase in the relative proportion of red cells circulating in the vascular volume. With the reduction in circulating blood volume in an exercising subject, the ability to adequately supply contracting muscle with oxygen and to move a sufficient amount of blood through the cutaneous vascular bed for body cooling is compromised. The immediate and obvious result is an increase in heart rate accompanied by a decrease in stroke volume of the heart since the reduction in blood volume lowers venous return for a given work load. In addition, because of the increase in the proportion of red cells to plasma, the viscosity of blood increases thus increasing the work of the heart. With the reduction in volume flow to muscle and skin, heat transport will diminish and when combined with the influence of increased osmolarity upon the sweat glands, body temperature will increase.[69]

2. Osmolarity and Sweating

Resting subjects undergoing progressive hypohydration exhibit a reduction in sweat rates.[70] The reduction has been correlated with an increase in osmolarity as well as an increase in [Na].[70] The latter cannot be separated from its osmotic role. In exercise, sweat rate appears to depend upon body water loss: the greater the water loss, the lower the sweat rate.[71,72] However, some subjects do not decrease their sweat rates though dehydrated. This would appear to indicate that the increase in osmolarity did not influence sweating, but that is not true. The stimulus for sweating is an increase in core or body temperature as noted above, and a given rise in body temperature for an individual will cause sweat to be produced at a given rate. If one examines the hypohydrating exercising subject, the constant sweating is driven by an ever increasing body temperature.[73] In a well-hydrated subject, the increase in temperature would be matched with an increased rate of sweating. With hypohydration, the sweat mechanism loses sensitivity and requires increased levels of stimulation in order to simply maintain sweating.

There are individuals that are unable to produce an adequate amount of sweat no matter how well hydrated they are and who cannot participate in athletic events in warm weather. If they do participate, they run the risk of heat injury.

3. Hypohydration and Performance

Hypohydration decreases the ability of athletes to perform. A body water loss equal to 1% of body weight diminishes the ability to perform a set task.[71] The problem to be faced here is that, as noted above, athletes will not ingest a sufficient amount of fluid to balance sweat losses. When a heterogenous group of marathon runners were weighed at the beginning and end of the race, their body weight loss averaged about 3%.[74] It is not unusual for marathon runners to lose between 3 and 5% of their body weight during runs in temperate climates. As pointed out by Maughan,[75] an elite marathon runner may sweat at a rate of 2 l/hr. This rate of sweating exceeds the absorbative power of the intestinal tract. Also, taking in large quantities of fluid leads to a sensation of fullness and for many, this is discomforting. An individual athlete engaged in training should have an appreciation of his/her weight loss for a given task in several climates and thus adjust their fluid intake accordingly. While the ideal is complete fluid and electrolyte replacement, a balance has to be struck between comfort and necessity.

4. Hypohydration and Temperature Regulation

The regulation of body temperature is centered in the preoptic area of the hypothalamus. Input from receptors located in the spinal cord, abdominal cavity, skin, and other organs is received and integrated in this area of the brain.[76,77] If needed, the appropriate stimuli to heat dissipating mechanisms are sent then to the periphery of the body leading to cutaneous vasodilatation and sweating. In the hypohydrated individual the sensitivity of the preoptic area is reduced and this reduction has been linked to the increase in [Na].[78] Considering exercising individuals, those undergoing short-term (<30 min) activity, the increase in body temperature would fit the description of Stitt[76] wherein the rise is a measure of the heat storage necessary to stimulate heat dissipation. Osmolarity and increase in [Na] make their presence felt when water loss from the body approaches 1% of body weight.

The influence of ionic changes upon the temperature regulating apparatus is complicated by the increased release of interleukin-1 in exercise. This cytokine and others have a number of actions depending on their concentrations.[79] At the low concentration produced during exercise, interleukin-1 raises the "set point" at which body temperature is maintained. What then is the effect of an increase in the [Na] superimposed upon the interleukin change in "set point"? The answer is not evident. Body temperatures recorded at the end of endurance exercise events wherein participants have lost 3–5% of body weight via sweating have exceeded 40°C in many instances.[75] How much of this increase is due to increased ionic concentrations of body fluids and how much can be assigned to interleukin has not been sorted out. Indeed, the role of interleukin in post-exercise metabolic rates has not been examined. We do not know how much of the post-exercise elevation of oxygen consumption is due to the exercise per se and how much is due to the demands of maintaining an interleukin-elevated body temperature.

This discussion has focused upon the central nervous system influences of increases in the ionic concentrations of body fluids. Peripheral events are also influenced by dehydration. Fortney et al.[80] have shown that decreases in blood volume and increases in osmolarity reduce the blood flow to forearm skin. For some subjects, there is a reduction in sweat rates with hypohydration. It may be that the elevations in central temperature cannot be assigned to a rigid order of events in all persons because the central events may not be uniform. In addition, the peripheral responses may also be individualized. For example, in one person, elevation of central temperature may bring about a decrease in skin blood flow with little change in sweat rate and in another person, the skin blood flow may not change but the sweat rate decreases. When experiments are reported, average responses are emphasized and individual responses are lost yet we know that individual responses to heat and exercise do differ from individual to individual.

5. Practical Aspects of Salt and Water Loss

How one trains for an athletic event is determined by the event itself. Sprinters and marathon runners do not adhere to identical training regimens nor do wrestlers spend time "ghosting" as do badminton players. For some athletes salt and water intake may not be a serious concern but for others, the amount of water and salt loss in sweat is critical and should determine pre- and post-exercise dietary requirements. This discussion will employ the example of a long distance runner training in a climate whose dry bulb temperature varies between 10 and 25°C. More generally, the discussion is easily applied to those persons engaged in football, soccer, basketball, or any other sport that exposes the individual to environmental temperatures and clothing requiring high rates of sweating.

A runner in training may exercise for 1–3 hr/day. Depending upon the runner's metabolic rate, the environmental temperature, solar radiation, and relative humidity, he/she may lose from 1 to 6 l of body water via the sweat glands. A primary requirement for this athlete is the replenishment of body water. As noted above, water loss in sweat is also accompanied by loss of ions particularly Na, K, and Cl. With the above sweat rates, the losses of these ions can range from 50 to 300 meq for Na and Cl and 5 to 30 meq of K. These losses can be compared with average dietary intakes determined in the United States. Dietary intake of Na ranges from 78 to 300 meq/day and the variation appears to depend upon salt added to the diet.[81] For K, the amount consumed per day depends upon the caloric intake. In the United States the K content ranges from 60 to 115 meq per 1000 calories of dietary intake.[81] Given an adequate caloric diet, there appears to be little reason to supplement K intake in athletes. For Na (and Cl), this is probably not the case. For individuals losing more than 200 meq/day in sweat, it may be prudent for these individuals to be certain that salt intake is adequate. For the average athlete, accurate supplementation is difficult to determine without analyzing urine for Na. However, given normal renal function[82] and adequate fluid intake, adding 50–100 meq of Na per day to the diet of an individual suffering sweat losses in the range noted above would probably solve any exercise-induced salt deficiency. If the salt were superfluous, the kidney would simply excrete the surplus. Again, it must be emphasized that fluid intake must be adequate to allow the kidney to correctly determine the rate of Na excretion or reabsorption. In household terms, 50 meq of Na is contained in 2.9 g of salt, an amount slightly in excess of one-fourth teaspoon.

Why worry about Na replacement during training? If Na replacement is neglected and Na depletion occurs, the ECV has to diminish. The other alternative, the acceptance of hyponatremia and/or hypoosmolality requires that ADH and ALD not act upon body fluid contents in their usual manner. In any case, the reduction in ECV is to be avoided for the reasons noted above, i.e., reduced blood volume, temperature regulation, sweating, etc. If a person trains and neglects proper body fluid balance, the performance during the actual competition will undoubtedly suffer.

6. Kidney Function During Exercise

Very little can be added to the observations of Robinson et al.[64] and of Rowell et al.[83] The former established that renal blood flow was reduced in exercise and the latter group found that splanchnic blood flow reduction was inversely related to the intensity of exercise. The reduction in renal blood flow is caused by a decrease in diameter of the resistance vessels within the kidney in response to sympathetic nervous system activity. The reduction in blood flow leads to a reduction in urine formation and hence is a method of maintaining body fluid volume during the exercise. With the end of exercise, kidney function is modified by the particular presence of ADH and ALD both of which increase in exercise. The secretion of ADH is a function of two modalities; reduction in blood volume and the increase in osmolarity.[84] Oddly enough, ALD secretion is probably related to the increase in the concentration of extracellular K during exercise and the decrease in blood pressure within the kidney.[85] When exercise ceases these two hormone levels remain elevated until there has been an increase in blood volume and a decrease in body fluid osmolarity. The attainment of normal resting osmolarity and volume requires the appropriate adjustment of the circulating levels of both hormones. With increasing volume and decreasing osmolarity, the amount of ADH will diminish but ALD will not return to "normal" levels until the correct proportion of Na to K is present.

VIII.   HEAT ACCLIMATION

Those athletes and workers exposed to annual changes in climate are said to become acclimatized to the natural shifts in temperature. However, in order to discuss the process of heat acclimation, we greatly depend upon studies wherein subjects were acclimated to heat. The exposure to heat was artificial and did not depend upon seasonal variation.

Traditionally, the signs of heat acclimation have been: (1) a decrease in heart rate; (2) an increase in sweat rate; and (3) a reduction in body temperature when a fixed task is performed in the heat. These results are also seen in acclimatization studies where individuals exercise in the heat for at least 90 min/day.[86] Most of the improvement in heart rate, sweat rate, and body temperature reduction occurs within a week but improvement slowly continues with continuing heat exposure.

Athletes who train become acclimated to heat and the degree of acclimation will depend upon the environmental temperature at which the athlete trains.[87,88] As noted earlier, training enlarges the plasma volume and this step is thought to be the basic reason for the decrease in heart rate during the performance of a fixed task.[89] Convertino et al.[31] showed that increases in plasma volume could be ascribed to two causes. The first is the effect of exercise itself while the second is the elevation in body temperature. Subjects who rested in the heat showed an increase in PV when their body temperatures were passively increased to equal that in exercising subjects. The combination of exercise and elevated body temperatures increased PV more than did passive heat exposure.

The increase in body temperature acting on and through the preoptic area of the hypothalamus initiates sweating to increase evaporative heat loss. With daily exercise bouts, the sweat mechanism is activated at a lower body temperature, and in addition, the amount of sweat for any given temperature elevation increases.[55] There is also evidence that functions of the sweat glands are also modified by increased skin temperature.[55] The increase in evaporative heat loss added to the increase in PV allows for better body cooling and thus for a given task, the body temperature will be reduced.

With the increase in sensitivity and gain of the sweating mechanism a change in the sweat contents takes place. The amount of Na and Cl in sweat diminishes to levels that may be 20% or less of the original sweat contents of a nontrained individual.[90] Levels of Na, and indirectly Cl, in sweat of persons serially exposed to heat first depends upon the amount of Na in the diet. Robinson et al.[64] have shown that increasing salt intake in heat decreases the reduction in sweat Na. Next, the amount of Na that is reabsorbed in the duct of the sweat gland is influenced by the presence of increased circulating level of aldosterone (see kidney function above).

All these responses to exercise at cooler temperatures can be increased in most endurance athletes (tennis, football, soccer, runners, cyclists, etc.) by exposing them to heat as they train. The key here is that exposure to elevated ambient temperatures must be accompanied by adequate fluid and salt intake.

The advantages of maintaining a lower body temperature in exercise is to reduce the danger of heat illness. Conservation of Na and Cl by the sweat glands increase the osmolarity of the ECV. As pointed out by Nose et al.[61] the increase in osmolarity causes an increase in fluid movement from the ICV to the ECV thus protecting plasma volume. The advantages of protecting or increasing blood volume has already been addressed as has the manner in which such increases are brought about. The mechanisms at work in exercise plus heat exposure are basically the same as in exercise alone.

Finally, one of the more interesting findings in acclimatization research has been an increase in efficiency in performing a fixed task after heat acclimatization takes place. Oxygen consumption appears to be approximately 3–5% less for a given exercise task.[91]

IX. FLUID REPLACEMENT

Noted earlier was the fact that athletes engaged in endurance exercises suffer from loss of body water via the sweat glands. These deficits are seldom made up during the actual exercise. Historically, water intake during prolonged athletic events was frowned upon.[63] For example, marathon runners in the United States were not allowed a water station until the

10 mile (16 km) mark. This situation has radically improved over the past 10–15 yr and water stations occur at interval as frequent as every 2–3 km.

The type of fluid and frequency of ingestion has been addressed in the most recent position statement of the American College of Sports Medicine on Exercise and Fluid Replacement.[5] The suggestions in this statement are based on present knowledge and should be considered by anyone coaching or participating in long-term exercises. Individual athletes should posses a reasonable idea as to their rate of water loss; indeed, it also should be the responsibility of the coaching staff or team trainer to gather the appropriate data by simply recording body weights at intervals during training.

A. CONTENTS OF REPLACEMENT FLUIDS[1,2,5]

For contests lasting less than 1 hr, water is the preferred drink. In 1 hr an athlete would rarely lose more than 2 l of sweat though higher rates have been recorded and increases in body fluid osmolarity and decreases in blood volume would not be of concern. In contests lasting longer than 1 hr, the ingested fluid should not only contain water but should also contain carbohydrate. While water ingestion helps to avoid dehydration and thermal injury, delivery of carbohydrate maintains concentrations of blood glucose and fatigue is delayed. The choice of carbohydrate is usually limited to sucrose, glucose, or complex carbohydrates, and 4–8 g are added to each deciliter of water. If fructose is taken in these concentrations, intestinal distress usually results. If fructose is to be added to the ingested fluid, the concentration should not be above 1–2%. When carbohydrates are added to water and the solution ingested, the rate at which the carbohydrate solution leaves the stomach decreases with the increase in carbohydrate concentration.[92-94] The concentrations recommended here leave the stomach at a rate somewhat less than pure water. The slower stomach emptying does not appear to seriously impair eventual fluid addition to the body water.

Recent studies have shown that fluid movement out of the stomach is primarily dependent upon the volume of fluid in the stomach, i.e., the greater the volume the greater the amount of fluid moving into the intestine.[92,93] Maintaining a large volume of fluid in the stomach, while physiologically ideal, is difficult to do. Feelings of discomfort or fullness generally are noted. Perhaps individuals can be trained to accept these conditions.

Stomach emptying is also influenced by the exercise intensity. If a person exercises at rates of oxygen consumption above 75% VO_2max, stomach emptying is slowed.[94] All things considered, ingestion of a 4–8% carbohydrate solution should be routine during prolonged exercise with sweat loss and the amount ingested should be short of discomfort.

1. Electrolytes and Fluid Replacement

For full volume replacement, the ions lost in sweat, particularly Na and Cl, must be replaced. Both of these ions are necessary for the maintenance of ECV. Should these ions be replaced in exercise? Because sweat is a hypotonic fluid, the remaining body fluids become more concentrated and osmotic pressure rises. Simple delivery of water will return ionic concentrations toward normal, but volume loss remains.[42] In short-term exercise, the prevention of ionic concentration is not important. There is support for the inclusion of Na (and attendant Cl) in fluids ingested during prolonged contests such as ultramarathons. Two potential problems may be addressed by salt inclusion; plasma volume reduction and hyponatremia (see below).[95,96] The grey area for salt inclusion in athletic drinks is in those contests lasting between 1 and 4 hr. Limited studies have not shown serious decreases in plasma Na for the majority of examined long distance runners. Where the advice to ultra-marathon runners is to include 0.5–0.7 g Na per liter in their rehydration drinks, the advice to standard marathon runners is that Na is not necessary.[5] This is a very narrow view point, for many athletes do not run marathons but lose large volumes of body water through sweat (ice-hockey players, baseball catchers). It would seem the lesser of two evils to also include the advised salt in the drinks of anyone exercising in the heat.

The dangers of inadequate fluid intake during athletic competition of any length have been well publicized. This apparently has stimulated a small group of runners to conscientiously ingest great quantities of fluid. The ECV [Na] is lowered below 130 meq/l, and the hyponatremic persons have collapsed or exhibited central nervous system disorders such as disorientation. The runners are usually hospitalized and treated with diuretics and recovery occurs. Noakes and co-workers[97] first described these events and the curious findings in these individuals. For example, even though large amounts of fluid were ingested, urine loss was quite small. Plasma volume was found to be reduced by 25% in some subjects. Noakes[98] has suggested that the water was sequestered in the gastrointestinal tract. Na would then move into the GI tract and thus lower the ECV and the ECV [Na]. While fluid intake during marathons, football practice, etc. is necessary to avoid dehydration, the possibility of overhydration also exists. How much fluid should be ingested in order to avoid dehydration and not produce hyperhydration and attendant hyponatremia? The first answer has already been given. During training the athlete should acquire knowledge as to his/her rate of weight loss during exercise under several climatic conditions through the year. During the contest, the athlete should then return a volume of fluid that should not exceed their maximum rate of weight loss. Failing this knowledge, then the advice presented in the statement of the American College of Sports Medicine should be followed where an intake of 600–1200 ml/h of a 4–8% carbohydrate solution should be ingested.[5] Whatever the intake, it should be ingested at sufficient intervals during the contest to avoid nausea or stomach discomfort from ingesting too much volume.

X. SUMMARY

Exercise increases the metabolic rate, and because 75–80% of the energy is converted to heat, provision has to be made to dissipate heat.[53] In cold climates, much of the heat can be lost via radiation and convection, but at moderate temperatures the avenue of heat loss increasingly becomes production and evaporation of sweat. The accommodation of the body to exercise and/or heat exposure is the increase in blood volume and an increase in the sensitivity of the sweating mechanism.[86-88] Athletes then must guard against two events: dangerous elevations of body temperatures and reductions in circulating blood volume accompanied by increases in osmolarity. The elevations in temperature are related to blood volume reduction, and performance in turn is related to both conditions.[71,74] In order to avoid or temper the changes in temperature, blood volume, and osmolarity, fluid ingestion is required. The amount needed should be related to loss of sweat and is best determined by weight loss during training. The ingested fluid should be water for short term exercise (<1 hr), while the solution should contain 4–8% carbohydrate and 0.5–0.7 g of Na (1.2–1.8 g of NaCl) per liter of solution.[5] Finally, if such a mixture is not available, water is the preferred drink. While lacking an ergogenic aid, it will reduce body fluid osmolarity and return blood volume toward normal thus avoiding damaging elevations in body temperatures.

REFERENCES

1. Maughan, R. J., Fluid and electrolyte loss and replacement in exercise, *J. Sports Sci.*, 9, 117, 1991.
2. Noakes, T. D., Fluid replacement during exercise, in *Exercise and Sport Sciences Reviews*, Vol. 21, Holloszy, J. O., Ed., Williams and Wilkins, Baltimore, 1993.
3. American College of Sports Medicine, Position statement on prevention of heat injuries during distance running, *Med. Sci. Sports Exer.*, 7, vii, 1975.

4. American College of Sports Medicine, Position stand on prevention of thermal injuries during distance running, *Med. Sci. Sports Exer.*, 16, ix, 1984.
5. American College of Sports Medicine, Position stand on exercise and fluid replacement, *Med. Sci. Sports Exer.*, 28, i, 1996.
6. Pitts, R. F., *Physiology of the Kidney and Body Fluids*, 3rd ed., Year Book, Chicago, 1974, Chap. 2.
7. Bland, J. H., Basic physiologic considerations of body water and electrolytes, in *Clinical Metabolism of Body Water and Electrolytes*, Bland, J. H., Ed., Saunders, Philadelphia, 1963, Chap. 2.
8. Valtin, J. and Schafer, J., *Renal Function*, 3rd ed., Little, Brown and Co., Boston, 1995, Chap. 2.
9. Judy, W. V., Body temperature regulation, in *Physiology*, 5th ed., Selkurt, E. E., Ed., Little, Brown, Boston, 1984, Chap. 28.
10. Guyton, A. C., *Textbook of Medical Physiology*, 8th ed., W. B. Saunders, Philadelphia, 1991, 799.
11. Guyton, A. C., *Textbook of Medical Physiology*, 8th ed., W. B. Saunders, Philadelphia, 1991, Chap. 5.
12. Edelman, I. S. and Leibman, J., Anatomy of water and electrolytes, *Am. J. Med.*, 27, 256, 1959.
13. Starling, E. H., Physiological factors involved in the causation of dropsy, *Lancet*, 1, 1405, 1896.
14. Schultze, H. E. and Heremans, J. F., *Molecular Biology of Human Proteins*, Vol. 1, Elsevier, New York, 1966, Chap. 2.
15. Schneeberger, E. E., Proteins and vesicular transport in capillary endothelium, *Fed. Proc.*, 42, 2419, 1972.
16. Senay, L. C., Jr., Changes in plasma volume and protein content during exposure of working men to various temperatures before and after acclimatization to heat: separation of the roles of cutaneous and skeletal muscle circulation, *J. Physiol.* (London), 224, 61, 1972.
17. Guyton, A. C., Taylor, A. E., and Granger, H. J., *Circulatory Physiology II: Dynamics and Control of the Body Fluids*, W. B. Saunders Co., Philadelphia, 1975.
18. Guyton, A. C., Interstitial fluid pressure II. Pressure-volume curves of interstitial space, *Circ. Res.*, 16, 452, 1965.
19. Eisenman, A. J., MacKenzie, L. B., and Peters, J. P., Protein of serum and cells of human blood with a note on the measurement of red blood cell volume, *J. Biol. Chem.*, 116, 33, 1936.
20. Oscai, L. B., Williams, B. T., and Hertig, B. A., Effect of exercise on blood volume, *J. Appl. Physiol.*, 24, 622, 1968.
21. Convertino, V. A., Blood volume: its adaptation to endurance training, *Med. Sci. Sports Exer.*, 23, 1338, 1991.
22. Senay, L. C., Jr. and Pivarnik, J. M., Fluid shifts during exercise, in *Exercise and Sport Sciences Reviews*, Vol. 13, Terjung, R. L., Ed., MacMillan, New York, 1985.
23. Saltin, B., Blomqvist, G., Mitchell, J. H., Johnson, R. L., Jr., Wildenthal, K., and Chapman, C. B., Response to exercise after bed rest and after training, *Circulation*, 38, Suppl. VII, 1, 1968.
24. Gillen, C. M., Lee, R., Mack, G. W., Tomaselli, C. M., Nishezasa, T., and Nadel, E. R., Plasma volume expansion in humans after a single intense exercise protocol, *J. Appl. Physiol.*, 71, 1914, 1991.
25. Carroll, J. F., Convertino, V. A., Wood, C. C., Lowenthal, D. T., and Pollock, M. L., Effect of training on blood volume and plasma hormone concentrations in the elderly, *Med. Sci. Sports Exer.*, 27, 79, 1995.
26. Avellini, B. A., Kamon, E., and Krajewski, J. T., Physiological responses of physically fit men and women to acclimation to humid heat, *J. Appl. Physiol.*, 49, 254, 1980.
27. Frye, A. J. and Kamon, E., Responses to dry heat of men and women with similar aerobic capacities, *J. Appl. Physiol.*, 50, 65, 1980.
28. Rocker, L., Kirsch, K. A., Heyduck, B., and Altenkirch, H. U., Influence of prolonged physical exercise on plasma volume, plasma proteins, electrolytes and fluid — regulating hormones, *Int. J. Sports Med.*, 10, 270, 1989.
29. Schmidt, W., Brabant, G., Kroger, C., Strauch, L., and Hilgendorf, A., Atrial natriuretic peptide during and after maximal and submaximal exercise under normoxic and hypoxic conditions, *Eur. J. Appl. Physiol.*, 61, 398, 1990.
30. El-Sayed, M. S., Davies, B., and Morgan, D. B., Vasopressin and plasma volume response to submaximal and maximal exercise in man, *J. Sports Med. Phys. Fitness*, 30, 420, 1990.
31. Convertino, V. A., Greenleaf, J. E., and Bernauer, E. M., Role of thermal and exercise factors in the mechanism of hyper volemia, *J. Appl. Physiol.*, 48, 657, 1980.
32. Convertino, V. A., Keil, L. C., Bernauer, E. M., and Greenleaf, J. E., Plasma volume, osmolality, vasopressin and renin activity during graded exercise in man, *J. Appl. Physiol.*, 50, 23, 1981.
33. Senay, L. C., Jr., Rogers, G., and Jooste, P., Changes in blood plasma during progressive treadmill and cycle exercise, *J. Appl. Physiol.*, 49, 59, 1980.
34. Olszewski, W., Engeset, A., Jaeger, P. M., Sokolowski, J., and Theodorsen, L., Flow and composition of leg lymph in normal men during venous stasis, muscular activity and local hyperthermia, *Acta Physiol. Scand.*, 99, 149, 1977.
35. Senay, L. C., Jr., Effects of exercise in the heat on body fluid distribution, *Med. Sci. Sports Exer.*, 11, 42, 1979.
36. Scatchard, G., Batchelder, A. C., and Brown, A., Chemical, clinical, and immunological studies on the products of human plasma fractionation. VI. The osmotic pressure of plasma and serum albumin, *J. Clin. Invest.*, 23, 458, 1944.

37. Sjostrand, T., Blood volume, in *Handbook of Physiology*. Sect. 2. *Circulation*, Hamilton, W. F. and Dow, P., Eds., Vol. 1, American Physiological Society, Washington, D.C., 1966, 55.

38. Gillen, C. M., Nishiyasu, T., Langhans, G., Weseman, C., Mack, G. W., and Nadel, E. R., Cardiovascular and renal function during exercise induced blood volume expansion in man, *J. Appl. Physiol.*, 76, 2602, 1994.

39. Pivarnik, J. M. and Senay, L. C., Jr., The effects of exercise detraining and deacclimation to the heat on plasma volume dynamics, *Eur. J. Appl. Physiol.*, 55, 222, 1986.

40. Pivarnik, J. M., Goetting, M. P., and Senay, L. C., Jr., The effects of body position and exercise on plasma volume dynamics, *Eur. J. Appl. Physiol.*, 55, 450, 1986.

41. Astrand, P. O. and Rodahl, K., *Textbook of Work Physiology*, McGraw Hill, New York, 1977, Chap. 12.

42. Nose, H., Mack, G. W., Shi, X., and Nadel, E. R., Shift in body fluid compartments after dehydration in man, *J. Appl. Physiol.*, 65, 318, 1988.

43. Lundvall, J., Mellander, S., Westling, H., and White, T., Fluid transfer between blood and tissues during exercise, *Acta Physiol. Scand.*, 85, 258, 1972.

44. Lundvall, J., Tissue hyperosmolality as a mediator of vasodilatation and transcapillary fluid flux in exercising skeletal muscle, *Acta Physiol. Scand.*, 86, Suppl. 379, 1, 1972.

45. Greenleaf, J. E., van Beaumont, W., Brock, P. J., Morse, J. T., and Mangseth, G. R., Plasma volume and electrolyte shifts with heavy exercise in sitting and supine positions, *Am. J. Physiol.*, 236, R206, 1979.

46. Powers, S. K., Howley, E. T., and Cox, R., A differential catecholamine response during prolonged exercise and passive heating, *Med. Sci. Sports Exer.*, 14, 435, 1982.

47. Guyton, A. C., *Textbook of Medical Physiology*, 8th ed., W. B. Saunders, Philadelphia, 1991, 759, 863.

48. Sjogaard, G. and Saltin, B., Extra- and intracellular water spaces in muscles of man at rest and with dynamic exercise, *Am. J. Physiol.*, 253, R271, 1982.

49. Medbo, J. I. and Sejersted, O. M., Plasma potassium changes with high intensity exercise, *J. Physiol.* (London), 421, 105, 1990.

50. Vollestad, N. K., Hallen, J., and Sejersted, O. M., Effect of exercise intensity on potassium balance in muscle and blood of man, *J. Physiol.* (London), 475, 359, 1994.

51. Carter, J. E. and Gisolfi, C. V., Fluid replacement during and after exercise in the heat, *Med. Sci. Sports Exer.*, 21, 532, 1989.

52. Viinamaki, O., The effect of hydration status on plasma vasopressin release during physical exercise in man, *Acta Physiol. Scand.*, 139, 133, 1990.

53. Werner, J., Temperature regulation during exercise: an overview, in *Perspectives in Exercise Science and Sports Medicine*, Vol. 6, *Exercise, Heat and Thermoregulation*, Gisolfi, C., Lamb, D. R., and Nadel, E. R., Eds., Brown and Benchmark, Dubuque, IA, 1993, Chap. 2.

54. Costill, D. L., Sweating: its composition and effects on body fluids, in *The Marathon: Physiological, Medical, Epidemiological, and Psychological Studies*, Vol. 301, Milvey, P., Ed., New York Academy of Sciences, New York, 1977, 160.

55. Sato, K., The mechanism of eccrine sweat secretion, in *Perspectives in Exercise Science and Sports Medicine*, Vol. 6, *Exercise, Heat, and Thermoregulation*, Gisolfi, C., Lamb, D. L., and Nadel, E. R., Brown and Benchmark, Dubuque, IA, 1993, Chap. 3.

56. Adolph, E. F. and Associates, *Physiology of Man in the Desert*, Interscience, New York, Chap. 10.

57. Senay, L. C., Jr., Plasma volumes and constituents of heat exposed men before and after acclimatization, *J. Appl. Physiol.*, 38, 570, 1975.

58. Costill, D. L., Cote, R., and Fink, W., Muscle water and electrolytes during varied levels of dehydration in man, *J. Appl. Physiol.*, 40, 6, 1976.

59. Kozlowski, S. and Saltin, B., Effect of sweat loss on body fluids, *J. Appl. Physiol.*, 19, 1119, 1964.

60. Morimoto, T., Miki, K., Nose, H., Yamada, S., Hirakawa, K., and Matsubara, C., Changes in body fluid volume and its composition during heavy sweating and the effect of fluid and electrolyte replacement, *Jpn. J. Biometerol.*, 18, 31, 1988.

61. Nose, H., Mack, G. W., Shi, X., and Nadel, E. R., Shift in body fluid compartments after dehydration in humans, *J. Appl. Physiol.*, 65, 318, 1988.

62. Astrand, P. O. and Saltin, B., Plasma and red cell volume after prolonged severe exercise, *J. Appl. Physiol.*, 19, 829, 1964.

63. Noakes, T. D., Dehydration during exercise: what are the real dangers?, *Clin. J. Sport Med.*, 5, 123, 1995.

64. Robinson, S., Maletich, R. T., Robinson, W. S., Rohrer, B., and Kung, A. L., Output of Na Cl by sweat glands and kidneys in relation to dehydration and salt depletion, *J. Appl. Physiol.*, 8, 615, 1956.

65. Pearcy, M., Robinson, S., Miller, D. I., Thomas, J. T., Jr., and DeBrota, J., Effects of dehydration, salt depletion and pitressin on sweat rate and urine flow, *J. Appl. Physiol.*, 8, 621, 1956.

66. Nose, H., Mack, G. W., Shi, X., and Nadel, E. R., The role of osmolality and plasma volume during rehydration in humans, *J. Appl. Physiol.*, 65, 325, 1988.

67. Francesconi, R. P., Sawka, M. N., and Pandolph, K. B., Hypohydration and heat acclimation: plasma renin and aldosterone during exercise, *J. Appl. Physiol.*, 55, 1790, 1983.

68. Greenleaf, J. E., Problem: thirst, drinking behavior, and involuntary dehydration, *Med. Sci. Sports Exer.*, 24, 645, 1992.
69. Rowell, L. B., Human cardiovascular adjustments to exercise and thermal stress, *Physiol. Rev.*, 54, 75, 1974.
70. Senay, L. C., Jr., Relationship of evaporative rates to serum [Na+], [K+], and osmolarity in acute heat stress, *J. Appl. Physiol.*, 25, 149, 1968.
71. Sawka, M. N., Physiological consequences of hypohydration: exercise performance and thermoregulation, *Med. Sci. Sports Exer.*, 24, 657, 1992.
72. Strydom, N. B. and Holdsworth, L. D., The effects of different levels of water deficit on physiological responses during heat stress, *Int. Z. angew. Physiol. einschl. Arbeitsphysiol.*, 26, 95, 1968.
73. Coyle, E. F. and Montain, S. J., Thermal and cardiovascular responses to fluid replacement during exercise, in *Perspectives in Exercise Science and Sports Medicine,* Vol. 6, *Exercise, Heat, and Thermoregulation,* Gisolfi, C. V., Lamb, D. R., and Nadel, E. R., Eds., Brown and Benchmark, Dubuque, IA, 1993, 193.
74. Whiting, P. H., Maughan, R. J., and Miller, J. D. B., Dehydration and serum biochemical changes in marathon runners, *Eur. J. Appl. Physiol.*, 52, 183, 1984.
75. Maughan, R. J., Fluid and electrolyte loss and replacement in exercise, *J. Sports Sci.*, 9, 117, 1991.
76. Stitt, J. T., Central regulation of body temperature, in *Perspectives in Exercise Science and Sports Medicine*, Vol. 6, *Exercise, Heat, and Thermoregulation*, Gisolfi, C. V., Lamb, D. R., and Nadel, E. R., Eds., Brown and Benchmark, Dubuque, IA, 1993, 14.
77. Dontas, S., Uber den Mechanisms der Warm Regulation, *Arch. Ges. Physiol.*, 241, 612, 1939.
78. Nielsen, B., Effect of change in plasma Na+ and Ca++ ion concentration on body temperature during exercise, *Acta Physiol. Scand.*, 91, 123, 1989.
79. Dinarello, C. A., Interleukin-1 and its biologically related cytokines, *Adv. Immunol.*, 44, 153, 1989.
80. Fortney, S. M., Wenger, C. B., Bove, J. R., and Nadel, E. R., Effect of hyperosmolality on control of blood flow and sweating, *J. Appl. Physiol.*, 57, 1688, 1984.
81. Scientific Tables, in *Documenta Geigy*, 6th ed., Diem, K., Ed., Geigy Pharmaceuticals, Ardsley, NY, 1962, 498.
82. Castenfors, J., Renal function during exercise, *Acta Physiol. Scand.*, 70, Suppl. 293, 1967.
83. Rowell, L. B., Blackman, J. R., and Bruce, R. A., Indocyanine green clearance and estimated hepatic blood flow during mild to maximum exercise, *J. Clin. Invest.*, 43, 1677, 1964.
84. Valtin, J. and Schafer, J., *Renal Function,* 3rd ed., Little, Brown and Co., Boston, 1995, 172.
85. Guyton, A. C., *Textbook of Medical Physiology,* 8th ed., W. B. Saunders, Philadelphia, 1991, 327.
86. Lind, A. R. and Bass, D., Optimal exposure time for development of acclimatization to heat, *Fed. Proc.*, 22, 704, 1963.
87. Gisolfi, C. V., Work — heat tolerance derived from interval training, *J. Appl. Physiol.*, 35, 349, 1973.
88. Adams, W. C., Fox, R. H., Fry, A. J., and MacDonald, I. C., Thermoregulation during marathon running in cool, moderate, and hot environments, *J. Appl. Physiol.*, 38, 1030, 1975.
89. Senay, L. C., Mitchell, D., and Wyndham, C. H., Acclimatization in a hot, humid environment: body fluid adjustments, *J. Appl. Physiol.*, 40, 786, 1976.
90. Allan, J. R. and Wilson, C. G., Influence of acclimatization on sweat sodium concentration, *J. Appl. Physiol.*, 30, 708, 1971.
91. Sawka, M. N., Pandolph, K. B., Avellini, B. A., and Shapiro, Y., Does heat acclimation lower the rate of metabolism elicited by muscular exercise?, *Aviat. Space Environ. Med.*, 54, 27, 1983.
92. Mitchell, J. B. and Voss, K. W., The influence of volume of fluid ingested on gastric emptying and fluid balance during prolonged exercise, *Med. Sci. Sports Exer.*, 23, 314, 1991.
93. Rehrer, N. J., The maintenance of fluid balance during exercise, *Internat. J. Sports Med.*, 15, 122, 1994.
94. Costill, D. L. and Saltin, B., Factors limiting gastric emptying during rest and exercise, *J. Appl. Physiol.*, 37, 679, 1974.
95. Brouns, F., Heat — sweat — dehydration — rehydration: a praxis oriented approach, *J. Sports Sci.*, 9, 143, 1991.
96. Brouns, F., Saris, W., and Schneider, H., Rationale for upper limits of electrolyte replacement during exercise, *Int. J. Sport Nutr.*, 2, 229, 1992.
97. Noakes, T. D., Norman, R. J., Buck, R. H., Godlonton, J., Stevenson, K., and Pittaway, D., The incidence of hyponatremia during prolonged ultra-endurance exercise, *Med. Sci. Sports Exer.*, 22, 165, 1990.
98. Noakes, T. D., Hyponatremia during endurance running: a physiological and clinical interpretation, *Med. Sci. Sports Exer.*, 24, 403, 1992.

Chapter **12**

NUTRIENT BEVERAGES
FOR PHYSICAL PERFORMANCE

Susan M. Puhl
Elsworth R. Buskirk

CONTENTS

0-8493-8560-1/97/$0.00+$.50
© 1998 by CRC Press LLC

I.　INTRODUCTION

Beverages containing various mixtures of nutrients such as carbohydrates and electrolytes are often used by athletes and exercise enthusiasts in an effort to enhance physical performance. Currently there are many such nutrient beverages commercially available. These solutions are consumed by individuals involved in organized professional and amateur competition as well as those who participate recreationally in activities for fun or fitness.

Several authors have reviewed topics of interest in the area of nutritional supplements ingested before, during, or after physical performance. Table 1[1-26] provides a listing of such reviews. The reader is encouraged to secure those of interest. All are well written and informative about the topic indicated.

A.　HOMEOSTATIC DISTURBANCES DURING EXERCISE

A bout of exercise results in changes which affect the homeostasis of the exercising individual. The beneficial effects of consuming nutritional beverages are attained if use of such products minimizes or ameliorates the exercise-induced changes which could detrimentally affect performance. Homeostatic disturbances which may result in decreased physical performance during exercise include but are not limited to: decreased plasma volume, increased deep body or core temperature, altered plasma and muscle electrolyte concentrations, and decreased nutrient fuel availability to the active skeletal muscle. The degree to which each of these disturbances results in a decrease in physical performance is a function of both the magnitude of the disturbance and the concomitant alterations in other homeostatic conditions. Several comprehensive reviews of the homeostatic disturbances associated with exercise are available, including that offered in the former edition of this volume.[27] The reader is encouraged to secure those of interest.

B.　ROLE OF REPLACEMENT BEVERAGES

In light of the exercise-induced alterations in homeostasis mentioned above, the possibility that ingestion of an appropriate nutrient solution may enhance physical performance is indeed welcome. However, the benefit of any such beverage comes only if it is capable of diminishing the detrimental effects of changes in plasma volume, body core temperature, blood and muscle electrolyte concentrations, and/or energy stores. If such diminishment is possible, then it can be expected that judicious use of appropriate nutrient beverages may lead to enhanced performance, i.e., support an increase in speed of movement or an extension of effort.

TABLE 1 Reviews of the Effects of Nutrient Use and Replacement on Physical Performance

Ref.	Authors	Information Reviewed
1	Brooks and Mercier, 1994	carbohydrate and lipid use during exercise
2	Brouns and Beckers, 1993	gastric emptying and nutrient absorption during exercise
3	Burke and Read, 1993	dietary supplements in sport
4	Coggan and Coyle, 1991	carbohydrate use during prolonged exercise
5	Consolazio and Johnson, 1972	carbohydrate use at rest and during exercise
6	Costill, 1985	carbohydrate ingestion before, during, and after activities of various durations and intensities
7	Costill, 1988	carbohydrate use during, and glycogen resynthesis following, intense exercise
8	Costill and Hargreaves, 1992	carbohydrates and fatigue
9	Coyle, 1991	carbohydrate metabolism and fatigue
10	Coyle and Coggan, 1984	carbohydrate ingestion during prolonged exercise
11	Dodd et al., 1993	caffeine and exercise performance
12	Gisolfi and Duchman, 1993	replacement beverages for exercise and sport
13	Hawley et al., 1995	carbohydrate, fluid, and electrolyte requirements during prolonged exercise
14	Ivy, 1991	muscle glycogen synthesis before and after exercise
15	Johnson, 1995	fluid, carbohydrate, and electrolyte requirements during heavy sweating
16	Kreider, 1993	amino acid supplementation
17	Lamb and Brodowicz, 1986	carbohydrate/electrolyte beverages ingested before, during, and/or after exercise
18	Maughan and Noakes, 1991	fluid replacement during exercise
19	Meyer and Bar-Or, 1994	fluid and electrolyte balance in children during exercise
20	Murray, 1987	carbohydrate/electrolyte consumption and gastrointestinal activity during and following exercise
21	Noakes, 1993	fluid replacement during exercise
22	Powers and Dodd, 1985	caffeine and endurance exercise
23	Sparling et al., 1993	fluid replacement during marathon running
24	Stanley and Connett, 1991	carbohydrate metabolism in muscle during exercise
25	Valeriani, 1991	carbohydrate needs during exercise
26	Wasserman and Cherrington, 1991	hepatic fuel metabolism during exercise

II. GENERAL CONSIDERATIONS
FOR NUTRIENT BEVERAGE UPTAKE

A. GASTRIC EMPTYING

The effectiveness of any ingested solution in maintaining plasma volume, electrolyte balance, or blood glucose during exercise is dependent on the ability of the ingested solution to traverse the stomach and be absorbed in the intestines. Relatively little is absorbed directly from the stomach; the small intestine is the primary site of nutrient absorption. Water is absorbed readily once it reaches the small intestine, and various nutrients are absorbed from the intestine at different rates.[28] Since nutrients are not absorbed from the stomach, the rate at which they empty into the intestines is an important limit to the benefit of any nutrient solution. Several excellent reviews of factors affecting gastric emptying and intestinal absorption have been written.[20,28-30]

Gastric emptying of water is primarily due to the pressure gradient between the stomach and duodenum.[29,30] Thus, a larger volume will empty faster than a smaller volume.[31] However, volumes greater than 600 ml do not appear to result in additional increases in emptying rate. Maintaining a relatively large volume of fluid in the stomach does not impair the rate of gastric emptying.[32] Cool water, at a temperature of from 5 to 15°C empties quicker than warmer solutions.[31,33-35]

The addition of carbohydrates and/or other nutrients to a beverage slows gastric emptying in proportion to the caloric content of the solution.[30,36-39] Once in the duodenum, nutrients act through neural feedback mechanisms to affect the rate of subsequent gastric emptying, resulting in a rate of gastric emptying which is approximately isocaloric regardless of the nature of the gastric contents.[29,36,40] Carbohydrate solutions empty in relative proportion to the solute concentration,[35,41,42] but such differences are not observed when the concentration differences are small (e.g., from 5 to 7%). The effect of osmolality on rate of gastric emptying has not yet been definitively demonstrated, with some authors reporting a slowing of gastric emptying as osmolality increases above isotonic[29,30,41] while others show no effect of osmolality aside from its association with calorie-laden nutrients.[38,43,44] Carbonating the beverage appears to have no effect on the rate of gastric emptying.[39]

An essential element to the discussion of nutrient beverages is the effect which differences in gastric emptying rates of various beverages may have on actual performance. As discussed above, there is ample evidence to show that the composition of a beverage may affect the rate at which the beverage empties from the stomach. However, such differences may have little effect on eventual exercise performance.[45]

B. INTESTINAL ABSORPTION

Absorption of water, carbohydrates, and electrolytes occurs largely in the duodenum and jejunum of the small intestine. Net absorption of water is increased via the active transport of glucose and sodium.[46-48] The capacity for water absorption is apparently unlimited so long as there exists an osmotic gradient which favors movement of water out of the intestinal lumen.[20] The introduction of hypertonic solutions into the intestines rapidly draws water into the intestinal lumen.[30,36] Thus, ingestion of hypertonic solutions, which empty from the stomach into the intestine with no significant alteration in osmolality, may result in decreases in plasma volume.[30]

Carbohydrates are absorbed primarily as monosaccharides along the duodenal and jejunal epithelia.[28] Sodium is essential for operation of the facilitated glucose transport system in the intestine.[46] Indeed, sodium-dependent transport is the rate-limiting step in glucose uptake.[28] However, altering the sodium content of a carbohydrate solution may not alter the rate of intestinal glucose absorption.[49] Additionally, as was noted in the discussion of gastric emptying, differences in rate of intestinal absorption for various nutrient solutions have not been demonstrated to result in differences in physical performance.

C. EXERCISE INTENSITY

Most investigations of the gastric emptying and/or intestinal absorption characteristics of nutrient beverages have been conducted on individuals at rest. The extent to which physical activity may modify those characteristics is important to athletes. Moderate intensity exercise (up to 70% VO_2max) does not hinder gastric emptying of water or hypotonic nutrient beverages,[31,35,45,50-52] even when the exercise continues for up to 3 h.[53] Intestinal absorption of water, glucose, and/or electrolytes is likewise unaffected by moderate cycling or running exercise.[48,50,54] Indeed, physical activities such as running may aid gastric emptying due to mechanical movement of the fluids or increases in intragastric pressure.[36,52] However, addition of heat and/or hypohydration stress during an exercise bout may impair gastric emptying,[51,55] probably because of the marked reduction in splanchnic blood flow.

D. METABOLIC AVAILABILITY OF INGESTED NUTRIENTS

The degree to which ingested carbohydrates or other nutrients are made available for metabolic activity will determine the efficacy of the use of such beverages as a fuel replacement source. Several investigators have shown that a significant portion of ingested carbohydrate is oxidized during exercise. Up to 98% of glucose and glucose polymers ingested during prolonged moderate-intensity exercise is metabolized, as demonstrated using labeled carbon.[56-58] Indeed, exercise increases the rate of oxidation of exogenous carbohydrate.[59] The amount of exogenous carbohydrate oxidized during prolonged, moderate-intensity exercise is relatively independent of time of ingestion[57] or beverage osmolality.[56] However, the type of carbohydrate ingested may affect metabolic availability, with ingested fructose less efficiently available for oxidation than glucose.[58,60,61] Some authors have suggested that the ability of the intestine to absorb fructose is limited because the ingestion of fairly low amounts of fructose may saturate absorption channels and that exercise may exacerbate the absorption of fructose by reducing intestinal transit time.[62] Ingestion of glucose polymers appears to provide no metabolic advantage over the ingestion of glucose.[58]

E. SUMMARY

Nutrient beverages must be absorbed to be of value. Once absorbed, the nutrients must be used by the body if they are to be of benefit to physical performance. The rate at which the ingested beverage empties from the stomach coupled with the rate of intestinal absorption determines the availability of ingested nutrients. Gastric emptying is largely a function of the volume and caloric content of the beverage ingested. Cool beverages, which increase gastric motility, empty more quickly than warmer beverages and have the added advantage of increasing palatability.[33] The addition of carbohydrates to a beverage slows its emptying in proportion to the caloric content. Osmolality itself, in the absence of the caloric influence, may not be an important determinant of gastric emptying. Intestinal absorption is a complex event involving many passive and active transport mechanisms. Different carbohydrates are absorbed via different mechanisms which may affect the rate of absorption. Addition of sodium to an ingested beverage should theoretically facilitate the sodium-dependent transport of glucose across the intestinal wall, however this has not been clearly documented. Moderately intense aerobic activity does not impair gastrointestinal transport of water or nutrients. Finally, most ingested carbohydrate is oxidized by active tissues. There is, then, ample evidence to suggest that ingestion of appropriate nutrient beverages may enhance performance during exercise.

III. PRE-EXERCISE INGESTION OF NUTRIENT BEVERAGES

A. RATIONALE

Nutrient beverages may be ingested prior to exercise in an attempt to prevent or delay the detrimental homeostatic disturbances which can accompany exercise. Pre-event use of such beverages seeks to accomplish two things: maintenance of plasma volume and optimization of nutrient availability to the exercising muscle. Fluid is ingested in an attempt to ensure adequate plasma volume at the onset of exercise and to provide a small "reservoir" of fluid in the gastrointestinal lumen which will be absorbed during the early phases of the exercise bout. Net movement of water out of the vascular space and the concomitant increase in plasma osmolality which normally occur during exercise may thereby be reduced. The desired result is an increase in performance time prior to hypohydration-induced compromises in cardiovascular and thermoregulatory functions. A second reason for the pre-exercise use of nutrient beverages is to optimize nutrient availability. Optimizing blood glucose may enhance performance by increasing carbohydrate oxidation in the later stages of endurance exercise, thereby increasing time to exhaustion in prolonged moderate- and high-intensity exercise. Table 2[63-92] presents an overview of the efficacy of various nutrient beverages ingested before exercise.

B. PRE-EXERCISE CARBOHYDRATE INGESTION
1. Effect of Time of Ingestion

The time prior to the onset of exercise at which carbohydrate is ingested may affect subsequent performance by altering blood glucose profiles during the exercise bout. At rest, ingestion of glucose results in an initial rise in blood glucose peaking approximately 30–45 min after ingestion.[74,78,79,90,91] Subsequent insulin-dependent uptake of the glucose may cause the blood glucose to fall below normal resting levels. However, the effect which these alterations in blood glucose may have on subsequent performance is not so clear.

Glucose or glucose polymers ingested in the 5 min period immediately prior to exercise result in a prolonged period of maintenance of blood glucose during moderate- to high-intensity exercise to exhaustion.[7,65,66] However, performance time to exhaustion may[66] or may not[65] be increased. The addition of sodium to the nutrient beverage has no effect on the bioavailability of the ingested glucose.[63]

Ingestion of carbohydrates from 20 to 15 min prior to exercise results in an increase in plasma glucose[67-69] with no significant effect on performance of high-intensity exercise.[67]

Ingestion of glucose in the period of from 1 h to 30 min prior to exercise results in the expected initial elevation of plasma glucose and is followed by a fall in plasma glucose during the early stages of exercise.[71,73-75,77,79,81,91,93] However, plasma glucose returns to normal concentrations within approximately 30 min of the onset of exercise in such glucose ingestion regimens.[73,78] Some investigators have indicated that during moderately-high intensity exercise (75–85% VO_2max), muscle glycogen utilization is greater[76] and endurance time is decreased[73,75,86] following glucose ingestion during the 60 to 30 min pre-exercise period. However, others have shown that muscle glycogen utilization during the first 30 min of exercise[71,75] or during prolonged exercise[75,77,78] is not affected by glucose ingested 30 min to 1 h prior to exercise. Time to exhaustion in moderately intense exercise may[82,93] or may not[74] be increased as a result of carbohydrate ingestion during this time period, while total carbohydrate oxidation is not affected.[75] Plasma free fatty acid concentration is decreased during the exercise when glucose is ingested from 1 h to 30 min prior to exercise.[73,74,78,79,81]

Glucose ingested 3–4 h prior to exercise results in the initial elevation and subsequent drop in blood glucose discussed above.[90-92] However, subsequent low- (45% VO_2max)[90] or moderate- (70% VO_2max)[91] intensity exercise is enhanced following ingestion of the glucose

TABLE 2   Effects of Ingesting Nutrient Beverages Prior to Exercise

Ref.	Authors	Time of Ingestion (min before exercise)	Nutrients Ingested	Exercise	Results
63	Hargreaves et al., 1994	0	glucose (400 ml of 10%) with a. 0 mmol/l Na b. 25 mmol/l Na c. 50 mmol/l Na	cycling — 30 min 75% VO_2max	no difference in plasma glucose
64	Melin et al., 1994	0 only, or 0, then 15 min intervals	water — 50% of that lost during dehydration	walking — treadmill to exhaustion 50% VO_2max	a. increased time to exhaustion with all water given at time 0 b. increased sweating with either replenishment c. increased plasma volume with rehydration
65	Segal et al., 1985	0	glucose (90 g)	cycling — intermittent to exhaustion 74% VO_2max	a. no difference in time to exhaustion b. increased blood glucose early but not later in exercise
66	Snyder et al., 1983	5	mixed CHO (150 g)	cycling — to exhaustion 68% VO_2max	a. increased time to exhaustion b. increased plasma glucose throughout exercise
67	Snyder et al., 1993	15	glucose polymer, 5 ml/kg of 19.7% solution	cycling — 4 intervals of 1.6 km time trials separated by steady state rides of 80–90% VO_2max	a. increased blood glucose b. no difference in performance time
68	Brouns et al., 1989	20	a. glucose b. sucrose c. fructose d. glucose polymer (300 or 600 ml)	cycling — 45 min HR = 150	increase in blood glucose with all beverages
69	Criswell et al., 1992	20, then 0, then 15 min intervals	glucose polymer/fructose (400 ml of 7%) with electrolytes	cycling — 115 min 65% VO_2max	a. better maintenance of plasma volume b. no difference in plasma osmolality, oxygen consumption, or respiratory exchange ratio
70	MacLean and Graham, 1993	20 and 45	branched-chain amino acids (77 mg/kg)	cycling — 60 min 75% VO_2max	a. increased plasma branched-chain amino acids throughout exercise b. increased plasma ammonia c. no difference in plasma glucose

TABLE 2   Effects of Ingesting Nutrient Beverages Prior to Exercise *(continued)*

Ref.	Authors	Time of Ingestion (min before exercise)	Nutrients Ingested	Exercise	Results
71	Fielding et al., 1987	30	a. glucose (75 g) b. fructose (75 g)	running — 30 min 70% VO$_2$max	a. increased initial blood glucose with glucose b. no change in blood glucose with fructose c. no difference in rate of muscle glycogen use
72	Ventura et al., 1994	30	a. glucose (75 g) b. fructose (75 g)	running — to exhaustion 82% VO$_2$ peak	a. increased time to exhaustion with glucose b. increased initial plasma glucose with glucose
73	Foster et al., 1979	30	a. glucose (75 g) b. liquid mixed meal	cycling — to exhaustion 80% VO$_2$max	a. decreased time to exhaustion with glucose b. increased initial blood glucose with glucose c. decreased serum FFA with glucose
74	Gleeson et al., 1986	45	a. glucose (1 g/kg) b. glycerol (1 g/kg)	cycling — to exhaustion 73% VO$_2$max	a. increased initial blood glucose with glucose b. increased CHO oxidation with glucose c. no change in blood glucose during exercise with glucose
75	Hargreaves et al., 1987	45	a. glucose (75 g)	cycling — to exhaustion 75% VO$_2$max	a. no difference in time to exhaustion b. increased initial blood glucose with glucose c. no difference (as compared to control) in blood glucose with fructose d. no difference in muscle glycogen utilization with glucose or fructose
76	Hargreaves et al., 1985	45	a. glucose (50 g) b. fructose (50 g)	cycling — 30 min 75% VO$_2$max	a. increased initial blood glucose with glucose b. no change in blood glucose with fructose c. no difference in muscle glycogen use (as compared to placebo) with fructose d. increased muscle glycogen use with glucose
77	Hughes et al., 1984	45	a. glucose (0.75 g/kg) b. fructose (0.75 g/kg)	cycling — 4 h 50% VO$_2$max	a. increased initial blood glucose with glucose b. no difference in muscle glycogen use
78	Koivisto et al., 1985	45	a. glucose (75 g) b. fructose (75 g)	cycling — 2 h 55% VO$_2$max	a. increased initial blood glucose with glucose b. no difference in glycogen use with glucose or fructose c. decreased plasma FFA with fructose

79	Koivisto et al., 1981	a. glucose (75 g) b. fructose (75 g)	cycling — 30 min 75% VO₂max	a. increased initial blood glucose with glucose b. decreased blood glucose during exercise with glucose c. attenuated blood glucose response with fructose d. decreased plasma FFA with glucose or fructose
80	Levine et al., 1983	a. glucose (75 g) b. fructose (75 g)	running — 30 min 75% VO₂max	a. increased initial blood glucose with glucose b. decreased muscle glycogen utilization with fructose
81	McMurray et al., 1983	a. glucose (100 g) b. fructose (100 g)	running — to exhaustion 80% VO₂max	a. increased time to exhaustion with glucose or fructose b. increased CHO oxidation with glucose or fructose
82	Anderson et al., 1994	a. glucose (70 g) b. oatmeal (70 g CHO, 20 g protein, 7 g fat)	cycling — to exhaustion 75–80% VO₂max	increased time to exhaustion with oatmeal but not glucose
83	Casal and Leon, 1985	caffeine (400 mg)	running — 45 min 75% VO₂max	a. increased plasma FFA with caffeine b. no difference in respiratory exchange ratio
84	Erickson et al., 1987	a. fructose (1 g/kg) b. caffeine (5 mg/kg)	cycling — 90 min 70% VO₂max	a. increased muscle glycogen use with caffeine b. increased plasma FFA with caffeine or fructose
85	Graham and Spriet, 1991	caffeine (9 mg/kg)	running/cycling to exhaustion 85% VO₂max	a. increased time to exhaustion b. no change in plasma FFA at rest or during exercise
86	Keller and Schwarzkopf, 1984	glucose (100 g)	cycling — intermittent to exhaustion 85% VO₂max	a. decreased time to exhaustion with glucose b. increased initial blood glucose with glucose
87	Okano et al., 1988	fructose (60 g, 85 g)	cycling — to exhaustion 60–80% VO₂max	a. increased time to exhaustion with fructose b. no change in blood glucose with fructose
88	Sasaki et al., 1987	a. sucrose (45 g) b. caffeine (300 mg)	running — to exhaustion 80% VO₂max	a. increased time to exhaustion with sucrose or caffeine b. increased CHO use with sucrose c. increased FFA use with caffeine
89	Tarnopolsky et al., 1988	caffeine (6 mg/kg)	running — 90 min 70% VO₂max	a. increased plasma FFA b. no change in plasma glucose or respiratory exchange ratio

TABLE 2 Effects of Ingesting Nutrient Beverages Prior to Exercise *(continued)*

Ref.	Authors	Time of Ingestion (min before exercise)	Nutrients Ingested	Exercise	Results
90	Jandrain et al., 1984	180	glucose (100 g) (labeled)	walking — 4 h 45% VO$_2$max	exogenous glucose accounted for 68 of the 253 g of CHO used during the exercise
91	Wright et al., 1991	180	mixed CHO (5 g/kg) (glucose polymers and sucrose)	cycling — to exhaustion 70% VO$_2$max	a. increased time to exhaustion b. increased rate of CHO use
92	Sherman et al., 1989	240	a. mixed CHO (45 g) b. mixed CHO (156 g) c. mixed CHO (312 g)	cycling—intermittent 70% VO$_2$max	a. increased performance with 312 g CHO (as compared to placebo) b. greater CHO oxidation with 312 g CHO c. maintenance of blood glucose with 312 g CHO

as compared to the same exercise following placebo. The ingested glucose presumably acts as a readily available energy source during the exercise bout.

2.   Effect of Type of Carbohydrate

Because different carbohydrates are absorbed via different mechanisms, ingestion of beverages which contain a mixture of carbohydrates may result in different rates of intestinal water absorption.[94] Additionally the rate at which specific carbohydrates are digested and absorbed varies[28] as indicated in the glycemic index.[95] The effects of pre-exercise ingestion of carbohydrates on blood glucose and eventual performance may therefore differ for the different carbohydrates.

Fructose has often been suggested as an alternative to glucose in nutritional beverages since it results in smaller alterations in both blood glucose and plasma insulin.[96] Several investigators have shown that ingestion of a fructose beverage 1 h to 30 min prior to moderate-intensity exercise (55–75% VO_2max) does not produce the blood glucose transients associated with glucose ingestion.[71,75-80,87,93,97] However, no differences in total glycogen use[71,75-78] or time to exhaustion[75,98] are observed for moderate-intensity exercise when comparing pre-exercise fructose ingestion to glucose ingestion. Exercise of high intensity (>80% of VO_2max) may benefit from the ingestion of fructose rather than glucose,[93] presumably because the time for which such exercise can be sustained is relatively short. Ingestion of fructose, however, has been associated with an increase in gastric distress relative to ingestion of glucose,[84] although such distress may be highly individual.

Results of pre-exercise ingestion of mixed carbohydrates (sucrose, fructose, and glucose combinations) have varied. Some investigators have shown increased time for performance of moderate-intensity endurance exercise[88] and increased carbohydrate oxidation during exercise,[99] while others have shown no effect of the ingested nutrients on endurance times or total carbohydrate oxidation during exercise.[100]

C.   PRE-EXERCISE INGESTION OF NONCARBOHYDRATE NUTRIENTS
1.   Water

Hypohydration can adversely affect exercise performance.[101] Reversing the hypohydrated state by replacing lost body water before exercise begins may increase plasma volume, decrease plasma osmolality, and result in increased time to exhaustion of moderately intense exercise.[64] These changes are most notable when the water is ingested immediately prior to exercise, as compared to at intervals throughout the exercise session.

2.   Glycerol

Ingestion of glycerol 45 min before high-intensity cycling exercise may decrease[74] or increase[102] time to exhaustion and decreased glucose oxidation when compared to glucose ingestion. It has been suggested that the rate at which glycerol is used as a gluconeogenic substrate is not fast enough to allow it to serve as a significant energy source during exercise. Its main effect may simply be associated with temporary expansion and/or maintenance of plasma volume.[102]

3.   Branched-Chain Amino Acids

Recent investigations have linked alterations in the ratio of plasma free trytophan to branched-chain amino acids as a contributing factor to the fatigue experienced during prolonged endurance exercise.[103,104] Ingestion of branched-chain amino acids prior to exercise increases the plasma branched-chain amino acid concentrations[70,104] and may improve running performance in some runners.[104]

4.   Caffeine

Ingestion of caffeine may enhance performance by altering endogenous energy supplies, principally by increasing lipolysis.[22] Investigations of the effect of pre-exercise ingestion of caffeine on subsequent plasma free fatty acids (FFA) and eventual exercise performance are varied. Some investigators have shown an advantage resulting from pre-exercise ingestion of caffeine[85] while others have shown little or no such advantage.[83,84,88,89]

5.   Buffering Agents

Ingestion of sodium bicarbonate approximately 1 h prior to short duration (1–2 min), very high-intensity exercise results in increased blood pH and bicarbonate concentration. Significant improvements in time to exhaustion of bicycle sprinting and time to run a fixed distance have been observed.[105,106] The increased performance is most probably associated with an increased buffering capacity of the blood. One side effect of the ingestion of sodium bicarbonate prior to an exercise bout is the development of diarrhea in approximately 50% of subjects.[106] The use of sodium citrate as a substitute for sodium bicarbonate apparently results in similar performance benefits without the gastric distress associated with sodium bicarbonate.[107]

IV.   INGESTION OF NUTRIENT BEVERAGES DURING EXERCISE

Alterations in plasma volume, plasma electrolytes, and nutrient fuels which may occur during a bout of exercise can eventually modify physical performance. Athletes may ingest nutrient beverages in an effort to prevent or delay the exercise-induced alterations in homeostasis and consequent decline in performance. Attempts to evaluate the effectiveness of nutrient beverages ingested during exercise are hampered by the lack of consistency in investigations of such beverages. Varying exercise durations and intensities, solution volumes, feeding frequencies, and environmental conditions preclude definitive statements as to the global efficacy of specific nutrient solutions in enhancing physical performance. Additionally, appropriate comparisons among the various commercially available nutrient beverages is difficult owing to the various investigative protocols. There are, though, characteristics of both the exercise and the nutrient beverage which may be examined to determine the best use of such beverages during exercise.

A.   EXERCISE CONSIDERATIONS
1.   Duration

Labeled carbon from exogenous glucose appears in the expired air within 7 min of ingestion,[54] indicating the metabolic availability of the carbohydrate during even short duration events. However, while the ingested carbohydrate may be available for use, it may be of little or no benefit to the performance of short duration events[6] presumably because endogenous glycogen stores will not be depleted in most individuals during events which are of less than 2 h in duration. In contrast, during events lasting longer than 2 h, there may be a failure of hepatic glucose production to keep up with muscle glucose uptake.[10] Plasma glucose may, in fact, measurably decrease by 90 min of moderate exercise.[108] Most investigations of the effect of ingested carbohydrates during low- and moderate-intensity exercise have demonstrated a delay in fatigue and improved performance.[91,108-117] However, other investigators have shown no increase in time to fatigue when subjects consumed carbohydrate drinks vs. placebo.[118-121]

Ingestion of carbohydrate during endurance exercise results in maintenance of blood glucose levels and a concomitant increase in the rate of carbohydrate oxidation during the later stages of the exercise.[91,109-112,114-119,121-127] This, rather than a sparing of muscle glycogen, appears to be the mechanism by which ingestion of carbohydrate-containing beverages during endurance exercise enhances performance, since carbohydrate ingestion does not decrease the rate of muscle glycogen use.[9,110,113,119,128] Carbohydrate ingestion does, however, reduce liver glycogen depletion.[129]

2. Intensity

Ingestion of nutrient beverages has been shown to enhance performance of low- (below 60% VO_2max),[114,130] moderate- (60–80% VO_2max),[91,108-110,115-117] and high- (greater than 80%, as in a sprint task at the end of moderate-intensity exercise)[113,123] intensity exercise. Thus, it appears that duration rather than intensity is the more important element in determining whether or not ingested nutrient beverages will result in improved performance.

B. BEVERAGE CONSIDERATIONS
1. Voluntary Fluid Ingestion

Laboratory-based investigations of nutrient beverage consumption have the advantage of allowing control of the volume of fluid ingested. However, during exercise bouts in "the real world," athletes are free to consume as much, or as little, as they desire. Consequently, characteristics of a beverage which influence voluntary consumption may affect eventual performance. As with pre-exercise nutrient beverage ingestion, the temperature of a beverage is important in determining the total quantity of beverage consumed. Cool beverages are voluntarily consumed in greater quantities than are warm beverages during exercise.[33,34] Flavoring the beverage further enhances voluntary ingestion.[34,122,131] When flavor is nondistinguishable between beverages, no difference exists in voluntary ingestion of isotonic vs. hypotonic beverages.[132]

2. Carbohydrates

Because the various carbohydrates vary in their gastric emptying and intestinal absorption characteristics, they may vary in their effectiveness in ameliorating exercise-induced changes in homeostatis. Table 3[57,58,111,116,121,125,133-140] presents the results of studies investigating the effects of glucose ingested during exercise; Table 4[58,91,108-110,112,114,115,117,119-121,124-127,136,141-147] presents information regarding ingestion of glucose polymers; and Table 5[60-62,91,111,113,115,118,119,121-123,146,148-155] presents the results of studies investigating the effects of ingesting beverages containing fructose, sucrose, and mixed carbohydrates on exercise performance.

a. Glucose

The hyper- followed by hypo-glycemic response often observed with pre-exercise ingestion of glucose has not been demonstrated with glucose feedings during exercise.[7] The major effect of ingestion of glucose beverages during prolonged exercise of low-[58] or moderate-[111,116,121,156] intensity appears to be a maintenance of blood glucose in the later stages of the exercise, although some investigators have shown no difference in blood glucose when comparing carbohydrate beverages to placebo.[136] Along with the increase in blood glucose is an increased oxidation of carbohydrate.[58,111] Maintenance of blood glucose, and the concomitant increase in carbohydrate oxidation, late in prolonged exercise appears to be the means by which carbohydrate ingestion enhances performance. It must be noted, however, that maintenance of blood glucose merely delays rather than prevents fatigue. Fatigue, usually defined as the inability to continue a prescribed intensity of exercise, occurs even though blood glucose may be well within normal limits.

An additional benefit of the ingestion of glucose beverages during prolonged, moderate-intensity exercise is the maintenance of plasma volume and/or cardiac output.[133,135] The

TABLE 3   Effects of Consuming Glucose Beverages During Prolonged Exercise

Ref.	Authors	Nutrients Ingested	Time of Ingestion	Volume Ingested	Exercise	Results
133	Bothorel et al., 1979	a. glucose/electrolyte isosmotic, acidic b. glucose/electrolyte isosmotic, neutral c. water	after 1 h and at 10 min intervals	120 ml	cycling, intermittent 3 h 90 W	a. maintenance of plasma volume with water and acid beverage b. increased plasma volume with neutral beverage c. no difference in plasma osmolality with acidic vs. neutral beverage
138	Davis et al., 1988	a. glucose (6%) with electrolytes b. glucose (12%) with electrolytes	20 min intervals	275 ml	cycling, intermittent 2 h 65% VO₂max	a. decreased rate of fluid absorption with 12% glucose b. increased nausea with 12% glucose c. no difference in plasma volume
111	Davis et al., 1988	a. glucose/electrolyte (2.5% glucose, Na, K) b. mixed CHO and electrolyte (2% glucose, 4% sucrose, Na, K)	20 min intervals	275 ml	cycling, timed ride	a. decreased time to perform task with high CHO b. increased blood glucose with high CHO c. increased respiratory exchange ratio with high CHO
134	Francis, 1979	a. glucose/electrolyte (13 g/l glucose, Na, K) b. water	20 min intervals	volume to replace water loss	cycling, intermittent 160 min 50% VO₂max	a. no difference in plasma volume, heart rate, or core temperature b. no difference in losses of Na⁺ or K⁺
135	Hamilton et al., 1991	a. glucose infusion b. water ingestion	20 min intervals	a. to maintain euglycemia b. to replace water loss	cycling 2 h 70% VO₂max	a. maintenance of cardiac output, heart rate, and VO₂ during exercise with glucose b. attenuation of decreased cardiac output and stroke volume with water

	Study	Beverage composition	Interval	Volume	Exercise	Results
139	Hawley et al., 1994	a. infusion, 25% glucose b. ingestion, 15% glucose		a. 0.29 ml/min b. 400 ml immediately prior to, then 100 ml every 10 min	cycling 125 min 70% VO₂ peak	a. increased plasma insulin with CHO ingestion b. increased plasma and total CHO oxidation during the midportion of the exercise with CHO ingestion
57	Krzentowski et al., 1984	glucose (100 g)	a. 15 min b. 120 min		walking 4 h 45% VO₂max	a. 55% of endogenous glucose was oxidized b. no difference in glucose oxidation based on time of ingestion
140	Leese et al., 1996	a. glucose (18.5%) b. sucrose (18.5%) c. maize syrup solids (18.5%)		330 ml	walking 1 h 75% VO₂max	a. no difference in CHO oxidation during exercise b. decreased maize syrup solid oxidation post-exercise
58	Massicotte et al., 1989	a. glucose (1.33 g/kg) b. glucose polymer (1.33 g/kg) c. fructose (1.33 g/kg)	20 min intervals	about 234 ml	cycling 120 min 53% VO₂max	a. increased oxidation of exogenous glucose and glucose polymer as compared to fructose b. increased initial blood glucose with glucose c. decreased plasma FFA, but not FFA use, with all CHO beverages
136	Maughan et al., 1987	a. glucose/electrolyte b. glucose polymer	10 min intervals	100 ml	cycling 60 min 68% VO₂max	a. no difference in blood glucose or CHO oxidation b. decreased plasma volume with glucose polymer
116	Murray et al., 1991	a. glucose (26 g/h) b. glucose (52 g/h) c. glucose (78 g/h)	15 min intervals		cycling 2 h 65–75% VO₂max then timed 4.8 km	a. decreased time to complete 4.8 km with all CHO beverages b. increased plasma glucose with all CHO beverages c. decreased plasma FFA with all CHO beverages

TABLE 3 Effects of Consuming Glucose Beverages During Prolonged Exercise *(continued)*

Ref.	Authors	Nutrients Ingested	Time of Ingestion	Volume Ingested	Exercise	Results
125	Owen et al., 1986	a. glucose (10%) b. glucose polymer (10%) c. water	20 min intervals	200 ml	running 2 h 65% VO$_2$max	a. increased plasma glucose with glucose or glucose polymer b. no differences in loss of plasma volume
137	Wells et al., 1985	a. glucose/electrolyte (0.93 g glucose/dl, Na, K, Cl) b. caffeine (5 mg/kg)	initial dose, then at 2.5 mile intervals	400 ml then doses of 100 ml	running 20 miles (32 km)	a. no difference in plasma FFA b. increased VO$_2$ during exercise with caffeine c. increased respiratory exchange ratio with caffeine
121	Williams et al., 1990	a. glucose polymer with glucose (50 g) b. glucose polymer with fructose (50 g) c. water	5 km intervals	150 ml	running 30 km as fast as possible	a. no difference in running time b. maintenance of blood glucose with either CHO beverage

Note: All investigations included a placebo.

TABLE 4 Effects of Consuming Beverages Containing Glucose Polymers During Exercise

Ref.	Authors	Nutrients Ingested	Time of Ingestion	Volume Ingested	Exercise	Results
141	Burstein et al., 1994	glucose polymer		a. ad libitum b. 900 ml/h	4 d march, average 33.5 km/d 5–6 km/h	a. no difference in fluid ingested b. no difference in plasma volume change c. no difference in plasma glucose
109	Coggan and Coyle, 1989	glucose polymer (3 g/kg)	at min 135		cycling to exhaustion 70% VO_2max	a. increased time to exhaustion b. increased plasma glucose following CHO ingestion c. increased respiratory exchange ratio following CHO ingestion
110	Coyle et al., 1986	glucose polymer (2 g/kg, then 0.4 g/kg)	20 min intervals		cycling to exhaustion 71% VO_2max	a. increased time to exhaustion b. maintenance of blood glucose c. maintenance of CHO use d. no difference in rate of muscle glycogen use
108	Coyle et al., 1983	glucose polymer (1 g/kg, then 0.25 g/kg)	min 20, then 60, 90, 120	300 ml	cycling to exhaustion 74% VO_2max	a. increased time to exhaustion b. decreased loss of plasma volume
144	Criswell et al., 1990	glucose polymer (7%) with electrolytes	6 rest periods	170 ml	football scrimmage	a. no difference in change in plasma electrolytes b. increased loss of plasma volume with glucose polymer
112	Edwards and Santeusanio, 1984	a. glucose polymer b. glucose polymer with fructose	25 min intervals		cycling 55.2 mile (88.7 km)	a. decreased time to finish with either CHO beverage b. increased blood glucose with either CHO beverage
142	Fayer et al., 1991	a. glucose ploymer (7%) b. polylactate with sodium lactate (4:1 in 7% solution)	5 min pre then 20 min intervals		cycling 180 min 50% VO_2max	a. no differences in plasma electrolytes, heart rate, or oxygen consumption between beverages b. increased pH and bicarbonate with polylactate

TABLE 4 Effects of Consuming Beverages Containing Glucose Polymers During Exercise *(continued)*

Ref.	Authors	Nutrients Ingested	Time of Ingestion	Volume Ingested	Exercise	Results
119	Flynn et al., 1987	a. glucose polymer (5%) with fructose (5%) b. glucose polymer (7.7%) with fructose (2.3%) c. glucose polymer (3%) with glucose (2%)	20 min intervals	150 ml	cycling 2 h 90 rpm isokinetic	a. no difference in work b. increased blood glucose with all CHO beverages c. no difference in muscle glycogen use
145	Ivy et al., 1979	a. glucose polymer (90 g) b. caffeine (500 mg)	15 min intervals	25 ml	cycling 2 h 80 rpm isokinetic	a. increased work and VO$_2$ with caffeine vs. placebo b. increased blood glucose with glucose polymer c. no difference in CHO use d. increased FFA use during later stages of exercise with caffeine
114	Ivy et al., 1983	glucose polymer (120 g total)	min 60, 90, 120, 150		walking to exhaustion 45% VO$_2$max	a. increased time to exhaustion b. increased CHO use c. increased blood glucose during exercise
124	Kingwell et al., 1989	glucose polymer (10%)	20 min intervals	200 ml	cycling 160 min 65% VO$_2$max	a. increased blood glucose and respiratory exchange ratio (as compared to control) b. no difference in plasma volume change
143	Langenfeld, 1983	glucose polymer (6.5%)	ad libitum		cycling 270 km 25 km/h	a. longer maintenance of blood glucose with glucose polymer b. increased respiratory exchange ratio with glucose polymer

58	Massicotte et al., 1989	a. glucose (1.33 g/kg) b. glucose polymer (1.33 g/kg) c. fructose (1.33 g/kg)	20 min intervals	about 234 ml	cycling 120 min 53% VO_2max	a. increased oxidation of exogenous glucose and glucose polymer as compared to fructose b. increased initial blood glucose with glucose c. decreased plasma FFA, but not FFA use, with all CHO beverages
136	Maughan et al., 1987	a. glucose/electrolyte b. glucose ploymer	10 min intervals	100 ml	cycling 60 min 68% VO_2max	a. no difference in blood glucose or CHO oxidation b. decreased plasma volume with glucose polymer
115	Millard-Stafford et al., 1990	carbohydrate/electrolyte (5% glucose polymer, 2% fructose, Na^+, K^+, Cl^-)	post-swim, 8 km intervals cycle, 3.2 km intervals run	2 ml/kg	triathlon 1.5 km swim 40 km cycle 10 km run	a. decreased time to complete task with CHO beverage b. increased blood glucose with CHO beverage c. increased respiratory exchange ratio with CHO beverage
146	Murray et al., 1987	a. glucose polymer (5%) b. glucose polymer (5%), with fructose (2%) c. glucose (2%), with sucrose (4%)	15 min (approx.) intervals	2 ml/kg	cycling, intermittent 140 min 55 or 65% VO_2max	a. increased plasma glucose with all CHO beverages b. no difference in plasma volume change, plasma electrolytes, or respiratory exchange ratio
125	Owen et al., 1986	a. glucose (10%) b. glucose polymer (10%) c. water	20 min intervals	200 ml	running 2 h 65% VO_2max	a. increased plasma glucose with glucose or glucose polymer b. no differences in loss of plasma volume
147	Peters et al., 1993	a. hypotonic solution with glucose polymer (33.3 g/100 ml) b. semisolid CHO	intermittent	varying	2 bouts of cycling and 2 bouts of running, intermittent 3 h 75% VO_2max	a. decreased nausea with semisolid CHO b. decreased bloating with either CHO
120	Powers et al., 1990	a. glucose polymer with electrolytes b. electrolytes c. water	15 min intervals		cycling to exhaustion 85% VO_2max	a. no difference in time to exhaustion b. no difference in blood electrolytes

TABLE 4   Effects of Consuming Beverages Containing Glucose Polymers During Exercise (continued)

Ref.	Authors	Nutrients Ingested	Time of Ingestion	Volume Ingested	Exercise	Results
126	Seidman et al., 1991	a. glucose polymer (7.2%) with electrolytes b. water	a. ad libitum b. 1000 ml/5 km		walking, intermittent 30 km 5 km/h	a. increased blood glucose with glucose polymer b. no differences in plasma osmolality c. increased plasma FFA with water
117	Wilber and Moffatt, 1991	glucose polymer	15 min intervals	125 ml	running to exhaustion 80% VO_2max	a. increased time to exhaustion b. increased plasma glucose c. increased respiratory exchange ratio
121	Williams et al., 1990	a. glucose polymer with glucose (50 g) b. glucose polymer with fructose (50 g) c. water	5 km intervals	150 ml	running 30 km as fast as possible	a. no difference in running time b. maintenance of blood glucose with either CHO beverage
91	Wright et al., 1991	mixed carbohydrates (5% glucose polymer, 3% fructose)	20 min intervals	2 g CHO/kg	cycling to exhaustion 70% VO_2max	a. increased time to exhaustion b. increased CHO use
127	Yaspelkis and Ivy, 1991	a. glucose polymer (2%) b. glucose polymer (8.5%)	15 min intervals	3 ml/kg	cycling 2 h 49% VO_2max	a. increased blood glucose with 8.5% solution b. increased CHO oxidation with 8.5% solution

Note: All investigations included a placebo.

TABLE 5 Effects of Consuming Beverages Containing Fructose, Sucrose, and Mixed Carbohydrates During Exercise

Ref.	Authors	Nutrients Ingested	Time of Ingestion	Volume Ingested	Exercise	Results
148	Adopo et al., 1994	a. glucose, 50 g b. glucose, 100 g c. fructose, 50 g d. fructose, 100 g e. glucose, 50 g with fructose, 50 g	5 min	500 ml	cycling 2 h 61% VO_2max	a. increased exogenous glucose oxidation with high glucose b. increased oxidation of exogenous CHO with glucose as compared to fructose c. increased oxidation of exogenous CHO with glucose/fructose mix
118	Brodowicz et al., 1984	carbohydrate/electrolyte: a. 6.6% CHO, 316 mOsmol/l b. 6% CHO, 113 mOsmol/l c. 2.5% CHO, 187 mOsmol/l d. 0% CHO, 16 mOsmol/l	20 min intervals	250 ml	cycling to exhaustion 74% VO_2max	a. no difference in time to exhaustion, plasma volume change, or plasma electrolytes b. increased plasma glucose with 6% or 6.6% CHO
122	Carter and Gisolfi, 1989	mixed CHO/electrolyte (4.8% glucose polymer, 2.6% fructose, Na, K, Ca, Cl)	ad libitum		cycling 3 h 60% VO_2max	a. increased plasma volume and plasma electrolytes b. increased plasma glucose c. increased voluntary ingestion
111	Davis et al., 1988	a. glucose/electrolyte (2.5% glucose, Na, K) b. mixed CHO/electrolyte (2% glucose, 4% sucrose, Na, K)	20 min intervals	275 ml	cycling, time trial	a. decreased time to perform task with high CHO b. increased blood glucose with high CHO c. increased respiratory exchange ratio with high CHO
150	Deuster et al., 1992	carbohydrate/electrolyte (7% CHO as glucose polymer/fructose)	30 min intervals	200 ml	running 2 h 60–65% VO_2max	a. no difference in plasma electrolytes b. decreased plasma FFA
113	Fielding et al., 1985	a. sucrose (10.75 g) b. sucrose (21.5 g)	a. 30 min intervals b. 1 h intervals	a. 200 ml b. 400 ml	cycling, intermittent 4 h 50–100% VO_2max	a. no difference in muscle glycogen use with CHO b. improved blood glucose with CHO c. increased respiratory exchange ratio with CHO d. improved performance on end-test maximal sprint with CHO

TABLE 5   Effects of Consuming Beverages Containing Fructose, Sucrose, and Mixed Carbohydrates During Exercise *(continued)*

Ref.	Authors	Nutrients Ingested	Time of Ingestion	Volume Ingested	Exercise	Results
119	Flynn et al., 1987	a. glucose polymer (5%) with fructose (5%) b. glucose polymer (7.7%) with fructose (2.3%) c. glucose polymer (3%) with glucose (2%)	20 min intervals	150 ml	cycling 2 h 90 rpm isokinetic	a. no difference in work b. increased blood glucose with all CHO beverages c. no difference in muscle glycogen use
62	Fujisawa et al., 1993	50 g of CHO as: a. fructose, 100% b. fructose/glucose 95%/5% c. fructose/glucose 70%/30% d. glucose, 100%	following first 30 min exercise bout	860 ml	walking, treadmill, intermittent two 30 min bouts increasing intensity to 70–75% VO₂max	a. decreased relative absorption of fructose as % fructose increased b. decreased relative absorption of fructose during exercise
123	Hargreaves et al., 1984	sucrose (43 g)	1 h intervals	400 ml	cycling, intermittent 4 h 50–100% VO₂max	a. decreased muscle glycogen with CHO b. increased blood glucose with CHO c. increased respiratory exchange ratio with CHO d. increased performance in end-test maximal sprint with CHO
61	Jandrain et al., 1993	a. glucose (25 g) b. fructose (25 g)	30 min intervals	100 ml	walking, treadmill 3 h 45% VO₂max	a. increased oxidation of exogenous glucose as compared to fructose b. increased total CHO oxidation with glucose c. no difference in blood glucose
149	Mason et al., 1993	a. rice-based liquid (5% CHO solution) b. CHO bar	0, 30, 60, 90 min	500 ml	cycling, intermittent to exhaustion 65% VO₂max	a. no difference in VO₂, HR, or respiratory exchange ratio b. increased blood glucose with either CHO c. no difference in blood glucose between CHOs

Ref	Author	Solution	Interval	Amount	Exercise	Results
60	Massicotte et al., 1994	a. glucose (1.33 g/kg) b. fructose (1.33 g/kg)	20 min intervals	about 234 ml	cycling 120 min 60% VO$_2$max	increased oxidation of exogenous glucose as compared to fructose
115	Millard-Stafford et al., 1990	carbohydrate/electrolyte (5% glucose polymer, 2% fructose, Na$^+$, K$^+$, Cl$^-$)	post-swim, 8 km intervals cycle, 3.2 km intervals run	2 ml/kg	triathlon 1.5 km swim 40 km cycle 10 km run	a. decreased time to complete task with CHO beverage b. increased blood glucose with CHO beverage c. increased respiratory exchange ratio with CHO beverage
151	Murray et al., 1991	a. glucose/electrolyte (6% glucose, Na$^+$, K$^+$, Cl$^-$) b. glycerol (10%) c. glucose/electrolyte (as in a.), with glycerol (4%)	15 min intervals to min 60	3 ml/kg	cycling 90 min 50% VO$_2$max	a. increased plasma osmolality with glycerol b. increased gastrointestinal distress with glycerol c. no difference in core temperature or sweat rate
146	Murray et al., 1987	a. glucose polymer (5%) b. glucose polymer (5%), with fructose (2%) c. glucose (2%), with sucrose (4%)	15 min (approx.) intervals	2 ml/kg	cycling, intermittent 140 min 55 or 65% VO$_2$max	a. increased plasma glucose with all CHO beverages b. no difference in plasma volume change, plasma electrolytes, or respiratory exchange ratio
152	Murray et al., 1989	a. glucose (6%) b. fructose (6%) c. sucrose (6%)	15 min (approx.) intervals	3 ml/kg	cycling, intermittent 115 min 65–80% VO$_2$max	a. no difference in CHO use b. decreased plasma glucose and volume with fructose c. decreased speed with fructose d. increased plasma FFA and gastric distress with fructose
153	Murray et al., 1989	in a solution with electrolytes: a. sucrose (6%) b. sucrose (8%) c. sucrose (10%)	20 min intervals	2.5 ml/kg	cycling, intermittent three 20 min bouts 65% VO$_2$max followed by timed task	a. decreased time to complete timed task with 6% sucrose b. increased plasma glucose and respiratory exchange ratio with all CHOs c. no difference in plasma volume, thirst, or gastrointestinal distress
121	Williams et al., 1990	a. glucose polymer with glucose (50 g) b. glucose polymer with fructose (50 g) c. water	5 km intervals	150 ml	running 30 km as fast as possible	a. no difference in running time b. maintenance of blood glucose with either CHO beverage

TABLE 5   Effects of Consuming Beverages Containing Fructose, Sucrose, and Mixed Carbohydrates During Exercise *(continued)*

Ref.	Authors	Nutrients Ingested	Time of Ingestion	Volume Ingested	Exercise	Results
91	Wright et al., 1991	mixed carbohydrates (5% glucose polymer, 3% fructose)	20 min intervals	2 g CHO/kg	cycling to exhaustion 70% VO$_2$max	a. increased time to exhaustion b. increased CHO use
154	Yaspelkis et al., 1993	liquid CHO polymer (25%, 1 g CHO/kg), then: a. liquid CHO polymer (10%) b. solid CHO (fructose/glucose polymer)	CHO (a.) at 20 min intervals CHO (b.) at 30 min intervals	ad libitum water throughout 180 ml of (a.) 270 ml water with (b.)	cycling, intermittent two bouts at 45–75% VO$_2$max then to exhaustion at 80% VO$_2$max	a. increased plasma glucose with liquid CHO b. increased time to exhaustion with either CHO c. increased muscle glycogen during exercise with liquid CHO
155	Zachwieja et al., 1993	mixed carbohydrates (3.8% glucose, 5.7% fructose)	15 min intervals	215 ml	cycling 2 h 70% VO$_2$max	a. increased respiratory exchange ratio with CHO b. increased CHO oxidation with CHO c. increased plasma glucose with CHO d. no difference in muscle glycogen utilization e. no difference in muscle glycogen resynthesis 2 h after exercise

Note: All investigations included a placebo.

enhanced hydration status occurs presumably through an enhanced uptake of fluid in the intestine.

b.   Glucose Polymers

There has been much interest in the past decade in the use of glucose polymers in nutrient beverages. Glucose polymers have the advantage of increasing the carbohydrate content of a solution with less increase in osmolality than would result from addition of the same amount of carbohydrate in the form of glucose or other monosaccharides. Since beverage osmolality may affect gastric emptying,[29,30,41] the use of a carbohydrate source which minimizes alterations in osmolality was thought to be advantageous. While the rate of gastric emptying of solutions containing glucose polymers may exceed that of solutions containing similar amounts of glucose,[41] there appears to be no physiological or performance advantage to the addition of glucose polymers, rather than glucose, to a nutrient beverage.[58,136,146,156]

Just as with ingestion of glucose, ingestion of glucose polymer during prolonged, low-[127,146] or moderate-[109,110,112,114,115,117,119,121,124,126,127,141,143,145,146,156] intensity exercise maintains blood glucose during the exercise. Carbohydrate oxidation is thus maintained at a higher level during the exercise.[58,91,109,110,114,115,117,124,127,143] The result is an increase in performance of prolonged, moderate-intensity exercise.[91,108-110,112,114,115,117]

c.   Fructose

Fructose empties from the stomach more quickly than a similar amount of glucose.[35] Additionally, the inclusion of fructose in a nutrient beverage prevents the glycemic response associated with glucose ingestion.[96] For these reasons, the inclusion of fructose in nutrient beverages ingested during exercise has been proposed as a means of minimizing the glucose-induced alterations in blood glucose which occur during the early stages of exercise. While pre-exercise ingestion of fructose does reduce the glucose transients associated with glucose ingestion,[75-78,80,87,97,119,157] there appears to be no such advantage to fructose ingested during exercise.[112,119,146] Neither does ingestion of fructose result in an increase in performance when compared to the ingestion of glucose or glucose polymers.[112,119,121,152] However, just as with glucose and glucose polymers, ingestion of fructose may improve prolonged, moderate-intensity exercise performance when compared to placebo.[91,112,115] One potential disadvantage to the inclusion of fructose in a nutrient beverage is a potential increase in gastric distress.[84,152]

d.   Mixed Carbohydrate Sources

Nutrient beverages which contain a mixture of carbohydrates may offer advantages over solutions containing a single carbohydrate.[84] Such solutions may capitalize on any advantages incurred in either gastric emptying or maintenance of blood glucose offered by single carbohydrates while minimizing disadvantages such as gastric distress. Investigations of the efficacy of mixed carbohydrate beverages in enhancing prolonged, moderate-intensity exercise performance have indicated no differences when using mixed carbohydrates as compared to single carbohydrate solutions.[118,119,121] However, as with single carbohydrate beverages, mixed carbohydrate beverages maintain blood glucose during prolonged, moderate-intensity exercise[111,113,115,118,119,121-123,146] which may result in improved performance when compared to placebo.[18,111,113,115,123]

3.   Noncarbohydrate Nutrients
a.   Electrolytes

Ingestion of a glucose/electrolyte solution during exercise may result in a maintenance[118,133] or increase[122,123,134,158] in plasma volume. Plasma osmolality during exercise may[118,122,133,159] or may not[120,126,130,134,144,150,158] be enhanced during exercise following ingestion of isotonic electrolyte solutions. Table 6[111,115,118,120,122,126,130,133,134,137,144,150,151,159] presents the results of investigations of the efficacy of electrolyte beverages ingested during exercise.

TABLE 6   Effects of Consuming Beverages Containing Specific Electrolytes During Exercise

Ref.	Authors	Nutrients Ingested	Time of Ingestion	Volume Ingested	Exercise	Results
130	Barr et al., 1991	a. saline (25 mmol/l) b. water	15 min intervals	sufficient to replace water loss	cycling, intermittent up to 6 h 55% VO_2max	a. increased performance time with saline or water b. no difference in plasma Na^+ with saline vs. water
133	Bothorel et al., 1979	a. glucose/electrolyte isosmotic, acidic b. glucose/electrolyte isosmotic, neutral c. water	after 1 h and at 10 min intervals	120 ml	cycling, intermittent 3 h 90 W	a. maintenance of plasma volume with water and acid beverage b. increased plasma volume and neutral beverage c. no difference in plasma osmolality with acidic vs. neutral beverage
118	Brodowicz et al., 1984	carbohydrate/electrolyte: a. 6.6% CHO, 316 mOsmol/l b. 6% CHO, 113 mOsmol/l c. 2.5% CHO, 187 mOsmol/l d. 0% CHO, 16 mOsmol/l	20 min intervals	250 ml	cycling to exhaustion 74% VO_2max	a. no difference in time to exhaustion, plasma volume change, or plasma electrolytes b. increased plasma glucose with 6% or 6.6% CHO
159	Candas et al., 1986	a. hypertonic b. isotonic c. hypotonic d. water	10 min intervals after min 70	1/18 of total water loss during control	cycling, intermittent 4 h 50% of W needed to achieve a HR of 170	a. increased plasma volume with isotonic b. decreased plasma osmolality with water
122	Carter and Gisolfi, 1989	mixed CHO/electrolyte (4.8% glucose polymer, 2.6% fructose, Na^+, K^+, Ca^{2+}, Cl^-)	ad libitum		cycling 3 h 60% VO_2max	a. increased plasma volume and plasma electrolytes b. increased plasma glucose c. increased voluntary ingestion
144	Criswell et al., 1990	glucose polymer (7%) with electrolytes	6 rest periods	170 ml	football scrimmage	a. no difference in change in plasma electrolytes b. increased loss of plasma volume with glucose polymer
111	Davis et al., 1988	a. glucose/electrolyte (2.5% glucose, Na^+, K^+) b. mixed CHO and electrolyte (2% glucose, 4% sucrose, Na^+, K^+)	20 min intervals	275 ml	cycling, time trial	a. decreased time to perform task with high CHO b. increased blood glucose with high CHO c. increased respiratory exchange ratio with high CHO

	Reference	Beverage	Interval	Volume	Exercise	Results
150	Deuster et al., 1992	carbohydrate/electrolyte (7% CHO)	30 min intervals	200 ml	running 2 h 60–65% VO_2max	a. no difference in plasma electrolytes b. decreased plasma FFA
134	Francis, 1979	a. glucose/electrolyte (13 g/l glucose, Na^+, K^+) b. water	20 min intervals	volume to replace water loss	cycling, intermittent 160 min 50% VO_2max	a. no difference in plasma volume, heart rate, or core temperature b. no difference in losses of Na or K
115	Millard-Stafford et al., 1990	carbohydrate/electrolyte (5% glucose polymer, 2% fructose, Na^+, K^+, Cl^-)	post-swim, 8 km intervals cycle, 3.2 km intervals run	2 ml/kg	triathlon 1.5 km swim 40 km cycle 10 km run	a. decreased time to complete task with CHO beverage b. increased blood glucose with CHO beverage c. increased respiratory exchange ratio with CHO beverage
151	Murray et al., 1991	a. glucose/electrolyte (6% glucose, Na^+, K^+, Cl^-) b. glycerol (10%) c. glucose/electrolyte (as in a.) with glycerol (4%)	15 min intervals to min 60	3 ml/kg	cycling 90 min 50% VO_2max	a. increased plasma osmolality with glycerol b. increased gastrointestinal distress with glycerol c. no difference in core temperature or sweat rate
120	Powers et al., 1990	a. glucose polymer with electrolytes b. electrolytes c. water	15 min intervals		cycling to exhaustion 85% VO_2max	a. no difference in time to exhaustion b. no difference in blood electrolytes
126	Seidman et al., 1991	a. glucose polymer (7.2%) with electrolytes b. water	a. ad libitum b. 1000 ml/5 km		walking, intermittent 30 km 5 km/h	a. increased blood glucose with glucose polymer b. no differences in plasma osmolality c. increased plasma FFA with water
137	Wells et al., 1985	a. glucose/electrolyte (0.93 g glucose/dl, Na^+, K^+, Cl^-) b. caffeine (5 mg/kg)	initial dose, then at 2.5 mile intervals	400 ml then doses of 100 ml	running 20 miles (32 km)	a. no difference in plasma FFA b. increased VO_2 during exercise with caffeine c. increased respiratory exchange ratio with caffeine

Note: All investigations included a placebo.

b.   Caffeine

Ingestion of caffeine during prolonged, intense exercise may result in an increase in total work performed,[145] an increase in free fatty acid utilization[145] or serum free fatty acid concentrations,[160] and an increase in VO_2.[137] However, caffeine ingestion by itself has no significant effect on performance during endurance events when compared to ingestion of glucose/electrolyte solutions during exercise.[137,160]

C.   SUMMARY

Several factors affect the influence which ingestion of nutrient beverages may have during exercise. Of most significance among these are the duration of the exercise and the composition of the beverage. For exercise lasting less than 90 min, addition of carbohydrates to a nutrient beverage is of little consequence to performance. However, during events lasting 2 h or more, carbohydrate ingestion delays fatigue by maintaining adequate blood glucose levels and thereby a high rate of carbohydrate oxidation during the later stages of the exercise. While carbohydrate solutions do not appear to affect the rate of muscle glycogen use, liver glycogen reserves may be spared.

Ingestion of carbohydrate during exercise does not result in the hypoglycemic response associated with some pre-exercise regimens of carbohydrate ingestion. While the form of carbohydrate ingested may lead to different plasma glucose responses, muscle glycogen use and performance may be the same regardless of the type of carbohydrate ingested. Ingestion of carbohydrate solutions of glucose, fructose, sucrose, and/or glucose polymer all seem to result in increased plasma glucose, when compared to water ingestion, during prolonged moderate-intensity exercise. Except for those individual athletes subject to hyponatremia, addition of electrolytes to nutrient beverages is not justified on the basis of the small changes which occur in blood osmolality. However, the addition of sodium to a beverage aids fluid and glucose absorption in the intestine and may thus be a beneficial component of a nutrient beverage solution. In regards to the electrolyte composition of nutrient beverages, hypotonic solutions are probably best for most endurance athletes.

While ingestion of appropriate nutrient beverages during exercise may delay fatigue, it is important to note that it does not prevent fatigue. Fatigue occurs in spite of the maintenance of plasma volume and blood glucose brought about through appropriate nutrient beverage ingestion.

V.   INGESTION OF NUTRIENT BEVERAGES FOLLOWING EXERCISE

A.   RATIONALE

The benefit of postexercise ingestion of nutrient beverages occurs if the beverages improve the recovery of plasma volume, electrolytes, and/or fuel stores following the exercise stress. Unfortunately, the use of nutrient beverages to enhance recovery from exercise has not been addressed to the same extent as the use of such beverages to enhance performance during exercise. The advantage of quick recovery from a prolonged bout of exercise can readily be seen for athletes competing in tournaments in which a performer is expected to participate in several endurance activities within one or very few days time. In addition, rapid recovery of water, electrolyte, and fuel storage is essential to continued high performance during day-to-day exercise training. Ingestion of appropriately formulated nutrient drinks during exercise does not appear to affect the rate of recovery of fuel stores following the exercise.[155] Thus, ingestion of nutrient beverages post-exercise may be beneficial if the rate of recovery is enhanced as compared to the recovery resulting from adjustments in normal meal consumption.

B. EFFECTS OF POSTEXERCISE CONSUMPTION OF NUTRIENT BEVERAGES

The effects of postexercise ingestion of various nutrient beverages are presented in Table 7.[122,161-171] Muscle glycogen resynthesis is enhanced if carbohydrate beverages are ingested immediately following an exercise bout.[161,162,164,167,170] The rate of glycogen resynthesis is dependent on the amount of carbohydrate in the ingested beverage.[162,164] Replenishment of muscle glycogen is greater when glucose or sucrose rather than fructose is the primary carbohydrate included in the beverage.[162] Glucose added to postexercise beverages may result in more rapid recovery of plasma volume,[166] due perhaps to enhanced voluntary fluid ingestion.[122] The addition of sodium to carbohydrate solutions results in increased replenishment of muscle glycogen.[168] Sodium may also act to enhance the rehydration process by maintaining a slightly hypertonic plasma and thereby enhancing dipsogenic stimuli.[168,169] Men and women appear to have similar responses to rehydration when water is the ingested nutrient.[171]

VI. DISCUSSION AND SUMMARY

Nutrient beverages are ingested before, during, and/or after exercise in an attempt to ameliorate the exercise-induced changes which may affect homeostasis and thereby diminish performance. The homeostatic disturbances associated with exercise include a decrease in plasma volume, an increase in deep body or core temperature, an increase in plasma osmolality, and a decrease in nutrient fuels available to the muscle. Each of these changes may be affected through judicious use of beverages containing various amounts and types of nutrients. Since the homeostatic disturbances, and consequent alteration in performance, vary with the intensity, duration, and type of exercise, no one nutrient beverage is best for all exercise situations. Rather, the informed exerciser should evaluate the different beverages in terms of the desired outcome of beverage ingestion.

In exercise bouts lasting less than 90 min, the availability of nutrient fuels to the working muscles is usually adequate to meet the demands of the exercise for most athletes consuming a well-balanced diet. In such exercise sessions, prevention of hypohydration and thermal stress through maintenance of plasma volume and osmolality, rather than enhancement of nutrient stores, would appear to be the important consideration. Ensuring optimal hydration is best accomplished through ingestion of cool, flavored beverages. Cool (5–15°C) beverages enhance gastric emptying by increasing gastric motility. Adding a flavoring agent, including carbohydrate and electrolytes, to the cool beverage results in increased voluntary consumption of the beverage. Additionally, active transport of sodium and glucose in the intestine increases the net absorption of water. However, since the caloric and perhaps osmotic characteristics of a beverage do affect the rate at which the fluid is emptied from the stomach, limiting the addition of carbohydrates and/or electrolytes would most beneficially affect hydration status. Volumes of fluid up to approximately 600 ml are emptied from the stomach in proportion to the volume. Since volumes greater than this do not add any gastric-emptying benefit, it would appear that volumes of 600 ml, with some adjustment for body size, would be the most beneficial in optimizing fluid maintenance during exercise.

During exercise events lasting longer than 90 min, blood glucose and muscle glycogen stores may be inadequate to meet the demands of the exercising tissues. Appropriate ingestion of carbohydrate may enhance performance of prolonged exercise of moderate to high intensity by maintaining blood glucose concentrations and thereby delaying, but not preventing, fatigue. Cool, flavored beverages, which are voluntarily consumed in greater quantities than warm, unflavored beverages, are again the most beneficial in meeting the needs of the exercise. This is particularly important during ultra-endurance events during which substantial loss of water may occur. Since blood glucose falls during prolonged exercise, the addition of carbohydrates

TABLE 7 Effects of Consuming Nutrient Beverages After Exercise

Ref.	Authors	Nutrients Ingested	Time of Ingestion	Volume Ingested	Exercise	Results
162	Blom et al., 1987	as a 30% solution: a. glucose (0.35 g/kg) b. glucose (0.7 g/kg) c. glucose (1.4 g/kg) d. sucrose (0.7 g/kg) e. fructose (0.7 g/kg)	immediately post, 2 h, 4 h		cycling, intermittent to exhaustion 75% VO_2max	a. increased muscle glycogen synthesis with glucose or sucrose vs. fructose b. increased muscle glycogen synthesis with higher concentration glucose beverages
161	Burke et al., 1993	a. CHO with glycemic index of 50 b. CHO with glycemic index of 108	immediately post, 4 h, 8 h, 21 h	10 g/kg body mass	cycling, 2 h 75% VO_2max then four 30 sec sprints	increased muscle glycogen at 24 h post with high glycemic CHO as compared to low glycemic CHO
122	Carter and Gisolfi, 1989	mixed CHO/electrolyte (4.8% glucose polymer, 2.6% fructose, Na^+, K^+, Ca^{2+}, Cl^-)	ad libitum		cycling 3 h 60% VO_2max	a. increased plasma volume and plasma electrolytes b. increased plasma glucose c. increased voluntary ingestion
163	Costill et al., 1975	a. glucose/electrolyte (13 g glucose, Na^+, K^+, Cl^-) b. water	ad libitum		cycling 5 days until daily loss of 3% body mass 55–60% VO_2max	a. no difference in electrolyte balance b. increased extracellular fluid with water
164	Costill et al., 1981	a. simple sugars (glucose, fructose, sucrose) b. complex carbohydrates (starches) c. low CHO (188 g/day) d. mixed CHO (375 g/day) e. high CHO (525 g/day)			running 16.1 km 80% VO_2max	a. no difference in muscle glycogen resynthesis 24 h post, simple vs. complex CHO b. increased muscle glycogen 48 h post with complex CHO c. increased muscle glycogen resynthesis 24 h post with increased CHO
166	Glace et al., 1994	glucose polymer/fructose	a. immediately post b. immediately post, then 2 h	1 l of a. 200 g b. 1.5 g/kg	cycling, 1 h	a. increased blood glucose with CHO b. decreased serum potassium with CHO c. increased rate of aldosterone decline with CHO d. decreased urine volume with CHO

	Study	Beverage	Timing	Amount	Exercise	Results
165	Lambert et al., 1992	a. 10% glucose/fructose, carbonated b. 10% glucose/fructose, noncarbonated c. carbonated noncaloric d. noncarbonated, noncaloric	15 min intervals for 4 h	equal to loss of body mass	cycling to lose 4.1% body mass 50% VO_2max	a. no difference in plasma volume at 6 h post b. increased plasma glucose with CHO c. increased respiratory exchange ratio with CHO d. carbonation had no effect
167	Neufer et al., 1991	glucose, 400 g	15 h a. following rehydration b. with no rehydration		cycle, intermittent 2 h 40–80% VO_2max	a. no difference in muscle glycogen resynthesis b. increased muscle water with rehydration
168	Nielsen et al., 1986	a. high K^+ (2.5% glucose, 51 mmol K/l) b. high Na^+ (2.5% glucose, 128 mmol NaCl/l) c. high CHO (9%)	15 min intervals for 2 h	300 ml	cycling 2 h 50% VO_2max	a. increased plasma volume with high Na^+ beverage b. increased intracellular rehydration with high K^+ and high CHO beverages
169	Nose et al., 1988	NaCl (capsules, 0.45 g/100 ml)	after 60 min, ad libitum for 3 h		cycling 90–110 min 40% VO_2max	a. increased restoration of water loss with NaCl b. increased plasma osmolality (and therefore dipsogenic stimulation) with NaCl
170	Reed et al., 1989	a. liquid CHO b. solid CHO c. CHO infusion	a. at 0 and 2 h b. at 0 and 2 h c. constant from 0 to 235 min		cycling 2 h	a. no difference in muscle glycogen resynthesis b. increased blood glucose with infusion
171	Stachenfeld et al., 1996	water	immediately post	1% body mass	cycling to lose 3% body mass anaerobic threshold	a. recovery of plasma volume within 60 min b. recovery of plasma osmolality within 60 min c. generally similar responses for men and women

in concentrations of 4–8% to the nutrient beverage will serve a useful purpose. Addition of carbohydrates within this concentration range has been shown to maintain blood glucose during the later stages of the exercise, and thereby increase performance time during exhaustive efforts.

The nutrients added to the ingested beverage may affect the efficacy of the solution in optimizing performance. Addition of carbohydrate to a beverage may delay the gastric emptying and intestinal absorption of the nutrients in proportion to the carbohydrate caloric content. However, there has been no evidence to suggest that such differences in emptying and absorption characteristics adversely affect performance. Addition of glucose, glucose polymers, sucrose, fructose, or mixed carbohydrates to a nutrient solution results in equally effective maintenance of blood glucose during prolonged exercise. Addition of fructose, however, may result in increased gastric distress in susceptible individuals. Small quantities of sodium in a nutrient solution enhance absorption of the carbohydrate component and would thus be beneficial. Caffeine may or may not increase the availability of nutrient fuels to working muscle. Consequently, its effectiveness in enhancing exercise performance, based on its ability to increase availability of nutrient fuels, is questionable.

Time of ingestion of a nutrient beverage has been shown to affect blood glucose and insulin. Ingestion of carbohydrate solutions, especially those which contain glucose, more than 30 min prior to an exercise bout may result in a transient increase in plasma glucose and insulin during the early stages of the exercise. However, plasma glucose normalizes within the first hour of exercise; eventual performance time is not adversely affected.

Following exercise, appropriate use of nutrient beverages may enhance the recovery of plasma volume, plasma osmolality, and muscle glycogen stores. Ingestion of a carbohydrate solution immediately following exercise leads to an increase in muscle glycogen resynthesis proportional to the amount of carbohydrate in the beverage. Glucose or sucrose is more effective than fructose in enhancing muscle glycogen resynthesis. Sodium increases the uptake of both the carbohydrate and water, and thus is a beneficial addition to the post-exercise nutrient beverage.

In summary, the following guidelines are offered for the selection of an appropriate nutrient beverage for physical performance:

1. Cool (5–15°C), flavored water is voluntarily ingested in greater quantities than plain, warm water. Therefore, for most exercise and sporting events, cool, flavored water is the optimal beverage for consumption both before and during the event.
2. Volumes of water of approximately 600 ml/h are most beneficial in terms of gastric emptying. However, since ingestion of such a large volume is impractical for most sport or exercise situations, ingestion of approximately 200 ml every 20 min appears optimal.
3. Addition of small amounts of glucose and sodium (30–50 mmol/l) to a nutrient beverage increases the net water absorption and thereby helps to maintain plasma volume and osmolality.
4. Carbohydrates (750–1250 ml/h of a 4–8% solution) added to a beverage consumed during prolonged exercise help to maintain blood glucose and thereby delay fatigue in exhaustive efforts.
5. The type of carbohydrate added to a beverage consumed prior to or during exercise does not affect exercise performance. However, addition of fructose to a nutrient beverage may increase gastric distress in some individuals.
6. Postexercise consumption of a beverage containing both carbohydrate (glucose rather than fructose) and electrolytes speeds the recovery of plasma volume, plasma osmolality, and muscle glycogen.

REFERENCES

1. Brooks, G. A. and Mercier, J., Balance of carbohydrate and lipid utilization during exercise: the crossover concept, *J. Appl. Physiol.*, 76, 2253, 1994.
2. Brouns, F. and Beckers, E., Is the gut an athletic organ?, *Sports Med.*, 4, 242, 1993.
3. Burke, L. M. and Read, R. S. D., Dietary supplements in sport, *Sports Med.*, 15, 43, 1993.
4. Coggan, A. R. and Coyle, E. F., Carbohydrate ingestion during prolonged exercise: Effects on metabolism and performance, in *Exercise and Sport Sciences Reviews*, Vol. 19, Holloszy, J. O., Ed., Williams & Wilkins, Baltimore, 1991, 1.
5. Consolazio, C. F. and Johnson, H. L., Dietary carbohydrate and work capacity, *Am. J. Clin. Nutr.*, 25, 85, 1972.
6. Costill, D. L., Carbohydrate nutrition before, during, and after exercise, *Fed. Proc.*, 44, 364, 1985.
7. Costill, D. L., Carbohydrates for exercise: dietary demands for optimal performance, *Int. J. Sports Med.*, 9, 1, 1988.
8. Costill, D. L. and Hargreaves, M., Carbohydrate nutrition and fatigue, *Sports Med.*, 13, 86, 1992.
9. Coyle, E. F., Carbohydrate metabolism and fatigue, in *Muscle Fatigue: Biochemical and Physiological Aspects*, Atlan, G., Beliveau, L., and Bouissou, P., Eds., Masson, Paris, 1991, 153.
10. Coyle, E. F. and Coggan, A. R., Effectiveness of carbohydrate feeding in delaying fatigue during prolonged exercise, *Sports Med.*, 1, 446, 1984.
11. Dodd, S. L., Herb, R. A., and Powers, S. K., Caffeine and exercise performance, *Sports Med.*, 15, 14, 1993.
12. Gisolfi, C. V. and Duchman, S. M., Guidelines for optimal replacement beverages for different athletic events, *Med. Sci. Sports Exer.*, 24, 679, 1992.
13. Hawley, J. A., Dennis, S. C., and Noakes, T. D., Carbohydrate, fluid, and electrolyte requirements during prolonged exercise, in *Sports Nutrition: Minerals and Electrolytes*, Kies, C. V. and Driskell, J. A., Eds., CRC Press, Boca Raton, FL, 1995, 235.
14. Ivy, J. L., Muscle glycogen synthesis before and after exercise, *Sports Med.*, 11, 6, 1991.
15. Johnson, H. L., The requirements for fluid replacement during heavy sweating and the benefits of carbohydrates and minerals, in *Sports Nutrition: Minerals and Electrolytes,* Kies, C. V. and Driskell, J. A., Eds., CRC Press, Boca Raton, FL, 1995, 215.
16. Kreider, R. B., Miriel, V., and Bertun, E., Amino acid supplementation and exercise performance: analysis of the proposed ergogenic value, *Sports Med.*, 16, 190, 1993.
17. Lamb, D. R. and Brodowicz, G. R., Optimal use of fluids of varying formulations to minimize exercise-induced disturbances in homeostasis, *Sports Med.*, 3, 247, 1986.
18. Maughan, R. J. and Noakes, T. D., Fluid replacement and exercise stress, *Sports Med.*, 12, 16, 1991.
19. Meyer, F. and Bar-Or, O., Fluid and electrolyte loss during exercise: the paediatric angle, *Sports Med.*, 18, 4, 1994.
20. Murray, R., The effects of consuming carbohydrate-electrolyte beverages on gastric emptying and fluid absorption during and following exercise, *Sports Med.*, 4, 322, 1987.
21. Noakes, T. D., Fluid replacement during exercise, in *Exercise and Sport Sciences Reviews,* Vol. 21, Holloszy, J. O., Ed., Williams & Wilkins, Baltimore, 1993, 297.
22. Powers, S. K. and Dodd, S., Caffeine and endurance performance, *Sports Med.*, 2, 165, 1985.
23. Sparling, P. B., Nieman, D. C., and O'Conner, P. J., Selected scientific aspects of marathon running: an update on fluid replacement, immune function, psychological factors and the gender difference, *Sports Med.*, 15, 116, 1993.
24. Stanley, W. C. and Connett, R. J., Regulation of muscle carbohydrate metabolism during exercise, *FASEB J.*, 5, 2155, 1991.
25. Valeriani, A., The need for carbohydrate intake during endurance exercise, *Sports Med.*, 12, 349, 1991.
26. Wasserman, D. H. and Cherrington, A. D., Hepatic fuel metabolism during muscular work: role and regulation, *Am. J. Physiol.*, 260, E811, 1991.
27. Puhl, S. M. and Buskirk, E. R., Nutritional beverages: exercise and sport, in *Nutrition in Exercise and Sport,* Wolinsky, I. and Hickson, J. F., Eds., CRC Press, Boca Raton, FL, 1994, 201.
28. Caspary, W. F., Physiology and pathophysiology of intestinal absorption, *Am. J. Clin. Nutr.*, 55, 299S, 1992.
29. Burks, T. F., Galligan, J. J., Porreca, F., and Barber, W. D., Regulation of gastric emptying, *Fed. Proc.*, 44, 2897, 1985.
30. Minami, H. and McCallum, R. W., The physiology and pathophysiology of gastric emptying in humans, *Gastroenterology*, 86, 1592, 1984.
31. Costill, D. L. and Saltin, B., Factors limiting gastric emptying during rest and exercise, *J. Appl. Physiol.*, 37, 679, 1974.
32. Lambert, G. P., Chang, R. T., Joensen, C., Shi, X., Summers, R. W., Schedl, H. P., and Gisolfi, C. V., Simultaneous determination of gastric emptying and intestinal absorption during cycle exercise in humans, *Int. J. Sports Med.*, 17, 48, 1996.

33. Armstrong, L. E., Hubbard, R. W., Szlyk, P. C., Matthew, W. T., and Sils, I. V., Voluntary dehydration and electrolyte losses during prolonged exercise in the heat, *Aviat. Space Environ. Med.*, 56, 765, 1985.

34. Hubbard, R. W., Sandick, B. L., Matthew, W. T., Francesconi, R. P., Sampson, J. B., Durkot, M. J., Maller, O., and Engell, D. B., Voluntary dehydration and alliesthesia for water, *J. Appl. Physiol.: Respirat. Environ. Exer. Physiol.*, 57, 868, 1984.

35. Neufer, P. D., Costill, D. L., Fink, W. J., Kirwan, J. P., Fielding, R. A., and Flynn, M. G., Effects of exercise and carbohydrate composition on gastric emptying, *Med. Sci. Sports Exer.*, 18, 658, 1986.

36. Brener, W., Hendrix, T. R., and McHugh, P. R., Regulation of the gastric emptying of glucose, *Gastroenterology*, 85, 76, 1983.

37. Rehrer, N. J., Wagenmakers, A. J. M., Beckers, E. J., Halliday, D., Leiper, J. B., Brouns, F., Maughan, R. J., Westerterp, K., and Saris, W. H. M., Gastric emptying, absorption, and carbohydrate oxidation during prolonged exercise, *J. Appl. Physiol.*, 72, 468, 1992.

38. Shafer, R. B., Levine, A. S., Marlette, J. M., and Morley, J. E., Do calories, osmolality, or calcium determine gastric emptying?, *Am. J. Physiol.*, 17, R479, 1985.

39. Zachwieja, J. J., Costill, D. L., Widrick, J. J., Anderson, D. E., and McConell, G. K., Effects of drink carbonation on the gastric emptying characteristics of water and flavored water, *Int. J. Sport Nutr.*, 1, 45, 1991.

40. Hunt, J. N. and Stubbs, D. F., The volume and energy content of meals as determinants of gastric emptying, *J. Physiol.*, 215, 209, 1975.

41. Foster, C., Costill, D. L., and Fink, W. J., Gastric emptying characteristics of glucose and glucose polymer solutions, *Res. Quart. Exer. Sport*, 51, 299, 1980.

42. Rehrer, N. J., Beckers, E., Brouns, F., Ten Hoor, F., and Saris, W. H. M., Exercise and training effects on gastric emptying of carbohydrate beverages, *Med. Sci. Sports Exer.*, 21, 540, 1989.

43. Fink, W. J., Costill, D. L., and Steven, C. F., Gastric-emptying characteristics of complete nutritional liquids, in *Nutrient Utilization During Exercise*, Fox, E. L., Ed., Ross Laboratories, Columbus, OH, 1983, 112.

44. McHugh, P. R. and Moran, T. H., Calories and gastric emptying: a regulatory capacity with implications for feeding, *Am. J. Physiol.*, 236, R254, 1979.

45. Cole, K. J., Grandjean, P. W., Sobszak, R. J., and Mitchell, J. B., Effect of carbohydrate composition on fluid balance, gastric emptying, and exercise performance, *Int. J. Sport Nutr.*, 3, 408, 1993.

46. Ferrannini, E., Barrett, E., Bevilacqua, S., Dupre, J., and Defronzo, R. A., Sodium elevates the plasma glucose response to glucose ingestion in man, *J. Clin. Endocrinol. Metab.*, 54, 455, 1982.

47. Gisolfi, C. V., Exercise, intestinal absorption, and rehydration, *Sports Sci. Exchange*, 4, 32, 1991.

48. Gisolfi, C. V., Spranger, K. J., Summers, R. W., Schedl, H. P., and Bleiler, T. L., Effects of cycle exercise on intestinal absorption in humans, *J. Appl. Physiol.*, 71, 2518, 1991.

49. Gisolfi, C. V., Summers, R. D., Schedl, H. P., and Bleiler, T. L., Effect of sodium concentration in a carbohydrate-electrolyte solution on intestinal absorption, *Med. Sci. Sports Exer.*, 27, 1414, 1995.

50. Fordtran, J. S. and Saltin, B., Gastric emptying and intestinal absorption during prolonged severe exercise, *J. Appl. Physiol.*, 23, 331, 1967.

51. Neufer, P. D., Young, A. J., and Sawka, M. N., Gastric emptying during exercise: effects of heat stress and hypohydration, *Eur. J. Appl. Physiol.*, 58, 433, 1989.

52. Neufer, P. D., Young, A. J., and Sawka, M. N., Gastric emptying during walking and running: effects of varied exercise intensity, *Eur. J. Appl. Physiol.*, 58, 440, 1989.

53. Ryan, A. J., Bleiler, T. L., Carter, J. E., and Gisolfi, C. V., Gastric emptying during prolonged cycling exercise in the heat, *Med. Sci. Sports Exer.*, 21, 51, 1989.

54. Costill, D. L., Bennett, A., Branam, G., and Eddy, D., Glucose ingestion at rest and during prolonged exercise, *J. Appl. Physiol.*, 34, 764, 1973.

55. Rehrer, N. J., Beckers, E. J., Brouns, F., Ten Hoor, F., and Saris, W. H. M., Effects of dehydration on gastric emptying and gastrointestinal distress while running, *Med. Sci. Sports Exer.*, 22, 790, 1990.

56. Jandrain, B. J., Pirnay, F., Lacroix, M., Mosora, F., Scheen, A. J., and Lefebvre, P. J., Effect of osmolality on availability of glucose ingested during prolonged exercise in humans, *J. Appl. Physiol.*, 67, 76, 1984.

57. Krzentowski, G., Jandrain, B., Pirnay, F., Mosora, F., Lacroix, M., Luyckx, A. S., and Lefebvre, P. J., Availability of glucose given orally during exercise, *J. Appl. Physiol.*, 56, 315, 1984.

58. Massicotte, D., Peronnet, F., Brisson, G., Bakkouch, K., and Hillaire-Marcel, C., Oxidation of a glucose polymer during exercise: comparison with glucose and fructose, *J. Appl. Physiol.*, 66, 179, 1989.

59. Perot, C. and Goubel, F., Effect of antagonistic contractions on the reflex response of a bifunctional muscle, *Eur. J. Appl. Physiol.*, 48, 51, 1982.

60. Massicotte, D., Peronnet, F., Adopo, E., Brisson, G. R., and Hillaire-Marcel, C., Effect of metabolic rate on the oxidation of ingested glucose and fructose during exercise, *Int. J. Sports Med.*, 15, 177, 1994.

61. Jandrain, B. J., Pallikarakis, N., Normand, S., Pirnay, F., Lacroix, M., Mosora, F., Pachiaudi, C., Gautier, J. F., Scheen, A. J., Riou, J. P., and Lefebvre, P. J., Fructose utilization during exercise in men: rapid conversion of ingested fructose to circulating glucose, *J. Appl. Physiol.*, 74, 2146, 1993.

62. Fujisawa, T., Mulligan, K., Wada, L., Schumacher, L., Riby, J., and Kretchmer, N., The effect of exercise on fructose absorption, *Am. J. Clin. Nutr.,* 58, 75, 1993.

63. Hargreaves, M., Costill, D., Burke, L., McConell, G., and Febbraio, M., Influence of sodium on glucose bioavailability during exercise, *Med. Sci. Sports Exer.,* 26, 365, 1994.

64. Melin, B., Cure, M., Jimenez, C., Koulmann, N., Savourey, G., and Bittel, J., Effect of ingestion pattern on rehydration and exercies performance subsequent to passive dehydration, *Eur. J. Appl. Physiol.,* 68, 281, 1994.

65. Segal, K., Nyman, A., Kral, J. G., Bjorntorp, P., Kotler, D. P., and Pi-Sunyer, F. X., Effects of glucose ingestion on sub maximal intermittent exercise, *Med. Sci. Sports Exer.,* 17, 205, 1985.

66. Snyder, A. C., Lamb, D. R., Baur, T., Connors, D., and Brodowicz, G., Maltodextrin feeding immediately before prolonged cycling at 62% VO_2max increases time to exhaustion, *Med. Sci. Sports Exer.,* 15, 126, 1983.

67. Snyder, A. C., Moorhead, K., Luedtke, J., and Small, M., Carbohydrate consumption prior to repeated bouts of high-intensity exercise, *Eur. J. Appl. Physiol.,* 66, 141, 1993.

68. Brouns, F., Rehrer, N. J., Saris, W. H., Beckers, E., Menheere, P., and ten Hoor, F., Effect of carbohydrate intake during warming-up on the regulation of blood glucose during exercise, *Int. J. Sports Med.,* 10, S68, 1989.

69. Criswell, D., Renshler, K., Powers, S. K., Tulley, R., Cicale, M., and Wheeler, K., Fluid replacement beverages and maintenance of plasma volume during exercise: role of aldosterone and vasopressin, *Eur. J. Appl. Physiol.,* 65, 445, 1992.

70. MacLean, D. A. and Graham, T. E., Branched-chain amino acid supplementation augments plasma ammonia responses during exercise in humans, *J. Appl. Physiol.,* 74, 2711, 1993.

71. Fielding, R. A., Costill, D. L., Fink, W. J., King, D. S., Kovaleski, J. E., and Kirwan, J. P., Effects of pre-exercise carbohydrate feedings on muscle glycogen use during exercise in well-trained runners, *Eur. J. Appl. Physiol.,* 56, 225, 1987.

72. Ventura, J. L., Estruch, A., Rodas, G., and Segura, Effect of prior ingestion of glucose or fructose on the performance of exercise of intermediate duration, *Eur. J. Appl. Physiol.,* 68, 345, 1994.

73. Foster, C., Costill, D. L., and Fink, W. J., Effects of preexercise feedings on endurance performance, *Med. Sci. Sports,* 11, 15, 1979.

74. Gleeson, M., Maughan, R. J., and Greenhaff, P. L., Comparison of the effects of pre-exercise feeding of glucose, glycerol and placebo on endurance and fuel homeostasis in man, *Eur. J. Appl. Physiol.,* 55, 645, 1986.

75. Hargreaves, M., Costill, D. L., Fink, W. J., King, D. S., and Fielding, R. A., Effect of pre-exercise carbohydrate feedings on endurance cycling performance, *Med. Sci. Sports Exer.,* 19, 33, 1987.

76. Hargreaves, M., Costill, D. L., Katz, A., and Fink, W. J., Effect of fructose ingestion on muscle glycogen usage during exercise, *Med. Sci. Sports Exer.,* 17, 360, 1985.

77. Hughes, V. A., Edwards, J. E., Meredith, C. N., Evans, W. J., Martin, R., and Young, V. R., Muscle glycogen utilization during low intensity endurance exercise following glucose or fructose ingestion, *Med. Sci. Sports Exer.,* 16, 190, 1984.

78. Koivisto, V. A., Harkonen, M., Karonen, S.-L., Groop, P. H., Elovainio, R., Ferrannini, E., Sacca, L., and Defronzo, R. A., Glycogen depletion during prolonged exercise: influence of glucose, fructose, or placebo, *J. Appl. Physiol.,* 58, 731, 1985.

79. Koivisto, V. A., Karonen, S.-L., and Nikkila, E. A., Carbohydrate ingestion before exercise: comparison of glucose, fructose, and sweet placebo, *J. Appl. Physiol.: Respirat. Environ. Exer. Physiol.,* 51, 783, 1981.

80. Levine, L., Evans, W. J., Cadarette, B. S., Fisher, E. C., and Bullen, B. A., Fructose and glucose ingestion and muscle glycogen use during submaximal exercise, *J. Appl. Physiol.: Respirat. Environ. Exer. Physiol.,* 55, 1767, 1983.

81. McMurray, R. G., Wilson, J. R., and Kitchell, B. S., The effects of fructose and glucose on high intensity endurance performance, *Res. Quart. Exer. Sport,* 54, 156, 1983.

82. Anderson, M., Bergman, E. A., and Nethery, V. M., Preexercise meal affects ride time to fatigue in trained cyclists, *J. Am. Diet. Assoc.,* 94, 1152, 1994.

83. Casal, D. C. and Leon, A. S., Failure of caffeine to affect substrate utilization during prolonged running, *Med. Sci. Sports Exer.,* 17, 174, 1985.

84. Erickson, M. A., Schwarzkopf, R. J., and McKenzie, R. D., Effects of caffeine, fructose, and glucose ingestion on muscle glycogen utilization during exercise, *Med. Sci. Sports Exer.,* 19, 579, 1987.

85. Graham, T. E. and Spriet, L. L., Performance and metabolic responses to a high caffeine dose during prolonged exercise, *J. Appl. Physiol.,* 71, 2292, 1991.

86. Keller, K. and Schwarzkopf, R., Preexercise snacks may decrease exercise performance, *Physician Sportsmed.,* 12, 89, 1984.

87. Okano, G., Takeda, H., Morita, I., Katoh, M., Mu, Z., and Miyake, S., Effect of pre-exercise fructose ingestion on endurance performance in fed men, *Med. Sci. Sports Exer.,* 20, 105, 1988.

88. Sasaki, H., Maeda, J., Usui, S., and Ishiko, T., Effect of sucrose and caffeine ingestion on performance of prolonged strenuous running, *Int. J. Sports Med.,* 8, 261, 1987.

89. Tarnopolsky, M. A., Atkinson, S. A., MacDougall, J. D., Sutton, J., and Sale, D. G., Caffeine as a potential ergogenic aid in endurance running, *Can. J. Sport Sci.,* 13, 89P, 1988.

90. Jandrain, B., Krzentowski, G., Pirnay, F., Mosora, F., Lacroix, M., Luyckx, A., and Lefebvre, P., Metabolic availability of glucose ingested 3 h before prolonged exercise in humans, *J. Appl. Physiol.: Respirat. Environ. Exer. Physiol.,* 56, 1314, 1984.

91. Wright, D. A., Sherman, W. M., and Dernbach, A. R., Carbohydrate feedings before, during, or in combination improve cycling performance, *J. Appl. Physiol.,* 71, 1082, 1991.

92. Sherman, W. M., Brodowicz, G., Wright, D. A., Simonsen, J., and Dernbach, A., Effects of 4 h preexercise carbohydrate feedings on cycling performance, *Med. Sci. Sports Exer.,* 21, 598, 1989.

93. Vukovich, M. D., Costill, D. L., Hickey, M. S., Trappe, S. W., Cole, K. J., and Fink, W. J., Effect of fat emulsion infusion and fat feeding on muscle glycogen utilization during cycle exercise, *J. Appl. Physiol.,* 75, 1513, 1993.

94. Shi, X., Summers, R. W., Schedl, H. P., Flanagan, S. W., Chang, R., and Gisolfi, C. V., Effects of carbohydrate type and concentration and solution osmolality on water absorption, *Med. Sci. Sports Exer.,* 27, 1607, 1995.

95. Thomas, D. E., Brotherhood, J. R., and Brand, J. C., Carbohydrate feeding before exercise: effect of glycemic index, *Int. J. Sports Med.,* 12, 180, 1991.

96. Bohannon, N. V., Karam, J. H., and Forsham, P. H., Endocrine responses to sugar ingestion in man, *J. Am. Diet. Assoc.,* 76, 555, 1980.

97. Geske, B. B. and Sharp, R. L., Pre-exercise ingestion of glucose and fructose: effects on exercise performance when exercise is begun at predetermined time of peak blood concentration of the sugar, *Med. Sci. Sports Exer.,* 16, 190, 1984.

98. Calles-Escandon, J., Devlin, J. T., Whitcomb, W., and Horton, E. S., Pre-exercise feeding does not affect endurance cycle exercise but attenuates post-exercise starvation-like response, *Med. Sci. Sports Exer.,* 23, 818, 1991.

99. Coyle, E. F., Coggan, A. R., Hemmert, M. K., Lowe, R. C., and Walters, T. J., Substrate usage during prolonged exercise following a preexercise meal, *J. Appl. Physiol.,* 59, 429, 1985.

100. Devlin, J. T., Calles-Escandon, J., and Horton, E. S., Effects of preexercise snack feeding on endurance cycle exercise, *J. Appl. Physiol.,* 60, 980, 1986.

101. Armstrong, L. E., Costill, D. L., and Fink, W. J., Influence of diuretic-induced dehydration on competitive running performance, *Med. Sci. Sports Exer.,* 17, 456, 1985.

102. Montner, P., Stark, D. M., Riedesel, M. L., Murata, G., Robergs, R., Timms, M., and Chick, T. W., Pre-exercise glycerol hydration improves cycling endurance time, *Int. J. Sports Med.,* 17, 27, 1996.

103. Blomstrand, E., Celsing, F., and Hewsholme, E. A., Changes in plasma concentrations of aromatic and branch-chain amino acids during sustained exercise in man and their possible role in fatigue, *Acta Physiol. Scand.,* 133, 115, 1988.

104. Blomstrand, E., Hassmen, P., Ekblom, B., and Newsholme, E. A., Administration of branch-chain amino acids during sustained exercise — effects on performance and on plasma concentration of some amino acids, *Eur. J. Appl. Physiol.,* 63, 83, 1991.

105. Costill, D. L., Verstappen, F., Kuipers, H., Janssen, E., and Fink, W., Acid-base balance during repeated bouts of exercise: influence of HCO_3, *Int. J. Sports Med.,* 5, 228, 1984.

106. Wilkes, D., Gledhill, N., and Smyth, R., Effect of acute induced metabolic alkalosis on 800-m racing time, *Med. Sci. Sports Exer.,* 15, 277, 1983.

107. McNaughton, L. R., Sodium citrate and anaerobic performance: implications of dosage, *Eur. J. Appl. Physiol.,* 61, 392, 1990.

108. Coyle, E. F., Hagberg, J. M., Hurley, B. F., Martin, W. H., Ehsani, A. A., and Holloszy, J. O., Carbohydrate feeding during prolonged strenuous exercise can delay fatigue, *J. Appl. Physiol.: Respirat. Environ. Exer. Physiol.,* 55, 230, 1983.

109. Coggan, A. R. and Coyle, E. F., Metabolism and performance following carbohydrate ingestion late in exercise, *Med. Sci. Sports Exer.,* 21, 59, 1989.

110. Coyle, E. F., Coggan, A. R., Hemmert, M. K., and Ivy, J. L., Muscle glycogen utilization during prolonged strenuous exercise when fed carbohydrate, *J. Appl. Physiol.,* 61, 165, 1986.

111. Davis, J. M., Lamb, D. R., Pate, R. R., Slentz, C. A., Burgess, W. A., and Bartoli, W. P., Carbohydrate-electrolyte drinks: effects on endurance cycling in the heat, *Am. J. Clin. Nutr.,* 48, 1023, 1988.

112. Edwards, T. L., Jr. and Santeusanio, D. M., Field test of the effects of carbohydrate solutions on endurance performance, selected blood serum chemistries, perceived exertion, and fatigue in world class cyclists, *Med. Sci. Sports Exer.,* 16, 190, 1984.

113. Fielding, R. A., Costill, D. L., Fink, W. J., King, D. S., Hargreaves, M., and Kovaleski, J. E., Effect of carbohydrate feeding frequencies and dosage on muscle glycogen use during exercise, *Med. Sci. Sports Exer.,* 17, 472, 1985.

114. Ivy, J. L., Miller, W., Dover, V., Goodyear, L. G., Sherman, W. M., Farrell, S., and Williams, H., Endurance improved by ingestion of a glucose polymer supplement, *Med. Sci. Sports Exer.,* 15, 466, 1983.

115. Millard-Stafford, M., Sparling, P. B., Rosskopf, L. B., Hinson, B. T., and Dicarlo, L. J., Carbohydrate-electrolyte replacement during a simulated triathlon in the heat, *Med. Sci. Sports Exer.,* 22, 621, 1990.

116. Murray, R., Paul, G. L., Seifert, J. G., and Eddy, D. E., Responses to varying rates of carbohydrate ingestion during exercise, *Med. Sci. Sports Exer.,* 23, 713, 1991.

117. Wilber, R. L. and Moffat, R. J., Influence of glucose polymer ingestion on plasma glucose concentration and performance in male distance runners, *Int. J. Sports Med.,* 12, 251, 1991.

118. Brodowicz, G. R., Lamb, D. R., Baur, T. S., and Connors, D. F., Efficacy of various drink formulations for fluid replenishment during cycling exercise in the heat, *Med. Sci. Sports Exer.,* 16, 138, 1984.

119. Flynn, M. G., Costill, D. L., Hawley, J. A., Fink, W. J., Neufer, P. D., Fielding, R. A., and Sleeper, M. D., Influence of selected carbohydrate drinks on cycling performance and glycogen use, *Med. Sci. Sports Exer.,* 19, 37, 1987.

120. Powers, S. K., Lawler, J., Dodd, S., Tulley, R., Landry, G., and Wheeler, K., Fluid replacement drinks during high intensity exercise: effects on minimizing exercise-induced disturbances in homeostasis, *Eur. J. Appl. Physiol.,* 60, 54, 1990.

121. Williams, C., Nute, M. G., Broadbank, L., and Vinall, S., Influence of fluid intake on endurance running performance: a comparison between water, glucose, and fructose solutions, *Eur. J. Appl. Physiol.,* 60, 112, 1990.

122. Carter, J. E. and Gisolfi, C. V., Fluid replacement during and after exercise in the heat, *Med. Sci. Sports Exer.,* 21, 532, 1989.

123. Hargreaves, M., Costill, D. L., Coggan, A., Fink, W. J., and Nishibata, I., Effect of carbohydrate feedings on muscle glycogen utilization and exercise performance, *Med. Sci. Sports Exer.,* 16, 219, 1984.

124. Kingwell, B., McKenna, M. J., Sandstrom, E. R., and Hargreaves, M., Effect of glucose polymer ingestion on energy and fluid balance during exercise, *J. Sports Sci.,* 7, 3, 1989.

125. Owen, M. D., Kregel, K. C., Wall, P. T., and Gisolfi, C. V., Effects of ingesting carbohydrate beverages during exercise in the heat, *Med. Sci. Sports Exer.,* 18, 568, 1986.

126. Seidman, D. S., Ashkenazi, I., Arnon, R., Shapiro, Y., and Epstein, Y., The effects of glucose polymer beverage ingestion during prolonged outdoor exercise in the heat, *Med. Sci. Sports Exer.,* 23, 458, 1991.

127. Yaspelkis, B. B., III and Ivy, J. L., Effect of carbohydrate supplements and water on exercise metabolism in the heat, *J. Appl. Physiol.,* 71, 680, 1991.

128. Hargreaves, M. and Briggs, C. A., Effect of carbohydrate ingestion on exercise metabolism, *J. Appl. Physiol.,* 65, 1553, 1988.

129. Bosch, A. N., Noakes, T. D., and Dennis, S., Carbohydrate ingestion during prolonged exercise: a liver glycogen sparing effect in glycogen loaded subjects, *Med. Sci. Sports Exer.,* 23, S152, 1991.

130. Barr, S. I., Costill, D. L., and Fink, W. J., Fluid replacement during prolonged exercise: effects of water, saline, or no fluid, *Med. Sci. Sports Exer.,* 23, 811, 1991.

131. Johnson, H. L., Nelson, R. A., and Consolazio, C. F., Effects of electrolyte and nutrient solutions on performance and metabolic balance, *Med. Sci. Sports Exer.,* 20, 26, 1988.

132. Decombaz, J., Gmunder, G., Daget, N., Munoz-Box, R., and Howald, H., Acceptance of isotonic and hypotonic rehydrating beverages by athletes during training, *Int. J. Sports Med.,* 13, 40, 1992.

133. Bothorel, B., Follenius, M., Gissinger, R., and Candas, V., Physiological effects of dehydration and rehydration with water and acidic or neutral carbohydrate electrolyte solutions, *Eur. J. Appl. Physiol.,* 60, 209, 1979.

134. Francis, K. T., Effect of water and electrolyte replacement during exercise in the heat on biochemical indices of stress and performance, *Aviat. Space Environ. Med.,* 50, 115, 1979.

135. Hamilton, M. T., Gonzalez-Alonso, J., Montain, S. J., and Coyle, E. F., Fluid replacement and glucose infusion during exercise prevent cardiovascular drift, *J. Appl. Physiol.,* 71, 871, 1991.

136. Maughan, R. J., Fenn, C. E., Gleeson, M., and Leiper, J. B., Metabolic and circulatory responses to the ingestion of glucose polymer and glucose/electrolyte solutions during exercise in man, *Eur. J. Appl. Physiol.,* 56, 356, 1987.

137. Wells, C. L., Schrader, T. A., Stern, J. R., and Krahenbuhl, G. S., Physiological responses to a 20-mile run under three fluid replacement treatments, *Med. Sci. Sports Exer.,* 17, 364369, 1985.

138. Davis, J. M., Burgess, W. A., Slentz, C. A., Bartoli, W. P., and Pate, R., Effects of ingesting 6% and 12% glucose/electrolyte beverages during prolonged intermittent cycling in the heat, *Eur. J. Appl. Physiol.,* 57, 563, 1988.

139. Hawley, J. A., Bosch, A. N., Weltan, S. M., Dennis, S. C., and Noakes, T. D., Effects of glucose ingestion or glucose infusion on fuel substrate kinetics during prolonged exercise, *Eur. J. Appl. Physiol.,* 68, 381, 1994.

140. Leese, G. P., Thompson, J., Scrimgeour, C. M., and Rennie, M. J., Exercise and the oxidation and storage of glucose, maize-syrup solids and sucrose determined from breath $^{13}CO_2$, *Eur. J. Appl. Physiol.,* 72, 349, 1996.

141. Burstein, R., Seidman, D. S., Alter, J., Moram, D., Shpilberg, O., Shemer, J., Wiener, M., and Epstein, Y., Glucose polymer ingestion — effect on fluid balance and glycemic state during a 4-d march, *Med. Sci. Sports Exer.,* 26, 360, 1994.

142. Fahey, T. D., Larsen, J. D., Brooks, G. A., Colvin, W., Henderson, S., and Lary, D., The effects of ingesting polylactate or glucose polymer drinks during prolonged exercise, *Int. J. Sport Nutr.*, 1, 249, 1991.

143. Langenfeld, M. E., Glucose polymer ingestion during ultraendurance bicycling, *Res. Quart. Exer. Sport*, 54, 411, 1983.

144. Criswell, D., Powers, S., Lawler, J., Tew, J., Dodd, S., Iryiboz, Y., Tulley, R., and Wheeler, K., Influence of a carbohydrate-electrolyte beverage on blood homeostasis during football, *Physiologist*, 33, A73, 1990.

145. Ivy, J. L., Costill, D. L., Fink, W. J., and Lower, R. W., Influence of caffeine and carbohydrate feedings on endurance performance, *Med. Sci. Sports Exer.*, 11, 6, 1979.

146. Murray, R., Eddy, D. E., Murray, T. W., Seifert, J. G., Paul, G. L., and Halaby, G. A., The effect of fluid and carbohydrate feedings during intermittent cycling exercise, *Med. Sci. Sports Exer.*, 19, 597, 1987.

147. Peters, H. P., Van Schelven, F. W., Verstappen, P. A., De Boer, R. W., Bol, E., Erich, W. G., Van Der Togt, C. R., and De Vries, W., Gastrointestinal problems as a function of carbohydrate supplements and mode of exercise, *Med. Sci. Sports Exer.*, 25, 1211, 1993.

148. Adopo, E., Peronnet, F., Massicotte, D., Brisson, G. R., and Hillaire-Marcel, C., Respoective oxidation of exogenous glucose and fructose given in the same drink during exercise, *J. Appl. Physiol.*, 76, 1014, 1994.

149. Mason, W. L., McConell, G., and Hargreaves, M., Carbohydrate ingestion during exercise: liquid vs. solid feedings, *Med. Sci. Sports Exer.*, 25, 966, 1993.

150. Deuster, P. A., Singh, A., Hofmann, A., Moses, F. M., and Chrousos, G. C., Hormonal responses to ingesting water or a carbohydrate beverage during a 2 h run, *Med. Sci. Sports Exer.*, 24, 72, 1992.

151. Murray, R., Eddy, D. E., Paul, G. L., Seifert, J. G., and Halaby, G. A., Physiological responses to glycerol ingestion during exercise, *J. Appl. Physiol.*, 71, 144, 1991.

152. Murray, R., Paul, G. L., Seifert, J. G., Eddy, D. E., and Halaby, G. A., The effect of glucose, fructose, and sucrose ingestion during exercise, *Med. Sci. Sports Exer.*, 21, 275, 1989.

153. Murray, R., Seifert, J. G., Eddy, D. E., Paul, G. L., and Halaby, G. A., Carbohydrate feeding and exercise: effect of beverage carbohydrate content, *Eur. J. Appl. Physiol.*, 59, 152, 1989.

154. Yaspelkis, B. B., III, Patterson, J. G., Anderla, P. A., Ding, Z., and Ivy, J. L., Carbohydrate supplementation spares muscle glycogen during variable-intensity exercise, *J. Appl. Physiol.*, 75, 1477, 1993.

155. Zachwieja, J. J., Costill, D. L., and Fink, W. J., Carbohydrate ingestion during exercise: effects on muscle glycogen resynthesis after exercise, *Int. J. Sport Nutr.*, 3, 418, 1993.

156. Owen, M. D., Kregel, K. C., Wall, P. T., and Gisolfi, C. V., Effects of carbohydrate ingestion on thermoregulation, gastric emptying and plasma volume during exercise in the heat, *Med. Sci. Sports Exer.*, 17, 185, 1985.

157. Kolka, M. A. and Stephenson, L. A., Plasma volume loss during maximal exercise in females, *Physiologist*, 33, A73, 1990.

158. Brandenberger, G., Candas, V., Follenius, M., Libert, J. P., and Kahn, J. M., Vascular fluid shifts and endocrine responses to exercise in the heat: effect of rehydration, *Eur. J. Appl. Physiol.*, 55, 113, 1986.

159. Candas, V., Libert, J. P., Brandenberger, G., Sagot, J. C., Amoros, C., and Kahn, J. M., Hydration during exercise: effects on thermal and cardiovascular adjustments, *Eur. J. Appl. Physiol.*, 55, 113, 1986.

160. Giles, D. and Maclaren, D., Effects of caffeine and glucose ingestion on metabolic and respiratory functions during prolonged exercise, *J. Sports Sci.*, 2, 35, 1984.

161. Burke, L. M., Collier, G. R., and Hargreaves, M., Muscle glycogen storage after prolonged exercise: effect of the glycemic index of carbohydrate feedings, *J. Appl. Physiol.*, 75, 1019, 1993.

162. Blom, P. C. S., Hostmark, A. T., Vaage, O., Kardel, K. R., and Maehlum, S., Effect of different post-exercise sugar diets on the rate of muscle glycogen synthesis, *Med. Sci. Sports Exer.*, 19, 491, 1987.

163. Costill, D. L., Cote, R., Miller, E., Miller, T., and Wyer, S., Water and electrolyte replacement during repeated days of work in the heat, *Aviat. Space Environ. Med.*, 46, 795, 1975.

164. Costill, D. L., Sherman, W. M., Fink, W. J., Maresh, C., Witten, M., and Miller, J. M., The role of dietary carbohydrates in muscle glycogen resynthesis after strenuous running, *Am. J. Clin. Nutr.*, 34, 1831, 1981.

165. Lambert, C. P., Costill, D. L., McConell, G. K., Benedict, M. A., Lambert, G. P., Robergs, R. A., and Fink, W. J., Fluid replacement after dehydration: influence of beverage carbonation and carbohydrate content, *Int. J. Sports Med.*, 13, 285, 1992.

166. Glace, B. W., Gleim, G. W., Zabetakis, P. M., and Nicholas, J. A., Systemic effects of ingesting varying amounts of a commercial carbohydrate beverage postexercise, *J. Am. Coll. Nutr.*, 13, 268, 1994.

167. Neufer, P. D., Sawka, M. N., Young, A. J., Quigley, M. D., Latzka, W. A., and Levine, L., Hypohydration does not impair skeletal muscle glycogen resynthesis after exercise, *J. Appl. Physiol.*, 70, 1490, 1991.

168. Nielsen, B., Sjogaard, G., Ugelvig, J., Knudsen, B., and Dohlmann, B., Fluid balance in exercise dehydration and rehydration with different glucose-electrolyte drinks, *Eur. J. Appl. Physiol.*, 55, 318, 1986.

169. Nose, H., Mack, G. W., Shi, X., and Nadel, E. R., Role of osmolality and plasma volume during rehydration in humans, *J. Appl. Physiol.*, 65, 325, 1988.

170. Reed, M. J., Brozinick, J. T., Jr., Lee, M. C., and Ivy, J. L., Muscle glycogen storage postexercise: effect of mode of carbohydrate administration, *J. Appl. Physiol.*, 66, 720, 1989.

171. Stachenfeld, N. S., Gleim, G. W., Zabetakis, P. M., and Nicholas, J. A., Fluid balance and renal response following dehydrating exercise in well-trained men and women, *Eur. J. Appl. Physiol.*, 72, 468, 1996.

Chapter 13

DIETARY SUPPLEMENTS AS ERGOGENIC AIDS

Luke R. Bucci

CONTENTS

I. INTRODUCTION

Ergogenic, derived from the Greek word for work (*ergon*), is defined as to increase work or potential for work.[1] Nutritional ergogenic aids are defined as substances found in the diet or cells that are ingested in an effort to produce improved or enhanced sport, exercise, and physical performance. The first half of this decade has seen a steady increase in substances tested for their ergogenic potential. Enaction and enforcement of laws designed to reduce ergogenic drug usage among athletes has increased usage and interest in nutritional ergogenic aids.

This chapter has been rearranged from the two previous editions in an effort to condense the huge amount of information available on nutritional ergogenic aids. Number of human clinical trials with micronutrient supplements has doubled within the past three years. New trends in effects of nutrient supplementation are becoming apparent which may explain the dichotomy between widespread public use of supplements and perceived widespread lack of scientific support for such use. A common theme of feeling better mentally after supplementation above and beyond a placebo effect has become apparent,[2] especially for micronutrients such as vitamins, minerals, antioxidants, amino acids, caffeine, and herbal preparations. The implication is that regardless of any physiological effects, consumers continue ingesting supplements because they simply *feel* better. This avenue will be considered in this chapter as an ergogenic property, since it is well known that psychological factors greatly affect exercise performance. This is the very reason for using double-blind, placebo-controlled study designs in human trials. Scope of nutritional ergogenic aids is widening to add psychological, mental, cognitive, neuromuscular, immunological, and hormonal effects to the customary metabolic or bioenergetic mechanisms.

II.   ALTERATIONS OF DIETARY MACRONUTRIENTS

A.   WATER AND ELECTROLYTES

Water and electrolytes in body fluids are important to exercise performance by:

1. maintaining blood volume and osmolality in order to transport and transfer oxygen, fuels, cellular waste products, and regulatory molecules;
2. thermoregulation to prevent dangerous overheating;
3. shock-absorbing and lubricating properties; and
4. homeostasis of enzymic and neuromuscular functions.[3-7]

When compared to limited or no fluid intake during exercise, ingestion of water and/or electrolytes often improved performance.[3-7] Thus, it appears that water administration during exercise can maintain optimal performance or prevent fatigue until other factors initiate fatigue. Can supranormal amounts of water (hyperhydration, superhydration, or overhydration) offer further increases in performance? Several studies found that hyperhydration during exercise in heat (48.8°C, 120°F) found improved performance and decreased body temperature.[8-14] These changes should prevent or delay adverse effects of dehydration.

Other results demonstrated that hyperhydration is not universally applicable. Consumption of 1–1.5 l of water immediately before a 200-yard (183 m) swimming medley actually slowed race times significantly.[15] Several individuals consuming large amounts of water (without electrolytes) during an ultramarathon experienced hyponatremia (loss of sodium), with a serious detriment to both performance and health.[16]

The American College of Sports Medicine has published a position statement for prevention of thermal injury (heat stroke) during distance running (or other sports activities such as football practice) in the heat.[3] Guidelines are listed in Table 1.

Electrolyte depletion is only a problem when high rates of sweating occur, usually over several days of vigorous exercise in the heat, after several events in one day (e.g., tennis tournaments), or after daily training.[4-7] Exercise under other conditions may actually lead to higher electrolyte concentrations in the blood, since sweat is hypotonic. Losses of 5–6 lbs (>2 kg) of body weight may indicate electrolyte depletion and a need for increased dietary

TABLE 1   Guidelines for Prevention of Thermal Injury During Endurance Exercise in the Heat (>80°F, >30°C)

1. Drink 500 ml (1 pint) of cold water (or dilute electrolyte drink) 20–30 min before exercise.
2. During exercise, every 15–20 min (or 2–3 km) drink 100–200 ml (6–7 fl oz) of cold water (or dilute electrolyte drink).
3. A total of 1.4–4.2 l of water should be consumed every hour (amounts >2 l/h are difficult to consume in practice).

Notes: 1. Phrases in parentheses are inserted by author.
2. Thirst is not an adequate indicator of dehydration. Liquids must be consumed *before* thirst is noticed.
3. Choose water or dilute electrolyte solutions that are good-tasting in order to encourage liquid consumption.

intake of sodium, potassium, and chloride.[11] Individuals may vary widely in their sweating rates (more than four-fold),[4,5,7] and close attention must be given to those who seem to sweat more than others.

A consensus of research has agreed that adding small amounts of salt to meals from a salt shaker on the table, during cooking, or from fluid replacement beverages is sufficient to prevent losses of sodium chloride detrimental to performance during exercise or training.[5,6] Alternatively, conservative use of salt tablets (three to six 500 mg tablets daily with meals) will accomplish the same intake levels of salt for individuals who consume low amounts of dietary salt. Excessive use of salt tablets or salt (>10 g/d) is to be discouraged in average settings, since excess sodium may induce potassium excretion and loss.[17]

Potassium supplements have helped to prevent muscle cramping and heat stroke in susceptible individuals.[18] Daily doses of supplemental potassium ranged from 0.75–3 g/d. Again, similar to sodium, high intakes of potassium (>10 g/d) are known to be hazardous to health. Fresh fruits and vegetables are rich in potassium, and their consumption is to be encouraged before resorting to potassium supplements. Daily dietary intakes of ≥3 g of potassium appear to be adequate to replace potassium losses from exercise in the heat.[18]

In summary, water is an important and essential ergogenic aid for the conditions listed in Table 2. Hyperhydration is recommended for exercise of long duration in the heat. Electrolyte replenishment (sodium, potassium, and chloride) is important for large, repetitive losses of sweat, especially when subjects are not acclimatized. Other conditions may not exhibit improved performance after consumption of water and/or electrolytes, but at least a decrease in performance is unlikely.

TABLE 2   Conditions for Ergogenic properties of Water and Electrolytes

Condition	Parameters
Prior Dehydration	
High ambient temperature	>30°C (>80°F)
High body temperature	>39°C (>104°F)
High relative humidity	>80%
High solar radiation	sunshine, reflective surfaces (sand, snow, water, concrete)
Lack of air movement	no wind or light rear wind
High rate of sweating	>2 l/h
Lack of Heat Acclimatization	
Untrained Subjects	
Exercise intensity	>75% VO_2max
Exercise duration	>1 h
Exercise Intensity-Duration Product	
High body fat percentage	>25% body fat by weight
Heat-trapping or Excessive Clothing	
Underwater exercise	scuba-diving, snorkeling, swimming, water polo
Altitude	>1500 km (>1 mile)
Voluntary fluid restriction	making weight practices for wrestlers, boxers, bodybuilders, weightlifters
Diuretic drugs	caffeine overdoses, thiazides, furosemide, bumetanide, spironolactone, etc.
Certain diseases	diabetes, renal diseases

B. CARBOHYDRATES

Availability of carbohydrate to muscles is a limiting factor in exercise performance.[19-23] Since carbohydrates supply about 50% of energy sources during submaximal exercise (<70% VO_2max) and the majority of energy at intensities >70% VO_2max,[19-23] fatigue is closely related to carbohydrate availability. Depletion of carbohydrate sources (tissue glycogen and blood glucose) has been repeatedly documented to cause fatigue and reduce exercise performance.[19-23] Furthermore, carbohydrate storage is directly dependent on recent dietary history, since relatively little (approximately 2000 kcal or 8.4 MJ) is stored in the body.

Glucose is the carbohydrate currency of human metabolism and can be stored in branched-chain polymers called glycogen, primarily in muscle and liver. Blood glucose levels are carefully regulated by an elegant hormonal system including insulin, glucagon, catecholamines, glucocorticoids, somatotropin, and eicosanoids. Muscle glycogen stores are utilized preferentially during exercise.[19-23] If exercise is of sufficient duration and/or intensity (usually >2 hr), muscle glycogen becomes depleted and muscles become reliant upon blood glucose for carbohydrate supply.[19-23] Liver glycogen, gluconeogenesis (formation of glucose by breakdown of amino acids), and exogenous dietary sources of carbohydrate then maintain blood glucose levels as long as possible.[19-23] When blood glucose levels decrease below normal physiological levels (70 mg/dl or 3.9 mmol/l), performance deteriorates rapidly.

Studies on the role of carbohydrates as ergogenic aids are numerous, and detailed descriptions would demand more space than is necessary for an overview. At this time, there is no doubt that exogenous carbohydrate ingestion and/or supplementation benefits exercise performance under the proper conditions.[19-23] Thus, a focus on what exercise conditions have shown benefit from carbohydrate supplementation will be presented.

1. Glycogen Supercompensation (Carbohydrate Loading)

Two basic types of carbohydrate manipulation are used to enhance exercise performance: (1) increasing glycogen stores; and (2) consuming carbohydrate during exercise. The practice of glycogen supercompensation, popularly known as carbohydrate loading, can produce supranormal levels of muscle glycogen, which can lead to improved performance, compared to a typical diet.[19-24] Glycogen supercompensation is designed for optimal performance during a single endurance event, such as a triathlon, marathon, ultramarathon, long cycling road races, or competitive sports events. Any event lasting more than 90 min and leading to exhaustion signals a need for glycogen supercompensation.[19-23] However, glycogen supercompensation should not be performed more than two or three times per month.

The preferred method of glycogen supercompensation starts seven days before an event. During the next week, one should consume a large amount (70% of total calories) of foods rich in complex carbohydrates (starches). Up to 600 g of carbohydrates daily is considered to be a high-carbohydrate diet. In practical terms, 600 g of carbohydrates is equivalent to 2 loaves of bread, 3 cups of sugar, 15 medium baked potatoes, or 12 cups of rice. Every second day, exercise amount is cut in half, until no exercise is performed the day before the event. Carbohydrate consumption is continued throughout the pre-event period, culminating in a pre-exercise meal. A high-carbohydrate (>300 g), pre-exercise meal should be consumed 3–4 hr before the event. Pre-exercise carbohydrates should be low-fiber, low-fat, and rich in complex carbohydrates (starches) instead of sugars to avoid an insulin response with resulting hypoglycemia during exercise.

Glycogen supercompensation (carbohydrate loading) is recommended for the conditions listed in Table 3. In general, long-term endurance events lasting more than 90 min or repetitive events occurring in single or multiple days (such as cycling road races) are primary conditions for maintaining a high-carbohydrate diet.

**TABLE 3   Exercise Activities with Ergogenic Benefits
from Glycogen Supercompensation
(Carbohydrate Loading)**

More Benefits	Less Benefits
Soccer	Runs <10 km
Marathon	Sprinting
Triathlon	Weight lifting
Ultramarathon	Hockey games
Ultra-endurance events	Football games
Cross-country skiing	Baseball games
Cycling time trials	Basketball games
Long distance swimming	Most rowing events
Long distance canoe or kayak	Most track and field events
Rock climbing	Walking and hiking
Mountain climbing	Downhill ski runs

2.   Carbohydrate Supplementation During Exercise

Similar to the prodigious amount of information on glycogen supercompensation, a voluminous body of literature (more than 100 original articles) exploring the effects of exogenous carbohydrate supplementation ingested *during* exercise is available.[19-24] A consensus of research has shown that carbohydrate ingestion during exercise can improve long-term endurance performance (lasting 90 min or more) and delay fatigue 30–60 min. Endurance events lasting longer than 90 min (listed in Table 3) showed the most benefits from carbohydrate supplementation during exercise.

The most recent guidelines on carbohydrate supplementation during exercise gave the following recommendations:[19-24]

1. Immediately before exercise, consume 200–400 ml of a moderately concentrated (5–7%) carbohydrate drink, preferably as glucose polymers.
2. Continue consuming 100–150 ml of the same drink at 10–15 min intervals for the first 2 hr of exercise.
3. After 2 hr, switch to a more concentrated drink (15–20% carbohydrate). Consume 100–150 ml every 15 min. For exhaustive events lasting less than 2 hr, consume the more concentrated drink during the last quarter of exercise. At least 200–300 ml total of the more concentrated drink should be consumed. Mild gastric discomfort is acceptable; however, nausea indicates an excess has been consumed.
4. It is highly recommended that each individual choose a drink that tastes palatable, a matter of individual preference.
5. At this time, it is not certain if additional ingredients (vitamins, minerals, lactic acid, buffers) offer further benefits.
6. One alternative to purchasing sports drinks is to dilute any fruit juice 1:1 with water and add a teaspoon of salt per liter (quart). This should approximate carbohydrate, electrolyte, and osmolality values of commercial sports drinks.

3.   Carbohydrates and Recovery from Exercise

For those engaging in highly strenuous activities on successive days (such as cycling road races), rapid replenishment of carbohydrate stores is advisable, since insufficient time for carbohydrate loading is available. Again, a burst of recent research has suggested the following guidelines to maximize glycogen stores to support exhaustive, repetitive tasks:[19-25]

1. Initiate carbohydrate feeding immediately (within 2 hr) after exhaustive exercise.
2. Consume simple sugars (0.7 g glucose or sucrose/kg body weight or 50 g carbohydrate) rather than complex carbohydrates every 2 hr for the first 4–6 hr after exercise.

3. After 6 hr, complex carbohydrates may be consumed. In the 20–24 hr after exercise, a total of 500–700 g of carbohydrates should be consumed, preferably from low-fat, low-fiber foods (much like a pre-exercise meal).

Rapid replenishment with carbohydrates after exercise hastens recuperation, allowing a quicker return to training and maintenance of performance during strenuous daily events.

C. PROTEIN

Ergogenic properties of protein revolve around two interests: (1) enhance endurance; and (2) increase or maintain muscle mass to improve strength and/or size. The question of whether increasing protein intake or protein supplementation during resistance training (weightlifting) will enhance or accelerate accretion of muscle mass or strength is of considerable public and professional interest.

Protein supplementation to prolong endurance performance by acting as an accessory fuel has some rationale, because 5–10% of energy production during long-term endurance exercise is produced from protein catabolism via the glucose-alanine cycle and subsequent gluconeogenesis.[26,27] Several reviews suggest that high-protein diets or protein supplements do not enhance long-term endurance performance;[26-28] however, studies are sparse and not definitive. Unanswered questions include the differential catabolism of leucine compared to other amino acids, gender differences in protein metabolism, maintenance of muscle mass in endurance athletes by protein supplementation to prevent adverse immunological or musculoskeletal events, and does that 5–10% contribution of energy production from muscular amino acid catabolism have practical significance for long-term, intense endurance performance?

A consensus of research by different methodologies has found that endurance athletes have an intensity-dependent, dietary protein requirement of 1.2–1.4 g/kg/d (150–175% of the RDA for sedentary people, which is 0.8 g/kg/d) to achieve nitrogen balance.[27] This equates to a daily protein intake of almost 100 g for a 70 kg male. Food equivalents of 100 g of protein are:

1. one 15 oz (0.43 kg) steak;
2. four skinless chicken breasts (3 oz or 85 g each);
3. 17 eggs;
4. 17 slices of 100% whole wheat bread; or
5. 1.5 cups of protein powder.

Exercise over 55% VO_2max for more than 90 min increases protein requirements over the RDA, even with adequate energy intake.[27]

Enough research on protein requirements and effects of supplementation during resistance training has been reported to tentatively propose some guidelines for protein intake. A dose-response effect for protein intake and nitrogen balance during weightlifting exercise has become apparent.[26,27] A protein intake requirement of 1.4–2.4 g/kg/d for intense resistance training has been found by almost every study examining this issue.[26,27,29-37] Protein intakes over 2 g/kg/d in strength athletes usually resulted in improved protein metabolism, protein synthesis, body mass, muscle mass, or strength measurements during weight training,[29-32,35] but also reached a plateau of metabolic benefit by virtue of increased amino acid oxidation without further increases in protein synthesis.[27]

For a large weightlifter (100 kg), 2.4 g/kg/d of protein is equivalent to:

1. one 35 oz (1.0 kg) steak;
2. nine skinless chicken breasts;
3. 40 eggs;

4. 40 slices of whole wheat bread; or

5. 3.5 cups of protein powder.

These food intakes are still less than reported chronic dietary protein intakes of 4.0–6.2 g/kg/d for intense weightlifters.[27]

Safety of high dietary intakes of protein in absence of renal or liver failure is not a concern based on no findings of adverse effects to date in strength athletes consuming large amounts of protein for long time periods.[27] Of more concern is concomitant intake of fat from protein-rich food sources, which can be negated by careful food selection or protein powder supplements.

D. FATS

"Fat-loading" has been hypothesized to extend endurance performance, since even a lean human body stores about 600,000 kJ (100 times more kcal as fat than carbohydrate).[38] Fat (long-chain fatty acid triglycerides or LCTs) is the primary fuel for exercise intensities less than 50% VO_2max,[38,39] and when carbohydrates are depleted by exercise, fat remains as an energy source.[39] Fat loading (50-90 g oral or 9 g intravenous) just before exercise raised serum-free fatty acid (FFA) levels and reduced carbohydrate utilization,[40-42] but studies measuring performance found no advantages for high fat meals and found gastric distress from delayed stomach emptying times during exercise.[43-45] Chronic high-fat, low carbohydrate (ketogenic) diets for 14 or 20 d found endurance was unchanged[46] or improved,[47] indicating that careful manipulation of diet and exercise may force muscles to adapt to ketone bodies as fuel. Other studies lasting less than a week found no advantages for high fat diets compared to moderate or low fat diets,[48-50] although one study with design flaws found enhanced endurance after a diet with 38% of calories from fat.[51]

These sketchy results from studies with short duration and low subject numbers seem to agree with many other studies on endurance performance and glycogen supercompensation.[19-23] However, no studies looked at anaerobic exercise, such as weightlifting. Unpublished data by DiPasquale (DiPasquale, M., *The Anabolic Diet* videotape, Optimum Training Systems, 1995) has claimed improvements in strength and muscle mass without body fat increase with a long-term ketogenic diet.

Medium chain triglycerides (MCTs), appear theoretically promising to enhance performance, since they possess different metabolic effects than LCTs. MCTs are metabolized similar to carbohydrates,[52] raise metabolic rate,[53] spare lean muscle mass,[54] and are not atherogenic.[55] Preliminary human studies have found that MCTs administered before and during long-term endurance exercise are oxidized at a rate similar to equicaloric glucose supplements,[56,57] but muscle glycogen is not spared.[58] One study measured performance (40-km cycle race time) after 2 hr of cycling at 60% of VO_2max after administration during exercise of drinks containing either 10% glucose, 4.3% MCTs, or 10% glucose plus 4.3% MCTs.[59] Race times were significantly slower (increased) after only MCT supplementation (72.13 ± 3.97 vs 66.75 ± 0.98 min for 10% glucose), but were significantly faster (decreased) after glucose + MCT (65.06 ± 1.31 vs 66.75 ± 0.98 min). These results suggest that acute administration of MCTs in absence of carbohydrate do not enhance endurance, but addition of MCTs to carbohydrate-containing beverages during long-term endurance exercise contributes an additional energy source, leading to improved performance.

Supplementation of 16 males with menhaden fish oil capsules plus salmon steaks for 10 weeks led to improvements in aerobic metabolism, although benefits were quantitatively less than aerobic exercise programs.[60] In a series of unpublished studies, omega-3 fatty acid supplementation was associated with increased muscular strength and improved aerobic performance for collegiate and professional football teams.[61] Postulated mechanisms of omega-3 fatty acids include enhancement of somatotropin release, vasodilator properties, erythrocyte flexibility, and anti-platelet aggregatory effects, mediated by changes in eicosanoid production.

A purified membrane phospholipid, phosphatidyl serine (PS), was shown to significantly diminish the increase in exercise-induced ACTH and cortisol in normal, healthy males after intravenous (50 or 75 mg)[62] or oral (80 mg/d for 10 d)[63] administration. These results may have potential application for reducing exercise-induced muscle catabolism from post-exercise cortisol release. In at least 23 double-blind studies, oral PS improved brain EEG and PET measurements, cognitive function, memory, and other mental functions in persons >65 years old.[64] Whether these results would be applicable to young, healthy athletes is unknown.

The other component of fat, glycerol, enhanced endurance in rats by preventing hypoglycemia.[65] Human studies did not find enhancement of exercise performance after administration of large amounts of glycerol in place of carbohydrate.[66-68] At a dose of 1 g/kg, glycerol delayed the decline in blood glucose after timed cycle ergometer or treadmill runs, suggesting that glycerol can be converted into glucose during exercise (a potentially beneficial situation).[66] Two patents showed that addition of glycerol to Gatorade™ lowered perceived levels of exertion, maintained blood volume, lowered pulse rate, and delayed the rise in body temperature during endurance work.[69,70]

Thus, dietary manipulation of fat as an ergogenic aid has had little research. Future areas of research include long-term adaptation to ketogenic diets, fat loading with adequate carbohydrate status, effect of MCTs in addition to carbohydrates during exercise, effects of omega-3 oils, and anaerobic exercise trials with MCT or omega-3 fatty acid supplementation.

E. OTHER FOODSTUFFS

Several foodstuffs have been used at one time or another as ergogenic aids. Such foods include beef liver, wheat germ oil, pollen, gelatin, and alcoholic beverages. Beef liver became popular before vitamin B_{12} was discovered, and its reputation as an anti-fatigue food has been slow to wither. There is no published evidence that beef liver supplementation enhances any type of physical performance.

Wheat germ oil was extensively studied by Cureton,[71] who found a few small improvements in endurance performance. These findings have not been confirmed. Bee pollen has enjoyed considerable use as an ergogenic aid. European studies[72] did find increased work capacity and improved metabolism in weightlifters.[73] However, five other studies have not found any benefits for physical performance after bee pollen administration, with doses ranging from unstated to 2700 mg daily.[73-77] Although no study was definitive, bee pollen does not appear to have consistent ergogenic properties.

Gelatin was thought to be a precursor for creatine in the 1940s, but a consensus of research found no benefits for many types of physical performance after gelatin administration.[78]

Ethanol is considered to be a drug or substance of abuse, and its presence in body fluids may cause disqualification in some athletic competitions. Ethanol has important and conflicting impacts on exercise performance. Small amounts can reduce psychological tension and insecurity, leading to increased self-confidence and improved physical performance via strictly psychological, not physiological, means.[79] Larger doses of alcohol, corresponding to blood levels of 0.040–0.075%, compromise motor performance, coordination, reaction times, and judgement, even though physiological parameters such as VO_2max, heart rate, or peak lactate levels generally show little or no changes. However, higher blood levels of ethanol (>0.10%) are considered legally intoxicating and possess detrimental physiological properties that definitely deteriorate physical performance. Furthermore, ethanol can increase dehydration and hypothermia in cold temperatures. Chronic, excess ethanol consumption can lead to excess caloric intake with associated body fat increase or displacement of nutrient-rich foods. Individual variations in response to ethanol ingestion are large. However, in general, one alcoholic drink per day is not associated with physical harm or performance deficits. One drink is defined as 12 oz (360 ml) of beer, 4 oz or 120 ml (one small glass) of wine, or 1 oz (30 ml) of hard liquor (100 proof).

III. MICRONUTRIENTS AS ERGOGENIC AIDS

A. AMINO ACIDS

Each amino acid has unique metabolic properties in human physiology, and many of these have been hypothesized to enhance or improve human exercise performance. This section will provide a brief overview of potential uses and clinical trials of amino acids.

Arginine and its metabolic relatives, ornithine and citrulline, are involved in several physiological areas of interest to athletes:

1. protein synthesis;
2. release of somatotropin, insulin, and prolactin;
3. creatine synthesis;
4. removal of ammonia;
5. polyamine synthesis; and
6. nitric oxide synthesis.

Both arginine and ornithine have been used to elicit a large release of somatotropin after intravenous administration of 15–30 g.[80] Somatotropin release after large oral doses of arginine or arginine salts has been observed.[81-84] Arginine pyroglutamate (L-arginine-2- pyrrolidone-5-carboxylate) combined with L-lysine hydrochloride (1200 mg each) increased somatotropin levels 2–8 times, doubled insulin levels, and tripled somatomedin A levels.[84] This study has been repeatedly misinterpreted as using arginine plus lysine. A mixture of arginine, ornithine, and lysine (2 g each/d) administered for 4 d to 11 weightlifters did not affect secretion of somatotropin or insulin throughout a 24 hr cycle.[85] Acute administration of 2.4 g of arginine plus lysine to 7 weightlifters increased serum somatotropin in 5 out of 7 subjects for a nonsignificant average of 2.8 times placebo levels.[86] Calculation of statistical power from the published results showed only a 20–40% chance of finding a difference, given the low subject number and large variability of results. As a control, the same subjects received 20 g of Bovril® (protein, amino acids, and carbohydrate), previously known to elicit a somatotropin response. Similar to arginine/lysine, 5 out of 7 subjects exhibited an increase in serum somatotropin levels. When 10 mM arginine was perifused to rat pancreatic islet cell preparations, resistance-trained animals exhibited double the insulin output of untrained animals.[87] Physically active college males were given 123 mg/kg/d (8–10 g total amino acids daily) of a 50:50 mixture of arginine and lysine for 10 weeks.[88] Supplementation had no effect on a glucose tolerance test or insulin-like growth factor-1 (IGF-1) levels. However, expected changes in glucose tolerance from resistance training were not seen, and coupled with low subject number (7–8 per group), results are suspect.

Administration of arginine aspartate and arginine glutamate reduced plasma ammonia after endurance exercise.[89,90] Arginine or a mixture of arginine, ornithine aspartate, and citrulline improved endurance exercise performance in rats.[91,92] A mixture of arginine and ornithine (1 g each daily) given to middle-aged males starting a 5 week weight training program led to increases in strength and lean body mass, with decreases in body mass, body fat, and urinary hydroxyproline.[93,94]

Similar to arginine, oral ornithine hydrochloride (170 mg/kg) led to 4-fold increases in serum somatotropin in 12 bodybuilders.[95] However, insulin levels were not affected,[96,97] and osmotic diarrhea was encountered at the dose of 170 mg/kg.[95] Lower doses of ornithine (70 or 100 mg/kg) did not significantly affect somatotropin levels. Acute administration of 1.1 g ornithine, 0.75 g tyrosine, 750 mg vitamin B_6, and 125 mg ascorbic acid to 7 weightlifters led to increases in serum somatotropin in 5 out of 7 subjects (3.3 times placebo levels).[86] The authors concluded that lack of statistical significance was evidence that oral ingestion of amino acids failed to elicit a somatotropin response. However, calculation of statistical power showed the trial exhibited only a 20–40% chance of finding a significant difference, given the large variability in results and low subject number.

The available research suggests that chronic administration of arginine, arginine-containing dipeptides, and/or ornithine may have ergogenic effects for resistance training.

Aspartate has many metabolic uses:

1. transport of minerals to subcellular sites;
2. precursor for the tricarboxylic acid cycle via oxaloacetate (cellular energy);
3. part of urea cycle (removal of ammonia);
4. resynthesis of ATP after depletion (via purine nucleotide cycle); and
5. possible brain antifatigue effects (as excitatory neurotransmitter).

Early reports implicated a medical use for potassium and magnesium L-aspartate salts (Spartase™) as antifatigue agents,[98,99] but this use was refuted since fatigue estimation was erroneously thought to be purely psychological.[100]

Aspartate salts appear to possess some ergogenic benefits when given in high doses (>7g) before endurance exercise.[101-105] Times to exhaustion during endurance exercise were increased 14–50%). Benefits appeared in untrained subjects at lower doses than trained subjects. DL-aspartate salts appeared to be more effective than L-aspartate salts. Studies that measured blood ammonia levels found trends toward decreased plasma ammonia levels after aspartate administration, consistent with known mechanisms. Other reports that did not find ergogenic benefits after aspartate supplementation usually administered lower doses (<7g) or L-aspartate salts (instead of DL-salts) than positive studies.[106-110] The conditions necessary to reproduce ergogenic effects of aspartates need further clarification.

Asparagine, a direct precursor of aspartate in muscle and brain[111-113] and a direct precursor for glutamine synthesis in muscles at rest and during exercise,[114,115] is decreased in plasma but increased in muscle during exhaustive exercise.[115,116] Supplementation of rats with 45 mg/kg each of asparagine and aspartate increased time to fatigue by 40% for endurance exercise.[113,116] Asparagine increased utilization of fatty acids, sparing muscle glycogen.[113,116] Asparagine is involved with magnesium metabolism intracellularly, possibly interacting with ATP stability.[117] Since intramuscular concentration of aspartate limits resynthesis of ATP after intense contractions in humans,[118] asparagine supplementation may represent an overlooked means to resist muscular fatigue by supplying aspartate and glutamine on demand (sparing glutamine).

Branched-chain amino acids (BCAA) leucine, isoleucine, and valine have been hypothesized to improve endurance exercise performance by preventing the rise of free (unbound) plasma tryptophan during exercise, which elevates brain serotonin and fatigue (central fatigue hypothesis).[119] Elevations of brain serotonin levels or effects do increase fatigue in humans,[119] but an increase in plasma free tryptophan/BCAA ratio appears intensity-dependent.[119-122] Supplementation with BCAA in a variety of doses (0.5 g/h to 21 g) to exercising humans has produced improvements in endurance performance,[123-126] physiological or hormone changes during exercise,[127-129] protection against muscle damage,[130,131] and lean body mass in triathletes.[129] Other studies with similar protocols and doses of BCAAs found no effects on exercise performance.[127,132-134] Ergogenic effects of BCAA supplementation are possible, although the mechanism does not appear to be related to the central fatigue hypothesis. It is still less expensive to extend performance by carbohydrate supplementation. BCAA supplementation during resistance training requires further exploration.

Glutamate is hypothesized to prevent fatigue by reduction of exercise-induced ammonia levels.[135-137] Compared to saline infusion, monosodium glutamate (MSG) infusion (9 g at

200 mg/min) to 6 healthy, untrained men decreased post-exercise blood ammonia levels by half, although lactate, pyruvate, urate, glucose, and urea values were unchanged.[138] Unfortunately, MSG infusion produced nausea in most subjects, making further studies of MSG as an ergogenic aid questionable. Also, incidence of toxicity from MSG (but not glutamic acid or glutamate dipeptides), known as the "Chinese Restaurant Syndrome," means that future research should explore other forms of glutamate, such as dipeptides like arginine-glutamate.

Glutamine is the most common amino acid in muscle and plasma, and is hypothesized to:

1. prevent lactate accumulation during exercise;
2. enhance muscle protein synthesis;
3. limit protein catabolism;
4. provide neurotransmitter precursors;
5. prevent decline in immune function from overtraining;
6. increase somatotropin;
7. increase muscle glycogen recovery;
8. remove ammonia during exercise; and
9. provide precursors for nucleotide synthesis.[24,139]

Overtraining or short periods of intense exercise depress plasma and muscle glutamine levels, possibly decreasing immune functions.[139,140] However, no correlation was found with plasma glutamine levels and incidence of upper respiratory infections in swimmers[141] and supplementation with 10 g of glutamine after a marathon race had little effects on immune system parameters.[142] Although glutamine supplementation (2 g/d) was found to significantly elevate plasma somatotropin and bicarbonate[143] and infusion of glutamine post-exercise stimulated muscle glycogen synthesis,[144] research on effects of supplemental glutamine for exercise performance or recovery has lagged far behind the application for surgery, trauma, burns, and injuries.[145]

During the 1940s, several reports on the ergogenic effects of glycine administration (5–12 g/d) found enhancement of exercise[146,147] or not.[148-150] However, results are suspect because of lack of experimental controls. At least large oral doses of glycine were well tolerated. Similar to arginine, ornithine, and glutamine, glycine has been shown to elicit increases in serum somatotropin after intravenous[151] and oral (6.75 or 30 g)[152,153] administration to normal subjects. However, these effects have not been examined in association with exercise or in athletes. Combined with alanine, glycine infusions did not enhance muscle glycogen synthesis after exercise.[144] Thus, research on glycine as an ergogenic aid is still incomplete but does not appear to have dramatic effects.

No differences in the physical performance test scores of "sub-par" college males were noted after consumption of placebo or 790 mg of L-lysine/d with a multiple vitamin.[154] Serum somatotropin levels were not affected by 1200 mg L-lysine, but were increased when lysine was co-administered with 1200 mg of arginine pyroglutamate.[84] When combined with arginine and/or ornithine, lysine did not affect glucose tolerance[88] and contributed variable effects on somatotropin release.[85,86] However, a rationale for continued study of lysine as an ergogenic aid is lacking.

Although several reports have found increased levels of serum somatotropin after oral tryptophan administration, side effects of drowsiness and mellow feelings were noted..[155-159] Total exercise time and total work load performed were greatly increased (49%) after supplementation with 1200 mg of L-tryptophan 24 hr before a treadmill test, compared to a placebo.[160] Ratings of perceived exertion were lowered, suggesting a possible effect on endogenous levels of endorphins/enkephalins, increasing pain tolerance and work performance. Tryptophan sales and distribution have been banned by the Food and Drug Administration (except for parenteral feeding solutions and protein fortification of neonatal formulas)

TABLE 4 Potential Ergogenic Effects in Humans after Oral Dosing with Single Amino Acids

Amino Acid	Daily Dose	Findings Related to Exercise	Ref.
Arginine, Arginine Aspartate or Glutamate	5 g, 250 mg/kg	↑ somatotropin and insulin release or response ↑ creatine stores ↓ exercise-induced blood ammonia	81–83,86,89,90
Arginine pyroglutamate/Lysine	1.2 g each	↑ somatotropin release	84
Arginine / Ornithine	1 g each	↑ body fat and weight loss during resistance training program	93,94
Aspartate Salts	7–10 g	↑ time to exhaustion, untrained subjects	98,99,101–105
Asparagine	3–6 g?	↑ time to exhaustion ?	113,116
Branched Chain Amino Acids (Leucine, Isoleucine, Valine)	5–10 g?	↑ time to exhaustion ↑ anabolic hormone release prevent lean body mass loss protect against muscle damage	123-131
Glutamine	2-6 g	↑ somatotropin release, bicarbonate ↑ muscle glycogen replenishment	143,144
Glycine	6-30 g	↑ somatotropin release ↑ muscular strength, creatine stores	146,147,151–153
Ornithine	170 mg/kg	↑ somatotropin release (diarrhea)	86,95
Tryptophan	>5 g	↑ somatotropin release ↑ work load and exercise time ↓ perception of pain and fatigue	155–160

since December 1989 after outbreaks of Eosinophilia Myalgia Syndrome (EMS) were related to tryptophan supplement consumption.[161-164] EMS cases were ultimately connected to ingestion of products manufactured by one Japanese manufacturer. Aniline dye and endotoxin contamination was the likely culprit, not tryptophan itself or tryptophan condensation products.[165] Research and use of tryptophan as an ergogenic aid is not feasible at this time.

In summary, single amino acids have effects on levels of endogenous hormones and some aspects of muscle physiology during exercise. After amino acid supplementation, practical effects of hormonal changes after amino acid supplementation are unknown, but some studies found improved performance. Table 4 lists some of the ergogenic properties of amino acids.

B. ANTIOXIDANTS

Exercise increases oxidative processes of muscles in an intensity-dependent manner, leading to adverse alterations in antioxidant status and increased generation of free radicals and their by-products in humans.[166-170] Free radicals have been observed to be intimately associated with fatigue during exercise.[166-170] Therefore, a rationale for antioxidant supplementation to prevent free radical damage to muscles and delay fatigue during exercise has been examined.

Antioxidants in human tissues and diets are listed in Table 5. More antioxidants are commercially available each year, especially from plant extracts. Study of antioxidants in exercise performance has not kept pace with the study of antioxidants in cardiovascular disease or cancer prevention. Thus, virtually all research to date has focused on the essential nutrient antioxidants ascorbate, tocopherol, and selenium to the exclusion of thiols, bioflavonoids, carotenoids, other plant phytochemicals, and synthetic antioxidants. Coenzyme Q_{10}

TABLE 5   Antioxidants in Human Tissues

Endogenous Production	Dietary Source
Bilirubin	Anthocyanidins, procyanidolic oligomers
Catalase	Ascorbic acid (Vitamin C)[a]
Coenzyme Q_{10} (Ubiquinone)	Beta carotene (pro-vitamin A)[a] and other carotenoids
Cysteine	N-acetyl-L-cysteine
Glutathione	Bioflavonoids
Glutathione peroxidase	Curcumin (from turmeric)
Histidine	Mannitol
Protein sulfhydryl groups	Methionine[a]
Superoxide dismutase	Plant phenolic acids (gallates, ferulates, ellagates, etc.)
Taurine	Polyphenols (tannins)
Urate	Synthetic antioxidants (BHA, BHT, TBHQ, ethoxyquin)
	Synthetic spin trappers (DMPO, PBN, POBN)
	Tocopherols (Vitamin E)[a]
	Zinc salts[a]

[a]   Essential (indispensable) nutrients.

Note: BHA, butylated hydroxyanisole; BHT, butylated hydroxytoluene; TBHQ, *tert*-butyl hydroquinone; DMPO, 5,5-dimethyl-1-pyrrolyn-*N*-oxide; PBN, *N-tert*-butyl-α-phenylnitrone; POBN, α-4-pyridyl-1-oxide-*N-tert*-butyl-nitrone.

will be considered independently since its primary function is bioenergetics in addition to antioxidant properties.

1.   Ascorbic Acid (Vitamin C)

Few nutrients have attracted as much scientific and popular attention as vitamin C. Widespread availability, popularity, use, and low cost has prompted numerous studies on human physical performance, with mostly contradictory results.

Supplementation with doses of vitamin C between 500 and 3000 mg/d either acutely or for periods of up to 3 weeks found no effects for sprint times, long-distance run times, grip strength, muscular strength, muscular endurance, anaerobic capacity, cycle ergometer workloads, Harvard step test, walk-run test time, oxygen utilization, respiratory quotient, ventilation parameters, heart rate, or post-exercise antioxidant capacity of serum or serum ammonia, lactate, and malondialdehyde (MDA) levels.[171-180]

Some of the studies just reported and similar studies using equivalent doses (500–3000 mg/d) and administration periods found improved efficiency of submaximal workloads, increased peak work capacity, increased muscular strength, and prevention of exercise-induced oxidation of blood glutathione. These studies also found decreased post-exercise lactate, heart rate, total energy cost of work, oxygen debt, oxygen consumption, pulmonary ventilation, blood glucose, and post-race upper respiratory tract infections.[171,175,179,181-184]

In summary, although some improvements in exercise physiology measurements have been found after vitamin C supplementation at doses ranging from 0.5–3.0 g/d, no improvements in performance times have been found. These doses appeared safe, with no side effects noted. Only one study[172] lasted longer than 3 weeks, and bowel tolerance doses (maximally tolerated doses) have not been approached nor studied. Thus, the ergogenic potential of vitamin C has not been adequately explored.

2.   Tocopherols (Vitamin E)

The biological functions of vitamin E are almost entirely due to its function as the major fat-soluble antioxidant.[166-170,185-189] Swim and run racing times, VO$_2$max, pulmonary function, muscular strength, ECG readings, postexercise blood lactate, postexercise serum creatine kinase (CPK) levels, and other physical tasks were not changed after vitamin E supplementation.[180,190-202] Doses of vitamin E ranged from 400–1600 IU/d, which are generally regarded as levels sufficient to benefit antioxidant status in humans. Other studies found vitamin E supplementation was associated with enhanced effects of aerobic training[203] and lower post-exercise blood lactate levels, breath pentane, blood lipid peroxides, leakage of muscle enzymes (including CPK), interleukin-1 (IL-1) and interleukin-6 (IL-6) production, post-exercise DNA damage in lymphocytes, and muscle conjugated dienes.[198,201,204-212] At high altitudes, evidence of free radical damage (blood rheological changes, elevated breath pentane) was completely reversed by 400 IU/d of vitamin E supplementation, along with improvements in oxygen utilization and physical performance.[213-216]

In summary, vitamin E administration has reproducibly decreased free radical damage induced by intense exercise, or by other conditions causing free radical production during exercise in humans (high altitude, ozone exposure). These findings may promote long-term health benefits in exercising individuals. At high altitudes, vitamin E prevents degradation of physical performance, while at sea level, vitamin E supplements do not appear to enhance performance. Effective doses of vitamin E appear to be 400–800 IU/d of either d-α-tocopherol (nature-identical form) or dl-α-tocopheryl esters (less expensive synthetic forms).

3. Selenium

Selenium is a component of glutathione peroxidase (GPx), an enzyme that utilizes glutathione to reduce peroxides.[168] Like vitamin E, selenium supplementation (100–240 mcg/d) to athletes improved antioxidant status and decreased oxidative damage after exercise,[217-222] but time to exhaustion on a treadmill was unchanged in the single study that examined performance.[222]

4. Other Antioxidants

Glutathione (GSH) supplementation (1 g/d) along with 2 g/d of vitamin C for 7 d decreased the oxidized glutathione (GSSG)/GSH ratio after exhaustive exercise, indicating an improvement in antioxidant status.[183] Animal studies with intraperitoneal administration of GSH found both improved endurance performance[223] and no change in performance.[224] Interestingly, carbohydrate supplementation during cycling exercise to fatigue at 70% VO$_2$max prevented the usual changes in blood GSH.[225] Other thiols (lipoic acid, cysteine, N-acetyl-L-cysteine) remain unstudied in human exercise trials.

Similar to vitamin E findings, when 15 untrained subjects were given BHT (20 mg/kg every 48 hr for 15 d), breath pentane was greatly decreased after exhaustive cycling.[226] Performance was not studied.

Several herbs containing phenolic antioxidants (bioflavonoid derivatives), such as green tea (*Camellia sinensis*), *Ginkgo biloba*, and Pycnogenol® have been shown to possess potent antioxidant activity *in vivo* in humans.[227-230] Effects on exercise performance remain untested.

5. Combinations of Antioxidants

The administration of combined (rather than single) antioxidants to humans in ergogenic studies reflects the dynamic interactions of endogenous antioxidants in the body. Seven studies administered a combination of beta carotene (10–45 mg/d), vitamin C (600–1250 mg/d), and vitamin E (300–1000 mg/d) for 4–8 wk to athletes engaged in endurance exercise.[231-236] Three studies found decreased oxidative damage post-exercise,[231,232,235] two did not,[233,234] and one did not find an effect on oxygen utilization or knee flexion/extension peak torque, work, or power.[236] One study found no effect on endurance times after supplementation with vitamin E (200 IU), coenzyme Q$_{10}$ (100 mg), inosine, and cytochrome c.[237] Another study found improved lymphocyte functions after long-term supplementation with vitamins C and E.[238] Combining results, it appears that combinations of antioxidants are capable of improving antioxidant status and reducing muscle and oxidative damage after exercise in athletes, but results on performance indicate that submaximal exercise performance is not improved.

In summary, antioxidant supplementation (singly or in combination) to athletes has been associated with reproducible improvements in antioxidant status and amelioration of indicators of oxidative damage induced by exercise. Submaximal exercise did not appear to produce enough of an oxidative stress for antioxidant supplementation to have an effect. Exercise to exhaustion or at high altitudes did seem to produce sufficient oxidative stress to allow some ergogenic benefits from single-nutrient antioxidant supplementation. Effects on exhaustive performance from a mixture of antioxidants remains to be studied.

C. HERBS

Herbs are defined in this chapter as plants or plant extracts ingested for perceived noncaloric benefits. Scientific investigation of possible ergogenic effects of herbs has not kept pace with widespread use of herbs since antiquity to enhance physical performance. Table 6 lists some herbs that are currently being ingested by athletes for purported enhancements of different aspects of exercise performance. Perhaps the best studied (and most used) herb is the ginseng family.

1. Ginsengs (American, Chinese, Korean, Siberian)

Ginseng supplementation is an ancient and revered custom in many Asian countries. Traditional use of ginseng centers around promoting vitality and prolonging life by restoring deficient Qi (life energy).[239] Chinese and Korean ginseng (*Panax ginseng*), American ginseng (*Panax quinquefolium*), and Siberian ginseng (*Eleutherococcus senticosus*) are available in a wide variety of forms, including root extracts standardized to known ginsenoside concentration. Growing conditions, age of the root, soil quality, and other agricultural and processing factors all affect ginsenoside identity and content, making comparison of studies difficult (this is true for herbs in general). A mechanism of glucocorticoid agonism/antagonism (encompassing fuel homeostasis during exercise) has been proposed for ginsenosides,[239-241] although other mechanisms are likely.

Table 7 lists ergogenic effects found or not found in *Panax* ginseng studies.[239-242] A time and dose-response effect is evident, as studies exhibiting ergogenic effects tended to use higher doses, standardized extracts, greater subject numbers, and longer durations. These parameters alone can account for much of the controversy surrounding ginseng ergogenicity. It must also be stressed that "modern" research has not duplicated traditional use, since no study has approached the traditional Chinese medicine daily doses of 3–9 g of root extract.[239] It can be concluded that long-term (>8 wk) supplementation with standardized *Panax ginseng* extracts (≥200 mg/d) has potential to improve aerobic capacity, strength, and mental functions or prevent their decline from overtraining, especially in older (>40 years) or untrained subjects.

Siberian ginseng has shown modest improvements in strength in one controlled trial,[242] and one study finding no effects on endurance performance reported a statistical power of 0.16–0.52.[243] Thus, limited research on Siberian ginseng has found conflicting results on human exercise performance.

Ginseng safety is well-documented by toxicology studies and thousands of years of use by millions of people, many elderly or infirm.[239-241] A ginseng abuse syndrome (nervousness, sleeplessness, hypertension) was reported in 1979,[239-241] but subjects also were consuming very large doses of caffeine, which could easily account for the observed symptoms. Of more concern are possible estrogenic activities of ginseng, which have been observed in a few cases.[239-241] Spontaneous vaginal bleeding, insomnia, irritability, dizziness, chest discomfort, and depression are traditional signs of ginseng overdose, and red ginseng is not indicated for pregnant women.[239]

2. Ephedra (Ma Huang)

The herb Chinese Ephedra (*Ephedra sinensis*) and other ephedra species contain a mixture of closely related alkaloids (ephedrine, pseudoephedrine, norephedrine, pseudonorephedrine,

TABLE 6 Herbs and Physical Performance, Current Status of Uses, Mechanisms, and Effects

Herb	Uses[a]	Mechanisms[b]	Effects[c]
Ginseng (Chinese, Korean, red, white, Ren shen), (*Panax ginseng*); American (*P. quinquefolium*)	enhance endurance exercise antifatigue enhance anabolism improve immune function	corticosteroid interactions alter fuel homeostasis alter mental functions (supported)	mixed; dose-response effect evident improved mental functions
Siberian Ginseng, Ciwujia (*Eleutherococcus senticosus*)	enhance endurance exercise antifatigue improve immune function	adaptogenic[d] (hypothetical)	no effects on exercise performance in few controlled studies
Ma Huang, Chinese Ephedra (*Ephedra sinensis*)	weight loss enhance endurance exercise bronchodilator antihistamine mental stimulant	sympathomimetic stimulant increases mental functions (supported)	no effects on exercise performance stimulates mental functions ↑ heart rate, blood pressure ↑ weight loss with caffeine
Rhodiola crenulata	enhance endurance exercise	adaptogenic (similar to ginseng) (hypothetical)	one study found faster run times
Yohimbe (*Pausinystalia johimbe*)	stimulant anabolic steroid alternative	α-adrenergic agonist (supported)	NA
Shilajit (Mummio) rock exudate of juniper berries	enhance endurance exercise	adaptogenic anabolic (hypothetical)	NA
Wild Oats (*Avena sativa*) sometimes combined with Stinging Nettle (*Urticaria dioica*)	anabolic	↑ testosterone (hypothetical)	one study found increased serum testosterone in men; no studies with exercise
Smilax (*Smilax officinalis*)	anabolic	testosterone precursor (hypothetical)	NA, no evidence to show conversion to testosterone in body
Ecdysterone (insect molting hormone)	anabolic	testosterone precursor (hypothetical)	NA, no evidence to show conversion to testosterone in body; possible interaction with steroid receptors
Muira Puama (Potency wood)	anabolic	unknown	traditional use for male fertility; NA
Suma (*Pfaffia paniculata*)	anabolic	ecdysterone source (hypothetical)	traditional use for male fertility; NA
Tribestan (*Tribulus terrestris*)	anabolic	testosterone mimic (hypothetical)	one report of increased sperm count in rams
Saw Palmetto berries (*Serrenoa repens*)	anabolic	testosterone metabolism enhancer (hypothetical)	NA; useful in benign prostatic hypertrophy
Truffles	anabolic	testosterone precursor (hypothetical)	contain androst-16-en-3-ol (no anabolic or androgenic activity)
Beta Sitosterol and other sterols (found in many plant foods)	anabolic	testosterone precursor (hypothetical)	NA; phytoestrogenic properties found would be counterproductive to anabolism

TABLE 6　Herbs and Physical Performance, Current Status of Uses, Mechanisms, and Effects *(continued)*

Herb	Uses[a]	Mechanisms[b]	Effects[c]
Cordyceps fungus (*Cordyceps sinensis*)	anabolic enhance endurance exercise	adaptogen (hypothetical)	NA; nonspecific immune stimulant evidence *in vitro*

[a]　Uses refer to intended, perceived, or advertised benefits for improving some aspect of athletic performance, including muscle hypertrophy as anabolic steroid alternatives.

[b]　Mechanisms may be hypothetical or be supported by research evidence as indicated. See text for details.

[c]　Effects in humans are briefly reviewed. NA = Not Available (no controlled studies yet exist to support or deny hypothetical mechanisms or ergogenic effects). See text for further details.

[d]　Adaptogenic refers to an ability to normalize homeostasis, producing a non-specific amelioration to various stressors. Multiple mechanisms may account for hypothetical anti-stress effects, and in general, adaptogens exhibit little, if any, effects in normal or insufficiently stressed subjects.

and others) that are potent sympathomimetic agents, simulating epinephrine effects.[244] Although ephedrine alkaloids have not been associated with enhancements in performance or physiological parameters during exercise,[241] mental functions are clearly stimulated.[241,244] Heart rate and blood pressure may be elevated.[241,244] Ephedrine and caffeine combinations (with or without aspirin) are well-documented to enhance weight loss effects of diet and exercise,[241,245] which is a growing reason for use among exercising adults.

Ephedrine alkaloids are also common in many over-the-counter and prescription medications (antihistamines, decongestants, and antiasthmatics). Presence of ephedrine alkaloids in herbal products, over-the-counter, and prescription medications will cause disqualification in sporting events that are tested for drugs, since ephedrine and related alkaloids are banned by many sports governing agencies. Occasionally, herbal "energy" products will contain undisclosed ephedrine, an illegal practice which may disqualify an unaware athlete.

Ephedrine has potential for abuse and adverse side effects (anxiety, nervousness, light-headedness, heart palpitations, rapid heart rate, elevation of blood pressure, interference with monoamine oxidase inhibitor drugs, hyperthermia, and death).[244] In 1996, products labeled as dietary supplements containing very high levels of ephedrine, caffeine, and other stimulants marketed outside usual outlets as "legal highs" to young adults have been associated with severe adverse side effects and at least one death. These cases can likely be attributed to overdoses of combinations of stimulants (not simply ephedrine itself) and also to excessive consumption by users to achieve more of a high. Doses of 24 mg of ephedrine alkaloids daily have been proven generally safe in many clinical trials, as echoed by centuries of use in traditional Chinese medicine for lung ailments.[241,244] Doses higher than 25 mg daily may

TABLE 7　Ergogenic Properties of Ginseng (*Panax ginseng*) in Humans[239-242,476]

Increased run time to exhaustion (3 out of 7 studies)
Increased muscle strength (1 out of 2 studies)
Increased work load (1 study)
Decreased rating of perceived exertion (1 out of 3 studies)
Improved recovery from exercise (3 out of 4 studies)
Improved oxygen metabolism during exercise (7 out of 9 studies)
Improved aerobic capacity (8 out of 9 studies)
Reduced exercise-induced lactate (5 out of 9 studies)
Reduced exercise heart rate (6 out of 8 studies)
Improved auditory and visual reaction times (6 out of 7 studies)
Improved mental concentration (5 out of 9 studies)
Improved vitality and feelings of well-being (6 out of 9 studies)
Improved visual/motor coordination (2 out of 3 studies)
Improved mental accuracy (2 out of 3 studies)

produce adverse side effects, especially when combined with other stimulants and alcohol. Most legitimate dietary supplements not marketed specifically to young adults contain less than 24 mg of ephedrine alkaloids and should state so on labels.

3.   Other Herbs

Table 6 lists uses and known effects of herbs currently marketed for sports. Except for one controlled human study with *Rhodiola crenulata*, an herb similar to ginseng, there has been no study of ergogenic effects from herbs. VO$_2$max and work capacity were significantly improved after ingestion of 1.5 g/d for 75 d of *Rhodiola crenulata* compared to a placebo group.[246] One unexplored facet is the ability of herbs rich in antioxidants (*Ginkgo biloba*, Milk thistle, Pycnogenol®, grape seed extract, green tea) to affect exercise performance or recovery, similar to other antioxidants.[227-230]

In summary, long periods of ingestion of standardized *Panax ginseng* but not Siberian ginseng supplements have been associated with improved physical and mental performance. Ephedrine-containing products may aid in weight loss and enhance mental functions but do not enhance exercise performance by physiological means. Care must be taken when choosing and using ephedrine-containing products (both supplements and drugs) due to potential for side effects and disqualification in drug testing. Other herbs are virtually untested, especially hypothetical anabolic contenders.

4.   Substances Isolated from Plants

Several compounds have been isolated from plants and used as ergogenic aids that do not fit amino acid, antioxidant, or metabolite categories. Aspirin (acetyl salicylic acid) is derived from salicylic acid, found in a few plant species such as white willow bark (*Salix alba*). When combined with ephedrine and caffeine, aspirin has been used successfully as a weight loss aid (2.2 kg weight loss vs 0.7 kg weight loss for placebo without caloric restriction).[241,245]

a.   *Caffeine*

The best-studied plant product on exercise performance is caffeine, a methylxanthine found in coffee, tea, guarana, kola nut, chocolate, and synthesized for addition to soft drinks and over-the-counter medications. Presently, there is less of a question of caffeine having ergogenic effects than under what conditions the effects are manifest. A preponderance of studies have examined the metabolic and physiologic effects of caffeine rather than performance effects. Nevertheless, because of the large amount of literature concerning exercise and caffeine, this will be a review of reviews.

Does caffeine enhance exercise performance, and if so, under what conditions? A careful perusal of 10 recent reviews on caffeine and exercise performance has found 39 studies showing an ergogenic effect and 35 studies not finding an ergogenic effect.[24,78,247-254] Ergogenic effects were seen for endurance exercise performance (cross-country ski races, run times to exhaustion, cycle times to exhaustion, swim times to exhaustion, work capacity, work output), strength, sprints, repetitive anaerobic work, shooting precision, reaction time, and perception of fatigue. Contrarily, other studies did not find enhancements of performance by caffeine for similar events. Some studies noted a large individual variation, which may help to explain performance results. Indeed, some studies divided subjects into caffeine responders and non-responders.

Factors raising likelihood of caffeine enhancing performance include: abstaining from caffeine ingestion for 2–4 d before an event, and ingesting caffeine 3–4 hr before an event. Conclusions of earlier reviews that noted differences between trained and untrained subjects or gender differences have been superseded by later studies. Many studies discussed in the reviews cited in the previous paragraph have attempted to find metabolic or physiologic mechanisms for caffeine effects, and findings are contradictory. Only recently have attempts been made to ascertain the neurological or psychological effects of caffeine, and a consensus has been reached that caffeine does attenuate perception of fatigue regardless of fuel homeostasis or lactate levels. This may mean that caffeine's main effect is mental rather than physiological. In other words, caffeine may induce a positive placebo response in excess of a normal placebo response. This is very likely, given the widespread use of caffeine-containing beverages as a stimulant.

Another ergogenic use for caffeine is in combination with ephedrine and/or aspirin as an aid to body fat loss at doses of 200 mg/d.[241,245] Several reviews have suggested that combining caffeine with exercise may enhance body fat loss, but definitive guidelines for most effective use remain to be determined.[24,78,247-254]

Caffeine safety must be addressed, although almost universal experience means most subjects have already determined personal limits for safe use. Nevertheless, a potential for side effects from excess and chronic consumption of caffeine exists, and symptoms consist of nervousness, anxiety, insomnia, shaking of hands, and hyperkinesis[24,78] Very large doses (more than 10 mg/kg) may produce gastric upset, arrhythmias, and memory impairment, while even larger doses may produce hallucinations and delirium.[24,78] Diuretic properties of caffeine have been shown to be minor and insignificant at doses normally used for enhancement of performance.[254]

Caffeine in levels of more than 15 mcg/ml in urine is unacceptable for many sports governing agencies and will disqualify athletes. This level can be reached with doses of 9–10 mg/kg. Thus, care must be taken by athletes undergoing drug testing not to consume excessive amounts of caffeine before an event.

In summary, a wealth of data from humans confirms that caffeine at doses of 3–6 mg/kg may enhance almost any type of exercise performance. However, results are highly variable between individuals, and prediction of who will be responders is still unclear. Certainly, central nervous stimulation by caffeine may help performance regardless of alteration of metabolic substrates. In general, effectiveness of caffeine is accentuated by abstinence for 4 d, and ingestion 3–4 hr before an event. More research is needed on chronic use to assist body fat loss, and research on typical weightlifting or bodybuilding exercises is almost completely lacking. Widespread social acceptance, low cost, relative lack of side effects, universal availability, and positive research studies make caffeine an important ergogenic aid.

b. Ferulates (Gamma Oryzanol)

Ferulic acid is a ubiquitous plant phenolic with antioxidant properties and interactions with hypothalamic neurotransmitters due to structural similarity with normetanephrine.[255] Intravenous administration of ferulic acid to heifers was associated with increased serum somatotropin.[256] Body weight and one-repetition maximum strength were significantly increased in supplemented weightlifters (30 mg/d for 8 wk) compared to a placebo group.[257] Similar doses augmented postexercise serum beta endorphin levels, but not cortisol or testosterone, suggesting a possible enhancement of recovery from strenuous exercise.[258]

Gamma oryzanol is a combination of ferulate esters with sterols found in rice bran with antioxidant activity.[255] Like other sterols, gamma oryzanol was erroneously believed to have testosterone-like effects by virtue of its structure, but there is no evidence to indicate this is true.[259] Any possible effects from gamma oryzanol would be due to presence of ferulate.

c. Octacosanol

Octacosanol is a long-chain (C_{28}) waxy alcohol found in most plants, especially wheat germ oil. Cureton reported improvements in endurance and reaction times,[71] which were not replicated by other researchers until McNaughton reported improvements in reaction time and grip strength but not aerobic endurance performance after 1000 mcg/d of octacosanol for 8 wk.[260] Thus, suggestive evidence exists that octacosanol may be ergogenic for skill sports.

D. INTERMEDIARY METABOLITES

Non-vitamin compounds present in human cells (and most foods) represent a growing area of research as ergogenic aids. Examples include a diverse array of compounds such as bicarbonate, citrate, creatine, nucleotides, organic acids, carnitine, and coenzyme Q_{10}. These substances are not legally classified as essential nutrients since they are synthesized by the body, but they are essential for cellular function.

1. Alkalinizers (Buffering Agents)

a. *Bicarbonate*

The large number of studies concerning exercise performance and sodium bicarbonate necessitates a review of reviews, similar to the section on caffeine. Bicarbonate is the chief buffering system of the human body.[261] Acidosis (increased hydrogen ion concentration) is produced by exhaustive exercise, especially when lactate is formed during anaerobic muscular metabolism.[261] Research efforts have focused on increasing cellular and blood buffer capacity, in an effort to delay fatigue by delaying the decrease in pH caused by anaerobic exercise. In general, administration of bicarbonate in doses of 0.3–0.5 g/kg have consistently increased alkaline reserves of exercising subjects.[24,247,262-266]

Scrutiny of reviews and studies published since 1994 have revealed at least 46 studies showing enhancements of exercise performance and at least 37 studies showing no enhancement.[24,247,262-273] No studies found decreases in exercise performance. Doses of 0.3 g/kg or higher taken 2–3 hr before an event were required for reproducible ergogenic effects, which are limited to certain conditions. Any *exhaustive* exercise lasting 1–7 min, maximal effort races (sprints, 200 m, 400 m, 800 m, and 1500 m), and repetitive, short-term, maximal anaerobic exercise bouts all showed enhancements of performance by an average of 22% over placebo groups.[264] Cycling, running, swimming, rowing, and weightlifting are examples of exercise performance that has shown benefits after sodium bicarbonate ingestion.

Conditions where bicarbonate may not show ergogenic benefits are single-repetition maximal exercises and long-term endurance exercise (>3000 m). Many studies with similar study design, dosage, and performance measurements to positive studies did not find significant ergogenic effects.[24,247,262-266] However, few studies found no effects at all, and many studies found nonsignificant improvements in exercise performance on the order of magnitude of up to 20%. Given the low subject number in most studies with no effects, it is possible that statistical power was low and an ergogenic effect missed. Recently, a few studies have compared sodium bicarbonate to equimolar amounts of sodium as sodium chloride and have found that sodium itself may exert some of the ergogenic effects attributed to bicarbonate buffering.

Bicarbonate loading has generally been tolerated, even though doses of 14–21 g of baking soda for a 70 kg person are ingested. Some subjects experience nausea, bloating, intestinal cramping, and diarrhea at doses of more than 0.3 g/kg. Large volumes of water must be consumed to prevent possible osmotic diarrhea, and hypertensive persons sensitive to salt intake should consult their physician before attempting bicarbonate loading. It is also recommended to try bicarbonate loading during training, instead of an important event, in case intolerance results.

In summary, sodium bicarbonate loading (0.3–0.5 g/kg) taken 1–3 hr before an intense, short-term, anaerobic exercise event may enhance exercise performance, as supported by many positive outcome studies. This practice appears more suited to occasional use rather than daily dosing. There is no literature on chronic use of bicarbonate loading, and rationale for frequent, chronic use appears risky. Bicarbonate is widely available and very inexpensive, similar to caffeine.

b. *Citrate*

Although more appropriately classified as an organic acid, sodium citrate supplementation has also been studied for buffering effects.[266] Like bicarbonate, doses of sodium citrate

(0.3–0.5 g/kg) have usually improved alkaline reserve of blood in exercising individuals.[266] Like bicarbonate, some studies were plagued by low statistical power due to low subject number, which may have accounted for increases in performance being measurable but not statistically significant.[269,274-277] Other studies did find statistically significant improvements in performance of anaerobic and aerobic tasks, including ratings of perceived exertion, cycle sprints lasting longer than 120 s, and 30 km cycle times.[277-281] Citrate at doses of 0.5 g/kg taken may possess ergogenic properties for exercise, but further research with larger subject numbers to ensure adequate statistical power are needed before firm conclusions can be drawn. Citrate appeared to be much better tolerated than bicarbonate at high doses, which further argues for additional research on citrate. Like bicarbonate and caffeine, citrate is inexpensive because of widespread use as food flavorings and preservatives.

Hydroxycitrate, found in high levels in *Garcinia cambogia* fruit from India, has been well-documented to inhibit citrate lyase.[282] Such inhibition has been theorized to promote gluconeogenesis during exercise,[282] which may be ergogenic for long-term endurance exercise. Hydroxycitrate has been studied as a weight-loss aid in humans with some success,[283,284] suggesting a potential role in enhancing body fat loss in conjunction with exercise.

Other alkalinizers (such as Tris) have not had sufficient study to assess their ergogenic effects or safety.

In summary, alkalinizing agents have been well-studied as ergogenic aids, and at high doses (>0.3 g/kg 2 h before an event), can improve acid/base balance, and often, improve exercise performance of short-term, repetitive, exhaustive exercise.

2.   Carnitine

L-Carnitine's major role is to facilitate entry of long-chain fatty acids into mitochondria for subsequent oxidation and energy production.[24,169,262,285-289] Other metabolic roles in energy and lipid metabolism exist for carnitine, and these may have additional impacts on exercise as yet uncharacterized. A scan of recent reviews and articles for results of carnitine supplementation on human physical performance has found seven studies showing enhancement and five showing no effect.[24,169,262,285-289] A large number of carnitine supplementation studies have focused on measuring metabolic or physiological variables such as carnitine, lactate, pH, and fatty acid levels, or lipid utilization.[24,169,262,285-289] These studies show that carnitine supplementation elevates plasma carnitine but only with difficulty raises muscle carnitine levels, if at all. Likewise, ability of carnitine supplements to affect lactate or lipid metabolism during exercise has been controversial. At present, the major hypothetical mechanism of action for carnitine (facilitating lipid utilization) is still not conclusively proven.

Other mechanisms for ergogenic effects seen after acute administration of carnitine (which is difficult to rationalize on the basis of muscular lipid metabolism because of limited uptake into muscle) may include oxidation of fatty acids in vascular endothelial cells rather than muscle cells[290] or reduction of free radical damage from exercise (an apparent antioxidant effect).[291] Possible effects on coordination and mental processes may also be another putative mechanism.[292] Of potential interest to strength athletes is the ability of acetyl-L-carnitine supplements to increase plasma testosterone of male rats.[293]

Considerable agreement has been reached on ergogenic effects of L-carnitine, acetyl-L-carnitine, or propionyl-L-carnitine supplementation for patients with cardiovascular disease (congestive heart failure, angina), respiratory diseases, and kidney failure (hemodialysis).[24,262,286,289] These results mean that many patients who would otherwise not exercise may be able to enjoy health benefits from an exercise program.

Even long-term supplementation with L-carnitine or L-carnitine esters has been free of adverse side effects. However, DL-carnitine may be toxic and should be avoided.

In summary, much less information on carnitine's effect on exercise performance is available than would be suspected from the prodigious literature base on carnitine. There is enough positive evidence to suggest carnitine may have ergogenic effects, but conflicting information for timing and length of administration, dosage, form (acetyl- and propionyl-carnitine esters may have larger effects than L-carnitine), metabolic effects, training status of subjects, and unclear mechanisms, render the ergogenic ability of carnitine as undecided. Perhaps carnitine may be useful in overtrained athletes, who have the potential for reduced muscle levels of carnitine.

3. Coenzyme Q$_{10}$ (Ubiquinone)

A lipophilic quinone, coenzyme Q$_{10}$ (ubiquinone) is obligatory for production of ATP by oxidative phosphorylation in mitochondria and is also a potent antioxidant.[24,262] A large amount of human clinical evidence has been published, especially for cardiovascular disease treatment, showing proper doses for affecting mitochondrial functions and also showing almost complete safety.[262] Production of ATP is obviously important for both long-term endurance performance and anaerobic exercises, and the finding that normal mitochondrial ubiquinone levels are insufficient to saturate energy-producing enzymes[294] gives valid rationale for supplementation.

Doses of 60–100 mg/d for 4–8 wk (6 months in one study) have been administered in every study examining the effect of ubiquinone on exercise to date.[24,262,295-308] Six studies found significant enhancements of exercise performance (time to exhaustion for treadmill runs or cycling, total work capacity, anaerobic capacity),[295-300] and one study found an increased perception of vigor,[307] suggesting psychological components may play a role in ubiquinone ergogenicity. Twelve studies found enhancements of metabolic or physiologic variables associated with aerobic energy production and greater generation of ATP (increased VO$_2$max, improved cardiac functions, increased lipid utilization, decreased serum free fatty acids, decreased release of creatine kinase and lactate dehydrogenase enzymes after exercise, decreased ammonia/lactate ratio, and decreased muscle soreness).[295-304] Other studies found no enhancements of exercise performance (forearm strength, cycle ergometry time to exhaustion)[237,305,306] or no enhancements of metabolic or physiologic variables during exercise (VO$_2$max, ratings of perceived exertion, lactate, glucose, free fatty acids, or lipid peroxide levels).[237,305-307] One study found a nonsignificant increase (because of high interindividual variability) in time to exhaustion of 8% for 12 subjects, mostly from one subject who almost doubled his endurance time.[237] This amounted to a chance of finding a significant difference (statistical power) of less than 10%. All studies suffered from low subject numbers, which would tend to make negative results due to low statistical power less conclusive than positive studies.

Similar to carnitine, ubiquinone supplementation to subjects with cardiovascular diseases, angina, or congestive heart failure has generally shown improvements in exercise performance, exercise tolerance, peak work capacity, and cardiac function.[24,262]

In summary, ubiquinone, in doses of 100 mg/d for longer than 4 wk, has been associated with enhancements in maximal exercise performance after aerobic endurance exercise (running or cycling) in both trained and untrained individuals. Further research on ergogenic effects of ubiquinone for other types of exercise and actual field tests is warranted, given the positive results to date, known safety, and known pharmacokinetics.

4. Creatine

Even though the importance of creatine for muscle metabolism has been known for most of this century; until 1993, the only published reports on creatine supplementation were from Beard[146] in 1943, which found no consistent enhancements of aerobic exercise with doses and study design now known to be ineffective. In the short span since 1992, an explosion of studies on creatine supplementation and exercise performance has occurred, with three comprehensive reviews.[308-310] At this date, creatine represents a success story of determining optimal dosage and demonstrating metabolic mechanisms before moving to measurements of performance that would be most likely to show ergogenic effects.

Creatine is found in large amounts in skeletal muscle and nerves, where about 60% is phosphocreatine, a high-energy compound.[308] During short term muscular contractions, phosphocreatine restores rapidly diminishing ATP levels before glycolysis can take over by transferring its phosphate group to ADP via creatine kinase, delaying muscular fatigue.[308-310] However, this restoration is limited and is only applicable to short-term, intense exercise.

Several dose-response studies found that maximal saturation of human skeletal muscle can be obtained by oral administration of 5 g of creatine monohydrate 4 times daily (20 g/d) for 5 d.[308-310] Muscle levels of creatine average 125 mmol/kg dry weight, and saturation occurs at 150–160 mmol/kg dry weight.[310] Similar muscle levels of creatine can be reached after 30 d of 3 g/d creatine administration.[308] Submaximal exercise, insulin, and simultaneous carbohydrate intake all appear to optimize creatine uptake into muscle and improve percentage of responders (Greenhaff, P.L., unpublished data presented at NIH Conference on Dietary Supplements for Physically Active People, June 1996, Bethesda, MD).[308-310] Once in muscle, creatine levels remain elevated for several weeks after cessation of supplementation, which has serious implications for crossover studies and training effects. The optimal administration of creatine appears to be 5 g taken 4 times daily for 5 d, followed by a single 2 g daily dose indefinitely.

Twelve studies have reported significant improvements of short-term, intense exercise performance (improved power, force, torque, strength; maximum lift, work, times to exhaustion for repetitive cycle sprints, 300 m and 1000 m run times).[308-322] Six studies did not find improvements in similar exercises (cycle sprints; 60-m sprint velocity; 25-, 50-, 100-m swim times; bench press and squat power), but one study[323] had a lower dose.[323-328] Consistent with known mechanisms, creatine supplementation did not enhance long-term endurance performance (9-km roller skate time; 6-km cross-country run time).[329,330] A consensus from the available research indicates creatine supplementation benefits repetitive, short-term, exhaustive, anaerobic exercise performance instead of a single maximal event. Also, creatine enhances strength in weightlifters. Longer times of administration were more likely to produce significant results.

Creatine supplementation also leads to gains in body mass of about 1–2 kg, mostly as lean body mass.[308-310,322] This weight is thought to be intramuscular water, but creatine supplementation can also improve muscle protein synthesis.[308-310] Persons with gyrate atrophy of the retina (impaired creatine synthesis) exhibited weight gains and muscular hypertrophy of Type II fibers after long-term administration (1–5 years) of 1.5 g/d of creatine monohydrate.[331,332] Likewise, creatine supplementation after leg fractures[333] or knee surgery[334] improved recovery of leg muscle mass and strength. Whether long-term creatine supplementation with resistance training would lead to greater gains in strength and muscular hypertrophy in normal, healthy athletes is untested. Vegetarians seem to have less creatine stores and have benefited more than meat-eaters.[308-310]

In summary, creatine has catapulted in the space of a few years from obscurity into a premier position as a well-supported dietary supplement known to enhance muscular strength and size, in addition to enhanced performance in explosive sporting events. Apparent lack of toxicity at doses listed in this section mean that weightlifters now have a viable alternative to anabolic steroids to enhance strength and muscle mass.

5.   Methyl Donors

A neglected area of cellular metabolism is the methyl (one carbon) donor pathways. For example, the primary methyl donor in all cells, S-adenosylmethionine (SAM), participates in more reactions than any other compound except ATP itself.[335] Many compounds just mentioned (carnitine, creatine, nucleotides) require a methyl group for synthesis. Since SAM is unstable and commercially difficult and expensive to procure, other methyl donors have been used in an attempt to enhance exercise performance. Keep in mind that folate and vitamin B_{12} are intimately involved in methyl group metabolism.

a.   Dimethylglycine (DMG) or Pangamic Acid

After gaining cult status among runners in the 1960s based on rumors of Soviet use, three reports showing ergogenic effects of DMG were published.[336-338] Five well-controlled studies found no ergogenic effects from DMG in maximal or submaximal exercises after daily doses of 100–200 mg daily.[339-344] Thus, ergogenic effects of DMG for endurance exercise are not apparent.

b.   Choline and Lecithin (Phosphatidyl Choline)

Choline is an essential nutrient for humans and is present in the free form, as acetylcholine (a neurotransmitter), and as a component of phospholipids as phosphatidylcholine.[169] Choline has developed a reputation with consumers as a lipotropic, based on dietary depletion studies in rodents, although no evidence exists in humans that choline supplementation can reduce fatty liver or body fat. Interest in choline as an ergogenic aid was stimulated by reports of large declines in plasma choline levels after marathon races.[345,346] A recent presentation reviewed five studies on choline supplementation and human exercise performance.[347] Choline supplementation (1 g/d) attenuated the decline in serum choline during intense or long-term exercise, and by so doing, could improve 20-km run[348] and swim times.[347] In other trials, choline supplementation improved mood but not exercise performance (vertical leap, basketball shooting performance, treadmill run with loaded backpack, cycle ergometry) when serum levels did not change after exercise.[347,349] Choline supplementation (0.2 mmol/kg) to healthy adults appeared to promote conservation of L-carnitine (reduced urinary excretion) after L-carnitine supplementation.[350]

Early studies on large doses of lecithin (17–35% phosphatidyl choline) found no ergogenic effects.[262] Lecithin supplementation (0.2 g/kg of 90% phosphatidyl choline 1 h before exercise) prevented the decline in plasma choline after long-term cycling or running.[351] Thus, lecithin may be used to raise plasma choline levels.

In summary, choline supplementation appears ergogenic both for physical and mental performance in cases where depletion of serum levels by exercise is expected (long-term endurance events lasting >1.5 h). When choline levels are not affected by exercise, no apparent ergogenic effects from supplementation are likely. Choline effects may go beyond methyl donor possibilities and include interactions with carnitine, neurotransmitters, and/or cell membrane effects.

6.   Nucleotides (Inosine)

DNA and RNA precursors and their metabolites (including adenine, guanine, cytosine, thymidine, uracil, orotate, inosine, xanthine, hypoxanthine, uric acid, and phosphorylated species) help replenish or prevent decline of ATP levels during high-intensity exercise, protect ischemic tissues, promote angiogenesis, or improve oxygen utilization in erythrocytes.[262,352] However, human supplementation trials published in peer-reviewed journals have not found ergogenic effects after inosine supplementation.[237,353] Three-mile treadmill run times, time to exhaustion during VO_2peak testing, VO_2peak,[353] and time to exhaustion after a combined treadmill/cycle exercise[237] were not affected or worsened.

Increased intake of purine nucleotides may increase serum uric acid.[262,352] Also, inosine elevation in serum is a marker for ischemia, including after intense exercise.[262,352] Enhancement of xanthine oxidase activity (which generates superoxide free radicals while producing uric acid) by excess inosine is a possibility,[262] which has experimental support since an ergolytic effect of inosine supplementation (6 g/d for 2 d) was seen for endurance exercise.[353]

Although commercial use of nucleotides is increasing in infant formulas and hospital clinical nutrition settings[354] and medical uses in cardiovascular disease and geriatrics have been studied in Europe,[262] more data on composition, dose, duration of supplementation, and safety is needed before ergogenicity of nucleotides can be studied in a logical manner.

7.   Organic Acids (Lactate, Pyruvate, Hydroxybutyrates, Tricarboxylic Acid Cycle Intermediates, Ketoacids of Amino Acids)

In spite of common occurrence in energy production pathways of all cells, very little research has been devoted to studying possible ergogenic effects of organic acid supplementation. Citrate has already been discussed previously as a buffering agent, but its contribution to energy production in such studies has not been emphasized. Organic acids are desired by athlete consumers for two reasons: (1) enhancement of endurance by increased flux of muscular energy production and glycogen sparing; or (2) enhancement of muscular strength or hypertrophy via sparing of muscle protein by ketoacid analogues of amino acids.

a.   Lactate and Polylactate

Increased removal of lactate produced by intense exercise has been hypothesized to delay fatigue, since lactate accumulation with resulting decrease in pH is considered one cause of muscular fatigue. Perhaps chronic feeding of lactate would induce additional enzyme activity to remove lactate, or lactate itself would provide a fuel for energy production or gluconeogenesis, which may ultimately delay fatigue during exercise.

Acute administration of 250 ml of 7% polylactate/lactate liquid before and during long-term cycle ergometry maintained blood glucose better than placebo and as effectively as equivalent glucose polymer administration.[355] Polylactate increased pH more than glucose polymers or placebo. Adding polylactate to a glucose polymer liquid and consuming the drink before and during long-term cycle ergometry was not associated with changes in cycle time to exhaustion or physiological measurements.[356] Concentrations of polylactate of more than 0.75% were associated with gastrointestinal distress. Similarly, another study found no effects on performance or metabolism when 2% lactate with glucose polymers was compared to glucose polymers alone.[357] Chronic consumption of 10 g/d of lactate salts did not affect lactate levels during or after intense cycle exercise compared to a maltodextrin placebo.[358] Taken together, these results suggest that lactate supplementation may be equivalent to carbohydrate supplementation but may not have an additive effect with carbohydrates.

b.   Pyruvate

Pyruvate is a point of entry for carbon skeletons into the tricarboxylic acid cycle, which is intimately involved in aerobic energy production. Can muscle cell energy flux be enhanced by additional pyruvate? Three studies fed 100 g/d of pyruvate and dihydroxyacetone (a metabolite of pyruvate) to healthy men and found increased cycle time to exhaustion (79 vs. 66 min),[359] increased arm exercise endurance (160 vs. 133 min),[360] decreased ratings of perceived exertion,[361] and increased muscle uptake of glucose with glycogen sparing.[359-361]

Substitution of dietary carbohydrate with pyruvate salts further enhanced weight loss and fat loss during low calorie diets in obese women.[362-364] Pyruvate salts have reproducibly enhanced endurance exercise performance and body fat loss in humans.

c.   Alpha Ketoglutarate and Ornithine Alpha Ketoglutarate

Alpha ketoglutarate (AKG) is an intermediate in the tricarboxylic acid cycle. Administration as pyridoxine-AKG (PAK) at doses of 30 mg/kg body weight led to significantly increased VO_2max (6%) and decreased lactate accumulation after supramaximal treadmill exercise.[365] AKG administration had no effects.

Ornithine α-ketoglutarate (OKG) consists of two ornithine molecules bound to one α-ketoglutarate molecule and has been used with clinical success in Europe for treatment of burns, sepsis, postsurgical repair, malnutrition, liver disease, renal disease, immunosuppression, and wound healing at oral doses of 10–20 g/d.[366,367] Oral administration of OKG, but not equimolar amounts of AKG and ornithine, have been associated with elevated somatotropin, insulin, protein synthesis, glutamine production, polyamine synthesis, and collagen synthesis.[366,367] Although OKG has shown potent anabolic effects in humans of interest to strength athletes and endurance athletes, no studies with exercising individuals have been reported.

d. Gamma Hydroxybutyrate (Sodium Oxybate) and β-Hydroxy-β-Methylbutyrate (Hydroxyisovaleric Acid)

Gamma hydroxybutyrate (GHB) was promoted to strength athletes as a potent releaser of somatotropin.[368] However, its known anesthetic, hypnotic, and hallucinogenic effects were underplayed[24] and recreational use unrelated to athletic consumers forced a ban on GHB distribution; it remains unavailable.

Hydroxymethylbutyrate (HMB) is a rare metabolite of ketoisocaproate (leucine's ketoacid). Forty men undergoing resistance training were given either placebo or 3 g/d of calcium HMB for 4 wk.[369] Significant increases in bench press strength, lean mass, and body fat loss were seen.

e. Other Organic Acids

Organic acids commercially available to consumers include α-ketoisocaproate, succinates, malate, tartrate, and fumarate. However, these and other naturally occurring organic acids have yet to be tested for possible effects on exercise performance in humans.

E. MINERALS
1. Calcium, Magnesium, Zinc

Calcium supplementation has not been specifically studied for its ergogenic potential. Low doses (<10% of RDI) of calcium salts have been used as placebos for bicarbonate and pangamate studies, and compared to control groups, no ergogenic effects have been seen.[24] One report did not find any differences between calcium-supplemented (500 mg/d) or control groups of military recruits for incidence of stress fractures.[370] This suggests that prophylactic calcium supplementation did not prevent overtraining at that particular dose and form of calcium in young, healthy males.

Magnesium supplementation for enhancement of exercise performance has rationale based on evidence of subnormal status in athletes from some, but not all, studies.[24,371] In a case report, muscle cramps caused by magnesium depletion in a tennis player were alleviated by supplementation with 500 mg/d of magnesium gluconate.[372] Magnesium supplementation enhanced physical capacity in endurance athletes[373,374] and quadriceps torque after resistance training.[375] Post-exercise serum creatine kinase levels were reduced after magnesium supplementation in a group of women athletes with low normal levels of serum magnesium.[374] However, one study did not find any change in magnesium status of serum or muscle of marathon runners after 4 wk of supplementation with 385 mg magnesium daily.[376] Marathon run times, serum creatine kinase, muscle soreness, quadriceps torque, and urinary hydroxyproline measurements were unchanged between magnesium-supplemented and control groups.

Studies on ergogenic effects of potassium-magnesium aspartate salts used doses of 40–400 mg/d of magnesium.[101-110] Some of these studies found ergogenic benefits;[101-105] however, it is not clear if benefits could be solely attributed to magnesium. Thus, there is more evidence than not that supplemental magnesium (either as aspartate or oxide) may enhance different types of exercise performance.

Only one study examined effects of zinc supplementation (135 mg/d) on performance.[377] In a double-blind, crossover study, zinc increased muscle strength and endurance in 16 women.[377] Care must be taken when administering zinc in excess of the RDI (15 mg/d), since decreased serum HDL cholesterol and copper deficiency may result.[374]

2.   Iron

Iron deficiency is a major public health problem worldwide.[378] Iron status has been categorized into three stages: Grade I is depletion of iron stores only; Grade II adds deficient erythrocyte formation; and Grade III adds decreased blood hemoglobin levels (iron-deficiency anemias) (Table 8).[379] Iron is involved in delivery of oxygen to tissues via hemoglobin and myoglobin, cellular energy production via activation of cytochromes, and activation of enzymes involved in neurotransmitter synthesis, connective tissue synthesis, detoxification, immune function, and thyroid hormones.[378] Iron-deficiency anemia has repeatedly been proven to decrease almost every aspect of physical performance, especially endurance exercise.[371,378,380-383] Iron supplementation (repletion) in iron-deficiency anemia has reproducibly improved (normalized) exercise and work performance, sometimes before hemoglobin levels normalized.[24,247,371,378,380-384]

Exercising individuals with Grade I or II iron depletion (nonanemic iron deficiency) have exhibited decreased exercise performance in a minority of reports.[24,371,380-385] Usually, exercise performance is not affected by nonanemic iron deficiency, but some individuals may exhibit decreased performance.[24,371,380-384,386-388] Iron supplementation to exercising individuals with nonanemic iron deficiency almost always improved indicators of iron stores (serum ferritin levels), but only sometimes improved blood hemoglobin levels.[24,371,380-384,388] Exercise performance (run times to exhaustion) after iron supplementation was improved in at least four studies,[385,388-390] but was unchanged in a larger number of studies.[383,386,388,391] Changes in metabolic indices of exercise performance (VO_2max, blood lactate) also showed mixed results after iron supplementation for nonanemic iron depletion.

Only one report has examined exercise performance after iron supplementation in exercising individuals with normal iron status, and no benefits were seen.[392] Two other studies did find improvements in indicators of iron status,[393,394] but at least seven studies found no changes in iron status after iron supplementation in individuals with normal iron status.[382-384]

Iron deficiency with or without anemia may have effects on exercise performance through well-known deterioration of mental functions before physical capacity is affected.[378] Improvements in subjective feelings of fatigue, activity, and mood have been found for a majority of iron-supplemented women.[395,396] Future studies on iron and exercise performance should address mental performance parameters.

Recent research has suggested that elevated iron stores (more frequent in middle-aged and older men) may be associated with increased risk of death from chronic degenerative diseases (cardiovascular diseases and cancer).[397] Free iron is well-known to catalyze formation of more dangerous hydroxyl radicals from superoxide and hydrogen peroxide (Fenton and Haber-Weiss reactions).[166,170] Thus, accumulation of increased free radical damage over a lifetime from increased iron stores may increase risk of tissue damage and chronic degenerative disease. Hemochromatosis (a hereditary iron overload condition) can be detected by the same laboratory testing that assesses iron status.

Taken together, these observations indicate clear guidelines for ergogenicity of iron:

- Populations at greater risk for iron deficiency include female endurance athletes, athletic amenorrhea, anyone restricting caloric intake, anyone with "chronic" fatigue, or anyone initiating a strenuous training program.
- Iron deficiency, deficiency grading, or overload is easily identified or ruled out by interpretation of laboratory testing from a single blood sample, requested by a physician. Other reasons for anemia or fatigue should also be explored if iron status is normal or nonanemic.
- Iron supplementation over the RDI (10 mg for males and post-menopausal females; 15 mg for menstruating females) is only justified when laboratory testing has proven either anemia or deficient stores (see Table 8).

TABLE 8 Determinants of Iron Status and Dietary Practices to Replete Iron Stores

Clinical Laboratory Tests for Iron Status

CBC (Complete Blood Count) includes:
  Hemoglobin (Hb or Hgb in g/dl)
  Hematocrit (Hct in %)
  Erythrocyte count (RBC in 10^6 cells/mm^3)
  Leukocyte count (WBC in 10^3 cells/mm^3)
  Leukocyte differential (cell %)
  Mean corpuscular volume (MCV in fl)
  Mean corpuscular hemoglobin (MCH in $\mu\mu$g)
  Mean corpuscular hemoglobin concentration (MCHC in %)
  Platelet count (10^3/mm^3)
Serum ferritin
Serum iron (Fe)
Total iron-binding capacity (TIBC)
Transferrin saturation (calculated from Fe and TIBC)
Free erythrocyte protoporphyrin (Zinc ProtoPorphyrin or ZPP)
Reticulocyte count
Bone marrow cytology (usually not practical)

Interpretation of Laboratory Results (Iron Deficiency Grading)

Test	Grade I	Grade II	Grade III (Anemia)
Bone marrow cytology	deficient	deficient	deficient
Serum ferritin	low	low	low
ZPP	normal	high	high
Transferrin saturation	>15%	<15%	<15%
Hemoglobin	normal	normal	low

Additional Laboratory Tests to Rule Out Non-Iron Deficiency Anemias[a]

Serum and erythrocyte folate
Serum vitamin B_{12}
Erythropoietin
Microbial assays for vitamin B_6 levels
Functional vitamin B_6 assays (erythrocyte transaminase saturation indices)
Serum copper

Dietary Changes to Improve Iron Intake and Uptake

1. Increase ingestion of heme iron by increasing intake of cooked muscle meats or blood, preferably lean red meats.
2. Increase consumption of vitamin C at same time as iron-rich foods or iron supplements by increasing *fresh* citrus fruits and green leafy vegetable intakes (but not spinach). Vitamin C supplements (100–1000 mg/d) are also appropriate.
3. Iron supplements (optional 10–25 mg/d to replete nonanemic iron deficiency; or higher doses for shorter periods — determined by a health care professional — in iron deficiency anemia) should be considered, especially for strict or lacto-ovo vegetarians.
4. Better iron supplements: ferritin, ferrous glycinate, ferrous lactate, ferrous gluconate, ferrous fumarate, iron dextran. Less ideal iron supplements: ferrous sulfate, reduced iron, carbonyl iron, ferric orthophosphate.

[a] Reference ranges for each test may differ between laboratories.

• Repletion is easily accomplished by dietary changes *and* supplementation with 15–100 mg/d of iron as glycinate, lactate, fumarate, gluconate, or dextran. Less-tolerated salts such as sulfate, orthophosphate, reduced iron, or carbonyl iron should be avoided. Supplementation and resulting iron status should be monitored by a health care professional (physician, nurse practitioner, registered dietitian, clinical nutritionist) to avoid possibility of iron overload.

- Dietary changes include addition of vitamin C (ascorbic acid) from citrus fruits or supplements (500 mg/d), increased intake of lean red meats for heme groups, reduction of coffee and tea, or other advice from a health care professional.

- Iron supplementation over the RDI in cases of normal status (or unknown status) should be strongly discouraged since no ergogenic effects are likely; acute side effects are possible; elevation of risk for chronic degenerative diseases is possible; and rarely, hemochromatosis may be extant.

- In cases of iron deficiency anemia, iron repletion is almost universally ergogenic and will be ergogenic only for some, but not all, individuals with nonanemic iron deficiency.

3. Phosphates

Phosphate salt supplementation to enhance physical performance has been reported in scientific journals since the early 20th century.[384] These early studies suffered from deficient study design but did indicate safety of large doses of phosphate salts for long time periods. Phosphate salts are hypothesized to be ergogenic by:

1. stimulating glycolysis;
2. delaying anaerobic threshold;
3. increasing 2,3-diphosphoglycerate (2,3-DPG) for enhanced oxygen delivery to tissues;
4. increasing phosphate for ATP and creatine phosphate resynthesis;
5. buffering acidity during intense exercise;
6. improving cardiac function; and
7. improving respiratory capacity.[24,171,266,384,398]

Seven studies found significantly improved exercise performance (cycle ergometry to exhaustion, 5-mile (8.0 km) race times, 40-km race times, treadmill runs to exhaustion) after phosphate ingestion.[398-403] Ten studies did not find benefits for exercise performance after phosphate ingestion.[274,404-412] Trends were noticed that might explain the variance of results. Ergogenicity of phosphate supplements were associated more often with trained subjects, aerobic exercise, ≥4 g/d of phosphate, duration of phosphate loading >4 d, and trisodium phosphate ingestion. Lack of ergogenic effects were associated more often with untrained subjects, anaerobic exercise, phosphate doses <4 g/d, loading duration of <4 d or single dose, acute administration, and dicalcium phosphate ingestion (dicalcium phosphate is well-known to have poor bioavailability). Thus, under certain conditions, phosphate supplementation has reproducibly enhanced aerobic endurance performance.

4. Chromium

Ergogenic properties of chromium revolve around its primary function as the Glucose Tolerance Factor (GTF), rendering insulin actions more efficient.[24,384,413-418] Coupled with chronic low dietary intakes and losses of chromium associated with exercise,[24,384,413-418] a rationale for supplementation in athletes wishing to accentuate insulin actions (anabolism, strength, lean muscle mass gain) was apparent.

Encouraging work from animal feed efficiency studies and diabetic human repletion studies was transferred to healthy young athletes in weight training programs. Initial reports found reductions in body fat in sedentary, middle-aged subjects,[419,420] and a landmark study by Evans found decreased body fat and body weight gain in college athletes in a weight training program.[421] Chromium dosage was 200 mcg/d as the picolinate salt for 6 wk, which has been repeated in almost every subsequent study to date. This single study sparked immense public interest in chromium as an anabolic steroid alternative, prompting other groups to reproduce Evans' data. These findings were reproduced in female weightlifters (increase in body weight only), but both males and females showed no changes in body fat or strength.[422] Evans also reported increased muscle mass gain was greater for chromium picolinate than for chromium polynicotinate at a dose of 400 mcg/d.[423] Other similar studies with tighter experimental controls found no significant changes (although trends were seen in some studies) for body composition changes and strength.[424-427] Lukaski[427] raised the question of an adverse interaction of chromium with iron based on his finding of a nonsignificant trend ($P = 0.17$) for reduced transferrin saturation after chromium picolinate (but not from chromium chloride).

At this time, there are as many reviews as original studies on anabolic effects of chromium during weight training. Dose-response has not been properly addressed, as 200 mcg/d is below therapeutic doses of chromium (1000 mcg/d) used to reduce blood lipids and glucose levels in Type II diabetics.[428] Nevertheless, given the low dietary intakes of athletes and the U.S. population in general, ensuring adequate chromium intake (RDI = 120 mcg/d) seems sound for long-term health. Anabolic effects of chromium are still controversial, and it is apparent that daily doses of 200 mcg/d are insufficient to reproducibly elicit anabolic responses in young, healthy athletes. Further testing with higher doses (and close attention to iron status) is needed before definitive conclusions on chromium ergogenicity can be rationally maintained.

5. Other Minerals (Boron and Vanadium)

The only other trace minerals that have attracted the attention of consumers are boron and vanadium. Boron received a reputation as an anabolic steroid alternative that can raise serum testosterone levels based on incorrect interpretation of an excellent study by Nielsen in 1987.[429] Nielsen fed postmenopausal women a diet deficient in boron, and after hormone levels had remained steadily lower than the pre-diet period, a 3 mg/d supplement of boron (as sodium borate) was given. Serum testosterone and estrogen levels promptly returned to prediet levels. This was wrongly interpreted as boron raising serum testosterone levels, when a return to normal levels (already very low) was obvious. One fact conveniently left out of advertisements for boron as an anabolic steroid alternative was the equally large rise in serum estrogen, which is diametrically opposed to testosterone. Boron supplementation (2.5 mg/d for 7 wk) to bodybuilders did not affect serum testosterone, lean body mass, or strength compared to a placebo group, although serum boron levels were significantly increased by supplementation.[430] Healthy volunteers were fed a diet low (0.25 mg/2000 kcal or 8.4 MJ) or adequate (3.25 mg/2000 kcal or 8.4 MJ) in boron.[431] Low boron intake resulted in significantly poorer manual dexterity, eye-hand coordination, attention, perception, encoding, and memory. Boron supplementation (3 mg/d) for one year to female college athletes and sedentary subjects found increased serum magnesium levels, while urinary calcium losses increased over time for all subjects.[432] Boron may also have anti-osteoarthritis effects and play a role in cellular energy production (perhaps via augmentation of magnesium status).[433] These results indicate that a boron deficient diet (low in fruits, nuts, and seeds) may adversely affect exercise performance in skill sports via mental function and musculoskeletal deterioration.

Vanadium salts have shown insulin-potentiating actions *in vitro* and in diabetic animal models.[415,434] As soon as this information was available, vanadyl sulfate and bis[maltolato]oxovanadium supplements became available as anabolic steroid alternatives for consumers, based on putative potentiation of anabolic effects of insulin. Although vanadium salts appear promising for adjunct therapy of Type II diabetics,[415,434] there is no evidence in athletes that vanadium salts possess anabolic effects. Vanadium salts are not without toxicity, and possibility of toxicity from vanadium supplements is an unanswered question.

Other essential minerals, such as iodine, manganese, copper, and molybdenum have not been studied for any specific ergogenic effects in exercising individuals.

In summary, mineral supplements show promise as ergogenic aids under certain conditions. Iron status should be tested if performance is not satisfactory, and deficient status should be corrected to prevent known decrements in physical and mental performance from iron-deficiency anemia. Magnesium and chromium supplementation appear promising, if only to correct unsuspected deficiencies in a subset of exercising individuals. Phosphate salts (sodium, not calcium) have reproducibly enhanced endurance when consumed at doses of more than 4 g/d over 4 d. Selenium was previously considered in the antioxidant section and shows promise for protecting tissues against free-radical damage from intense exercise. Minerals deserve further study as ergogenic aids.

F. VITAMINS

1. Vitamins A, D, and K

Reviews of the few studies examining the ergogenic effects of vitamins A, D, and K found no effects.[2,24,247,382,435-438] Ingesting large doses of vitamin A, D, or K should be discouraged because of potential toxicity from overdoses. Thus, there is little rationale or evidence that supplemental vitamin A, D, or K possess ergogenic properties for exercising individuals.

2. B Vitamins

Application of single B vitamins (thiamin, riboflavin, niacin, pyridoxine, folate, cobalamins, pantothenate, and biotin) for enhancement of exercise performance has been studied since the 1920s. Many reviews have found that supplementation with single B vitamins with doses 1–10 times the RDI in well-controlled studies generally has not been associated with ergogenic benefits, with a few exceptions.[2,24,171,247,371,382,435-441]

Exceptions include large doses of thiamin (900 mg/d) improving anaerobic threshold, blood lactate, and heart rates after maximal cycle ergometry,[442] and improvement of reaction times after acute, but not chronic administration of 50 mg of thiamin.[443] Riboflavin supplementation (10 mg before exercise) led to lowering of neuromuscular irritability after electrical stimulation.[444]

Niacin (but not niacinamide), given in large doses (300–2000 mg) before exercise, has reproducibly been ergolytic (decreased aerobic performance), because of inhibition of free fatty acid release during exercise.[445-455] Also, ingestion of more than 50 mg of niacin (nicotinic acid) can cause flushing, an often irritating and unpleasant side effect in most people. Thus, large doses of nicotinic acid should be avoided. Interestingly, niacinamide (the form commonly used in dietary supplements) does not cause flushing or reduction of fatty acids and may improve joint function (range of motion, pain and swelling) in both osteoarthritis and rheumatoid arthritis after long-term (>1 y), high-dose (250 mg t.i.d.) supplementation.[456]

Vitamin B_6 (pyridoxine) supplementation has been associated with enhanced somatotropin release after maximal exercise[457] and increased carbohydrate usage during exercise at modest doses (8–10 mg).[458,459] These effects may benefit short-term, anaerobic exercises (such as weightlifting) which rely chiefly on rapid glycogenolysis.

Vitamin B_{12} supplementation as cobamamide, one coenzymatic form of cobalamin, and also known commercially as Dibencozide, was perceived to be an anabolic steroid alternative, based on reports of enhanced growth in malnourished children.[24,413] However, no evidence exists that cobamamide supplementation augments muscle gains. One report on injectable vitamin B_{12} found improvements in "general well-being," suggesting a mental effect for popularity of vitamin B_{12} supplements and injections (a positive, placebo-like effect).[460]

Decreased blood lactate and oxygen consumption during prolonged cycling was found after 2 g/d for 2 wk of pantothenate supplementation.[461]

Except for one study by Matter on folate supplementation (with no effect on run times),[386] folate and biotin remain unstudied for ergogenic effects in exercising individuals. Thus, some ergogenic effects from single B vitamin supplementation has been described for thiamin, riboflavin, pyridoxine, and pantothenate. However, large doses of niacin (but not niacinamide) may actually decrease long-term endurance exercise. The impact of these findings is still unclear, but given the safety of doses employed and widespread use of multiple vitamin products by exercising individuals, there may be a significant number of persons who subjectively feel benefits from vitamin supplementation, fostering continued use by consumers. Further research on effects of B vitamins on mental as well as physical performance is indicated.

Combinations of B vitamins have been studied repeatedly in many different doses and combinations, which makes conclusions on ergogenicity difficult.[2,24,171,247,371,382,435-441] No studies have examined effects of a combination of more than six of all eight B vitamins (except for multiple vitamin/mineral formulas). A dose-response is apparent, as studies administering higher doses found improvements in mental performance (but not physical performance),[462] improved neuromuscular motor control,[463] or running performance in heat.[464] Thus, there is some suggestive evidence that high but safe doses of mixtures of B vitamins reinforces findings from single B vitamin supplementation studies and may improve performance under certain conditions involving mental skills.

In summary, supplementation with single B vitamins or mixtures of B vitamins has shown some ergogenic effects, but only at doses substantially higher than the RDI (>10 times). More effects on mental or neuromuscular performance than physical performance have been reported, which supports a hypothesis that B vitamin supplementation, widely practiced by consumers, may make exercising individuals "feel" better subjectively, accounting for popularity of supplements.[2]

G. MULTIPLE VITAMIN/MINERAL COMBINATIONS

Similar to the situation for B complex vitamins, many different combinations of vitamins and minerals have recently been studied[440,465-479] and reviewed[2,24,171,247,371,382,435-441] for possible ergogenic effects. Many reviews have maintained that there is no evidence for performance-enhancing effects from multiple vitamin/mineral mixtures. However, a recent review[2] that actually scored the studies for methodological quality[480] and evaluated other reports routinely ignored by other reviews[475-479] has concluded that ergogenic effects have been reported and are possible. Furthermore, *all* studies evaluated suffered from one or more of the following limitations:

1. lack of sufficient statistical power to discern a significant difference;
2. use of nutrient doses that did not affect nutrient status (low doses);
3. poor compliance;
4. incomplete mixtures; and
5. insufficient duration.

It can be safely concluded that supplementation with relatively low doses of vitamins and minerals at or near the RDI does not enhance exercise performance. However, if deficient status is encountered for one or more nutrients, then a chance for normalization of performance is increased over taking a lesser number of nutrients. Individualized, moderate to high (but safe) doses of vitamins and minerals have some support for enhancement of exercise performance as shown by improvements in race times or strength, faster recovery, improvement of hematological parameters, reduction of injuries or infections, and improved feelings of well-being.[2,462-468]

These findings simply confirm results found by investigation of single nutrient effects reviewed earlier in this chapter, particularly for combined antioxidant vitamins/minerals (ascorbate, tocopherols, carotenoids, and selenium), B vitamins, magnesium, iron, trace minerals, and choline. Thus, findings of ergogenicity with increased dosages of combinations of essential vitamins and minerals is logical and consistent with known data.

These findings also extend information into areas to consider for future research. Table 9 lists the multiples of the RDI for each nutrient supplemented in several multiple vitamin/mineral supplements, along with tentative limits on safety and ergogenicity. It can be

TABLE 9 Comparative Doses of Selected Multiple Vitamin/Mineral Studies on Exercise Performance. Correlation with Known Ergogenic Doses, Safety, and Recommended Dietary Intakes

	RDI[a]	Ergogenic Dose (multiple of RDI)[b]	Safety Limit (multiple of RDI)[c]	Ref. 465–467	468	477	469	440	478	478	474	472	479
Kleijnen Score[d]				60	52	50	67		56	56	75	68	90
Ergogenicity[e]				yes	no	yes	no	no	no	yes	no	no	yes[f]
Vitamin A (IU)	5000	NA[g]	5	0	1	0.5–6.0	2	1	1	1	1	0.1	0.6
Vitamin D (IU)	400	NA	5	0	1	1–9	1	1	1	1	1	0	0
β-Carotene (mg)	—	>5	?	0	0		0	0	0	0	0	0	0
Vitamin C (mg)	60	>8	100	17	2	33–267	14	8	8	1	9	3	10
Vitamin E (IU)	30	>10	60	3	0.5	7–50	30	5	0.5	0.5	10	3	3
Selenium (mg)	0.070	>1	40	0	0.5	3–14	0.7	0	0	0.5	0	0	0
Thiamin (mg)	1.5	>30	10000	13	10	27–400	43	5	1	1	50	36	9
Riboflavin (mg)	1.7	>5?	10000	18	9	18–150	38	12	1	1	15	15	10
Niacin (mg)	20	>50?	10000	2	3	5–50	4	10	1	1	5	2	6
Vitamin B_6 (mg)	2.0	5	50	25	10	5–150	30	10	1	76	50	68	11
Vitamin B_{12} (mg)	0.06	?	NA	0	2	17–50	20	5	2	20	17	8	5
Folate (mg)	0.4	?	2000	4	1	5–75	10	10	6	1	0.5	0.7	10
Pantothenate (mg)	10	9–200	2000	4	4	5–100	10	10	0	0	10	6	0
Biotin (mg)	0.3	?	10000	0	0	7–33	0	7	0	0	0.3	1.3	0
Calcium (mg)	1000	?	2+	0.5	0	1–3.5	0.3	0	0	0	0.3	0	0
Phosphorus (mg)	1000	>4	5?	1	0	0.2–2.0	0.15	0	0	0	0	0	0
Magnesium (mg)	400	>1	5	0.8	0.1	2.5–5.0	0.3	0	0	0	0	0.15	0
Iron (mg)	15	>1	5?	0	2	2–4	1.3	5	1	6	0	0	0

TABLE 9 Comparative Doses of Selected Multiple Vitamin/Mineral Studies on Exercise Performance. Correlation with Known Ergogenic Doses, Safety, and Recommended Dietary Intakes *(continued)*

	RDI[a]	Ergogenic Dose (multiple of RDI)[b]	Safety Limit (multiple of RDI)[c]	Ref.									
				465–467	468	477	469	440	478	478	474	472	479
Zinc (mg)	15	10?	3	0	1	3–10	0.3	0	1	4	0.2	1	0
Manganese (mg)	2.0	?	?	0	1.5	10–50	600?	0	0	0	0	0	0
Copper (mg)	2.0	?	5	0	1.5	0–2.5	0.3	0	0	0	0	0	0
Iodine (mg)	0.15	?	?	0	1	1–7	0	0	1	1	0	0	0
Chromium (mg)	0.12	>3	40	0	0	3–10	0	0	0	0	0.1	0	0
Molybdenum (mg)	0.075	?	?	0	0	0–70	0	0	0	0	0	0	0
Potassium (mg)	3500	?	>2	0	0	0–1.5	0	0	0	0	0	0	0
Choline (mg)	NA	>1g	?	0	0.1	0–2	0	0	0	0	0	0	0

[a] RDI = Reference Daily Intake, 1995.

[b] Ergogenic doses were taken from studies cited in this chapter and converted to multiples of the RDI.

[c] Safety limits were taken from the author's previous estimates from a wide variety of sources.[2,24,247,384,438] (Bucci, L.R., *Nutrition Applied to Injury Rehabilitation and Sports Medicine*, CRC Press, Boca Raton, FL, 1994.)

[d] Kleijnen Score describes an assessment of methodological quality for human clinical trials, taking into account study design, subject numbers, suitability of measurements, and reporting.[480] Values range from 0–100, with 100 indicating the best-designed study.

[e] Ergogenicity indicates whether a statistically significant improvement in some type of exercise performance was described.

[f] Ergogenicity in this study is an improvement of mood, not physical performance.

[g] NA = Not Applicable.

seen that most studies did not administer doses known to be ergogenic, and many nutrients were not supplemented at all (especially chromium and carotenoids). In general, ergogenic effects were seen for greater numbers of nutrients administered, higher doses of antioxidants, and high doses of biotin and folate. This points out the need for further studies on doses of biotin and folate that are known to have therapeutic effects from other fields of study, such as inherited metabolic disorders or homocysteine metabolism studies (>10 times RDI). In particular, biotin, which is completely unstudied for its ergogenic effects, occupies a role that may allow greater flux of the tricarboxylic acid cycle by introducing more pyruvate via carboxlyation pathways, rather than decarboxylation pathways.

Can indiscriminate use of high-potency multiple vitamin/mineral supplements enhance exercise or subjective mental performance? Research findings support common usage by consumers (in spite of negative recommendations by most health care professionals) that perceived benefits do exist. Nevertheless, care must be taken not to exceed safe doses of essential nutrients for long time periods (see Table 9).

H. COMBINATIONS OF MICRONUTRIENTS

With an ever-increasing number of single nutrients commercially available, and with market pressures to produce unique products, an increasing number of combinations of essential with nonessential nutrients are available. Such combinations usually contain vitamins, minerals, metabolites, amino acids, carbohydrates, protein, buffers, herbs, and other nutrients. Testing of such products or combinations of nutrients will never catch up with the available number of products, but some reports have examined the ergogenic effects of supplementation with multi-category nutrient combinations.

In general, outcomes are mixed, with some studies showing improvements in exercise performance, and others not.[24,247,481] Like multiple vitamin/mineral studies, a dose- and time-response is apparent. Very recent reports not covered by previous reviews include two studies finding improvements in response to resistance training after consumption of carbohydrate/protein or carbohydrate/protein/vitamin/mineral/amino acid/creatine supplementation.[482,483] Interestingly, the latter combination outperformed another commercial product consisting of mostly carbohydrates with protein/vitamins/minerals/amino acids with respect to lean muscle mass gains. These results indicate that the popular weight gain powders consumed by weightlifters have some efficacy, a new finding with practical realizations for prevention of anabolic steroid use.

Other reports administering various mixtures of antioxidants and metabolites either found improvements in anaerobic exercise performance (Wingate test)[484] or no effect on endurance time to fatigue.[485] In general, testing of nutrient combinations is beginning to reflect the application of ergogenic effects from testing of single nutrients, with mostly positive results.

IV. GUIDELINES, SUMMARY, AND CONCLUSIONS

The study of nutritional ergogenic aids is accelerating, with each year finding almost exponential growth in reported studies and breadth of nutrients tested. Some general problems with study design still remain, especially with statistical power (low subject numbers frequently cause Type I errors given the large biological variability among subjects),[486] lack of dose-response, and insufficient duration. Double-blind studies are not fool-proof, especially when administered substances have mental affects not considered by investigators (such as caffeine, B vitamins, ephedrine). This means that many subjects know whether or not they receive a placebo or active supplement, and their performance may involve a placebo effect. This was illustrated by a study which administered decaffeinated coffee and led subjects to believe they were getting a placebo or caffeinated drink.[487] Subjects' performance varied with their belief about caffeine effects, suggesting that many studies may have spurious results.

This means that many ergogenic effects may be attributed to mental effects, rather than physiological effects. In any event, the bottom line is that humans performed better after supplementation. Other physiological and metabolic measurements are needed to rule out a strictly mental effect.

Most studies do not determine whether supplementation affects tissue or cellular status, which often leads to conflicting results between studies, creating confusion for consumers. Thus, an individual can select scientific literature to support a pro-ergogenicity or anti-ergogenicity stance on almost any nutrient tested.

Finally, guidelines for rational use of nutrients as ergogenic aids can now be updated, as illustrated in Table 10. It is becoming more apparent that sufficient dose and duration of many nutrients can enhance exercise performance and training of many subjects.

TABLE 10 Guidelines for Rational Use of Nutritional Ergogenic Aids with Documented Efficacy

Aerobic Exercise

running, cycling, swimming, skiing, rowing, sports events, or training lasting longer than 60 min

1. Carbohydrate-Electrolyte Drinks — 400–600 ml before event and 100–200 ml every 15 min during event.
2. Glycogen Supercompensation (Carbohydrate Loading) — single events: 60–70% carbohydrate diet started 1 wk before event; taper exercise down by 1/2 every 2nd day until event; consume >300 g carbohydrates (low fat, low fiber, complex) 3–4 hr before event; consume 500–700 mg carbohydrates (sugars) immediately after exercise.
3. Protein Intake — maintain 1.8–2.0 g protein/kg/d intake during strenuous training.
4. Iron — If anemic or iron-depleted, add 15–50 mg of supplemental iron from organic chelates; increase dietary heme iron (lean meats) and vitamin C (fresh fruits and vegetables). Laboratory testing is recommended before iron supplementation greater than the RDI is attempted.
5. Caffeine — 200–300 mg (2 or 3 fresh brewed cups of coffee or equivalent) 1 hr before event.
6. Multiple Vitamin/Mineral supplement with >10 times the RDI for B vitamins and RDI amounts of all essential minerals (excluding calcium and phosphorus).
7. Phosphate salts (trisodium phosphate, not dicalcium phosphate or monobasic sodium phosphate) — 4.0 g/d for > 4 d.
8. Coenzyme Q_{10} – 100 mg/d for at least 8 wk.
9. Antioxidant Mixture — Vitamin E: 400–800 IU/d; Vitamin C: 500–2000 mg/d; Beta Carotene and/or other carotenoids: 25,000–100,000 IU/d; Selenium: 100–250 mcg/d; N-acetyl-L-cysteine; 1500 mg/d; possibly proanthocyanidins and polyphenols from green tea, maritime pine bark, grape seeds, *Ginkgo biloba* or other herbs.

Anaerobic Exercise

weightlifting, bodybuilding, track and field, maximal intensity events (short-term, repetitive, or <60 min exhaustive exercise like football, hockey, wrestling, rowing, cycle sprints, volleyball)

1. Protein Intake — 100–200 g/d (2.0–2.5 g protein/kg/d).
2. Sodium bicarbonate (baking soda) — single events: 0.2–0.3 g/kg 2 hr before exercise; consume water ad libitum. Because of possible gastrointestinal intolerance, practice with dosing before an important event.
3. Antioxidant Mixture — (same as for aerobic exercise).
4. Creatine monohydrate — 20 g/d for 5 d in 4 divided doses of 5 g each, followed by 2 g/d indefinitely; or 3 g/d for 30 d, simultaneous carbohydrate intake improves uptake into muscle.
5. Weight Gain Powders — should contain protein (25 g/serving), carbohydrate (>25 g/serving), creatine (>3 g/serving), and possibly L-glutamine (6 g/serving), taurine (>2 g/serving); preferably ingested just after workouts.
6. Asian ginseng (*Panax ginseng*) standardized ginsenoside extracts — at least 400 mg/d for at least 8 wk, or 3–9 g/d of root powder.
7. Multiple Vitamin/Mineral supplement — (same as aerobic exercise).

Skill Sports

sports requiring fine motor control, coordination and reaction time (shooting, archery, baseball, basketball, gymnastics, diving, car racing)

1. Multiple Vitamin/Mineral supplement — (same as aerobic exercise).
2. Octacosanol — >1000 mcg/d for at least 8 wk.
3. Caffeine (200–300 mg/serving) — test dosage before important event, as some subjects may become jittery with fine tremors.

ACKNOWLEDGMENTS

I would like to thank Dr. Muhammed Majid of Sabinsa Corp. for providing reprints on herbs, Dr. Steve Nissen for providing preprints on hydroxymethylbutyrate, Dr. Bobby Sandage for providing preprints on choline, and Dr. Ron Stanko for providing pyruvate references.

REFERENCES

1. Thomas, C. L., Ed., *Taber's Cyclopedic Medical Dictionary*, 15th ed., F.A. Davis, Philadelphia, 1985, 568.
2. Bucci, L. R., Introduction, in *Sports Nutrition: Vitamins and Trace Minerals*, Wolinsky, I. and Driskell, J., Eds., CRC Press, 1996, in press.
3. American College of Sports Medicine, Position stand on prevention of thermal injuries during distance running, *Med. Sci. Sports Exer.*, 16, ix, 1984.
4. Maughan, R. J. and Noakes, T. D., Fluid replacement and exercise stress. A brief review of studies on fluid replacement and some guidelines for the athlete, *Sports Med.*, 12, 16, 1991.
5. Pivarnik, J. M. and Palmer, R. A., Water and electrolyte balance during rest and exercise, in *Nutrition in Exercise and Sport*, Wolinsky, I. and Hickson, J. F., Jr., Eds., CRC Press, Boca Raton, FL, 1994, 245.
6. Buskirk, E. R. and Puhl, S. M., Eds., *Body Fluid Balance: Exercise and Sport*, CRC Press, Boca Raton, FL, 1996.
7. Murray, R., Fluid needs in hot and cold environments, *Int. J. Sport Nutr.*, 5(Suppl.), S62, 1995.
8. Blyth, C. and Burt, J., Effect of water balance on ability to perform in high ambient temperatures, *Res. Q. Am. Assoc. Health Phys. Educ.*, 32, 301, 1961.
9. Nadel, E. R., Fortney, S. M., and Wenger, C. B., Effect of hydration state on circulatory and thermal regulations, *J. Appl. Physiol.*, 49, 715, 1980.
10. Moroff, S. V. and Bass, D. E., Effects of overhydration on man's physiological responses to work in the heat, *J. Appl. Physiol.*, 20, 267, 1965.
11. Greenleaf, J., Exercise and water electrolyte balance, in *Nutrition and Physical Activity*, Blix, G., Ed., Almqvist and Wiksells, Uppsala, 1967.
12. Greenleaf, J. and Castle, B., Exercise temperature regulation in man during hypohydration and hyperhydration, *J. Appl. Physiol.*, 30, 847, 1971.
13. Nielsen, B., Thermoregulation in exercising man during dehydration and hyperhydration with water and saline, *Int. J. Biometeorol.*, 15, 195, 1971.
14. Gisolfi, C. and Copping, J., Thermal effects of prolonged treadmill exercise in the heat, *Med. Sci. Sports*, 6, 108, 1974.
15. Foley, P., Effect of ingesting water in swimming, *Swimming Technique*, 8, 34, 1971.
16. Noakes, T. D., Goodwin, N., Rayner, B. L., Branken, T., and Taylor, R. K. N., Water intoxication: a possible complication during endurance exercise, *Med. Sci. Sports Exer.*, 17, 370, 1985.
17. Knochel, J. P. and Vertel, R. M., Salt loading as a possible factor in the production of potassium depletion, rhabdomyolysis, and heat injury, *Lancet*, 1, 659, 1967.
18. Lane, H. W. and Cerda, J., Potassium requirements and exercise, *J. Am. Diet. Assoc.*, 73, 64, 1978.
19. Valeriani, A., The need for carbohydrate intake during endurance exercise, *Sports Med.*, 12, 349, 1991.
20. Costill, D. L. and Hargreaves, M., Carbohydrate nutrition and fatigue, *Sports Med.*, 13, 86, 1992.
21. Liebman, M. and Wilkinson, J. G., Carbohydrate metabolism and exercise, in *Nutrition in Exercise and Sport*, Wolinsky, I. and Hickson, J. F., Jr., Eds., CRC Press, Boca Raton, FL, 1994, 15.
22. Miller, G. D., Carbohydrates in ultra-endurance exercise and athletic performance, in *Nutrition in Exercise and Sport*, Wolinsky, I. and Hickson, J. F., Jr., Eds., CRC Press, Boca Raton, FL, 1994, 65.
23. Walberg-Rankin, J., Dietary carbohydrate as an ergogenic aid for prolonged and brief competitions in sport, *Int. J. Sports Nutr.*, 5(Suppl.), S13, 1995.
24. Bucci, L. R., Nutritional ergogenic aids, in *Nutrition in Exercise and Sport*, Wolinsky, I. and Hickson, J. F., Jr., Eds., CRC Press, Boca Raton, FL, 1994, 295.
25. Friedman, J. E., Neufer, P. D., and Dohm, G. L., Regulation of glycogen resynthesis following exercise. Dietary considerations, *Sports Med.*, 11, 232, 1991.
26. Lemon, P. W. R. and Proctor, D. N., Protein intake and athletic performance, *Sports Med.*, 12, 313, 1991.
27. Lemon, P. W. R., Do athletes need more dietary protein and amino acids?, *Int. J. Sports Nutr.*, 5(Suppl.), S39, 1995.
28. Kaufmann, D. A., Protein as an energy substrate during intense exercise, *Ann. Sports Med.*, 5, 142, 1990.
29. Consolazio, C. F., Johnson, H. L., Nelson, R. A., Dramise, J. G., and Skala, J. H., Protein metabolism during intensive physical training in the young adult, *Am. J. Clin. Nutr.*, 28, 29, 1975.

30. Oddoye, E. B. and Margen, S., Nitrogen balance studies in humans: long-term effect of high nitrogen intake on nitrogen accretion, *J. Nutr.*, 1979, 109, 363.

31. Marable, N. L., Hickson, J. F., Korslund, M. K., Herbert, W. G., and Desjardins, R. F., Urinary nitrogen excretion as influenced by a muscle-building exercise program and protein intake variation, *Nutr. Rep. Int.*, 19, 795, 1979.

32. Dragan, G. I., Vasiliu, A., and Georgescu, E., Effects of increased supply of protein on elite weight lifters, in *Milk Proteins '84*, Galesloot, T. E. and Timbergen, B. J., Eds., Pudoc, Waningen, Netherlands, 1985.

33. Hecker, A. L. and Wheeler, K. B., Protein: a misunderstood nutrient for the athlete, *NSCA J.*, 7, 28, 1985.

34. Frontera, W. R., Meredith, C. N., O'Reilly, K. P., Knuttgen, G., and Evans, W. J., Strength conditioning in older men: skeletal muscle hypertrophy and improved function, *J. Appl. Physiol.*, 64, 1038, 1988.

35. Fern, E. B., Bielinski, R. N., and Schutz, Y., Effects of exaggerated amino acid and protein supply in man, *Experentia*, 47, 168, 1991.

36. Walberg, J. L., Leidy, M. K., Sturgill, D. J., Hinkle, D. E., Ritchey, S. J., and Sebolt, D. R., Macronutrient content of a hypoenergy diet affects nitrogen retention and muscle function in weight lifters, *Int. J. Sports Med.*, 9, 261, 1988.

37. Tarnopolsky, M. A., Atkinson, S. A., MacDougall, J. D., Chesley, A., Phillips, S., and Schwarcz, H. P., Evaluation of protein requirements for trained strength athletes, *J. Appl. Physiol.*, 73, 1986, 1992.

38. Bassett, D. R. and Nagle, F. J., Energy metabolism in exercise and training, in *Nutrition in Exercise and Sport*, Wolinsky, I. and Hickson, J. F., Jr., Eds., CRC Press, Boca Raton, FL, 1994, 139.

39. Sherman, W. M. and Lenders, N., Fat loading: the next magic bullet?, *Int. J. Sport Nutr.*, 5(Suppl.), 51, 1995.

40. Hargreaves, M., Kiens, B., and Richter, E. A., Effect of increased plasma free fatty acid concentrations on muscle metabolism in exercising men, *J. Appl. Physiol.*, 70, 194, 1991.

41. Dyck, D. J., Putman, C. T., Heigenhauser, G. J. F., Hultman, E., and Spriet, L. L., Regulation of fat-carbohydrate interaction in skeletal muscle during intense aerobic cycling, *Am. J. Physiol.*, 265, E852, 1993.

42. Vukovich, M. D., Costill, D. L., Hickey, M. S., Trappe, S. W., Cole, E. J., and Fink, W. J., Effect of fat emulsion infusion and fat feeding on muscle glycogen utilization during cycle exercise, *J. Appl. Physiol.*, 75, 1513, 1993.

43. Costill, D. L., Coyle, E., Dalsky, G., Evans, W., Fink, W., and Hoopes, D., Effects of elevated plasma FFA and insulin on muscle glycogen usage during exercise, *J. Appl. Physiol.*, 43, 695, 1977.

44. Ivy, J., Costill, D. L., Fink, W. J., and Maglischo, E., Contribution of medium and long chain triglyceride intake to energy metabolism during prolonged exercise, *Int. J. Sports Med.*, 1, 15, 1980.

45. Ivy, J., Costill, D. L., Van Handel, P. J., Essig, D. A., and Lower, R. W., Alteration in the lactate threshold with changes in substrate availability, *Int. J. Sports Med.*, 2, 139, 1981.

46. Phinney, S., Bistrian, B. R., Evans, W. J., Gervino, E., and Blackburn, G. L., The human metabolic response to chronic ketosis without caloric restriction: preservation of submaximal exercise capability with reduced carbohydrate oxidation, *Metabolism*, 32, 769, 1983.

47. Lambert, E. V., Speechly, D. P., Dennis, S. C., and Noakes, T. D., Enhanced endurance in trained cyclists during moderate intensity exercise following 2 weeks adaptation to a high fat diet, *Eur. J. Appl. Physiol.*, 69, 287, 1994.

48. Johannessen, A., Hagen, C., and Galbo, H., Prolactin, growth hormone, thyrotropin, 3,5,3'-triiodothyronine, and thyroxine responses to exercise after fat- and carbohydrate-enriched diet, *J. Clin. Endocrinol. Metab.*, 52, 56, 1981.

49. Sherman, W. M. and Wimer, G. S., Insufficient dietary carbohydrate during training: does it impair athletic performance?, *Int. J. Sport Nutr.*, 1, 28, 1991.

50. Sherman, W. H., Doyle, J. A., Lamb, D. R., and Strauss, R. H., Dietary carbohydrate, muscle glycogen, and exercise performance during 7 d of training, *Am. J. Clin. Nutr.*, 57, 27, 1993.

51. Muoio, D. M., Leddy, J. J., Horvath, P. J., Awad, A. B., and Pendergast, D. R., Effect of dietary fat on metabolic adjustments to maximal VO_2 and endurance in runners, *Med. Sci. Sports Exer.*, 26, 81, 1994.

52. Bach, A. S. and Babayan, V. K., Medium-chain triglycerides — an update, *Am. J. Clin. Nutr.*, 36, 950, 1982.

53. Seaton, T. B., Welle, S. L., Warenko, M. K., and Campbell, R. G., Thermic effect of medium-chain and long-chain triglycerides in man, *Am. J. Clin. Nutr.*, 44, 630, 1986.

54. Dias, V., Effects of feeding and energy balance in adult humans, *Metabolism*, 39, 887, 1990.

55. Blackburn, G. L., Kater, G., Mascioli, E. A., Kowalchuk, M., Babayan, V. K., and Bistrian, B. R., A reevaluation of coconut oil's effect on serum cholesterol and atherogenesis, *J. Phil. Med. Assoc.*, 65, 144, 1989.

56. Massicotte, D., Péronnet, F., Brisson, G. R., and Hillaire-Marcel, C., Oxidation of exogenous medium-chain free fatty acids during prolonged exercise: comparison with glucose, *J. Appl. Physiol.*, 73, 1334, 1992.

57. Jeukendrup, A. E., Saris, W. H. M., Schrauwen, P., Brouns, F., and Wagenmakers, J. M., Metabolic availability of medium-chain triglycerides coingested with carbohydrates during prolonged exercise, *J. Appl. Physiol.*, 79, 756, 1995.

58. Borghouts, L., Jeukendrup, A. E., Saris, W. H. M., Brouns, F., and Wagenmakers, A. J. M., No effect of medium chain triglyceride (MCT) ingestion during prolonged exercise on muscle glycogen utilization, *Med. Sci. Sports Exer.*, 27, S101, 1995.

59. Van Zyl, C., Lambert, E. V., Noakes, T. D., and Dennis, S. C., Effects of medium-chain triglyceride ingestion on carbohydrate metabolism and cycling performance, *Clin. Sci.*, 87 (Suppl.), 30, 1994.

60. Brilla, L. R. and Landerholm, T. E., Effect of fish oil supplementation and exercise on serum lipids and aerobic fitness, *J. Sports Med.*, 30, 173, 1990.

61. Sears, B., BIOSYN Training Manual, Marblehead, MA, 1990.

62. Monteleone, P., Beinat, L., Tanzillo, C., Maj, M., and Kemali, D., Effects of phosphatidylserine on the neuroendocrine response to physical stress in humans, *Neuroendocrinology.*, 52, 243, 1990.

63. Monteleone, P., Maj, M., Beinat, L., Natale, M., and Kemali, D., Blunting by chronic phosphatidylserine administration of the stress-induced activation of the hypothalamo-pituitary-adrenal axis in healthy men, *Eur. J. Clin. Pharmacol.*, 42, 385, 1992.

64. Kidd, P. M., *Phosphatidylserine (PS). A Remarkable Brain Cell Nutrient*, Lucas Meyer, Decatur, IL, 1995.

65. Terblanche, S. E., Fell, R. D., Juhlin-Dannfelt, A. C., Craig, B. W., and Holloszy, J. O., Effects of glycerol feeding before and after exhausting exercise in rats, *J. Appl. Physiol.*, 50, 94, 1981.

66. Miller, J., Coyle, E. F., Sherman, W. M., Hagberg, J. M., Costill, D. L., Fink, W. J., Terblanche, S. E., and Holloszy, J. O., Effect of glycerol feeding on endurance and metabolism during prolonged exercise in man, *Med. Sci. Sports Exer.*, 15, 237, 1983.

67. Gleeson, M., Maughan, R. J., and Greenhaff, P. L., Comparison of the effects of pre-exercise feeding of glucose, glycerol and placebo on endurance and fuel homeostasis in man, *Eur. J. Appl. Physiol.*, 55, 645, 1986.

68. Maughan, R. J. and Gleeson, M., Influence of a 36 h fast followed by refeeding with glucose, glycerol or placebo on metabolism and performance during prolonged exercise in man, *Eur. J. Appl. Physiol.*, 57, 570, 1988.

69. Fregly, M. J., Privette, R. M., and Cade, R., Compositions and methods for achieving improved physiological response to exercise, United States Patent 4,981,687, 1991.

70. Fregly, M. J., Privette, R. M., and Cade, R., Compositions and methods for achieving improved physiological response to exercise, United States Patent 5,147,650, 1992.

71. Cureton, T. K., Ed., *The Physiological Effects of Wheat Germ Oil on Humans in Exercise*, Charles C Thomas, Springfield, IL, 1972.

72. Jethon, Z., Szczurek, A. L., and Put, A., Effects of additional supply of minerals and vitamins on physical work capacity in strength sports, in *Symposium for Sportsmen*, Cernelle, A. B., Ed., Helsingborg, Sweden, 1972, 173.

73. Steben, R. E., Wells, J. C., and Harless, I. L., The effect of bee pollen tablets on the improvement of certain blood factors and performance of male collegiate swimmers, *J. Natl. Athletic Trainers Assoc.*, 11, 124, 1976.

74. Steben, R. E. and Boudreaux, P., The effects of pollen and protein extracts on selected factors and performance of athletes, *J. Sports Med.*, 18, 221, 1978.

75. Maughan, R. J. and Evans, S. P., Effects of pollen extract upon adolescent swimmers, *Br. J. Sports Med.*, 16, 142, 1982.

76. Chandler, J. V. and Hawkins, J. D., The effect of bee pollen on physiological performance, *Med. Sci. Sports Exer.*, 17, 287, 1985.

77. Williams, M. H., Ed., Ergogenic foods, in *Nutritional Aspects of Human Physical and Athletic Performance*, 2nd ed., Charles C Thomas, Springfield, IL, 1985, 312.

78. Bucci, L.R., Dietary substances not required in human metabolism, in *Nutrients as Ergogenic Aids for Sports and Exercise*, CRC Press, Boca Raton, FL, 1993, 83.

79. Williams, M. H., Drug foods — alcohol and caffeine, in *Nutritional Aspects of Human Physical and Athletic Performance*, 2nd ed., Charles C Thomas, Springfield, IL, 1985, 272.

80. Knopf, R. F., Conn, J. W., Falans, S. S., Floyd, J. C., Guntsche, E. M., and Rull, J. A., Plasma growth hormone responses to intravenous administration of amino acids, *Clin. Endocrinol.*, 25, 1140, 1965.

81. Mathieni, G., Growth hormone secretion by arginine stimulus: the effect of both low doses and oral arginine, *Boll. Soc. It. Sper. Biol.*, 56, 2254, 1980.

82. Besset, L., Increase in sleep related growth hormone and prolactin secretion after chronic arginine aspartate administration, *Acta Endocrinol.*, 99, 18, 1982.

83. Elsair, C., Effets de l'arginine, administrie par voie orale, *C. R. Soc. Biol.*, 179, 608, 1985.

84. Isidori, A., Lo Monaco, A., and Cappa, M., A study of growth hormone release in man after oral administration of amino acids, *Curr. Med. Res. Opinion*, 7, 475, 1981.

85. Fogelholm, G. M., Näveri, H. K., Kiilavuori, K. T. K., and Härkönen, Low-dose amino acid supplementation: no effects on serum growth hormone and insulin in male weightlifters, *Int. J. Sport Nutr.*, 3, 290, 1993.

86. Lambert, M. I., Hefer, J. A., Millar, R. P., and Macfarlane, P. W., Failure of commercial oral amino acid supplements to increase serum growth hormone concentrations in male body-builders, *Int. J. Sport Nutr.*, 3, 298, 1993.

87. Fluckey, J. D., Gordon, S. E., Kraemer, W. J., and Farrell, P. A., Arginine stimulated insulin secretion from pancreatic islets is increased following resistance exercise, *Med. Sci. Sports Exer.*, 26(5 Suppl.), S22, 1994.

88. Gater, D. R., Gater, D. A., Uribe, J. M., and Hunt, J. C., Effects of arginine/lysine supplementation and resistance training on glucose tolerance, *J. Appl. Physiol.*, 72, 1279, 1992.

89. Denis, C., Dormois, D., Linossier, M. T., Eychenne, J. L., Hauseux, P., and Lacour, J. R., Effect of arginine aspartate on the exercise-induced hyperammonemia in humans: a two periods cross-over trial, *Arch. Int. Physiol. Biochim. Biophys.*, 99, 123, 1991.

90. Eto, B., Peres, G., and Le Moel, G., Effects of an ingested glutamate arginine salt on ammonemia during and after long lasting cycling, *Arch. Int. Physiol. Biochim. Biophys.*, 102, 161, 1994.

91. Guarnieri, C., Fussi, F., Fanelli, D., Davalli, P., and Clo, C., RNA and protein synthesis in rat brain during exercise. Effect of arginine and some phosphorylated amino acids, *Pharmacology*, 19, 51, 1979.

92. Meneguello, M. O., Lancha, A. H., Costa Rosa, L. F. B. P., and Curi, R., Effect of the supplementation of ornithine, citrulline and arginine on metabolism of acute exercised rats, *Med. Sci. Sports Exer.*, 27(Suppl. 5), S147, 1995.

93. Elam, R. P., Morphological changes in adult males from resistance exercise and amino acid supplementation, *J. Sports Med.*, 28, 35, 1988.

94. Elam, R. P., Hardin, D. H., Sutton, R. A., and Hagen, L., Effects of arginine and ornithine on strength, lean body mass and urinary hydroxyproline in adult males, *J. Sports Med. Phys. Fitness*, 29, 52, 1989.

95. Bucci, L. R., Hickson, J. F., Pivarnik, J. M., Wolinsky, I., McMahon, J. C., and Turner, S. D., Ornithine ingestion and growth hormone release in bodybuilders, *Nutr. Res.*, 10, 239, 1990.

96. Bucci, L. R., Hickson, J. F., Wolinsky, I., and Pivarnik, J. M., Ornithine supplementation and insulin release in bodybuilders, *Int. J. Sports Nutr.*, 2, 287, 1992.

97. Cynober, L., Coudray-Lucas, C., de Bandt, J. P., Guechot, J., Aussel, C., Salvucci, M., and Giboudeau, J., Action of ornithine alpha-ketoglutarate, ornithine hydrochloride, and calcium alpha-ketoglutarate on plasma amino acid and hormonal patterns in healthy subjects, *J. Am. Coll. Nutr.*, 9, 2, 1990.

98. Kruse, C. A., Treatment of fatigue with aspartic acid salts, *Northwest Med.*, 60, 597, 1961.

99. Shaw, D. L., Chesney, M. A., Tullis, I. F., and Agersborg, M. P. K., Management of fatigue: a physiological approach, *Am. J. Med. Sci.*, 243, 758, 1962.

100. Council on Drugs, A.M.A., Potassium and magnesium aspartate (Spartase), *J. Am. Med. Assoc.*, 183, 362, 1963.

101. Ahlborg, B., Ekelund, L. G., and Nilsson, C. G., Effect of potassium-magnesium aspartate on the capacity for prolonged exercise in man, *Acta Physiol. Scand.*, 74, 238, 1968.

102. Gupta, J. S. and Srivastava, K. K., Effect of potassium-magnesium aspartate on endurance work in man, *Ind. J. Exp. Biol.*, 11, 392, 1973.

103. Von Franz, I. W. and Chintanaseri, C., Über die Wirkung des Kalium-Magnesium-Aspartates auf die Ausdauerleistung unter besonderer Berücksichtigung des Aspartates, *Sportarzt. Sportmed.*, 28, 37, 1977.

104. Nagle, F. J., Balke, B., Ganslen, R. V., and Davis, A. W., The mitigation of physical fatigue with "Spartase," *U.S. Civil Aeromed. Res. Inst.*, 11, 1963.

105. Wesson, M., McNaughton, L., Davies, P., and Tristram, S., Effects of oral administration of aspartic acid salts on the endurance capacity of trained athletes, *Res. Quart. Exer. Sport*, 59, 234, 1988.

106. Fallis, N., Wilson, W. R., Tetreault, L. L., and Lasagna, L., Effect of potassium and magnesium aspartate on athletic performance, *J. Am. Med. Assoc.*, 185, 129, 1963.

107. Consolazio, C. F., Nelson, R. A., Matoush, L. O., and Isaac, G. J., Effects of aspartic acid salts (Mg and K) on physical performance of men, *J. Appl. Physiol.*, 19, 257, 1964.

108. de Hann, A., van Doom, J. E., and Westra, H. G., Effects of potassium and magnesium aspartate on muscle metabolism and force development during intensive static exercise, *Int. J. Sports Med.*, 6, 44, 1985.

107. Hagen, R. D., Upton, S. J., Duncan, J. J., Cummings, J. M., and Gettman, L. R., Absence of effect of potassium-magnesium aspartate on physiologic response to prolonged work in aerobically trained man, *Int. J. Sports Med.*, 3, 177, 1982.

108. Maughan, R. J. and Sadler, D. J. M., The effects of oral administration of salts of aspartic acid on the metabolic response to prolonged exhausting exercise in man, *Int. J. Sports Med.*, 4, 119, 1983.

109. Hagen, R. D., Upton, S. J., Duncan, J. J., Cummings, J. M., and Gettman, L. R., Absence of effect of potassium-magnesium aspartate on physiologic response to prolonged work in aerobically trained man, *Int. J. Sports Med.*, 3, 177, 1982.

110. Maughan, R. J. and Sadler, D. J. M., Effects of the administration of salts of aspartic acid on the performance of prolonged exhausting exercise, *Med. Sci. Sports Exer.*, 14, 112, 1982.

111. Butterworth, R. F., Landreville, F., Hamel, E., Merkel, A., Giguere, F., and Barbeau, A., Effects of asparagine, glutamine and insulin on cerebral amino acid neurotransmitters, *Can. J. Neurol. Sci.*, 7, 447, 1980.

112. Reubi, J. C., Toggenburger, G., and Cuenod, M., Asparagine as precursor for transmitter aspartate in corticostriatal fibres, *J. Neurochem.*, 35, 1015, 1980.

113. Lancha, A. H., Recco, M. B., Abdalla, D. S. P., and Curi, R., Effect of aspartate, asparagine, and carnitine supplementation in the diet on metabolism of skeletal muscle during a moderate exercise, *Physiol. Behav.*, 57, 367, 1995.

114. Chang, T. W. and Goldberg, A. L., The metabolic fates of amino-acids and the formation of glutamine in skeletal muscle, *J. Biol. Chem.*, 253, 3685, 1978.

115. Graham, T. E., Turcotte, L. P., Kiens, B., and Richter, E. A., Training and muscle ammonia and amino acid metabolism in humans during prolonged exercise, *J. Appl. Physiol.*, 78, 725, 1995.

116. Lancha, A. H., Han, D. H., Hansen, P. A., and Holloszy, J. D., Effect of aspartate and asparagine supplementation in the glucose transport activity in epitrochlearis muscle, *Med. Sci. Sports Exer.*, 27 (Suppl. 5), S146, 1995.

117. Schmidbaur, H., Classen, H. G., and Helbig, J., Asparagine and glutamine as ligands for alkali and alkaline earth metals: structural chemistry contribution to the complex to magnesium therapy, *Angew. Chem.*, 102, 1122, 1990.

118. Soderlund, K. I., Energy metabolism in human skeletal muscle during intense contraction and recovery with reference to metabolic differences between type I and type II fibres, Doctoral dissertation, Karolinska Institute, Stockholm, 1991.

119. Davis, J. M., Carbohydrates, branched-chain amino acids, and endurance: the central fatigue hypothesis, *Int. J. Sport Nutr.*, 5, S29, 1995.

120. Jakeman, P. M., Hawthorne, J. E., Maxwell, S. R. J., and Kendall, M. J., Changes in circulating amino acid precursors of brain monoamine synthesis and prolactin during prolonged exhaustive endurance exercise in endurance-trained and un-trained subjects, *Clin. Sci.*, 87 (Suppl.), 52, 1994.

121. Lambert, M. I., Velloza, P. E., Wilson, G. R., and Dennis, S. C., The effect of carbohydrate and branch chain amino acid supplementation on cycling performance and mental fatigue, *Clin. Sci.*, 87 (Suppl.), 53, 1994.

122. Blomstrand, E., Celsing, F., and Newsholme, E. A., Changes in plasma concentrations of aromatic and branch-chain amino acids during sustained exercise in man and their possible role in fatigue, *Acta Physiol. Scand.*, 133, 115, 1988.

123. Blomstrand, E., Hassmen, P., Ekblom, B., and Newsholme, E. A., Administration of branched-chain amino acids during sustained exercise — Effects on performance and on plasma concentration of some amino acids, *Eur. J. Appl. Physiol.*, 63, 83, 1991.

124. Blomstrand, E., Hassmen, P., and Newsholme, E. A., Effect of branched-chain amino acid supplementation on mental performance, *Acta Physiol. Scand.*, 136, 473, 1991.

125. Hefler, S. K., Wideman, L., Gaesser, G. A., and Weltman, A., Branched-chain amino acid (BCAA) supplementation improves endurance performance in competitive cyclists, *Med. Sci. Sports Exer.*, 27 (Suppl. 5), S149, 1995.

126. Mittleman, K., Miller, C., Ricci, M., Fakhrzadeh, L., and Bailey, S. P., Branched-chain amino acid (BCAA) supplementation during prolonged exercise in heat: influence of sex, *Med. Sci. Sports Exer.*, 27(Suppl. 5), S148, 1995.

127. Galiano, F. J., Davis, J. M., Bailey, S. P., Woods, J. A., and Hamilton, M., Physiologic, endocrine and performance effects of adding branch chain amino acids to a 6% carbohydrate-electrolyte beverage during prolonged cycling, *Med. Sci. Sports Exer.*, 23, S14, 1991.

128. Carli, G., Bonifazi, M., Lodi, L., Lupo, C., Martelli, G., and Viti, A., Changes in the exercise-induced hormone response to branched chain amino acid administration, *Eur. J. Appl. Physiol.*, 64, 272, 1992.

129. De Palo, E. F., De Palo, C. B., Schiraldi, C., Gugelmetto, M., Gati, R., and Spinella, P., Branched chain amino acid (BCAA) chronic treatment and plasma human growth hormone (hGH) after physical exercise in triathlon athletes, *Clin. Sci.*, 87 (Suppl.), 51, 1994.

130. MacLean, D. A., Graham, T. E., and Saltin, B., Branched chain amino acid supplementation attenuates net muscle protein degradation during exercise, *Clin. Sci.*, 87 (Suppl.), 51, 1994.

131. Coombes, J. and McNaughton, L. R., The effects of branched chain amino acid supplementation on indicators of muscle damage after prolonged strenuous exercise, *Med. Sci. Sports Exer.*, 27 (Suppl. 5), S149, 1995.

132. Varnier, M., Sarto, P., Martines, D., Lora, L., Carmignoto, F., Leese, G., and Naccarato, R., Effect of infusing branched-chain amino acid during incremental exercise with reduced muscle glycogen content, *Eur. J. Appl. Physiol.*, 69, 26, 1994.

133. Madsen, K. and Christensen, D., Administration of glucose, glucose plus branched-chain amino acids or placebo during sustained exercise and their effects on a 100 km bike performance, *Clin. Sci.*, 87(Suppl.), 35, 1994.

134. van Hall, G., Raaymakers, J. S. H., Saris, W. H. M., and Wagenmakers, A. J. M., Supplementation with branched-chain amino acids (BCAA) and tryptophan has no effect on performance during prolonged exercise, *Clin. Sci.*, 87(Suppl.), 52, 1994.

135. Banister, E. W. and Cameron, B. J. C., Exercise-induced hyperammonemia: peripheral and central effects, *Int. J. Sports Med.*, 11, S129, 1990.

136. Mutch, B. J. C. and Banister, E. W., Ammonia metabolism in exercise and fatigue: a review, *Med. Sci. Sports Exer.*, 15, 41, 1983.

137. Banister, E. W., Rajendra, W., and Mutch, B. J. C., Ammonia as an indicator of exercise stress: implications of recent findings to sports medicine, *Sports Med.*, 2, 34, 1985.
138. Brodan, V., Kuhn, E., Pechar, J., Placer, Z., and Slabochova, Z., Effects of sodium glutamate infusion on ammonia formation during intense physical exercise in man, *Nutr. Rep. Int.*, 9, 223, 1974.
139. Rowbottom, D.G., Keast, D., and Morton, A.R., The emerging role of glutamine as an indicator of exercise stress and overtraining, *Sports Med.*, 21, 80, 1996.
140. Parry-Billings, M., Budgett, R., Koutedakis, Y., Blomstrand, E., Brooks, S., Williams, C., Calder, P. C., Pilling, S., Baigre, R., and Newsholme, E. A., Plasma amino acid concentrations in the overtraining syndrome: possible effects on the immune system, *Med. Sci. Sports Exer.*, 24, 1353, 1992.
141. Mackinnon, L. T. and Hooper, S. L., Plasma glutamine and upper respiratory tract infection during intensified training in swimmers, *Med. Sci. Sports Exer.*, 28, 285, 1996.
142. Poortmans, J. R., Castell, L. M., Leclercq, R., Brasseur, M., Duchateau, J., and Newsholme, E. A., Influence of glutamine supplementation in blood lymphocytes and plasma substrate levels after a marathon race, *Clin. Sci.*, 87(Suppl.), 25, 1994.
143. Welbourne, T. C., Increased plasma bicarbonate and growth hormone after an oral glutamine load, *Am. J. Clin. Nutr.*, 61, 1058, 1995.
144. Varnier, M., Leese, G. P., Thompson, J., and Rennie, M. J., Stimulatory effect of glutamine on glycogen accumulation in human skeletal muscle, *Am. J. Physiol.*, 269, E309, 1995.
145. Bucci, L. R., Single amino acids, in *Nutrition Applied to Injury Rehabilitation and Sports Medicine*, CRC Press, Boca Raton, FL, 1994, 33.
146. Beard, H. H., Ed., *Creatine and Creatinine Metabolism*, Brooklyn Chemical Publishers, Brooklyn, 1943.
147. Chaikelis, A. S., The effect of glycocoll (glycine) ingestion upon the growth, strength and creatinine-creatine excretion in man, *Am. J. Physiol.*, 132, 578, 1941.
148. Maison, G. L., Failure of gelatin or aminoacetic acid to increase the work ability, *J. Am. Med. Assoc.*, 115, 1439, 1940.
149. Horvath, S. M., Knehr, C. A., and Dill, D. B., The influence of glycine on muscular strength, *Am. J. Physiol.*, 134, 469, 1941.
150. King, E. Q., McCaleb, L. B., Kennedy, H. F., and Klumpp, T. G., Failure of aminoacetic acid to increase the work capacity of human subjects, *J. Am. Med. Assoc.*, 118, 594, 1942.
151. Kasai, K., Suzuki, H., Nakamura, T., Shiina, H., and Shimoda, S., Glycine stimulates growth hormone in man, *Acta Endocrinol.*, 93, 283, 1980.
152. Braverman, E. R. and Pfeiffer, C. C., Glycine, in *The Healing Nutrients Within. Facts, Findings and New Research on Amino Acids*, Keats Publishing, New Canaan, CT, 1986, 237.
153. Kasai, K., Kobayashi, M., and Shimoda, S., Stimulatory effect of glycine on human growth hormone secretion, *Metabolism*, 27, 201, 1978.
154. McCollum, R. H., The effect of L-lysine and a vitamin compound upon the physical performance of subpar college men, Ed.D. thesis, University of Oregon, Eugene, 1960.
155. Muller, E. E., Brambilla, F., Cavagnini, F., Peracchi, M., and Panerai, A., Slight effect of L-tryptophan on growth hormone release in normal human subjects, *J. Clin. Endocrinol. Metab.*, 39, 1, 1974.
156. Woolf, P. D. and Lee, L., Effect of the serotonin precursor, tryptophan, on pituitary hormone secretion, *J. Clin. Endocrinol. Metab.*, 45, 123, 1977.
157. Fraser, W. M., Tucker, H. S., Grubb, S. R., Wigand, J. P., and Blackard, W. G., Effect of L-tryptophan on growth hormone and prolactin release in normal volunteers and patients with secretory pituitary tumors, *Horm. Metab. Res.*, 11, 149, 1979.
158. Glass, A. R., Schaaf, M., and Dimond, R. C., Absent growth hormone response to L-tryptophan in acromegaly, *J. Clin. Endocrinol. Metab.*, 48, 664, 1979.
159. Koulu, M. and Lammintausta, R., Effect of methionine on L-tryptophan and apomorphine-stimulated growth hormone secretion in man, *J. Clin. Endocrinol. Metab.*, 49, 70, 1979.
160. Segura, R. and Ventura, J. L., Effect of L-tryptophan supplementation on exercise performance, *Int. J. Sports Med.*, 9, 301, 1988.
161. Slutsker, L., Eosinophilia-Myalgia Syndrome associated with exposure to tryptophan from a single manufacturer, *J. Am. Med. Assoc.*, 264, 213, 1990.
162. Belongia, R., An investigation of the cause of the Eosinophilia-Myalgia Syndrome associated with tryptophan use, *New Engl. J. Med.*, 323, 357, 1990.
163. Jaffe, R., Eosinophilia Myalgia Syndrome secondary to contaminated tryptophan — clinical experience, *J. Nutr. Med.*, 2, 195, 1991.
164. Aldhous, P., Yellow light on L-tryptophan, *Nature*, 353, 490, 1991.
165. Jaffe, R., Tryptophan update: helpful adjunct and innocent bystander, *J. Nutr. Med.*, 4, 133, 1994.
166. Dekkers, J. C., van Doornen, L. J. P., and Kemper, H. C. G., The role of antioxidant vitamins and enzymes in the prevention of exercise-induced muscle damage, *Sports Med.*, 21, 213, 1996.
167. Jenkins, R. R., Exercise, oxidative stress, and antioxidants: a review, *Int. J. Sport Nutr.*, 3, 356, 1993.
168. Kanter, M. M., Free radicals, exercise, and antioxidant supplementation, *Int. J. Sport Nutr.*, 4, 205, 1994.

169. Kanter, M. M. and Williams, M. H., Antioxidants, carnitine, and choline as putative ergogenic aids, *Int. J. Sport Nutr.*, 5, S120, 1995.

170. Aruoma, O. I., Free radicals and antioxidant strategies in sports, *J. Nutr. Biochem.*, 5, 370, 1994.

171. Keys, A., Physical performance in relation to diet, *Fed. Proc.*, 2, 164, 1943.

172. Gey, G. O., Cooper, K. H., and Bottenberg, R. A., Effect of ascorbic acid on endurance performance and athletic injury, *J. Am. Med. Assoc.*, 211, 105, 1970.

173. Bailey, D. A., Carron, A. V., Teece, R. G., and Wehner, H. J., Vitamin C supplementation related to physiological response to exercise in smoking and nonsmoking subjects, *Am. J. Clin. Nutr.*, 23, 905, 1970.

174. Bender, A. and Nash, A., Vitamin C and physical performance, *Plant Foods for Men*, 1, 217, 1975.

175. Howald, H., Segesser, B., and Korner, W. F., Ascorbic acid and athletic performance, *Ann. N.Y. Acad. Sci.*, 258, 458, 1975.

176. Inukai, M., The effect of vitamin C on anaerobic activities. Committee report on vitamin C., *Jpn. Phys. Educ. Assoc.*, No. 5, 1977.

177. Keren, G. and Epstein, Y., The effect of high dosage vitamin C intake on aerobic and anaerobic capacity, *J. Sports Med.*, 20, 145, 1980.

178. Keith, R. E. and Merrill, E., The effects of vitamin C on maximum grip strength and muscular endurance, *J. Sports Med.*, 23, 253, 1983.

179. Bramich, K. and McNaughton, L., The effects of two levels of ascorbic acid on muscular endurance, muscular strength and on VO$_2$max, *Int. Clin. Nutr. Rev.*, 7, 5, 1987.

180. Maxwell, S. R. J., Jakeman, P., Thomsen, H., Leguen, C., and Thorpe, G. H. G., Changes in plasma antioxidant status during eccentric exercise and the effect of vitamin supplementation, *Free Rad. Res. Commun.*, 19, 191, 1993.

181. Hoogerweif, A. and Hoitink, A., The influence of vitamin C administration on the mechanical efficiency of the human organism, *Int. Z. Angew. Physiol.*, 20, 164, 1963.

182. Spioch, F., Kobza, R., and Mazur, B., Influence of vitamin C upon certain functional changes and the coefficient of mechanical efficiency in humans during physical effort, *Acta Physiol. Pol.*, 17, 204, 1966.

183. Sastre, J., Asensi, M., Gasco, E., Pallardo, F. V., Ferrero, J. A., Furukawa, T., and Vina, J., Exhaustive physical exercise causes oxidation of glutathione status in blood: prevention by antioxidant administration, *Am. J. Physiol.*, 263, R992, 1992.

184. Peters, E. M., Goetzsche, J. M., Grobbelaar, B., and Noakes, T. D., Vitamin C supplementation reduces the incidence of postrace symptoms of upper-respiratory-tract infection in ultramarathon runners, *Am. J. Clin. Nutr.*, 57, 170, 1993.

185. Gerster, H., Function of vitamin E in physical exercise: a review, *Z. Ernahrungswiss*, 30, 89, 1991.

186. Packer, L., Protective role of vitamin E in biological systems, *Am. J. Clin. Nutr.*, 53, 1050S, 1991.

187. Papas, A. M., Vitamin E and exercise: aspects of biokinetics and bioavailability, *World Rev. Nutr. Diet.*, 72, 165, 1993.

188. Simon-Schnass, I., Vitamin requirements for increased physical activity: vitamin E, *World Rev. Nutr. Diet.*, 71, 144, 1993.

189. Tiidus, P. M. and Houston, M. E., Vitamin E status and response to exercise training, *Sports Med.*, 20, 12, 1995.

190. Sharman, I. M., Down, M. G., and Sen, R. N., The effects of vitamin E and training on physiological function and athletic performance in adolescent swimmers, *Br. J. Nutr.*, 26, 265, 1971.

191. Lawrence, J., Smith, J., Bower, R., and Riehl, W., The effect of alpha-tocopherol (vitamin E) and pyridoxine HCl (vitamin B6) on the swimming endurance of trained swimmers, *J. Am. Coll. Health Assoc.*, 23, 219, 1974.

192. Lawrence, J., Bower, R., Riehl, W., and Smith, J., Effects of alpha-tocopherol acetate on the swimming endurance of trained swimmers, *Am. J. Clin. Nutr.*, 28, 205, 1974.

193. Shephard, R. J., Campbell, R., Pimm, P., Stuart, D., and Wright, G., Vitamin E, exercise and the recovery from physical activity, *Eur. J. Appl. Physiol.*, 33, 119, 1974.

194. Shephard, R. J., Stuart, R., Campbell, R., Wright, G., and Pimm, P., Do athletes need vitamin E?, *Phys. Sportsmed.*, 2, 57, 1974.

195. Watt, T., Romet, T. T., McFarlane, I., McGuey, D., Allen, C., and Goode, R. C., Vitamin E and oxygen consumption, *Lancet*, 2, 354, 1974.

196. Sharman, I. M., Down, M. G., and Morgan, N. G., The effects of vitamin E on physiological function and athletic performance of trained swimmers, *J. Sports Med.*, 16, 215, 1976.

197. Talbot, D. and Jamieson, J., An examination of the effect of vitamin E on the performance of highly trained swimmers, *Can. J. Appl. Sci.*, 2, 67, 1977.

198. Dillard, C. J., Litov, R. E., Savin, W. M., Dumelin, E. E., and Tappel, A. L., Effects of exercise, vitamin E and ozone on pulmonary function and lipid peroxidation, *J. Appl. Physiol.*, 45, 927, 1978.

199. Helgheim, I., Hetland, O., Nilsson, S., Ingjer, F., and Stromme, S. B., The effects of vitamin E on serum enzyme levels following heavy exercise, *Eur. J. Appl. Physiol.*, 40, 283, 1979.

200. Hackney, J. D., Linn, W. S., Buckley, R. D., Jones, M. P., Wightman, L. H., Karuza, S. K., Blessey, R. L., and Hislop, H. J., Vitamin E supplementation and respiratory effects of ozone in humans, *J. Toxicol. Environ. Health*, 7, 383, 1981.

201. Cannon, J. C., Orencole, S. F., Fielding, R. A., Meydani, M., Meydani, S. N., Fiatarone, M. A., Blumberg, J. B., and Evans, W. J., Acute phase response in exercise: interaction of age and vitamin E on neutrophils and muscle enzyme release, *Am. J. Physiol.*, 259, R1214, 1990.

202. Lorino, A. M., Paul, M., Cocea, L., Scherrer-Crosbie, M., Dahan, E., Meignan, M., and Atlan, G., Vitamin E does not prevent exercise-induced increase in pulmonary clearance, *J. Appl. Physiol.*, 77, 2219, 1994.

203. Clausen, D. A., The combined effect of aerobic exercise and vitamin E upon cardiorespiratory endurance and measured blood variables, M.Sc. Thesis, University of Wyoming, Laramie, 1971.

204. Shephard, R. J., Vitamin E and athletic performance, *J. Sports Med.*, 23, 461, 1983.

205. Shephard, R. J., Athletic performance and urban air pollution, *Can. Med. Assoc. J.*, 131, 105, 1984.

206. Sumida, S., Tanaka, K., Kitao, H., and Nakadamo, F., Exercise-induced lipid peroxidation and leakage of enzymes before and after vitamin E supplementation, *Int. J. Biochem.*, 21, 835, 1989.

207. Goldfarb, A. H., Todd, M. K., Boyer, B. T., Alessio, H. M., and Cutler, R. G., Effect of vitamin E on lipid peroxidation at 80% VO_2max, *Med. Sci. Sports Exer.*, 21, S16, 1989.

208. Cannon, J. G., Meydani, S. N., Fielding, R. A., Fiatarone, M. A., Meydani, M., Farhangmehr, M., Orencole, S. F., Blumberg, J. B., and Evans, W. J., Acute phase response in exercise. II. Associations between vitamin E, cytokines, and muscle proteolysis, *Am. J. Physiol.*, 260, R1235, 1991.

209. Baldi, C., Sforzo, G., and Jenkins, R., The effect of vitamin E and iron supplementation on free radical production in response to exercise, *Med. Sci. Sports Exer.*, 19, S16, 1992.

210. Meydani, M., Evans, W., Handelman, G., Fielding, R. A., Meydani, S. N., Fiatarone, M. A., Blumberg, J. B., and Cannon, J. G., Antioxidant response to exercise-induced oxidative stress and protection by vitamin E, *Ann. N. Y. Acad. Sci.*, 669, 363, 1992.

211. Meydani, M., Evans, W. J., Handelman, G., Biddle, L., Fielding, R. A., Meydani, S. N., Burrill, J., Fiatarone, M. A., Blumberg, J. B., and Cannon, J. G., Protective effect of vitamin E on exercise-induced oxidative damage in young and older adults, *Am. J. Physiol.*, 264, R992, 1993.

212. Hartmann, A., Niess, A. M., Grunert-Fuchs, M., Poch, B., and Speit, G., Vitamin E prevents exercise-induced DNA damage, *Mutat. Res.*, 346, 195, 1995.

213. Kobayashi, Y., Effect of vitamin E on aerobic work performance in man during acute exposure to hypoxic hypoxia, Ph.D. dissertation, University of New Mexico, Albuquerque, 1974.

214. Simon-Schnass, I. and Pabst, H., Influence of vitamin E on physical performance, *Int. J. Vit. Nutr. Res.*, 58, 49, 1988.

215. Simon-Schnass, I. and Korniszewski, L., The influence of vitamin E on rheological parameters in high altitude mountaineers, *Int. J. Vit. Nutr. Res.*, 60, 26, 1990.

216. Simon-Schnass, I. M., Nutrition at high altitude, *J. Nutr.*, 122, 778, 1992.

217. Dragan, I., Ploesteanu, E., Cristea, E., Mohora, M., Dinu, V., and Troescu, V. S., Studies on selenium in top athletes, *Physiologie*, 25, 187, 1988.

218. Dragan, I., Dinu, V., Mohora, M., and Cristea, E., Studies regarding the antioxidant effects of selenium on top swimmers, *Rev. Rhoum. Physiol.*, 27, 15, 1990.

219. Olinescu, R., Talaban, D., Nita, S., and Mihaescu, G., Comparative study of the presence of oxidative stress in sportsmen in competition and aged people, as well as the preventive effect of selenium administration, *Rom. J. Int. Med.*, 33, 47, 1995.

220. Tessier, F., Hida, H., Favier, A., and Marconnet, P., Muscle GSH-Px activity after prolonged exercise, training, and selenium supplementation, *Biol. Tr. Elem. Res.*, 47, 279, 1995.

221. Zamora, A. J., Tessier, F., Marconnet, P., Margaritis, I., and Marini, J. F., Mitochondria changes in human muscle after prolonged exercise, endurance training and selenium supplementation, *Eur. J. Appl. Physiol.*, 71, 505, 1995.

222. Tessier, F., Margaritis, I., Richard, M. J., Moynot, C., and Marconnet, P., Selenium and training effects on the glutathione system and aerobic performance, *Med. Sci. Sports Exer.*, 27, 390, 1995.

223. Novelli, G. P., Falsini, S., and Bracciotti, G., Exogenous glutathione increases endurance to muscle effort in mice, *Pharmacol. Res.*, 23, 149, 1991.

224. Leeuwenburgh, C., Fiebig, R., Leichtweis, S., Hollander, J., and Ji, L. L., Effect of glutathione and glutathione ester supplementation during prolonged exercise, *Med. Sci. Sports Exer.*, 27 (Suppl. 5), S39, 1995.

225. Ji, L. L., Katz, A., Fu, R., Griffiths, M., and Spencer, M., Blood glutathione status during exercise: effect of carbohydrate supplementation, *J. Appl. Physiol.*, 74, 788, 1993.

226. Kagan, V. E., Spirichev, V. B., and Erin, A. N., Vitamin E in physical exercise and sport, in *Nutrition in Exercise and Sport*, Hickson, J. F., and Wolinsky, I., Eds., CRC Press, Boca Raton, 1989, 255.

227. Bors, W., Heler, W., Michel, C., and Stettmaier, K., Flavonoids and polyphenols: chemistry and biology, in *Handbook of Antioxidants*, Cadenas, E. and Packer, L., Eds., Marcel Dekker, New York, 1996, 409.

228. Weisburger, J. H., Tea antioxidants and health, in *Handbook of Antioxidants*, Cadenas, E. and Packer, L., Eds., Marcel Dekker, New York, 1996, 469.

229. Haramaki, N., Packer, L., Droy-Lefaix, M. T., and Christen, Y., Antioxidant actions and health implications of *Ginkgo biloba* extract, in *Handbook of Antioxidants*, Cadenas, E. and Packer, L., Eds., Marcel Dekker, New York, 1996, 487.

230. Elstner, E. F. and Kleber, E., Radical scavenger properties of leucocyanidine, in *Flavonoids in Biology and Medicine III*, Das, N. P., Ed., National University of Singapore, 1990, 227.

231. Viguie, C. A., Packer, L., and Brooks, G. A., Antioxidant supplementation affects indices of muscle trauma and oxidant stress in human blood during exercise, *Med. Sci. Sports Exer.*, 21, S16, 1989.

232. Kanter, M. M., Nolte, L. A., and Holloszy, J. O., Effects of an antioxidant supplement on expired pentane production following low and high intensity exercise, *Med. Sci. Sports Exer.*, 22(Suppl. 2), S86, 1990.

233. Kanter, M. M. and Eddy, D. E., Effect of antioxidant supplementation on serum markers of lipid peroxidation and skeletal muscle damage following eccentric exercise, *Med. Sci. Sports Exer.*, 24, S17, 1992.

234. Witt, E. H., Reznick, A. Z., Viguie, C. A., Starke-Reed, P., and Packer, L., Exercise, oxidative damage and effects of antioxidant manipulation, *J. Nutr.*, 122, 766, 1992.

235. Kanter, M. M., Nolte, L. A., and Holloszy, J. O., Effects of an antioxidant vitamin mixture on lipid peroxidation at rest and postexercise, *J. Appl. Physiol.*, 74, 965, 1993.

236. Kankaanpaa, M. J., Marin, E., Ristonmaa, U., Airaksinen, O., Hanninen, O., and Bray, T. M., Effect of vitamin C, vitamin E, β-carotene and selenium supplementation on exercise performance in humans, *Med. Sci. Sports Exer.*, 26, S67, 1994.

237. Snider, I. P., Bazzare, T. L., Murdoch, S. D., and Goldfarb, A., Effects of coenzyme athletic performance system as an ergogenic aid on endurance performance to exhaustion, *Int. J. Sport Nutr.*, 2, 272, 1992.

238. Ismail, A. H., Petro, T. M., and Watson, R. R., Dietary supplementation with vitamin E and C in fit and nonfit adults: biochemical and immunological changes, *Fed. Proc.*, 42, 335, 1983.

239. Hobbs, C., *The Ginsengs, A User's Guide*, Botanica Press, Santa Cruz, CA, 1996.

240. Bahrke, M.S. and Morgan, W.P., Evaluation of the ergogenic properties of ginseng, *Sports Med.*, 18, 229, 1994.

241. Bucci, L. R., Selected herbals and human exercise performance, *Am. J. Clin. Nutr.*, in press, 1997.

242. McNaughton, L., Egan, G., and Caelli, G., A comparison of Chinese and Russian ginseng as ergogenic aids to improve various facets of physical fitness, *Int. Clin. Nutr. Rev.*, 90, 32, 1989.

243. Dowling, E. A., Redondo, D. R., Branch, J. D., Jones, S., McNabb, G., and Williams, M. H., Effect of *Eleutherococcus senticosus* on submaximal and maximal exercise performance, *Med. Sci. Sports Exer.*, 28, 482, 1996.

244. Kalix, P., Pharmacology of psychoactive alkaloids from Ephedra and Catha, *J. Ethnopharmacol.*, 32, 201, 1991.

245. Daly, P., Krieger, D., Dulloo, A., Young, J., and Landsberg, L., Ephedrine, caffeine and aspirin: safety and efficacy for treatment of human obesity, *Int. J. Obesity*, 17, S73, 1993.

246. Qian, J., Zhang, H., Yang, G., and Wang, B., Protective effects of *Rhodiola crenulata* on rats under antiorthostatic position and professional athletes, *Space Med. Med. Engineering*, 6, 6, 1993.

247. Bucci, L. R., Nutritional ergogenic aids, in *Nutrition in Exercise and Sport*, Hickson, J. F. and Wolinsky, I., Eds., CRC Press, Boca Raton, FL, 107, 1989.

248. Clarkson, P. M., Nutritional ergogenic aids: caffeine, *Int. J. Sports Nutr.*, 3, 103, 1993.

249. Dodd, S. L., Herb, R. A., and Powers, S. K., Caffeine and exercise performance. An update, *Sports Med.*, 15, 14, 1993.

250. Graham, T. E., Rush, J. W. E., and VanSoeren, M. H., Caffeine and exercise: metabolism and performance, *Can. J. Appl. Physiol.*, 2, 111, 1994.

251. Nehlig, A. and Debry, G., Caffeine and sports activity: a review, *Int. J. Sports Med.*, 15, 215, 1994.

252. Tarnopolsky, M. A., Caffeine and exercise performance, *Sports Med.*, 18, 109, 1994.

253. Spriet, L. L., Caffeine and performance, *Int. J. Sports Nutr.*, 5, S84, 1995.

254. Graham, T. E. and Spriet, L. L., Caffeine and exercise performance, *Sports Sci. Exchange*, 9, 1, 1996.

255. Bruni, O. J., *Gamma Oryzanol — The Facts*, Claudell Publishing, Houston, TX, 1989.

256. Gorewit, R. C., Pituitary and thyroid hormone responses of heifers after ferulic acid administration, *J. Dairy Sci.*, 66, 624, 1983.

257. Bucci, L. R., Blackman, G., Defoyd, W., Kaufmann, R., Mandel-Tayes, C., Sparks, W. S., Stiles, J. C., and Hickson, J. F., Effect of ferulate on strength and body composition of weightlifters, *J. Appl. Sport Sci. Res.*, 4, 104, 1990.

258. Bonner, B., Warren, B., and Bucci, L., Influence of ferulate supplementation on postexercise stress hormone levels after repeated exercise stress, *J. Appl. Sport Sci. Res.*, 4, 110, 1990.

259. Wheeler, K. B. and Garleb, K. A., Gamma oryzanol-plant sterol supplementation: metabolic, endocrine, and physiologic effects, *Int. J. Sports Nutr.*, 1, 170, 1991.

260. Saint-John, M. and McNaughton, L., Octacosanol ingestion and its effects on metabolic responses to submaximal cycle ergometry, reaction time and chest and grip strength, *Int. Clin. Nutr. Rev.*, 6, 81, 1986.

261. Hultman, E. and Sahlin, K., Acid-base balance during exercise, *Exer. Sport Sci. Rev.*, 8, 41, 1980.

262. Bucci, L. R., Micronutrient supplementation and ergogenesis — metabolic intermediates, in *Nutrients as Ergogenic Aids for Sports and Exercise*, CRC Press, Boca Raton, FL, 1993, 41.

263. Linderman, J. and Fahey, T. D., Sodium bicarbonate ingestion and exercise performance. An update, Sports Med., 11, 71, 1991.

264. Matson, L. G. and Tran, Z. V., Effects of sodium bicarbonate ingestion on anaerobic performance: a meta-analytic review, *Int. J. Sport Nutr.*, 3, 2, 1993.

265. Linderman, J. K. and Gosselink, K. L., The effects of sodium bicarbonate ingestion on exercise performance, *Sports Med.*, 18, 75, 1994.

266. Horswill, C. A., Effects of bicarbonate, citrate, and phosphate loading on performance, *Int. J. Sport Nutr.*, 5, S111, 1995.

267. Kozak-Collins, K., Burke, E. R., and Schoene, R. B., Sodium bicarbonate ingestion does not improve performance in women cyclists, *Med. Sci. Sports Exer.*, 26, 1510, 1994.

268. Bird, S. R., Wiles, J., and Robbins, J., The effect of sodium bicarbonate ingestion on 1500-m racing time, *J. Sports Sci.*, 13, 399, 1995.

269. Nickel, G. L., Potteiger, J. A., Webster, M. L., Haub, M. D., and Palmer, R. J., The effects of sodium bicarbonate and sodium citrate ingestion on endurance running performance, *Med. Sci. Sports Exer.*, 27, S148, 1995.

270. Gladden, L. B., Portington, K. J., Pascoe, D. D., Webster, M. J., Anderson, L. H., and Rutland, R. R., Sodium bicarbonate ingestion does not improve resistance exercise performance, *Med. Sci. Sports Exer.*, 27, S148, 1995.

271. Aschenbach, W. G., Williams, J. H., Ocel, J. V., Craft, L. L., and Ward, C. W., Effect of $NaHCO_3$ and NaCl on high-intensity exercise in college wrestlers, *Med. Sci. Sports Exer.*, 27, S149, 1995.

272. Gaitanos, G. C., Williams, C., Boobis, L. H., Brooks, S., and Lakomy, H. K. A., Sodium bicarbonate ingestion, muscle metabolism and performance during intermittent maximal exercise, *Clin. Sci.*, 87 (Suppl.), 27, 1994.

273. Murphy, R. M., Stathis, C. G., Selig, S. E., McKenna, M. J., Febbraio, M. A., Carey, M. F., and Snow, R. J., The effects of sodium bicarbonate ingestion on adenine nucleotide metabolism during intermittent, high intensity exercise, *Clin. Sci.*, 87 (Suppl.), 119, 1994.

274. Johnson, W. R. and Black, D. H., Comparison of effects of certain blood alkalinizers and glucose upon competitive endurance performance, *J. Appl. Physiol.*, 5, 577, 1953.

275. Parry-Billings, M. and MacLaren, D. P. M., The effect of sodium bicarbonate and sodium citrate ingestion on anaerobic power during intermittent exercise, *Eur. J. Appl. Physiol.*, 55, 224, 1986.

276. Kowalchuk, J. M., Maltais, S. A., Yamaji, K., and Hughson, R. L., The effect of citrate loading on exercise performance, acid-base balance and metabolism, *Eur. J. Appl. Physiol.*, 58, 858, 1989.

277. Cox, G. and Jenkins, D. G., The physiological and ventilatory responses to repeated 60 s sprints following sodium citrate ingestion, *J. Sports Sci.*, 12, 469, 1994.

278. McNaughton, L. R., Sodium citrate and anaerobic performance: implications of dosage, *Eur. J. Appl. Physiol.*, 61, 392, 1990.

279. McNaughton, L. and Cedaro, R., Sodium citrate ingestion and its effects on maximal anaerobic exercise of different durations, *Eur. J. Appl. Physiol.*, 64, 36, 1992.

280. Pujol, P., Effect of citrate loading on muscle metabolism during isometric exercise as assessed by ^{32}P NMRS and NIRS, *Med. Sci. Sports Exer.*, 27, S144, 1995.

281. Potteiger, J. A., Nickel, G. L., Webster, M. J., Haub, M. D., and Palmer, R. J., Sodium citrate ingestion enhances 30 km cycling performance, *Int. J. Sports Med.*, 17, 7, 1996.

282. McCarty, M. F., Inhibition of citrate lyase may aid aerobic endurance, *Med. Hypotheses*, 45, 247, 1995.

283. Conte, A. A., A non-prescription alternative in weight reduction therapy, *The Bariatrician*, Summer, 17, 1993.

284. McCarty, M. F., Promotion of hepatic lipid oxidation and gluconeogenesis as a strategy for appetite control, *Med. Hypoth.*, 42, 215, 1994.

285. Heinonen, O. J., Carnitine and physical exercise, *Sports Med.*, 22, 109, 1996.

286. Cerretelli, P. and Marconi, C., L-Carnitine supplementation in humans. The effects on physical performance, *Int. J. Sports Med.*, 11, 1, 1990.

287. Wagenmakers, A. J. M., L-carnitine supplementation and performance in man, in *Advances in Nutrition and Top Sport: Medicine and Sport Science*, Vol. 32, Brouns, F., Ed., Karger, Basel, 1991, 110.

288. Clarkson, P. M., Nutritional ergogenic aids: carnitine, *Int. J. Sport Nutr.*, 2, 185, 1992.

289. Brass, E. and Hiatt, W., Carnitine metabolism during exercise, *Life Sci.*, 54, 1383, 1994.

290. Dubelaar, M. L., Lucas, C. M., and Hulsmann, W. C., Acute effect of L-carnitine on skeletal muscle force tests in dogs, *Am. J. Physiol.*, 260, E189, 1991.

291. Corbucci, G. G., Montanari, G., Mancinelli, G., and Diddio, S., Metabolic effects induced by L-carnitine and propionyl-L-carnitine in human hypoxic muscle tissue during exercise, *Int. J. Clin. Pharmacol. Res.*, 10, 197, 1990.

292. Cereda, G. and Scolari, M., Effect of an energy stimulator on the performance of a group of young people: evaluation of a videogame test, *Acta Vitaminol. Enzymol.*, 6, 63, 1984.

293. Bidzinka, B., Petraglia, F., and Angioni, S., Effect of different chronic stressors and acetyl-L-carnitine on hypothalamic beta-endorphin and GnRH and on plasma testosterone levels in male rats, *Neuroendocrinology*, 57, 985, 1993.

294. Lenaz, G., Fato, R., Castelluccio, C., Batino, M., Cavazzoni, M., Rauchova, H., and Castelli, G. P., Coenzyme Q saturation kinetics of mitochondrial enzymes: Theory, experimental aspects and biomedical implications, in *Biomedical and Clinical Aspects of Coenzyme Q*, Vol. 6, Folkers, K., Yamagami, T., and Littarru, G. P., Eds., Elsevier/North-Holland, Amsterdam, 1991, 11.

295. Vanfraechem, J. and Folkers, K., Coenzyme Q_{10} and physical performance, in *Biomedical and Clinical Aspects of Coenzyme Q*, Vol. 3, Folkers, K. and Yamamura, Y., Eds., Elsevier/North-Holland, Amsterdam, 1981, 235.

296. Wyss, V., Lubich, T., Ganzit, G. P., Cesaretti, D., Fiorella, P. L., Dei Rocini, C., Bargossi, A. M., Battistoni, R., Lippi, A., Grossi, G., Sprovieri, G., and Battino, M., Remarks on prolonged ubiquinone administration in physical exercise, in *Highlights in Ubiquinone Research*, Lenaz, G., Barnabei, O., Rabbi, A., and Battino, M., Eds., Taylor and Francis, London, 1990, 303.

297. Fiorella, P. L., Bargossi, A. M., Grossi, G., Motta, R., Senaldi, R., Battino, M., Sassi, S., Sprovieri, G., and Lubich, T., Metabolic effects of coenzyme Q_{10} treatment in high level athletes, in *Biomedical and Clinical Aspects of Coenzyme Q*, Vol. 6, Folkers, K., Yamagami, T., and Littarru, G. P., Eds., Elsevier/North-Holland, Amsterdam, 1991, 513.

298. Zeppilli, P., Merlino, B., de Luca, A., Palmieri, V., Santini, C., Vannicelli, R., la Rosa Gangi, M., Caccese, R., Cameli, S., Servidei, S., Ricci, E., Silvestri, G., Lippa, S., Oradei, A., and Littarru, G. P., Influence of coenzyme Q_{10} on physical work capacity in athletes, sedentary people and patients with mitochondrial disease, in *Biomedical and Clinical Aspects of Coenzyme Q*, Vol. 6, Folkers, K., Yamagami, T., and Littarru, G. P., Eds., Elsevier/North-Holland, Amsterdam, 1991, 541.

299. Yamabe, H., and Fukuzaki, H., The beneficial effect of coenzyme Q_{10} on the impaired aerobic function in middle aged women without organic disease, in *Biomedical and Clinical Aspects of Coenzyme Q*, Vol. 6, Folkers, K., Yamagami, T., and Littarru, G. P., Eds., Elsevier/North-Holland, Amsterdam, 1991, 535.

300. Ostman, B., Foxdal, P., Sjodin, A., Branth, S., and Sjodin, B., The effect of vitamin E and ubiquinone-10 supplementation on physical performance and muscle metabolism, *Clin. Sci.*, 87, 80, 1984.

301. Guerra, G. P., Ballardini, E., Lippa, S., Oradel, A., and Littarru, G. P., Effetto della somministrazione di Ubidearenone sul consumo massimo di ossigeno e sulla performance fisica in un gruppo di giovani ciclisti, *Med. Sport*, 40, 359, 1987.

302. Zuliani, U., Bonetti, A., Campana, M., and Cerioli, G., The influence of ubiquinone (CoQ_{10}) on the metabolic response to work, *J. Sports Med.*, 29, 57, 1989.

303. Cerioli, G., Tirelli, G., and Musiani, L., Effect of CoQ_{10} on the metabolic response to work, in *Biomedical and Clinical Aspects of Coenzyme Q*, Vol. 6, Folkers, K., Yamagami, T., and Littarru, G. P., Eds., Elsevier/North-Holland, Amsterdam, 1991, 521.

304. Amadio, E., Palermo, R., Peloni, G., and Littarru, G. P., Effect of CoQ_{10} administration on VO$_2$max and diastolic function in athletes, in *Biomedical and Clinical Aspects of Coenzyme Q*, Vol. 6, Folkers, K., Yamagami, T., and Littarru, G. P., Eds., Elsevier/North-Holland, Amsterdam, 1991, 525.

305. Braun, B., Clarkson, P. M., Freedson, P. S., and Kohl, R. L., Effects of coenzyme Q10 supplementation on exercise performance, VO2max, and lipid peroxidation in trained cyclists, *Int. J. Sport Nutr.*, 1, 353, 1991.

306. Porter, D. A., Costill, D. L., Zachwieja, J. J., Krzeminski, K., Fink, W. J., Wagner, E., and Folkers, K., The effect of oral coenzyme Q10 on the exercise tolerance of middle-aged, untrained men, *Int. J. Sports Med.*, 16, 421, 1995.

307. Roberts, J., The effects of coenzyme Q10 on exercise performance, *Med. Sci. Sports Exer.*, 22, S87, 1990.

308. Balsom, P. D., Söderlund, K., and Ekblom, B., Creatine in humans with special reference to creatine supplementation, *Sports Med.*, 18, 268, 1994.

309. Maughan, R. J., Creatine supplementation and exercise performance, *Int. J. Sport Nutr.*, 5, 94, 1995.

310. Greenhaff, P. L., Creatine and its application as an ergogenic aid, *Int. J. Sport Nutr.*, 5, S100, 1995.

311. Greenhaff, P. L., Casey, A., Short, A. H., Harris, R. C., Söderlund, K., and Hultman, E., Influence of oral creatine supplementation on muscle torque during repeated bouts of maximal voluntary exercise in man, *Clin. Sci.*, 84, 565, 1993.

312. Balsom, P. D., Ekblom, B., Söderlund, K., Sjodin, B., and Hultman, E., Creatine supplementation and dynamic high-intensity intermittent exercise, *Scand. J. Med. Sci. Sports*, 3, 143, 1993.

313. Harris, R. C., Viru, M., Greenhaff, P. L., and Hultman, E., The effect of oral creatine supplementation on running performance during maximal short term exercise in man, *J. Physiol.*, 467, 74P, 1993.

314. Harridge, S. D. R., Balsom, P. D., and Söderlund, K., Creatine supplementation and electrically evoked human muscle fatigue, *Clin. Sci.*, 87 (Suppl.), 124, 1994.

315. Birch, R., Noble, D., and Greenhaff, P. L., The influence of dietary creatine supplementation on performance during repeated bouts of maximal isokinetic cycling in man, *Eur. J. Appl. Physiol.*, 69, 268, 1994.

316. Söderlund, K., Balsom, P. D., and Ekblom, B., Creatine supplementation and high intensity exercise: influence on performance and muscle metabolism, *Clin. Sci.*, 87(Suppl.), 120, 1994.

317. Ziegenfuss, T., Bredle, D., Rogers, M., Newcomer, B., Boska, M., and Lemon, P., Effect of creatine on repeated maximal muscle contraction, *Can. J. Appl. Physiol.*, 19, 36, 1994.

318. Lemon, P., Boska, M., Bredle, D., Rogers, M., Zeigenfuss, T., and Newcomer, B., Effect of oral creatine supplementation on energetics during repeated maximal muscle contraction, *Med. Sci. Sports Exer.*, 27, S148, 1995.

319. Grindstaff, P., Kreider, R., Weiss, L., Fry, A., Wood, L., Bullen, D., Miyaji, M., Ramsey, L., Li, Y., and Almada, A., Effects of ingesting a supplement containing creatine monohydrate for 7 days on isokinetic performance, *Med. Sci. Sports Exer.*, 27, S146, 1995.

320. Almada, A., Kreider, R., Weiss, L., Fry, A., Wood, L., Bullen, D., Miyaji, M., Grindstaff, P., Ramsey, L., and Li, Y., Effects of ingesting a supplement containing creatine monohydrate for 28 days on isokinetic performance, *Med. Sci. Sports Exer.*, 27, S146, 1995.

321. Balsom, P. D., Söderlund, K., Sjödin, B., and Ekblom, B., Skeletal muscle metabolism during short duration high-intensity exercise: influence of creatine supplementation, *Acta Physiol. Scand.*, 154, 303, 1995.

322. Earnest, C. P., Snell, P. G., Rodriguez, R., Almada, A. L., and Mitchell, T. L., The effect of creatine monohydrate ingestion on anaerobic power indices, muscular strength, and body composition, *Acta Physiol. Scand.*, 153, 207, 1995.

323. Odland, L. M., MacDougall, J. D., Tarnopolsky, M., Elorriaga, A., Borgmann, A., and Atkinson, S., The effect of oral Cr supplementation on muscle (PCr) and power output during a short-term maximal cycling task, *Med. Sci. Sports Exer.*, 26, S23, 1994.

324. Earnest, C. P., Snell, P. G., Mitchell, T. L., Rodriguez, R., and Almada, A. L., Effect of creatine monohydrate on peak anaerobic power, capacity and fatigue index, *Med. Sci. Sports Exer.*, 26, S39, 1994.

325. Redondo, D., Williams, M., Dowling, E., Graham, B., Jones, S., and Almada, A., The effect of oral creatine monohydrate supplementation on running velocity, *Med. Sci. Sports Exer.*, 27, S146, 1995.

326. Burke, L. M., Pyne, D. B., and Telford, R. D., Oral creatine supplementation does not improve sprint performance in elite swimmers, *Med. Sci. Sports Exer.*, 27, S146, 1995.

327. Febbraio, M. A., Flanagan, T. R., Snow, R. J., Zhao, S., and Carey, M. F., Effect of creatine supplementation on intramuscular TCr, metabolism and performance during intermittent, supramaximal exercise in humans, *Acta Physiol. Scand.*, 155, 387, 1995.

328. Cooke, W. H., Grandjean, P. W., and Barnes, W. S., Effect of oral creatine supplementation on power output and fatigue during bicycle ergometry, *J. Appl. Physiol.*, 78, 670, 1995.

329. Balsom, P. D., Harridge, S. D. R., Söderlund, K., Sjödin, B., and Ekblom, B., Creatine supplementation *per se* does not enhance endurance exerciser performance, *Acta Physiol. Scand.*, 149, 521, 1993.

330. Östberg, K. and Söderlund, K., Kreatin, *Skidskytte*, 5, 16, 1993.

331. Sipilä, I., Rapola, J., Simell, O., and Vannas, A., Supplementary creatine as a treatment for gyrate atrophy of the chorioid and retina, *New Engl. J. Med.*, 304, 867, 1981.

332. Vannas-Sulonen, K., Sipilä, I., Vannas, A., Simell, O., and Rapola, J., Gyrate atrophy of the choroid and retina — a five year follow-up of creatine supplementation, *Ophthalmology*, 92, 1719, 1985.

333. Pirola, V., Pisani, L., and Teruzzi, P., Evaluation of the recovery of muscular trophicity in aged patients with femoral fractures treated with creatine phosphate and physiokinesitherapy, *Clin. Ter.*, 139, 115, 1991.

334. Satolli, F. and Marchesi, G., Creatine phosphate in the rehabilitation of patients with muscle hyponotrophy of the lower extremity, *Curr. Ther. Res.*, 46, 67, 1989.

335. Stramentinoli, G., Pharmacological aspects of S-adenosylmethionine. Pharmacokinetics and pharmacodynamics, *Am. J. Med.*, 83 (Suppl. 5A), 35, 1987.

336. Gray, M. E. and Titlow, L. W., B_{15}: myth or miracle?, *Phys. Sportsmed.*, 10, 107, 1982.

337. Pipes, T. V., The effects of pangamic acid on performance in trained athletes, *Med. Sci. Sports Exer.*, 12, 98, 1980.

338. Kemp, G. L., A clinical study and evaluation of pangamic acid, *J. Am. Osteopath. Assoc.*, 58, 714, 1959.

339. Girandola, R. N., Wiswell, R. A., and Bulbulian, R., Effects of pangamic acid (B-15) ingestion on metabolic response to exercise, *Med. Sci. Sports Exer.*, 12, 98, 1980.

340. Girondola, R. N., Wiswell, R. A., and Bulbulian, R., Effects of pangamic acid (B-15) ingestion on metabolic response to exercise, *Biochem. Med.*, 24, 218, 1980.

341. Black, D. G. and Suec, A. A., Effects of calcium pangamate on aerobic endurance parameters. A double-blind study, *Med. Sci. Sports Exer.*, 13, 93, 1981.

342. Gray, M. E. and Titlow, L. W., The effect of pangamic acid on maximal treadmill performance, *Med. Sci. Sports Exer.*, 14, 424, 1982.

343. Harpaz, M., Otto, R. M., and Smith, T. K., The effect of N_1N_1-dimethylglycine ingestion upon aerobic performance, *Med. Sci. Sports Exer.*, 17, 287, 1985.

344. Bishop, P. A., Smith, J. F., and Young, B., Effects of N,N-dimethylglycine on physiological response and performance in trained runners, *J. Sports Med. Phys. Fit.*, 27, 53, 1987.

345. Conaly, L.A., Wurtman, R. J., Blusztaijn, K., Coviella, I. L. G., Maher, T. J., and Evoniuk, G. E., Decreased plasma choline concentrations in marathon runners, *New Engl. J. Med.*, 315, 892, 1986.

346. Conlay, L. A., Sabounjian, L. A., and Wurtman, R. J., Exercise and neuromodulators: choline and acetyl-choline in marathon runners, *Int. J. Sports Med.*, 13 (Suppl. 1), S141, 1992.

347. Sandage, B. W., Choline, in Workshop on Dietary Supplements for Physically Active People, National Institutes of Health, Office of Dietary Supplements, Bethesda, MD, June 1996.

348. Sandage, B. W., Sabounjian, L., White, R., and Wurtman, R. J., Choline citrate may enhance endurance athletic performance, *Physiologist*, 35, 236, 1992.

349. Spector, S. A., Jackman, M. R., Sabounjian, L. A., Sakkas, C., Landers, D. M., and Willis, W. T., Effect of choline supplementation on fatigue in trained cyclists, *Med. Sci. Sports Exer.*, 27, 668, 1995.

350. Dodson, W. L. and Sachan, D. S., Choline supplementation reduces urinary carnitine excretion in humans, *Am. J. Clin. Nutr.*, 63, 904, 1996.

351. von Allworden, H. N., Horn, S., Kahl, J., and Feldheim, W., The influence of lecithin on plasma choline concentrations in triathletes and adolescent runners during exercise, *Eur. J. Appl. Physiol.*, 67, 87, 1993.

352. DiPasquale, M. G., Inosine, *Drugs Sports*, 3, 6, 1995.

353. Williams, M. H., Kreider, R. B., Hunter, D. W., Somma, C. T., Shall, L. M., Woodhouse, M. L., and Rokitski, L., Effect of inosine supplementation on 3-mile treadmill run performance and VO$_2$peak, *Med. Sci. Sports Exer.*, 22, 517, 1990.

354. Bucci, L. R., Normal cellular components: proteases, nucleic acids, and antioxidant enzymes, in *Nutrition Applied to Injury Rehabilitation and Sports Medicine*, CRC Press, Boca Raton, FL, 1994, 175.

355. Fahey, T. D., Larsen, J. D., Brooks, G. A., Colvin, W., Henderson, S., and Lary, D., The effect of ingesting polylactate or glucose polymer drinks during prolonged exercise, *Int. J. Sport Nutr.*, 1, 249, 1991.

356. Swensen, T., Crater, G., Bassett, G. R., and Howley, E. T., Adding polylactate to a glucose polymer solution does not improve endurance, *Int. J. Sports Med.*, 15, 430, 1994.

357. Bryner, R., Hornsby, G., Chetlin, R., Ullrich, I., and Yeater, R., Effect of lactate consumption on exercise performance, *Med. Sci. Sports Exer.*, 27, S148, 1995.

358. Brouns, F., Fogelholm, M., van Hall, G., Wagenmakers, A., and Saris, W.H.M., Chronic oral lactate supplementation does not affect lactate disappearance from blood after exercise, *Int. J. Sport Nutr.*, 5, 117, 1995.

359. Stanko, R. T., Robertson, R. J., Galbreath, R. W., Reilly, J. J., Greenawalt, K. D., and Goss, F. L., Enhanced leg exercise endurance with a high carbohydrate diet and dihydroxyacetone and pyruvate, *J. Appl. Physiol.*, 69, 1651, 1991.

360. Stanko, R. T., Robertson, R. J., Spina, R. J., Reilly, J. J., Greenawalt, K. D., and Goss, F. L., Enhancement of arm exercise endurance capacity with dihydroxyacetone and pyruvate, *J. Appl. Physiol.*, 68, 119, 1990.

361. Robertson, R. J., Stanko, R. T., Goss, F. L., Spina, R. J., Reilly, J. J., and Greenawalt, K. D., Blood glucose extraction as a mediator of perceived exertion during prolonged exercise, *Eur. J. Appl. Physiol.*, 61, 100, 1990.

362. Stanko, R. T., Tietze, D. L., and Arch, J. E., Body composition, energy utilization, and nitrogen metabolism with a severely restricted diet supplemented with dihydroxyacetone and pyruvate, *Am. J. Clin. Nutr.*, 55, 771, 1992.

363. Stanko, R. T., Tietze, D. L., and Arch, J. E., Body composition, energy utilization, and nitrogen metabolism with a 4.2 MJ/d low energy diet supplemented with pyruvate, *Am. J. Clin. Nutr.*, 56, 630, 1992.

364. Stanko, R. T., Reynolds, H. R., Hoyson, R., Janosky, J. E., and Wolf R., Pyruvate supplementation of a low-cholesterol, low-fat diet: effects on plasma lipid concentrations and body composition in hyperlipidemic patients, *Am. J. Clin. Nutr.*, 59, 423, 1994.

365. Marconi, C., Sassi, G., and Cerretelli, P., The effect of an alphaketoglutarate-pyridoxine complex on human maximal aerobic performance, *Eur. J. Appl. Physiol.*, 49, 307, 1982.

366. Cynober, L., Ornithine α-ketoglutarate in nutritional support, *Nutrition*, 7, 1, 1991.

367. Silk, D. B. A. and Payne-James, J. J., Novel substrates and nutritional support: possible role of ornithine α-ketoglutarate, *Proc. Nutr. Soc.*, 49, 381, 1990.

368. Takahara, J., Yunoki, S., Yakushiji, W., Yamauchi, J., Yamane, Y., and Ofuji, T., Stimulatory effects of gamma-hydroxybutyric acid on growth hormone and prolactin release in humans, *J. Clin. Endocrinol. Metab.*, 44, 1014, 1977.

369. Nissen, S., Panton, L., Wilhelm, R., and Fuller, J. C., Effect of β-hydroxy-β-methylbutyrate (HMB) supplementation on strength and body composition of trained and untrained males undergoing intense resistance training, *FASEB J.*, 10, A287, 1996.

370. Schwellnus, M. P. and Jordaan, G., Does calcium supplementation prevent bone stress injuries? A clinical trial, *Int. J. Sport Nutr.*, 2, 165, 1992.

371. Fogelholm, M., Indicators of vitamin and mineral status in athletes' blood: a review, *Int. J. Sport Nutr.*, 5, 267, 1995.

372. Liu, L., Borowski, G., and Rose, L. I., Hypomagnesemia in a tennis player, *Phys. Sportsmed.*, 11, 79, 1983.

373. Steinacker, J. M., Grünert-Fuchs, M., Steininger, K., and Wodick, R. E., Effects of long-time administration of magnesium on physical capacity, *Int. J. Sports Med.*, 8, 151, 1987.

374. Lukaski, H. C., Micronutrients (magnesium, zinc, and copper): are mineral supplements needed for athletes?, *Int. J. Sport Nutr.*, 5, S74, 1995.

375. Brilla, L. and Haley, T., Effect of magnesium supplementation on strength training in humans, *J. Am. Coll. Nutr.*, 11, 326, 1992.

376. Terblanche, S., Noakes, T. D., Dennis, S. C., Marais, D. W., and Eckert, M., Failure of magnesium supplementation to influence marathon running performance or recovery in magnesium-replete subjects, *Int. J. Sport Nutr.*, 2, 154, 1992.

377. Krotkiewski, M., Gudmundsson, M., Backsrtrom, P., and Mandroukas, K., Zinc and muscle strength and endurance, *Acta Physiol. Scand.*, 116, 309, 1982.

378. Fairbanks, V. F., Iron in medicine and nutrition, in *Modern Nutrition in Health and Disease*, 8th ed., Shils, M. E., Olson, J. A., and Shike, M., Eds., Vol. 1, Lea and Febiger, Philadelphia, 1994, 185.

379. Hastka, J., Lasserre, J. J., Schwarzbeck, A., Reiter, A., and Hehlmann, R., Laboratory tests of iron status: correlation or common sense?, *Clin. Chem.*, 42, 718, 1996.

380. Williams, M. H., The role of minerals in physical activity, in *Nutritional Aspects of Human Physical Performance*, 2nd ed., Charles C Thomas, Springfield, IL, 1985, 186.

381. Sherman, A. R. and Kramer, B., Iron nutrition and exercise, in *Nutrition in Exercise and Sports*, Hickson, J. F. and Wolinsky, I., Eds., CRC Press, Boca Raton, FL, 1989, 291.

382. Clarkson, P. M., Vitamins and trace minerals, in *Perspectives in Exercise Science and Sports Medicine. Volume 4: Ergogenics — Enhancement of Performance in Exercise and Sport*, Lamb, D. R. and Williams, M. H., Eds., Brown & Benchmark, Ann Arbor, MI, 1991, 123.

383. Haymes, E. M., Trace minerals and exercise, in *Nutrition in Exercise and Sports*, 2nd ed., Wolinsky, I. and Hickson, J. F., Eds., CRC Press, Boca Raton, FL, 1994, 223.

384. Bucci, L. R., Micronutrient supplementation and ergogenesis — minerals, in *Nutrients as Ergogenic Aids for Sports and Exercise*, CRC Press, Boca Raton, FL, 1993, 63.

385. Rowland, T. W., Deisroth, M. B., Green, G. M., and Kelleher, J. F., The effect of iron therapy on exercise capacity of nonanemic iron-deficient adolescent runners, *Am. J. Dis. Child*, 142, 165, 1988.

386. Matter, M., Stittfall, T., Graves, J., Myburgh, K., Adams, B., Jacobs, P., and Noakes, T. D., The effect of iron and folate therapy on maximal exercise performance in female marathon runners with iron and folate deficiency, *Clin. Sci.*, 72, 415, 1987.

387. Newhouse, I. J., Clement, D. B., Taunton, J. E., and McKenzie, D. C., The effects of prelatent/latent iron deficiency on work capacity, *Med. Sci. Sports Exer.*, 21, 263, 1989.

388. Telford, R. D., Bunney, C. J., Catchpole, E. A., Catchpole, W. R., Deakin, V., Gray, B., Hahn, A. G., and Kerr, D. A., Plasma ferritin concentration and physical work capacity in athletes, *Int. J. Sport Nutr.*, 2, 335, 1992.

389. Lamanca, J. and Haymes, E., Effects of dietary iron supplementation on endurance, *Med. Sci. Sports Exer.*, 21, S77, 1989.

390. Yoshida, T., Udo, M., Chida, M., Ichioka, M., and Makiguchi, K., Dietary iron supplement during severe physical training in competitive distance runners, *Sports Training Med. Rehab.*, 1, 279, 1990.

391. Schoene, R. B., Escourrou, P., Robertson, H. T., Nilson, K. L., Parsons, J. R., and Smith, N. J., Iron repletion decreases maximal exercise lactate concentrations in female athletes with minimal iron deficiency anemia, *J. Lab. Clin. Med.*, 102, 306, 1983.

392. Davies, C. T. M. and van Haaren, J. P. M., Effect of treatment on physiological responses to exercise in East African industrial workers with iron deficiency anaemia, *Br. J. Indust. Med.*, 30, 335, 1973.

393. Barry, A., Cantwell, J. T., Doherty, F., Folan, J. C., Ingoldsby, M., Kevany, J. P., O'Brien, J. D., O'Conner, H., O'Shea, B., Ryan, B. A., and Vaughan, J., A nutritional study of Irish athletes, *Br. J. Sports Med.*, 15, 99, 1981.

394. Nilson, K., Schoene, R. B., Robertson, H. T., Escourrou, P., and Smith, N. J., The effect of iron repletion on exercise-induced lactate production in minimally iron-deficient subjects, *Med. Sci. Sports Exer.*, 13, 92, 1981.

395. Buetler, E., Iron therapy in chronically fatigued non-anemic women: a double blind study, *Ann. Int. Med.*, 52, 378, 1960.

396. Kuleschova, E. A. and Riabova, N. V., Effect of iron deficiency of the body on the work capacity of women engaged in mental work, *Ter. Arkh.*, 61, 92, 1989.

397. Ames, B. N., Shigenaga, M. K., and Hagen, T. M., Oxidants, antioxidants, and the degenerative diseases of aging, *Proc. Natl. Acad. Sci.*, 90, 7915, 1993.

398. Kreider, R. D., Miller, G. W., Schenck, D., Cortes, C. W., Miriel, V., Somma, C. T., Rowland, P., Turner, C., and Hill, D., Effects of phosphate loading on metabolic and myocardial responses to maximal and endurance exercise, *Int. J. Sport Nutr.*, 2, 20, 1992.

399. Cade, R., Conte, M., Zauner, C., Mars, D., Peterson, J., Lunne, D., Hommen, N., and Packer, D., Effects of phosphate loading on 2,3-diphosphoglycerate and maximal oxygen uptake, *Med. Sci. Sports Exer.*, 16, 263, 1984.

400. Farber, M., Sullivan, T., Fineberg, N., Carlone, S., and Manfredi, F., Effect of decreased O_2 affinity of hemoglobin on work performance during exercise in healthy humans, *J. Lab. Clin. Med.*, 104, 166, 1984.

401. Farber, M., Carlone, S., Palange, P., Serra, P., Paoletti, V., and Fineberg, N., Effect of inorganic phosphate in hypoxemic chronic obstructive lung disease patients during exercise, *Chest*, 93, 310, 1987.

402. Stewart, I., McNaughton, L., Davies, P., and Tristram, S., Phosphate loading and the effects of VO$_2$max in trained cyclists, *Res. Quart.*, 61, 80, 1990.

403. Kreider, R. B., Miller, G. W., Williams, M. H., Somma, C. T., and Nasser, T., Effects of phosphate loading on oxygen uptake, ventilatory anaerobic threshold, and run performance, *Med. Sci. Sports Exer.*, 22, 250, 1990.

404. Ahlberg, A., Weatherwax, R., Deady, M., Perez, H., Otto, R., Cooperstein, D., Smith, T., and Wygand, J., Effect of phosphate loading on cycle ergometer performance, *Med. Sci. Sports Exer.*, 18, S11, 1986.

405. Weatherwax, R., Ahlberg, A., Deady, M., Perez, H., Otto, R., Cooperstein, D., Smith, T., and Wygand, J., Effect of phosphate loading on cycle ergometer performance, *Med. Sci. Sports Exer.*, 18, S11, 1986.

406. Duffy, D. J. and Conlee, R. K., Effects of phosphate loading on leg power and high intensity treadmill exercise, *Med. Sci. Sports Exer.*, 18, 674, 1986.

407. Bredle, D., Stager, J., Brechue, W., and Farber, M., Phosphate supplementation, cardiovascular function, and exercise performance in humans, *J. Appl. Physiol.*, 65, 1821, 1988.

408. Mannix, E. T., Stager, J. M., Harris, A., and Farber, M. O., Oxygen delivery and cardiac output during exercise following oral phosphate-glucose, *Med. Sci. Sports Exer.*, 22, 341, 1990.

409. Thompson, D. L., Grantham, S., Hall, M., Johnson, J., McDaniel, J., Servidio, F., Thompson, W. C., and Thompson, W. R., Effects of phosphate loading on erythrocytic 2,3-diphosphoglycerate, adenosine-5'-triphosphate, hemoglobin, and maximal oxygen uptake, *Med. Sci. Sports Exer.*, 22, S36, 1990.

410. Roberts, C. J., Galloway, S. D., Sexsmith, J. R., and Tremblay, M. S., Effects of acute dibasic calcium phosphate supplementation on ventilatory and lactate metabolic thresholds, *Med. Sci. Sports Exer.*, 26, S23, 1994.

411. Galloway, S. D. R., Sexsmith, J. R., Tremblay, M. S., and Roberts, C. J., The effects of acute phosphate supplementation in subjects of different aerobic fitness levels, *Med. Sci. Sports Exer.*, 26, S23, 1994.

412. Kraemer, W. J., Gordon, S. E., Lynch, J. M., Pop, M. E. M. V., and Clark, K. L., Effects of a multibuffer supplementation on acid-base balance and 2,3-diphosphoglycerate following repetitive anaerobic exercise, *Int. J. Sport Nutr.*, 5, 300, 1995.

413. Wagner, J. C., Use of chromium and cobamamide by athletes, *Clin. Pharm.*, 8, 832, 1989.

414. Clarkson, P. M., Nutritional ergogenic aids: chromium, exercise, and muscle mass, *Int. J. Sports Nutr.*, 1, 289, 1991.

415. Moore, R. J. and Friedl, K. E., Physiology of nutritional supplements: chromium picolinate and vanadyl sulfate, *Natl. Strength Cond. Assoc. J.*, 14, 47, 1992.

416. Lefavi, R. G., Anderson, R. A., Keith, R. E., Wilson, G. D., McMillan, J. L., and Stone, M. H., Efficacy of chromium supplementation in athletes: emphasis on anabolism, *Int. J. Sport Nutr.*, 2, 111, 1992.

417. Clarkson, P. M. and Haymes, E. M., Trace mineral requirements for athletes, *Int. J. Sport Nutr.*, 4, 104, 1994.

418. Evans, G., The role of chromium in sports, in *Chromium Picolinate. Everything You Need to Know*, Avery Publishing, New York, 1996, 99.

419. Riales, R. and Albrink, M. J., Effect of chromium chloride supplementation on glucose tolerance and serum lipids including high-density lipoprotein of adult men, *Am. J. Clin. Nutr.*, 34, 2670, 1981.

420. Kaats, G. R., Fisher, J. A., Blum, K., and Adelman, J. A., The effects of chromium picolinate supplementation on body composition in different age groups, *Age*, 14, 138, 1991.

421. Evans, G. W., The effect of chromium picolinate on insulin controlled parameters in humans, *Int. J. Biosoc. Med. Res.*, 11, 163, 1989.

422. Hasten, D. L., Rome, E. P., Franks, B. D., and Hegsted, M., Effects of chromium picolinate on beginning weight training students, *Int. J. Sport Nutr.*, 2, 343, 1992.

423. Evans, G. W. and Pouchnik, D. J., Composition and biological activity of chromium- pyridine carboxylate complexes, *J. Inorg. Biochem.*, 49, 177, 1993.

424. Anderson, R. A., Polansky, M. M., Bryden, N. A., Roginski, E. E., Mertz, W., and Glinsmann, W., Chromium supplementation of human subjects: effects on glucose, insulin, and lipid parameters, *Metabolism*, 32, 894, 1983.

425. Hallmark, M. A., Reynolds, T. H., DeSouza, C., Dotson, C. O., Anderson, R. A., and Rogers, M. A., Effects of chromium and resistive training on muscle strength and body composition, *Med. Sci. Sports Exer.*, 28, 139, 1996.

426. Clancy, S. P., Clarkson, P. M., DeCheke, M. E., Nosaka, K., Freedson, P. S., Cunningham, J. J., and Valentine, B., Effects of chromium picolinate supplementation on body composition, strength, and urinary chromium loss in football players, *Int. J. Sport Nutr.*, 4, 142, 1994.

427. Lukaski, H. C., Bolonchuk, W. W., Siders, W. A., and Milne, D. B., Chromium supplementation and resistance training: effects on body composition, strength, and trace element status of men, *Am. J. Clin. Nutr.*, 63, 954, 1996.

428. Anderson, R., Cheng, N., Bryden, N., Polansky, M., Cheng, N., Chi, J., and Feng, J., Beneficial effects of chromium for people with Type II diabetes, *Diabetes*, 45 (Suppl. 2), 454, 1996.

429. Nielsen, F., Hunt, C., Mullen, L., and Hunt, J., Effect of dietary boron on mineral, estrogen, testosterone metabolism in postmenopausal women, *FASEB J.*, 1, 394, 1987.

430. Ferrando, A. A. and Green, N. R., The effect of boron supplementation on lean body mass, plasma testosterone levels, and strength in male bodybuilders, *Int. J. Sport Nutr.*, 3, 140, 1993.

431. Penland, J. G., Dietary boron, brain function, and cognitive performance, *Environ. Health Perspect.*, 102(Suppl. 7), 65, 1994.

432. Meacham, S. L., Taper, L. J., and Volpe, S. L., Effects of boron supplementation on bone mineral density and dietary, blood, and urinary calcium, phosphorus, magnesium, and boron in female athletes, *Environ. Health Perspect.*, 102(Suppl. 7), 79, 1994.

433. Bucci, L. R., Boron and sports medicine: update, *Drugs Sports*, 2, 5, 1993.

434. Brichard, S. M. and Henquin, J. C., The role of vanadium in the management of diabetes, *Trends Pharmacol. Sci.*, 16, 265, 1995.

435. Williams, M. H., The role of vitamins in physical activity, in *Nutritional Aspects of Human Physical and Athletic Performance*, 2nd ed., Charles C Thomas, Springfield, IL, 1985, 147.

436. Keith, R. E., Vitamins in sport and exercise, in *Nutrition in Exercise and Sport*, Hickson, J. F., Jr. and Wolinsky, I., Eds., CRC Press, Boca Raton, 1989, 233.

437. Keith, R. E., Vitamins and physical activity, in *Nutrition in Exercise and Sport*, 2nd ed., Wolinsky, I. and Hickson, J. F., Eds., CRC Press, Boca Raton, FL, 1994, 159.

438. Bucci, L. R., Micronutrient supplementation and ergogenesis — vitamins, in *Nutrients as Ergogenic Aids for Sports and Exercise*, CRC Press, Boca Raton, FL, 1993, 23.

439. Williams, M. H., Vitamin supplementation and athletic performance, *Int. J. Vit. Nutr. Res.*, Suppl. 30, 163, 1989.

440. van der Beek, E. J., Vitamin supplementation and physical exercise performance, *J. Sports Sci.*, 9, 77, 1991.

441. Haymes, E. M., Vitamin and mineral supplementation to athletes, *Int. J. Sport Nutr.*, 1, 146, 1991.

442. Knippel, M., Mauri, L., Belluschi, R., Bana, G., Galli, C., Pusterla, G. L., Spreafico, M., and Troina, E., The action of thiamin on the production of lactic acid in cyclists, *Med. Sport*, 39, 11, 1986.

443. Goswami, S. and Dhara, P. C., Effect of vitamin B1 supplementation on reaction time in adult males, *Med. Sci. Res.*, 22, 279, 1994.

444. Haralambie, G., Vitamin B2 status in athletes and the influence of riboflavin administration on neuromuscular irritability, *Nutr. Metabol.*, 20, 1, 1976.

445. Carlson, L., Havel, R., Ekelund, L., and Holmgren, A., Effect of nicotinic acid on the turnover rate and oxidation of the free fatty acids of plasma during exercise, *Metabolism*, 12, 837, 1963.

446. Jenkins, D. J. A., Effects on nicotinic acid on carbohydrate and fat metabolism during exercise, *Lancet*, 1, 1307, 1965.

447. Bergstrom, J., Hultman, E., Jorfeldt, L., Pernow, B., and Wahren, J., Effect of nicotinic acid on physical working capacity and on metabolism of muscle glycogen in man, *J. Appl. Physiol.*, 26, 170, 1969.

448. Pernow, B. and Saltin, B., Availability of substrates and capacity for prolonged heavy exercise in man, *J. Appl. Physiol.*, 31, 416, 1971.

449. Lassers, B. W., Wahlqvist, M. L., Kauser, L., and Carlson, L. A., Effect of nicotinic acid on myocardial metabolism in man at rest and during exercise, *J. Appl. Physiol.*, 33, 72, 1972.

450. Galbo, H., Holst, J. J., Christensen, N. J., and Hilsted, J., The effect of nicotinic acid and propanolol on glucagon and plasma catecholamine responses to prolonged exercise in man, *Diabetologia*, 11, 343, 1975.

451. Norris, B., Schade, D. S., and Eaton, R. P., Effects of altered free fatty acid mobilization on the metabolic response to exercise, *J. Clin. Endocrinol. Metab.*, 46, 254, 1978.

452. Gilman, W. D. and Lemon, P. W. R., Effects of altered free fatty acid levels and environmental temperature on lactate threshold, *Med. Sci. Sports Exer.*, 14, 113, 1982.

453. Heath, E. M., Wilcox, A. R., and Quinn, C. M., Effects of nicotinic acid on respiratory exchange ratio and substrate levels during exercise, *Med. Sci. Sports Exer.*, 25, 1018, 1993.

454. Trost, S. G., Wilcox, A., and Gillis, D., The effect of nicotinic acid on excess post-exercise consumption (EPOC), *Med. Sci. Sports Exer.*, 26, S71, 1994.

455. Murray, R., Bartoli, W. P., Eddy, D. E., and Horn, M. K., Physiological and performance responses to nicotinic-acid ingestion during exercise, *Med. Sci. Sports Exer.*, 27, 1057, 1995.

456. Bucci, L. R., B vitamins, in *Nutrition Applied to Injury Rehabilitation and Sports Medicine*, CRC Press, Boca Raton, FL, 1994, 79.

457. Moretti, C., Fabbri, A., Gnessi, L., Bonifacio, V., Fraioli, F., and Isidori, A., Pyridoxine (B6) suppresses the rise in prolactin and increases the rise in growth hormone induced by exercise, *New Engl. J. Med.*, 307(7), 444, 1982.

458. deVos, A. M., Leklem, J. E., and Campbell, D. E., Carbohydrate loading, vitamin B6 supplementation, and fuel metabolism during exercise in man, *Med. Sci. Sports Exer.*, 14, 137, 1982.

459. Manore, M. M. and Leklem, J. E., Effect of carbohydrate and vitamin B6 on fuel substrates during exercise in women, *Med. Sci. Sports Exer.*, 20, 233, 1988.

460. Ellis, F. R. and Nasser, S., A pilot study of vitamin B12 in the treatment of tiredness, *Br. J. Nutr.*, 30, 277, 1973.

461. Litoff, D., Scherzer, H., and Harrison, J., Effects of pantothenic acid supplementation on human exercise, *Med. Sci. Sports Exer.*, 17, 287, 1985.

462. Simonson, E., Enzer, N., Baer, A., and Braun, R., The influence of vitamin B (complex) surplus on the capacity for muscular and mental work, *J. Indust. Hyg. Toxicol.*, 24, 83, 1942.

463. Boncke, D. and Nickel, B., Improvement of fine motoric movement control by elevated dosages of vitamin B_1, B_6, and B_{12} in target shooting, *Int. J. Vit. Nutr. Res.*, 30S, 198, 1989.

464. Early, R. G. and Carlson, R. B., Water-soluble vitamin therapy in the delay of fatigue from physical activity in hot climactic conditions, *Int. Z. Angew. Physiol.*, 27, 43, 1969.

465. Keul, J., Haralambie, G., Winker, K. H., Baumgartner, A., and Bauer, G., Die Wirkung eines Multivitamin-Elektrolytgranulats auf Kreislauf und Stoffwechsel bei langwährender Körperarbeit, *Schweiz. Z. Sportmed.*, 22, 169, 1974.

466. Haralambie, G., Keul, J., Baumgartner, A., Winker, K. H., and Bauer, G., Die Wirkung eines Multivitamin-Elektrolytpräparates auf Elektrodermalreflex une neuromuskuläre Erregbarkeit bei langwährender Körperarbeit, *Schweiz. Z. Sportmed.*, 23, 113, 1975.

467. van Dam, B., Vitamins and sport, *Br. J. Sports Med.*, 12, 74, 1978.

468. Barnett, D. W. and Conlee, R. K., The effects of a commercial dietary supplement on human performance, *Am. J. Clin. Nutr.*, 40, 586, 1984.

469. Weight, L. M., Noakes, T. D., Labadarios, D., Graves, J., Jacobs, P., and Berman, P. A., Vitamin and mineral status of trained athletes including the effects of supplementation, *Am. J. Clin. Nutr.*, 47, 186, 1988.

470. Guilland, J. C., Penaranda, T., Gallet, C., Boggio, V., Fuchs, F., and Klepping, J., Vitamin status of young athletes including the effects of supplementation, *Med. Sci. Sports Exer.*, 21, 441, 1989.

471. Singh, A., Moses, F. M., and Deuster, P. A., Vitamin and mineral status in physically active men: effects of a high-potency supplement, *Am. J. Clin. Nutr.*, 55, 1, 1992.

472. Singh, A., Moses, F. M., and Deuster, P. A., Chronic multivitamin-mineral supplementation does not enhance physical performance, *Med. Sci. Sports Exer.*, 24, 726, 1992.

473. Telford, R. D., Catchpole, E. A., Deakin, V., McLeay, A. C., and Plank, A. W., The effect of 7 to 8 months of vitamin/mineral supplementation on the vitamin and mineral status of athletes, *Int. J. Sport Nutr.*, 2, 123, 1992.

474. Telford, R. D., Catchpole, E. A., Deakin, V., Hahn, A. G., and Plank, A. W., The effect of 7 to 8 month vitamin/mineral supplementation on athletic performance, *Int. J. Sport Nutr.*, 2, 135, 1992.

475. Dragan, G. I., Ploesteanu, E., and Selejan, V., Studies concerning the ergogenic value of Cantamega-2000 supply in top junior cyclists, *Rev. Rhoum. Physiol.*, 28, 13, 1991.

476. Pieralisi, G., Ripari, P., and Vecchiet, L., Effects of a standardized ginseng extract combined with dimethylaminoethanol bitartrate, vitamins, minerals, and trace elements on physical performance during exercise, *Clin. Ther.*, 13, 373, 1991.

477. Colgan, M., Effects of multinutrient supplementation on athletic performance, in *Sport, Health, and Nutrition*, Katch, F.I., Ed., Human Kinetics Publishers, Champaign, IL, 1986.

478. Colgan, M., Micronutrient status of endurance athletes affects hematology and performance, *J. Appl. Nutr.*, 43, 16, 1991.

479. Benton, D., Haller, J., and Fordy, J., Vitamin supplementation for 1 year improves mood, *Neuropsychobiology*, 32, 98, 1995.

480. Kleijnen, J. and Knipschild, P., *Ginkgo biloba* for cerebral insufficiency, *Br. J. Clin. Pharmacol.*, 34, 352, 1992.

481. Bucci, L. R., Specific combinations of nutrients, in *Nutrients as Ergogenic Aids for Sports and Exercise*, CRC Press, Boca Raton, FL, 1993, 79.

482. Chandler, R. M., Byrne, H. K., Patterson, L. G., and Ivy, L. J., Dietary supplements affect the anabolic state after weight-training exercise, *J. Appl. Physiol.*, 76, 839, 1994.

483. Kreider, R. B., Klesges, R., Harmon, K., Grindstaff, P., Ramsey, L., Bullen, D., Wood, L., Li, Y., and Almada, A., Effects of ingesting supplements designed to promote lean tissue accretion on body composition during resistance training, *Int. J. Sport Nutr.*, 6, 234, 1996.

484. Maresh, C. M., Armstrong, L. E., Hoffman, J. R., Hannon, D. R., Gabaree, C. L. V., Bergeron, M. F., Whittlesey, M. J., and Deschenes, M. R., Dietary supplementation and improved anaerobic performance, *Int. J. Sport Nutr.*, 4, 387, 1994.

485. Snider, I. P., Bazzare, T. L., Murdoch, S. D., and Goldfarb, A., Effects of coenzyme athletic performance system as an ergogenic aid on endurance performance to exhaustion, *Int. J. Sport Nutr.*, 2, 272, 1992.

486. Zar, J. H., *Biostatistical Analysis*, Prentice-Hall, Englewood Cliffs, NJ, 1972, 44.

487. Kirsch, I. and Weixel, L. J., Double-blind versus deceptive administration of placebo, *Behav. Neurosci.*, 102, 319, 1988.

Chapter 14

NUTRITION AND STRENGTH

_____ Terry L. Bazzarre

CONTENTS

0-8493-8560-1/97/$0.00+$.50
© 1998 by CRC Press LLC

I. INTRODUCTION

The focus of this update on nutrition and strength training includes research on both male and female athletes who engage in some aspect of resistance training. The individuals included in these studies include elite, world class athletes, "recreational athletes," and previously inactive individuals. Because of the increased interest in the potential benefits of strength training for people of all ages, an effort has been made to include as many recent studies in this review as possible, including several case studies.

Most of the studies reported in this chapter are based on populations such as bodybuilders, weight lifters, power lifters, and football players; however, strength training has become a major component of many fitness programs offered in a variety of settings. In fact, many other athletes, such as gymnasts, skiers, basketball players, and tennis players now devote a significant portion of their training program to weight-training activities. Many trainers now recognize the importance of strong muscles in the prevention of fatigue and injuries and in the promotion of muscular endurance. Consequently, strength training has become an integral component of the training program for athletes from a wide variety of sports.

It is important to recognize that while some athletes engage only in strength-training activities, many other athletes have balanced their gains in strength by incorporating stretching and flexibility exercises into their training programs. Other strength-trained athletes also include aerobic training into their schedules. For example, some bodybuilders now use aerobic training such as cycling as a means of increasing muscular definition in the final stages of their preparation for competition. Thus, the overall training programs of the populations cited in this review reflect observations based on individuals who presumably devote a considerable part of their training to the development of muscular strength, but may also engage in other beneficial forms of physical training.

While most of the sports nutrition research has focused on aerobically trained athletes, more and more studies are being published on the food/nutrient intakes of athletes engaged in strength-training activities. The health benefits of strength training are becoming more widely recognized, and special strength training programs are being developed for special target audiences including the elderly, individuals who have had a heart attack or stroke, and individuals who want to improve their health by reducing their level of obesity. Considerable interest has developed on the effects of resistance training on lipid levels, especially among athletes using hormones to achieve their body composition goals.

II. METHODOLOGICAL CONSIDERATIONS

In reviewing the literature on the food and nutrient intake of strength-trained athletes, it is important to recognize that the measurement of food intake is only one component of evaluating the nutritional status of an individual or a population.[1] The four major components of nutritional assessment include the measurement of food intake, anthropometric assessment of body composition and other physical dimensions of the body, the evaluation of clinical signs and symptoms of poor nutritional status, and, finally, biochemical or laboratory assessments of various tissues of the body. Functional measures of nutritional status are also available.[1]

The adequacy of evaluations of nutritional status is always dependent upon the use of ancillary information on the demographic characteristics of an individual and relevant knowledge about both the personal and family medical history of the individual or population. This information is particularly useful in selecting normative data or reference standards that are used to evaluate the data obtained from individuals or populations being screened for nutrition problems.

To date, there are no known population standards for athletes in general, nor for any specific group of athletes. Not only are population standards needed for athletes in general, but standards are needed that reflect variations in training and body composition that impact metabolic requirements. Data collected on groups undergoing basic military training or even more intensive training such as Navy SEALS represent an excellent starting point. Caution is warranted in the selection and use of population-based reference standards obtained from various segments of the general population with individual data for athletes. The body mass index (BMI) for example, which is often used as an index of excess adiposity in the general population, is not appropriate for all athletes, especially strength-trained athletes, for whom high BMI values may reflect increased lean body mass (LBM) rather than increased adiposity. Also, the use of the BMI or body weight in calculating correlations between body composition and selected risk factors or performance variables may result in the identification of relationships which are opposite to those observed in the general population or in obese populations.

The collection of food intake information may be achieved by using various methods which generally reflect the need to collect data for a specific day or period of time (i.e., food records or 24-h dietary recalls) while other methods such as diet histories and food frequency questionnaires can be used to assess usual food intake.[2,3] The methods used to assess food intake information in studies of athletes have not always been described, and the lack of familiarity with the various methods/terminology has occasionally resulted in false information about the method that was actually used (e.g., some investigators have reported using a diet history when they actually used a food record or a 24-h recall). Generally, 3- to 7-d food records are considered more valid and reliable estimates of actual food intake for individuals and groups than 24-h recalls and diet histories, which are subject to problems related to memory.[2,3] Diet histories are generally a more reliable estimate of usual intake than the 24-h recall, because a single day's food intake may not be representative of the wide variety of food choices than an individual makes during the period of a year.[2,3] Therefore, caution is warranted in generalizing about the information collected on small samples, especially when the data are based on the 24-h recall method. Fortunately, in this series of studies, most investigators used either 3- or 7-d food records. Thus, methodologic variation in the collection of food intake data is minimal for this group of studies and is an unlikely explanation for differences in the results between studies.

The interpretation of nutrient intakes must also be made with caution if little or no information is provided about the food composition data base used in analyzing the nutrient content of an athlete's diet. Some food composition tables/software have a limited number of food items, while other tables may not be complete for all nutrients.[2] Thus, it is possible that the amount of a nutrient ingested by an individual may be greater than the reported intake because the amount of the nutrient present in all foods consumed was not accounted for. Care must also be taken in interpreting the data because food tables generally use a weighted average for the value listed for a specific food; however, the actual amount of nutrient present in the food may vary widely depending on differences in soil and water content (especially minerals). Food preparation methods may affect the biological availability of nutrients. For example, vitamin C levels may decrease rapidly as a result of exposure to heat from cooking or from light. Thus, measures of variability are also important considerations in interpreting mean intakes.

Some investigators report the distribution of nutrient intakes among populations as well as mean values in order to provide a more comprehensive evaluation of nutritional status. Investigators also use a wide variety of descriptive information in reporting their findings which has prevented a direct comparison of the data from one study to another. For example, some investigators report energy intakes provided by protein, fat, and carbohydrate in total grams per day or in total grams per kilogram body weight, while other investigators may report intakes as a percent of total calories consumed. Studies on the nutrient intakes of athletes or other groups of individuals who have unusual body proportions, such as 7-ft-tall basketball players or 5-ft-tall jockeys, may need to adjust their values to reflect the effects of these differences in body composition. An evaluation of dietary intakes of bodybuilders is an example of the need to consider differences in body types within a group of athletes, as competitive male bodybuilders in the lightweight division are frequently under 5'6" while those in the heavyweight division are often well over 6'0". The relatively low body fat, high lean body mass of competitive bodybuilders represents another reason for carefully considering the descriptive units used to report nutrient intakes.

The interpretation of data collected from athletes living in foreign countries is also an important consideration. Food composition tables and reference standards such as dietary allowances vary from country to country. Cultural food practices and differences in food availability may also account for differences in nutrient intakes among athletes in different countries. Fresh fruits and vegetables are not always available or economical for many populations. Individuals evaluated in institutional settings or sports academies may also consume foods based on what is available rather than individual food preferences.

In evaluating biochemical indices of nutritional status of athletes, it is important to recognize that the effects of hemoconcentration due to excessive sweating or as a potential reflection of consuming "excessive" intakes of protein and other constituents of the blood may alter the interpretation of blood values. The hypervolemia of endurance training which is associated with an increase in total blood volume represents a pseudo-dilutional anemia in endurance-trained athletes; however, an expansion of blood volume due to increased strength training has not been reported. Thus, the interpretation of blood concentrations of nutrients' metabolites may vary from one population of athletes to the next and may vary with changes in the training program of a given individual. Care must also be taken in the collection of plasma and serum samples as hemolysis of red blood cells (RBC) may significantly increase plasma/serum concentrations. The concentration of constituents in erythrocytes may be falsely elevated because of the increased concentrations in RBC compared to plasma or serum.[1]

Finally, it is important to recognize that blood concentrations of many nutrients do not generally change until tissue stores are either depleted or, alternatively, until tissue stores become saturated. Thus, the inadequate or excessive intake of foods and nutrients may be the only component of nutritional assessment that would reflect the potential development of nutrition problems in the future.

III. FOOD INTAKE AND NUTRITIONAL STATUS OF STRENGTH-TRAINED ATHLETES

A. OVERVIEW OF ALL STUDIES

The report by Short and Short[4] on the nutrient intakes of Syracuse University athletes represents one of the earliest efforts to measure food intake of athletes in a comprehensive and systematic manner. Their report, based on measuring dietary intakes of 554 male and female athletes who averaged at least 2 h of training on a daily basis, included data for 6 male bodybuilders and 66 football players. Anthropometric, biochemical, and training information about this population, which would be helpful in evaluating the nutrient intakes of this population and in comparing these results, were not included in their 4-year study. The data are, nevertheless, useful as a starting point for a review and discussion of nutrient intakes.

This review of the literature on nutrient intakes of strength-trained athletes has been expanded from 7 studies on male bodybuilders[4-10] and 3 studies of female bodybuilders[5,6,11] to a total of 26 studies: 15 on bodybuilders, 6 on weightlifters and wrestlers, 3 on football players, and 2 of individuals engaged in strength training programs (Table 1). Fogleholm et al.[12] evaluated dietary, anthropometric, and biochemical data for 25 Finnish weightlifters and 34 wrestlers; however, all of these data were reported in a larger sample of 147 athletes classified as "moderate energy expenditure" athletes. Unfortunately, because of collapsing their data into the larger sample which included athletes engaged in "sprinting" and "throwing," none of their results are reported in this section.

TABLE 1   Nutrient Intakes of Athletes Engaged in Strength-Training Activities

Investigators	Sample	Age (Years)	Method	% Body Fat	Energy (Kcal)[a]	PRO (g, % kcal)	Fat (g, % kcal)	CHO (g, % kcal)	P/S Ratio	Cholesterol (mg)	Fiber (g)
Female Bodybuilders (BB) and Weightlifters (WL)											
Bazzarre et al., 1990[5]	8 comp BB	28 ± 4	7-d FR	9.8 ± 1.5%	2260 ± 2660	162 ± 93 37 ± 16%	33 ± 41 13 ± 9%	332 ± 525 49 ± 18%	3.8 ± 1.9	462 ± 631	13 ± 7
Bazzarre et al., 1992[6]	11 comp BB	29	3-d FR	9.1 ± 1.4%	1597 ± 614	143 ± 45 39 ± 13%	22 ± 17 12 ± 5%	206 ± 120 48 ± 16%	1.0 ± 1.0	223 ± 138	7 ± 5
Heyward et al., 1989[14] (longitudinal)	12 precomp BB	29 ± 7	3-d FR	16.8 ± 4.5% 58.3 ± 5.2 kg	1630 ± 550	102 26%	42 ± 30 21%	208 ± 60 53%	—	320 ± 317	—
	12 comp BB			9.5 ± 3.3% 52.3 ± 4.5 kg	1453 ± 652	77 g 21%	15 ± 7 10%	261 ± 112 72%	—	152 ± 121	—
LaMar-Hildebrand, 1989[15] (longitudinal)	6 comp BB	18–30	3-d FR	53 ± 6 kg	2228 ± 1192	67 ± 25 17%	49 ± 48 20%	359 ± 194 64%	—	148 ± 104	—
	4 noncomp BB			60 ± 5 kg	1873 ± 393	82 ± 25 18%	56 ± 28 27%	284 ± 48 61%	—	332 ± 316	—
Morgan et al., 1986[11]	9 WL	36	3-d FR	21.3 ± 1.5 BMI	1549 ± 430	85 ± 30 23 ± 8%	57 ± 34 32 ± 13%	182 ± 63 47 ± 10%	1.2 ± 0.7	317 ± 124	—
Sandoval et al., 1989[19]	6 comp BB	28 ± 4	3-d FR	8.4 ± 1.4% 52.5 kg	1535 ± 596	105 ± 59 26%	25 ± 12 14%	242 ± 87 64%	0.4	236 ± 185	36 ± 17
Walberg-Rankin et al., 1993[16] (longitudinal)	6 comp BB	27 ± 5	3-d FR	12.7 ± 1.7% 54.3 kg	pre: 1630 ± 478 comp: 1839 ± 647 post: 2790 ± 1321	29 ± 6 17 ± 7% 72 19 ± 6%	17 ± 12% 6 ± 5% 29 ± 16%	54 ± 11% 78 ± 16% 53 ± 13%	—	—	—
X ± SD/comp[b]	**Total: 53 BB/9 WL**	**29.5 ± 3.3**		**9.9 ± 1.7**	**1875 ± 364**	**103 ± 42 27 ± 9%**	**29 ± 13 11 ± 3%**	**280 ± 64 62 ± 13%**	**1.7 ± 1.8**	**244 ± 128**	**19 ± 15**
Male Bodybuilders											
Bazzarre et al., 1990[5]	19 comp	28 ± 4	7-d FR	6.0 ± 1.8%	2015 ± 1060	169 ± 94 34 ± 12%	40 ± 51 15 ± 9%	243 ± 121 50 ± 13%	2.4 ± 1.1	513 ± 582	18 ± 12
Bazzarre et al., 1992[6]	19 comp	30	3-d FR	4.9 ± 1.6%	2620 ± 803	247 ± 105 40 ± 15%	33 ± 19 11 ± 5%	334 ± 194 49 ± 21%	1.0 ± 1.0	444 ± 318	9 ± 7
Faber et al., 1986[7]	76	27 ± 6	7-d FR	16.0 ± 2.6%	3187 ± 1027[c]	19%	36%	42%	0.62 ± 0.24	509 ± 151	17 ± 10
				14.9 ± 2.5%	4143 ± 1088[d]	31%	46%	20%	0.55 ± 0.19	2823 ± 542	18 ± 11

TABLE 1 Nutrient Intakes of Athletes Engaged in Strength-Training Activities *(continued)*

Investigators	Sample	Age (Years)	Method	% Body Fat	Energy (Kcal)[a]	PRO (g, % kcal)	Fat (g, % kcal)	CHO (g, % kcal)	P/S Ratio	Cholesterol (mg)	Fiber (g)
Ferando and Green, 1993[20]	10 comp	23.2 ± 3.3	3-d FR	8.8 ± 1.8%	3556 ± 2013	18 ± 8%	20 ± 9%	60 ± 15%	—	—	—
	9 comp	23.8 ± 2.9		11.7 ± 2.2%	3804 ± 1063	19 ± 8%	22 ± 11%	49 ± 10%		—	—
Heyward et al., 1989[14] (longitudinal)	7 precomp	28 ± 6	3-d FR	9.7 ± 3.1% / 91.5 ± 9.2 kg	3590 ± 1159	215 g / 25%	110 ± 71 / 26%	457 ± 148 / 52%		702 ± 417	—
	7 comp			5.9 ± 3.2% / 81.6 ± 9.5 kg	2331 ± 259	163 g / 28%	32 ± 18 / 13%	365 ± 76 / 63%		310 ± 110	—
Hurley et al., 1984[9]	8	29 ± 1	24 hr R, diet history	12.0 ± 1.0%	—	20%	40–50%	30–35%		—	—
Kleiner et al., 1989[8] (longitudinal)	18 SU	30	3-d FR	13.1%	5739 ± 2500	324 ± 163 / 22%	214 ± 109 / 34%	637 ± 259 / 44%	0.6 ± 0.3	1413 ± 1151	—
	17 NSU	26	8-wk FR	13.8%							
Manore et al., 1993[13] (longitudinal)	1 comp	31	w/o MCT	6.9–9.0%	3674 ± 279	19% / 1.9 g/kg BW	5%	76%		182 ± 61	—
			w/MCT		4952 ± 279	14%	30%	56%		182 ± 61	—
Sandoval et al., 1989[19]	5 comp	25 ± 3	3-d FR	7.2 ± 1.6%	2347	199 ± 65 g / 34%	41 ± 19 / 16%	305 ± 91 / 52%	0.6	427 ± 215	40 ± 17
Short and Short, 1983[4]	6	—	3-d FR	—	3962	197 / 19%	176 / 39%	350 / 36%	0.27	1271	—
Spitler et al., 1980[10]	10 comp	30	NR	9.9%	—	85%	10%	5%		—	—
Tarnopolsky et al., 1992[21]	noncomp	NR		80.0 kg	4802	216 g / 19%	32%	49%			—
X ± SD/comp[d]	**Total: 196**	**28 ± 2**		**8.0 ± 2.6%**	**3089 ± 1057**	**195 ± 38[e] / 28 ± 10%**	**37 ± 5[e] / 18 ± 7%**	**312 ± 52[e] / 54 ± 5%**	**1.3 ± 0.9**	**362 ± 147**	**22 ± 16**
Male Weightlifters (WL) and Wrestlers (WRE)											
Chen et al., 1989[24]	10 elite WL	21 ± 2	3–5-d FR	80 ± 19 kg	4597 ± 604 / 57 6/kg BW	257 ± 47 / 22 ± 4%	205 ± 33 / 40 ± 7%	431 ± 96 / 38 ± 8%		—	—
	5 amateur WL	16 ± 1	3–5-d FR	71 ± 2 kg	4113 ± 555 / 58 8/kg BW	143 ± 20 / 14 ± 2%	203 ± 21 / 44 ± 5%	430 ± 115 / 42 ± 11%		—	—
Fry et al., 1993[26]	28 WL / 13 AA[c]		FR	—	3714 ± 436	15 ± 1%	33 ± 1%	53 ± 2%		—	—
	15 Placebo		Cafeteria	—	3841 ± 275	15 ± 1%	31 ± 2%	54 ± 2%		—	—

Study	Subjects	Age (yr)	Diet method	Body weight	Energy (kcal)	Protein	Fat	CHO			
Heinemann and Zerbes 1989[25]	15 WL	15–19	3-d FR	95 kg	79/kg BW	15%	46%	39%	—	—	—
	20 WRE	19–22		85 kg	52/kg BW	18%	38%	44%	—	—	—
Hurley et al., 1984[9]	8 PL	31±1	24-hr R diet history	94 ± 5 kg 14 ± 2% BMI: 32	—	20%	30–35%	45–50%			
Steen and McKinney, 1986[18]	42 WRE	18–23	various 24 hr R 4-d FR 24 hr R	preseason: 14% midseason: 11% post-season: 14%	4.6–25.7% data presented graphically; actual means not presented						
Warren et al., 1991[27]	28 Olympic WL	17 ± 1			3714 ± 1573	>2.0g/kg	—	—			
X ± SD[b]	**58 WL/62 WRE**	**16–23**		**83 ± 10**	**4066 ± 391**	**17 ± 3%**	**39 ± 6%**	**45 ± 6%**			
					62 ± 12/kg BW						

Football Players

Study	Subjects	Age (yr)	Diet method	Body weight	Energy (kcal)	Protein	Fat	CHO			
Hickson et al., 1987[29]	46 Jr. H.S.	12–14	NR	61 ± 12 kg	2523 ± 936 43 ± 16/kg BW	91 ± 34 14% 1.5 g/kg	109 ± 59 39%	302 ± 125 47%	—	—	
	88 H.S.	15–18	1-d FR	76 ± 14 kg	3365 ± 1592 48 ± 21/kg BW	133 ± 77 16% 1.9 g/kg	154 ± 90 40%	366 ± 170 44%	—	—	
Hickson et al., 1987[30]	11 College	20 ± 0.4	3-d FR	108 ± 3 kg	3593 ± 217 33/kg BW	190 ± 10 22 ± 1% 1.8 g/kg	158 ± 12 39 ± 1%	329 ± 26 39 ± 1%	—	—	
Short and Short, 1983[4]	10 def. backs	NR	3-d FR	NR	3306	130 16%	146 40%	374 45%	0.13	626	
	23 defense				4823	191 16%	218 41%	528 43%	0.20	927	
	33 offense				4853	201 16%	206 38%	550 44%	0.23	970	
X ± SD[b]	**Total: 211**	**16 ± 4**		**82 ± 24**	**3744 ± 921**	**156 ± 44 17 ± 3%**	**165 ± 40 40 ± 1%**	**408 ± 105 44 ± 3**	**0.19 ± 0.05**	**841 ± 187**	
					41 ± 8/kgBW	**1.7 g/kg**					

TABLE 1   Nutrient Intakes of Athletes Engaged in Strength-Training Activities *(continued)*

Investigators	Sample	Age (Years)	Method	% Body Fat	Energy (Kcal)[a]	PRO (g, % kcal)	Fat (g, % kcal)	CHO (g, % kcal)	P/S Ratio	Cholesterol (mg)	Fiber (g)
Resistance Trained Males											
Bazzarre et al., 1986[17]	26 Triathletes	30 ± 7	7-d FR	11 ± 5	2628 ± 526	103 ± 23 / 15 ± 2%	95 ± 25 / 33 ± 7%	337 ± 100 / 50 ± 10%		366 ± 189	
	12 Endurance	31 ± 7		13 ± 5	2423 ± 677	92 ± 33 / 15 ± 2%	86 ± 21 / 32 ± 4%	298 ± 102 / 48 ± 8%		352 ± 143	
	11 RT	25 ± 5		14 ± 4	2709 ± 632	104 ± 32 / 15 ± 4%	105 ± 30 / 34 ± 3%	313 ± 72 / 46 ± 5%		353 ± 162	
Gater et al., 1992[31]	37 RT	23 ± 3	Avg of 10	9–18%						—	
	7 P/C	21 ± 0	1-d FR	17 ± 2%	1699 ± 167	64.8 ± 6.5 / 15%	57.1 ± 7.9 / 30.2%	231.3 ± 28.1 / 54.5%			
	8 P/RT	21 ± 1		17 ± 2%	2275 ± 207	92.9 ± 10.7 / 16%	85.0 ± 8.9 / 33.6%	286.8 ± 31.7 / 50.1%			
	7 AL/C	24 ± 1		15 ± 1%	2283 ± 254	104.4 ± 13.0 / 18%	92.4 ± 11.7 / 36.4%	258.4 ± 37.3 / 45.3%			
	8 AL/RT	23 ± 1		16 ± 1%	2321 ± 294	113.2 ± 14.9 / 20%	91.9 ± 12.2 / 35.6%	260.3 ± 36.0 / 44.9%			
	7 EX/RT	23 ± 1		16 ± 2%	2835 ± 436	115.4 ± 20.6 / 16%	88.7 ± 16.7 / 28.2%	353.8 ± 61.2 / 55.5%			

Note: Abbreviations — FR, Food Record; NR, Not Recorded; comp, during competitive training period; precomp, prior to competitive training period; post-comp, after competitive training period; SU, Steroid Users; NSU, Non-Steroid Users; P/C, Placebo/Control; AL/C, Arginine-Lysine/Control; EX/RT, Exceed/Resistance Training.

a   Multiply by 4.184 joules/kcal to convert to kilojoules.

b   Mean ± Standard Deviation for all studies without adjustment for differences in sample size.

c   Consumed <1.5 eggs per day.

d   Consumed >6 eggs per day.

e   Data for Spitler et al.[10] excluded.

f   Attending National Training Camp.

The sample size of most studies has been quite small. The total sample in most studies ranged from a case study by Manore et al.[13] to 35 subjects.[8] However, data on several larger populations such as a group of 76 South African bodybuilders[7] and a report on young football players (46 junior high school students and 88 high school students)[15,16] have been reported in the literature. The series of studies included in this review represent data on a total of 53 female and 196 male bodybuilders, 9 female and 58 male weightlifters, 62 wrestlers, 211 football players, and 49 individuals engaged in resistance training programs. The data base on nutrition and strength athletes could be much improved if researchers were encouraged to use larger samples, and if professional athletes were encouraged to work with nutrition scientists through professional bodybuilding associations. In addition, editors of nutrition journals could discourage publication of "pilot studies" using small sample sizes.

Most subjects were between 18 and 30 years of age. The average age for women in the studies was 30 ± 3 years and 28 ± 2 years for men. With the increased popularity of strength training among both youth and older adults and the growth of "masters level" bodybuilding competition, researchers should be encouraged to study these unique populations.

Most of the studies on bodybuilders were cross-sectional in design; however, Heyward et al.,[14] Lamar-Hildebrand et al.,[15] Walberg-Rankin et al.,[16] Kleiner et al.,[8] and Manore et al.[13] conducted longitudinal studies. Lamar-Hildebrand et al.[15] monitored 6 competitive and 4 noncompetitive female bodybuilders during a 12-week period. Walberg-Rankin et al.[16] measured food intakes at 28 d prior to competition, the week of competition and 28 d post competition. Kleiner et al.[8] conducted a 6-month longitudinal study of 18 steroid-using and 17 non-steroid-using male bodybuilders while Manore et al.[13] conducted an 8-week case study of an elite, world class bodybuilder. Bazzarre et al.[17] conducted a 24-week study of changes in nutritional status of male and female endurance athletes which included a control group of 12 males who engaged in resistance training more than 2 times per week.

Measures of food intake were generally based on food records collected by subjects ranging in length from 3- to 7-d. Hurley et al.[9] used both the 24-h recall and diet history methods, while Spitler et al.[10] included a "recall diet history." The case study by Manore et al.[13] involved measuring nutrient intake by the weighed food record methodology. Different versions of food composition information were used in these studies. None of the data reported on nutrient intake in the tables in this chapter include intakes reflecting supplement use, although supplements are widely used by bodybuilders.

Heyward et al.,[14] Kleiner et al.,[8] Lamar-Hildebrand et al.,[15] and Walberg-Rankin et al.[16] demonstrated that significant changes in food intake can occur during the training period leading up to competition. The nutrient intakes reported in most studies represent data collected at the time of competition or during the period immediately prior to competition. Thus, differences in reported intakes among these studies, and the high level of interindividual variation observed within studies may reflect differences in food intake associated with changes in food selection, training, and metabolism. One recommendation for future published reports may be to encourage investigators to include individual data in tabular form as well as to report mean values. Investigators should be encouraged to look for patterns in changes among their total sample using relevant criteria for subcatetories (e.g., those subjects who lost, maintained, or gained body weight and/or body fat, altered their training program, etc.).

The cyclical nature of training among highly competitive athletes such as bodybuilders, wrestlers, and even endurance athletes clearly suggests alterations in neuro-hormonal regulators of body composition and metabolism which represent tremendous opportunities for future research. These same changes may increase the risk of nutrition problems, lead to alterations in functional measures of nutritional status, and/or result in changes in risk factors for disease such as lipid profiles and blood pressure.

The data reported by Bazzarre et al.[5,6] and Manore et al.[13] represent information on elite bodybuilders at the time of national competition. In comparison to surveys of food intake and nutritional status of other groups of athletes, the literature on bodybuilder populations is unique in that individuals who are world class as well as individuals who have competed at the national and state level have been included in some of these studies.

Some of the reported dietary information obtained from male bodybuilders is very limited. For example, Spitler et al.[10] and Hurley et al.[9] only reported the distribution of energy intake provided by protein, fat, and carbohydrate but did not report mean energy intake. Some investigators have elected to present their data in graph format only (e.g., Steen and McKinney[18]). Since it was not possible to accurately quantitate the actual nutrient values in these graphs, their data were not included in the summary tables.

In general, the nutrient intakes of the strength-trained athletes in each of the studies listed in Table 1 show wide interindividual variability. Investigators in this series of studies were more likely to report the vitamin and mineral intakes of women than men as vitamin-mineral intakes were reported in 6 of 7 studies on women compared to only 12 of the 19 studies on men. Few investigators reported any information about the prevalence of vitamin/mineral supplement use among these populations.[8] Thus, in many of these studies the dietary intakes for vitamins and minerals are underestimates of total intakes.

B. NUTRIENT INTAKES OF BODYBUILDERS

Nutrient intakes for female bodybuilders[5,6,11,14-20] and weightlifters[11] are presented in Table 1 while nutrient intakes for male bodybuilders[4-10,13,14,17,19-21] are presented in Table 1. Since most data were collected at the time of competition or during the competitive training period, means for those studies were averaged and are summarized in the last row of data at the bottom of each table. The averages/means were not adjusted for differences in sample size. Energy intake is expressed in kilocalories; however, the intake can be converted to kilojoules by multiplying the kcal value by 4.184.

Mean energy intakes of competitive female bodybuilders were quite similar among the studies with an average of 1875 ± 364 kcal (7845 kilojoules). Energy intakes in these studies ranged from 1453 ± 652 kcal (6079 kilojoules)[14] to a high of 2260 ± 2660 kcal (9456 kilojoules).[5] The average energy intakes of competitive male bodybuilders (3089 ± 1057 kcal [12924.376 kilojoules]) was twice that of competitive female bodybuilders. Mean energy intakes among the studies of competitive male bodybuilders ranged from 2015 ± 1060 kcal (8431 kilojoules)[5] to 4952 ± 279 kcal (20719 kilojoules) in an 8-week case study of an elite, world class bodybuilder consuming MCT oil in addition to his food intake.[13]

Variations in energy intakes within studies were quite large which may reflect differences in these athletes' efforts to maintain lean body mass while other athletes continued their efforts to reduce their body fat levels or prevent gains in body fat. The variation in energy intakes between the different studies on competitive male bodybuilders was much greater than that observed among the studies conducted on competitive female bodybuilders. Variations in energy intakes are also a reflection of dramatic differences in body weight among the different weight classes. The range of energy intakes for both female and male bodybuilders appears to be similar to that reported for other populations of athletes and nonathletes.

Mean energy intake was lower among elite male bodybuilders at the time of national competition[5,6,14,19] than those measured during some phase of the training season.[4,7,8,14] These data are in contrast to those reported for female bodybuilders. Heyward et al.[14] reported a decrease in energy intake among 12 female bodybuilders from 1630 ± 550 kcal (6820 kilojoules) before competition to 1453 ± 652 kcal (6079 kilojoules) whereas Walberg-Rankin et al.[16] reported an increase in energy intake from 1630 ± 478 kcal (6820 kilojoules) 28 days prior to competition to 1839 ± 647 kcal (7694 kilojoules) in 6 competitive female bodybuilders. Of interest in the latter study was the increase in energy intake to 2790 ± 1321 kcal (11673 kilojoules) 28 days after competition.

Lamar-Hildebrand et al.[15] conducted the only study of competitive female bodybuilders that included a comparison group of noncompetitive bodybuilders. The mean energy intake of the six competitive female bodybuilders in this study was 2228 ± 1192 kcal (9322 kilojoules) as compared to a mean intake of 1873 ± 393 kcal (7837 kilojoules). One might speculate that some of this difference was due to the greater training regimens of the competitive group as their average body weight was 7 kg less than their noncompetitive counterparts. Future research is needed to account for the dramatic differences in energy/food intake and training programs of individual bodybuilders. Unfortunately for this series of studies, it is not possible to accurately assess or evaluate some of the reasons for the differences in the data reported either between studies or even within a specific study.

Energy intakes of 76 South African bodybuilders reported by Faber et al.[7] were quite variable; however, the intake of those bodybuilders, who consumed no eggs (3187 ± 1027 kcal [13334 kilojoules]), was considerably less than that of bodybuilders who consumed an average of 12 eggs daily (4143 ± 1088 kcal [17334 kilojoules]). Differences in egg intake appeared to alter significantly the distribution of energy intake provided by protein, fat, and carbohydrate in these South African bodybuilders, accounting for a 12% increase in the proportion of calories provided by both protein and fat and a 22% decrease in the proportion of calories provided by carbohydrate. These differences illustrate the important contribution of differences in food selection on the nutrient composition on these athlete's diets.

Averages for those studies of bodybuilders during the competitive training period reflect a high protein, low fat diet pattern. In fact the distribution of energy intake provided by protein, fat, and carbohydrate was relatively similar for both male and female bodybuilders at the time of national competition.[5,6] These data may suggest that both male and female bodybuilders tend to develop similar goals in regulating the qualitative energy content of their diets as they prepare for competition.

A more detailed review of the individual studies, however, illustrates the large variability between studies and a high level of interindividual variability. Protein intake as a percent of total kilocalories ranged from 17% in two studies[15,16] to a high of 39% for competitive female bodybuilders;[6] and from 14% in the case study by Manore et al.[13] to a high of 85% by Spitler et al.[10] for male bodybuilders. The kilocalorie contribution from protein was so high in the latter study that these data were not used in calculating the averages for the energy distribution from protein, fat, and carbohydrate for competitive male bodybuilders (Table 1).

Protein as a percent of total energy intake was considerably higher in most studies of both female and male bodybuilders as compared to the U.S. population, while fat intake was reduced to remarkably low levels of about 6–22% of total energy intake.

The carbohydrate content of the diet of bodybuilders at the time of competition (as a percent of total kilocalories) appears to be quite similar to the high carbohydrate content of the diet of endurance athletes during their "carbohydrate-loading" regimens. Based on my research, bodybuilders during competitive training appear to consume a higher percent of their carbohydrate intake in the form of complex carbohydrates such as baked potatoes, pasta, and rice while endurance athletes tend to also consume more bread as well as carbohydrate foods containing liberal quantities of simple sugars.

Protein intake in these studies was in excess of the Recommended Dietary Allowances (RDA),[22] averaging 103 ± 42 g daily for female bodybuilders during competitive training and 195 ± 38 g for competitive male bodybuilders. These intakes are about two times the RDA for females, and three times the RDA for males, respectively. Mean protein intake was greater than 100 g per day in all studies of male bodybuilders; however, some studies[15,16] of competitive female bodybuilders reported relatively modest protein intakes of 67–72 g per day. Male and female bodybuilders at the more senior competitive level[6] consumed more protein and less fat than their "junior"-level counterparts.[5] While male bodybuilders appear to increase total protein intake and protein intake as a percent of total energy, this trend may not be consistent for females. For example, the competitive female bodybuilders studied longitudinally by Heyward et al.[14] and Walberg-Rankin et al.[16] decreased their absolute protein intake, and their protein intake as a percent of total kilocalories when they changed from their precompetition diet to the diet they consumed at the time of competition. In the latter study,[16] protein intake increased from 17 to 19% of total kilocalories 1 month after competition even though the women consumed almost 1000 kcal (4184 kilojoules) more per day.

At the time of competition, the average dietary fat intake was quite low for female (11 ± 3%) and male (18 ± 7%) bodybuilders, ranging from a total of 32 ± 18 to 41 ± 19 g daily for males compared to a range of 15 ± 7 to 49 ± 48 g daily for females. Competitive bodybuilders consumed very little fat as a percent of total calories (6–20% for females, and 11–22% for males with the exception of the case study by Manore et al.[13] in which the use of MCT [Medium Chain Triglycerides] oil increased the fat intake from 5 to 30% of total kcal). Fat, as a percent of total calories, provided 20 and 27% of total calories for competitive and noncompetitive female bodybuilders, respectively, evaluated by Lamar-Hildebrand et al.[15] In the longitudinal studies for competitive female bodybuilders,[15,16] fat intake decreased significantly. Walberg-Rankin et al.[16] noted a five-fold increase in fat intake at the time of competition from 6 ± 5% of total kilocalories to 29 ± 16% of kilocalories 1 month later.

These data clearly illustrate the dramatic shifts in total energy intake as well as in the distribution of energy intake as bodybuilders make dietary changes prior to competition, at the time of competition, and during the recovery period after competition. These changes in dietary consumption patterns, training volume and intensity, and body composition, under-score the need to also conduct research on neuro-hormonal regulators of energy metabolism including possible alterations in risk factors for chronic diseases. They also suggest that alterations in nutritional status may increase if the nutrient density of those foods providing protein, fat, and carbohydrate is not adequate.

The polyunsaturated-saturated fat (P/S) ratio in the diets of bodybuilders is quite variable among the reported studies ranging from 0.4 to 3.8 for competitive female bodybuilders and from 0.6 to 2.4 for competitive male bodybuilders. P/S ratios averaged 1.7 ± 1.8 for competitive female bodybuilders and 1.3 ± 0.9 for competitive male bodybuilders. The wide variation in P/S ratios reported in these studies suggests wide variation in the source and contribution of fats derived from animal and plant products. It is unfortunate that most studies provided little, if any, information on the kinds and amounts of fats being consumed. Few of the studies on lipids of individuals involved in strength training provided adequate infor-mation on dietary fat intake.

The average daily cholesterol intake was 244 ± 128 mg for competitive female body-builders and 362 ± 147 mg for competitive male bodybuilders. Mean dietary cholesterol intakes have ranged from 148 ± 104[15] to 462 ± 631[5] mg daily for competitive female bodybuilders. Mean dietary cholesterol intakes for male bodybuilders ranged from 182 ± 61 in the case study by Manore et al.[13] in which most of the fat was provided in the form of MCT oil to 513 ± 582 mg daily.[5] Thus, dietary cholesterol intakes tend to be higher among males than females, and many bodybuilders appear to consume higher amounts of cholesterol than recommended according to the National Cholesterol Education Program Guidelines (NCEP).[23] Kleiner et al.[8] reported a mean intake of 1413 ± 1151 mg per day while Faber et al.[7] reported a mean intake as high as 2823 ± 542 mg per day in a group of bodybuilders who ate more than six whole eggs per day. One subject consumed as many as 81 eggs per week.[7] Eggs appear to be an important source of protein for many bodybuilders and consequently are the major contributor to total cholesterol intake in these athletes. Some bodybuilders are shifting from the use of whole eggs to the use of egg whites or cholesterol-free egg products.

Dietary fiber intake (Table 1) among "senior"-level elite male and female bodybuilders[5] was approximately half that of their "junior"-level male and female counterparts.[6] The low intakes of 7 ± 7 and 7 ± 5 g daily among the senior-level males and females, respectively, in comparison to the junior-level males and females reflect differences in food choices. Since carbohydrate intake as a percent of total calorie intake was relatively similar among both groups while total energy intake was approximately 600 calories (2.5 joules) less among senior-level vs. junior-level competitors, these differences may simply reflect differences in absolute carbohydrate intake. Dietary fiber intake among 76 South African bodybuilders averaged 18 ± 9 g daily and did not vary significantly between bodybuilders who consumed a large quantity of eggs per week compared to those bodybuilders who consumed few eggs.[7] Longitudinal data are needed in order to determine if the usual fiber intakes of elite bodybuilders are also low. Such data combined with other biochemical data would be needed in order to assess the physiological consequences of a low fiber intake. Data are also needed on the types (soluble and insoluble) of fiber and the amounts of each in order to evaluate the potential role of fiber on blood lipids and blood pressure of bodybuilders as well as other populations of athletes.

Vitamin and mineral intakes (Table 2) were not reported in several of the studies in which food intake information was collected.[9-11,21] Vitamins A and C intakes were generally well above the RDA. Intakes for thiamin and other B vitamins also appear to be above the RDA. Vitamin D intake was nil for competitive female bodybuilders evaluated by Bazzarre et al.[5] The vitamin D intake varied widely among competitive male bodybuilders in the same study, which reflected differences in the consumption of dairy products. Avoidance of dairy products is commonplace among bodybuilders as they prepare for competition; however, there is no apparent scientific basis for this practice. The lack of dietary vitamin D among competitive bodybuilders may be offset by the suntanning practices of this group of athletes.

The average calcium intake among female bodybuilders during competitive training in this series of studies was 408 ± 170 mg per day while the average intake for male bodybuilders was 631 ± 219 mg. Dietary calcium intakes varied among the studies ranging from 272 ± 140[14] to 709 ± 662[15] mg among competitive female bodybuilders and from 416 ± 209[14] to 917 ± 953[6] mg among competitive male bodybuilders (Table 2). Low calcium intakes were consistently observed for bodybuilders evaluated at the time of competition compared to reports for bodybuilders conducted at other time periods. These cross sectional study comparisons were consistent with changes in dietary calcium intake in the longitudinal studies of competitive female bodybuilders.[14-16] Walberg-Rankin et al.[16] reported even higher calcium intakes (1046 ± 600 mg) at recovery 1 month after competition than either precompetition (667 ± 493 mg) and competition (280 ± 121 mg). Heyward et al.[14] demonstrated the dramatic influence of restricting the intake of milk in their longitudinal study of seven male bodybuilders whose mean calcium intake declined from 2141 ± 1673 mg daily prior to competition to 416 ± 209 mg during the time of competition.

Low calcium intakes in this series of studies reflect the restriction of milk and dairy products. While low calcium intakes among female endurance athletes with amenorrhea has created concern about their increased risk of osteoporosis, it is not clear if reduced bone density is a problem for strength-trained female athletes who also have low calcium and vitamin D intakes. Since competitive female bodybuilders can achieve body fat levels less than 10%, which is associated with menstrual disturbances, and because more and more women are participating in this sport, research on the consequences of low body fat in association with low dietary calcium and vitamin D intake on osteoporosis are urgently needed.

The average magnesium intake for female bodybuilders during competitive training was 314 ± 76 mg per day while the average for male bodybuilders was 569 ± 156 mg. Mean magnesium intakes among the studies of female bodybuilders varied by 175 mg. Mean magnesium intake decreased from 304 ± 103 mg during the precompetition period to 280 ± 168 mg at the time of competition in the longitudinal study of 12 female bodybuilders by Heyward et al.[14] while the mean intake increased slightly from 249 ± 113 mg to 298 ± 112 mg in six female bodybuilders studies by Walberg-Rankin et al.[16] and rose significantly to 341 ± 122 mg 1 month after competition. The changes in magnesium intakes in these studies[14,16] parallel those observed for energy intake in the respective studies.

Magnesium intake among male bodybuilders competing at a national "senior-level" competition[6] (424 ± 198 mg) were 43% more than that reported for male bodybuilders at a

TABLE 2   Mineral and Vitamin Intakes of Athletes Engaged in Strength-Training Activities

Investigators	Sample	Minerals					Vitamins			
		Calcium (mg)	Magnesium (mg)	Iron (mg)	Zinc (mg)	Copper (mg)	A (RE)[b]	C (mg)	D (mg)	Thiamin (mg)
Female Bodybuilders										
Bazzarre et al., 1990[5]	8 comp	293 ± 231	254 ± 107	24 ± 40	9 ± 5	1.9 ± 1.6	—	—	—	—
Bazzarre et al., 1992[6]	11 comp	418 ± 198	424 ± 158	17 ± 10	9 ± 5	1.1 ± 0.6	—	196 ± 168	0	1.3 ± 0.6
Heyward et al., 1989[14] (longitudinal)	12 precomp	705 ± 390	304 ± 103	14 ± 4	9 ± 4	—	—	133 ± 80	—	1.3 ± 0.5
	12 comp	272 ± 140	280 ± 168	11 ± 5	7 ± 5	—	—	187 ± 109	—	3.4 ± 7.7
Lamar-Hildebrand 1989[15] (longitudinal)	6 comp	709 ± 662	—	12 ± 6	—	—	—	—	—	—
	4 noncomp	962 ± 544	—	15 ± 5	—	—	—	—	—	—
Sandoval et al., 1989[19] (longitudinal)	6 comp	478 ± 339	—	14 ± 5	—	—	—	166 ± 103	—	1.7 ± 0.8
Walberg-Rankin, 1993[16] (longitudinal)	6 precomp	667 ± 493	249 ± 113	14 ± 4	7 ± 3	1.3 ± 0.7	4666 ± 2915	74 ± 35	—	1.4 ± 0.5
	6 comp	280 ± 121	298 ± 112	18 ± 6	5 ± 2	1.8 ± 1.2	3247 ± 4478	151 ± 106	—	2.3 ± 2.0
	6 post-comp	1046 ± 600	341 ± 122	19 ± 9	9 ± 6	2.1 ± 2.0	5451 ± 1501	149 ± 80	—	3.3 ± 2.7
X ± SD/comp[a]	**(53 total)**	**408 ± 170**	**314 ± 76**	**16 ± 5**	**8 ± 2**	**1.6 ± 0.4**	—	**175 ± 20**	—	**2.2 ± 0.9**
Male Bodybuilders										
Bazzarre et al., 1990[5]	19 comp	605 ± 586	385 ± 214	16 ± 9	11 ± 6	2.5 ± 1.8	—	—	—	—
Bazzarre et al., 1992[6]	19 comp	917 ± 953	700 ± 318	24 ± 6	14 ± 5	2.1 ± 1.4	—	272 ± 258	93 ± 287	2.1 ± 0.7
Faber et al., 1986[7]	76	1508 ± 664	447 ± 153	24 ± 8	24 ± 9	2.9 ± 1.4	3476 ± 2364	178 ± 112	—	2.8 ± 0.8
Heyward et al., 1989[14]	7 precomp	2141 ± 1673	631 ± 204	29 ± 10	24 ± 12	—	—	154 ± 94	—	2.1 ± 0.7
	7 comp	416 ± 209	494 ± 146	19 ± 7	12 ± 6	—	—	171 ± 82	—	9.0 ± 14.0
Kleiner et al., 1989[8]	18 SU	2987 ± 1825	—	44 ± 31	40 ± 31	—	5366 ± 9087	493 ± 326	—	—
	17 NSU									
Manore et al., 1993[13]	1 comp	786 ± 172	697 ± 189	20 ± 3	11 ± 2	—	6186 ± 3117	145 ± 49	—	4.5 ± 0.4
Sandoval et al., 1989[19]	5 comp	433 ± 189	—	19 ± 6	—	—	—	137 ± 71	—	2.0 ± 1.0
Short and Short, 1983[4]	6	1786	—	29	—	—	1210	185	—	—
X ± SD[a]	**Total: 168**	**631 ± 219[a]**	**569 ± 156[a]**	**19 ± 3[a]**	**12 ± 1[a]**	**2.3 ± 0.3[a]**	**5776 ± 580[a]**	**181 ± 62[a]**	**93 ± 287**	—

Male Weightlifters (WL), Wrestlers (WRE), and Football Players (FB)

Chen et al., 1989[24]	10 elite WL	1597 ± 195	50 ± 9	—	777 ± 304	—	1547 ± 99	93 ± 35	—	1.8 ± 0.3
	5 amateur WL	908 ± 144	46 ± 6	36 ± 11	374 ± 141	5.5 ± 1.2	1199 ± 172	52 ± 13	—	2.4 ± 0.4
Heinemann and Zerbes, 1989[25]	15 WL	—	—	—	—	—	—	260	—	—
	20 WRE	—	—	—	—	—	—	230	—	—
Hickson et al., 1987[29]	46 Jr. HS FB	1261 ± 655	15 ± 11	13 ± 8	482 ± 287	—	6063 ± 6130	103 ± 93	—	1.5 ± 1.0
	88 HS FB	1737 ± 1359	20 ± 12	17 ± 12	634 ± 437	—	8025 ± 8658	180 ± 239	—	2.2 ± 1.6
Hickson et al., 1987[30]	11 College FB	110% RDA	231% RDA	166% RDA	79% RDA	—	108% RDA	265% RDA	—	133% RDA
Short and Short, 1983[4]	10 def. backs	1876	15	—	—	—	1444	244	—	2
	23 defense	1818	28	—	—	—	2694	297	—	3.1
	33 offense	2084	29	—	—	—	2133	300	—	3.5
X ± SD[a]	Total: 195	1378 ± 370	33 ± 18	22 ± 12	567 ± 176	5.5 ± 1.2	4209 ± 3373	153 ± 83	—	2.0 ± 0.4

Note: Abbreviations — comp, during competitive training period; precomp, prior to competitive training period; post-comp, after competitive training period; SU, Steroid Users; NSU, Non-Steroid Users.

a   Means ± Standard Deviation for studies without adjustment for differences in sample size.
b   Retinol equivalents. 1 retinol equivalent = 1 μg retinol or 6 μg β-carotene.

national "junior-level" competition[5] (293 ± 107 mg). In a longitudinal study of seven male bodybuilders,[14] mean magnesium intake decreased substantially from 631 ± 204 mg per day before competition to 494 ± 146 mg at the time of competition. Magnesium intakes for competitive male bodybuilders were at or above the RDA for men while magnesium intakes for competitive female bodybuilders tended to be near the RDA for women.

The average dietary iron intake in this series of studies was 16 ± 5 mg per day for female bodybuilders during their competitive training and 19 ± 3 mg for male bodybuilders. Iron intakes were well above RDA for male bodybuilders and for competitive female bodybuilders. Iron intake decreased in both male and female bodybuilders from their precompetition training periods to their intakes at the time of competition in the longitudinal study by Heyward et al;[14] however, iron intake increased from 14 ± 4 mg per day in six female bodybuilders studied by Walberg-Rankin et al.[16] to 18 ± 6 mg at the time of competition. The high dietary intakes of iron in these studies reflects the liberal intake of red meat. Iron intakes can be excessive as illustrated by a mean dietary intake of 44 ± 31 mg per day in the bodybuilders studied by Kleiner et al.[8] Studies of excessive iron and protein intake in bodybuilders warrant future investigation on the effects of these dietary constituents on blood clotting factors, thrombogenic regulation, and blood lipids as well as their potential to elevate blood homocysteine levels.

The average intake for dietary zinc in this series of studies was 8 ± 2 mg per day for female bodybuilders and 12 ± 1 mg for competitive male bodybuilders. Zinc intakes were lower than the RDA for all studies of male and female bodybuilders during the competitive training period and for female bodybuilders regardless of the time of data collection. High intakes of dietary zinc in male bodybuilders have been reported by Kleiner et al.[8] (40 ± 31 mg daily) and in South African bodybuilders who averaged 24 ± 9 g daily compared to 31 ± 17 g daily when supplements were included in estimating daily intakes.[7] High intakes of zinc have been associated with low HDL-cholesterol levels. Thus, the low HDL-cholesterol levels observed in bodybuilders could be related to excessively high intakes of zinc as well as other dietary factors.

Estimates of dietary copper intake are limited to just a few investigations in this series of studies.[5-7,16] Intakes for competitive male bodybuilders[5,6] were well within the Estimated Safe and Adequate Daily Dietary Intake (ESADDI).[22] Copper intakes ranged from 1.1 ± 0.6[6] to 1.9 ± 1.4[5] mg daily for competitive female bodybuilders. Copper intake among South African bodybuilders was 2.9 ± 1.4 mg daily and 4.2 ± 2.6 mg daily when supplements were included.[7]

Lower vitamin/mineral intakes among females tend to reflect lower calorie/food intakes compared to males, which follows the general patterns usually observed between males and females. The lower intakes of vitamins and minerals among the competitive male bodybuilders[5,6] compared to other bodybuilders also reflect lower energy/food intakes.

C. WEIGHTLIFTERS AND WRESTLERS

Six studies on the dietary intakes of male weightlifters and wrestlers,[9,18,24-27] representing a total of 58 male weightlifters and 62 wrestlers (Table 1), and one study on nine female weightlifters[11] have been reported in the literature (Table 1). The data by Short and Short[4] in their 4 year study of collegiate athletes included wrestlers; however, the data are not reported here because no means or average intakes for the wrestlers studied over the 4 year period were provided and because the sample size changed from year to year.

The males in these studies ranged in age from 16 to 23 years while the mean age of the female weightlifters was 36 years. The latter study[11] is significant in the sports nutrition literature because this is one of the older groups of athletes that have been studied. Body weights for the males in these studies ranged from 71 kg[24] to 95 kg.[25] Steen and McKinney[18] reported body fat levels which were 14% pre- and post-season as compared to 11% during mid-season. Body fat levels of 14% were reported by Hurley et al.[9] in eight powerlifters who had their lipid levels measured. The body fat levels in these studies were greater than that reported for national level female as well as male bodybuilders.[5,6] Short and Short[4] did not provide any age, body composition, or training information in their study of college athletes.

The data reported by Chen et al.[24] are based on a comparison of the intakes of ten elite weightlifters 21 ± 2 years of age compared to five amateur weightlifters 16 ± 1 year of age. It is important to recognize that the latter data reflect the cultural food patterns of Chinese athletes. Elite weightlifters weighed 10 kg more than the amateur weightlifters. The impact of differences in training dose (volume and intensity) between the amateur and elite groups on nutrient intake and body composition were not evaluated in this report.

Using the 24-h recall method of estimating nutrient intake, Warren et al.[27] reported average daily energy intake greater than 3714 ± 1573 kcal d^{-1} and protein intakes above 2.0 g/d^{-1} in a group of 28 male Olympic weightlifters. Hurley et al. compared the dietary intakes of eight male bodybuilders to that of eight male powerlifters[9] while Heinemann and Zerbes[25] measured the dietary intakes of 15 weightlifters and 20 wrestlers. The latter study included data obtained for other groups of athletes not reported here and also reflects cultural food practices of German athletes.[25] In addition to the need to consider the potential impact of differences in the training regimens of wrestlers vs. weightlifters, it is also important to recognize that the weightlifters' body weight averaged 95 kg compared to 85 kg for the wrestlers. Morgan et al.[11] reported the only data for a group of nine females engaged in a wide variety of strength-training regimens which were compared to a control group of nine sedentary females and a group of nine female endurance athletes.

Energy intake among elite Chinese weightlifters was approximately 500 calories (2.092 joules) more per day than their amateur counterparts.[24] The lower intake among the amateur weightlifters might be explained by their lower body weights and/or by a presumed decrease in physical training effort in comparison to their elite counterparts. Similarly, the 27 calorie (0.112968 joules) per kilogram body weight (BW) difference between the wrestlers and weightlifters may be accounted for by differences in training volume and intensity.[25] Energy intake per kilogram BW was fairly similar among Chinese amateur and elite wrestlers and German wrestlers (52–58 kcal/kg BW [217.568 kilojoules]), but much less than that of German weightlifters (79 kcal/kg BW [330.536 kilojoules]).

The amount and categories of nutrient intake information in many of these studies was very limited. Based on the data available for this series of studies, the average distribution of energy intake as a percent of total kilocalories for males engaged in weightlifting, power lifting, or wrestling was $17 \pm 3\%$ protein; $39 \pm 6 \%$ fat; and $45 \pm 6 \%$ carbohydrate. The mean intake for the nine females engaged in weighlifting study by Morgan et al.[11] as a percent of total kilocalories consumed was $23 \pm 9\%$ protein; $32 \pm 13 \%$ fat; and $47 \pm 10\%$ carbohydrate. Thus, average protein intake as a percent of kilocalories was in the range that would be expected for the U.S. male population in general. Protein intake as a percent of total kilocalories for women in the study by Morgan et al.[11] was higher than that for the U.S. population of adult women but lower than the average observed for female bodybuilders at the time of competition.

Average fat intake as a percent of total kilocalories in this group of studies of male weightlifters and wrestlers at 39% was significantly higher than the average of 11% for male bodybuilders during the competitive training period. Fat intake as a percent of total kilocalories in female[11] at 32% was also significantly higher than the average of 11% for female bodybuilders during competitive training.

Carbohydrate as a percent of total kcal consumed was similar for female weightlifters compared to female bodybuilders during their competitive training period. The average carbohydrate intake of the male weightlifters and wrestlers (45%) in this series of studies was 19% less than that observed for male bodybuilders (64%) during competitive training.

Hurley et al.[9] combined the data for both bodybuilders and weightlifters and only reported information on the percent of total calories provided by protein, fat, and carbohydrate. These combined intakes were similar to the distributions reported by Chen et al.[24] for elite weightlifters (20–22% of kcal by protein). Protein intake as a percent of total kilocalories among amateur Chinese weightlifters (14%) was similar to that of German weightlifters and wrestlers (15–18%).

Data for male weightlifters and wrestlers intakes of vitamins and minerals (Table 2) is limited to three studies: 15 Chinese weightlifters,[24] 35 weightlifters and wrestlers from Germany,[25] and 42 American wrestlers.[18] Unfortunately, the data for the U.S. athletes is more limited because these investigators presented their data only in bar graph format as a percent of the RDA. Consequently, it is not possible to provide any information of the absolute intakes of specific vitamins and minerals nor to easily compare these data with other data reported in the literature. Researchers should be encouraged to fill in this gap in the literature as alterations in weight-cycling by diet and weightloss practices involving dehydration are likely to significantly impact the nutritional status of many minerals.

Calcium and magnesium intakes of elite Chinese weightlifters were almost twice that of their amateur weightlifting counterparts; however, no explanations for these differences were provided by the authors.[24] Differences in food choices represent one explanation for these differences in nutrient intakes as energy intakes were quite similar on a per kilogram BW basis. Chinese weightlifters had the highest iron intakes of any of the populations studied (50 ± 9 and 46 ± 6 mg daily for elite and amateurs, respectively). Unusually high zinc and copper intakes were also reported for amateur Chinese weightlifters (no data were reported for elite weightlifters). Vitamin C intakes were lower for Chinese strength-trained athletes than for any other population evaluated and averaged only 52 ± 13 mg daily for amateur weightlifters.

Steen and McKinney[18] reported the percent of wrestlers who did not consume at least two-thirds of the RDA for selected vitamins and minerals during the preseason, midseason, and postseason periods. They also evaluated the contribution of supplements to total intakes for these nutrients in their report. The data also support previous comments in this chapter suggesting that athletes do modify their food/nutrient intakes during the training season. Fewer wrestlers did not consume at least two-thirds of the RDA postseason compared to preseason and midseason for all nutrients reported (i.e., vitamin A, vitamin C, vitamin B$_6$, thiamin, iron, zinc, and magnesium). A higher percentage of wrestlers did not consume two-thirds of the RDA for vitamin A and vitamin C (about 45 and 22%, respectively) as compared to the preseason measures. About 65% of the wrestlers did not consume at least two-thirds of the RDA for vitamin B$_6$ during the preseason period as compared to about 59% midseason and 50% postseason. About 25, 52, and 64% of wrestlers did not consume at least two-thirds of the RDA for iron, zinc, and magnesium during the midseason period.

D. OTHER STRENGTH-TRAINED POPULATIONS (FOOTBALL PLAYERS)

Hickson et al. studied 11 collegiate football players, 88 high school football players, and 46 junior high school football players (Table 1).[29,30] Short and Short[4] studied the dietary intakes of football players over a 4-year period during which the sample ranged from as few as 10 players to as many as 34 subjects). Their data for 10 defensive backs, 23 defensive players, and 33 offensive players collected in a single season are reported in Table 1. Readers should refer to the original paper for additional information collected on players during the other years in the 4-year study. Information on the dietary intakes of professional football players is lacking and represents an area for future research.

The average energy intake for the 211 football players in these four studies was 3744 ± 921 kcal (15,665 kilojoules). Energy intakes in the 4000–6000 kcal (16,736 kilojoules) range and higher do not appear to be uncommon in football players. Although this range is much higher than that observed for male bodybuilders during competitive training, intakes of 5739 ± 2500 kcal (24,012 kilojoules) per day were reported by Kleiner et al.[8] in 35 male bodybuilders. Manore et al.[13] reported an intake of 4952 ± 279 kcal (20,719 kilojoules) per day in a case study of a world class bodybuilder consuming MCT oil as part of his diet.

Energy intake increased with age and body size in the series of studies on junior high, high school, and collegiate football players reported by Hickson et al.[29,30] Mean energy intakes among the Syracuse University Football team ranged from 4470 to 6149 calories (18,702 to 25,727 joules) during the 4-year period.[4] Individual intakes ranged from as low as 1990 (8.32616 joules) to as much as 11,020 calories (46,108 joules).[4] Energy intakes were about 1500 kcal (6276 kilojoules) more per day among offensive and defensive players as compared to defensive backs. Although no data on body weight were reported, some of the differences in energy intakes in the latter study may be due to differences in the bodyweight of those athletes playing line positions compared to those playing in the backfield.

The average distribution of protein, fat, and carbohydrate as a percent of total kilocalories intakes in this series of studies was 17, 40, and 44%, respectively. These distributions are similar to the averages reported for weightlifters and wrestlers but are clearly at variance with the averages observed for competitive male bodybuilders during competitive training. It is interesting to note that many collegiate players develop a strong interest in bodybuilding after their collegiate playing period and consequently may alter their food intake patterns accordingly.

Mean dietary cholesterol intakes among Syracuse University football players (Table 1) were extremely high, ranging from 626 to 1425 mg daily.[4] The average intake for the 66 players during one year was 841 ± 187 mg per day. Individual intakes ranged from a low of 296 mg daily to a high of 3584 mg. The P/S ratio of the diets consumed by these same football players was exceptionally low, ranging from a mean of 0.23 to a high of 0.38. The average P/S ratio was 0.19 ± 0.05 for the 66 players and was quite low for individual players reaching values of 0.07, 0.08, and 0.09 among different groups of players. The highest P/S ratios among individual football players were 0.50, 0.57, and 0.72. The P/S ratios of the diets of these athletes were not even close to a 1:1 ratio. A significant number of athletes apparently consumed more than 300 g of fat on a daily basis.

Clearly, the dietary intakes of these football players would place some athletes into a high risk group for cardiovascular disease. Data on the blood lipid profiles, blood pressure, and body fat levels are clearly needed. Since many collegiate lineman also demonstrated considerable abdominal obesity, the assessment of cardiovascular risks among this group is warranted. Since the body weights and presumably the body fat levels and girths of offensive and defensive linemen at both the collegiate and professional level has continued to rise over the past decade or longer, the relative impact of such extreme weights on cardiovascular and diabetes risk factors should be examined, particularly as these players get older.

Mean dietary intakes for calcium, magnesium, and iron (Table 2) were greater than the RDA for junior high school, senior high school, and collegiate football players studied by Hickson et al.[29,30] Mean zinc intakes were above the RDA for senior high school and collegiate players but not for their junior high school counterparts. The higher food/energy intakes of the older players contributed to the high intakes of vitamins and minerals among these groups. The high food/energy intakes reported by Short and Short[4] for college football players also contributed to the high level of adequacy for vitamins and minerals among this group.

E. RECREATIONAL STRENGTH-TRAINED ATHLETES

Little information has been reported on the nutritional status of individuals involved in "recreational" strength training. The term "recreational" is used here to imply that these individuals were not professionals. However, it is clear from working with many "recreational" athletes that many of them are quite serious about their training and competitive experiences. In fact, some of them have aspired to become professional athletes.

Lamar-Hildebrand et al.[15] reported data on six noncompetitive females involved in bodybuilding who might be classified as recreational, strength-trained athletes. The nine females evaluated by Morgan et al.[11] might also be classified as recreational athletes. Because of the sparsity of data on females, the data from all studies for females engaged in any form of strength training were grouped together (Table 1).

Bazzarre et al.[17] conducted a 24-week longitudinal study of endurance athletes which included a group of 12 control males who regularly engaged in strength training and who maintained a relatively constant training program during the 24-wk study. Age, heights, body weights, and body fat levels (11–14%) were not significantly different between the recreational strength trained males, a group of 26 male triathletes and a group 12 endurance athletes (note that the body fat levels in this group of males classified as recreational athletes was within the range for bodybuilders during their noncompetitive training period). Although the male strength trained athletes (controls) consumed about 150 kcal more per day than the endurance athletes, these differences were not statistically significant. The protein, fat, and carbohydrate intakes were relatively similar between these two groups at 14, 31–34, and 46–50%, respectively. The distribution of energy intakes was somewhat similar to that reported by Gater et al.[31] who studied the effects of resistance training and amino acid supplementation on 37 males about 23 years of age. The percent body fat in these males, 16–17%, was higher than that reported by Bazzarre et al.[17] The distribution of protein, fat, and carbohydrate in the study by Gater et al.[31] was 15–20, 28–36, and 45–56%, respectively.

The energy intake of these recreational strength athletes[17] was similar to that of bodybuilders at the time of competition but less than the reported for other bodybuilders, wrestlers, and weightlifters, as well as high school and college age football players. Protein as a percent of total kilocalories was similar to that of amateur Chinese athletes (14%) evaluated by Chen et al.[24] but much less than that reported in other studies (Table 1). These data may suggest that more highly trained strength athletes consume more energy and more protein than their recreational or amateur counterparts.

Dietary cholesterol (453 ± 57 mg) intake in these recreational strength trained athletes[17] was within the range reported for competitive male bodybuilders[5,6] but much less than reported by Kleiner et al.[8] and Faber et al.[7] Fiber intake (6.2 ± 0.9 g) was lower than reported for competitive male bodybuilders (9–18 g daily).

The mean intakes for these recreational strength trained athletes for vitamins A, C, pyridoxine, B_{12}, thiamin, and riboflavin (but not niacin) were above RDA levels.[22] Mean intakes for calcium, phosphorus, magnesium, and iron were also at or above RDA levels, while dietary zinc and copper intakes (13.9 ± 1.4 and 1.3 ± 0.6 mg daily, respectively) were below RDA levels. Thus, low zinc intakes appear to be common among both recreational strength-trained athletes as well as male and female bodybuilders at the time of competition.

F.   BIOCHEMICAL INDICES OF NUTRITIONAL STATUS

Few of the investigators of studies of strength-trained athletes measured biochemical indices of nutritional status in the populations surveyed.[5,6,17,24] Since the mean dietary intakes of these subjects appeared to be adequate, it is not surprising that the mean biochemical indices for iron (hemoglobin, hematocrit, and serum ferritin), zinc, copper, magnesium, and calcium were all within normal ranges. Vitamin C levels were low in five recreational strength trained athletes[17] which was consistent with relatively low vitamin C intakes in this group.

A secondary set of data analyses was conducted by Bazzarre et al.[32] who evaluated the impact of vitamin-mineral supplement use, former use, and nonuse in a sample of 91 athletes. Supplements were used by 100% of female athletes but only 51% of male athletes used supplements. Both male and female supplement users tended to have lower body fat levels, but these differences were not statistically significant. The distribution of dietary fat, protein, and carbohydrate as a percent of total kilocalories intake was not significantly different between supplement users and nonusers. Dietary intakes (excluding supplements) of supplement users tended to be higher than that for nonusers (vitamin C, thiamin, riboflavin, niacin,

B$_6$, B$_{12}$, folate, calcium, iron, and magnesium), but again these differences were not statistically significant. Blood levels of vitamin C were significantly higher (p <0.05) among supplement users than nonusers; however, there were no significant differences in biochemical measures of iron, zinc, or copper status.

The lack of any strong evidence of nutrition problems based on biochemical measures of nutritional status was consistent with the findings of Fogelholm et al.[12] who conducted an extensive series of biochemical tests of nutritional status in a large sample of Finnish athletes. The incidence of nutritional deficiency was between 0 and 5% of the population for hemoglobin, ferritin, magnesium, zinc, and vitamin C. Of these Finnish athletes, 3–4% had low erythrocyte transketolase activity, suggesting marginal or deficient thiamin status.

IV. STUDIES OF PROTEIN REQUIREMENTS OF STRENGTH-TRAINED ATHLETES

While much research has been conducted to determine the amount of energy required to perform different types and amounts of work, relatively few investigations have examined the impact of increased amounts of work (i.e., increased energy expenditure) on other nutrient requirements. The protein requirements of athletes or military personnel has been the focus of most studies that have examined the effects of physical training on nutrient needs. Results for at least 25 investigations on the protein requirements of athletes have been published in the literature.[35-38] Many investigators have examined the effects of protein requirements on sedentary or untrained subjects, while other investigators have examined the protein needs of endurance-trained athletes.

Most published review articles on the nutrient needs of athletes include sections on protein and energy. Most authors of review papers cited prior to 1975 drew conclusions based on assumptions about the protein needs of athletes. Unfortunately, the assumptions made in these early review papers (i.e., the protein needs of athletes/laborers are no different than the protein needs of the general population) were not based on any specific research conducted on athletes. The authors of these review articles simply made extrapolations based on the Recommended Dietary Allowances (RDA).[22] These review articles have, unfortunately, been cited all too frequently. The lack of awareness of the existing research data base may explain why so little research has been conducted on this topic.

This discussion has been organized according to the kinds of methods used to evaluate the protein needs of individuals including athletes engaged in strength training. These methods include complete nitrogen balance (NBAL) investigations (i.e., investigations which collected 24-h urine, fecal, and sweat excretions), investigations which measured only urinary output, and a single investigation in which only sweat nitrogen (N) losses were measured.[58]

Major limitations of many investigations include the extremely small sample size and the large interindividual variation. Kraut et al.[47] and Mole and Johnson[51] studied only two and three subjects, respectively, while Gontzea et al.[44] evaluated 30 subjects. Most investigators evaluated the N needs/metabolism of six or fewer subjects. We are unaware of any reports in the literature which contain complete NBAL data for females engaged in high levels of physical energy output, and little research has been conducted to date on the potential effects of differences in age on N needs relative to similar levels of work performance. Thus, important research questions on the role of gender and age on the protein needs of strength-trained athletes remain to be examined.

A. NITROGEN BALANCE STUDIES

At least 25 investigations are known in the literature which provide NBAL data on subjects performing various kinds of work/physical activity. Some of these investigations are reported in journals for which either complete bibliographic information and/or results were not available.

Increased physical training/increased energy expenditure appears to increase protein needs regardless of the form of exercise (i.e., muscular vs. endurance) although increased requirements appear to be greater for endurance-trained athletes than strength-trained athletes. Recent research by Murdoch and colleagues[57] suggests that the protein needs of highly trained endurance athletes were well above the RDA of 0.8 g/kg BW per day, as only 78% of subjects were in NBAL while consuming diets that provided at least 1.6 g protein per kilogram body weight per day and at least 2800 kcal (11,715.2 kilojoules) daily. These findings are consistent with reports by Tarnopolsky et al.[54] and others.[50,51] On the basis of multiple regression analysis, Tarnopolsky et al.[54] calculated that endurance athletes would be in NBAL at an intake of 1.4 g protein/kg BW/day and a daily intake of approximately 4500 kcal (18,828 kilojoules). In this same study, Tarnopolsky et al. reported that the protein needs of endurance athletes and bodybuilders were 1.67 and 1.12 times greater, respectively, than sedentary control subjects consuming 0.7 g protein/kg BW/day and 3200 kcal (13,388.8 kilojoules) daily.

Consolazio et al.[41] reported marginal NBAL data for eight subjects during a rigorous physical training program. These subjects were participating in two 40-d NBAL studies separated into four 10-d periods each. In the first experiment, subjects received 3084 kcal (12,903.456 kilojoules) and 1.4 g protein/kg BW daily, whereas in the second experiment, the subjects received 3500 kcal (14,644 kilojoules) and 2.8 g protein/kg BW daily. Although no measures of variance were reported, mean NBAL during the four 10-d periods ranged from +0.26 to +0.71 g daily in experiment A and from +0.14 to +3.24 g daily in experiment B. Assuming that the variance in these subjects was similar to that observed in other studies, it does not appear that all subjects in these two series of experiments were in NBAL. Consolazio et al.[41] noted that failure to measure or correct for "sweat [N] losses could seriously invalidate the accuracy of metabolic balance studies." Furthermore, these investigators recommended that individuals engaged in vigorous physical training programs consume at least 100 g protein daily.

Gontzea et al.[44,45] conducted two studies on NBAL of athletes cycling approximately 2-h daily. In the first study, 29 of 30 athletes were in NBAL at a daily intake of 1.0 g protein/kg BW, whereas only two of six subjects were in NBAL at a daily intake of 1.5 g protein/kg BW. It is not clear if the energy intake and exercise prescriptions in these two studies were the same.

Mole and Johnson[51] reported that three untrained subjects were in NBAL (N intake was 7% greater than N excretion) when consuming a diet that provided 2.0 g protein and 46 kcal/kg (192.464 kilojoules) BW daily. When these subjects were exercised on a treadmill in which the workouts expended 500 and 1000 kcal (2092 kilojoules) (which were balanced by increased energy intake of 500 and 1000, respectively), N retention increased. Mole and Johnson[51] did not account for either sweat or miscellaneous N losses, and they included rest and exercise days within each 9-d study period, thus the validity of their observations is questionable.

Relatively recent studies on the protein requirements of bodybuilders suggest that muscular strength training increased protein needs, but the exact lower limits have not been clearly established. Tarnopolsky et al.[54] and Celejowa and Homa[40] reported positive NBAL among bodybuilders receiving between 1.05 and 2.77 g protein/kg BW daily. However, four of the ten weightlifters studied by Celejowa and Homa[40] were in negative NBAL even when fed 2.0 g protein/kg BW/day. Marable et al.[50] reported marginal NBAL among bodybuilders consuming 2.0 g protein/kg BW daily while Laritcheva et al.[48] reported negative NBAL data for athletes consuming 2700 kcal (11,296.8 kilojoules) and 2.7 g protein/kg BW or 1800 kcal and 1.3 g protein/kg BW daily.

Tarnopolsky et al.[59] estimated that the protein intake for zero NBAL in seven athletes (22 ± 2 years of age; 10 ± 3% body fat) who engaged in strength training less than four times per week was 1.41 g/kg BW/day compared to 0.89 g/kg BW for 6 sedentary males 25 ±

4 years of age with an average body fat of 21 ± 5%. The athletes included two football players, two rugby players, and three men who were involved in resistance training exclusively for 3 months before the study. Except for the final three days of each NBAL study period, there was no apparent effort to control the frequency, duration, and volume of work/resistance training among all athletes. Thus, without further information it is not clear if the resistance training performed during the study period was consistent with the prescriptions achieved by competitive bodybuilders who presumably train using a higher total workload than performed in this study. The resistance training performed by the subjects in this study was associated with a 98% greater protein need compared to the sedentary subjects (1.41 vs. 0.69 g/kg). The safety margin for determining recommended protein intakes was based on the Canadian standard of ± 1 SD rather than the 2 SD used by the National Academy of Sciences Food and Nutrition Board in estimating the U.S. RDA for protein.[22] Using the Canadian standard, the authors estimated that protein intake of individuals engaged in resistance training was 1.76 g/kg BW which is more than two times the U.S. RDA for men. These recommendations[59] are considerably higher than previous recommendations by Tarnopolsky et al.[54]

Walberg et al.[56] reported that seven bodybuilders were in negative NBAL (–3.19 g) while consuming 0.8 g/kg BW protein daily, but they achieved a positive NBAL when protein intake was increased to 1.6 g protein. These bodybuilders trained 90–120 min daily, 6-d each week. The negative NBAL observed in these bodybuilders reflected the importance of total energy intake as well as the importance of the protein content. Both groups of bodybuilders consumed hypoenergetic diets (18 kcal/kg [75.312 kilojoules] BW). Even though the low energy intake was held constant, a twofold increase in protein intake was associated with positive NBAL.

There has been some question as to whether individuals can maintain large positive NBAL over long periods of time. Oddoye and Margen[33] demonstrated that individuals placed on high-protein diets (following a prolonged period of negative NBAL) do indeed maintain large positive NBAL for prolonged periods of time (i.e., 20–50 days). These data suggest the potential for individuals involved in strength training to theoretically benefit from high protein intakes. Nitrogen retention was higher in strength- and endurance-trained subjects (32.4 vs. 7.1 g, respectively) consuming 2.8 vs. 1.4 g protein/kg BW/day during a 40-d study conducted by Consolozio et al.[34] The men consuming the higher protein intake also increased their body weight (3.3 kg) more than the men on the lower intake (1.2 kg).

The outcome of increased NBAL on increased body weight (and preferentially, increased lean body mass, LBM) has been evaluated in some, but not all, NBAL studies of strength-trained athletes. Marable et al.[50] did not observe any significant differences in weight gains of men consuming 300% of the RDA for protein compared to men consuming the RDA. Dragan et al.[35] reported 6% gains in LBM (and 5% gains in strength) in Romanian weight-lifters when they increased their dietary protein intake from 275 to 438% of the RDA over a period of several months. Frontera et al.[36] reported that 0.33 g protein/kg BW/day consumed daily for a period of 12 weeks resulted in significant increases in thigh muscle mass and urinary creatinine compared to strength training alone. Lemon and colleagues[37] have also reported increased muscle mass among participants consuming a high-protein diet (334% RDA) compared to 124% RDA among novice bodybuilders during a 6-d/week intensive training program; however, the increased nitrogen retention did not significantly affect increased muscle mass or muscle strength during the initial month of training. The latter studies also suggest the potential benefits of prolonged use of a high-protein diet on increased muscle mass and strength by maintaining a high NBAL during periods of adaptation to intensive training.

Butterfield[60] has criticized many NBAL studies of athletes because researchers failed to provide adequate calories or they did not allow for an adequate period of adjustment to the diet and/or training regimens. Ideally, investigators should provide at least 7- to 10-d for adjustments for changes in diet and/or training prescription. Many NBAL studies were conducted for periods of only 2–3 d each.

Not all studies have demonstrated increased protein needs of athletes. Polykov[52] reported that an unknown number of athletes went into positive NBAL after 15-d of a 30-d NBAL study in which the subjects consumed 0.57 g protein/kg BW/day while participating in a 500-kcal (2092 kilojoules) workout training program.

Butterfield and Calloway,[39] Todd et al.,[55] and Goranzon and Forsum[43] conducted studies in which subjects were fed 0.57 g protein/kg BW. Todd et al.[55] reported that subjects were in positive NBAL when energy intake exceeded energy expenditure, but subjects were in negative NBAL when energy intake was either low or when energy intake was less than expenditure. Goranzon and Forsum[43] reported that their subjects were in negative NBAL.

The subjects evaluated by Todd et al.[55] were not given a high work load (e.g., cycling at 40% of VO_2 max for 1-h) and were previously untrained. It is unlikely that these subjects received any significant training effect from the exercise prescription used in this study. Thus, it seems inappropriate to use these data for drawing inferences about the protein needs of strength-trained athletes or highly trained endurance athletes.

The large group variation reported in these subjects[55] whose mean NBAL was positive also merits consideration. For example, at a level of 0.85 g protein/kg BW/day, the subjects' mean NBAL was 0.42 ± 0.73 g. The large standard deviation suggests that some of the subjects were in negative NBAL. These subjects were in more positive NBAL at higher levels of energy intake, i.e., 0.82 ± 0.58 g N/day.

The research by Todd et al.[55] is also unique because the only protein source used in this study was egg white fed in a liquid purified diet. Since egg white has the highest biological value of all food proteins, and since most individuals in a free-living population do not subsist on this kind of diet, it is important to note that more protein would be needed to achieve NBAL if the subjects were fed a mixed diet. The amount of protein would be approximately 25% higher if the subjects were fed a vegetarian diet in comparison to a mixed diet containing meat and dairy products. Other researchers have also used liquid formula diets or liquid formula diets in conjunction with solid foods.[54,56]

The differences in the data reported and the apparent lack of a rigorous design in some of these studies are reflected in the research reported in the literature. These investigations demonstrate the need to carefully examine the details of each study as these design factors may account for many of the differences observed across the studies. For example, some investigations did not account for or measure the amount of work performed, the energy intake of the subjects was not reported in other investigations, variable levels of energy were used relative to energy expenditure, and the source of dietary protein has varied weekly.

The previous training status of strength athletes may also affect the protein needs as a reflection of the process of adaptation to the training load/stimulus. For example, Tarnopolsky et al.[38] showed that protein requirements of bodybuilders with more than 3 years of training experience averaged 0.9 g/kg BW/day in contrast to 1.5 g for novice bodybuilders during their first month of training.

Future investigations of the protein requirements of athletes may need to examine the protein/energy requirements relative to the potential confounding effects of increased adiposity. As noted in the study by Murdoch et al.,[57] the subjects with the lowest energy needs had higher body fat levels than all of the other subjects, and two of those individuals had the highest NBAL data observed. Thus, it is conceivable that untrained subjects such as those used by Todd et al.[55] and others might have lower protein needs as a result of increased energy efficiency concomitant with greater levels of adiposity. This relationship may be relative, as none of the research subjects studied by Murdoch et al.[57] would be considered obese. The inverse associations between energy intake and NBAL ($r = -0.39$) and between energy intake and percent body fat support the hypothesis that relative adiposity concomitant with increased energy efficiency (i.e., decreased energy needs) might contribute to decreased protein needs. The extremely low body fat levels achieved by highly competitive bodybuilders and the large fluctuations in body fat levels that occur during the year among bodybuilders suggest that the protein needs of those athletes may shift during the year in response to changes in training, body fat levels, and with variations in the amount and source of protein-energy foods as well as supplements.

Recent research on the benefits of resistance training on older subjects' functional capacity and metabolism has created considerable interest among healthcare professionals who want to improve the quality of life of older citizens. Fielding[61] reviewed the literature on the benefits of progressive resistance training on the preservation of lean body mass in older subjects. In seven studies in which the training programs ranged from 12 to 26 weeks, strength increased from a range of 5–65% in one study to levels of 72% in males and 66% in females in another study. Body weight did not change in five studies, however, various measures of body fat declined 2–7% in most studies.

Research by Campbell et al.[62] on 12 older men and women between 56 and 80 years of age suggests that a 12-week resistance training program improves NBAL. Subjects were fed either a low protein diet providing 0.80 ± 0.02 g/kg BW or a high protein diet containing 1.62 ± 0.02 g/kg BW daily. Following the diet adjustment period, NBAL was -4.6 ± 3.4 g on the low protein diet and 13.6 ± 1.0 g on the high protein diet. Resistance training increased NBAL 12.8 and 12.7% in the low and high protein diets, respectively. In comparison to the high protein diet, the low protein diet was associated with an increase in N retention efficiency, a decrease in leucine flux and leucine oxidation ($p < 0.001$) and a decrease in leucine uptake for protein synthesis. An increase in leucine flux ($p < 0.05$) was associated with resistance training in both diet treatment groups; however, the increase in the efficiency of N retention was greater in the group fed the low protein diet compared to the high protein diet. This study is consistent with other research published by Campbell et al.[63] who recommend that protein intakes of older individuals be in the range of 1.0–1.25 g/kg BW/day of high-quality protein. Another study by Campbell et al.[64] indicated that energy needs increased about 15% in older participants participating in a resistance training program.

Older subjects participating in a 12-week resistance training program conducted by Frontera et al.[65] exhibited impressive gains in total muscle mass and urinary creatinine excretion, a measure of total muscle mass, when consuming a 23 g protein supplement daily. Muscle thigh area increased 14.6 ± 1.5 cm^2 in the supplement group compared to 6.1 ± 2.4 cm^2 in the control group although gains in 1-RM (maximum resistance load/weight that can be lifted one time) were not significantly different between the groups. Measures of 1-RM represent only one index of strength. Perhaps other measures such as the number of repetitions at 70% of 1-RM would be a more functional measure of improvements in muscular endurance. Protein when fed at a level of 3.3 vs. 1.3 g/kg BW increased protein synthesis five-fold, and resulted in a total increase in body weight gain of 2.8 ± 0.9 kg compared to 1.5 ± 0.6 kg during a 4-week resistance training program conducted by Fern et al.[66] These data suggest that protein intakes above those levels needed to achieve NBAL may result in additional increments in LBM when combined with resistance training programs. Such benefits are important not only for bodybuilders but also for maintaining LBM in older populations.

In summary, athletes and older individuals engaged in resistance training both appear to benefit from increased protein intakes during periods of resistance training. The increases in lean body mass as well as the maintenance of lean body mass in both groups may be achieved with regular resistance training provided that the dietary intakes of protein and energy are adequate to meet protein requirements. Individual needs may be quite variable based on differences in body composition, age, and training status including level of adaptation to the training stimulus.

B. NITROGEN NEEDS OF ATHLETES BASED ON URINARY EXCRETION STUDIES

Several investigations have been reported in the literature which assessed the N/protein needs of athletes based on urinary excretion. The primary assumption in using 24-h urine samples is based on the premise that fecal N losses are relatively constant on a controlled diet and that changes in urinary N excretion accurately reflect a decrease or increase in protein utilization if diet and other sources of N losses are kept constant.

Mole and Johnson[51] estimated that the protein needs of athletes could be met by a diet containing 2.0 g protein and 46 kcal/kg BW/day. Marable et al.[50] noted that urinary N excretion decreased 7% when subjects consumed 0.8 g protein/kg BW/day but decreased 22% when subjects were fed 2.4 g protein/kg BW/day, suggesting that the subjects were in more positive NBAL at the higher level of protein intake.

In a well-controlled study, Hickson et al.[46] reported that a single bout of strength training of 1-h duration did not significantly alter urinary N excretion. Given the need for a biologically significant dose of work and the short duration of the latter study combined with the limitations of the NBAL technique, it was not surprising that the single hour of strength training had no apparent effect on 24-h urinary N excretion or on urinary excretion measured during any portion of the 24-h period following the training stimulus. Furthermore, there may have been a lag period between the exercise stimulus and the time at which a change in urinary N excretion would be observed (i.e., more than 24 h of time).

Other investigators have attempted to evelute the effects of a single bout of resistance exercise on protein metabolism. Chesley et al.[67] evaluated the effects of a single session of heavy resistance exercise in 12 males about 24 years of age divided into two groups with body fat levels averaging 11 and 15%, respectively who had been training on average about 4 years or longer. The investigators used exercised and control (resting from the opposite arm) biceps brachii as the muscle source for biopsy samples. Muscle protein synthesis was significantly elevated in the exercised biceps at four and 24 h post exercise. RNA activity but not RNA capacity was also significantly elevated. The authors interpreted these findings as the result of post-transcriptional events.

C. STUDIES ON AMINO ACIDS

Dohm et al.[68] and Evans et al.[69] suggest that protein probably contributes 5–15% of total energy needs during exercise. This assumption is based on studies of relatively short duration (e.g., about 1 h) and reflects the effects of aerobic work. Similar studies based on individuals engaged in strength training have not been reported to date.

Evans et al.[69] reported that a single bout of exercise performed at 55% of VO_2 max for 2 h increased total leucine oxidation 240% over the values observed during a 2-h rest period. In this study, which used stable leucine, the investigators estimated that the amount of work performed during this 2-h period at a relatively low intensity of effort represented the oxidation of 853 mg of leucine (i.e., approximately 90% of the total daily requirement for this amino acid). Matthews et al., cited by Evans et al.,[69] reported that greater increases in energy expenditure increase both the rate and total amount of leucine oxidation. The work of Evans et al.[69] is consistent with the data reported by Hagg et al.,[70] who also reported an increase in leucine oxidation and a decrease in the rate of leucine utilization to support net protein synthesis. The twofold increase in leucine oxidation was paralleled by a twofold increase in plasma lactate and alanine, although blood concentrations of leucine and other amino acids as energy substrates might lead to an imbalance in the ratio of essential to nonessential amino acids, and consequently increase an athlete's risk of negative NBAL when energy and protein intakes are marginal. It is not clear if strength training would result in similar levels of leucine oxidation to that observed among subjects performing aerobic exercises.

Although the number of reports in the literature is relatively few, and although much of the research reported to date is based on relatively small samples, the data collected thus far suggest that protein needs may be increased in response to increased energy expenditure or work. Unfortunately, little research has been reported that has evaluated the effects of work on the protein needs of females. Efforts to explore the potential benefits of resistance training and diet on the functional capacity of the elderly has stimulated research on the effects of age on the protein needs of individuals performing similar levels of work. Variations on the effects of different amounts and types of strength training (i.e., powerlifting vs. bodybuilding), differences in body fat, and energy source are needed. Since many bodybuilders often consume liquid protein supplements, the effects of liquid supplements vs. diets based on mixtures of solid foods are also needed.

More research is also needed in order to develop guidelines for dietary planning of individuals and groups of individuals who are performing large volumes of work. Many highly dedicated bodybuilders and powerlifters train 3 h/day or longer for 5- to 7-d each week. Thus, in developing guidelines, nutrition scientists must recognize that most of the research reported to date does not make an allowance for the potential effects of the large training prescriptions achieved by these elite athletes. In addition to reporting means for NBAL for groups being studied, investigators should also be encouraged to report the percent of those subjects who are actually in NBAL since much of the literature suggests that not all subjects were in NBAL when fed diets containing low or moderate levels of protein. Researchers should also monitor differences in responses based on differences in body fat levels.

Lemon[71] suggests that on the basis of present data, strength athletes should be consuming at least 12–15% of their total energy requirements as protein. This amount would translate to about 1.5–2.0 g protein/kg BW/day, which is at least two times the RDA.

Nutritionists and athletes should also recognize that even though the RDAs are based on protein intakes, the requirement is a reflection of the biological metabolism of specific amino acid needs. Young et al.[72] published provocative findings on their estimates of amino acids using metabolic tracer techniques, noting that the requirements for some amino acids may be 23–178% greater than the estimates based on balance studies.

Bazzarre et al.[73] measured changes in plasma amino acids in response to two successive bouts of exercise to exhaustion in triathletes using high-performance liquid chromatography analysis. Alanine, glycine, isoleucine, serine, valine, threonine, and tyrosine decreased significantly ($p \leq 0.05$) in response to the initial exercise to exhaustion challenge while taurine increased significantly. At the end of the 20-min recovery period following the first exhaustion, leucine, isoleucine, ornithine, phenylalanine, tyrosine, urea, and valine increased significantly. Alanine, glycine, isoleucine, leucine, valine, ornithine, serine, phenylalanine, threonine, and tyrosine decreased significantly in response to the second exercise to exhaustion. Using adjusted mean change scores, carbohydrate replacement had no effect on any amino acid from exhaustion to the end of recovery; however, from the end of the recovery period to the end of the second exhaustion, the changes in serine, glycine, and threonine were significantly different from the placebo (artificially sweetened water). Unfortunately, data on the effects of changes in amino acids in response to prolonged periods of resistance training or strength training to exhaustion have not been conducted.

V. NUTRITIONAL ERGOGENIC AIDS AND STRENGTH PERFORMANCE

Although considerable anecdotal evidence, such as muscle/strength magazine articles and advertisements, suggests that bodybuilders use a wide variety of nutrition supplements, little research has been published on the effects of specific supplements on muscular performance and development. The potential benefits, if any, of many of the supplements consumed by bodybuilders and powerlifters may be difficult to evaluate if nutrient intake (and hence, nutritional status) is adequate. An assessment of the potential benefits of supplements would also be exacerbated by the fact that many athletes engaged in strength training use more than one kind of supplement.

Supplement use was reported infrequently in the studies cited in the section on food intake of strength-trained athletes.[9,15,74] A wide range of supplements were used in the studies that evaluated supplement use. Supplement use generally ranged from about 60 to 100% of the athletes evaluated.

Sobal and Marquart[75] reviewed 51 studies reported in the literature that provided quantitative data on 10,274 male and female athletes representing 15 different sports. Supplements were used by 46% of the athletes in these studies with the prevalence of use ranging from 6 to 100% in specific groups. Elite athletes had a greater prevalence of supplement use than college or high school athletes, and female athletes used supplements more frequently than their male counterparts. Supplement use varied by sport, and athletes engaged in sports involving strength had high rates of prevalence use. Prevalence rates were 100, 69, 43, and 39% for weightlifters, bodybuilders, football players, and wrestlers, respectively. The authors also noted limitations in the data collected on supplement use and problems in comparing the results between various studies. For example, only 32 of the 51 studies reviewed provided information about the types of supplements used, and only 20 studies provided data on the types of supplements used by a specific percent of athletes. Little information was provided in most studies on the costs of the supplements used by athletes which can be as high as $100 or more per month. Some athletes reportedly took as many as 87 pills on a daily basis.

Sobal and Marquart[76] reported that 59% of 44 wrestlers and 39% of 83 football players in a survey of 742 high school athletes used supplements. Parents, doctors, coaches, and friends were listed by 36, 26, 14, and 10%, respectively, of these high school athletes as being very important influences on vitamin/mineral supplement use. In another report on this same sample Marquart and Sobal[77] reported that 90% of the athletes said that muscular development was either very important or somewhat important. The majority felt that nutrition and genetics were important contributors to muscle development. Grandjean et al.[78] reported that 98% of college athletes believed that a high protein diet improved performance, and 80% believed that "large" amounts of protein were necessary to increase muscle mass.

Bucci[79] and Williams,[80] among others, have extensively reviewed the literature on the effects of various nutritional ergogenic aids on athletic performance. Both authors have indicated that much of the research conducted to date has not been rigorously designed. The small sample size of many studies, combined with failure to use double-blind, cross-over designs, and failure to use control subjects or to account for possible training effects has made it difficult to interpret many of the reported findings. Many of the studies that have demonstrated favorable benefits were based on animal or human studies in which the subjects were deficient in the nutrient under investigation.

A. FLUID/ELECTROLYTE REPLACEMENT AND STRENGTH PERFORMANCE

Studies on the effects of large fluid losses among wrestlers and bodybuilders who are attempting to "make weight" for competition is one area of particular concern since fluid losses can impair performance and increase risk for heat injury. Fluid and electrolyte losses associated with heavy sweat losses are associated with increased muscular fatigue and decreased performance. Large imbalances affect the nervous system and can lead to ventricular fibrillation and even death.

Steen and McKinney[18] noted that 58% of their population of 42 college wrestlers used fluid restriction to lose weight as well as other dehydration practices such as saunas, wearing a plastic suit, laxatives, and diuretics. Bodybuilders attempting to make their weight category also use these practices prior to the official weigh-in. Steen and McKinney noted that in addition to fluid restriction, energy intake averaged 334 kcal (1397.456 kilojoules) the day before the match, 4214 kcal (17,631.376 kilojoules) the evening after the match, and 5235 kcal (21,903.24 kilojoules) the next day resulting in a weekly weight loss and regain of about 12 pounds (5.45 kg).

B. PROTEIN/AMINO ACID SUPPLEMENTATION AND STRENGTH PERFORMANCE

With the exception of amino acid supplements, most studies on the effects of various nutrient supplements on measures of athletic performance have been conducted on athletes other than bodybuilders or powerlifters. The results of such studies are reported elsewhere in this book. Grunewald and Bailey[81] published a report on the health claims of 624 commercially available supplements targeted at bodybuilders, noting that many performance claims were not supported by research. Amino acids (mixtures or individual amino acids) were the most commonly marketed products. Of 87 mixtures, more than 50% claimed to promote weight or muscle gain while more than 25% claimed to have anabolic or growth promoting properties.

Following publication of a paper on human growth hormone (GH) changes with aging by Bazzarre et al.[82] and the availability of synthetic GH in more recent years, articles and books appearing in the popular press promoted GH as a possible ergogenic aid for enhancing muscular development as well as for reducing body fat levels (GH is often referred to as the hormone of lipolysis). Bazzarre et al.[82] suggested that increased adiposity and reduced levels of physical activity associated with the aging process might account for the observation of diminished GH response to standard provocative stimuli as well as lower 24-h integrated GH concentrations. In the older men evaluated in this study, peaks in GH during sleep appeared only in those older men who were physically active. Administration of GH was associated with increased N retention in older men consuming a diet providing 0.8 g/kg BW daily.

Numerous studies[28,31,83-92] have been published in the literature that are based on investigators' efforts to evaluate specific benefits of protein and/or amino acid supplementation on body composition, strength, and/or measures of growth hormone activity (Table 3). More research is needed on the potential anabolic effects of GH on body composition and strength performance. The results of the studies published to date provide no clear consensus about the effects of GH, and many of the studies were poorly designed. Few studies have provided adequate control of all of the variables known to affect GH. The pulsatile nature of natural GH release combined with GH regulation and counter-regulation by diet, physical activity, body fat and various stressors makes it difficult to effectively control for variables known to affect GH action. For example, body fat levels and increased age are associated with reductions in GH. High fat diets appear to blunt GH response to provocative stimuli while a high protein meal and specific amino acids such as arginine and ornithine stimulate GH release. In fact, high fat meals have been shown to blunt GH response to arginine infusion[93] underscoring the importance of controling both long-term and acute dietary factors. Since obesity and physical activity alter GH response and because hormonal responsiveness may change with adaptation to exercise according to Newsholme's hypothesis,[94] special precautions should be taken in the selection and screening of subjects.

In addition to direct measurement of GH to provocative stimuli such as exercise and pharmacoligical stimuli, investigators have attempted to use surrogate measures of GH such as other hormones (e.g., somatostatin, insulin-like growth factor, growth hormone releasing factor) and other indices of GH metabolism such as changes in urinary nitrogen, hydroxyproline, and creatinine excretion. Insulin-like growth factor appears to be a better measure of daily GH activity than measures of GH levels at one time or even a series of carefully selected times. Thus, given the array and complexity of issues related to evaluating the effects of GH

TABLE 3   Effects of Amino Acid and Protein Supplementation in Strength Trained Athletes

Investigators	Design	Subjects	Age (Years)	Dose	Diet	% Body Fat	Body Composition	Strength	Hormone
Bucci et al., 1990[84]		9 males	28	2–12 g 40 mg/kg BW					90 min hGH: <4 ng/ml
		3 females	34	100 mg/kg BW 170 mg/kg BW					<4 ng/ml 9.2 ± 3.0 ng/ml (p <0.05)
Elam et al., 1989[85]	DB 5-wk RT; p-test only	22 males	37	2 g ea Arg + Orn 1 g vit. C (placebo)		—	73 ± 6 kg LBM 65 ± 5 kg LBM p <0.05	563 ± 123 kg 468 ± 76 kg p <0.05	10.6 ± 5.5 mg/l UH 16.9 ± 8.6 p >0.05
Elam, 1988[86]	DB 5-wk RT	10 males 8 males	38	2 g ea Arg + Orn placebo, unknown		−0.9 ± 2.4% −0.2 ± 2.1 p <0.01 12%			
Fogelholm et al., 1993[87]	DB-XO 4 days 4-wk WO R-??	11 WL trained	25	2 g/day: 1g Orn 1g Lys in two divided doses	no control except on day of study 19% PRO				no SD GH 24 hrs insulin @ 5:00 p.m. <w/AA 3.2 ± 0.3 m IU/L vs placebo 5.0 ± 0.7 m IU/L

Post Exercise hGH (ng/ml)

Investigators	Design	Subjects	Age (Years)	Dose	Diet	% Body Fat	Body Composition	5 min	15 min
Fry et al., 1993[88]	DB/R	13 AA 15 Placebo Nat'l WL Training Camp	17		FRs cafeteria	6 ± 1% 7 ± 1%		29.5 ± 2.5 30.7 ± 1.8	30.5 ± 1.8 27.4 ± 2.1
Gater et al., 1992[31]	3 × 2 10-wk RT	37 RT 7 P/C 8 P/RT 7 AL/C	23 ± 3 20–30 21 ± 0 21 ± 1 24 ± 1	132 mg · kg⁻¹	See Table 1	9–18% 17 ± 2% 17 ± 2% 15 ± 1%	FFB: decrease (p <0.05) increase (p <0.01) no change	NS 1-RM Total (p <0.01) NS	no signif. increase in resting IGF-1 in any group

Reference	Design	Subjects	Age	Supplement/dose	Diet	% BF pre	% BF post	Results	Comments
Hawkins et al., 1991[83]	13 WL	8 AL/RT	23 ± 1	1–1½ cans daily; 1 g Arg/kg BW		16 ± 1%		increase (p <0.01); BF decrease (p <0.01)	IGF-1 = index of 24 hr integrated GH status
		7 EX/RT	23 ± 1			16 ± 2%		increase (p <0.01)	
Isidori et al., 1981[89]		15 untrained	15–20	1.2 g Lys; 1.2 g Arg		61–108 kg BW; 53–67 kg BW			hGH peak @ 90 min 180 ± 7 ng/ml; 180 min I-hGH: 284 ± 117, 326 ± 133, 646 ± 277, 104 ± 57, 1206 ± 511
Lambert et al., 1993[90]	single dose 180″	7 BB 5–10 hr/wk fasted	23	• 2.4 g Arg/Lys • 1.1 g Orn • 20 g Bovril® • placebo • GH-RF	7-d FR	12%			
Papadakis et al., 1996[91]		52 males	75	1.56 g/day				1-RM Total (p <0.01); 1-RM Total (p <0.01)	
Walberg-Rankin, 1994[92]		18							IGF-1 not signif. diff. A vs. P pre or post diet; GH not signif. diff. A vs. P pre GH signif. > A vs. P during low energy no effect of A on N bal
		6 C	22 ± 2	Ad lib		—	—		
		6 A	22 ± 2	1 g protein $\cdot$ kg^{-1}, 55% CHO, 30% Fat		12.5 ± 2.7	10.5 ± 2.9		
		6 P	21 ± 1	+ 10 day low E (22 kcal $\cdot$ kg^{-1})		10.5 ± 0.8	8.4 ± 1.0		
Kraemer et al., 1992[28]	DB-OX	28 Olympic PL	17 ± 1					snatch perf: NS	NS effect on supplements on: lactate, ammonia, testosterone, cortisol, or GH; although blood levels increased significantly with exercise
Total:		**128**	17–34			**6–17%**			

Note: Abbreviations — DB, Double Blind; P/C, Placebo/Control; P/RT, Placebo/Resistance Training; AL/C, Arginine-Lysine/Control; AL/RT, Alanine-Lysine/Resistance Training; EX/RT, Exceed/Resistance Training; FFB, Fat-Free Body Weight; 1-RM, 1 Repetition Maximum; R, Randomized; UB, Urinary Hydroxyproline; W/O, Wash out; XO, Cross-over.

on body composition and strength performance, it is understandable that the results reported in the literature to date provide no consistent information. Before the effects of protein or amino acid supplementation are evaluated any further, investigators need to determine the dose-threshold required to induce alterations in GH. The absence of any changes in body composition, performance, or GH activity may be a reflection of using doses below the threshold required to stimulate biological activity of this hormone.

According to Bucci,[79] the stimulation of growth hormone and prolactin by arginine may have an anabolic effect on muscular development. Arginine may also increase creatine stores and may reduce ammonia levels. Bucci[79] reported anecdotal findings, stating that ingestion of 4–8 g of a 50:50 mixture of ornithine and arginine was associated with decreased muscular fatigue and post-workout muscle soreness in well-trained and steroid-free bodybuilders.

Elam et al.[85] reported significant improvement in total strength performance (563 ± 123 kg vs. 468 ± 76 kg) in a 5-week double-blind placebo study of 22 males about 37 years of age as well as significant differences in lean body mass (73 ± 6 kg vs. 65 ± 5 kg LBM) and urinary hydroxyproline excretion (10.6 ± 5.5 mg/l vs. 16.9 ± 8.6 mg/l) between the treatment group receiving 2 g each ornithine and arginine daily compared to the placebo group which received 1 g vitamin C). The design of this study was unusual in that no measurements were made at baseline. In another double-blind study of 18 males participating in a 5-week resistance training program, Elam[86] reported a significantly greater decrease in body fat (–0.9% vs. –0.2%) in the group receiving 2 g each of arginine and ornithine compared to the placebo group.

Gater et al.[31] reported significant improvement in 1-RM measures of strength as a result of a 10-week resistance training program compared to control groups but did not observe any significant effects of either arginine/lysine supplementation (132 mg/kg BW) or a nutrition supplement (1 ± 1/2 cans of Exceed) on increased strength in 37 men 23 ± 3 years of age randomly assigned to one of five subgroups. Resistance training was associated with significant increases in fat-free body mass; however, the increase was significantly greater in the group receiving Exceed compared to the other groups. Body fat levels decreased in all resistance-trained groups, but the decrease was significant only in the group receiving the arginine/lysine supplement. There were no significant differences in resting insulin-like growth factor-1.

Kraemer et al.[28] did not find any significant improvement as a consequence of amino acid supplementation in snatch performance or other biochemical indices (lactate, ammonia, testosterone, cortisol, and growth hormone) in a group of 28 male Olympic-style weightlifters divided into experimental and placebo groups using a double-blind, cross-over design. The authors postulated that the absence of any significant effect may have been masked by the high protein intake (more than 2.0 g/kg BW/day) of the subjects.

Using a double-blind design, Hawkins et al.[83] did not observe any benefit of oral arginine supplementation (1.0 g arginine/kg BW/day) in a group of 13 experienced male weightlifters divided into placebo and experimental groups on body composition changes during a weight loss program or on peak torque and endurance. During the 10-d low-calorie diet period, subjects lost an average of 3.2 kg BW and 2.0% body fat, peak torque declined ($p < 0.5$) while muscle endurance increased (significantly for biceps but not quadriceps).

Fogelholm et al.[87] conducted a 4-d double-blind, cross-over trial on the effects of 1 g each of arginine, ornithine, and lysine administered twice daily on 24-h GH and insulin levels in 11 weightlifters 8–20% bodyfat. There was no diet control during the 3 d prior to administration of the study protocol, and little control of physical activity (no more than 2 h of intensive training allowed daily). Subjects were fed a control diet on the day of the test but not on any of the previous days. Given the acute nature of the study design and the lack of any rigorous control of variables known to affect GH and insulin levels, it was not surprising that the authors did not observe any significant differences between the amino acid and placebo treatments relative to either GH or insulin levels over a 24-h period.

Lambert et al.[90] did not observe any significant effect of oral amino acid supplements on seven male bodybuilders who trained between 5–10 h each week. Subjects were permitted a relatively wide range in protein intake: 1.2–2.2 g/kg BW. Subjects received a 2.4 g arginine/lysine supplement, a 1.85 g ornithine/tyrosine supplement, 20 g Bovril (a protein drink), or a placebo in random order on four separate occasions with at least 1 wk between tests. Body fat levels ranged between 9.5 and 18.5% among the seven subjects. Responses of individual subjects to each of the treatments were highly variable, and responses of all individuals to a specific test were also highly variable. Serum GH variation of individuals to the four tests were more than 15 times the response to the placebo treatment (13.5 vs. 249 ng/ml), and variation in response to a specific test among the seven subjects was as much as 52 times (33.0 vs. 1725 ng/ml). The data from these studies clearly illustrate the tremendous variability in GH response within and between individuals and the difficulty of designing studies to evaluate the biological effects of GH alone or in combination with diet and resistance training on body composition and performance of strength-trained athletes. In this study, the 20 g Bovril protein-drink resulted in an integrated GH concentration of 646 ± 277 ng/ml which was six times the mean concentration for the placebo trial of 104 ± 57 ng/ml and approximately twice that of the two amino acids trials. Yet these differences were not statistically significant. More rigorous screening of subjects and control of factors known to alter GH response may have reduced the large individual variability observed in studies like this and increased the probability of identifying true biological effects. Researchers also need to recruit a sufficiently large sample to detect statistically significant differences. The standard errors reported in this study were about half of the mean values.

Fry et al.[88] conducted a short-term study (1 wk) on the effects of high volume weight-lifting and amino acid supplementation (2.4 g amino aicds immediately prior to each of three daily meals as well as 2.1 g of branched-chain amino acids supplemented with L-glutamine and L-carnitine immediately prior to each workout) on a sample of 28 elite junior weightlifters (6–7% body fat) participating in a national training camp. The investigators did not observe any statistically significant effects of amino acid supplementation on resting or post-exercise GH levels.

Research by Isidori et al.[89] suggests that the effects of amino acids on GH release may not be due to specific amino acids but due to specific combinations of amino acids. They noted that 1.2 mg each of L-lysine and L-arginine administered in combination significantly increased GH levels; however, administration of each amino acid alone did not result in any appreciable increase in GH. The study population was based on 15 males 15–20 years of age, but no additional information on the training status, dietary intake, or body composition of this population was provided.

Walberg-Rankin et al.[92] did not observe any significant effect of arginine administration in a double blind study in which 18 males were randomized to a control, placebo, or supplement group. Arginine was administered at a dose of about 1–2 g daily (0.1 g/kg BW administered twice daily). Subjects were asked to adhere to a similar training program. Body weight and body fat decreased significantly in both groups during a 10-d hypocaloric diet phase. The arginine supplement group had about 2% more body fat on average compared to the placebo group, which may have been a confounding factor. Peak torque decreased significantly for both the biceps and quadriceps in both groups. During the weight maintenance phase, there was no significant effect of oral arginine administration in comparison to the placebo (casein); however, at the end of the 10-d hypocaloric diet period, arginine administration resulted in consistently higher GH levels during the 90-min period following arginine ingestion compared to the placebo, but these differences were not statistically significant. There was no significant effect of arginine supplementation on resting insulin-like growth factor-1 (IGF-1) levels during either diet period. The absence of any significant effect of low-dose arginine supplementation on GH, IGF-1 levels, and nitrogen retention is consistent with most other studies; however, the increase in GH levels in response to arginine supplementation during the hypocaloric phase during which the subjects also lost weight and body fat suggests that even small doses of some amino acids may enhance the body's efforts to preserve LBM during periods of dietary inadequacy. Future research is needed to identify a physiological dose of specific amino acids or protein that could be administered that would not only increase GH levels but would also increase IGF-1 levels. These data illustrate the exquiste balance, as well as counter-regulatory effects of dietary constituents including adequacy of energy intake, between diet and the endocrine system.

Although most studies on the effects of GH on muscular development and performance have been based on young groups of males, some research has been done on older subjects.[82,91] Little, if any, research on the effects of GH on muscular development and strength performance has been conducted on female athletes. Papadakis et al.[91] conducted a double-blind, randomized study on the effect of GH administered at a dose of 0.03 mg/kg BW three times a week for a 6-m period to a group of 52 males with a mean age of 75 years. GH administration was associated with increased LBM (+4.3%), reduced fat mass (−13.1%), and increased bone mineral content (+0.9%), but no improvements in measures of functional ability were observed. The authors also reported side effects and possible long-term adverse effects of GH administration. Furthermore, they presented four possible reasons for the lack of a GH effect on functional measures but did not include the possibility that the most important factor in improving functional capacity is direct training of muscle groups. Coaches focus on providing the proper intensity, duration, and frequency of the training program rather than dietary regimens to improve athletic performance. Thus, researchers should evaluate the additive effects of improving diet or hormone levels to training studies intended to improve functional measures of performance but should not design studies that do not include a training stimulus.

In summary, larger doses of amino acids administered at doses of 8 g or more daily or protein supplements/drinks like Bovril administered at doses of 20 g or more may increase lean body mass, reduce body fat, and perhaps even improve measures of muscular performance by enhancing GH activity. Lower doses of protein and/or amino acids administered over relatively short periods of time such as a week or less do not appear to have any statistically significant effect above that which can be achieved by resistance training alone. The variability in GH responsiveness among and between individuals to a variety of provocative stimuli represent a challenge in designing studies that will help to elucidate the interrelationships between diet, physical activity, and the neuro-hormonal mechanisms that regulate body composition and muscular performance.

C.   CARBOHYDRATE SUPPLEMENTATION AND STRENGTH PERFORMANCE

Walberg-Rankin[95] has reviewed the literature on the benefits of increased carbohydrate intake on athletic performance. While most of the literature represents research on the benefits of glycogen loading regimens on endurance performance, some investigators have examined the effects of glycogen replacement on high power activities of relatively brief duration. Muscle glycogen levels during training involving explosive resistance activities generally do not decrease to levels associated with prolonged endurance exercise.

Pascoe et al.[97] demonstrated that carbohydrate replacement compared to water resulted in muscle glycogen replacement to 91% of initial glycogen levels vs. 75% for water after 1 h of high power activities that reduced muscle glycogen levels approximately 30% from resting levels. Houston et al.[98] and Walberg-Rankin et al.[99] have demonstrated decreased muscular performance in wrestlers in response to either food restriction or a reduction in carbohydrate intake. Recommendations for muscle glycogen replacement include the consumption of approximately 40–60 g carbohydrate per hour during recovery. Chan et al.[100] showed that glucose-potassium loading (20 mmol [mEq]/500 ml glucose) of eight undernourished, hospitalized patients significantly increased the force-frequency characteristics and the maximal relaxation rate of the adductor pollicis muscle.

Steen and McKinney[18] reported that the low energy and carbohydrate intakes of wrestlers contribute to the development of reduced muscle glycogen levels and chronic fatigue during the competitive season. Steen et al.[96] reported that wrestlers with a history of weight cycling have significantly lower energy requirements, and hence, lower metabolic rates than noncylcers. Thus, wrestlers and bodybuilders who frequently alter their weight in preparation for competition may find that they need to reduce their energy intake from previous levels during their recovery or noncompetitive period as a result of reducing their metabolism.

D. VITAMIN C SUPPLEMENTATION AND STRENGTH PERFORMANCE

Howald et al.[101] found no significant difference in PWC (Physical Work Capacity) 170 work performance (total amount of work performed) between placebo and vitamin C treatments (1 g/d in the morning) of 13 athletes, but heart rates were significantly lower in this double-blind, cross-over study. Blood glucose concentrations were significantly lower while free fatty acid concentrations were significantly higher during the PWC test for the vitamin C vs. the placebo treatments. An acute double-blind, cross-over study on the effects of 600 mg vitamin C or placebo administered 4 h prior to testing by Keith and Merrill[102] revealed no significant differences between placebo and experimental treatments on maximum grip strength nor on muscular endurance using a hand dynamometer.

Bramich and McNaughton[103] conducted a double-blind test on the muscular strength of pectoral and quadriceps muscles, muscle endurance, and VO_2max of 24 subjects given acute doses of vitamin C (500 or 2000 mg 4 h prior to testing) and after 1 wk of supplementation. No significant changes in response to the 2000-mg acute dose were observed for muscular strength, endurance, or VO_2max; however, the 500-mg acute dose was associated with a significant increase in quadriceps strength and a decrease in VO_2max. At the end of the 7-d supplementation periods, the 2000-mg dose was associated only with a significant reduction in VO_2max, while the 500-mg dose was associated with significant increases in both quadriceps and pectoral strength, but decreased muscular endurance of both muscle groups as well as a significant decrease in VO_2max.

Tuttle et al.[104] conducted an interesting double-blind, crossover investigation in which a mega-dose of vitamin C (administered at 150 mg/kg BW) was used as a placebo in comparison to an equal quantity of potassium-magnesium aspartate administered at the same dose. It was not surprising that these investigators found no statistically significant effects of aspartate on blood ammonia concentrations, blood lactate levels or ratings, or perceived exertion during or after a controlled resistance training workout in 12 males 18–30 years of age who had been weight training for a period of at least 1 year.

E. TRACE MINERAL SUPPLEMENTATION AND STRENGTH PERFORMANCE

A number of trace mineral supplements have appeared on the market during the 90s claiming to increase strength and lean body mass while at the same time reducing body fat levels. Grunewald and Bailey[81] reported that 5 of 10 commercially available boron supplements claimed to promote weight or muscle gain while two supplements were marketed as promoting growth or increased strength. In the same report, 9 of 14 chromium supplements claimed to promote increased weight or muscle gain while 13 of the 14 supplements claimed to have anabolic or growth promoting properties, and 5 of the 14 chromium supplements maintained claims promoting body fat reduction.

Ferrando and Green[20] reported the effects of 2.5 mg boron supplementation in 10 males over a 7-week period compared to 9 males consuming a placebo. While plasma boron levels increased significantly in the treatment group from 20.1 ± 7.7 to 32.6 ± 27.6 parts per billion (ppb) in the treatment group and declined from 15.1 ± 14.4 to 6.3 ± 5.5 ppb in the placebo group, the researchers did not observe any significant differences between the treatment and placebo groups during the study. Resistance training in both groups was associated with increases in total testosterone, LBM, 1-RM squat, and 1-RM bench even though both groups were asked to maintain their current training programs. Particpants were asked to maintain 3-d food records and not to use supplements during the study period in order to reduce any potential effects of dietary changes on the study results.

Hasten et al.[105] evaluated the effects of 200 μg chromium supplementation on 59 college students (37 males and 22 females) in a 12-wk weight training program for beginners using a double blind, randomized design. Males and females were randomized into treatment or placebo groups. Resistance training was associated with significant increases in body circumferences and in reductions in the sum of skinfold measurements in all groups. Chromium supplementation significantly increased weight gain in females (+2.5 kg) compared to females receiving the placebo (+0.6 kg). There was no significant difference in weight gain between the males receiving the chromium supplementation (+0.8 kg) compared to males receiving the placebo (+1.3 kg).

Clancy et al.[106] also conducted a double blind study of the effects of 200 ug chromium picolinate on 38 football players but did not observe any statistically significant effect of chromium on any measure of strength, body weight, or body fat. Three-day diet records were maintained by 13 of 36 subjects who completed the 9-wk study, however, no dietary information was actually reported. Activity logs were maintained by subjects to monitor the subjects' strength training activities. Urinary chromium excretion (24 h), used as a measure of compliance with chromium supplementation, was significantly higher among the supplement group than the placebo group.

F.　OTHER SUPPLEMENTS AND STRENGTH PERFORMANCE

Bucci[79] has summarized research on the potential ergogenic benefits of alkalinizers. Alkalinizers theoretically reduce fatigue associated with anaerobic performance by maintaining blood and muscle pH. Decreased pH inhibits phosphofructokinase, the rate-limiting step in glycolysis. The majority of investigators who have measured anaerobic, short-term exercise performance times after large doses of biocarbonate of about 0.2–0.3 g/kg BW approximately 1–3 h before exercise have reported increased time to fatigue. Bucci[79] cautions about the possible adverse effects of excessive bicarbonate use, which include nausea, vomiting, flatulence, diarrhea, and muscle cramps. Although carbonate loading is not currently banned by any sports government agency, this form of loading can be detected easily by urinalysis.

Apparently, little or no research has been reported to date that evaluated the effects of alkalinizers of anaerobic performance of weightlifters. Bucci[79] also notes the need to explore the potential benefits of nutrient antioxidants on the reduction of free radical damage associated with exercise. Supplements containing superoxide dismutase and catalase have been marketed for athletes, but the research on their benefits is lacking.

VI.　HEALTH STATUS OF STRENGTH-TRAINED ATHLETES: NUTRITIONAL IMPLICATIONS

A.　RAPID WEIGHT LOSS

Rapid weight loss among wrestlers and bodybuilders prior to competition in order to make their weight class is commonplace. Rapid weight loss, generally achieved by various methods of dehydration, may produce multiple problems for these athletes.[107,108] The short-term negative side effects include reduced muscular strength and endurance, increased fatigue, decreased plasma volume, which is associated with impaired cardiac function (i.e., higher heart rate, decreased stroke volume, and reduced cardiac output), decreased glomerular blood flow and, consequently, reduced fibrillation rate, liver and muscle glycogen depletion, increased electrolyte losses, decreased oxygen consumption, and impaired thermoregulation. Heat exhaustion and heat stroke are possible outcomes, particularly when fluid loss exceeds 5% or more of total body water.

Professional bodybuilders are well aware of the fact that their success in competition requires them to reduce their body fat to a minimum while preserving the maximum in lean body mass. Some bodybuilders strive for a reduction in all body fat without realizing that some body fat is essential. Although the data are somewhat limited, minimum body fat levels appear to be about 4–6% as reported by Friedl et al.[109] who evaluated 55 of 261 men who completed a rigorous, 8-wk training course involving muscular endurance and food restriction (no information was provided on the food composition of the diet fed during the training course). The authors noted that the reduction of body fat to levels of 4–6% were associated with a 16% average reduction in body weight. The authors were impressed with the individual variation in the changes in this group. The investigators illustrated the individual variation by reporting on the responses of the two men with the lowest body fat levels initially (6 and 8%, respectively), body weights of 75 and 77 kg; and BMIs of 24.5. These two men completed the course with body fat levels in the 4–5% range; however, one man lost 9% of his body weight while the other lost 23%! The subject with the highest weight loss also lost the most body mass (40%). These data illustrate the importance of establishing individual weight and body fat loss goals for both bodybuilders and wrestlers, especially younger athletes, and the need to monitor body weights and other measures of body composition on an individual basis. These data also illustrate the motivation of bodybuilders to achieve extremely low body fat levels since the body fat levels of competitive bodybuilders are in the range of 4–6%.

Weight losses during the competitive season compared to pretraining weights are typically 7–21 lb (3.2–9.5 kg) or more and represent a difference of about three weight classes.[107,108] Acute weight loss cycles may occur 15–30 times or more during the competitive season for wrestlers and do vary considerably among wrestlers and bodybuilders, depending upon the number of competitions and other training/competition factors. Lamar-Hildebrand et al.[15] reported that four female competitive bodybuilders gained 20 lb while two others gained 10 lb or less within a 4-wk period following competition, suggesting that weight fluctuations in females approach those observed among male bodybuilders. Weight loss is generally achieved by restricting fluid and food intake, as well as other dehydrating practices, which include the use of saunas, sweat suits, laxatives, and diuretics, and even spitting.

Much of the research on the physiological effects of weight cycling has been conducted on obese subjects, especially females.[107] However, less work has been conducted on the effects of weight cycling of athletes, in whom fluctuations in body weight largely reflect changes in body water and carbohydrate availability (as compared to the changes in body weight among obese subjects in whom the fluctuations presumably reflect changes in adiposity). Additionally, it is not clear how differences in energy expenditure and types of training (e.g., aerobic vs. strength) affect fluctuations in body weight/composition in comparison to the effects of adjusting energy intake and the source of energy substrate (percent of total kilocalories provided by fat, carbohydrate, and protein).

Recent research on the potential benefits of using medium-chain triglycerides (MCT) in promoting weight loss have been reviewed by Bach et al.[110] MCT are promoted as energy-yielding substrates and apparently have been promoted for the past three decades for reducing BW. The benefits, or lack thereof, of MCT in promoting weight/fat loss appear to depend on the energy intake, nature of ingredients, MCT/LCT ratio, octanoate/decanoate ratio, and the duration of the regimen. Physiological factors of MCT that would promote weight/fat loss include: lower energy density, satiety, rapid intrahepatic delivery and oxidation rate, and poor rates of incorporation into adipose tissue. These factors, however, may be opposed by other factors such as the stimulation of insulin secretion, increased de novo fatty acid synthesis, and the induction of hypertriglyceridemia. In order to promote weight and fat loss, about 50% of energy needs must be supplied by MCT. Although long-term compliance with MCT would probably be poor, Manore et al.[13] have demonstrated that an elite professional bodybuilder was able to incorporate a diet high in MCT into the diet regimen for an 8-wk period in which MCT provided about 1300 kcal (5439.2 kilojoules) and increased fat intake from about 5% of total kilocalories (not MCT) to 30% of total kilocalories. Percent body fat in this case study decreased from 9.0 to 6.9%. The benefits of MCT in promoting weight loss may be limited to lean subjects, as a study by Yost and Eckel[111] with 16 obese women did not show any benefit on weight loss compared to the use of LCT.

B. RESISTANCE TRAINING AND WEIGHT LOSS

Little attention has been given to the potential role of resistance strength training on weight loss of obese females. Ballor et al.[112] studied the effects of a 3-d/wk resistance-training program on weight loss and the maintenance of LBM in obese women who averaged 35.9 ± 0.9% body fat. The 40 obese women were randomly assigned to one of four treatment groups: control, diet alone, exercise alone, or diet plus exercise. Significant increases in muscle area and strength were observed among the groups receiving the 8-wk resistance training program. Weight training in combination with energy restriction was associated with the preservation of LBM in comparison to energy restriction alone. The investigators concluded that energy restriction and weight training acted independently on weight loss, since they did not observe any statistically significant interaction of diet and exercise. The energy intake of subjects was theoretically reduced by about 1000 kcal/d (4184 kilojoules) , although no data were reported to validate this assumption. Protein supplements were provided to ensure that protein intake was ≥1.0 g/d. Thus, it is not clear if protein supplementation has any potential role in maintaining LBM. It is also unclear if blood lipids and blood pressure were favorably affected among any of the treatment groups compared to the control group. The benefits of resistance training on glucose tolerance is considered at the end of this section. Many of the studies in this later section include populations of elderly males who also have higher than desirable body fat levels.

C. BLOOD LIPID PROFILES

Since 1984, 17 investigations on the blood lipid profiles of individuals engaged in some form of strength training have been published (Table 4).[5,6,8,9,11,113-123] The populations studied included 40 female bodybuilders and 216 male bodybuilders or powerlifters, 53 males engaged in some form of resistance training, and three case studies of males. All of these studies were cross-sectional, except for those conducted by Kleiner et al.,[8] Peterson and Fahey,[119] Warber and Bazzarre,[122] and Webb et al.[116] Morgan et al.[11] studied females only, whereas Cohen et al.[113] and Bazzarre et al.[5,6] included both females and males in their surveys. All other studies were based on populations of males only. The sample size in most of the cross-sectional studies was relatively small, ranging from 5 males evaluated by Peterson and Fahey[119] to 76 South African male bodybuilders assessed by Faber et al.[7] Kleiner et al.[8] studied 35 males over a 6-month period. The average age of females in these studies was 30 ± 4 years while the average age of the male bodybuilders was 28 ± 3 years. The average percent body fat for females was 11.1% while that for male bodybuilders was 10.8%.

Powerlifters were included in the studies by Cohen et al.[113] and by Hurley et al.,[9] whereas bodybuilders were evaluated by other investigators. The bodybuilders studied by Elliot et al.[114] were competitors in a regional competition of natural bodybuilders, whereas Bazzarre et al.[5,6] studied bodybuilders at national championships. Data for male subjects placed in some form of a resistance training program are reported separately in Table 4.

TABLE 4 Lipid Profiles, Energy Intake, and Anthropometric Data of Male and Female Bodybuilders and Weightlifters

Investigators	Study Design	Sample Size	Age (Years)	% Body Fat	Dietary Methods	Energy Intake (kcal)[a]	TC (mg %)	HDL-C (mg %)	HDL2 (mg %)	HDL3 (mg %)	HDL-C/TC
Female Bodybuilders											
Bazzarre et al., 1990[5]	Cross-sectional	2	28	9.8	FR	2260	198	56	15	41	0.28
Bazzarre et al., 1992[6]	Cross-sectional	11	29	9.1	FR	1597	145 ± 38	56 ± 9	7 ± 6	49 ± 7	0.39
Cohen et al., 1986[113]	Cross-sectional	3 SU	—	—	None	—	216	31	0	31	0.14
Elliot et al., 1987[114]	Cross-sectional	15	27	14.4	—	—	166	55	—	—	0.33
Females Strength Training											
Morgan et al., 1986[11]	Cross-sectional	9 RT	36	BMI: 21.7	3-d weighted	1549	180	56	—	—	0.31
		9 Runners	27	BMI: 20.0	FR	1888	182	72	—	—	0.39
		9 Controls	34	BMI: 24.3	—	2132	183	58	—	—	0.32
		Total: 40									
		18 others									
X ± SD[b]			30 ± 4	11.1 ± 3		1802 ± 397	172 ± 22	56 ± 1	—	—	0.32 ± 0.05
Male Bodybuilders											
Bazzarre et al., 1990[5]	Cross-sectional	19	28	6.0	7-d FR	2015	187 ± 11	37 ± 6	13 ± 4	24 ± 4	0.20
Bazzarre et al., 1992[6]	Cross-sectional	13	30	4.9	3-d FR	2620	154 ± 30	48 ± 17	4 ± 6	45 ± 16	0.31
Cohen et al., 1986[113]	Cross-sectional	9 SU	—	—	—	—	291	24	2	22	0.08
Cohen et al., 1996[115]	Cross-sectional	10 SU	27	11.2	3-d FR	1169 ± 392					
		8 SU	23	10.7		503 ± 166 mg dietary cholesterol					
Elliot et al., 1987[114]	Cross-sectional	16	25	7.2	None	—	158	45	—	—	0.28
Faber et al., 1986[7]	Cross-sectional	76	27	15.4	7-d FR	3187	176 ± 25	50 ± 7	—	—	0.28
						4143	189 ± 23	56 ± 13	—	—	0.30
Hurley et al., 1984[9]	Cross-sectional	8 BB	29	12.0	24-hr R	NR	172	55	12	—	0.32
		8 PL	31	14.0	24-h R	NR	195	38	6	—	0.19
Kleiner et al., 1989[8]	Longitudinal	18 SU	30	13.1	3-d FR and FFQ	5739	214	16	2	17	0.07
		17 NSU	26	13.8			178	46	16	32	0.26

TABLE 4 Lipid Profiles, Energy Intake, and Anthropometric Data of Male and Female Bodybuilders and Weightlifters (continued)

Investigators	Study Design	Sample Size	Age (Years)	% Body Fat	Dietary Methods	Energy Intake (kcal)[a]	TC (mg %)	HDL-C (mg %)	HDL2 (mg %)	HDL3 (mg %)	HDL-C/TC
Webb et al., 1984[116]	Longitudinal	11 BB + 3 PL SU NSU	31 ± 8	85 ± 14 87 ± 15	BMI: 27 ± 0.5 28 ± 0.6	—	209 ± 55 210 ± 46	29 ± 8 61 ± 14	LDL-C: 150 ± 44 125 ± 38	—	0.14 0.29
X ± SD		Total: 216	28 ± 3	10.8 ± 3.6		3146 ± 1624	NSU: 180 ± 18 NS: 238 ± 46	48 ± 8 23 ± 7	10 ± 5 2 ± 0	34 ± 11 20 ± 4	0.27 ± 0.05 0.10 ± 0.04
Male Strength Training											
Bazzarre et al., 1990[117]	Cross-sectional	26 Triathletes	30	11		3500 kcal wk 0 wk 24	172 ± 28 175 ± 30	45 ± 11 49 ± 10			0.27 ± 0.08 0.29 ± 0.08
		12 Endurance	31	33		wk 0 wk 24	185 ± 36 180 ± 15	47 ± 17 57 ± 15			0.26 ± 0.08 0.32 ± 0.09
		11 RT	25	14		wk 0 wk 24	175 ± 28 162 ± 23	42 ± 10 42 ± 6			0.24 ± 0.08 0.27 ± 0.05
Costill et al., 1984[117]	Cross-sectional	9 SU 13 NSU 12 untrained	31 32 34	— — —	None		218 204 210	17 45 46			0.08 0.22 0.22
Higuchi et al., 1991[118]	Cross-sectional	15 WL 13 untrained	19 19	BMI: 25.0 BMI: 22.0	None		147 146	50 61			0.34 0.42
Peterson and Fahey, 1984[119]	Longitudinal	5: SU NSU	29	—	None		223 200	16 52			0.07 0.26
X ± SD		Total: 53 RT 38 others					NSU: 182 ± 26 SU: 221 ± 4	47 ± 5 17 ± 1			0.27 ± 0.05 0.08 ± 0.01
Case Studies											
Frankle et al., 1988[120]	Case study Stroke	34-year-old male		12.3 mg % with a stroke			—	12	—		
McNutt et al., 1988[121]	Case study MI	22-year-old male		worldclass powerlifter, 330 lb			596	14	513		
Warber and Bazzarre, 1991[122]	Case study Hyperlipidemic	Baseline: Detraining RT Running RT	6 wk 10 wk 10 wk 10 wk	9.7 10.5 10.5 10.3 9.9		3257 kcal 20% fat 4% sat fat 145 mg chol 61% CHO	265 228 215 218 216	53 43 42 48 46	— — — —	— — — —	0.20 0.21 0.19 0.22 0.22

Note: Abbreviations — SU, Steroid Users; RT, Resistance Trained; NSU, Non-Steroid Users; FR, Food Record; R, Recall; DH, Diet History; FFQ, Food Frequency Questionnaire.

[a] Multiply by 4.184 joules/kcal to convert to kilojoules.

[b] Means ± Standard Deviations for females involved in RT while not using steroids.

The average total cholesterol (TC) for female bodybuilders in this series of studies was 172 ± 22 mg%, and the average for high-density lipoprotein cholesterol (HDL-C) was 56 ± 1 mg%. For male bodybuilders who were not using steroids, the average total cholesterol was 182 ± 26 mg% compared to 221 ± 4 mg% for those using steroids. HDL-C averaged 47 ± 5 mg% for male bodybuilders not using steroids in contrast to an average of 17 ± 1 mg% for those using steroids.

In most studies (Table 4), mean TC levels were generally below 200 mg%; however, TC values were consistently above 200 mg% in association with steroid use[8,115,117,119] (Table 4). Total cholesterol was 36 mg% higher among steroid-using bodybuilders compared to nonsteroid users studied by Kleiner et al.,[8] but only 14 mg% higher among steroid-using vs. nonsteroid-using strength-trained athletes evaluated by Costill et al.[117] TC declined from 223 to 200 mg% among five males studied by Peterson and Fahey.[119] TC levels for control subjects included in three investigations were within the same range as the strength-trained groups.[11,17,117,118]

Mean HDL-C among males ranged from 56 ± 13 mg% among eight bodybuilders with a high egg consumption compared to 50 ± 7 mg% for male bodybuilders with a low egg intake.[7] Mean HDL-C ranged from 31 mg% among three female powerlifters[113] who used steroids to 56 mg% among two populations of female bodybuilders at the time of national competition.[5,6] Mean HDL2 cholesterol (HDL2-C) ranged from zero among three female powerlifters who used steroids to 15 mg% among two female bodybuilders.[5] HDL2-C values of 0 mg% observed among competitive bodybuilders and other strength-trained athletes apparently reflect the use of steroids. Mean HDL3 cholesterol (HDL3-C) ranged from 31 mg% among female powerlifters using steroids to 41 and 49 mg% among competitive female bodybuilders.[5,6] Mean HDL3-C among strength-trained males ranged from 17[8] to 22 mg%[12] among those who used steroids; and, from 32[8] to 45mg%[6] among bodybuilders who did not use steroids.

Dietary intake was measured in nine of the studies that measured blood lipid profiles of strength-trained athletes (Table 4). Food records were the most commonly used method to estimate nutrient intake in these studies. Hurley et al.,[9] who used the 24-h recall and diet histories to evaluate nutrient intake, only reported the distribution of energy intake provided by protein, fat, and carbohydrate, while the other investigators provided more complete nutrient information. The nutrient content of these diets is summarized in an earlier section of this chapter. Kleiner et al.[8] and Bazzarre et al.[5,6] evaluated the relationships between dietary and anthropometric variables, and the lipid profiles of bodybuilders. None of these anthropometric or dietary variables were significantly associated with TC in the first study by Bazzarre et al.[5] However, percent body fat levels were positively and significantly associated with HDL-C ($r = 0.63$; $p = 0.04$) and HDL3-C ($r = 0.65$; $p = 0.03$). Saturated fat intake (which was quite low) was the only nutrient variable associated with any lipid variable, HDL2-D ($r = 0.60$; $p = 0.05$). Correlations reported by Kleiner et al.[8] were saturated fat intake with HDL3-C ($r = -0.59$; $p = 0.05$); total fat intake and HDL3-C ($r = -0.62$; $p = 0.04$); and, polyunsaturated fat intake with very low-density lipoprotein (VLDL)-C ($r = 0.69$; $p = 0.01$). The differences between the dietary and lipid correlations reported in these two studies may reflect large differences in energy and fat intakes between the two study populations, combined with large differences in body fat levels (6.0 vs. 13.5%) between the groups (Table 4).

Although no significant correlations were observed between TC and any dietary variable in the former studies,[5,8] Bazzarre et al.[6] more recently observed significant correlations between TC and dietary fat among competitive female, but not male, bodybuilders. The significant association in the more recent study may reflect the effect of gender. Dietary fiber intake was significantly associated with HDL-C in both competitive male and female bodybuilders and with HDL3-C in competitive male, but not female, bodybuilders.[6] Vitamin C intake was significantly associated with HDL-C, HDL2-C, and HDL3-C in competitive male bodybuilders and with HDL3-C in competitive female bodybuilders. Positive associations between dietary vitamin C intake and HDL-C have been reported in farmers and in other populations.[123]

Kohl et al.[124] evaluated the relationships between measures of musculoskeletal fitness and blood lipids in 5463 males 20–69 years of age attending a preventive medicine clinic between 1980 and 1987. On the basis of multiple regression analysis in which the effects of age and cardiorespiratory fitness were controlled, they found that HDL-C levels were significantly associated (p <0.0001) with both the leg press and bench press. No significant associations were observed between TC and any of the four measures of musculoskeletal fitness.

Few of the studies that have been conducted on bodybuilders or other groups involved in resistance training have included comparison groups (Table 4). In a 6-month study of changes in training status, body composition, and diet, Bazzarre et al.[17] noted that the TC and HDL-C levels of 11 males involved in resistance training (average age: 25 years; 14% body fat) more than two times per week were similar to those of 26 triathletes (30 years; 11% body fat) and 12 other endurance athletes (31 years; 13% body fat). TC levels were similar between 15 weightlifters studied by Higuchi et al.[118] and 13 untrained males, although HDL-C levels were substantially higher among the untrained group (61 mg%; BMI = 22) compared to the weightlifters (50 mg%; BMI = 25). It is possible that the lower body fat levels in the untrained group may have been associated with the higher HDL-C levels. The mean age for both groups was 19 years. Peterson and Fahey[119] conducted a longitudinal study of 5 males 29 years of age whose TC (223 mg%) and HDL-C (16 mg%) while taking steroids. The TC was 200 mg% and HDL-C was 52 mg% when this group of males was not using steroids. In a cross-sectional study by Costill et al.,[117] TC levels were only slightly lower in a group of 13 males engaged in a resistance training program (204 mg%) and a group of 12 untrained males (210 mg%) compared to a group of 9 males involved in a resistance training program who used steroids. HDL-C were significantly lower in the steroid using group (17 mg%) compared to the other two groups (45–46 mg%).

Two case studies in the literature clearly demonstrate the potential life-threatening effect of steroids on blood lipids, myocardial infarction, and stroke.[120,121] Frankle et al.[120] reported a case study of a 34-year-old male bodybuilder who had a HDL-C level of 12 mg%. The authors noted the potential increase in hypercoagulability and increased risk of thrombosis associated with some anabolic-androgenic steroids but did not examine potential dietary constituents such as high dietary zinc intakes which could also suppress HDL-C and high dietary iron intakes which could have also increased coagulation and thrombosis. McNutt et al.[121] reported a case study of a 22-year-old male world-class power lifter weighing 330 lb who suffered an acute myocardial infarction (MI). At the time of admission his TC was 596 mg%, his LDL-C was 513 mg%, and his HDL-C was 14 mg%. The patient was released 24 d post MI with a TC of 283 mg%, an LDL-C of 220 mg%, and an HDL-C of 35 mg%. Lipid studies of the patient's parents and two siblings were performed: TC was <200 mg% in all immediate family members, and HDL-C levels were within the "normal" range. Platelet aggregation studies revealed hyperaggregability upon admission but not at 12 d post MI. The authors did not totally exclude diet and power lifting as contributing factors to the patient's hypercholesterolemia, but presumably were referring to dietary intake and not the potential effects of excessive dietary zinc and iron intakes.

Warber and Bazzarre[122] conducted a 38-wk case study to evaluate the independent effects of diet, resistance training, and endurance training on the lipid profiles and body fat of a 32-year-old hypercholesterolemic male dietitian whose serum TC was in the 98th percentile for high risk TC. The patient followed the same menu every day for the entire 38-wk period. The 3257 kcal diet was 20% fat, 4% saturated fat, 61% carbohydrate, and contained 145 mg cholesterol per day. A 2-wk baseline period was used to adjust energy intake needed to maintain body weight, followed by a 6-wk detraining period. The detraining period was followed by three, 10-wk periods of resistance training, aerobic training (running), and resistance training.

Data for percent body fat, TC, HDL-C, and the HDL-C/TC ratio are presented in Table 4. Diet had the most profound effect on the patient's TC and HDL-C which decreased 37 and 10 mg%, respectively, from baseline to the end of the detraining period. TC declined further 10–13 mg% during the 30-wk training periods with little effect of training modality. HDL-C was highest (48 mg%) during the aerobic training period as compared to the two resistance training periods (42 and 46 mg%, respectively). The male dietitian in this study was a highly trained subject as evidenced by his low body fat level which ranged from 9.7 to a high of 10.5% during the study period, and he was highly motivated to follow the diet because of his high risk status for CVD.

As an anecdotal comment based on working with this recreational athlete and many other bodybuilders and endurance athletes, health care professionals should not assume that these athletes are not at risk for abnormal lipids or even elevated blood pressure simply because they are highly trained and have little bodyfat. Having screened the blood lipids and blood pressures of many athletes, those who have high risk levels often report little surprise upon receiving their results noting that they have a strong family history of heart disease and/or stroke. Many indicate that one of the motivating factors in their training program is to hopefully reduce their risk of death associated with these major causes of mortality.

To date, there does not appear to have been any prospective long-term study on the impact of resistance training on blood lipid levels and blood pressure. Since resistance training may be an important contributor to the maintence of lean body mass and functional capacity, and because resistance training may be an effective component of weight reduction programs, future research is needed to examine the impact of resistance training on body composition and lipid profiles. Some researchers have suggested that some of the benefit of aerobic training is due to the contributions of such training regimens on reductions in body fat levels, especially abdominal adipose tissue. Perhaps some of the benefits of resistance training may also be derived indirectly through decreases in body fat levels.

Within the scope of evaluating the potential benefits of resistance training on risk for cardiovascular disease and stroke, special care must be taken to consider other training practices, diet, and health behaviors. Drug use among bodybuilders and other athletes is one of the areas of major concern. Surveys of college and high school athletes suggest that the frequency of use is of sufficient magnitude to create a public health concern. Melia et al.[125] conducted a survey of anabolic-androgenic steroid use in 16,169 Canadian students 12–18 years of age who were randomly selected from 107 schools. Almost 3% of students (83,000) admitted steroid use either to enhance athletic performance or to improve their body image. Of those students injecting steroids, almost 30% admitted sharing needles.

D. GLUCOSE TOLERANCE AND RESISTANCE TRAINING

Recent research on the potential benefits of resistance training on glucose tolerance and the role of resistance training in the treatment of individuals with adult onset diabetes has been published. Miller et al.[126] conducted a 16-wk resistance training program in 11 males 58 ± 1 year who demonstrated a 47% increase in total strength (total weight lifted increased from 575 ± 30 to 846 ± 42 kg; p <0.001), and a decrease in body fat from 27.2 ± 1.8 to 25.6 ± 1.9 % (p <0.001). Plasma insulin also decreased significantly from 85 ± 25 to 55 ± 10 pmol/l (p <0.05). These changes were attributed primarily to the effects of the resistance training program and the decline in body fat as body weight remained stable. The study design should be considered as a model for studies investigating the effects of diet and resistance training on growth hormone metabolism and body composition. For example, the investigators placed the subjects on an American Heart Association diet containing about 30% fat, 51–52% carbohydrate, and 18–19% protein for 6 wk and fed the subjects a controlled isocaloric diet prior to each testing period. The authors noted that changes in fasting and 2-hr glucose responses were related to intial glucose levels (i.e., the higher the initial glucose levels, the greater the reduction in glucose levels following training). The authors suggested that this relationship may account for differences in the results reported between some studies (i.e., studies in which subjects had relatively low glucose levels did not demonstrate any statistically significant reduction in glucose levels whereas studies in which subjects had higher glucose levels noted significant reductions).

A wide range of responses have been reported in various studies. Smutock et al.[127] showed improvement in glucose tolerance whereas Craig et al.[128] and Miller et al.[129] showed no change. Insulin responses were generally lower in most[127-129] but not all studies.[130] A cross-sectional study of young bodybuilders compared to sedentary, age-matched controls by Fluckey et al.[131] suggested that resistance training increases insulin action. These effects appear to be similar to those achieved with aerobic training. Fluckey et al.[131] conducted a study on the effects of a single bout of resistance training (three sets of exercises of 10 repetitions each) on glucose tolerance in three groups: seven young control males 27 ± 1 years, $19 \pm 1\%$ body fat; three older control males 51 ± 2 years, $19 \pm 3\%$ body fat; and, seven older males with noninsulin dependent diabetes mellitus (NIDDM) 53 ± 2 years, $23 \pm 2\%$ body fat. Young and older males had significantly lower glucose levels than older males with NIDDM both before and after resistance training. Insulin levels were also significantly lower before and after resistance training in younger and older males compared to NIDDM males. Thus, resistance training appears to increase the ability to clear insulin from the circulation in association with lower glucose levels. Although more research is needed on the benefits of resistance training on individuals with diabetes, the data published to date suggest that resistance training as well as aerobic training may improve glucose tolerance and reduce circulating insulin levels. The effects of resistance training on reducing elevated triglyceride levels in diabetics need further investigation.

VII. SUMMARY

Strength-trained athletes represent a wide variety of sports and may engage in other forms of physical conditioning besides strength training. The evaluation of the nutritional status of any individual or group of athletes is based on a comprehensive evaluation of food intake, anthropometric measurements, laboratory tests, and an assessment of any signs and symptoms combined with the appropriate use of selected demographic and medical information. A wide range of specific methods are available for assessing each of the four components of nutritional assessment, and each method has certain advantages and limitations that tend to be characteristic of that method. Because of the homeostatic regulation of the constituents of the blood, serum and/or plasma values may not be indicative of nutritional problems until tissue stores are either developed or saturated. Thus, special attention should be given to the potential development of nutrition problems associated with reliable and valid measures of food intake.

Coaches, trainers, health professionals, and athletes need to recognize the value of a complete nutritional assessment before using individual or group data as opposed to relying on the data obtained for a single component of the nutritional assessment process. The use of all four components of nutrition assessment increases the probability of detecting a nutrition problem when one usually does exist and reduces the probability of assuming that an athlete has a nutrition problem when he or she really does not have one. Furthermore, the use of all four components of nutrition assessment may help to identify potential problems that would be considered marginal before a true deficiency state has a chance to develop. Dietary interventions to prevent deficient states are more likely to be successful if instituted early.

On the basis of the investigations published in the literature on strength-trained athletes, there clearly is considerable variability in the nutrient intakes among athletes. The individual variability reflects differences in gender, body mass, energy expenditure, and training status, as well as cultural differences and individual food preferences.

The few longitudinal studies that have been published on bodybuilders consistently demonstrate dramatic changes in energy intake and the distribution of energy substrates in the diet as these athletes prepare for competition. Moderate increases in protein intake and dramatic decreases in dietary fat intake as a percentage of total calories suggest that bodybuilders developed dietary strategies which, combined with intensive, high-volume training, result in exquisitely low body fat levels in elite bodybuilders. Changes in food consumption patterns among bodybuilders reflect an avoidance of milk and other dairy products which results in marginal intakes of both calcium and vitamin D. No studies have been conducted to date that demonstrate an impact of these food preference cycles on reduced bone density in either female or male strength-trained athletes.

The composition of fat intake reported in the studies cited in the literature reflects a wide range of intakes regarding the polyunsaturated to saturated fat ratios in the diets of strength-trained athletes. Dietary cholesterol intake is above recommended levels for prevention of heart disease even when energy intakes have been curtailed in preparation for competition. Dietary cholesterol intake varies widely among bodybuilders, reflecting differences in the consumption of whole eggs vs. the consumption of egg whites. High intakes of tuna fish and other seafood are common among bodybuilders and may have some potential benefit on both lipid profiles as well as blood pressure. Dietary fiber has not been reported in most dietary studies but appears to be well below guidelines associated with healthy diets.

Dietary vitamin and mineral intakes of both male and female strength-trained athletes tend to be at, or well above, recommended levels, with the exception of dietary zinc intake, which is marginal, and dietary copper intake for females. Biochemical measures of nutritional status for selected vitamins and minerals among athletes have not been commonly reported but generally suggest a low prevalence of marginal or deficient levels. Problems of RBC hemolysis can dramatically elevate concentrations for some minerals, and special care should be taken to avoid the use of hemolyzed samples. The apparently widespread use of vitamin/mineral supplements which have not been accounted for in most dietary studies of strength-trained athletes would theoretically increase the nutrient availability relative to the already adequate (or perhaps more than adequate) intakes among the individuals who use supplements (provided that the specific vitamin/mineral formulations represent the biologically active forms of each nutrient).

Functional improvements in body composition or other measures of strength performance as a consequence of dietary supplements have not been impressive, although several studies on the protein requirements of strength-trained athletes have noted increased measures of lean body mass with increased dietary protein intakes.

Although older review articles on the protein needs of athletes have commonly reported no difference in protein requirements of athletes compared to "general" population, many of the studies suggest that the protein needs of highly trained athletes tend to fall within a range of 1.2–1.6 g/kg BW/d. At the lower limit, the differences in increased protein intake among athletes would represent an increase of at least 50% above the RDA and perhaps as much as 200% above the RDA. Protein requirements of strength-trained athletes also appear to be less than that of endurance-trained athletes, but more research is needed.

The protein requirements of athletes should be met by the usual diets consumed by athletes. Thus, there is little need for alarm regarding the possibility of protein deficiency among athletes, and no convincing data that protein supplements are needed to meet requirements. The data do suggest that the level of protein adequacy is clearly dependent upon an adequate energy intake. Consequently, protein needs of strength-trained athletes and other highly trained athletes probably change during the course of the training, competitive, and recovery seasons. It is also important to recognize that given a sufficient period of time to allow for adaptation to training/competition stresses, most athletes should eventually achieve an equilibrium at which they will be in nitrogen balance.

Considerable interest has been expressed in evaluating the potential benefits of low doses of amino acids on stimulating increased GH activity as part of an overall strategy to increase lean body mass while simultaneously reducing body fat levels. Much of the research published on these efforts has been poorly designed and has not adequately controlled for a wide variety of factors that are known to alter GH activity.

A positive energy balance associated with progressive increases in relative adiposity may also be associated with increased energy and protein efficiency, even among relatively lean athletes, and strength-trained athletes such as wrestlers who experience a high frequency of weight loss and regain may be prone to increased energy efficiency in association with a lower metabolic rate. Energy intakes of about 3000 calories (12.552 joules) per day may be sufficient to achieve/maintain nitrogen balance in some athletes, provided they have adequate fat stores to meet the energy cost of training, while energy intakes of 5000–6000 calories (20.92 kilojoules) may not be sufficient to maintain nitrogen balance if the athlete has reduced adipose tissue depots to levels below their usual body fat levels. The relationship of body fat levels to protein/energy needs of highly trained athletes is speculative at best, but future research on this issue may help explain some of the differences in protein needs of athletes (and body composition changes among athletes) as they physiologically adjust to different training demands. Until such data become available, it would be wise to obtain serial measurements of changes in body fat and lean body mass when evaluating the dietary adequacy of strength-trained athletes. A dramatic decrease in body fat levels, especially if combined with an absolute decrease in lean body mass, might be used as a guideline for caution in evaluating the adequacy of both energy and protein intakes. Based on personal diet counseling experiences, energy/food intakes of many athletes may be low because the athlete simply does not schedule time for eating.

The health status of strength-trained athletes is an important area of nutrition research. Weight loss practices in an effort to achieve competitive weight classes may place an athlete at risk of severe dehydration, electrolyte imbalances, thermoregulatory problems, and impaired kidney function, as well as a decline in performance associated with decreased strength and endurance.

The blood lipid profiles of strength-trained athletes reported in the literature have varied widely, ranging from values associated with an increased risk of cardiovascular heart disease to levels associated with good health. A wide range of values is present among athletes similar to the wide range observed for the population at large. While total cholesterol levels among highly trained competitive bodybuilders appear to be relatively low, HDL cholesterol levels tend to be lower than those reported for highly trained endurance athletes. HDL2 cholesterol levels appear also to be low and frequently undetectable among steroid users. Steroid use has consistently been associated with elevated TC, and extremely low HDL-C, which also reflect training and dietary practices, may account for the favorable lipid profiles observed among this group. Additionally, the intakes of vitamin C which tend to be about three to four times the RDA may also contribute to the HDL-C, HDL2-C, and HDL3-C observed among competitive bodybuilders.

Although more research is needed, resistance training may improve glucose tolerance and enhance insulin action, especially among individuals who have higher glucose levels initially. Little research has been conducted on the effects of resistance training on blood pressure. Athletes with a strong family history of cardiovascular disease, stroke, or diabetes should be screened and followed-up appropriately. Older individuals who are at an increased risk of chronic diseases including obesity may benefit from a balanced exercise program that includes resistance training as well as endurance training and activities which promote flexibility.

REFERENCES

1. Gibson, R., *Principles of Nutritional Assessment*, Oxford University Press, New York, 1990.
2. Bazzarre, T. L. and Myers, M. P., The collection of food intake data in cancer epidemiology studies, *Nutr. Cancer*, 1, 22, 1979.
3. Bazzarre, T. L. and Yuhas, J. A., Comparative evaluation of methods of collecting food intake data for cancer epidemiology studies, *Nutr. Cancer*, 5, 201, 1983.
4. Short, S. and Short, W. R., Four-year study of university athletes' dietary intake, *J. Am. Diet. Assoc.*, 82, 632, 1983.
5. Bazzarre, T. L., Kleiner, S. M., and Litchford, M. D., Nutrient intake, body fat and lipid profiles of competitive male and female bodybuilders, *J. Am. Coll. Nutr.*, 9, 136, 1990.
6. Bazzarre, T. L., Kleiner, S. M., and Ainsworth, B. E., Vitamin C intake and lipid profiles of competitive male and female bodybuilders, *Int. J. Sport Nutr.*, 2, 260, 1992.
7. Faber, M., Benade, A. J. S., and van Eck, M., Dietary intake, anthropometric measurements, and blood lipid values in weight training athletes, *Int. J. Sports Med.*, 7, 342, 1986.
8. Kleiner, S. M., Calabrese, L. H., Fiedler, K. M., Naito, H. K., and Skibinski, C. I., Dietary influences on cardiovascular disease risk in anabolic steroid-using and non-using bodybuilders, *J. Am. Coll. Nutr.*, 8, 109, 1989.
9. Hurley, B., Seals, D. R., Hagberg, J. M., Goldberg, A. C., Ostrove, S. M., Holloszy, J. O., Weist, W. G., and Goldberg, A. P., High-density lipoprotein cholesterol in bodybuilders vs. powerlifters, *J. Am. Med. Assoc.*, 252, 507, 1984.
10. Spitler, D., Diaz, F. J., Horvath, S. M., and Wright, J. E., Body composition and maximal aerobic capacity of bodybuilders, *J. Sports Med. Phys. Fitness*, 20, 181, 1980.
11. Morgan, D. W., Cruise, R. J., Girardin, B. W., Lutz-Schneider, V., Morgan, D. H., and Qi, W. M., HDL-C concentrations in weight-trained, endurance-trained, and sedentary females, *Phys. Sportsmed.*, 14, 166, 1986.
12. Fogleholm, G. M., Himberg, J.-J., Alopaeus, K., Gref, C.-G., Laadso, J. T., Letho, J. J., and Mussalo-Rauhamaa, H., Dietary and biochemical indices of nutritional status in male athletes and controls, *J. Am. Coll. Nutr.*, 11, 181, 1992.
13. Manore, M. M., Thompson, J., and Russo, M., Diet and exercise strategies of a world-class bodybuilder, *Int. J. Sport Nutr.*, 3, 76, 1993.
14. Heyward, V. H., Sandoval, W. M., and Colville, B. C., Anthropometric, body composition and nutritional profiles of bodybuilders during training, *J. Appl. Sports Sci. Res.*, 3, 22, 1989.
15. Lamar-Hildebrand, N., Saldanha, L., and Endres, L., Dietary and exercise practices of college-aged female bodybuilders, *J. Am. Diet. Assoc.*, 89, 1308, 1989.
16. Walberg-Rankin, J., Edmonds, C. E., and Gwazdauskas, F. C., Diet and weight changes of female body-builders before and after competition, *Int. J. Sport Nutr.*, 3, 87, 1993.
17. Bazzarre, T. L., Marquart, L. F., Izurieta, I. M., and Jones, A., Incidence of poor nutrition status among triathletes and control subjects, *Med. Sci. Sports Exer.*, 18, 590, 1986.
18. Steen, S. N. and McKinney, S., Nutrition assessment of college wrestlers, *Phys. Sportsmed.*, 14, 100, 1986.
19. Sandoval, W. M., Heyward, V. H., and Lyons, T. M., Comparison of body composition, exercise and nutritional profiles of female and male body builders at competition, *J. Sports Med. Phys. Fitness*, 29, 63, 1989.
20. Ferrando, A. A. and Green, N. R., The effect of boron supplementation on lean body mass, plasma testerone levels and strength in male bodybuilders, *Int. J. Sport Nutr.*, 3, 140, 1993.
21. Tarnopolsky, M. A., Atkinson, S. A., MacDougall, J. D., Chesley, A., Phillips, S., and Schwarcz, H. P., Evaluation of protein requirements for trained strength athletes, *J. Appl. Physiol.*, 73, 1986, 1992.
22. Food and Nutritional Board, National Academy of Sciences, *Recommended Dietary Allowances*, 10th ed., National Academy Press, Washington, D.C., 1989.
23. National Cholesterol Education Program, Report of the National Cholesterol Education Program expert panel on detection, evaluation and treatment of high blood cholesterol in adults, *Arch. Intern. Med.*, 148, 36, 1988.
24. Chen, J. D., Wang, J. F., Zhao, Y. W., Wang, S. W., Jiao, Y., and Hou, X. Y., Nutritional problems and measures in elite and amateur athletes, *Am. J. Clin. Nutr.*, 49, 1084, 1989.
25. Heinemann, L. and Zerbes, H., Physical activity, fitness, and diet: behavior in the population compared with elite athletes in the GRD, *Am. J. Clin. Nutr.*, 49, 1007, 1989.
26. Fry, A. C., Kraemer, W. J., Stone, M. H., Warren, B. J., Kearney, J. T., Maresh, C. M., Weseman, C. A., and Fleck, S. J., Endocrine and performance responses to high volume training and amino acid supplementation in elite junior weightlifters, *Int. J. Sport Nutr.*, 3, 306, 1993.
27. Warren, B. J., Stone, M. H., Kearny, J. T., Fleck, S. J., Kraemer, W. J., and Johnson, R. L., The effect of amino acid supplementation of physiological and performance responses of elite junior weightlifters, *Med. Sci. Sports Exer.*, 23, S15, 1991.

28. Kraemer, W. J., Fry, A. C., Warren, B. J., Stone, M. H., Fleck, S. J., Kearney, J. T., Conroy, B. P., Maresh, C. M., Weseman, C. A., and Triplett, N. T., Acute hormonal responses in elite junior weightlifters, *Int. J. Sports Med.*, 13, 103, 1992.

29. Hickson, J., Duke, M. A., Risser, W. L., Johnson, C. W., Palmer, R., and Stockton, J. E., Nutritional intake from food sources of high school football athletes, *J. Am. Diet. Assoc.*, 87, 1656, 1987.

30. Hickson, J., Wolinsky, K., Pivarnik, J. M., Neuman, E. A., Itak, J. F., and Stockton, J. E., Nutritional profile of football athletes eating from a training table, *Nutr. Res.*, 7, 27, 1987.

31. Gater, D. R., Gater, D. A., Uribe, J. M., and Bunt, J. C., Impact of nutritional supplements and resistance training on body composition, strength and insulin-like growth factor-1, *J. Appl. Sports Sci. Res.*, 6, 66, 1992.

32. Bazzarre, T. L., Scarpino, A., Sigmon, Marquart, L. F., Wu, S. L., and Izurieta, M., Vitamin-mineral supplement use and nutritional status of athletes, *J. Am. Coll. Nutr.*, 12, 162, 1993.

33. Oddoye, E. B. and Margen, S., Nitrogen balance studies in humans: long-term effect of high nitrogen intake on accretion, *J. Nutr.*, 109, 363, 1979.

34. Consolozio, C. F., Nelson, R. A., Matoush, L. O., Harding, R. S., and Canham, J. E., Nitrogen excretion in sweat and its relationship to nitrogen balance experiments, *J. Nutr.*, 79, 399, 1963.

35. Dragan, G. I., Vasiliu, A., and Georgescu, E., Effects of increased supply of protein on elite weightlifters, in *Milk Proteins '84*, Galesloot, T. E. and Tinbergen, B. J., Eds., Pudoc, Wageningen, The Netherlands, 1985, 99.

36. Frontera, W. R., Meredith, C. N., and Evans, W. J., Dietary effects on muscle strength gain and hypertrophy during heavy resistance training in older men, *Can. J. Sports Sci.*, 13, 13P, 1988.

37. Lemon, P. W. R., MacDougall, J. D., Tarnopolsky, M. A., and Atkinson, S. A., Effect of dietary protein and body building exercise on muscle mass and strength gains, *Can. J. Sport Sci.*, 15, 14S, 1990.

38. Tarnopolsky, M. A., Lemon, P. W. R., MacDougall, J. D., and Atkinson, S. A., Effect of body building exercise on protein requirements, *Can. J. Sports Sci.*, 15, 22S, 1990.

39. Butterfield, G. and Calloway, D. J., Physical activity improves protein utilization in young men, *Br. J. Nutr.*, 51, 171, 1984.

40. Celejowa, I. and Homa, M., Food intake, N and energy balance in Polish weightlifters during a training camp, *Nutr. Metab.*, 12, 259, 1970.

41. Consolazio, C. F., Johnson, H. L., Nelson, R. A., Dramise, J. G., and Skala, J. H., Protein metabolism during intensive physical training in the young adult, *Am. J. Clin. Nutr.*, 28, 29, 1979.

42. Decombaz, J., Reinhardt, R., Anantharaman, K., von Glutz, G., and Poortmans, J. R., Biochemical changes in a 100 km run: free amino acids, urea, and creatinine, *Eur. J. Appl. Physiol.*, 41, 61, 1979.

43. Goranzon, H. and Forsum, E., Effect of reduced energy intake versus increased physical activity on the outcome of nitrogen balance experiments in man, *Am. J. Clin. Nutr.*, 41, 919, 1985.

44. Gontzea, I. P., Sutzescu, P., and Dumitrache, S., The influence of muscular activity on nitrogen balance and on the need of man for proteins, *Nutr. Rep. Int.*, 10, 35, 1974.

45. Gontzea, I. P., Sutzescu, P., and Dumitrache, S., The influence of adaptation to physical effort on nutrition balance in man, *Nutr. Rep. Int.*, 11, 231, 1975.

46. Hickson, J. F., Wolinsky, I., Rodriquez, G. P., Pivarnik, J. M., Kent, M. C., and Shier, N. W., Failure of weight training to affect urinary indices of protein metabolism in men, *Med. Sci. Sports Exer.*, 18, 563, 1986.

47. Kraut, H., Muller, E. A., and Muller-Wecker, H., Influence of the composition of dietary protein on nitrogen balance and muscle training, *Int. Z. Angew. Physiol., Einschl., Arbeitsphysiol.*, 17, 378, 1958.

48. Laritcheva, J. A., Yalovaya, N. I., Shubin, V. I., and Smirnov, P. V., Study of energy expenditure and protein needs of top weightlifters, in *Nutrition, Physical Fitness, and Health*, Parizkova, J. and Rogozkin, V. A., Eds., University Park Press, Baltimore, 1978, 155.

49. Lemon, P. W. R. and Mullin, J. P., Effect of initial muscle glycogen levels on protein catabolism during exercise, *J. Appl. Physiol. Respir. Environ. Exer. Physiol.*, 48, 624, 1980.

50. Marable, N. L., Hickson, J. K., Korslund, M. K., Herbert, G., Desjardins, R. F., and Thye, F. W., Urinary nitrogen excretion as influenced by a muscle-building exercise program and protein variation, *Nutr. Rep. Int.*, 19, 795, 1979.

51. Mole, P. and Johnson, R. E., Disclosure by dietary modification of an exercise-induced protein catabolism in man, *J. Appl. Physiol.*, 31, 185, 1971.

52. Polykov, V. V., Nitrogen balance in man during reduced and increased energy expenditure, *Kosm. Biol. Aviakosm. Med.*, 8, 82, 1974.

53. Refsum, H. E. and Stromme, S. B., Urea and creatinine production and excretion in urine during and after prolonged heavy exercise, *Scan. J. Clin. Lab. Invest.*, 33, 247, 1974.

54. Tarnopolsky, M. A., MacDougall, J. D., and Atkinson, S. A., Influence of protein intake and training status on nitrogen balance and lean body mass, *J. Appl. Physiol.*, 64, 187, 1988.

55. Todd, K. S., Butterfield, G., and Calloway, D. H., Nitrogen balance in men with adequate and deficient energy intake at three levels of work, *J. Nutr.*, 114, 2107, 1984.

56. Walberg, J. L., Leedy, M. K., Sturgill, D. J., Hinkle, D. E., Ritchey, S. J., and Sebolt, D. R., Macronutrient content of a hypoenergy diet affects nitrogen retention and muscle function in weightlifters, *Int. J. Sports Med.*, 9, 261, 1988.

57. Murdoch, S. D., Bazzarre, T. L., Wu, S. L., Herr, D., and Snider, I. P., Nitrogen balance in highly trained athletes, *Med. Sci. Sports Exer.*, 24, S178, 1992.

58. Liappes, N., Kelderbacher, S. D., Kesseler, K., and Bantzer, P., Quantitative study of free amino acids in human eccrine sweat excreted from the forearms of healthy trained and untrained men during exercise, *Eur. J. Appl. Physiol.*, 42, 227, 1979.

59. Tarnopolsky, M. A., Atkinson, S. A., MacDougall, J. D., Chesley, A., Phillips, S., and Schwarcz, Evaluation of protein requirements for trained strength athletes, *J. Appl. Physiol.,* 73, 1986, 1992.

60. Butterfield, G. E., Whole-body protein utilization in humans, *Med. Sci. Sports Exer.*, 19, S157, 1987.

61. Fielding, R. A., The role of progressive resistance training and nutrition in the preservation of lean body mass in the elderly, *J. Am. Coll. Nutr.,* 14, 587, 1995.

62. Campbell, W. W. , Crim, M. C., Young, V. R., Joseph, L. J., and Evans, W. J., Effects of resistance training and dietary protein intake on protein metabolism in older adults, *Am. J. Physiol.*, 268, 1143, 1995.

63. Campbell, W. W., Crim, M. C., Young, V. R., and Evans, W. J., Increased energy requirements and changes in body composition with resistance training in older adults, *Am. J. Clin. Nutr.*, 60, 167, 1994.

64. Campbell, W. W., Crim, M. C., Dallas, G. E., Young, V. R., and Evans, W. J., Increased protein requirement in elderly people: new data and retrospective reassessments, *Am. J. Clin. Nutr.*, 60, 501, 1994.

65. Frontera, W. R., Meredith, C. N., and Evans, W. J., Dietary effect on muscle strength gain and hypertrophy during heavy resistance training in older men, *Can. J. Sport Sci.,* 13, 13P, 1988.

66. Fern, E. B., Bielinski, R. N., and Schutz, Y., Effects of exaggerated amino acid and protein supply in man, *Experientia,* 47, 168, 1991.

67. Chesley, A., MacDougall, J. D., Tarnopolsky, M. A., Atkinson, S. A., and Smith, K., Changes in human muscle protein synthesis after resistance exercise, J. Appl. Physiol., 73, 1383, 1992.

68. Dohm, G. L., Kasparek, G. J., Tapscott, E. B., and Barakat, H. A., Protein metabolism during endurance exercise, *Fed. Proc.*, 44, 348, 1985.

69. Evans, W. J., Fisher, E. C., Hoerr, R. A., and Young, V. R., Protein metabolism and endurance exercise, *Phys. Sportsmed.*, 11, 63, 1983.

70. Hagg, S. A., Morse, E. L., and Adibi, S. A., Effect of exercise on rate of oxidation, turnover, and plasma clearance of leucine in human subjects, *Am. J. Physiol. Endocrinol. Metab.,* 5, E407, 1982.

71. Lemon, P. W. R., Protein and amino acid needs of the strength athlete, *Int. J. Sport Nutr.*, 1, 127, 1991.

72. Young, V. R., Bier, D. M., and Pellet, P. L., A theoretical basis for increasing current estimates for the amino acid requirements in adult man with experimental support, *Am. J. Clin. Nutr.*, 50, 80, 1989.

73. Bazzarre, T. L., Murdoch, S. D., Wu, S. L., and Snider, I. P., Amino acid response to two successive exhaustion trials and carbohydrate feeding, *J. Am. Coll. Nutr.,* 11, 501, 1992.

74. Kleiner, S. M., Bazzarre, T. L., and Litchford, M. D., Metabolic profiles, diet and health practices of championship male and female bodybuilders, *J. Am. Diet. Assoc.*, 90, 962, 1990.

75. Sobal, J. and Marquart, L. F., Vitamin/mineral supplement use among athletes: a review of the literature, *Int. J. Sport Nutr.,* 4, 320, 1994.

76. Sobal, J. and Marquart, L. F., Vitamin/mineral supplement use among high school athletes, *Adolescence,* 29, 835, 1994.

77. Marquart, L. F. and Sobal, J., Beliefs and information sources of high school athletes regarding muscle development, *Ped. Exer. Sci.,* 5, 377, 1993.

78. Grandjean, A. C., Hursh, L. M., Majure, W. C., and Hanley, D. F., Nutrition knowledge and practices of college athletes, *Med. Sci. Sports Exer.,* 13, 82, 1981.

79. Bucci, L., Nutritional ergogenic aids, in *Nutrition in Exercise and Sport*, 2nd ed., Wolinsky, I. and Hickson, J.F., Jr., Eds., CRC Press, Boca Raton, FL, 1994.

80. Williams, M. H., Ergogenic aids, in *Sports Nutrition for the 90s: The Health Professionals Handbook*, Berning, J. R. and Steen, S. N., Eds., Aspen Publishers, Gaithersburg, MD, 1991.

81. Grunewald, K. K. and Bailey, R. S., Commercially marketed supplements for bodybuilding athletes, *Sports Med.,* 15, 90, 1993.

82. Bazzarre, T. L., Johanson, A. J., Huseman, C. A., Varma, M. M., and Blizzard, R. M., Human growth hormone changes with age, *Excerpta Medica*, 381, 261, 1975.

83. Hawkins, C. E., Walberg-Rankin, J., and Sebolt, D. R., Oral arginine does not affect body composition or muscle function in male weightlifters, *Med. Sci. Sports Exer.*, 23, S15, 1991.

84. Bucci, L., Hickson, J. F., Pivarnik, J. M., Wolinsky, I., McMahon, J. C., and Turner, S. D., Ornithine ingestion and growth hormone release in bodybuilders, *Nutr. Res.*, 10, 239, 1990.

85. Elam, R. P., Hardin, D. H., Sutton, R. A. L., and Hagen, L., Effects of arginine and ornithine on strength, lean body mass and urinary hydroxyproline in adult males, *J. Sports Med. Phys. Fitness*, 29, 52, 1989.

86. Elam, R. P., Morphological changes in adult males from resistance exercise and amino acid supplementation, *J. Sports Med. Phys. Fitness,* 28, 35, 1988.

87. Fogelholm, G. M., Naveri, H. K., Kiilavuori, K. T. K., and Harkonen, M. H. A., Low-dose amino acid supplementation: no effects on serum human growth hormone and insulin in male weightlifters, *Int. J. Sport Nutr.,* 3, 290, 1993.

88. Fry, A. C., Kraemer, W. J., Stone, M. H., Warren, B. J., Kearney, J. T., Maresh, C. M., Weseman, C. A., and Fleck, S. J., Endocrine and performance responses to high volume training and amino acid supplementation in elite junior weightlifters, *Int. J. Sport Nutr.,* 3, 306, 1993.

89. Isidori, A., Monaco, A. L., and Cappa, M., A study of growth hormone release in man after oral administration of amino acids, *Curr. Med. Res. Opin.,* 7, 475, 1981.

90. Lambert, M. I., Hefer, J. A., Millar, R. P., and Macfarlane, P. W., Failure of commercial oral amino acid supplements to increase serum growth hormone concentration in male bodybuilders, *Int. J. Sport Nutr.,* 3, 298, 1993.

91. Papadakis, M. A., Grady, D., Black, D., Tierney, M. J., Gooding, G. A. W., Schambelan, M., and Grunfeld, C., Growth hormone replacement in healthy older men improves body compostion but not functional ability, *Ann. Intern. Med.,* 124, 708, 1996.

92. Walberg-Rankin, J., Hawkins, C. E., Fild, D. S., and Sebolt, D. R., The effect of oral arginine during energy restriction in male weight trainers, *J. Strength Condition. Assoc.,* 8, 170, 1994.

93. Fineberg, S. E., Horland, A. A., and Merimee, T. J., Free fatty acid concentrations and growth hormone secretion in man, *Metabolism,* 21, 491, 1972.

94. Newsholme, E., The regulation of intracellular and extra cellular fuel supply during sustained exercise, *Ann. NY Acad. Sci.,* 301, 81, 1977.

95. Walberg-Rankin, J., Dietary carbohydrate as an ergogenic aid for prolonged and brief competitions in sport, *Int. J. Sport Nutr.,* 5, S13, 1995.

96. Steen, S. N., Oppliger, R. A., and Brownell, K. D., Metabolic effects of repeated weight loss and regain in adolescent wrestlers, *J. Am. Med. Assoc.,* 260, 47, 1988.

97. Pascoe, D. D., Costill, D. L., Robergs, R. A., Davis, J. A., Fink, W. J., and Pearson, D. R., Effects of exercise mode on muscle glycogen restorage during repeated days of exercise, *Med. Sci. Sports Exer.,* 22, 593, 1990.

98. Houston, M. E., Marrin, D. A., Green, H. J., and Thomson, J. A., The effect of rapid weight loss on physiological functions in wrestlers, *Phys. Sportsmed.,* 9, 73, 1981.

99. Walberg-Rankin, J., Ocel, J., Craft, L., VanGeluwe, S., Williams, J., and Aschenbach, W., Effect of weight loss and carbohydrate content of recovery diet on anaerobic performance in wrestlers, *Med. Sci. Sports Exer.,* 26(Suppl.), S53, 1994.

100. Chan, S. T. F., McLaughlin, S. J., Ponting, G. A., Biglin, J., and Dudley, H. A.F., Muscle power after glucose-potassium loading in undernourished patients, *Br. Med. J.,* 293, 1055, 1986.

101. Howald, C. E., Segesser, B., and Korner, W. F., Ascorbic acid and athletic performance, *Ann. NY Acad. Sci.,* 258, 458, 1975.

102. Keith, R. D. and Merrill, E., The effects of vitamin C on maximum grip strength and muscular endurance, *J. Sports Med.,* 23, 145, 1980.

103. Bramich, K. and McNaughton, L., The effects of two levels of ascorbic acid on muscular endurance, muscular strength and VO₂max, *Int. Clin. Nutr. Rev.,* 7, 5, 1987.

104. Tuttle, J. L., Potteiger, J. A., Evans, B. W., Ozmun, J. C., Effect of acute potassium-magnesium aspartate supplementation on ammonia concentrations during and after resistance training, *Int. J. Sport Nutr.,* 5, 102, 1995.

105. Hasten, D. L., Rome, E. P., Franks, B. D., and Hegsted, M., Effects of chromium picolinate on beginning weight training students, *Int. J. Sport Nutr.,* 2, 343, 1992.

106. Clancy, S. P., Clarkson, P. M., DeCheke, M. E., Nosaka, K., Freedson, P. S., Cunningham, J. J., and Valentine, B., Effects of chromium picolinate supplementation on body composition, strength, and urinary chromium loss in football players, *Int. J. Sport Nutr.,* 4, 142, 1994.

107. Saris, W. H. M., Physiological aspects of exercise in weight cycling, *Am. J. Clin. Nutr.,* 49, 1099, 1989.

108. Freischlag, J., Weight loss, body composition, and health of high school wrestlers, *Phys. Sportsmed.,* 12, 121, 1984.

109. Friedl, K. E., Moore, R. J., Martinez-Lopez, L. E., Vogel, J. A., Askew, E. W., Marchitelli, L. J., Hoyt, R. W., and Gordon, C. C., Lower limit of body fat in healthy active men, *J. Appl. Physiol.,* 77, 933, 1994.

110. Bach, A. C., Ingenbleek, Y., and Frey, A., The usefullness of dietary medium-chain triglycerides in body weight control: fact or fancy?, *J. Lipid Res.,* 37, 708, 1996.

111. Yost, T. J. and Eckel, R. H., Hypocaloric feeding in obese women: metabolic effects of medium-chain triglyceride substitution, *Am. J. Clin. Nutr.,* 49, 326, 1989.

112. Ballor, D. L., Katch, V. L., Becque, M. D., and Marks, C. R., Resistance weight training during exercise restriction enhances lean body weight maintenance, *Am. J. Clin. Nutr.,* 47, 19, 1988.

113. Cohen, J. C., Faber, W. M., Benade, A. J. S., and Noakes, T. D., Altered serum lipoprotein profiles in male and female powerlifters ingesting anabolic steroids, *Phys. Sportsmed.,* 14, 131, 1986.

114. Elliot, D. L., Goldberg, L., Kuehl, K. S., and Catlin, D. H., Characteristics of anabolic-androgenic steroid-free male and female bodybuilders, *Phys. Sportsmed.*, 15, 169, 1987.

115. Cohen, L. I., Hartford, C. G., and Rogers, G. G., Lipoprotein (a) and cholesterol in body builders using anabolic androgenic steroids, *Med. Sci. Sports Exer.,* 28, 176, 1996.

116. Webb, O. L., Laskarzewski, P. M., and Glueck, C. J., Severe depression of high-density lipoprotein cholesterol levels in weight lifters and body builders by self-administered exogenous testosterone and anabolic-androgenic steroids, *Metabolism,* 33, 971, 1984.

117. Costill, D. L., Pearson, D. R., and Fink, W. J., Anabolic steroid use among athletes: changes in HDL-C levels, *Phys. Sportsmed.*, 12, 113, 1984.

118. Higuchi, M., Iwaoka, K., Ishii, K., and Kobayashi, S., Plasma lipoprotein and apolipoprotein in male weightlifters, *Med. Sci. Sports Exer.*, 23, S22, 1991.

119. Peterson, G. E. and Fahey, T. D., HDL-C in five elite athletes using anabolic-androgenic steroids, *Phys. Sportsmed.*, 12, 120, 1984.

120. Frankle, M. A., Eichberg, R., and Zachariah, S. B., Anabolic androgenic steroids and a stroke in an athlete: case report, *Arch. Phys. Med. Rehabil.,* 69, 632, 1988.

121. McNutt, R. A., Ferenchick, G. S., Kirlin, P. C., and Hamlin, N. J., Acute myocardial infarction in a 22-year-old world class weight lifter using anabolic steroids, *Am. J. Cardiol.,* 62, 164, 1988.

122. Warber, J. and Bazzarre, T., A comparison between running and weight lifting on fasting plasma lipids of a well-conditioned hypercholesterolemic male, *Int. J. Sport Nutr.,* 3, 265, 1991.

123. Bazzarre, T. L., Wu, S. L., Murdoch, S. D., and Hopkins, R. G., Nutritional status, energy expenditure, body fat, stress and cardiovascular disease risk factors of North Carolina farm families, *Nutr. Res.,* 11, 1119, 1991.

124. Kohl, H. W., Gordon, N. F., Vaandrager, H., and Blair, S. N., Musculoskeletal fitness and serum lipid levels in men, *Med. Sci. Sports Exer.*, 23, S22, 1991.

125. Melia, P., Pipe, A., and Greenberg, G., The use of anabolic-androgenic steroids by Canadian students, *Clin. J. Sport Med.,* 6, 9, 1996.

126. Miller, J. P., Pratley, R. E., Goldberg, A. P., Gordon, P., Rubin, M., Treuth, M. S., Ryan, A. S., and Hurley, B. F., Strength training increases insulin action in healthy 50- to 65-yr-old men, *J. Appl. Physiol.,* 77, 1122, 1994.

127. Smutock, M. A., Reece, A. C., Kokkinos, P. F., Farmer, C., Dawson, P., Shulman, R., DeVane-Bell, J., Patterson, J., Charabogos, C., Goldberg, A. D., and Hurley, B. F., Aerobic versus strength training for risk factor intervention in middle-aged men at high risk for coronary heart disease, *Metabolism,* 42, 177, 1993.

128. Craig, B. W., Everhart, J., and Brown, R., The influence of high-resistance training on glucose tolerance in young and elderly subjects, *Mech. Ageing Dev.,* 49, 147, 1989.

129. Miller, W. J., Sherman, W. M., and Ivy, J. L., Effect of strength training on glucose tolerance and post-glucose insulin response, *Med. Sci. Sport Exer.,* 16, 539, 1984.

130. Gater, D. R., Gater, D. A., Uribe, J. M., and Bunt, J. C., Effects of agrinine/lysine supplementation and resistance training on glucose tolerance, *J. Appl. Physiol.,* 72, 1279, 1992.

131. Fluckey, J. D., Hickey, M. S., Brambrink, J. K., Hart, K. K., Alexander, K., and Craig, B. W., Effects of resistance exercise on glucose tolerance in normal and glucose-intolerant subjects, *J. Appl. Physiol.,* 77, 1087, 1994.

Chapter 15

DIETARY HABITS OF OLYMPIC ATHLETES

Ann C. Grandjean
Kristin J. Reimers
Jaime S. Ruud

CONTENTS

I. INTRODUCTION

What are the dietary habits of Olympic athletes? Are their nutritional needs different from nonelite athletes? Do they adhere to any special dietary regimens? What, if any, are the nutritional problems and dietary hurdles of these athletes? This chapter will attempt to answer these questions.

One of the difficulties in discussing "Olympic" athletes is distinguishing between Olympic, elite, and nonelite athletes. According to *The American Heritage Dictionary of the English Language*, Olympic has been defined as "of or belonging to the game ...," whereas elite means "the best or most skilled." Olympic athletes, therefore, are rightfully considered elite. And while one can find elite athletes at all levels of competition, most people consider the elite athlete as one who is successful in national or international competition, such as the Olympics.[1]

There are certain characteristics that exemplify the subpopulation of athletes referred to as Olympians. A century ago, they were lightly trained amatuers with natural athletic ability. However, today's athletes approach their sports as professionals and work full-time at developing their skills.[2] They may live with their immediate family, a spouse, other roommates, or alone. They may be adolescents or parents of adolescents. Olympic sports cover a wider variety of sports than seen in professional, college, or high school athletics. For example, while swimming, basketball, and wrestling are common at all levels, sports such as orienteering, team handball, luge, and equestrian are not.

Olympic athletes represent a group of very dedicated and hard-working individuals who are training at the limit of their physical capacity,[3] which sets them apart from their less successful counterparts. Even though the "experienced" marathon runner may average 46 km/wk,[4] the elite runner is training between 90 and 150 km/wk.[3] Road cyclists may ride 644–965 km during a training week.

Olympic athletes, among other qualities, possess a positive self-concept, function with a strong sense of personal autonomy, and have a high expectancy of success.[5] Winning a gold medal in international competition, such as the Winter or Summer Olympics, is a common goal for these athletes.

II. HISTORICAL PERSPECTIVE

Considerable interest has always been taken in the dietary habits of Olympic athletes. Early writings on the training and dietary regimens of well-known ancient athletes are among the most fascinating texts to survive from antiquity.[6,7] Throughout history, athletes have pursued optimal performance by eating specific foods and taking certain substances. In the Ancient Games of the 7th century B.C., competitors consumed a vegetarian diet consisting mainly of cheese, figs, and bread. Meat was introduced about the middle of the 5th century B.C. by Stymphalos, a long-distance runner who had won two Olympic victories.[8]

Perhaps the most referenced account of diet, training, and athletic prowess dates back to the 6th century B.C. in Greece. Milo of Croton, a famous wrestler whose achievements of feats of strength became legendary, won five successive Olympic titles from 532 to 516 B.C. As the story goes, Milo trained by carrying a bull across his shoulders and as the animal grew so did Milo's strength. His diet is said to have consisted of 9 kg of meat, 9 kg of bread, and 8.5 l of wine a day.[9] Although undoubtedly Milo possessed a hearty appetite, the validity of these dietary reports must be suspect, as basic estimations reveal that if he trained on such a volume of food, Milo would have consumed approximately 238,500 kJ (57,000 kcal) per day!

The last Olympiad of the ancient period was in 393 A.D. and for 15 centuries no Olympic games took place.[6] In 1896, the first modern Olympic games were held in Athens, Greece. A total of 311 athletes, all men, participated in 10 sports and 42 events. The 1996 Summer Olympic Games in Atlanta marked the 100th anniversary of the modern era and a century of great progress. An estimated 10,000 athletes, 3779 women, participated in 26 sports, 34 disciplines, and 271 events. Since 1896, each Olympiad has served as a measure of human potential, a barometer of how much faster and higher athletes have gone and how much stronger they have become.[2]

Despite the fascination in the eating habits and training rituals of Olympic athletes, dietary data are sparse. This comes as no surprise given the small number of Olympians who have participated in the Games over the years.

One of the first studies to appear on the diets of Olympic athletes was conducted in association with the 1948 London Olympic Games. Berry et al.[10] collected 4-d food intakes of 28 Olympic athletes representing different countries and a variety of sports. Berry writes:

The athletes collected their food on the cafeteria system; a dietitian followed and was served with duplicates of the meal. At the end of each meal the food left by the athletes was collected. The duplicate meals and the left-overs thus obtained were put separately into kilner jars for eventual chemical analysis.

The average daily intake for protein was 139 g (range 65–231 g); for carbohydrate, 390 g (range 128–572 g); and for fat, 137 g (range 92–223 g). Total energy intakes of the athletes ranged from 8841 kJ/d (2113 kcal/d) to 19,828 kJ/d (4739 kcal/d) with an average of 14,016 kJ/d (3350 kcal/d). Several of the athletes were interviewed about eating habits during training and before competition. Results showed that food habits varied considerably during training. Generous helping of steak, eggs, and milk were often consumed. Some athletes took glucose, vitamin preparations, or large amounts of salt. The majority of athletes reported consuming a light meal 3–4 h before competition; a guideline followed by many athletes today. However, the composition of the pregame meal was primarily protein (i.e., eggs and bacon) in contrast to the high-carbohydrate meal advocated today.[11]

During the 1952 games in Helsinki, a survey was conducted comparing the diets of Olympic athletes with the average American diet, the "ideal diet" as defined by Ancel Keys and the diets of nonindustrialized populations.[12] Compared to the average U.S. intake, the Olympic athletes had a higher mean calorie intake at 18,828 (4500 kcal), a higher percentage of calories from protein (20%) and lower percentage of calories from carbohydrate (Figure 1). The author also presented summary data that compared national Olympic achievement with different levels of caloric consumption and determined that a higher caloric intake related to better athletic performance and vice versa. This study may have been the genesis of the oft repeated statement that the only nutritional difference between athletes and nonathletes is the increased need for calories. Current knowledge in sports nutrition, however, indicates a more complex relationship.[13]

In 1968, Steel et al.[14] studied 66 male and 14 female athletes at the Olympic games in Mexico City. Seven-day dietary records were collected and analyzed by means of food composition tables. Included in the analysis were food supplements such as Ovaltine, Sustagen, and wheat germ. Results of this study showed a wide range of energy intakes, from 8368 kJ/d (2000 kcal/d) to 25,104 kJ/d (6000 kcal/d). The percentage of calories from protein, carbohydrate, and fat were 14, 41, and 43% for the men and 15, 39, and 44% for the women athletes. Mean intakes of vitamins and minerals studied were greater than the recommended allowances. The majority of athletes consumed a high-protein meal 1.5–4 h before competition.

de Wijn et al.[15] collected dietary information on champion rowers from the Netherlands during training for the 1968 Olympic Games in Mexico City and again 3 months after the Games. Food intake was analyzed from 7-d food intake records. The athletes' mean energy intake and percent of total calories from protein was greater during training than 3 months later. Protein intake during training averaged 1.6 g/kg bw/d.

III. DIETARY INTAKES OF ELITE ATHLETES

While recent scientific data on the nutritional habits of athletes participating in Olympic Games are limited, studies on elite athletes from several countries have been reported. Grandjean and Ruud[16] colleted data on 103 Olympians representing a variety of sports (Table 1). Daily energy intakes ranged from 10,598 kJ/d (2533 kcal/d) to 17,861 kJ/d (4269 kcal/d) for the male Olympians and from 7807 kJ/d (1866 kcal/d) to 12,590 kJ/d (3009 kcal/d) for female Olympians. Considering the majority of these athletes train heavily on a daily basis, group mean carbohydrate intakes were lower than current recommendations, ranging from

Diet of Olympic Athletes - Helsinki Games 1952

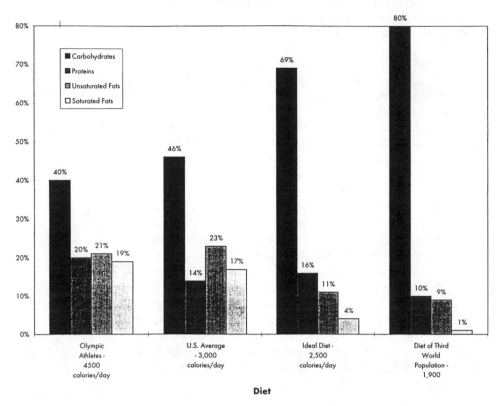

FIGURE 1 Comparison of diets of Olympic Athletes, average American diet, ideal diet, and diet of third world populations. (From Jokl, E., in *Physiology of Exercise*, Charles C. Thomas, Springfield, IL, 1964, 13. With permission.)

4.2 g/kg bw for male hockey players to 6.5 g/kg bw for male cyclists, and 4.4 g/kg bw for female judo players to 7.1 g/kg bw for female cyclists. Mean protein intakes for male groups ranged from 1.5 g/kg bw for judo players to 2.2 g/kg bw for cyclists, supplying 14–19% of energy. For female athletes, protein intake ranged from 1.0 g/kg bw in judo players to 1.7 g/kg bw in cyclists, supplying 12–15% of energy. Fat intakes as percent of total calories ranged from means of 29% in male distance runners to 41% for male cyclists and 29% for female tennis players to 34% for female judo players.

Mean intakes of vitamins and minerals for all male elite athletes studied by Grandjean and Ruud[16] met or exceeded the Recommended Dietary Allowance (RDA).[17] Elite female athletes, on the other hand, consumed less than 100% of the RDA for iron, calcium, zinc, and vitamin B_6. Vitamin C intakes from food alone were high in male and female cyclists, representing 586 and 425% of the RDA, respectively. Vitamin B_{12} intakes were also high (499% of the RDA) for the group of weight lifters.

Food intake data have also been reported on 419 athletes competing primarily on an international level, including several European, world, and Olympic medal winners.[18,19] Eating habits varied greatly with gender and sport. As was also true of athletes in Grandjean and Ruud's[16] study, energy intakes were highest in male endurance sports and the lowest in female athletes where body weight and/or composition is a major concern. Only five sport groups

TABLE 1 Nutrient Intake of 103 Olympic Athletes

	n	kJ/d	kJ/kg	Protein			Carbohydrate			Fat		
				Per Day (g/d)	Per Weight (g/kg)	Percent of Total Energy (%)	Per Day (g/d)	Per Weight (g/kg)	Percent of Total Energy (%)	Per Day (g/d)	Per Weight (g/kg)	Percent of Total Energy (%)
Males												
Cycling	9	17,861	247	160	2.2	15	471	6.5	43	196	2.7	41
Distance running	11	13,000	188	124	1.8	16	420	6.1	53	106	1.5	29
Figure skating	7	10,598	180	103	1.8	16	336	5.8	52	88	1.5	31
Hockey	8	14,510	180	156	1.9	18	343	4.2	39	155	1.9	39
Judo	7	13,217	176	114	1.5	14	358	4.9	45	127	1.7	36
Weightlifting	21	15,723	172	178	1.9	19	372	4.2	39	165	1.8	38
Females												
Cycling	10	12,590	218	100	1.7	13	409	7.1	53	111	1.9	31
Distance running	9	8962	176	82	1.6	15	275	5.4	50	74	1.4	30
Figure skating	8	7807	167	66	1.4	14	248	5.3	52	69	1.5	33
Judo	4	8226	134	62	1.0	12	264	4.4	53	77	1.2	34
Tennis	9	8535	146	80	1.4	15	279	4.8	54	68	1.2	29

Note: 1 kilojoule (kJ) = 0.239 kilocalories (kcal).

(namely Tour de France cyclists, Tour de l'Avenir cyclists, amateur cyclists, marathon skaters, and runners) reached the level of 55% of total calories from carbohydrate.[18]

In general, vitamin intakes for the total group studied by van Erp-Baart and colleagues[19] were adequate with the exception of low vitamin B_6 and thiamin intakes in professional cyclists. The authors attributed this to high intake of refined foods, such as sweet cakes or soft drinks. With respect to mineral intake, the authors concluded that calcium and iron may be problematic for young female athletes who are dieting. The major differences in food choices between the sport groups were in meat intake; endurance athletes tended toward a vegetarian diet.

IV. DIETARY SUPPLEMENTS

Elite athletes are generally knowledgeable and sophisticated in regard to nutrition and its effect on performance. Because the field of nutrition and performance is in its infancy, misinformation sometimes outweighs the scientific information that these athletes are exposed to. Thus, despite the scientific data disproving the ergogenic effects of most dietary supplements, many Olympians and Olympic hopefuls ingest a variety of nutrient and non-nutrient supplements. Of the aforementioned Olympians, 52% reported routine use of dietary supplements.[16] Patterns emerge when the data are analyzed by sport (Table 2), with male and female cyclists being the largest consumers of nutritional supplements. Similar results were reported by van Erp-Baart et al.,[19] who found a high supplement use by professional cyclists and body builders. Tour de France cyclists studied by Saris et al.[20] took several concentrated vitamin/mineral supplements, particularly iron and vitamin B_{12}.

Although little is known about the rationale for supplement use by Olympic athletes, one would assume it is to improve performance, to gain a competitive edge, and to be the best. Burke and Read,[21] who studied the eating habits of elite Australian football players, found the most frequently reported reasons for taking vitamins were to compensate for poor nutrition and lifestyle or in response to respiratory infections and excess alcohol consumption. Some players also felt dietary supplements would compensate for tiredness and loss of appetite due to heavy training.

TABLE 2   Percent of Athletes
Reporting Routine Use of
Supplements by Sport

Sport	Percent
Males	
Cycling	66
Distance running	54
Weightlifting	47
Judo	42
Hockey	37
Figure skating	14
Females	
Cycling	100
Distance running	66
Tennis	55
Figure skating	37

V. DIETARY CONCERNS

The Olympic athlete's nutritional program is comprised of four phases: training, pre-competition, during competition, and postcompetition. The importance of each of these phases and the specific dietary recommendations vary with the individual and the sport. For example, during competition, nutrition for a marathon runner or road cyclist is much different than for the gymnast or figure skater. The energy expenditure of Tour de France cyclists is the highest recorded for an athletic event. To maintain body weight, these athletes have to eat more than 25,104 kJ/d (6000 kcal/d) during competition.[20] They depend on easily digested foods and beverages such as sport drinks, energy bars, and fruit to supply additional calories during races.

Often, the stress of hard training can suppress appetite, making it increasingly difficult for the athlete to consume adequate calories and carbohydrate on a regular basis. In fact, many Olympic-level athletes are unable to maintain a regular meal schedule. Training for several hours a day leaves little time for preparing and ingesting meals, a dilemma shared by many professional and collegiate athletes. As a result, small meals and/or snacks contribute significantly to total calorie intake. In a study by Lindeman,[22] triathletes ate an average of nine times a day. However, one should not assume that adequate caloric intake ensures adequate nutrient intake. Green et al.[23] reported that female triathletes consuming an average of 17,359 kJ/d (4149 kcal/d) had low intakes of several vitamins and minerals. The athletes selected mostly high-calorie, low nutrient dense foods.

In addition to long training hours, travel is another disruption for athletes who compete on an international level. Many athletes travel to different countries to train and compete. Food intake often depends on local restaurant facilities and thus access to familiar foods may be limited. This can be a dilemma, especially for athletes with high calorie requirements. Additionally, eating atypical foods for long periods of time may have negative emotional and psychological effects.

Most Olympians have devoted the better part of their lives to intense training in hopes of being the best in the world. And for many, there is only one moment in time to achieve their ultimate dream. One of an Olympian's greatest fears is to become sick or sustain an injury just prior to or during the Olympic Games. Food-borne illness and GI distresses of other etiology can prohibit competing or diminish performance, thus a safe food supply at the Games is a major concern of all host countries and one of many reasons why years of planning and training food service employees precede the Games.

The challenge for food service at the Olympic Games, in addition to a safe food supply, is to satisfy the desires and preferences of a diverse group of athletes. Host countries do an excellent job of meeting these needs by providing a wide variety of foods in a buffet setting and the use of box lunches for athletes whose competition venues are away from the Village.

VI. DIETARY RECOMMENDATIONS

The relationships of various nutrients to athletic performance have been studied, and dietary recommendations have been made.[24-26] This section provides a brief overview of current dietary recommendations. Other chapters in this volume provide a more comprehensive discussion of specific nutrients.

A. CARBOHYDRATE

It is well established that dietary carbohydrate contributes directly to maintenance of muscle glycogen stores and may delay fatigue during endurance exercise. As such, athletes participating in prolonged (>60 min), intense exercise (65–70% VO$_2$max) are advised to consume a diet containing approximately 8–10 g carbohydrate/kg bw/d.[24] This amount of dietary carbohydrate has been shown to adequately restore skeletal glycogen within 24 h.[27] However, it is unknown whether athletes consuming less than this amount will have impaired performance. For athletes training aerobically for durations less than 60 min daily, performance can likely be maintained with a lower carbohydrate intake.[28] Although optimal carbohydrate intake will vary depending on body size, sport, and training routine, a minimum of 200 g carbohydrate/d is required to maintain liver glycogen.

B. PROTEIN

Research suggests that athletes have increased protein requirements compared to the general population. According to Lemon,[25] both endurance and strength training athletes will benefit from diets providing more protein than the current RDA of 0.8 g/kg bw/d. Strength athletes should consume between 1.4 to 1.8 g/kg and endurance athletes 1.2 to 1.4 g/kg bw/d.[25] In most cases, the additional amount of protein can be easily covered by a normal mixed diet as long as adequate amounts of food are consumed. Energy intake is a primary consideration, as protein requirement increases as energy intake decreases. Thus, weight-conscious athletes may require a more protein-dense diet to cover needs. The strict vegetarian also needs to consume higher levels of protein to maintain nitrogen balance than athletes who eat meat, dairy products, or eggs. This is due primarily to differences in the amino acid composition of vegetable protein and animal protein.

C. FAT

The USDA's Dietary Guidelines for Americans recommend that individuals consume no more than 30% of total calories from fat.[29] However, the "ideal" fat intake of elite athletes is not defined. Fat intakes will vary depending on the athletes' health, current eating habits, and performance goals. In a review of the nutritional habits of elite athletes, Economos[30] reported that during training, total fat intake for male endurance athletes ranged from 20 to 40% and for elite female endurance athletes, 26 to 38% of total calories. Obviously, athletes with a family history of heart disease, cancer, or obesity should follow a prudent diet for disease prevention. However, among healthy athletes, fat intakes greater than 30% are sometimes necessary to meet high caloric needs.

D. VITAMINS AND MINERALS

The RDA is the standard currently used in the United States for evaluating the adequacy of nutrient intakes of groups of people.[17] It represents a level of intake sufficient to meet the nutrient needs of most healthy people. While intakes less than the RDA are not necessarily considered inadequate, the more a mean intake falls below this standard, the greater is the number of people for which it is potentially inadequate.[31]

Taken in excess, vitamins and minerals provide no advantage, can be toxic, and may interfere with the absorption and metabolism of other nutrients. On the other hand, minerals that affect peak bone mass and exercise endurance, such as calcium, iron, and zinc, may require special attention among athletes who are low energy consumers, e.g., figure skaters and gymnasts.

VII. CONCLUSIONS

Olympic athletes are a very dedicated group of individuals with a high expectancy of success. Although the available research indicates that their eating habits are not unique compared to other groups of athletes, consumption of dietary supplements is prevalent and their dietary concerns are performance-related. Two factors that interfere with adequate food consumption in these athletes are long training hours and travel. Although the relationship between nutrition and performance has been studied for several years, methodologies are not always consistent; sample sizes are often small; level of accomplishment, type of sport, and training season vary from study to study; and data are not collected, analyzed, and reported in a consistent manner. Only when a substantial pool of data accumulates will more accurate profiles emerge and allow for more specific recommendations to be made.

REFERENCES

1. Butts, N. K., Profile of elite athletes: physical and physiological characteristics, in *The Elite Athlete*, Butts, N. K., Gushiken, T. T., and Zarins, B., Eds., Spectrum Publications, Jamaica, NY, 1985, 183.
2. McDonald, M., Pushing the envelope, *Civilization*, May/June, 40, 1996.
3. Holmich, P., Darre, E., Jahnsen, F., and Hartvig-Jense, T., The elite marathon runner: problems during and after competition, *Br. J. Sports Med.*, 22, 19, 1988.
4. Nieman, D. C., Butler, J. V., Pollett, L. M., Dietrich, S. J., and Lutz, R. D., Nutrient intake of marathon runners, *J. Am. Diet. Assoc.*, 89, 1273, 1989.
5. Parsons, T. W., Bowden, D., Garrett, M., McDonald, J., Schrock, M., Tesnow, D., and Wright, R., Profile of the elite athlete, *Coaching Rev.*, 9, 62, 1986.
6. Messinesi, X. L., *A Branch of Wild Olive, The Olympic Movement and the Ancient and Modern Olympic Games,* Exposition Press, New York, N.Y., 1973.
7. Kieran, J., Daley, A., and Jordan, P., *The Story of the Olympic Games: 776 B. C., to 1976,* J.B. Lippincott, Philadelphia, 1977.
8. Simopoulos, A. P., Opening Address. Nutrition and fitness from the first Olympiad in 776 B.C., to 393 A.D., and the concept of positive health, *Am. J. Clin. Nutr.*, 49, 921, 1989.
9. Harris, H. A., Nutrition and physical performance: the diet of Greek Athletes, *Proc. Nutr. Soc.*, 25, 87, 1966.
10. Berry, W. T. C., Beveridge, J. B., Bransby, E. R., Chalmers, A. K., Needham, B. M., Magee, H. E., Townsend, H. S., and Daubney, C. G., Diet, haemoglobin, and blood pressures of Olympic athletes, *Br. Med. J.*, 4598, 300, 1949.
11. Position of The American Dietetic Association and The Canadian Dietetic Association, Nutrition for physical fitness and athletic performance for adults, *J. Am. Diet. Assoc.*, 93, 691, 1993.
12. Jokl, E., The nutrition of athletes, in *Physiology of Exercise*, Charles C. Thomas, Springfield, IL, 1964, 13.
13. Grandjean, A. C., Diet of elite athletes. Has the discipline of sports nutrition made an impact?, *J. Nutr.*, 127, 8745, 1997.
14. Steel, J. E., A nutritional study of Australian Olympic athletes, *Med. J. Australia*, 2, 119, 1970.
15. de Wijn, J. F., Leusink, J., and Post, G. B., Diet, body composition and physical condition of champion rowers during periods of training and out of training, *Biblthea. Nutr. Dieta.*, 27, 143, 1979.
16. Grandjean, A. C. and Ruud, J. S., Olympic athletes, in *Nutrition and Exercise in Sport*, 2nd ed., Wolinsky, I. and Hickson, J. F., Eds., CRC Press, Boca Raton, FL, 1994, 447.
17. Food and Nutrition Board, *Recommended Dietary Allowances*, 10th rev. ed., National Academy of Sciences, Washington, D.C., 1989.
18. van Erp-Baart, A. M. J., Saris, W. H. M., Binkhorst, R. A., Vos, J. A., and Elvers, J. W. H., Nationwide survey on nutritional habits in elite athletes. Part I. Energy, carbohydrate, protein, and fat intake, *Int. J. Sports Med.*, 10, S3, 1989.
19. van Erp-Baart, A. M. J., Saris, W. H. M., Binkhorst, R. A., Vos, J. A., and Elvers, J. W. H., Nationwide survey on nutritional habits in elite athletes. Part II. Mineral and vitamin intake, *Int. J. Sports Med.*, 10, S11, 1989.
20. Saris, W. H. M., van Erp-Baart, M. A., Brouns, F., Westerterp, K. R., and ten Hoor, F., Study on food intake and energy expenditure during extreme sustained exercise: the Tour de France, *Int. J. Sports Med.*, 10, S26, 1989.
21. Burke, L. M. and Read, R. S. D., A study of dietary patterns of elite Australian football players, *Can. J. Sport Sci.*, 13, 15, 1988.
22. Lindeman, A. K., Eating and training habits of triathletes: a balancing act, *J. Am. Diet. Assoc.*, 90, 993, 1990.
23. Green, D. R., Gibbons, C., O'Toole, M., and Hiller, W. B. O., An evaluation of dietary intakes of triathletes: are RDA's being met?, *J. Am. Diet. Assoc.*, 89, 1653, 1989.
24. Sherman, W. M. and Wimer, G. S., Insufficient dietary carbohydrate during training: does it impair athletic performance?, *Int. J. Sport Nutr.*, 1, 28, 1991.

25. Lemon, P. W. R., Do athletes need more dietary protein and amino acids?, *Int. J. Sport Nutr.*, 5, S39, 1995.

26. Leaf, A. and Frisa, K. B., Eating for health or for athletic performance?, *Am. J. Clin. Nutr.*, 49, 1066, 1989.

27. Costill, D. L., Sherman, W. M., Fink, W. J., Maresh, C., Witten, M., and Miller, J. M., The role of dietary carbohydrate in muscle glycogen resynthesis after strenuous running, *Am. J. Clin. Nutr.*, 34, 1831, 1981.

28. Sherman, W. M., Doyle, J. A., Lamb, D. R., and Strauss, R. H., Dietary carbohydrate, muscle glycogen, and exercise performance during 7 d of training, *Am. J. Clin. Nutr.,* 57, 27, 1993.

29. U.S. Department of Agriculture, Nutrition and your Health: Dietary Guidelines for Americans, 4th ed., Home and Garden Bulletin No. 232, 1995.

30. Economos, C. D., Bortz, S. S., and Nelson, M. E., Nutritional practices of elite athletes, *Sports Med.,* 16, 381, 1993.

31. Guthrie, H. A., Interpretation of data on dietary intake, *Nutr. Rev.*, 47, 33, 1989.

Chapter 16

NUTRITIONAL CONCERNS
OF FEMALE ATHLETES

Jaime S. Ruud
Ann C. Grandjean

CONTENTS

0-8493-8560-1/97/$0.00+$.50
© 1998 by CRC Press LLC

I. INTRODUCTION

As the number of women participating in athletics continues to grow, issues associated with the female athlete become increasingly important. Nutrition is one of the more important factors but is often surrounded by myths and misconceptions. Nutrition can impact performance in many ways. The well-nourished athlete has the energy and stamina to train hard and perform her best. She is also less likely to suffer from illness and injury. Among comparable athletes, the one with the knowledge and practice of good nutrition most likely will have the competitive advantage.

While men and women should observe the same basic dietary principles, there are nutritional concerns unique to active women, such as low energy intakes, amenorrhea, eating disorders, and premenstrual syndrome. This chapter provides a nutritional review of these issues.

II. ENERGY REQUIREMENTS

The energy requirement of an athlete depends on many factors, including age, gender, body composition, type of sport, and intensity and duration of the sport. Ideally, energy intake should balance energy expenditure. If energy intake is consistently above or below an athlete's requirement, weight gain or weight loss can be expected, both of which may compromise health and performance.

The World Health Organization[1] defines energy requirement as "that level of energy intake from food which will balance energy expenditure when the individual has a body size and composition, and level of physical activity, consistent with long-term health; and that will allow for the maintenance of economically necessary and socially desirable physical activity." The energy requirement of an athlete must include the energy needs associated with her sport and level of training.

Energy intake is the energy associated with food consumed in the diet and is influenced by hunger, appetite, and satiety. Energy expenditure is the energy released by the body as heat and consists of three major components: basal metabolic rate (BMR), the thermic effect of food (TEF), and the energy expended in physical activity. To understand how energy requirements are determined, a brief explanation of these factors is necessary.

A. BASAL METABOLIC RATE

Basal metabolism is the energy level required to maintain life-sustaining activities like breathing, circulation, and heart beat. It is measured in terms of basal metabolic rate, the rate at which the body uses energy to keep all these life-supporting processes going.

Basal metabolic rate is the largest contributor to total energy expenditure, accounting for 60–70% of daily energy needs[2] and is affected by many factors such as age, fat-free mass, gender, body temperature, and conditions such as pregnancy and menstruation. Basal metabolic rate is approximately 3% lower in women than men, independent of body composition and activity level.[3] According to Tataranni et al.[4] women expend as many as 4464–11,937 kJ/d (1067–2853 kcal/d) to support basal metabolism.

B. THERMIC EFFECT OF FOOD

The second component of energy expenditure is the energy required for the body to digest, absorb, metabolize, and store food. When food is consumed, the activity in the cells increases. This increase in cellular activity is known as the thermic effect of food (TEF) or diet-induced thermogenesis. The thermic effect of food is relatively small, accounting for about 7–10% of total energy needs, or about 502–711 kJ/d (120–170 kcal/d) for women.[5] The energy cost associated with TEF is determined by the macronutrient composition of a meal. Carbohydrate and protein increase TEF, while fat intake has relatively little effect.[6] Some data have shown that female athletes have a lower TEF than nonathletes, indicating that athletes may be more energy efficient.[7] However, other studies fail to support this theory.[8-10]

Although the thermic effect of food has been examined extensively, its role in energy balance is still controversial. Studies examining the TEF in humans have reported conflicting results, which may be due to methodological differences, particularly differences in the time taken to measure TEF. Weststrate[11] concluded that the TEF can be accurately assessed within 3 h for meals providing approximately 2508 kJ (600 kcal). Reed and Hill[12] analyzed 131 TEF tests from a wide range of subjects ingesting meals of varying sizes and composition to determine how long TEF should be measured. Results of their study indicated that the TEF is a response lasting ≥6 h in most people and thus they recommend that measurements last ≥5 h.

C. PHYSICAL ACTIVITY

The final component influencing energy expenditure is physical activity. Of all the components, it is the most variable among individuals.[13] The amount of energy used by an athlete depends greatly on the type of sport and the frequency, intensity, and duration of the activity. Among well-trained female athletes, energy expended in physical activity can be as high as 36–38% of daily energy expenditure.[14,15] Body size impacts energy expenditure more than any other single factor. Tall athletes with a large, lean body mass use more energy to perform a given task than do smaller, less muscular athletes.

Why has it been so difficult to firmly establish concepts related to energy expenditure in humans? According to Heymsfield et al.[16] part of the answer may be that energy requirements in humans have been, until recently, very difficult, if not impossible, to measure. To date, the most common methods of estimating energy requirements have been through direct or indirect calorimetry and dietary assessment. Although both direct and indirect calorimetry yield excellent accuracy in laboratory settings, the relevance for subjects under normal living conditions is questionable. The introduction of the doubly labeled water technique is now finally allowing scientists to accurately measure the total energy expenditure of subjects in a free-living environment.[17]

The doubly labeled water method is based on the principle that carbon dioxide production can be estimated by the difference in elimination rates of body hydrogen and oxygen.[18] This technique has been validated for measuring energy expenditure in free-living subjects, and, as a result, may serve as a reference for validating the accuracy of energy intake.[19]

In female athletes, comparisons between reported energy intake and energy expenditure using the doubly labeled water technique have been made and large discrepancies have been found.[15,20,21] Edwards et al.[20] reported a 32% difference in the mean daily values for energy expenditure compared to energy intake in highly trained female runners. As several researchers have suggested, the differences reported for energy intake and energy expenditure are probably due to restricted eating during the recording period[15] or under-reporting by subjects.[20] While the doubly labeled water method offers potential for studying subjects in free-living situations, it is a relatively new and expensive technique requiring technical expertise.

D. ENERGY INTAKE OF FEMALE ATHLETES

The average daily energy intake for the referenced 19- to 24-year-old female is 9211 kJ (2200 kcal) or 159 kJ/kg/d (38 kcal/kg/d).[22] For the serious competitive female athlete, further adjustments in energy intakes must be made. For example, elite female runners training twice a day may need an additional 2929–4184 kJ/d (700–1000 kcal/d) to support activity levels.

Results of surveys examining the energy intakes of female athletes are shown in Table 1. There is a wide range of energy intakes between and within sport groups. Female triathletes,

TABLE 1 Summary of Energy Intakes of Female Athletes

Sport Group	No. of Subjects	Age	kJ	kJ/kg
Runners				
Beidleman et al.[8]	10	22	8163	152
Bergen-Cico and Short[23]	44	13	10,410	—
van Erp-Baart et al.[24]	18	31	—	167
Nieman et al.[25]	56	38	7816	142
Kaiserauer et al.[26]	9	26	10,418	—
Manore et al.[27]	10	34	9506	—
Singh et al.[28]	14	32	9753	—
Haymes and Spillman[29]	11	20	7627	—
Pate et al.[30]	103	30	6707	117
Tanaka et al.[131]	10	19	8318	155
Swimmers				
Vallieres et al.[32]	6	22	10,343	167
Barr[33]	10	16	8636	146
Tilgner and Schiller[34]	19	19	10,431	—
Barr[35]	14	19	9606	—
Lukaski et al.[36]	16	—	9176	—
Berning et al.[37]	21	15	14,945	255
Cyclists				
Grandjean[38]	12	26	12,673	213
van Erp-Baart et al.[24]	21	23	—	163
Keith et al.[39]	8	22	7452	—
Triathletes				
Green et al.[40]	34	—	17,359	—
Khoo et al.[41]	10	39	10,351	—
Gymnasts				
Grandjean[38]	10	16	8096	184
Reggiani et al.[42]	26	12	6494	180
van Erp-Baart et al.[24]	11	15	—	159
Benardot et al.[43]	22	11–14	7138	—
Kirchner et al.[44]	26	19	5778	—
Dancers				
Dahlstrom et al.[45]	14	24	8322	142
Benson et al.[46]	92	14	7908	—
Evers[47]	21	21	7427	—
Heavyweight Rowers				
Steen et al.[48]	16	21	11,016	—
Bodybuilders				
Heyward et al.[49]	25	28	6079	—
Kleiner et al.[50]	8	28	9456	—
Lamar-Hildebrand et al.[51]	10	18–30	5226	—

Note: One kilojoule (kJ) is equal to 0.239 kilocarlories (kcal).

swimmers, and heavyweight rowers had among the highest mean energy intakes ranging from 11,016 to 17,359 kJ/d (2633 to 4149 kcal/d). The lowest mean energy intakes were noted for female bodybuilders (5226 kJ/d; 1249 kcal/d), gymnasts (5778 kJ/d; 1381 kcal/d), and dancers (7427 kJ/d; 1775 kcal/d). Mean energy intakes of female runners ranged from 6707 to 10,410 kJ/d (1603 to 2488 kcal/d). It is difficult, however, to make comparisons, due to differences in research design, age, body size, level of competition, and way in which the data were reported.[52] Additionally, athletes' energy intakes may vary due to weight control practices. Nutter[53] reported that the desire to be thin influences the energy and nutrient intakes of many young female athletes. Furthermore, when assessing energy intakes, one should consider the different stages of the menstrual cycle. Studies have reported higher energy intakes during the luteal phase than the follicular phase of the menstrual cycle.[54,55]

Researchers have been puzzled as to why some athletes are not losing weight if reported energy intakes really reflect normal eating habits. One explanation may be that lean female athletes are more energy efficient as evidenced by a decrease in basal metabolic rate. This hypothesis has recently been tested by Beidleman et al.[8] They examined energy balance in female distance runners and untrained control subjects of similar age, body weight, and fat-free mass (FFM). Energy intake was estimated from 3-d diet records and energy expenditure was determined from individual heart rate oxygen uptake (HR/VO$_2$) curves during rest and exercise, 24-h HR records, and the thermic effect of meals (TEF). Results of the study showed that energy intakes were similar for both groups. The female runners averaged 8163 ± 507 kJ/d or 152 kJ/kg/d (1951 ± 121 kcal/d or 36 kcal/kg/d) and the control subjects, 7656 ± 389 or 134 kJ/kg/d (1830 ± 93 kcal/d or 32 kcal/kg/d). There were no significant differences between groups in absolute BMR or BMR adjusted for FFM, nor TEF. However, energy expenditure was higher for the runners (12,294 kJ/d; 2938 kcal/d) compared with the control subjects (9308 ± 511 kJ/d; 2225 ± 122 kcal/d), resulting in an energy deficit of -4131 ± 1185 kJ/d (987 ± 283 kcal/d). The runners, who averaged 11.6 km/d, had maintained body weight for 6 months before the study. The authors concluded that the large energy deficit experienced by these runners was not a result of an enhanced metabolic efficiency but rather may have been due to restricted eating and under-reporting during the study.

Horton et al.[14] also found no significant increase in energy efficiency of female cyclists compared to a control group. They measured usual energy intake from self-selected diets and determined energy expenditure using indirect calorimetry. The athletes maintained energy balance by consuming more calories on cycling days compared with noncycling days.

Future studies assessing the energy requirements of athletes need to address the issue of underestimating or under-reporting energy intake. This has been a problem in the athletic population as well as the general population. de Vries et al.[56] calculated self-reported energy intakes from 3-d dietary records with actual intakes needed to maintain body weight and found that subjects underestimated their energy intake by 10%. Mertz et al.[57] also found under-reporting to be common; 81% of the subjects in Mertz's study reported energy intakes below the amount required to maintain body weight.

To summarize, surveys assessing energy intakes show that many female athletes are in negative caloric balance. One major suspect is under-reporting of food intake. Nevertheless, women who are very active in their sport and have low calorie intakes should be evaluated for adequate nutrient intake and the possibility for eating disorders.

III. EATING DISORDERS

Today, there is enormous pressure for young girls to be attractive and achieve a certain body weight. In athletics, this influence may be even greater. Concerns about body weight are very prevalent among female athletes.[58-61] This is especially true for athletes who must maintain a low body weight or low body fat for their sport. Davis and Cowles[61] reported that athletes in "thin-build" sports (gymnastics, figure skating, distance running, ballet) had greater concerns, more body dissatisfaction, and more persistent dieting than athletes in normal-build sports such as field hockey, basketball, sprinting, and volleyball.

The inability to control weight and body shape can lead to a multitude of nutrition-related health problems, the most severe of which are anorexia and bulimia nervosa. Restrictive eating can, in and of itself, result in nutritional inadequacies, amenorrhea, iron deficiency, and low bone mineral density.

Coaches, team physicians, and sports nutritionists need to be aware of athletes with weight concerns and help them achieve a body weight that promotes optimal health and performance. This section presents an overview of eating disorders in athletes, including definition and diagnostic criteria, prevalence, risk factors, and effects on health and performance.

A. DIAGNOSTIC CRITERIA

According to the revised fourth edition of *Diagnostic and Statistical Manual of Mental Disorders (DSM-IV)*,[62] eating disorders are characterized by severe disturbances in eating behavior. The term eating disorder typically refers to anorexia nervosa or bulimia nervosa. However, "eating disorder" has recently been applied to eating disorders not otherwise specified, such as anorexia athletica and binge-eating disorder, categories for disorders of eating that do not meet the criteria for anorexia or bulimia.

Up to 1% of adolescent and young adult women have anorexia nervosa, and 2–4% have bulimia nervosa.[62] Many cases go unnoticed. Coaches, trainers, team physicians, and sports nutritionists need to be aware of the early signs of eating disorders so that preventive steps can be taken. The death of U.S. gymnast Christy Heinrich in 1994 increased awareness of anorexia nervosa and how it can totally consume the life of an athlete.[63] Fortunately, most athletes do not reach extreme levels of eating disorders. Instead, they exhibit fewer severe or subclinical forms of eating disorders.[64]

B. PREVALENCE OF EATING DISORDERS IN ATHLETES

Information on the prevalence of eating disorders in athletes varies with the diagnostic tool used to measure eating disorders and with the sport.[65] The majority of studies examining the prevalence of eating disorders have employed the Eating Attitudes Test (EAT) or the Eating Disorder Inventory (EDI). Both are standardized self-report instruments with demonstrated reliability and validity. However, one must use discretion when making conclusions based on the use of these instruments alone.[65] The EAT and the EDI were developed for use in nonclinical settings to assess attitudes and behaviors of individuals consistent with those exhibited by persons with eating disorders.[66,67]

Sundgot-Borgen[65] used the EDI and a self-developed questionnaire to identify individuals at risk for eating disorders. Results of her survey showed that athletes under-reported use of purging methods such as laxatives, diuretics, and vomiting and over-reported binging behaviors. Reasons why athletes may not accurately report weight control behaviors and attitudes include fear of being discovered by coaches, trainers, or teammates, and/or fear of losing their position on the team.[65]

The literature continues to support the theory that eating disorders occur more often in sports that emphasize leanness.[65,68-70] Sundgot-Borgen[65] examined the prevalence of eating disorders in 522 Norwegian elite female athletes representing 35 different sports. The prevalence of eating disorders and the use of pathogenic weight control practices were significantly higher among athletes in aesthetic (34%) and weight dependent (27%) sports compared to endurance (20%), technical (13%), and team sports (11%). Furthermore, the prevalence of eating disorders within sport groups varied significantly. For instance, among the endurance athletes in Sundgot-Borgen's study,[65] runners and cross-country skiers were at higher risk of eating disorders than cyclists, swimmers, and women rowers.

C. RISK FACTORS FOR EATING DISORDERS

Many sociocultural, biological, and psychological factors are known to contribute to the development of eating disorders. Some individuals with eating disorders have easily identifiable signs, and others do not.

Females are at greater risk, because society places greater demands on women to be thin. Studies show that even young girls who are underweight for their height are dieting to combat their fears of being overweight.[71] For many girls, weight and dieting concerns surface as early as the age of nine.[72]

Another factor contributing to the development of eating disorders relates to family dynamics. Families of women with eating disorders may present a history of alcoholism, sexual abuse, and emotional stress.

Low self-esteem is another well-known trait of eating disorder patients and may be a motivating factor in the development of anorexia and bulimia.[73] Mallick et al.[74] studied the behavioral and psychological traits of weight-conscious teenagers and reported a history of low self-esteem and difficulty with problem solving and coping with stress as well as emotional instability and withdrawl from social relationships.

The association between body image and athletic performance makes athletes especially vulnerable to an over-emphasis with weight. Although sports that emphasize leanness place athletes at greater risk of weight control problems, it is important to note that eating disorders occur in athletes in all sports. One study[75] that involved sport-by-sport comparisons between track, volleyball, basketball, and softball showed that softball players scored highest on five of the eight EDI subscales and three of four pathogenic weight control behaviors.

Although many factors can account for an athlete's predisposition for eating disorders, peronality characteristics of athletes and pressure from coaches and parents to lose weight for competition are important issues. More than one survey has demonstrated that athletes score higher on perfectionism, body dissatisfaction, and binge-purge behavioral subscales than non-athletes.[75,76] In a study examining risk factors for eating disorders, Williamson et al.[77] concluded that pressure from coaches and peers to be thin, combined with anxiety about athletic performance, were the factors most associated with concerns about body size and shape.

Other factors known to trigger eating disorders are dieting at an early age, frequent weight fluctuations, a sudden increase in training volume, and emotional circumstances such as injury or loss of a coach.[78]

D. WARNING SIGNS FOR ANOREXIA NERVOSA AND BULIMIA NERVOSA

According to Grandjean et al.,[79] there is a distinct difference between being thin and having anorexia, and between vomiting to reach a desired weight and having bulimia. For example, athletes may exhibit concerns about body weight and display aberrant eating behaviors but resume normal eating habits and gain weight after the season is over.[80] However, an assessment is warranted if the athlete displays noticeable weight loss or weight gain, depressive moods, or an unusual preoccupation with food.[81]

Experience shows that an important clue to the presence of an eating disorder may be the athlete's response to injury. Many female athletes use excessive exercise as a means of controlling weight and become very anxious when an injury prevents them from participating in their regular exercise regimens.[82,83]

E. EFFECTS OF EATING DISORDERS ON HEALTH AND PERFORMANCE

The general medical signs and symptoms of anorexia nervosa and bulimia nervosa have been described and discussed at length elsewhere.[84,85] This section will briefly review some of the nutrition and performance-related issues affecting athletes with eating disorders.

Athletes with eating disorders typically consume diets low in energy and essential nutrients. In one of the few studies to assess the nutrient intake of female athletes with eating disorders, Sundgot-Borgen[86] reported low dietary intakes of carbohydrate, calcium, vitamin D, and iron. Athletes often cautiously watch the amount of fat they eat, striving for intakes less than 10% of total calories. Dairy foods and quality protein sources, such as red meat, are often eliminated from the diet.[87]

Prolonged energy restriction and/or restrictive eating behaviors can lead to serious health and performance consequences. Low carbohydrate intakes can deplete muscle glycogen stores and result in a deterioration in performance. Binge-purge behaviors, such as vomiting, laxative use, and diuretic use, can cause fluid and electrolyte loss and risk of dehydration.

F. EVALUATION AND TREATMENT

While coaches, trainers, nutritionists, and parents can help identify symptoms of anorexia nervosa or bulimia nervosa, a diagnosis can only be made by a physician or professional who specializes in eating disorders. The complex multifaceted nature of anorexia and bulimia suggests that an interdisciplinary team is the best approach. The physician monitors the athlete's medical condition, the psychologist focuses on family and peer issues as well as body image and eating disordered behaviors, the nutritionist provides appropriate nutritional guidance, and the coach and trainer provides emotional support and an understanding of the sport environment.[79] For many athletes, their sport is their whole life and maintaining a scholarship or winning a gold medal may be pursued at any cost.[84]

One of the first issues likely to occur in treatment is whether or not the athlete should continue to train and compete. Some experts believe the decision should be based on the risk of injury or significant health problems to the athlete.[88] Some athletes binge and purge only occasionally, while others, several times a day. Restrictive eating behaviors or compulsive exercise may not be severe enough to cause serious risk to the athlete. However, prolonged starvation, laxative abuse, and compulsive vomiting can have a devastating effect on the athlete's health and performance. In the end, it may simply be a matter of compliance. If the athlete is not willing to follow treatment guidelines, she should not be allowed to stay on the team.[88]

When counseling the eating-disordered athlete, remember that each athlete's recovery process is unique and treatment plans and goals should be individualized.[89] Weight gain is a priority because many of the existing symptoms of an eating disorder are secondary to starvation.[79] A weight gain of 2.2 kg/wk is advised until the athlete achieves her goal weight.[83]

Eating disorders are easier to prevent than to treat. Early detection and intervention are essential to the athlete's health and career in sports. The preparticipation exam provides an opportunity to screen for unusual eating behaviors. The athlete suspected of an eating disorder should receive an in-depth evaluation by a physician or be referred to a nutritionist for dietary counseling.

IV. ATHLETIC AMENORRHEA

In 1991, the American College of Sports Medicine established a task force on women's issues in sports to address an area of growing concern in sports medicine: a triad of disorders observed in adolescent and young female athletes.[90] This triad includes three major health problems: amenorrhea, eating disorders, and osteoporosis. Some groups of female athletes, such as runners, gymnasts, and dancers, exercise and diet to the point where they develop eating problems and menstrual irregularities. This section will briefly focus on one aspect of the triad, amenorrhea.

Amenorrhea is the absence of menstruation and is defined as no more than one period for 6 months in a woman who has established menstrual cycles. Amenorrhea can be divided into two categories:

1. Primary amenorrhea — women who have never had a menstrual period
2. Secondary amenorrhea — the absence of menstruation in women who have previously had a regular menstrual cycle. It is characterized by low to normal levels of gonadotropin and estradiol.

A. PREVALENCE AMONG ATHLETES

It is estimated that up to 5% of sedentary females have amenorrhea. The prevalence of amenorrhea among female athletes is reportedly higher and varies both between and within sport groups. In a study of 226 elite athletes, gymnasts had the highest incidence of amenorrhea (71%), followed by lightweight rowers (46%), and runners (45%).[91] Among professional ballet dancers, the reported incidence ranges from 9.8 to 52%.[91-94]

Several factors have been associated with the higher incidence of amenorrhea among athletes: low body weight or percent body fat, low energy intake, vegetarian eating habits, and strenuous training.[95] Putukian[95] believes exercise-associated amenorrhea is the most frequent cause of amenorrhea among athletes and is considered a hypothalamic disorder.

More recently, Perry et al.[96] added aberrant eating behaviors to the list of potential causes of amenorrhea. They assessed nutrient intakes and psychological parameters of eumenorrheic and amenorrheic female athletes. Subjects completed a 3-d food intake record and the EAT. No significant differences in nutrient intakes were reported. Both groups consumed less than 8786 kJ/d (2100 kcal/d). However, EAT scores were significantly ($p < 0.05$) higher for amenorrheic athletes than the eumenorrheic athletes, 26.3 and 12.4, respectively. A score greater than 30 indicates eating attitudes similar to those found in anorexia nervosa. Myerson et al.[9] also found that amenorrheic athletes scored higher than regularly menstruating female athletes on the EAT.

The primary health concern of amenorrheic athletes has been infertility. However, research has shown that one of the long-term consequences of exercise-induced amenorrhea is premature osteoporosis.[97] Compared to regularly menstruating women, amenorrheic athletes have lower bone mineral density.[98,99] Some data have also reported a greater incidence of scoliosis and stress fractures in amenorrheic athletes.[87,100,101] A comprehensive review of bone health in physical activity and sport is covered elsewhere in this volume.

B. TREATMENT

In managing exercise-associated amenorrhea, professionals should encourage athletes to resume menstrual cycles by training less intensely.[101] It is also recommended that athletes receive nutrition counseling. Studies comparing the diets of regularly menstruating athletes to amenorrheic athletes indicate that amenorrheic athletes tend to consume fewer calories[10,26] and have lower dietary fat intakes,[87,99] both of which can negatively impact nutritional status. Nutritional strategies for the amenorrheic athlete include weight gain (if the athlete is underweight) and guidelines on proper food choices.

Dueck et al.[102] examined the effect of a 15-wk diet and exercise intervention program on energy balance, body composition, and menstrual function of a 19-year-old amenorrheic runner. The athlete ran twice a day, 4 d/wk and lifted weights the other 3 d. At the start of the competitive season she weighed 48 kg (106 lb). She had difficulty maintaining body weight and had complained of fatigue, poor performance, and recurring injury. The athlete's energy intake was 12,740 kJ/d (3045 kcal/d) at baseline with an estimated energy expenditure of 13,389 kJ/d (3200 kcal/d), which resulted in an energy deficit of approximately 649 kJ/d (155 kcal/d). The athlete was instructed to follow her usual diet and supplement with a liquid beverage containing 1506 kJ (360 kcal) per 11-oz (312 g) serving (59 g carbohydrates, 17 g protein, and 7 g fat). To help the athlete achieve energy balance, her training load was decreased from 7 d/wk to 6 d/wk. By the end of the 15-wk program, the subject had increased her energy intake to 15,410 kJ/d (3683 kcal/d) and reduced daily energy expenditure to 12,552 kJ/d (3000 kcal/d), resulting in positive energy balance. She gained 2.7 kg in body weight and increased body fat from 8.2 to 14.4%. Although she did not resume menstruation during the intervention period, she did so 3 months following the study. The results of this study demonstrate that dietary modification and a reduction in training are effective methods of treating athletic amenorrhea.

V. PREMENSTRUAL SYNDROME

Premenstrual syndrome (PMS) is of particular interest to athletes and coaches because symptoms may potentially affect athletic performance. According to Reid,[103] PMS is the "cyclic recurrence in the late luteal phase of the menstrual cycle of a combination of distressing physical, psychological, and/or behavioral changes of sufficient severity to result in deterioration of interpersonal relationships and/or interference with normal activities."

In 1987, the American Psychiatric Association (APA) concluded that severe PMS is actually a psychiatric disorder. They introduced a new definition entitled "late luteal phase dysphoric disorder" (LLPDD) to the appendix of the *Diagnostic and Statistical Manual of Mental Disorders*.[104] In DSM-IV, the terminology was changed to "Premenstrual Dysphoric Disorder."[105] According to the APA's definition, the essential features are symptoms such as markedly depressed mood, marked anxiety, marked affective lability, and decreased interest in activities. It is estimated that 20–50% of women experience minor or isolated premenstrual symptoms and that 3–5% meet the criteria for premenstrual dysphoric disorder.[105]

More than 150 symptoms have been attributed to PMS.[106,107] The symptoms, which usually occur 7–10 d prior to the onset of menses, can be divided into three categories: psychological, physical, and behavioral. The most common symptoms are abdominal bloating and/or pain, backache, headache, constipation, breast tenderness, food cravings (carbohydrates, sweets, chocolate, salt), fatigue, irritability, and symptoms related to depression. However, there can be considerable overlap in a number of symptoms.[108] Health professionals should be aware that PMS complaints can also be the result of an underlying disease. Thyroid disease, hyperprolactinemia, diabetes mellitus, and hypoglycemia can cause physical and psychological symptoms similar to PMS.[109]

A. PREVALENCE

The prevalence of PMS varies depending on the diagnostic tool used to measure symptoms. There are several types of questionnaires used to rate PMS symptoms. Questionnaires can be retrospective, based on past events and experiences, or prospective, based on actual events as they occur. The Moos' Menstrual Distress Questionnaire (MDQ)[110] has been one of the most widely used self-rating instruments for diagnosis of PMS. It requires women to rate 47 symptoms on a scale of one to six, with six being "acute or partially disabling." Woods et al.[111] administered the MDQ to a group of women and found that 30% or more reported common PMS symptoms such as weight gain, cramps, anxiety, fatigue, painful breasts, mood swings, or tension, although only 2–8% of women described these symptoms as severe or disabling.

B. ETIOLOGY

The etiology of PMS remains unknown, however, the fact that it is a female disorder makes hormones a major suspect. Estrogen and progesterone levels change dramatically the week before menstruation and thus can affect many psychological and physiological functions. This may explain why progesterone therapy has been widely prescribed for PMS even though there are few well-controlled studies demonstrating its efficacy.

1. Serotonin Theory

According to recent theories, serotonin, the neurotransmitter synthesized from the amino acid tryptophan may play an important role in PMS. Rapkin et al.[112] found that compared to a control group, serotonin levels of women with PMS were significantly (p <0.05) lower during the midluteal, late luteal, and premenstrual phases which may account for some of the psychological symptoms of PMS such as depression, anxiety, sleeplessness, headaches, and mental confusion. Low serotonin levels may also trigger early ovulation and a shift in estrogen and progesterone patterns, which could account for some of the physical symptoms of PMS such as breast tenderness, abdominal bloating, water retention, acne, and food cravings.

Although it is not known exactly how a deficiency of serotonin relates to PMS symptoms, the amino acid tryptophan may play an important role. Tryptophan and other large neutral amino acids such as valine, leucine, and phenylalanine compete for the same saturable carrier protein for transport across the blood-brain barrier.[113] Research suggests that the ratio of plasma tryptophan to the sum of those competing amino acids predicts the level of tryptophan and thus serotonin levels in the brain.[113]

Increased hunger and food cravings are symptoms frequently reported by women who suffer from PMS. It has been suggested that these food cravings are related to deficiencies of serotonin activity in the brain which, in turn, may affect mood and appetite. The approach has been to reduce the intake of refined carbohydrates especially during the late luteal phase of the menstrual cycle. However, research now suggests that consuming carbohydrates may help reduce PMS symptoms and improve moods.

Sayegh et al.[114] tested the efficacy of a carbohydrate-rich beverage designed to increase the serum ratio of tryptophan to other large neutral amino acids, on mood, appetite, and cognitive function in women with PMS. Over a duration of three menstrual cycles, 24 subjects participated in a double-blind, crossover study. Results showed that the carbohydrate beverage significantly decreased self-reported depression, anger, confusion, and food cravings .

C. EFFECTS ON PERFORMANCE

Of greater concern to the female athlete is the effect of PMS on performance. The good news is that women who are physically active tend to suffer less from PMS. Prior et al.[115] conducted a 3-month controlled study involving six sedentary women and eight women who began an exercise training program. The exercising women reported significant decreases in breast tenderness and fluid retention after 3 months of gradual training. In another study, Steege and Blumenthal[116] found that women who participated in aerobic exercise for 60 min three times a week showed significant improvements in PMS symptoms, especially premenstrual depression.

The most convincing evidence linking exercise to PMS involves beta-endorphin, a chemical in the brain associated with emotion and behavior. Chuong et al.[117] showed that PMS subjects had lower levels of plasma beta-endorphin during the luteal phase of the menstrual cycle. Because exercise stimulates endorphin production,[118] being active may provide some relief from PMS symptoms. Further research is needed to confirm this observation.

D. TREATMENT

PMS symptoms can be physical, psychological, and/or behavioral. Thus, treatment must address all three areas. Female athletes with mild symptoms may respond well to diet and lifestyle changes. However, for those with severe PMS symptoms, drug therapy and psychiatric counseling may be necessary. Treatment depends on the individual and the severity of her symptoms.

E. DIETARY RECOMMENDATIONS

A variety of therapeutic approaches have been recommended for PMS, but none have been entirely accepted. The nutritional factors that have been studied include vitamin B_6, magnesium, vitamin E, caffeine, tryptophan, and food cravings.[119] Most dietary recommendations include simple modifications such as limiting caffeine, salt, and sugar. These recommendations, however, are empirically based and may or may not work for everyone.

A diet high in complex carbohydrates, such as whole grains, vegetables, breads, pasta, and cereals is encouraged. These foods contain important vitamins and minerals, such as vitamin B_6, and magnesium, as well as dietary fiber, which help prevent constipation. Eating carbohydrates may also reduce PMS symptoms by increasing serotonin levels in the brain. Equally important is the fact that carbohydrates are the primary energy source during exercise and thus consuming adequate amounts will benefit performance.

VI. NUTRIENTS OF SPECIAL CONCERN

Several studies have reported inadequate dietary intakes of calcium, iron, and zinc among female athletes.[30,34,39,44,49] These three minerals perform specific functions in the body and thereby play important roles in health and performance. Inadequate dietary calcium can contribute to low bone density and risk for osteoporosis.[120] Athletes who do not consume enough dietary iron risk iron depletion and impaired performance.[121] Generally when dietary iron intake is low, so is zinc, because food sources of these two minerals are similar (Table 2).

TABLE 2   Nutrients of Special Concern in Female Athlete's Diet

Nutrient	RDA[a]	Functions	Absorption and Utilization	Food Sources
Calcium	1200 mg/d	Builds bones and teeth. Needed for muscle contraction, normal heart rhythm, nerve functioning, blood clotting	**Enhancers:** vitamin D, phosphorus **Inhibitors:** sodium, oxalates, protein phytates	Milk, yogurt, cheese, turnip greens, broccoli, kale, small fish with bones, calcium-fortified orange juice
Iron	15 mg/d	Constituent of hemoglobin and myoglobin; carries oxygen in the blood; involved in blood formation; necessary for the utilization of energy	**Enhancers:** Heme iron (meat, fish, poultry), vitamin C **Inhibitors:** Tannins in tea, coffee, bran, calcium supplements	Lean meats, fish, poultry, eggs, legumes, dried fruit
Zinc	12 mg/d	Component of carbonic anhydrase and several enzymes; part of the hormone insulin; involved in genetic material, immune function, and wound healing	**Enhancers:** Meat, liver, seafood, eggs **Inhibitors:** Phytates, fiber	Oysters, lean meats, seafood, eggs, poultry, vegetables, grains

[a]   RDA reflects daily amounts established for 11- to 24-year-old females.

The body's ability to absorb and utilize calcium, iron, and zinc is greatly affected by the presence of other nutrients and dietary substances as well as physiological factors. These topics are reviewed more extensively in other chapters in this book.

Female athletes who are dieting are encouraged to include low-fat dairy products and lean meat in the diet. Those who do not consume significant amounts of calcium, iron, and zinc through foods may benefit from a multivitamin/mineral providing no more than 100% of the recommended amount for these nutrients.

VII. CONCLUSIONS

Dietary surveys show that many female athletes are not consuming enough energy to support their training and competitive schedule. Adequate energy intake is essential to optimal health and performance. Researchers have questioned why some athletes are not consistently losing weight if reported energy intakes truly reflect daily eating habits. Part of the answer may be that female athletes are underestimating or under-reporting food intake, which may reflect concerns about weight and body image. Coaches, trainers, and support staff should be aware of the nutritional problems associated with low energy intakes. Indiscriminate reduction in total food intake, or exclusion of major food groups, and disordered eating behaviors can have adverse effects on health and performance. Female athletes who train vigorously and consume a low-energy diet are at risk for amenorrhea. These are typically athletes who maintain a very lean body for esthetic and/or athletic reasons. Amenorrhea is associated with decreased bone mineral density and risk for osteoporosis. It is also one of the diagnostic criteria for anorexia nervosa. Although many factors can account for an athlete's predisposition for eating disorders, pressure from coaches and parents to lose weight for competition and personality characteristics of athletes are important issues. Early detection and intervention are important to the athlete's health and career in sports. Eating disorders may be prevented if warning signs are recognized and athletes are provided with realistic expectations about body weight and performance.

REFERENCES

1. World Health Organization, Energy and protein requirements, Report of Joint FAO/WHO/UNO Expert Consultation, Technical Report Series, 724, Geneva: World Health Organization, 1985.
2. Poehlman, E. T., A review: exercise and its influence on resting energy metabolism in man, *Med. Sci. Sports Exer.,* 21, 515, 1989.
3. Arciero, P. J., Goran, M. I., and Poehlman, E. T., Resting metabolic rate is lower in women than in men, *J. Appl. Physiol.,* 75, 2514, 1993.
4. Tataranni, P. A. and Ravussin, E., Variability in metabolic rate: biological sites of regulation, *Int. J. Obesity,* 19, S102, 1995.
5. Ravussin, E., Lillioja, S., Anderson, T. E., Christin, L., and Bogardus, C., Determinants of 24-hour energy expenditure in man. Methods and results using a respiratory chamber, *J. Clin. Invest.,* 78, 1568, 1986.
6. Schultz, Y., Bessard, T., and Jequier, E., Diet-induced thermogenesis measured over a whole day in obese and nonobese women, *Am. J. Clin. Nutr.,* 40, 542, 1984.
7. LeBlanc, J., Diamond, P., Cote, J., and Labrie, A., Hormonal factors in reduced postprandial heat production of exercise-trained subjects, *J. Appl. Physiol.,* 56, 772, 1984.
8. Beidleman, B. A., Puhl, J. L., and De Souza, M. J., Energy balance in female distance runners, *Am. J. Clin. Nutr.,* 61, 303, 1995.
9. Myerson, M., Gutin, B., Warren, M. P., May, M. T., Contento, I., Lee, M., Pi-Sunyer, F. X., Pierson, R. N., and Brooks-Gunn, J., Resting metabolic rate and energy balance in amenorrheic and eumenorrheic runners, *Med. Sci. Sports Exer.,* 23, 15, 1991.
10. Wilmore, J. H., Wambsgan, K. C., Brenner, M., Broeder, C. E., Paijmans, I., Volpe, J. A., and Wilmore, K. M., Is there energy conservation in amenorrheic compared with eumenorrheic distance runners?, *J. Appl. Physiol.,* 72, 15, 1992.

11. Weststrate, J. A., Resting metabolic rate and diet-induced thermogenesis: a methodological reappraisal, *Am. J. Clin. Nutr.*, 58, 592, 1993.

12. Reed, G. W. and Hill, J. O., Measuring the thermic effect of food, *Am. J. Clin. Nutr.*, 63, 164, 1996.

13. Hill, J. O., Melby, C., Johnson, S. L., and Peters, J. C., Physical activity and energy requirements, *Am. J. Clin. Nutr.*, 62, 1059S, 1995.

14. Horton, T. J., Drougas, H. J., Sharp, T. A., Martinez, L. R., Reed, G. W., and Hill, J. O., Energy balance in endurance-trained female cyclists and untrained controls, *J. Appl. Physiol.*, 76, 1937, 1994.

15. Schultz, L. O., Alger, S., Harper, I., Wilmore, J. H., and Ravussin, E., Energy expenditure of elite female runners measured by respiratory chamber and doubly labeled water, *J. Appl. Physiol.*, 72, 23, 1992.

16. Heymsfield, S. B., Darby, P. C., Muhlheim, L. S., Gallagher, D., Wolper, C., and Allison, D. B., The calorie: myth, measurement, and reality, *Am. J. Clin. Nutr.*, 62, 1034S, 1995.

17. Schoeller, D. A. and van Santen, E., Measurement of energy expenditure in humans by doubly labeled water method, *J. Appl. Physiol.*, 53, 955, 1982.

18. Hildreth, H. G. and Johnson, R. K., The doubly labeled water technique for the determination of human energy requirements, *Nutr. Today*, 30, 254, 1995.

19. Schoeller, D.A., How accurate is self-reported dietary energy intake?, *Nutr. Rev.*, 48, 373, 1990.

20. Edwards, J. E., Lindeman, A. K., Mikesky, A. E., and Stager, J. M., Energy balance in highly trained female endurance runners, *Med. Sci. Sports Exer.*, 25, 1398, 1993.

21. Sjodin, A. M., Andersson, A. B., Hogberg, J. M., and Westerterp, K. R., Energy balance in cross-country skiers: a study using doubly labeled water, *Med. Sci. Sports Exer.*, 26, 720, 1994.

22. Food and Nutrition Board, National Academy of Sciences, *Recommended Dietary Allowances*, National Academy Press, Washington, D. C., 1989, 33.

23. Bergen-Cico, D. K. and Short, S. H., Dietary intakes, energy expenditures, and anthropometric characteristics of adolescent female cross-country runners, *J. Am. Diet. Assoc.*, 92, 611, 1992.

24. van Erp-Baart, A. M. J., Saris, W. H. M., Binkhorst, R. A., Vos, J. A., and Elvers, J. W. H., Nationwide survey on nutritional habits in elite athletes, Part I. Energy, carbohydrate, protein, and fat intake, *Int. J. Sports Med.*, 10, S3, 1989.

25. Nieman, D. C., Bulter, J. V., Pollet, L. M., Dietrich, S. J., and Lutz, R. D., Nutrient intake of marathon runners, *J. Am. Diet. Assoc.*, 89, 1273, 1989.

26. Kaiserauer, S., Snyder, A. C., Sleeper, M., and Zierath, J., Nutritional, physiological, and menstrual status of distance runners, *Med. Sci. Sports Exer.*, 21, 120, 1989.

27. Manore, M. M., Besenfelder, P. D., Wells, C. L., Carroll, S. S., and Hooker, S. P., Nutrient intakes and iron status in female long-distance runners during training, *J. Am. Diet. Assoc.*, 89, 257, 1989.

28. Singh, A., Deuster, P. A., Day, B. A., and Moser-Veillon, P. B., Dietary intakes and biochemical markers of selected minerals: comparison of highly trained runners and untrained women, *J. Am. Coll. Nutr.*, 9, 65, 1990.

29. Haymes, E. M. and Spillman, D. M., Iron status of women distance runners, sprinters, and control women, *Int. J. Sports Med.*, 10, 430, 1989.

30. Pate, R. R., Sargent, R. G., Baldwin, C., and Burgess, M. L., Dietary intake of women runners, *Int. J. Sports Med.*, 11, 461, 1990.

31. Tanaka, J. A., Tanaka, H., and Landis, W., An assessment of carbohydrate intake in collegiate distance runners, *Int. J. Sport Nutr.*, 5, 206, 1995.

32. Vallieres, F., Tremblay, A., and St-Jean, L., Study of the energy balance and the nutritional status of highly trained female swimmers, *Nutr. Res.*, 9, 699, 1989.

33. Barr, S. I., Energy and nutrient intakes of elite adolescent swimmers, *J. Can. Diet. Assoc.*, 50, 20, 1989.

34. Tilgner, S. A. and Schiller, M. R., Dietary intakes of female college athletes: the need for nutrition education, *J. Am. Diet. Assoc.*, 89, 967, 1989.

35. Barr, S. I., Relationship of eating attitudes to anthropometric variables and dietary intakes of female collegiate swimmers, *J. Am. Diet. Assoc.*, 91, 976, 1991.

36. Lukaski, H. C., Hoverson, B. S., Gallagher, S. K., and Bolonchuk, W. W., Physical training and copper, iron, and zinc status of swimmers, *Am. J. Clin. Nutr.*, 51, 1093, 1990.

37. Berning, J. R., Troup, J. P., VanHandel, P. J., Daniels, J., and Daniels, N., The nutritional habits of young adolescent swimmers, *Int. J. Sport Nutr.*, 1, 240, 1991.

38. Grandjean, A. C. et al., unpublished data.

39. Keith, R. E., O'Keeffe, K. A., Alt, L. A., and Young, K. L., Dietary status of trained female cyclists, *J. Am. Diet. Assoc.*, 89, 1620, 1989.

40. Green, D. R., Gibbons, C., O'Toole, M., and Hiller, W. B. O., An evaluation of dietary intakes of triathletes: are RDAs being met?, *J. Am. Diet. Assoc.*, 89, 1653, 1989.

41. Khoo, C., Rawson, N. E., Robinson, M. L., and Stevenson, R. J., Nutrient intake and eating habits of triathletes, *Ann. Sports Med.*, 3, 144, 1987.

42. Reggiani, E., Arras, G. B., Trabacca, S., Senarega, D., and Chiodini, G., Nutritional status and body composition of adolescent female gymnasts, *J. Sports Med.*, 29, 285, 1989.

43. Benardot, D., Schwarz, M., and Heller, D. W., Nutrient intake in young, highly competitive gymnasts, *J. Am. Diet. Assoc.*, 89, 401, 1989.
44. Kirchner, E. M., Lewis, R. D., and O'Connor, P. J., Bone mineral density and dietary intake of female college gymnasts, *Med. Sci. Sports Exer.*, 27, 543, 1995.
45. Dahlstrom, M., Jansson, E., Nordevang, E., and Kaijser, L., Discrepancy between estimated energy intake and requirement in female dancers, *Clin. Physiol.*, 10, 11, 1990.
46. Benson, J. E., Allemann, Y., Theintz, G. E., and Howald, H., Eating problems and calorie intake levels in swiss adolescent athletes, *Int. J. Sports Med.*, 11, 249, 1990.
47. Evers, C. L., Dietary intake and symptoms of anorexia nervosa in female university dancers, *J. Am. Diet. Assoc.*, 87, 66, 1987.
48. Steen, S. N., Mayer, K., Brownell, K. D., and Wadden, T. A., Dietary intake of female collegiate heavyweight rowers, *Int. J. Sport Nutr.*, 5, 225, 1995.
49. Heyward, V. H., Sandoval, W. M., and Colville, B. C., Anthropometric, body composition, and nutritional profiles of bodybuilders during training, *J. Appl. Sport Sci. Res.*, 3, 22, 1989.
50. Kleiner, S. M., Bazzarre, T. L., and Litchford, M. D., Metabolic profiles, diet, and health practices of championship male and female bodybuilders, *J. Am. Diet. Assoc.*, 90, 962, 1990.
51. Lamar-Hildebrand, N., Saldanha, L., and Endres, J., Dietary and exercise practices of college-aged female bodybuilders, *J. Am. Diet. Assoc.*, 89, 1308, 1989.
52. Grandjean, A. C. and Ruud, J. S., Energy intake of athletes, in *Oxford Textbook of Sports Medicine,* Harries, M., Williams, C., Stanish, W. D., and Micheli, L. J., Eds., Oxford University Press, New York, 1994, 53.
53. Nutter, J., Seasonal changes in female athlete's diets, *Int. J. Sport Nutr.*, 1, 395, 1991.
54. Martini, M. C., Lampe, J. W., Slavin, J. L., and Kurzer, M. S., Effect of the menstrual cycle on energy and nutrient intake, *Am. J. Clin. Nutr.*, 60, 895, 1994.
55. Tarasuk, V. and Beaton, G. H., Menstrual-cycle patterns in energy and macronutrient intake, *Am. J. Clin. Nutr.*, 53, 442, 1991.
56. de Vries, J. H. M., Zock, P. L., Mensink, R. P., and Katan, M. B., Underestimation of energy intake by 3-d records compared with energy intake to maintain body weight in 269 nonobese adults, *Am. J. Clin. Nutr.*, 60, 855, 1994.
57. Mertz, W., Tsui, J. C., Judd, J. T., Reiser, S., Hallfrisch, J., Morris, E. R., Steele, P. D., and Lashley, E., What are people really eating? The relation between energy intake derived from estimated diet records and intake determined to maintain body weight, *Am. J. Clin. Nutr.*, 54, 291, 1991.
58. Werblow, J. A., Fox, H. M., and Henneman, A., Nutritional knowledge, attitudes, and food patterns of women athletes, *J. Am. Diet. Assoc.*, 73, 242, 1978.
59. Perron, M. and Endres, J., Knowledge, attitudes, and dietary practices of female athletes, *J. Am. Diet. Assoc.*, 85, 573, 1985.
60. Welch, P. K., Zager, K. A., Endres, J., and Poon, S. W., Nutrition education, body composition, and dietary intake of female college athletes, *Phys. Sportsmed.*, 15, 63, 1987.
61. Davis, C. and Cowles, M., A comparison of weight and diet concerns and personality factors among female athletes and nonathletes, *J. Psychosomatic. Res.*, 33, 527, 1989.
62. American Psychiatric Association, *Diagnostic and Statistical Manual of Mental Disorders*, 4th ed., Washington, D. C., American Psychiatric Association, 539, 1994.
63. Thomas, D., Athletes, Coaches, Wise Up, *Omaha World-Herald,* August 15, 1994.
64. Beals, K. A. and Manore, M. M., The prevalence and consequences of eating disorders in female athletes, *Int. J. Sport Nutr.*, 4, 175, 1994.
65. Sundgot-Borgen, J., Prevalence of eating disorders in elite female athletes, *Int. J. Sport Nutr.*, 3, 29, 1993.
66. Garner, D. M. and Garfinkel, P. E., The eating attitudes test, an index of the symptoms of anroexia nervosa, *Psych. Med.*, 9, 273, 1979.
67. Garner, D. M., Olmstead, M. P., and Polivy, J., Development and validation of a multidimensional eating disorder inventory for anorexia nervosa and bulimia, *Int. J. Eating Disorders*, 2, 15, 1983.
68. O'Connor, P. J., Lewis, R. D., and Kirchner, E. M., Eating disorder symptoms in female college gymnasts, *Med. Sci. Sports Exer.*, 27, 550, 1994.
69. Rosen, L. W., McKeag, D. B., Hough, D. O., and Curley, V., Pathogenic weight control behavior in female athletes, *Phy. Sportsmed.*, 14, 79, 1986.
70. Rucinski, A., Relationship of body image and dietary intake of competitive ice skaters, *J. Am. Diet. Assoc.*, 89, 98, 1989.
71. Koff, E. and Rierdan, J., Perceptions of weight and attitudes toward eating in early adolescent girls, *J. Adolescent Health*, 12, 307, 1991.
72. Mellin, L. M., Irwin, C. E., and Scully, S., Prevalence of disordered eating in girls: a survey of middle-class children, *J. Am. Diet. Assoc.*, 92, 851, 1992.
73. Lindeman, A. K., Self-esteem: its application to eating disorders and athletes, *Int. J. Sport Nutr.*, 4, 237, 1994.

74. Mallick, M. J., Whipple T. W., and Huerta, E., Behavioral and psychological traits of weight-conscious teenagers: a comparison of eating-disordered patients and high- and low-risk groups, *Adolescence,* 22, 157, 1987.

75. Taub, D. E. and Blinde, E. M., Eating disorders among adolescent female athletes: influence of athletic participation and sport team membership, *Adolescence,* 27, 833, 1992.

76. Sundgot-Borgen, J. and Corbin, C. B., Eating disorders among female athletes, *Phys. Sportsmed.,* 15, 89, 1987.

77. Williamson, D. A., Netemeyer, R. G., Jackman, L. P., Anderson, D. A., Funsch, C. L., and Rabalais, J. Y., Structural equation modeling of risk factors for the development of eating disorder symptoms in female athletes, *Int. J. Eating Disorders,* 17, 387, 1995.

78. Sundgot-Borgen, J., Risk and trigger factors for the development of eating disorders in female elite athletes, *Med. Sci. Sports Exer.,* 26, 414, 1994.

79. Grandjean, A. C., Woscyna, G., and Ruud, J. S., Eating disorders in athletes, in *Office Sports Medicine,* Mellion, M. B., Ed., Hanley & Belfus, Philadelphia, 1996, 113.

80. Leon, G. R., Eating disorders in female athletes, *Sports Med.,* 12, 219, 1991.

81. Wilmore, J. H., Eating and weight disorders in female athletes, *Int. J. Sport Nutr.,* 1, 104, 1991.

82. Squire, D. L., Eating disorders, in *Sports Medicine Secrets,* Mellion, M.B., Ed., Hanley & Belfus, Philadelphia, 136, 1994.

83. Clark, N., How to help the athlete with bulimia: practical tips and a case study, *Int. J. Sport Nutr.,* 3, 450, 1993.

84. Thompson, R. A. and Sherman, R. T., *Helping Athletes With Eating Disorders,* Human Kinetic Publishers, Champaign, 1993.

85. Johnson, M. D., Disordered eating in active and athletic women, *Clin. Sports Med.,* 13, 355, 1994.

86. Sundgot-Borgen, J., Nutrient intake of female elite athletes suffering from eating disorders, *Int. J. Sport Nutr.,* 3, 431, 1993.

87. Frusztajer, N. T., Dhuper, S., Warren, W. P., Brooks-Gun, J., and Fox, R. P., Nutrition and the incidence of stress fractures in ballet dancers, *Am. J. Clin. Nutr.,* 51, 779, 1990.

88. Harris, S. S. and Nattiv, A., Controversies in sports medicine: should women with eating disorders be allowed to participate in athletics?, *Sports Med. Digest,* 17, 1, 1995.

89. Position of the American Dietetic Association: Nutrition intervention in the treatment of anorexia nervosa, bulimia nervosa, and binge eating, *J. Am. Diet. Assoc.,* 92, 902, 1995.

90. Yeager, K. K., Agostini, R., Nattiv, A., and Drinkwater, B., The female athlete triad: disordered eating, amenorrhea, osteoporosis, *Med. Sci. Sports Exer.,* 25, 775, 1993.

91. Wolman, R. L. and Harries, M. G., Menstrual abnormalities in elite athletes, *Clin. Sports Med.,* 1, 95, 1989.

92. Fogelholm, M., Lichtenbelt, W. V. M., Ottenheijm, R., and Westerterp, K., Amenorrhea in ballet dancers in the Netherlands, *Med. Sci. Sports Exer.,* 28, 545, 1996.

93. Holderness, C. C., Brooks-Gunn, J., and Warren, M. P., Eating disorders and substance use: a dancing vs a nondancing population, *Med. Sci. Sports Exer.,* 26, 297, 1994.

94. Benson, J. E., Geiger, C. J., Eiserman, P. A., and Wardlaw, G. M., Relationship between nutrient intake, body mass index, menstrual function, and ballet injury, *J. Am. Diet. Assoc.,* 89, 58, 1989.

95. Putukian, M., The female triad: eating disorders, amenorrhea, and osteoporosis, *Med. Clin. N. Amer.,* 78, 345, 1994.

96. Perry, A. C., Crane, L. S., Applegate, B., Marquez-Sterling, S., Signorile, J. F., and Miller, P. C., Nutrient intake and psychological and physiological assessment in eumenorrheic and amenorrheic female athletes: a preliminary study, *Int. J. Sport Nutr.,* 6, 3, 1996.

97. Fisher, E. C., Nelson, M. E., Frontera, W. R., Turksoy, R. N., and Evans, W. J., Bone mineral content and levels of gonadotropins and estrogens in amenorrheic running women, *J. Clin. Endocrinol. Metab.,* 62, 1232, 1986.

98. Myburgh, K. H., Bachrach, L. K., Lewis, B., Kent, K., and Marcus, R., Low bone mineral density at axial and appendicular sites in amenorrheic athletes, *Med. Sci. Sports Exer.,* 25, 1197, 1993.

99. Drinkwater, B. L., Bruemner, B., and Chesnut, C. H., Menstural history as a determinant of current bone density in young athletes, *J. Am. Med. Assoc.,* 263, 545, 1990.

100. Warren, M. P., Brooks-Gunn, J., Hamilton, L. H., Warren, L. F., and Hamilton, W. G., Scoliosis and fractures in young ballet dancers, *N. Engl. J. Med.,* 314, 1348, 1986.

101. Sutton, J. R. and Nilson, K. L., Repeated stress fractures in an amenorrheic marathoner, *Phys. Sportsmed.,* 17, 65, 1989.

102. Dueck, C. A., Matt, K. S., Manore, M. M., and Skinner, J. S., Treatment of athletic amenorrhea with a diet and training intervention program, *Int. J. Sport Nutr.,* 6, 24, 1996.

103. Reid, R. L., Premenstrual syndrome, *N. Engl. J. Med.,* 324, 1208, 1991.

104. American Psychiatric Association, *Diagnostic and Statistical Manual of Mental Disorders- DSM-III-R,* 3rd ed., American Psychiatric Association, Washington, D. C., 1987, 367.

105. American Psychiatric Association, *Diagnostic and Statistical Manual of Mental Disorders-DSM-IV,* 4th ed., American Psychiatric Association, Washington, D. C., 1994, 715.

106. Reid, R. L., Premenstrual Syndrome, *Curr. Probl. Obstet. Fertil.*, 8, 1, 1985.
107. Smith, S. and Schiff, I., The premenstrual syndrome-diagnosis and management, *Fertil. Steril.*, 52, 527, 1989.
108. Bancroft, J., Williamson, L., Warner, P., Rennie, D., and Smith, S. K., Perimenstrual complaints in women complaining of PMS, menorrhagia, and dysmenorrhea: toward a dismantling of the premenstrual syndrome, *Psychosom. Med.*, 55, 133, 1993.
109. Chuong, C. J., Pearsall-Otey, L. R., and Rosenfeld, B. L., Revising treatments for premenstrual syndrome, *Contemp. Ob/Gyn,* January, 1994, 66.
110. Moos, R. H., The development of menstrual distress questionnaire, *Phychosom. Med.*, 30, 853, 1968.
111. Woods, N. F., Most, A., and Dery, G. K., Prevalence of perimenstrual symptoms, *Am. J. Public Health*, 72, 1257, 1982.
112. Rapkin, A. J., Reading, A. E., Woo, S., and Goldman, L. M., Tryptophan and neutral amino acids in premenstrual syndrome, *Am. J. Obstet. Gynecol.*, 165, 1830, 1991.
113. Fernstrom, J. D., Role of precursor availability in control of monoamine biosynthesis in brain, *Physiol. Rev.,* 63, 484, 1983.
114. Sayegh, R., Schiff, I., Wurtman, J., Spiers, P., McDermott, J., and Wurtman, R., The effect of a carbohydrate-rich beverage on mood, appetite, and cognitive function in women with premenstrual syndrome, *Obstet. Gynecol.,* 86, 520, 1995.
115. Prior, J. C., Vigna, Y., and Alojada, N., Conditioning exercise decreases premenstrual symptoms, *Eur. J. Appl. Physiol.,* 55, 349, 1986.
116. Steege, J. F. and Blumenthal, J. A., The effects of aerobic exercise on premenstrual symptoms in middle-aged women: a preliminary study, *J. Psychosom. Res.*, 37, 127, 1993.
117. Chuong, C. J., Coulam, C. B., and Kao, P. C., Neuropeptide levels in premenstrual syndrome, *Fertil. Steril.*, 44, 760, 1985.
118. Thoren, P., Floras, J. S., Hoffmann, P., and Seals, D. R., Endorphins and exercise: physiological mechanisms and clinical implications, *Med. Sci. Sports Exer.*, 22, 417, 1990.
119. Ruud, J. S., Premenstrual syndrome-nutritional implications, in *Nutritional Concerns of Women*, Wolinsky, I. and Klimis-Tavantzis, D. J., Eds., CRC Press, Boca Raton, FL, 1996, Chap. 8.
120. Optimal Calcium Intake. NIH Consens Statement 1994, Jun 6–8; 12(4):1–31.
121. Davies, K. J. A., Maguire, J. J., Brooks, G. A., Dallman, P. R., and Packer, L., Muscle mitochondrial bioenergetics, oxygen supply, and work capacity during dietary iron deficiency and repletion, *Am. J. Physiol.*, 242, E418, 1982.

Chapter 17

THE VEGETARIAN ATHLETE

_____ Rosemary A. Ratzin

CONTENTS

I. INTRODUCTION

Fueling the body becomes an important issue and critical component of a training regimen for the athlete. A competitive athlete is one whose goal is winning, while a recreational athlete is one whose goal is exercise for health and wellness and not necessarily competition. Questions consistently arise with respect to diet; particularly, what nutritional practices will improve performance and perhaps enhance competition but, most importantly, what practices will meet and support short- and long-term goals of various levels of competitive and recreational athletics. The dilemma regarding diet, then, is unique and complex for both the recreational and competitive athlete.

One such unique and healthful approach to a diet is vegetarianism. This chapter will explore this meatless dietary regimen, which has become increasingly popular in the American population. Areas that will be covered are:

1. a brief background of meatless eating;
2. what is and what is not a vegetarian;
3. nutritional status of vegetarians;
4. a brief history of the vegetarian athlete;

5. how to go about eating a healthy meatless diet; and
6. dietary considerations for the vegetarian athlete.

II. BACKGROUND

The nutritional needs of individuals have been met by various forms of vegetarianism for longer than is often recognized. Majumder[1] stated that vegetarianism was perceived as a fad diet in the 1960s, and its advocates were identified as followers of various cults. Interestingly, the fad diet so identified has a history of nearly 2000 years; vegetarian historians usually agree that the founder of the philosophical vegetarian movement was Pythagoras, the Greek mathematician.[2] In fact, up until 1847 vegetarians referred to themselves as "Pythagoreans."[3]

Vegetarianism has faded in and out of history since the time of ancient Greece. However, in the United States, vegetarian practices are usually traced back to an English minister, William Metcalfe, who emigrated to Philadelphia in 1817 with a number of his followers. A Presbyterian minister, Sylvester Graham, was converted to vegetarianism by a member of Metcalfe's church.[4] The Reverend Graham went on to become a well-known health reform lecturer advocating vegetarianism and is most remembered for inventing the graham cracker. While the American Vegetarian Society was established in 1850, it is noted that vegetarianism experienced a decline in the 1860s. It has been suggested by Roe[5] that this decline in enthusiasm was due to involvement in the American Civil War.

An individual influenced by Graham was John Harvey Kellogg, M.D., a Seventh-day Adventist and a vegetarian. In 1876, Dr. Kellogg became the first administrator of a type of health spa known as the Battle Creek Sanitarium in Michigan. It was here that the breakfast cereal industry emerged as an outgrowth of Dr. Kellogg's experimentation to provide a healthful and palatable vegetarian dietary program for the sanitarium patrons and workers.[6]

Since the Civil War, vegetarianism largely faded out and had not been widely publicized until the Woodstock generation. The attraction for this regimen did not subside after Woodstock but rather continues to increase. A position paper of the American Dietetic Association that addressed vegetarianism stated:

> The attention focused today on personal health habits is unprecedented, as more and more Americans adopt health-promoting life-styles that include alterations in diet and exercise patterns. Simultaneously, there has been an increased interest in vegetarian diets.[7]

As meatless eating gains popularity, the question arises: what exactly is a vegetarian? It appears that there are as many different kinds of vegetarians as there are types of individuals. Therefore, to avoid confusion, the term "vegetarian" warrants definition.

III. WHAT A VEGETARIAN IS

Every individual is on a diet as "diet" is loosely defined as food and drink consumed each day. However, vegetarianism is classically defined as a dietary practice of abstaining from the ingestion of animal flesh which includes red meat, poultry, fish, and seafood. This dietary regimen is usually divided into three to five types of adherents, and the definitions that follow are those that are usually accepted among vegetarians. The following three types are the most common:

1. Lacto-ovo vegetarian — A vegetarian who combines milk products and eggs with a diet of vegetables, fruits, nuts, seeds, legumes, and grains.

2. Lacto vegetarian — A vegetarian who consumes milk products but no eggs with a diet of vegetables, fruits, nuts, seeds, legumes, and grains.
3. Vegan — This type of vegetarian excludes both milk products and eggs and consumes a diet derived exclusively from plant protein.

The latter or vegan diet is based on a philosophy of life that promotes the desire to minimize exploitation and suffering of nonhuman animals. The vegan avoids foods of animal origin, which includes honey, and products from animals such as leather, wool, fur, down, silk, ivory, and pearl. Additionally, cosmetics and household items that contain animal ingredients or that are tested on animals are avoided.

The two less common types of vegetarians are:

1. Ovo vegetarian — A vegetarian who consumes eggs but no milk products with a diet of vegetables, fruits, nuts, seeds, legumes, and grains.
2. Fruitarian — A vegetarian who extends the philosophy of nonexploitation to plants as well as animals. The fruitarian diet usually consists of consuming those parts of the plant that are cast off or dropped from the plant and that do not involve the destruction of the plant itself.[8]

Mention should be made of the dietary known as macrobiotics, formerly known as "Zen" Macrobiotics. It is a philosophy that includes and revolves around a nutritional system that claims to prevent and cure many diseases. The diets prescribed, of which there are ten, are largely vegetarian, with heavy emphasis on whole-grain cereals and avoidance of sugar and fluids. Fish and fowl are included in the lower five levels of this diet. The highest diet, which is diet seven, is composed of 100% cereal. This diet is based on the teachings of the movement's founder, George Ohsawa (1893–1966), who combined Zen Buddhism and Chinese philosophies to create the macrobiotic movement.[9]

In the 1960s, macrobiotics became very popular. Because of problems resulting from the restrictive nature of macrobiotics when practiced at the extreme levels, the American Medical Association strongly opposed this diet:

… when a diet has been shown to cause irreversible damage to health and ultimately lead to death, it should be roundly condemned as a threat to human health.[10]

The followers of macrobiotics have revised and improved the diet since its inception. They have also dropped the term "Zen" from the name of this regimen. Depending on how it is followed, macrobiotics may or may not be a vegetarian diet.

Dwyer[11] investigated individuals following various forms of vegetarianism, and these individuals were referred to as "new" vegetarians. Also, the term "alternate life-style diet" describing vegetarianism surfaced in the literature around the same time. Additionally, the terms "semi-vegetarian" or "near vegetarian" (usually meaning one who ingests fish and fowl but no red meat but can also refer to infrequent meat intake) and "pesco-vegetarian" (ingests fish but no chicken or red meat) emerged. All these terms refer to type or quantity and frequency of flesh foods consumed. Perhaps a better descriptor for several of these regimens would have been "low-meat diet" or "restrictive meat diet" and not vegetarian.

Vegetarianism appears to be on a continuum of a diet consisting solely of plant foods to a diet restricting certain kinds of flesh foods or limiting the frequency of flesh foods. Unfortunately, it is not a singly defined diet. However, when perplexed as to what is and what is not a vegetarian, Dr. Harvey Kellogg's definition can be used: when patrons of the Battle Creek Sanitarium put the question, he would reply something to the effect that if what you want to eat can get away from you, don't eat it — that's a vegetarian.[12]

IV. NUTRITIONAL STATUS OF VEGETARIANS

A survey conducted in 1992 demonstrated that nearly 7% of the American public (approximately 12.4 million people) regarded themselves as vegetarians. Prevalence of this dietary was previously reported as almost 4% of the American population.[13] As the numbers of vegetarians continue to increase, reasons for adopting this meatless diet include: focus on health, budgetary constraints, religious affiliation, ecological concerns, and other moral and ethical issues revolving around treatment of nonhuman animals. Whatever the motive for embracing and adhering to a vegetarian diet, certainly, the most critical topic which needs to be addressed is whether an individual following this regimen can maintain adequate growth and ultimate health. The American Dietetic Association,[7,14,15] the American Academy of Pediatrics Committee on Nutrition,[16] and the National Academy of Sciences Committee on Nutritional Misinformation[17] all acknowledged that a vegetarian diet can adequately meet nutritional needs.

Recent research indicated that supplemental to health benefits (to be addressed later in this chapter) vegetarians also exhibit a lower mortality rate than the general population due to a lower death rate from ischemic heart disease and certain cancers. Additionally, "substantial public health and environmental benefits would likely result from a more widespread adoption of vegetarianism."[18]

In one of the earliest investigations involving one of the most restrictive vegetarian dietaries, Jaffa[19] followed a California fruitarian family for approximately 2 years (2 females, 30 and 33 years; and 3 children, 6, 9, and 13 years). He reported that all appeared to be in good health aside from the children being below average in height and weight. A fruitarian diet was maintained by this family for a period of 5–7 years. This study demonstrated that it was possible to exist on the most restricted plant-based diet.

The research that has been conducted on the less restrictive lacto-ovo form of vegetarianism[20-24] and on the more restrictive vegans[25-29] indicated that vegetarians presented with normal blood findings, lower body weights, and lower skinfold measurements. Energy intake was reported as adequate to low. Macronutrient intake was usually sufficient, and the protein content of vegetarian diets was successful in meeting nutritional needs. The scientific literature showed that inadequate protein intake was not a concern in this type of diet.

Vitamin intake was usually adequate in vegetarians. However, the B vitamins and in particular vitamin B_{12} have been reported as being low.[20] Vitamin B_{12} generally causes concern among vegetarians as the information that is popular in the press indicates that vitamin B_{12} can only be derived from animal sources. Immerman[30] disagrees with this popular notion and reported that this vitamin might be found in root vegetables or in the soil of poorly washed root vegetables, mung beans and mung bean sprouts, comfrey leaves, peas and whole wheat, ground nuts, lettuce, alfalfa, some batches of turnip greens, and fermented soybean products. Immerman stated that although a vegetarian diet is generally thought to be low in vitamin B_{12} intake, a review of the literature indicated that most studies that have found vitamin B_{12} deficiency have been unconvincing. He further stated that vegans that have been evaluated usually have had a normal vitamin B_{12} status. In studies where deficiency was discovered, the vegetarians also presented with other complications such as tropical sprue, hookworms, partial gastrectomy — conditions which would affect vitamin B_{12} status. Therefore, it was concluded that vitamin B_{12} intake should not be a problem among the majority of healthy, adult vegetarians.

The area of mineral intake should, however, present concern among vegetarians. The literature reveals those minerals that are generally indicated as being low are calcium, iron, phosphorus, and zinc.[31,32] Because vegetarians were so consistently low in certain mineral intake, complementing a meatless diet with a mineral supplement might be a consideration to ensure adequate mineral intake.

In the area of disease, a vegetarian lifestyle is associated with risk reduction for a number of chronic, degenerative diseases such as obesity, coronary artery disease, hypertension, diabetes, certain cancers,[7] and possibly osteoporosis, kidney stones, and diverticular disease.[33] Other researchers[34-41] have demonstrated lower rates of cancer, hypertension, and coronary heart disease among the vegetarian population. Serum cholesterol levels were repeatedly reported as being low in vegetarians as compared to controls.[42-47]

In summary, research did support those adult individuals who were practicing a meatless dietary regimen. The potential problem areas most frequently reported were low energy intake along with low levels of certain minerals and vitamins. Mineral intake represented the most serious potential hindrance for following vegetarian diets. The low weights and low skinfolds described in vegetarians are not a major concern as this would tend to be a more desirable state of health than obesity. Low blood pressures and low levels of serum cholesterol were reported, and again, this would generally be considered a desirable state of health. Low incidence of certain diseases would be advantageous as well. Research on the various forms of vegetarianism generally indicated that these individuals were healthy and vegetarianism may be beneficial in certain health states where lower weight, blood cholesterol, and blood pressure levels are sought.

A recent review by Dwyer[48] concluded that vegetarianism is an option that certain individuals freely choose and that the health consequences of this diet are neutral and may even be positive. She further stated that nutrition professionals have an obligation to take vegetarians seriously.

V. THE VEGETARIAN ATHLETE

Heavy meat eating for enhanced performance became a training diet with ancient Greek athletes. Consider the following:

> Ever since the ancient Greek Olympic hero Milo of Croton won fame on a reputed training diet of twenty pounds of meat and eighteen pints of wine a day (as well as twenty pounds of bread), it had been popularly assumed that athletes required flesh for victory.[49]

The early history of diet and performance is summarized by Whorton.[50] The standard diet for collegiate teams in the late 1800s consisted of two kinds of meat served at all three meals. Also, most training guides recommended that beef be served rare. This resulted in meat being so rare that at some training tables it was referred to as "red rags." These primitive thoughts regarding training diets appear at times to continue to permeate certain sports even today.

Still, early vegetarian athletes followed a stricter dietary and training regimen than did their meat-eating contemporaries in spite of jokes being made about them. Also at this time alcoholic beverages were considered ergogenic aids and their consumption around competition was considered appropriate behavior. In the 1908 Olympics, for example, some marathoners drank cognac to enhance performance while a walker in a 100-km race in Germany in the same year reportedly consumed 22 glasses of beer and a half bottle of wine.[51] Again, vegetarian athletes exhibited a different standard of practice, and because they were exposed to the health practices of the day and reportedly did not imbibe, their performance most likely was exemplary.

Fisher[52] conducted experiments that were designed to investigate the effects of thorough mastication of food upon endurance while allowing his subjects, nine male Yale University students, choice in their diets during the length of the experiment. All types of food were available, and the subjects were encouraged to eat meat. Some of the subjects gravitated toward a meatless diet. In one of the seven endurance tests, Fisher noted that a vegetarian was able to perform 1000 deep knee bends, whereas none consuming meat were able to meet or exceed that record.

In 1934 Wishart[53] reported the results of a dietary study on a 48-year-old male vegetarian Olympic cyclist who was tested on a bicycle ergometer. Four experimental meatless diets with different levels of protein were used in this study; however, none represented a typical mixed diet. The subject was reported to have excelled on a high protein intake provided mainly by eggs and milk. This high protein diet was not initially a part of the experiment but was a diet of the subject's choice.

Not many studies have surfaced since 1934. Meyer et al.[54] investigated the effect of a predominantly fruit diet on the athletic performance of nine university and high school students (six males and three females, 17–24 years old). The subjects exercised for 1 h daily in addition to running at least 20 km/d. The training program lasted for 1 year prior to the experiment. The subjects were then asked to run 8 km as fast as possible, their times were recorded, and different diets then followed. After 14 days on a predominantly fruit diet, the best times were recorded and compared for all subjects; however, the results were not statistically significant.

Hanne, Dlin, and Rostein[55] investigated physical fitness and anthropometric and metabolic parameters in 29 male vegetarian athletes and 29 controls (17–60 years). These athletes trained from 5–8 h/wk and participated in a variety of activities. No significant difference in heart rate, blood pressure, aerobic capacity, predicted VO_2max or in anaerobic capacity was found between vegetarians and age-matched nonvegetarian controls.

Few modern studies have compared athletic ability of vegetarian vs. meat-eating subjects. Nieman[56] stated that the fact that vegetarianism is not a single-defined diet, coupled with the impact that training and lifestyle may have on the individual, makes definition of specific influences of the diet on performance unclear. Although this is apparently true, many individuals who exercise regularly are adopting heart healthy diets and, in particular, meatless diets because of the apparent health benefits. Therefore, the next topic emerges: how should one eat when following a vegetarian diet?

VI. HOW TO EAT A HEALTHY MEATLESS DIET

Before proceeding to recommendations regarding existing vegetarian diets or for those desiring to change their diets to that of a vegetarian, three areas with respect to impressions of vegetarians and the dietary regimens that they follow will be briefly discussed:

1. How do vegetarians fare regarding nutrition knowledge?
2. Are vegetarians at increased risk for disordered eating?
3. Are vegetarians accepted and supported by professionals in the field of nutrition?

Three studies will be mentioned that address these topics.

Freeland-Graves et al.[57] conducted a study in which 106 vegetarians and 106 nonvegetarians, who were matched for age, gender, residence, and nutrition training, were tested in relation to general principles of nutrition and concepts related to vegetarianism. The results indicated that the vegetarians scored significantly higher in the total test as well as the general and vegetarian nutrition subtests than did the nonvegetarians.

Janelle and Barr[58] compared nutrient intake between vegetarian (n = 23) and nonvegetarian women (n = 22) who observed similar health practices. The subjects also completed a questionnaire which assessed relationships with eating behaviors. The results of this research indicated that the diets of all women adhered closely to current nutrient recommendations.

Also, vegetarians exhibited lower restraint scores on the questionnaire which suggested that they were not at increased risk for disordered eating.

In another study conducted by Strobl and Groll,[59] a questionnaire was mailed to a random sample of 312 members chosen from the current membership list of the California Dietetic Association. The goal of the questionnaire was to assess present knowledge of vegetarianism, to reveal prevailing attitudes toward vegetarians, and to identify present counseling practices with vegetarians. It was found that knowledge was below the predicted mean score and attitudes were slightly above neutral in support of vegetarianism. Although respondents recognized that there were economic and health benefits to vegetarianism, they did not support the client's choice to eliminate meat from their diet.

While the studies by Freeland-Graves et al.[57] and Strobl and Groll[59] were conducted in the early 1980s, they are significant in that these data showed that individuals following vegetarian diets were generally nutritionally aware, however, they were unsupported by professionals in the nutrition community. Additionally, the more recent work of Janelle and Barr[58] demonstrated that vegetarians are also not at risk for disordered eating.

The American Dietetic Association has since responded to the needs of the vegetarian population by formation of the Vegetarian Nutrition Practice Group within its organization[60] and publication of a daily food guide for vegetarians.[61] However, having been given a brief history of vegetarianism, is it not time for recognition that this is not a fad diet? Additionally, is it not time for acknowledgment that the majority of those who choose to follow various patterns of meatless dietary regimens are healthy individuals cognizant of healthy eating patterns? With this in mind, the following are guidelines to eating a healthy meatless diet.

For the transition to a vegetarian diet simply continuing the same eating pattern except for eliminating meat and/or increasing consumption of high-fat dairy products in place of meat would seem to be misguided and an unhealthy approach to change. If an individual is going to make lifestyle changes in their diet, it would seem that improving their present diet to a healthier eating pattern would be a first step. Once this is accomplished, alterations to an existing healthy diet can usually occur without comprising nutritional status. The manner in which an individual makes the movement to vegetarianism is very individual; some stop eating red meat, then fowl, and finally fish and seafood. Others proceed less gradually and exclude flesh foods all at once. However one chooses to change over to a meatless diet, the process of change should include guidelines for healthy eating based on current recommendations from reputable sources. Therefore, three sets of guidelines are recommended; they are as follows: (1) Dietary Guidelines for Americans[62] (general dietary recommendations), (2) Food Guide Pyramid[63] (general daily food guide), and (3) Eating Well — The Vegetarian Way[61] (specific daily food guide for vegetarians).

A comparison between the Food Guide Pyramid and daily food guide for vegetarians will be presented. Both sets of recommendations are similar, and Table 1 contrasts and compares them for healthy adults.

In making the transition to a vegetarian diet follow the Food Guide Pyramid and eat a healthy, regular, mixed diet. Once a healthy eating pattern is established, one can then make changes to a meatless regimen following the food guide for vegetarians, eating at least the minimum number of servings.

As outlined above, the food guide for vegetarians was developed by the American Dietetic Association and represents a preferred diet-planning tool. There are, however, other food guides and pyramids[64] that have been devised for vegetarian diets and the Vegetarian Food Pyramid available through The Health Connection (Figure 1) is also a helpful guide to follow. Serving sizes in the Vegetarian Food Pyramid are similar to the two previously mentioned guides.

Table 2 lists three selected days from an economical 4-week lacto-ovo vegetarian meal plan that was developed by the Vegetarian Resource Group.[65] These menus were designed

TABLE 1   Comparison of Food Guide Pyramid[63] to Food Guide for Vegetarians[61]

Food Guide Pyramid	Food Guide for Vegetarians
6–11 servings bread, cereal, rice, pasta	6 or more servings
3–5 servings vegetable group	4 or more servings
2–4 servings fruit group	3 or more servings
2–3 servings milk, yogurt, and cheese	up to 3 servings, optional
2–3 servings meat, poultry, fish, dry beans, eggs and nuts	2–3 servings legumes and meat substitutes

Note: Both guides recommend limited calories from fats and sweets. Serving sizes are the same for both guides except for the meat/legume group, and I serving counts as the following:

Grain Group	I slice bread (30 g), 1/2 cup cooked rice, pasta, cereal (100 g), or 1 oz dry cereal
Vegetable Group	1/2 cup cooked (50 g) or 1 cup raw (50 g)
Fruit Group	1 piece fruit (100 g), 3/4 cup juice (180 g), or 1/2 cup canned fruit (125 g)
Milk Group	1 cup nonfat or low-fat milk (245 g), 1 cup nonfat or low-fat yogurt (225 g), 1-1/2 oz natural cheese (45 gm), or 2 oz process cheese
Meat/legume Group	
Pyramid	2-1/2 to 3 oz cooked lean meat, poultry or fish, and 1/2 cup cooked beans (100 g), 1 egg or 2 tbsp (30 g) peanut butter counts as 1 oz lean meat (1-1/2 cup cooked beans count as 3 oz meat or 1 serving)
Vegetarian	1/2 cup cooked beans (100 g), 1/2 cup tofu (100 g), 8 oz soy milk, 2 tbsp nuts or seeds (eggs are optional — 1 egg or 2 egg whites equal 1 serving, 3–4 limit of yolks per week)

as follows: week 1 uses ordinary foods that can be prepared quickly and easily; week 2 introduces common recipes; week 3 uses new foods requiring longer preparation; and week 4 eliminates animal products.

In addition to the suggestions in Table 2, other nutrition information pertaining to vegetarian diets should be mentioned. There are two basic nutrition concepts which are necessary to emphasize at this point. They apply equally to healthy eating in general and vegetarianism in particular:

1. Caloric (energy) intake must be adequate to meet activity requirements.
2. Eat a wide variety of foods.[15]

Based on the findings in the scientific literature, the vegetarian needs to be aware of the importance of adequate caloric intake. On a vegetarian diet, where meat intake is eliminated, a decrease in fat kilocalories generally occurs. Therefore, meeting energy needs can be problematic. Most adults require between almost 2000 and 3000 kcal/d (8360 and 12,540 kJ) with women needing around 2000 (8360) and men requiring closer to 3000 (12,540).[66] Again, the vegetarian must be mindful of adequate caloric intake, and foods consumed should constitute a wide variety of nutrients. If vegetarians follow these two recommendations, then the possibility of nutrient deficiencies decreases.

Perhaps most concern on meatless regimens centers around adequate protein intake and the notion that proteins need to be complemented at every meal. Research has shown that

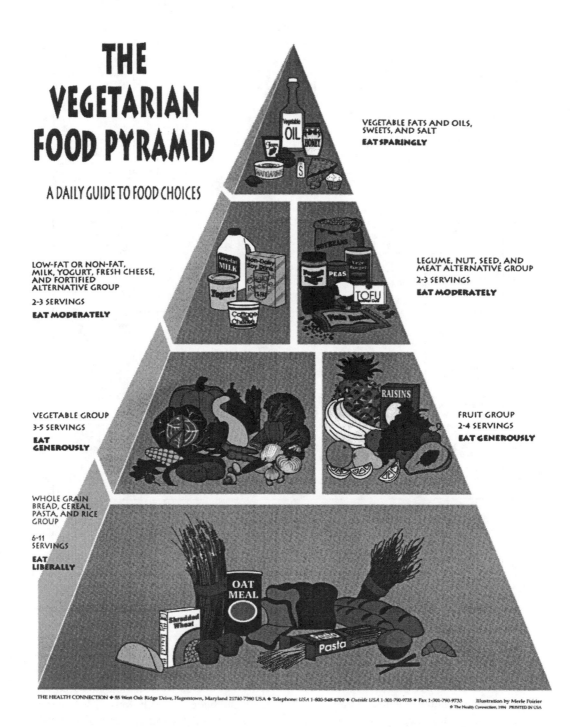

Figure 1 The vegetarian food pyramid. (From The General Conference Nutrition Council, Stoy Proctor, chair, and Merle Poirier, designer, copyright The Health Connection, 1-800-548-8700 or 301-790-9735. With permission.)

Left margin (top to bottom): Limit foods high in fat, cholesterol, sugar, and salt. — Select relative portions to meet your caloric need. — Choose from a variety of whole grains, fruits, and vegetables.

Food Groups	One Serving Equals One Item	Nutrient Contributions	Calories			Food Choice Examples
			1600 (Many Women and Older Adults)	2200 (Children, Teen Girls, Active Women, and Most Men)	2800 (Teen Boys and Active Men)	
Eat Liberally 6-11 Servings daily **Whole Grain Group**	1 slice bread (30 gm) ½ cup hot cereal (100 gm) 1 cup dry cereal (30 gm) ¼ cup granola (30 gm) ½ cup rice or pasta (100 gm) 1 tortilla (30 gm) 1 chapati (30 gm) ½ bagel or English Muffin (30 gm) 3-4 crackers (30 gm) ½ muffin (30 gm) ½ cup cooked beans (100 gm)	Complex CHO Fiber Protein Vitamin B_1 (Thiamine) Vitamin B_2 (Riboflavin) Vitamin B_6 and Niacin Iron Magnesium Calcium Trace minerals	6	9	11	Grains: oats, brown rice, barley, millet, bulgar wheat, rye, corn, whole wheat, multi-grain, etc.
Eat Generously 3-5 Servings daily **Vegetable Group**	1 cup raw, leafy vegetable salad (50 gm) ½ cup chopped raw vegetables (50 gm) ½ cup cooked vegetables (80 gm) ¾ cup vegetable juice (180 gm)	Fiber Potassium Beta-Carotene Folate Vitamin C Calcium Magnesium	3	4	5	Vegetables: broccoli, kale, cabbage, collards, spinach, pumpkin, carrots, winter squash, sweet potatoes, potatoes, parsnips, rutabagas, turnips, tomatoes, beets, eggplant, okra, summer squash, cauliflower
Eat Generously 2-4 Servings daily **Fruit Group**	1 medium, whole fruit (100 gm) ½ cup canned fruit (125 gm) ¼ cup dried fruit (100 gm) 1 cup berries (100 gm) ¾ cup fruit juice (180 gm)	Vitamin C Beta-Carotene Fiber Potassium Folate Magnesium	2	3	4	Fruits: oranges, grapefruit, lemons, apricots, peaches, nectarines, plums, persimmons, apples, pears, kiwi, papaya, mango, pineapple, bananas, strawberries, raspberries, blueberries Dried Fruits: raisins, dates, pears, pineapple, prunes, peaches, figs
Eat Moderately 2-3 Servings daily **Legume, Nut, Seed, and Meat Alternative Group**	½ cup cooked beans or peas (100 gm) ½ cup tofu (100 gm) ¼ cup seeds (30 gm) ¼ cup (1 oz.) nuts (30 gm) 2 Tbs (1 oz.) nut butter (30 gm) ¼ cup meat alternative (30 gm) 2 egg whites (50 gm)	Protein Zinc Iron Fiber Calcium Vitamin B_6 Vitamin E Niacin (B_3) Linoelic Acid	2	2-3	3	Legumes: pinto, black, white, navy, soybeans, garbanzoes, lentils, blackeye, green pea, split pea, peanuts Nuts: almonds, walnuts, filberts, chestnuts, brazil, pecans, cashews Seed: pine nuts, sesame, sunflower, pumpkin Alternatives: tofu, meat alternatives
Eat Moderately 2-3 Servings daily **Low-Fat Dairy Group**	1 cup milk, nonfat or lowfat (245 gm) 1 cup soymilk (fortified) (245 gm) ½ cup lowfat cottage cheese (100 gm) ½ cup soy cheese (100 gm) 1 ½ oz. fresh cheese (45 gm) 1 cup low-fat or non-fat yogurt (225 gm) 1 Tbs (½ oz.) cream cheese (15 gm)	Calcium Protein Vitamins A and D Riboflavin (B_2) Vitamin B_{12}	2	2-3	3	Dairy: milk, yogurt, cottage cheese, ricotta, other fresh cheeses Fortified Alternatives: soy or tofu milk, soy cheese

Eat Sparingly — Vegetable Fats and Oils, Sweets, and Salt

The small tip of the Pyramid shows vegetable fats and oils, salt, and sweets. These foods such as salad dressings and vegetable oils, cream, butter, margarine, sour cream, cream cheese, sugars, soft drinks, candies, and sweet desserts provide calories and are low in nutrients. Vegetable oils contain essential fatty acids, but use these sparingly because they are high in calories. For every tablespoon of fat added to a 2200 calorie diet, you increase the percentage of calories as fat by approximately five percent. Every tablespoon of sugar adds two percent calories as sugar.

- Use visible fats sparingly.
- Limit desserts to two or three per week.
- Use honey, jams, jelly, corn syrups, molasses, sugar sparingly
- Use soft drinks and candies very sparingly, if at all.
- Limit foods high in salt.

1 Tbs margarine	= 11.4 gm fat	102 calories	0 mg, cholesterol
1 Tbs butter	= 12.0 gm fat	108 calories	33 mg, cholesterol
1 Tbs mayonnaise	= 11.0 gm fat	99 calories	4 mg, cholesterol
1 Tbs sour cream	= 3.0 gm fat	30 calories	5 mg, cholesterol
1 Tbs cream cheese	= 5.0 gm fat	52 calories	15 mg, cholesterol
1 Tbs cream	= 15.0 gm fat	52 calories	21 mg, cholesterol

1 tsp salt (5 gm table salt) = 2000 mg sodium
1 Tbs oil = 13.6 gm fat 120.0 calories
1 tsp oil = 4.5 gm fat 40.1 calories

1 Tbs sugar = 12 gm 48 calories
1 tsp sugar = 4 gm 16 calories
1 Tbs honey = 21 gm 64 calories

FIGURE 1 *Continued.*

vegetarian diets are adequate in protein intake and it is no longer necessary to complement proteins at the same meal.[15] As long as a wide variety of foods is consumed, all essential amino acids should be provided in the diet. As a matter of course, most individuals complement proteins without paying attention to them, i.e., peanut butter and jelly sandwiches, bean-based soups with a slice of bread, combining beans and rice, or eating a bean burrito. Still, the vegetarian should be aware of good sources of plant protein, and they include: grains, legumes (beans, lentils, peas, and peanuts), nuts, seeds, low-fat dairy products, and foods such as tofu.

The intake of mineral elements should be of concern to vegetarians, especially calcium, iron, and zinc. Good sources of calcium are broccoli, greens (kale, collard, mustard, and turnip), low-fat dairy products, and fortified soy milk. Sources of iron include dried fruit,

TABLE 2   Menu Suggestions for Transition to a Vegetarian Diet

Day 1 (Week 1)

Breakfast	Sliced cheese, toast, orange juice
Lunch	Peanut butter and jelly on whole wheat bread, celery/carrot sticks, apple
Dinner	Spaghetti with mushrooms or other vegetable, parmesan cheese, spinach, fruit salad
Snack	Popcorn

Day 2 (Week 2)

Breakfast	Oatmeal, raisins, milk
Lunch	Broiled cheese toast, potato salad, tomato slices, watermelon
Dinner	Pasta with frozen vegetables, green salad, garlic bread
Snack	Ice cream

Day 3 (Week 4)

Breakfast	Potato pancakes, applesauce
Lunch	Pasta salad, pita bread, vegetable juice, watermelon
Dinner	Baked beans, Spanish rice, carrots, fresh pear
Snack	Nut/seed/raisin mix

Note: A heart-healthy suggestion is to use low-fat or nonfat dairy products.

From Vegetarian J., IV, 3, 1985. With permission.

prune juice, spinach, and dried beans. Including a good source of vitamin C such as orange or tomato juice, citrus fruit, or broccoli at meal time will enhance iron absorption. Sources of zinc include peas, lentils, and wheat germ.

Vitamin B_{12} intake will be adequate if low-fat dairy products and/or eggs are included in a vegetarian diet. However, if one follows the vegan regimen, then fortified foods such as breakfast cereals or soy milk should be consumed. Also, on the vegan regimen, attention should be paid to riboflavin and vitamin D. Vegetarian sources of riboflavin include broccoli, asparagus, and almonds. Where exposure to sunlight is adequate, vitamin D status should be adequate as well.[32]

To make vegetarian meal planning healthful and nutritionally sound it is important to take in adequate calories and eat a wide variety of foods. Also, limiting the amount of sweets and fatty foods will help enhance the quality of the diet. To make the transition to vegetarianism, follow the guidelines and recommendations as mentioned to insure a healthy diet. However, when activity level increases, what modifications to a vegetarian diet should an athlete make?

VII.   DIETARY CONSIDERATIONS FOR THE VEGETARIAN ATHLETE

Since vegetarian diets are usually higher in carbohydrate intake, many endurance athletes choose to follow this dietary regimen. It is well known that when glycogen stores are depleted, activity stops and that the higher carbohydrate intake of a vegetarian diet enhances glycogen stores. Endurance athletes such as runners, bicyclists, and distance swimmers who train at a high level for approximately an hour or more a day might find that a vegetarian regimen is of greater benefit to them rather than a regular, mixed diet.[67]

Few recent investigations relating vegetarian diet to performance have been published, and prevalence of vegetarianism among athletes has not been well researched.[68] One recent study investigated sedentary vegetarian and nonvegetarian males who were placed on an aerobic conditioning program. Prior to and after 6 weeks of exercising, there was no significant difference in aerobic power between both groups of subjects.[8] In another study, male endurance athletes were placed on a lacto-ovo vegetarian diet for 6 weeks and then on a mixed, meat-rich diet for 6 weeks. No significant changes in performance were reported at the end of the study.[69] These data suggest that there is no effect of a vegetarian diet on performance.

There is a question as to whether or not the recommendations for the vegetarian athlete should be similar to those of the meat-eating athlete. One of the issues in meatless diets is the known low caloric intake of vegetarians. Low energy increases the possibility of nutrient deficiencies. It was previously mentioned that the energy requirement for adult women is about 2000 kcal (8360 kJ)/d and for adult men closer to 3000 kcal (12,540 kJ)/d. Age, body size, and activity level will all affect the actual number of kilocalories needed in a day. An athlete will most certainly require more energy, and the vegetarian athlete needs to account for the additional amount. Active individuals usually consume between 2000 (8360 kJ) to 5000 kcal (20,900 kJ)/d. To estimate energy intake for individuals who participate in low to moderate exercise activities, use Table 3, based on the 1989 Recommended Dietary Allowances (RDA).[66] If the activity level increases, then the calculations for additional energy expenditure can be found elsewhere.[70]

TABLE 3   How to Estimate Daily Energy Intake for Light to Moderate Activity

Age Category by Gender	kcal/kg
Males	
11–14	55
15–18	45
19–24	40
25–50	37
51+	30
Females	
11–14	47
15–18	40
19–24	38
25–50	36
51+	30

Note: (1) Calculation: First determine your weight in kg. Then find your age category by gender and estimated kcal equivalent. Multiply this number times your weight to determine approximate daily energy intake. (2) Example: A 110 lb (50 kg) female who is 22 would divide 110 by 2.2 and multiply 50 kg × 38 kcal/kg = 1900 kcal/d for moderate level of activity. Higher levels need additional kcals. (3) To convert to joules: 1 kcal = 4.18 kJ.

From *Recommended Dietary Allowance,* 10th ed., National Academy Press, Washington, D.C., 1989.

TABLE 4   Example of a 1-d, 2400 kcal (10,032 kJ) Meal Plan for a Lacto Vegetarian

Food	Serving Size	Calories
Breakfast		
Grapefruit juice	1 cup	94
Whole wheat bread	1 slice	67
Peanut butter	2 tbsp	l88
Skim milk	1 cup	86
Snack		
Tangerines	2 medium	74
Lunch		
Split pea soup	1 cup	190
Pita bread	1	203
Low-fat cottage cheese	1/2 cup	82
Grated carrots	1 cup	47
Canned cherries	1/2 cup	39
Banana	1 medium	105
Orange juice	1/2 cup	56
Snack		
Dried apricots	7 halves	58
Dried dates	2-1/2	57
Dinner		
Cheese pizza	1/4 of 10 in.	280
Tossed green salad	1 cup	36
Italian dressing	2 tbsp	137
Sourdough bread	2 slices	203
Margarine	2 tsp	68
Apple	1 medium	81
Snack		
Plain low-fat yogurt	1 cup	144
Strawberries	1/4 cup	11
Granola	1/4 cup	149
Totals		2455

Note: Breakdown of the above 2455 kcals (10,261 kJ): 62% carbohydrate; 25% fat; 15% protein. To convert to joules: 1 kcal = 4.18 kJ.

From *Sports Nutrition, A Guide for the Professional Working with Active People,* 2nd ed., p. 199.

Consuming adequate calories to support activity can be challenging to the vegetarian athlete, and the Sports and Cardiovascular Nutritionists (SCAN), a practice group of the American Dietetic Association, offers a meal plan based on 2400 kcal (10,032 kJ)/d (Table 4).[71] This meal plan can easily be expanded to include more calories by increasing portion sizes or by adding fruit juices and low-fat dairy products to this diet. If eggs are included, it is recommended that no more than three to four yolks be consumed on a weekly basis.

Because of the need for increased energy in the diet, vegetarian individuals tend to develop an eating pattern called "grazing" in which they consume small quantities of food at frequent intervals throughout the day in order to consume enough calories. Some practical suggestions which might help "grazers" increase calories follows:

1. Instead of three meals per day, try eating five or six smaller meals.
2. Increase the number of snacks.
3. Eat higher energy foods.

To meet the need for increasing caloric intake, Clark[72] offers vegetarian athletes suggestions such as eating two peanut butter sandwiches at lunch time. She also includes many meatless recipes in her book, which are fast to prepare as well as nutritious to consume.

In addition to the need for adequate caloric intake, are there other issues that vegetarian athletes need to be cognizant of? A few considerations the vegetarian athletes should address follows:

1. Mineral intake
2. Protein intake
3. Athletic amenorrhea

In the area of mineral intake, iron and zinc are the two nutrients most often deficient in the diets of all athletes. Kleiner[73] recommends including vitamin C sources with meals to enhance iron absorption. She also advises athletes to avoid constituents that block iron and zinc absorption. A few examples of absorption blockers include: coffee and tea (regular and decaffeinated), whole grains, bran, dried beans and peas, and spinach, as well as a high-fiber intake. Again, to enhance absorption of these foods include a rich source of vitamin C at meal time.

Vegetarian athletes must also pay close attention to their protein intake as they utilize more protein to produce energy during the activity. It has also been suggested that strength athletes would benefit from a slightly higher intake of protein above the RDA. However, the research is conflicting as to recommendations for protein intake for athletes. In general, Americans tend to exceed the recommendations of the RDA of 0.8–1.0 g of protein per kilogram body weight, while vegetarians more closely approximate this requirement. Consequently, where very strenuous training occurs, a vegetarian athlete might consider an increased protein intake.

Lastly, amenorrhea in female vegetarians will be addressed. Messina and Messina[64] give current information on this topic and state that the data on vegetarian diet and menstrual cycle patterns in athletes are conflicting. It is further stated that the etiology on amenorrhea among athletes includes many variables with diet being only one factor that may increase risk for this condition. The female vegetarian athlete may be advised to include higher levels of fat and high levels of calcium in her diet. Guidelines for this are: increasing milk products and calcium-fortified soymilk as well as increasing consumption of grains, dried beans and peas, green leafy vegetables, vegetables in general, fruit, and nuts and seeds. Again, the athlete might pay attention to the amount of fat in her diet.

In addition to the above, the vegetarian athlete can also follow several simpler practices to monitor the conditioning response. Weight can be monitored, and there should not be great fluctuations in weight gain and loss over the longer term. As adequate hydration needs are important, weight can be taken before and after a workout. More detailed information on the important topic of hydration is given elsewhere in this volume. In addition to paying attention to weight, another area that can be monitored is the level of fatigue during a workout. Fatigue is a good indicator of glycogen stores, and undue tiredness usually indicates that glycogen levels are low. Lastly, performance should also be monitored and, particularly if no improvements are seen or there are decrements, steps can be taken to ensure that the vegetarian athlete's daily dietary intake is adequate and balanced. By following these simple practices and observing the body's response to exercise, the vegetarian athlete is better able to determine if any dietary modifications should be made, which in turn should allow the athlete to become a better competitor either at the recreational or more elite levels.

VIII. SUMMARY

In summary, general recommendations for the vegetarian athlete present a challenge because:

1. There are various types of vegetarians.
2. There are other forms of flesh-restricted diets that are labelled vegetarian.
3. Few research studies have been conducted on the vegetarian athlete, especially recently.

Therefore, the general recommendations for the vegetarian athlete include those of the meat-eating athlete. However, where an individual is a classical vegetarian, then it is recommended that they follow the daily food guide given for nonexercising vegetarians. Another option is the Vegetarian Food Pyramid. In addition to these guidelines, vegetarian athletes were given an example of a 2400 kcal (10,032 kJ) diet. This meal plan could easily be expanded to accommodate additional calories in the diet. However, the vegetarian athlete must pay close attention to the importance of adequate caloric intake to support the additional energy expenditure of increased exercise. The vegetarian athlete must be aware of the need for adequate intake of the mineral elements in general and calcium, iron, and zinc, in particular. Iron and zinc represent the greatest risk of inadequate intake for athletes in general. Consequently, a mineral supplement may be considered for the vegetarian in general and vegetarian athletes in particular. When planned correctly, following the suggestions given, the diet of the vegetarian athlete should be nutritionally adequate.

In closing, the meatless dietary regimen known as vegetarianism is a choice. The real issue regarding an alternate lifestyle diet is not, should one eat meat or not eat meat. Indeed, the most important issue is adequate caloric intake to support the level of activity of an athlete while maintaining a balanced diet (with or without meat).

REFERENCES

1. Majumder, S. K., Vegetarianism: fad, faith, or fact?, *Am. Sc.*, 60, 175, 1972.
2. Dombrowski, D. A., *The Philosophy of Vegetarianism*, The University of Massachusetts Press, Amherst, 1984, 35.
3. Ireland, C., Vegetarian timeline, *Vegetarian Times*, February, 56, 1992.
4. Giehl, D., *Vegetarianism, A Way of Life*, Harper and Row, Publishers, New York, 1979, 208.
5. Roe, D. A., History of promotion of vegetable cereal diets, *J. Nutr.*, 116, 1355, 1986.
6. Hardinge, M. G. and Crooks, H., Non-flesh dietaries, I. Historical background, *J. Am. Diet. Assoc.*, 43, 545, 1963.
7. American Dietetic Association, A.D.A. reports, position of the American Dietetic Association: Vegetarian diets — technical support paper, *J. Am. Diet. Assoc.*, 88, 351, 1988.
8. Ratzin, R. A., Effect of aerobic conditioning on resting serum testosterone levels and muscle fiber types in vegetarian and nonvegetarian sedentary males. Doctoral dissertation, University of Northern Colorado, Greeley, CO, 1990.
9. Erhard, D., The new vegetarians, Part two — The Zen macrobiotic movement and other cults based on vegetarianism, *Nutr. Today*, 20, 1974.
10. American Medical Association, Council on Foods and Nutrition, Zen macrobiotic diet, *J. Am. Med. Assoc.*, 218, 397, 1971.
11. Dwyer, J. T., Mayer, L. D. V. H., Kandel, R. F., and Mayer, J., The new vegetarians, Who are they?, *J. Am. Diet. Assoc.*, 62, 503, 1973.
12. Sussman, V. S., *The Vegetarian Alternative*, Rodale Press, Emmaus, PA, 1978, 10.

13. Havala, S., Vegetarian diets — clearing the air, *West. J. Med.*, 160, 483, 1994.
14. American Dietetic Association, Position paper on the vegetarian approach to eating, *J. Am. Diet. Assoc.*, 77, 61, 1980.
15. American Dietetic Association, Position of The American Dietetic Association: vegetarian diets, *J. Am. Diet. Assoc.*, 93, 1317, 1993.
16. American Academy of Pediatrics, Committee on Nutrition, Nutritional aspects of vegetarianism, health foods and fad diets, *Pediatrics*, 59, 460, 1977.
17. National Academy of Sciences, Committee on Nutritional Misinformation, *Vegetarian diets, A statement of the Food and Nutrition Board, Division of Biological Sciences, Assembly of Life Sciences, National Research Council*, U.S. Government Printing Office, Washington, D.C., May, 1974.
18. White, R. and Frank E., Health effects and prevalence of vegetarianism, *West. J. Med.*, 160, 465, 1994.
19. Jaffa, M. E., Nutrition investigations among fruitarians and Chinese, *USDA Agric. Bull.*, 107, 1901.
20. Hardinge, M. and Stare, F. J., Nutritional studies of vegetarians, 1. Nutritional, physical, and laboratory studies, *J. Clin. Nutr.*, 2, 73, 1954.
21. Harland, B. F. and Peterson, M., Nutritional studies of lacto-ovo vegetarian Trappist monks, *J. Am. Diet. Assoc.*, 72, 259, 1978.
22. Simons, L. A., Gibson, C., Paino, C., Hosking, M., Bullock, J., and Trim, J., The influence of a wide range of absorbed cholesterol on plasma cholesterol levels in man, *Am. J. Clin. Nutr.*, 31, 1334, 1978.
23. Armstrong, B., Clarke, H., Martin, C., Ward, W., Norman, N., and Masarei, J., Urinary sodium and blood pressure in vegetarians, *Am. J. Clin. Nutr.*, 32, 2472, 1979.
24. Taber, L. A. L. and Cook, R. A., Dietary and anthropometric assessment of adult omnivores, fish-eaters, and lacto-ovo vegetarians, *J. Am. Diet. Assoc.*, 76, 21, 1980.
25. Ellis, F. R. and Montegriffo, V. M. E., Veganism, clinical findings and investigations, *Am. J. Clin. Nutr.*, 23, 249, 1970.
26. Abdulla, M., Andersson, I., Asp, N., Berthelsen, K., Birkhed, D., Decker, I., Johansson, C., Jagerstad, M., Kolar, K., Nair, B., Nilsson-Ehle, P., Norden, A., Rassner, S., Akesson, B., and Ockerman, P., Nutrient intake and health status of vegans. Chemical analysis of diets using the duplicate portion sampling technique, *Am. J. Clin. Nutr.*, 34, 2464, 1981.
27. Burslem, J., Schonfeld, G., Howald, M. A., Weidman, S. W., and Miller, J. P., Plasma apoprotein and lipoprotein lipid levels in vegetarians, *Metabolism*, 27, 711, 1978.
28. Sanders, T. A. B., Ellis, F. R., and Dickerson, J. W. T., Studies of vegans: the fatty acid composition of plasma choline phosphoglycerides, erythrocytes, adipose tissue, and breast milk, and some indicators of susceptibility to ishcemic heart disease in vegans and omnivore controls, *Am. J. Clin. Nutr.*, 31, 805, 1978.
29. Freeland-Graves, J. H., Bodzy, P. W., and Eppright, M.A., Zinc status of vegetarians, *J. Am. Diet. Assoc.*, 77, 655, 1980.
30. Immerman, A. M., Vitamin B_{12} status on a vegetarian diet, a critical review, *World Rev. Nutr. Diet*, 37, 38, 1981.
31. Ratzin, R. A., *Vegetarianism: A review and critique of the scientific literature*, Unpublished master's research project, University of CO, Boulder, Colorado, 1982.
32. University of California at Berkeley Wellness Letter, *The new vegetarianism*, 9, March, 1993.
33. Guthrie, H. A., *Introductory Nutrition*, 7th ed., Times Mirror/Mosby College Publishing, St. Louis, 1989.
34. Lemon, F. R., Walden, R., and Woods, R. W., Cancer of the lung and mouth in Seventh Day Adventists, *Cancer*, 17, 486, 1964.
35. Phillips, R. L., Role of life-style and dietary habits in risk of cancer among Seventh-day Adventists, *Cancer Res.*, 35, 3513, 1975.
36. Phillips, R. L., Lemon, F. R., Beeson, L., and Kuzma, J. W., Coronary heart disease mortality among Seventh-day Adventists with differing dietary habits: a preliminary report, *Am. J. Clin. Nutr.*, 31, S191, 1978.
37. Haines, A. P., Chakrabarti, R., Fisher, D., Meade, T. W., North, W. R. S., and Stirling, Y., Haemostatic variables in vegetarians and non-vegetarians, *Thrombosis Res.*, 19, 139, 1980.
38. Armstrong, B., van Merwyk, A. J., and Coates, H., Blood pressure in Seventh-day Adventist vegetarians, *Am. J. Epidemiol.*, 105, 444, 1977.
39. Armstrong, B., Clarke, H., Martin, C., Ward, W., Norman, N., and Masarei, J., Urinary sodium and blood pressure in vegetarians, *Am. J. Clin. Nutr.*, 32, 2472, 1979.
40. Beilin, L. J., Rouse, I. L., Armstrng, B. K., Margetts, B. M., and Vandongen, R., Vegetarian diet and blood presdure levels: incidental or causal association?, *Am. J. Clin. Nutr.*, 48, 806, 1988.
41. Fraser, G. E., Determinants of ischemic heart disease in Seventh-Day Adventists: a review, *Am. J. Clin. Nutr.*, 48, 833, 1988.
42. Walden, R. T., Schaefer, L. E., Lemon, F. R., Sunshine, A., and Wynder, E. L., Effect of environment on the serum cholesterol-triglyceride distribution among Seventh-Day Adventists, *Am. J. Med.*, 36, 269, 1964.
43. West, R. O. and Hayes, O. B., A comparison between vegetarians and non-vegetarians in a Seventh-Day Adventist group, *Am. J. Clin. Nutr.*, 21, 853, 1968.
44. Burslem, J., Schonfeld, G., Howald, M. A., Weidman, S. W., and Miller, J. P., Plasma apoprotein and lipoprotein lipid levels in vegetarians, *Metabolism*, 27, 711, 1978.

45. Sanders, T. A. B., Ellis, F. R., and Dickerson, J. W. T., Studies of vegans: the fatty acid composition of plasma choline phosphoglycerides, erythrocytes, adipose tissue, and breast milk, and some indicators of susceptibility to ishcemic heart disease in vegans and omnivore controls, *Am. J. Clin. Nutr.*, 31, 805, 1978.

46. Simons, L. A., Gibson, C., Paino, C., Hosking, M., Bullock, J., and Trim, J., The influence of a wide range of absorbed cholesterol on plasma cholesterol levels in man, *Am. J. Clin. Nutr.*, 31, 1334, 1978.

47. Ornish, D., Brown, S., Scherwitz, L., Billings, J., Armstrong, W. Ports, T., McLanahan, S., Kirkeeide, R., Brand, R, and Gould, K. L., Can lifestyle changes reverse coronary heart disease?, *Lancet*, 336, 129, 1990.

48. Dwyer, J. T., Nutritional Consequences of Vegetarianism, *Annu. Rev. Nutr.*, 11, 61, 1991.

49. Whorton, J. C., *Crusaders for Fitness, the History of American Health Reforms*, Princeton University Press, Princeton, NJ, 1982, 227.

50. Whorton, J. C., Muscular vegetarianism: the debate over diet and athletic performance in the progressive era, *J. Sport History*, 8, 58, 1981.

51. Whorton, J. C., *Crusaders for Fitness, the History of American Health Reforms*, Princeton University Press, Princeton, NJ, 1982, 233.

52. Fisher, I., The effect of diet on endurance, based on an experiment with nine healthy students at Yale University, *Conn. Acad. Arts Sci.*, 13, 1, 1906.

53. Wishart, G. M., The efficiency and performance of a vegetarian racing cyclist under different dietary conditions, *J. Physiol.*, 82, 189, 1934.

54. Meyer, B. J., de Bruin, E. J. P., Brown, J. M. M., Bieler, E. U., Meyer, A. C., and Grey, P. R., The effect of a predominantly fruit diet on athletic performance, *Plant Foods for Man*, 1, 239, 1975.

55. Hanne, N., Dlin, R., and Rostein, A., Physical fitness, anthropometric and metabolic parameters in athletes, *J. Sports Med.*, 26, 180, 1986.

56. Nieman, D. C., Vegetarian dietary practices and endurance performance, *Am. J. Clin. Nutr.*, 48, 754, 1988.

57. Freeland-Graves, J. H., Greninger, S. A., Vickers, J., Bradley, C. L., and Young, R. K., Nutrition knowledge of vegetarians and non-vegetarians, *J. Nutr. Educ.*, 14, 21, 1982.

58. Janelle, K. C. and Barr, S. I., Nutrient intakes and eating behavior scores of vegetarian and nonvegetarian women, *J. Am. Diet. Assoc.*, 95, 180, 1995.

59. Strobl, C. M. and Groll, L., Professional knowledge and attitudes on vegetarianism: implications for practice, *J. Am. Diet. Assoc.*, 79, 568, 1981.

60. VEGEDINE, Association of Vegetarian Dietitians and Nutrition Educators, *Issues in vegetarian dietetics*, IV, 1, 1990.

61. American Dietetic Association, *Eating well — The Vegetarian Way*, Chicago, 1992.

62. U.S. Department of Agriculture and U.S. Department of Health and Human Services, *Nutrition and Your Health: Dietary Guidelines for Americans*, 3rd ed., Washington, D.C., 1990.

63. U.S. Department of Agriculture and U.S. Department of Health and Human Services, *Food Guide Pyramid, A Guide to Daily Food Choices*, 1991.

64. Messina, M. and Messina, V., *The Dietitian's Guide to Vegetarian Diets*, Aspen Publication, Gaithersburg, MD, 1996.

65. Four weeks of menus, *Vegetarian J.*, IV, 3, 1985.

66. Food and Nutrition Board, *Recommended Dietary Allowance*, 10th ed., National Academy Press, Washington, D.C., 1989.

67. Williams, M. H., *Nutrition for Fitness and Sport*, 3rd ed., Wm. C. Brown Publishers, Dubuque, 1992, chap. 12.

68. Ruud, J. S., *Vegetarianism — Implications for Athletes*, International Center for Sports Nutrition, Omaha, NE, 1990.

69. Raben, A., Kiens, B., Richter, E. A., Rasmussen, L. B., Svenstrup, B., Micic, S., and Bennett, P., Serum sex hormones and endurance performance after a lacto-ovo vegetarian and a mixed diet, *Med. Sci. Sports Exer.*, 24, 1290, 1992.

70. Jackson, C. G. R., *Nutrition for the Recreational Athlete*, CRC Press, Boca Raton, FL, 1995.

71. Sports and Cardiovascular Nutritionists, a Practice Group of The American Dietetic Association, *Sports Nutrition, A Guide for the Professional Working with Active People*, 2nd ed., 1993.

72. Clark, N., *Nancy Clark's Sports Nutrition Guidebook*, Leisure Press, Champaign, IL, 1990.

73. Kleiner, S. M., The role of meat in an athlete's diet: its effect on key macro-and micronutrients, *Sports Sci. Exchange*, Gatorade Sports Science Institute, 58, 8, 5, 1995.

Chapter 18

NUTRITION AND THE YOUNG ATHLETE

Susan M. Groziak
Gregory D. Miller

CONTENTS

I. INTRODUCTION

After birth, with the exception of infancy, the human body grows most rapidly during childhood and adolescence. During early puberty, children may gain up to 20% of their final adult height[1] and researchers estimate that roughly 45% of adult skeletal volume is formed during adolescence.[2] These rapid growth rates during childhood and adolescence exert a profound effect on nutrient needs. If these nutrient needs are not met, children and adolescents may suffer irreversible, harmful effects on growth and development.

Physical activity can exert a significant influence on nutrient needs, particularly calories, at all ages. However, additional nutritional needs imposed by sports training places a significantly greater stress on children and adolescents by augmenting the already existing high nutritional demands of rapid growth.[1] Sports training places extraordinary demands on the respiratory, cardiovascular, muscular, and skeletal systems. For example, at a high intensity

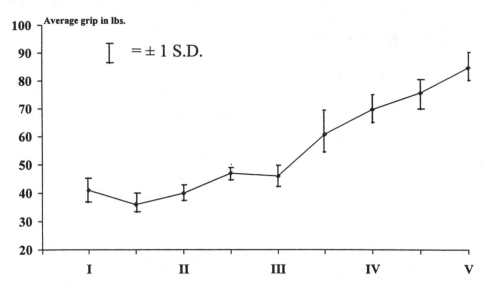

FIGURE 1 Grip strength related to sexual maturity (Tanner stages 1 to 5). (From Kreipe, R. and Gewanter, H., *Pediactrics,* 75, 6, 1985. With permission.)

of training, an adolescent swimmer may swim up to 16,000 m per day.[3] If dietary intake does not meet the exercise-induced increase in nutrient requirements, sports training may impair the growth and biological maturation of child and adolescent athletes.

More than 50% of children and adolescents in the United States participate in competitive athletics in either school- or community-based programs.[4] These numbers include more than 7 million boys and girls involved in high school sports and an additional 20 million boys and girls between 8 and 16 years of age who participate in nonschool, community-sponsored athletic programs.[5] Because of the significant number of children and adolescents involved in athletics and the important impact that sports training has on nutrient needs, it is critical that parents, coaches, adolescents, and children develop a good understanding of sports nutrition.

II. CHILDREN

Most children do not possess the neuromuscular skills to train in sports until about 5 years of age.[5] Capability to participate in contact sports is often assessed by a measure of physical maturity such as Tanner staging[6] or a combination of grip strength and Tanner stage[7] (see Figure 1).

A. NUTRITION KNOWLEDGE, ATTITUDES, AND BEHAVIOR

Children, in general, possess a rudimentary understanding of nutrition. A survey[8] conducted by the International Food Information Council on children 6–9 years of age found that 45% of the children were aware of the Basic Five Food Groups and more than 40% could identify all of the food groups. A separate study of 60 four- to seven-year-old children found that 55% believed that eating the right foods and exercising would make them healthier.[9]

U.S. children, on average, consume fairly nutritious diets. According to data from the 1989–91 Continuing Survey of Food Intake by Individuals (CSFII),[10] boys and girls 6 through 11 years of age, on average, consume 1811 and 1728 calories per day, respectively, and meet their Recommended Dietary Allowances (RDAs)[11] for vitamins A, B_6, B_{12}, and C; thiamin; riboflavin; niacin; folate; calcium; phosphorus; magnesium; iron; and zinc. Although U.S.

children, on average, meet their RDA for calcium, the calcium intake of children in the United States is a growing concern. Data from the U.S. National Health and Nutrition Examination Surveys (NHANES) indicates that calcium intakes among 6- to 11-year-olds decreased between 1988 and 1991.[12] Data from NHANES and other research studies also indicate that more than one-half of all U.S. children fail to consume their current RDA of 800 milligrams a day for calcium.[13] In addition, a 1994 Consensus Conference convened by the National Institutes of Health concluded that 6- to 10-year-old children need to consume 800–1200 mg of calcium per day to optimize bone health.[14]

Another nutritional concern facing youths today is the fact that obesity among children and teens has increased significantly during the past three decades.[15] According to the 1988–1991 NHANES survey,[15] 22% of children 6 through 17 years of age weighed more than the 85th percentile for their height and age (an increase of 5% since 1976). Many researchers attribute this weight gain over the decades to inactivity due to an increase in sedentary activities such as watching television.

Children, parents, and coaches should be taught both the principles of good nutrition and the specific nutritional demands of high levels of activity. For the most part, the nutritional needs of a child athlete are the same as the nutrient needs of a nonathletic child. However, individuals involved in child athletics need to pay particular attention to the child athlete's intakes of calories, water, and calcium.

B. ENERGY

Children are much less inefficient with their movements than adults. For this reason, children require 20–30% more oxygen per unit of body weight than adults to run at a set speed.[16] Consequently, children require more kilocalories per unit body weight than adults.[17]

Limited data exist on the effect of intense physical training on children's calorie needs. However, increasing calories to cover the child athlete's energy requirements is a primary concern.[18] Research indicates that, for most athletes, training and competition will impose the need for an additional 500–1500 calories (120–359 kilojoules) per day.[19] The current RDA for calories for children seven to ten years old is 2000 calories (478 kilojoules).[11] However, coaches and parents should not automatically assume that an athletic child will require 2500–3500 calories (598–837 kilojoules) per day. The RDAs are recommended intakes, not requirements, and are limited by the fact that they are based on chronological age rather than on maturational development.[20] Research also indicates that children have a fairly accurate ability to self-regulate their calorie intake based on energy needs. However, the effects of strenuous exercise on this self-regulation have not been determined.[18] Consequently, plotting a child athlete's growth pattern and comparing his or her weight for height to established standards may be one of the best methods to assess whether or not a child is consuming adequate calories to support growth and development.

Child athletes should be encouraged to consume three meals a day plus nutrient-dense snacks. Tissue glycogen stores will optimally meet the energy demands of training and competition only if replenished by regular, periodic food intakes.[21]

C. HYDRATION

Adequate hydration is critical for temperature regulation and performance for athletes of all ages.[22] Maintenance of adequate hydration is crucial to the prevention of heat stress, heat stroke, and death.[4,23] Roughly 80% of the energy released during exercise is released as heat.[4] For the exercising individual, the chief mechanism for heat dissipation is the evaporation of sweat from the skin.[4]

Ideally, the volume of water intake during exercise should match its overall loss from sweat, urine, and respiration. In hot or especially humid environments, an athlete can lose several pounds of water with a single practice.[18] Children are at a significant disadvantage compared to adults when it comes to dissipating heat. Children have a smaller absolute surface area but a 36% greater relative surface area (i.e., area per unit mass) than adults. Therefore, children experience greater heat transfer to and from the body, especially at temperature extremes.[16,20] In addition, children are limited by several factors: they produce more heat per kilogram of body weight, require a greater core temperature to initiate sweating, exhibit a lower sweating capacity (2.5 times less per gland), acclimatize more slowly to heat, have a lower cardiac output, and are less efficient at transferring heat from the muscles to the skin than adults.[20,24,25]

Sweat is a very hypotonic solution (80–185 mOsm/l), particularly in children.[4,21,22] Consequently, water is the best fluid replacement for children. Additionally, research does not support a benefit of adding carbohydrate and/or electrolytes to fluids consumed by children performing short-term, high-intensity exercise. One study[22] found no difference between a carbohydrate-containing beverage, carbohydrate-containing beverages with added electrolytes, and water on performance of 9- to 12-year-old children cycling for 2 hours in the heat. Concentrated or even isotonic beverages and salt tablets may actually contribute to hypernatremic dehydration in a child athlete engaged in vigorous exercise in a warm environment.[21] Because prepubescent children have a lower electrolyte loss in the sweat than adolescents or young adults, it is important to encourage consumption of cool water to restore fluids.[15,24]

Coaches, trainers, physicians, and parents should provide consistent encouragement to child athletes to drink fluids prior to the onset of thirst and encourage an intake of at least 4–6 oz (112–168 g) of fluid every 20–30 min during exercise to optimize performance and prevent adverse health effects.[4]

D. CALCIUM

In general, athletes have higher bone density than their less active peers.[26] Research indicates that children who engage in weight-bearing, impact sports such as running, gymnastics, tumbling, and dance have higher bone density than children whose major athletic activity is swimming, where unloading occurs.[27] Exercise can increase bone density by causing bones to work against gravity and providing mechanical stress.[26,28] Although exercise benefits bones, it cannot compensate for the adverse effects of an inadequate calcium intake. Consuming an adequate intake of calcium during childhood is not only critical to bone formation during childhood but also may play a substantial role in protecting bones against osteoporosis later in life.

As mentioned earlier, research indicates that more than one-half of all U.S. children fail to consume their current RDA for calcium and children may require even higher calcium intakes than the RDA to optimize bone health.[12] One prospective study found that 7- to 9-year-old children who consumed an additional three-quarters cup (184 g) of milk each day for 2 years exhibited higher bone density 14 years later than children who did not consume the additional calcium.[29] Similarly, a study of 9- to 12-year-old girls found that increasing calcium intake from 750 to 1370 mg a day for 1 year by consuming more dairy foods resulted in significantly higher total and spine bone density when compared to prepubescent girls who did not increase their dairy food intake.[30] In addition, a study of older adults in Germany links higher reported intakes of milk and milk products during childhood and adolescence with decreased risk of osteoporosis.[31] Because optimal bone health is critical to participation in sports and prevention of osteoporosis later in life, every effort should be made to educate young athletes about the importance of consuming adequate calcium from calcium-rich foods.[20]

III. TEENAGERS

A. NUTRITION KNOWLEDGE, ATTITUDES, AND BEHAVIOR

Research indicates that adolescent athletes are rarely interested in nutrition unless it is connected to a particular activity and/or hoped-for improvement in performance.[17] Most teenagers have a good understanding of general nutrition but often have misconceptions about specific nutrition issues, including sports nutrition.[32,33] A survey[34] called "How Are Kids Making Food Choices?" conducted by the International Food Information Council (IFIC) and The American Dietetic Association (ADA) on children 9 to 15 years of age found that 84% were aware of the Five Basic Food Groups and more than one-half (57%) could correctly identify all of the food groups. However, nine out of ten subjects in the IFIC/ADA study incorrectly believed that "to eat healthy you should avoid all high-fat foods" and 77% agreed with the statement that "you should never eat foods with large amounts of sugar."[34] Similarly, a study of 26 high school female volleyball players found that 46% of the subjects correctly answered general nutrition knowledge questions.[35] However, these subjects exhibited markedly less knowledge about sports nutrition.[35] A survey of 391 high school students participating in competitive or recreational sports found that 52% incorrectly believed that protein and protein supplements increased muscle size.[32]

Even when teenagers have accurate nutrition knowledge, they may not put this knowledge into practice. Although 92% of 26 high school female athletes knew that milk was a good source of calcium, only 12% of these subjects' diets met the RDA for calcium.[35] In addition, although 42% of these girls knew that a pre-event meal should be eaten three to four hours before competition to avoid gastrointestinal discomfort, 80% ate the pregame meal within one hour of an athletic event.[35]

Like many children, most teens are at least partly responsible for their food selection and preparation. The study of 26 high school female volleyball players found that 92% were responsible for the selection and preparation of some portion of their food.[35] Unfortunately, teenage athletes may not be making the most appropriate food choices. Teenage athletes, like many teens, frequently skip breakfast. A survey of 391 high school students who participated in competitive or recreational sports found that 13% did not eat breakfast.[32] In contrast, snacking is an ingrained food habit among all teens.[18] The National Adolescent Students Health Survey of more than 11,000 junior and senior high school students found that 91% reported eating at least one snack on the previous day. Fortunately, if selected wisely, snacks can contribute significantly to teenagers' nutrient intake. Data from the 1977–78 Nationwide Food Consumption Survey[36] indicates that snacks and meals provided comparable amounts of calcium, magnesium, and vitamin C for youths 11 to 18 years of age. The researchers conclude that, because of the frequency of snacking among teens, the nutritional quality of snacks can have an important impact on adolescents' total nutrient intake.[36] Unfortunately, teenagers frequently select low nutrient snacks.[37]

As children grow into their teen years, their average intake of vitamins and minerals on a per calorie basis decreases.[38] This fact, together with the fact that the RDAs for most nutrients increase during adolescence, makes it increasingly difficult for teenagers to meet their nutrient needs.[38] According to the 1989–91 CSFII,[10] males and females 12 through 19 years of age, on average, consume 2337 and 1731 calories (9778 and 7243 kilojoules) per day, respectively, and meet their RDAs for vitamins A, B_6, B_{12}, and C; thiamin; riboflavin; niacin; folate; and phosphorus. Calcium and iron are problem nutrients for teenagers. Both teenage boys and girls, on average, fail to meet their RDA of 1200 mg of calcium per day. According to the 1989–91 CSFII,[10] males and females 12 through 19 years of age consume, on average, only 1098 and 789 mg of calcium per day, respectively. Although, on average, teenage boys meet their RDA for iron, teenage girls, on average, consume only 12 mg of iron compared to their RDA of 15 mg per day.[10]

Only limited data exists on the nutrient intake of adolescent athletes. Available data indicates that male adolescent athletes tend to consume more calories and higher levels of nutrients than teenage boys who do not participate in athletics. Female athletes consume either higher or lower calorie and nutrient intakes than nonathletic girls depending on the sport they are participating in — with girls involved in gymnastics exhibiting lower calorie and nutrient intakes than the average teenage girl.

A study of 12- and 13-year-old male hockey players in Finland found that these individuals consumed more calories, protein, thiamin, riboflavin, niacin, vitamins C and E, calcium, iron, zinc, copper, and selenium than boys not involved in organized sports.[1] Similarly, a study of 22 teenage male 15 to 18 years of age and 21 female swimmers 14 to 17 years of age found that these boys and girls consumed, on average, 5222 and 3573 calories (21,849 and 14,949 kilojoules) per day, respectively — levels much higher than the average teenager.[3] This study also found that the average daily intakes of both male and female adolescent athletes exceeded the RDAs for vitamins A and C, thiamin, riboflavin, niacin, calcium, and iron.[3] The boys consumed an average of 1634 mg of calcium and 26 mg of iron per day, and the girls consumed, on average, 1235 mg of calcium and 18 mg of iron a day.[3] In contrast, a study of 26 high school female volleyball players 13 to 17 years of age found that these athletes consumed significantly fewer calories and slightly, but not significantly, less, calcium (772 vs 896 mg per day) than teenage girls participating in the National Health and Nutrition Examination Survey.[35] Similarly, a study of 97 competitive female gymnasts 11 to 17 years of age found that 40% consumed less than two-thirds of the RDA for calcium and 53% consumed less than two-thirds of the RDA for iron.[23] These data indicate that the nutritional concerns for adolescent athletes include calories, calcium, and iron. Other nutrition issues confronting teenage athletes include hydration, weight control sports, eating disorders, and vitamin and mineral supplements.

B. ENERGY

The rate of growth in adolescence is second only to that of infancy.[20] Consequently, similar to child athletes, ensuring adequate calorie intake is a significant concern for adolescent athletes. The RDA for energy for males and females 15 through 18 years of age is 3000 and 2200 calories per day, respectively.[19] Research indicates that the daily energy requirement for the moderately active teenager may be 1500–3000 calories (6276–12,552 kilojoules) beyond baseline needs.[23] However, teenage athletes' energy needs vary widely with gender and the specific sports they are involved in (Table 1) and also vary between individuals. Similar to children, plotting an adolescent athlete's growth pattern and comparing his or her weight for height to established standards is one of the best ways to ensure that an adolescent is consuming adequate energy. Additionally, because of the important contribution that snacks make to an adolescent's energy and nutrient intake, adolescent athletes should be encouraged to consume higher energy, nutrient-dense snacks.

C. HYDRATION

Although sweat rate and sweat composition approach adult levels in late puberty, most adolescents exhibit a lower sweat rate and more hypotonic sweat than adults.[39,40] Consequently, similar to children, the fluid needs of adolescent athletes should be carefully monitored. Many teenage athletes choose to drink sports beverages often based on the misperception that these drinks provide a performance advantage. To the contrary, although drinking carbohydrate solutions may enhance the performance of athletes participating in prolonged exercise (such as soccer, field hockey, rugby, and tennis), data indicates that the use of electrolyte/carbohydrate-containing beverages offers no advantage over water in maintaining

TABLE 1   Daily Energy Cost of Various Activities[a,b]

3000–4000		3000–5000	3000–6000	4000–6000
Discus	Hurdles	880-yd run (8 hm)	Football	Cross-country
Hammer throw	Long jump	1- and 2-mile	Basketball	running
Shot-put	Pole vault	(1.6–3.2 km) runs	Ice hockey	6-mile run
Javelin	Long horse vault	Swimming events	Lacrosse	(9.7 km)
High jump	Swimming events,	more than 100 yd	Tennis	Marathon running
Diving	50- and 100-yd	(0.9 hm)	Gymnastic, all	Soccer
Ski jumping	(0.5 and 0.9 hm)	Wrestling	around	Cross-country
Dashes — 440 yd	Baseball	Most gymnastic	Fencing	skiing
(4 hm)	Golf	events	3-mile run (4.8 km)	
		Downhill, slalom		
		skiing		

[a]   Assumes that body weight and size are similar among participants of the sport.
[b]   The energy cost of the activities listed would be approximately 10% less for females.

Adapted from McKeag, D. J., *Adolesc. Health Care*, 7, 1215, 1986.

plasma volume or electrolyte concentrations or in improving intestinal absorption of water.[4] Cold water remains the ideal replacement beverage for teenage athletes.[4] Teenage athletes should consume 8–12 oz of fluid every 20–30 min during exercise.[4] Adolescent athletes can easily replace any lost electrolytes with the consumption of food after exercise.[16] Salt tablets are *not* recommended for young athletes.[16]

D. CALCIUM

Adolescence is a critical time for developing bone mass.[26] On average, bones grow in length until about 18 years of age in females and 22 years of age in males.[41] Bone density of the spine, hip, and total skeleton peaks in boys at about 18 years of age.[42] Similarly, although peak bone mass is not achieved in females until the late 20s and early 30s, most bone is deposited in women by age 19.[43]

As mentioned earlier, due to mechanical loading, athletes in general exhibit higher bone density than their nonathletic peers.[26] The playing arm of a tennis player may be up to 30% more dense than the nonplaying arm.[28] Studies conducted on teenagers also indicate that exercise during adolescence may actually have a long-lasting positive effect on bone density. A study that followed more than 260 teenagers for 11 years linked exercising regularly with higher hip and spine bone density in men and higher hip bone density in women.[43] Similarly, a study of 204 minimally active young women 18 to 31 years of age linked higher estimated high school energy expenditure with higher total body bone mineral density, bone mineral content, femoral neck bone mineral density, and spine bone mineral content.[44] Although exercise, particularly weight-bearing exercise, promotes higher bone density, no research indicates that exercise will reverse the adverse effects of a low calcium intake on bone. Calcium intakes are critically low among both athletic and nonathletic teens and thereby warrant concern. Additionally, intense physical activity in female adolescent athletes may lead to a state of amenorrhea which can result in significantly decreased bone density.[26,43]

According to the 1989–91 U.S. Department of Agriculture's Continuing Survey of Food Intakes by Individuals,[10] 12- to 19-year-old males and females consume, on average, 1145 and 797 mg of calcium per day, respectively. The 1994 National Institute of Health (NIH) Consensus Panel on Optimal Calcium Intakes[13] concluded that teenagers should consume between 1200 and 1500 mg of calcium per day to optimize bone health. Research supports that increasing teenagers' calcium intakes to NIH recommended levels benefits bone density. A 2-year longitudinal study of 31 girls 14 years of age found that increasing calcium intake from 850 to 1640 mg per day with either milk or calcium carbonate increased bone mass and bone density on all sites measured.[45] However, adolescents should rely on calcium-rich foods rather than supplements to obtain the calcium they need. Calcium is not the only nutrient needed to optimize bone health. Other nutrients such as protein, phosphorus, and vitamin D also play important roles in enhancing bone health. Consequently, adding 700 mg of calcium a day in the form of dairy foods to adolescents' diets increased bone mineral accretion by up to 10%.[46,47] In contrast, increasing calcium intake 300–700 mg a day via calcium supplements resulted in only a 1–5% increase in bone mineral accretion.[47] Similar to exercise, consuming adequate calcium during adolescence may also exert long-term beneficial effects on bone. A study of older adults in Germany linked higher reported intakes of milk and milk products during childhood and adolescence with decreased risk of osteoporosis.[31] Similarly, a study of more than 500 older women found that women who reported drinking milk throughout their teen and adult years exhibited greater arm and spine bone density later in life than women who consumed little or no milk.[48] Adolescent athletes should make a special effort to consume adequate calcium-rich foods to ensure healthy bones for life as well as for ensuring strong bones for participation in sports.

Exercise-induced amenorrhea is an additional concern for teenage adolescent girls. Women competing in ballet and gymnastics exhibit a higher incidence of primary and secondary amenorrhea, lower bone density, and increased incidence of stress fractures compared to women not involved in these sports.[49] Amenorrhea may lead to decreased bone density due to a decrease in levels of the beneficial bone hormone, estrogen. Research further indicates that amenorrhea can cause irreversible bone loss if prolonged for two to three years.[28] Female athletes suffering from amenorrhea should seek advice from a physician to reestablish normal menses.

E. IRON

Research indicates that iron-depletion greatly limits exercise tolerance.[21] Adolescents' intake of iron is a particular concern because the high growth rate experienced during this time of development significantly increases the need for iron.[16] Additionally, teenage girls have a higher need for iron than teenage boys due to the onset of menses. Even when they consume similar intakes of iron (15 and 16 mg of iron a day), athletic teenage girls exhibit lower serum ferritin levels than athletic teenage boys.[50] An additional factor compounding this problem is the fact that teenage girls are more likely than boys to fail to consume their RDA for iron.[1]

Exercise may also increase the need for iron depending on the intensity of the exercise. Some investigators have documented that exercise compromises iron status in endurance-trained athletes or in individuals involved in vigorous exercise.[51,52] However, other researchers do not report such an effect for moderate exercise.[53] Although the effect of exercise on iron needs is debatable, an adequate iron intake remains a concern for adolescent female athletes because of their high iron need, low iron intake, and the potential adverse effects of low iron status on athletic performance. Adolescent female athletes should be counseled to consume good food sources of iron such as red meat and iron-fortified cereals on a regular basis.

F. WEIGHT CONTROL SPORTS

Weight loss is endemic to several sports including wrestling, boxing, and martial arts. Unfortunately, most adolescents participating in weight-conscious sports, especially wrestling, typically do not follow a planned weight management program. Instead, they frequently engage in frequent cycles of rapid weight reduction and weight gain.[54] With the intent to gain a competitive edge, adolescent athletes often employ fasting, vomiting, laxatives, diuretics, fluid deprivation, and induced sweating to meet a set weight limit[54,55] (Table 2). A survey of 197 high school wrestlers found that increased activity (i.e., running) and decreased food intake (eating less or nothing) were the most frequently reported weight loss methods.[54] 46% tried to lose weight by spitting, 42% avoided drinking fluids, 35% used rubber suits, 15%

TABLE 2   Wrestlers' Use of
           Various Methods for
           Weight Loss

Method	Reported Use, Percent (n)
Not eating	61 (119)
Spitting	46 (88)
Not drinking	42 (81)
Rubber suits	35 (67)
Saunas	24 (47)
Steam rooms	19 (36)
Laxatives	15 (29)
Vomiting	15 (28)
Diet pills	7 (13)
Other	18 (34)

Adapted from Marguart, L. and Sobal, J., *J.*
Adolesc. Health, 15, 410, 1994.

tried laxatives, 15% reported vomiting, and 7% used diet pills.[54] Some of these competitive athletes deliberately lose 3–5% of their body weight during the 1–2 days prior to competition. A survey of 713 high school wrestlers found that the average wrestler lost 3.2 kg to compete and fasted 20 hours prior to weigh-in.[55]

For the most part, adolescent athletes participating in weight-monitored sports remain blind to the facts that rapid weight loss techniques can have adverse effects on nutritional status, muscular strength, aerobic and anaerobic power, and athletic performance.[54] As little as 2% decrease in body weight through fluid loss results in an increase in heart rate and body temperature and a decrease in plasma volume.[4] Many researchers report that water loss resulting in a 3–5% decrease in body weight markedly decreases an athlete's capacity for muscle work and maximal physical work capacity.[56,57] Higher fluid losses can result in heat cramps, heat exhaustion, and heat stroke.[4] One article reports a massive pulmonary embolism in a high school wrestler who underwent rapid dehydration twice in one week.[58]

The importance of adequate nutrition and hydration should be stressed to wrestlers and all adolescents involved in weight-conscious sports. All adolescent athletes should be encouraged to eat three meals per day and nutrient-dense snacks and consume adequate fluids.[54] Coaches, trainers, physicians, and parents should counsel teenage athletes to maintain and compete at a healthy weight. To monitor fluid losses, adolescents participating in these sports should weigh themselves before and after training.[54] Researchers recommend that two cups of water should be consumed for each pound lost during a training session.[54] Adolescent athletes should try to maintain a clear, light yellow, odorless urine.[54]

G. EATING DISORDERS

Adolescents are at high risk for developing an eating disorder. Many adolescents have a distorted perception of their ideal body weight.[59] According to a national survey, 34% of adolescents consider themselves to be overweight[60] and 40% of teenagers are attempting to lose weight.[61] Teenage girls are more likely than teenage boys to consider themselves overweight.[62] A study of 497 senior high school students found that two-thirds of teenage girls and 15% of teenage boys were preoccupied with weight and dieting.[63] A study of 854 females 12 to 23 years of age found that 67% were dissatisfied with their weight and 54% were dissatisfied with their body shape.[64] A study of 326 high school girls 13 to 18 years of age found that 17% were underweight for their height.[59] However, 51% of these underweight girls described themselves as extremely fearful of fat and 36% were preoccupied with body fat.[59] This study also found that almost one-third (32%) of girls with a healthy weight were dieting to lose weight and 26% of all of the girls in this study reported bingeing.[59] One study found that, to lose weight, 31% of females 12 to 23 years of age had fasted, 9% had vomited, and 6% used diuretics.[64] Similarly, a study of 1728 tenth graders found that 11% of the girls reported vomiting, 7% used laxatives, and 4% used diuretics to lose weight.[65]

Eating disorders, anorexia nervosa, and bulimia are common among both athletic adolescents and adolescents not involved in athletics.[20] However, due to the stress of competition, erratic eating habits resulting from scheduled practices, and the pressure to compete in specific weight categories, adolescent athletes may be particularly vulnerable to developing eating disorders.[20,32] Researchers[66] report that the prevalence of anorexia and bulimia in adolescent athletes are increasing in frequency. A study of 26 high school female volleyball players found that the majority (92%) were concerned about their weight and 73% wanted to lose weight.[35] A survey of 713 high school wrestlers found that 1.7% met five established criteria for bulimia, a rate much higher than that expected for average adolescents.[55] An additional 43% engaged in weight-reducing practices common in bulimia, including self-induced vomiting, the use of laxatives or diuretics, and strict dieting or fasting.[57] Similarly, a study of 49 high school wrestlers found that a higher percentage (27%) of these subjects reported bingeing and vomiting (8%) to lose weight than control subjects (10% reported bingeing and none reported vomiting).[67]

Eating disorders are serious problems that not only have profound, adverse short-term health effects on adolescent athletes, including chronic fatigue, hypoglycemia, and an increased incidence of illness and heat injury, but potentially long-term adverse effects such as delayed growth and development and increased risk of osteoporosis.[18] A study that compared 18 girls 12 to 20 years of age suffering from anorexia nervosa to healthy girls of comparable age found that the anorexic girls exhibited significantly lower lumbar vertebral bone density and whole body bone mass than the controls[68] (Table 3). Adolescent athletes suspected of having an eating disorder should receive both nutrition and psychiatric counseling.

H. VITAMIN/MINERAL SUPPLEMENTS

Research indicates that fewer adolescents (20–25%) than adults (35–40%) use vitamin and mineral supplements.[69] However adolescent athletes may consume supplements more often than teenagers not actively involved in sports. Studies conducted on high school athletes estimate supplement use at 33%,[70] 38%,[71] 46%,[72] and 56%.[73]

Most adolescent athletes believe that supplements can improve athletic performance.[73] The belief that supplements improve athletic performance varies among sports and appears to be highest among gymnasts and wrestlers.[71] The supplements most frequently consumed by adolescent athletes include vitamin C, multivitamins, iron, calcium, vitamin A, and B vitamins.[71]

Even for the highly active adolescent athletes, nutritional supplements are not necessary. Consuming three meals a day plus nutrient-dense snacks can easily meet a teenage athlete's nutrient needs. Furthermore, unlike supplements, foods provide many other nutrients beneficial

TABLE 3   Bone Mineral Densities in Female Adolescents With and Without Anorexia Nervosa[a]

	Lumbar Vertebral	Radius	Whole Body
Control adolescents	1.054 ± 0.139	0.678 ± 0.067	0.955 ± 0.130
Patients with anorexia nervosa	0.830 ± 0.140	0.640 ± 0.060	0.700 ± 0.120

[a]   Results are given as a means ± standard deviations in grams per centimeter squared. Probability values were as follows: lumbar vertebral bone density, $P < 0.0001$; radius bone density, $P = 0.12$; whole body bone density, $P < 0.0001$.

Adapted from Bachrach, L., Guido, D., Katzman, D., Litt, I.F., and Marcus, R., *Pediatrics*, 86, 440, 1990. With permission.

to good health such as carbohydrate, protein, fiber, flavonoids, antioxidants, and sphingolipids. Foods are also a much safer source of nutrients than supplements. The risk of consuming excessive amounts of nutrients is far greater with supplements than with food.

Practitioners who work with adolescent athletes should assess supplement use with a vitamin/mineral supplement history.[71] Adolescent athletes consider parents, doctors, and coaches important sources of information concerning supplement use.[71] These individuals can teach young athletes that vitamins and minerals are not in themselves energy producing but help regulate the energy nutrients while foods, not supplements, are the best source of energy producing nutrients.[71] Athletes should also be taught that even the most rigorous and demanding sports training does not increase the body's need for any specific nutrients beyond calories and water.[21] A balanced and varied diet consisting of foods from all of the Five Food Groups and adequate in calories to meet the energy demands of training will provide all of the essential nutrients needed by active teens.[21]

IV. CONCLUSIONS

With the exception of primarily calories and water, the nutrient needs of child and adolescent athletes, in general, do not differ significantly from those of youths not involved in athletics. A well-balanced diet providing adequate calories and fluids will meet the nutritional needs of athletic children and teens. However, taking into consideration the rigors of a sports training schedule, specific recommendations for young athletes may include:

- Weigh children periodically to monitor whether energy needs are being met. Height and weight measures should be plotted on the growth chart. To estimate energy needs, one must consider rate of growth, age, and activity patterns.[72,74,75]
- Encourage young athletes to drink fluids before, during, and after exercise. Motivate young athletes to drink fluids prior to the onset of thirst.[3] Plain water is the best and most economical source of fluid for activity lasting less than an hour.[74,75]
- Encourage young athletes to eat breakfast. Breakfast helps replenish glycogen stores depleted during an overnight fast to ensure that a child has adequate energy stores for afternoon training.[7]
- Promote healthy snacking. Both child and adolescent athletes should be encouraged to frequently consume high calorie, nutrient-dense snacks throughout the day to meet their calorie and nutrient needs.[72,74,75] Children should be encouraged to distribute food intake over regular periods of time throughout the day. This will ensure the presence of readily available sources of energy to support training activity.[16]
- Do not restrict foods on basis of fat content.[74] Fat is a major, if not the most important, fuel for light to moderate intensity exercise and a valuable metabolic fuel for muscle activity during prolonged exercise.[3] In addition, foods from the Five Food Groups which contain fat are also good sources of other essential nutrients such as protein, iron, and calcium.[16]
- Provide young athletes with a high carbohydrate snack (pregame meal) at least two hours before competition. Children should be encouraged to consume a nutritious snack that is pleasing to the child in addition to at least 8 oz (224 g) of fluid (water or diluted juice).
- Rely on foods rather than supplements to provide needed nutrients to child and adolescent athletes.[74,75] There is no place in the diet of a healthy child or adolescent athlete for the vitamin, protein, or mineral supplements that are often vigorously promoted to athletes of all ages.[16,74,75]
- Consuming additional carbohydrates during a sports event may enhance the performance of teenage athletes participating in prolonged exercise that exceeds 90 min in

duration.[75] Adolescents involved in these activities may benefit by consuming a lowfat, high carbohydrate snack or fruit juice diluted to contain 5–10% carbohydrate.

- Be on guard for signs of eating disorders.[49,75] Child and adolescent athletes should be taught and motivated to achieve and maintain a healthy weight.

REFERENCES

1. Rankinen, T., Fogelhom, M., Kujala, U., Rauramaa, R., and Uusitupa, M., Dietary intake and nutritional status of athletic and nonathletic children in early puberty, *Intl. J. Sports Nutr.*, 5,136, 1995.
2. Matkovic, V., Calcium and peak bone mass, *J. Intern. Med.*, 231,151, 1992.
3. Berning, J., Troup, J. P., VanHandel, P. J., Daniels, J., and Daniels, N., The nutritional habits of young adolescent swimmers, *Intl. J. Sport Nutr.*, 1, 240, 1991.
4. Squire, D., Heat illness: fluid and electrolyte issues for pediatric and adolescent athletes, *Sports Med.*, 37, 1085, 1990.
5. McKeag, D., Adolescents and exercise, *J. Adolescent Health Care*, 7, 121S, 1986.
6. Garrick, J. G. and Smith, N. J., Pre-participation sports assessment, *Pediatrics*, 66, 803, 1980.
7. Kreipe, R. E. and Gewanter, H. L., Physical maturity screening for participation in sports, *Pediatrics*, 75, 6, 1076, 1985.
8. International Food Information Council, Kids Make the Nutritional Grade, Survey conducted by Youth Research, June 1992.
9. Singleton, J. C., Achterberg, C. L., and Shannon, B. M., Role of food and nutrition in the health perceptions of young children, *J. Am. Diet. Assoc.*, 92, 67, 1992.
10. Tippett, K. S., Mickle, S. J., and Golman, J. D., *Food and Nutrient Intakes by Individuals in the United States, 1 Day, 1989–1991. Continuing Survey of Food Intakes by Individuals 1989–1991*, Nationwide Food Surveys Rep. No. 91–2, September 1995.
11. Food and Nutrition Board, National Research Council, Recommended Dietary Allowances, 10th ed., National Academy Press, Washington, D.C., 1989.
12. Kennedy, E. and Goldberg, J., What are American children eating? Implications for public policy, *Nutr. Rev.*, 53, 111, 1995.
13. International Food Information Council, *Food Insight*, September/October, 1994.
14. NIH Consensus Conference, Optimal calcium intake, *J. Am. Med. Assoc.*, 272, 1942, 1994.
15. Troiano, R. P., Flegal, K. M., Kuczmarski, R. J., Campbell, S. M., and Johnson, C. L., Overweight prevalence and trends for children and adolescents, *Arch. Pediatr. Adolesc. Med.*, 149,1085, 1995.
16. Daniels, J., Differences and changes in VO_2 among runners 10–18 years of age, *Med. Sci. Sports Exer.*, 10, 200, 1978.
17. Steen, S. N., Nutritional assessment and management of the school-aged child athlete, in *Sports Nutrition for the 90s: the Health Professional's Handbook*, Berning, J. R. and Steen, S. N., Eds., Aspen Publishers, Gaithersburg, MD, 1991, 229.
18. Allen, J. and Overbaugh, K., The adolescent athlete. Part III: The role of nutrition and hydration, *J. Pediatr.*, 8, 250, 1994.
19. Harvey, J. S., Nutritional management of the adolescent athlete, *Clinics Sports Med.*, 3, 671, 1984.
20. O'Connor, H., Special needs: children and adolescents in sport, in *Clinical Sports Nutrition*, Burke, L. and Deak, V., Eds., McGraw-Hill, Sydney, Australia, 1994, 390.
21. Smith, N. J., Nutrition and the adolescent athlete, in *Adolescent Nutrition*, Winick, M., Ed., John Wiley & Sons, New York, 1982, 63.
22. Meyer, F., Bar-Or, O., MacDougall, D., and Heigenhauser, G. J. F., Drink composition and the electrolyte balance of children exercising in the heat, *Med. Sci. Sports Exer.*, 27, 882, 1995.
23. Loosli, A. R. and Benson, J., Nutritional intake in adolescent athletes, *Ped. Clinics N. Amer.*, 37, 1143, 1990.
24. Committee on Sports Medicine, American Academy of Pediatrics, Thermoregulation and fluid and electrolytes needs, in *Sports Medicine: Health Care for Young Athletes*, Smith, N.J., Ed., American Academy of Pediatrics, Evanston, IL, 1983, 17,143.
25. Bar-Or, O., Climate and the exercising child — a review, *Int. J. Sports Med.*, 1, 53, 1980.
26. Orr, S. M., Bone density in adolescents, *N. Engl. J. Med.*, 325, 1646, 1991.
27. Grimston, S. K., Willows, N. D., and Hanley, D. A., Mechanical loading regime and its relationship to bone mineral density in children, *Med Sci. Sports Exer.*, 25, 1203, 1993.
28. Wolman, R. L., ABC of sports medicine. Osteoporosis and exercise, *Br. Med. J.*, 309, 400, 1994.
29. Johnston, C. C., Jr., Miller, J. Z., Slemenda, C. W., Reister, T. K., Hui, S., Christian, J. C., and Peacock, M., Calcium supplementation and increases in bone mineral density in children, *N. Engl. J. Med.*, 327, 82, 1992.
30. Chan, G., Hoffman, K., Wiehke, G., and McMurray, M., Dairy products improve prepuberal girls' bone mineral and lean body mass status, *J. Am. Coll. Nutr.*, 587, (abst. 32) 1993.

31. Renner, E., Dairy calcium, bone metabolism, and prevention of osteoporosis, *J. Dairy Sci.,* 77, 3498, 1994.

32. Schmalz, K., Nutritional beliefs and practices of adolescent athletes, *J. Sch. Nursing,* 9, 18, 1993.

33. Borra, S., Schwartz, N. E., Spain, C. G., and Natchipolsky, M. M., Food, physical activity, and fun: inspiring America's kids to more healthful lifestyles, *J. Am. Diet. Assoc.,* 95, 816, 1995.

34. International Food Information Council and The American Dietetic Association, *How are Kids Making Food Choices?,* Prepared by the Gallup Organization, Inc., Princeton, NJ, July 1991.

35. Perron, M. and Endres, J., Knowledge, attitudes, and dietary practices of female athletes, *J. Am. Diet. Assoc.,* 85, 573, 1985.

36. Bigler-Doughten, S. and Jenkins, R.M., Adolescent snacks. Nutrient density and nutritional contribution to total intake, *J. Am. Diet. Assoc.,* 87, 1678, 1987.

37. Portnoy, B. and Christianson, G. M., Cancer knowledge and related practices: results from the National Adolescent Student Health Survey, *J. Sch. Health,* 59, 218, 1989.

38. Nicklas, T., Dietary studies of children: the Bogalusa Heart Study experience, *J. Am. Diet. Assoc.,* 95, 1127, 1995.

39. Falk, B., Bar-Or, O., and MacDougall, D. J., Thermoregulatory responses of pre-, mid-, and late-pubertal boys to exercise in dry heat, *Med. Sci. Sports Exer.,* 24, 688, 1992.

40. Meyer, F., Bar-Or, O., MacDougall, D., and Heigenhauser, G. J. F., Sweat electrolyte loss during exercise in the heat: effects of gender and maturation, *Med. Sci. Sports Exer.,* 24, 975, 1992.

41. Anderson, J. J., Calcium, phosphorus and human bone development, *J. Nutr.,* 126, 1253S, 1996.

42. Lu, P.-W., Briody, J. N., Ogle, G. D., Morley, K., Humphries, I. R., Allen, J., Howman-Giles, R., Sillence, D., and Cowell, C. T., Bone mineral density of total body, spine, and femoral neck in children and young adults: a cross-sectional and longitudinal study, *J. Bone Min. Res.,* 9, 1451, 1994.

43. Matkovic, V., Jelic, T., Wardlaw, G. M., Ilich, J. Z., Goel, P. K., Wright, J. K., Andon, M. B., Smith, K. T., and Heaney, R. P., Timing of peak bone mass in Caucasian females and its implications for the prevention of osteoporosis. Inference from a cross-sectional model, *J. Clin. Invest.,* 93, 799, 1994.

44. Teegarden, D., Proulx, W., Kern, M., Sedlock, D., Weaver, C., Johnston, C., and Lyle, R., Previous physical activity relates to bone mineral measures in young women, *Med. Sci. Sports Exer.,* 28, 105, 1996.

45. Matkovic, V., Fontana, D., Tominac, C., Goel, P., and Chesnut, C.H., III, Factors that influence peak bone mass formation: a study of calcium balance and the inheritance of bone mass in adolescent females, *Am. J. Clin. Nutr.,* 52, 878, 1990.

46. Chan, G. M., Hoffman, K., and McMurry, M., Effects of dairy products on bone and body composition in pubertal girls, *J. Pediatr.,* 126, 551, 1995.

47. Kerstetter, J. E. and Isogna, K., Do dairy products improve bone density in adolescent girls?, *Nutr. Rev.,* 53, 328, 1995.

48. Soroko, S., Holbrook, T. L., Edelstein, S., and Barrett-Connor, E., Lifetime milk consumption and bone mineral density in older women, *Am. J. Publ. Health,* 84, 1319, 1994.

49. Committee on Sports Medicine, Amenorrhea in adolescent athletes, *Pediatrics,* 84, 384, 1989.

50. Willows, N. D., Grimston, S. K., Roberts, D., Smith, D. J., and Hanley, D. A., Iron and hemotologic status in young athletes relative to puberty: a cross-sectional study, *Pediatr. Exer. Sci.,* 5, 367, 1993.

51. Lampe, J. W., Slavin, J. L., and Apple, F. S., Poor iron status of women runners training for a marathon, *Int. J. Sports Med.,* 7, 11, 1986.

52. Parr, R. B., Bachman, L. A., and Moss, R. A., Iron deficiency in female athletes, *Phys. Sports Med.,* 12, 81, 1984.

53. Pratt, C. A., Woo, V., and Chrisley, B., The effects of exercise on iron status and aerobic capacity in moderately exercising adult women, *Nutr. Res.,* 16, 1, 23, 1996.

54. Marquart, L. F. and Sobal, J., Weight loss beliefs, practices and support systems for high school wrestlers, *J. Adoles. Health,* 15, 410, 1994.

55. Oppliger, R. A., Landry, G. L., Foster, S. E., and Lambrecht, A. C., Bulimic behaviors among interscholastic wrestlers: a statewide survey, *Pediatrics,* 91, 826, 1993.

56. Caldwell, J. E., Ahonen, E., and Nousianinen, U., Differential effects of sauna-, diuretic- and exercise-induced hypohydration, *J. Appl. Physiol. Respir. Environ. Exer. Physiol.,* 57, 1018, 1984.

57. Torranin, C., Smith, D. P., and Byrd, R. J., The effect of acute thermal dehydration and rapid rehydration on isometric and isotonic endurance, *J. Sports Med. Phys. Fitness,* 19,1, 1979.

58. Croyle, P. H., Place, R. A., and Hilgenberg, A. D., Massive pulmonary embolism in a high school wrestler, *J. Am. Med. Assoc.,* 241, 827, 1979.

59. Moses, N., Banilivy, M.-M., and Lifshitz, F., Fear of obesity among adolescent girls, *Pediatrics,* 83, 393, 1989.

60. Story, M., Rosenwinkel, K., Himes, J. H., Resnick, M., Harris, L. J., and Blum, R. W., Demographic and risk factors associated with chronic dieting in adolescents, *Am. J. Dis. Child.,* 145, 994, 1991.

61. Serdula, M.K., Collins, M.E., Williamson, D.F., Anda, R.F., Pamuk, E., and Byers, T.E., Weight control practices of U.S. adolescents and adults, *Ann. Intern. Med.,* 119, 667, 1993.

62. Kann, L., Warren, C. W., Harris, W. A., Collins, J. C., Douglas, K. A., Collin, M. E., Williams, B. I., Ross, J. G., and Kolbe, L. J., Youth risk behavior surveillance — United States, 1993, *J. Sch. Health,* 65, 163, 1995.

63. Casper, R. C. and Offer, D., Weight and dieting concerns in adolescents, fashion or symptom?, *Pediatrics,* 86, 394, 1990.

64. Moore, D. C., Body image and eating behavior in adolescent girls, *Am. J. Dis. Child.,* 144, 475, 1990.

65. Killen, J., Taylor, C. B., Telch, M. J., Saylor, K. E., Maron, D. J., and Robinson, T. N., Self-induced vomiting and laxative and diuretic use among teenagers. Precursors of the binge-purge syndrome?, *J. Am. Med. Assoc.,* 255, 1447, 1986.

66. Burkes-Miller, M. E. and Black, D. R., Eating disorders: a problem in athletics?, *Health Ed.,* 9, 22, 1988.

67. Woods, E. R., Wilson, C. D., and Masland, R. P., Weight control methods in high school wrestlers, *J. Adolesc. Health Care,* 9, 394, 1988.

68. Bachrach, L., Guido, D., Katzman, D., Litt, I.F., and Marcus, R., Decreased bone density in adolescent girls with anorexia nervosa, *Pediatrics,* 86, 440, 1990.

69. Sobal, J. and Muncie, H.L., Vitamin/mineral supplement use among adolescents, *J. Nutr. Ed.,* 20, 314, 1988.

70. Krowchuck, D. P., Anglin, T. M., Goodfellow, D. B., Stancin, T., Williams, P., and Zimet, G. D., High school athletes and the use of ergogenic aids, *Am. J. Dis. Child.,* 143, 486,1989.

71. Sobal, J. and Marquart, L. F., Vitamin/mineral supplement use among high school athletes, *Adolescence,* 29, 835, 1994.

72. Parr, R. B., Porter, M. A., and Hodgson, S. C., Nutrition knowledge and practices of coaches, trainers, and athletes, *Phys. Sports Med.,* 12, 127, 1984.

73. Douglas, P. D. and Douglas, J. G., Nutrition knowledge and food practices of high school athletes, *J. Am. Diet. Assoc.,* 84, 1198, 1984.

74. The American Dietetic Association, Timely statement of The American Dietetic Association: nutrition guidance for child athletes in organized sports, *J. Am. Diet. Assoc.,* 96, 610, 1996.

75. The American Dietetic Association, Timely statement of The American Dietetic Association: nutrition guidance for adolescent athletes in organized sports, *J. Am. Diet. Assoc.,* 96, 611, 1996.

Chapter 19

NUTRITION AND THE OLDER ATHLETE

CONTENTS

I. INTRODUCTION

The older age groups comprise an increasing proportion of the population.[1] Mounting evidence demonstrates the benefits of exercise throughout the life span. Therefore, how exercise may affect the nutritional requirements and overall health of this subgroup of the population is of increasing importance. At present, approximately 12% of the U.S. population is 65 years of age or older,[1] and this percentage is expected to nearly double by the year 2030. The large cohort of "baby boomers," individuals born between 1946 and 1964, are now on the threshold of entering the older age groups, and they bring unique characteristics and lifestyle patterns to their older years when compared with those of preceding generations.[2] Survey data from the previous cohorts that now comprise the older age groups of U.S. adults suggest that the vast majority do not engage in regular leisure-time physical activity.[3] In contrast, the baby boomers are described as having a goal of wellness and being more uncomfortable with physical decline, so a greater proportion of this group is likely to continue, rather than discontinue, exercise patterns that were adopted during their adolescent and young adult years. Among the current older age groups, the master athletes who participate in regular training programs and compete in track and field and swimming events represent a model of continued exercise throughout the adult years.

As described by Lipschitz,[4] the aging process basically results from interaction between genetic factors and exposure to environmental factors, such as diet. Because of the variety of predetermining factors and exposures that may have occurred throughout infancy, childhood, adolescence, and early adulthood, the older age groups are, characteristically, a very heterogeneous group. Knowledge of the nutritional requirements of older adults in general has been notably limited, and the levels for the Recommended Dietary Allowances (RDA) in even the most recent edition[5] are based on an age division at 51 years as a rather arbitrary point to distinguish older from younger adults. Clearly, the physiologic characteristics of athletes aged 51–69 years are likely to differ a great deal from those of the very old or frail elderly. Thus, when considering nutritional needs of the older athlete, the wide interindividual differences, as well as the particularly large span of age that may be involved, must be recognized.

II. UNIQUE CHARACTERISTICS

A. CHANGES IN BODY COMPOSITION

Aging is associated with distinct changes in body composition, some of which may be modified by activity and exercise patterns in the older adult. Loss of muscle mass, attributed to both a loss of muscle fibers (especially Type II fibers) and a reduction in size, has been consistently demonstrated to occur with aging.[6,7] Various approaches to evaluating muscle mass, including examination of urinary creatinine excretion rates and computed tomography imaging of individual muscles, have shown a decline in muscle mass after age 30,[7] which declines more steeply after age 50.[8,9] Correlated with the loss of muscle mass is a reduction in muscle strength, which most dramatically differs from younger age groups after 70 years of age. As summarized by Evans,[7] current data suggest that muscle strength declines by about 15% per decade during the 60s and 70s and by about 30% in subsequent years, primarily due to loss of muscle mass. However, exercise or athletic training has been shown to be an important determinant of muscle mass and strength in aging. Male athletes aged 70–81 years participating in several types of physical training, including endurance exercise, were found to demonstrate preservation of muscle strength and mass when compared with these characteristics in the average male population of the same age.[6]

A reduction in the amount of skeletal muscle is the major determinant of reduced lean body mass, which has also been observed in association with aging.[10,11] A relative increase in the proportion of fat occurs concomitantly and is particularly characterized by the accumulation of abdominal fat (rather than subcutaneous or other depot fat), although this characteristic may also be modified by exercise patterns. Lower waist-to-hip ratio, an indicator of less abdominal fat, has been observed in master athletes who averaged 64 years of age when compared to age-matched sedentary controls.[12]

Bone mass declines from a peak concentration between 20 and 40 years of age and is estimated to occur at an overall rate of 6–10% decline per decade.[13,14] Numerous etiologic factors are known to contribute to the loss in bone mineral density in aging, such as gender, hormonal status, calcium and vitamin D intake, and heredity. However, high-intensity strength training in postmenopausal women has been shown to have a protective effect on this body compartment in addition to improving muscle mass and strength,[14] and regular exercise across the lifespan may also reduce the rate of loss in bone mass that has been observed with aging.

B.   OTHER PHYSIOLOGIC CHANGES

As a measure of physical fitness, maximal oxygen consumption (VO_2max) is commonly used to quantify the functional capacity of the cardiovascular system and the ability of the muscles to utilize oxygen. In numerous cross-sectional and a few longitudinal studies, VO_2max has been shown to decline in association with aging, reportedly at a rate that averages 10% decline per decade in the majority of the subjects that have been examined.[15,16] However, data collected from cross-sectional studies has suggested that regular exercise may reduce the rate of decline considerably, and results from recent longitudinal studies support this concept. For example, when VO_2max of 15 trained master endurance athletes and 14 sedentary control subjects (males 47–84 years of age) was compared before and after an 8-year interval, the rate of decline was calculated to be 5.5% vs 12% per decade for the athletes and sedentary controls, respectively.[17] A 15-year follow-up study of VO_2max in 36 male former elite athletes and 23 control subjects who were representative of the general population revealed that both a decrease in aerobic training and an increase in body fat strongly and independently influenced the rate of decline that was observed.[18] Similarly, 13 highly trained middle-aged and older female endurance athletes (aged 49–67 years) were found to exhibit levels of VO_2max that were 85% higher on average than age-matched healthy untrained controls, consistent with previous findings in men.[19]

Other characteristics of athletic performance in older athletes have also been previously examined. For example, anaerobic muscle power in 20 young (aged 17–26 years) and 115 older (aged 40–78 years) master athletes was compared with that of 36 healthy untrained subjects (aged 22–67 years).[20] In this cross-sectional study across a wide age range, lower peak muscle power was linearly associated with age even when corrected for muscle mass. Older athletes who were power trained (i.e., sprinters, jumpers) had slightly better anaerobic muscle power than the endurance trained athletes (i.e., long-distance runners, cyclists, cross-country skiers), although the difference between these two subgroups of athletes disappeared with increasing age. Among master swimmers, a decline in speed during sprint competitions (e.g., 50- and 100-yard [or 50- and 100-meter] events) with greater cohort age has been well-documented and is mainly attributed to a decline in muscle strength with aging.[21]

Age-associated changes in organ function may also affect athletic performance and the physical capabilities of the individual. With increasing age, a reduction in the contractility of the myocardium, along with other metabolic and physiologic changes that affect cardiac function, result in a decline in the maximal heart rate.[22] Systolic blood pressure increases in association with age, and a linear decrease in the glomerular filtration rate that occurs with aging may adversely affect renal concentrating ability.[23] With increasing age, the pancreas produces less insulin in response to glucose stimulation and the sensitivity of peripheral tissues to the metabolic effects of insulin is also reduced.[24] In some instances, regular exercise may reverse these age-related processes. For example, exercise training is known to enhance insulin sensitivity,[22] specifically preventing the increase in insulin resistance that is associated with aging. Older athletes (aged 60–70 years) have been observed to exhibit hormonal and metabolic profiles before and during exercise that are more similar to those of younger athletes (aged 20–32 years) than sedentary older subjects.[25]

C.   DISEASE AND MEDICATIONS

For many older athletes, the physiologic changes attributable to aging per se are superimposed on the pathologic changes of disease, which requires some modification in the exercise prescription. For example, osteoarthritis of the knee has a prevalence rate of 28% among individuals aged 55–64 years and increases to 39% among 65- to 74-year-olds.[26] Although there are a few contraindications to exercise in elderly patients (e.g., severe dementia) most older individuals are capable of some degree of regular exercise to maintain or improve their level of physical fitness.[22,27] The most common limitations that must be imposed due to the presence of disease consist of exercising at a lower intensity for a longer duration and doing activities that involve less impact on joints. With special attention to warm-up and technique, even individuals with osteoarthritis of the knee have been shown to benefit from supervised exercise programs, including walking.[28]

The exercise prescription for the older individual with coronary heart disease involves adaptations and modifications to adjust for the structural and functional cardiovascular changes.[29] Depending on the level of activity, a cardiologist may need to provide a specific exercise prescription, and safety can be further ensured if the individual exercises in a supervised setting.[22] Exercise and aerobic conditioning have a recognized role in enhancing recovery and functional capacity following a myocardial infarction or the diagnosis of ischemic heart disease in older individuals.

Older athletes are also more likely to be using prescribed and over-the-counter medications when compared with younger athletes, and chronic medication use can impose additional considerations when determining nutritional needs.[30] In addition to polypharmacy, i.e., the regular use of several prescription and over-the-counter medications, vitamin and other nutrient supplement use is quite common among older individuals.[31] Some have argued that nutrient supplementation may provide some benefits for the older age groups,[32] although this practice may result in nutrient imbalance or excess.[33]

D. EXERCISE PATTERNS

Recent reports from the Third National Health and Nutrition Examination Survey (NHANES III) indicate that walking and gardening or yard work, remain the most frequently reported leisure-time physical activities among all U.S. adults aged 20 years or older.[3] A decreasing proportion of the population participates in regular exercise in association with aging, which is evident when prevalence rates across the age groups are compared.[3] Among men aged 50–59 years, 18% report no leisure-time physical activity, which increases to 40% among those aged 80 years or older. Among women aged 50–59 years, 30% report no leisure-time physical activity, and this proportion steadily increases to 62% among those aged 80 years or older.

In a previous survey focused on older adults,[34] walking was specifically found to be the most common type of exercise in adults 65 years of age and older. Notably, large gender differences were present: 70% of the men vs 57% of the women reported that they walked regularly. In many urban communities, indoor shopping malls have been made available during non-retail business hours for older adults who may have substantial barriers to regular walking, such as climate, poor air quality, and personal safety.

Swimming and supervised water aerobics classes (which do not require swimming skills) are other alternatives for the older athlete with musculoskeletal limitations. Individuals in master swimming and track and field programs train against age-specific standards in a supportive atmosphere that encourages fitness exercise or training to compete with others of the same age and gender. Recent research has demonstrated that resistance training can effectively increase muscle mass and strength in the elderly individual (discussed below), although it has little or no effect on VO_2max.[35] For this reason, an exercise program that includes both aerobic exercise and strength training is probably ideal for the overall health of the older athlete.

Injuries, associated with either acute trauma or overuse syndromes, are a risk of sports activities and athletics in any age group, and risk for injury among older athletes has been investigated in a few previous studies. Musculoskeletal injuries are the most common type reported among older runners, but the rates in the older age groups are comparable to those of younger athletes who are running at the same mileage level.[36,37] In a recent comparison of injuries in 57 older (>60 years old) vs 457 younger (aged 21–25 years) athletes at a sports medicine clinic,[38] knee injuries were the most common type in both age groups. A greater proportion of injuries in the older age group, compared with the younger age group, were overuse injuries (70% vs 41%, respectively).

III. SPECIFIC NUTRITIONAL CONCERNS

A. ENERGY AND MACRONUTRIENTS

The average older individual, when compared with younger age groups, requires a lower level of energy intake for weight maintenance.[7,13,33] The two primary reasons for this observed difference are a lower level of lean body mass or skeletal muscle and reduced physical activity, rather than more efficient use of energy by the metabolically active tissue. Because the amount of lean body mass is the major determinant of energy expenditure, the size of this compartment in the older athlete is most important for defining the individual energy requirement. Most adults spontaneously consume lower amounts of energy in association with aging, often to the degree that nutritional needs may not be met if total dietary intake becomes increasingly limited.[32,33] However, many active older adults are specifically concerned with (and need guidance for) weight control, which may also be the motivating factor for their involvement in the exercise program.[39] The older athlete has the advantage of being able to consume relatively greater amounts of energy than sedentary peers, without causing unwanted weight gain. Evidence to suggest that increased exercise may promote a spontaneous increase in energy and nutrient intake in older adults is inconsistent.[7,13,33]

Balancing energy intake with energy expenditure is the key component of long-term weight control for adults of all ages.[40] Several methods of estimating energy needs have been developed, and the most commonly used are formulas based on height, body weight, age, and other factors such as general activity level or the presence of physiologic stress. The most classic of these is the Harris-Benedict equation:[42]

$$\text{Women:} \quad \text{BEE} = 655 + 9.6(W) + 1.8(H) - 4.7(A)$$
$$\text{Men:} \quad \text{BEE} = 66 + 13.7(W) + 5(H) - 6.8(A)$$

where BEE = Basal energy expenditure (kcal/day), W = weight (kg), H = height (cm), and A = age (yr). To estimate the average total daily energy expenditure, multiply BEE × 1.3. To convert to kJ/day, multiply by 4.184. In estimating the energy requirement, figures derived from this formula tend to overestimate the needs of sedentary women, underestimate the basal needs of athletic women, and may also underestimate energy requirements for older men (>65 years of age).[13,42,43] The energy cost of exercise is well known to have a potentially large effect on total daily energy expenditure; for example, a 155-pound (70.5 kg) man expends 1–1.2 kcal/min (4–5 kJ/min) while sitting quietly and 5–7.4 kcal/min (21–31 kJ/min) while walking.

The loss of one pound (2.2 kg) of body fat is estimated to result from an energy deficit of 3500 kcal (14,644 kJ), which can be achieved safely in one week by a daily deficit of 500 kcal (2092 kJ). Energy restricted diets for obese adults that promote a loss of 1% of body weight per week pose little health risk and may promote maintenance of weight loss.[44] A key characteristic of successful weight management is that the behavioral patterns and modification in food choices that are adopted to promote weight loss are continued as permanent and healthful lifestyle changes. Weight control programs with the potential for success and minimal risk for older adults are based on eating plans that satisfy all nutrient needs besides energy, include food choices that meet individual tastes and habits, and are conducive to improvement of overall health and permanent behavior change.[44]

The current dietary recommendations for the distribution of energy intake among the macronutrients (e.g., carbohydrate, protein, fat) in the diets of older athletes are similar to the recommendations for the general population.[45,46] Carbohydrates should contribute 50–60%, protein should contribute 10–20%, and fat should be limited to 30% of energy in a dietary pattern which is mainly comprised of grain products, vegetables, fruits, low-fat dairy products, and lower-fat sources of protein. In athletes who participate in prolonged and intense exercise, low muscle glycogen levels have been linked specifically to exhaustion and consumption of adequate amounts of carbohydrate facilitates restoration of depleted glycogen stores. For the average individual in the United States, dietary fat currently provides 34% of energy, so some modification in food choices may be advisable to achieve the recommended level. However, very-low-fat diets (<20% of energy) are not necessarily advantageous and are associated with some disadvantages for the older athlete, such as limited meal satiety and reduced absorption of possibly protective micronutrients such as carotenoids.[40,44]

Older individuals concerned with dietary fat intake and cardiovascular disease should be advised that saturated fat, rather than total fat or cholesterol, is the dietary factor that exerts the greatest influence on blood cholesterol levels, thus increasing disease risk. The eating pattern recommended by the National Cholesterol Education Program (NCEP) of the National Heart, Lung, and Blood Institute involves an intake of saturated fat of 8–10% of energy, 30% or less of energy from total fat, and cholesterol less than 300 mg/day.[45] In adults whose serum cholesterol does not respond to this degree of diet modification, the NCEP Step 2 guidelines (see Table 1), which involve a greater restriction of saturated fat and cholesterol intake, are recommended.

The current RDA for protein for adults is 0.8 g/kg/day, which may underestimate the protein requirements of the older athlete. Evans[7,47] has suggested that a level of protein intake more likely to promote nitrogen balance, particularly among elderly adults, is 1.00–1.25 g/kg/day, derived primarily from high quality protein sources (i.e., lean meat, poultry, fish, dairy products). Maintenance of lean body mass is dependent in part on overall nitrogen balance, although protein metabolism and nitrogen balance are highly dependent on adequate energy intake as well.

B. MICRONUTRIENTS: VITAMINS AND MINERALS

An increasing amount of evidence suggests that aging may affect the requirements for certain vitamins.[48] Influencing factors that may play a role in these changing needs include alterations in the capability of absorbing and metabolizing these compounds, differing baseline metabolic requirements, and specific age-related risk factors. Table 2 summarizes the current RDA for vitamins and minerals for older adults.

For vitamin D, the current RDA (5 µg/day) may be too low for many older individuals, who are at particular risk for adverse effects of poor vitamin D status, such as negative calcium balance. For example, a level of >5.5 µg/day was found to be necessary to maintain normal circulating concentrations of the active metabolite, 1,25-dihydroxyvitamin D, and

TABLE 1   Dietary Modifications for Hypercholesterolemia

Dietary Component	Step 1 Diet	Step 2 Diet
Total fat	<30% of kcal	<30% of kcal
Saturated fat	8–10% of kcal	<7% of kcal
Polyunsaturated fat	<10% of kcal	<10% of kcal
Monounsaturated fat	10–15% of kcal	10–15% of kcal
Carbohydrate	50–60% of kcal	50–60% of kcal
Protein	10–20% of kcal	10–20% of kcal
Cholesterol	<300 mg/day	<200 mg/day
Total energy intake	To achieve and maintain desirable weight	To achieve and maintain desirable weight

Adapted from Expert Panel on Detection, Evaluation, and Treatment of High Blood Cholesterol in Adults.[45]

TABLE 2 Recommended Dietary Allowances for Adults Aged 51 Years and Older

Micronutrient	Males	Females
Vitamin A (µg RE/day)	1000	800
Vitamin D (µg/day)	5	5
Vitamin E (mg α-TE/day)	10	8
Vitamin K (µg/day)	80	65
Vitamin C (mg/day)	60	60
Thiamin (mg/day)	1.2	1.0
Riboflavin (mg/day)	1.4	1.2
Niacin (mg/day)	15	13
Vitamin B_6 (mg/day)	2.0	1.6
Folate (µg/day)	200	180
Vitamin B_{12} (µg/day)	2.0	2.0
Calcium (mg/day)	800	800
Phosphorus (mg/day)	800	800
Magnesium (mg/day)	350	280
Iron (mg/day)	10	10
Zinc (mg/day)	15	12
Iodine (µg/day)	150	150
Selenium (µg/day)	70	55

Adapted from Food and Nutrition Board, Commission on Life Sciences, National Research Council.[5]

parathyroid hormone in 333 postmenopausal women.[49] Endogenous production of vitamin D during sunlight exposure has been shown to be less efficient in older vs younger individuals,[50] which increases the importance of the exogenous supply (dietary intake) of this micronutrient. Vitamin B_6 requirements of older individuals may also be higher than the current RDA (2.0 and 1.6 mg/day in males and females, respectively). Evidence from depletion and repletion studies using a highly bioavailable formulation indicates that a minimum intake of 1.96 and 1.90 mg/day for men and women, respectively, should be recommended.[51] The requirement for vitamin B_{12} may be higher in older vs younger individuals, in part due to the increased prevalence of atrophic gastritis (which reduces absorption efficiency) in association with aging. Current data suggest that an intake of 3.0 µg vitamin B_{12}/day may be more appropriate than the current RDA of 2.0 µg/day for older adults.[48] Some evidence suggests that the current RDA level for riboflavin may have little margin for error in older individuals, so an increase in the level recommended to that recommended for younger adults (1.7 and 1.3 mg/day for males and females, respectively) may be advisable.[48]

Increased amounts of other micronutrients have been recommended for older individuals based primarily on associations with risk for diseases associated with aging, such as vitamin C to reduce risk for cataracts and vitamin E and folate to reduce risk for cardiovascular disease.[32] Adequate amounts of all of these other essential micronutrients are required for the older athlete, but insufficient data are currently available to prescribe levels beyond those of the RDA. Several studies involving institutionalized elderly and other high risk groups suggest that some subgroups of the older population may not be consuming the recommended levels of vitamins, primarily due to overall dietary inadequacy.[32,33] Known risk factors for inadequate micronutrient intake are alcohol abuse, restricted energy intake (<1200 kcal/day [5021 kJ/day]), and socioeconomic factors, such as limited income and social isolation. In older athletes who are limiting total energy intake, increased nutrient density of the diet becomes an important consideration if the dietary requirements for vitamins are to be met.

Because dietary calcium plays a permissive role in age-related bone loss, adequate calcium intake is of great importance for optimal health of the older athlete.[52] Current evidence suggests that the RDA for older adults (800 mg/day) is lower than the level needed to facilitate calcium balance, suggested to be 1200–1500 mg/day for older athletes.[13] The interaction between estrogen status of the older female athlete and dietary calcium requirement is illustrated by calcium balance studies[53] in which 1000 mg calcium/day was shown to be necessary for estrogen-treated postmenopausal women vs 1500 mg/day for those not prescribed hormone replacement therapy.

Iron is another mineral of interest in the older athlete, and issues of both inadequacy and excessive intake are current considerations. Because of increased iron losses, the dietary iron requirement for male distance runners (and postmenopausal female runners) has been suggested to be nearly 18 mg/day,[54] rather than the current RDA of 10 mg/day. From another perspective, however, results from recent epidemiologic studies suggest that excessive iron may actually increase risk for cardiovascular disease and cancer,[55] so hematologic evidence of inadequacy of the body stores (i.e., serum ferritin concentration) should be the basis for considering the need for iron supplementation.

Similar to vitamins, inadequate intake of essential minerals may occur as a result of overall dietary inadequacy in the older athlete. Excessive amounts of several micronutrients, including both vitamins and minerals, are known to cause adverse effects and toxicities. For older athletes who choose to use supplements or who may have dietary inadequacies, recommending a low-dose vitamin and mineral supplement at RDA levels (with exceptions described above) is a low-risk approach.

C. FLUID REPLACEMENT

Adequate fluid consumption is important for athletes of all ages, because sufficient water is crucial for body temperature regulation. Several physiologic changes associated with aging, such as reduced thirst and poor renal responsiveness to limited fluid intake, may increase risk for dehydration in the older athlete.[56] Reduced heat tolerance has been reported to be more common among older vs younger individuals.[57] In addition to increased risk for dehydration, another factor that may contribute to altered thermoregulatory response to heat in older athletes is reduced skin blood flow, which has been suggested to be 25–40% lower in older vs younger athletes.[58] Some reports also indicate that aging is associated with reduced sweating capabilities,[56] but whether or not this difference is of functional significance for the older athlete is unclear.[59]

To reduce risk for dehydration, older athletes need encouragement to consume sufficient water before, during, and after exercise. A common approach is to prescribe the consumption of two cups (473 ml) of water before the exercise and 200–400 ml of water every 20 min of activity.[40] The water should be cool (40–50°F [4–10°C]), which may help to stabilize the core body temperature. If fluid replacement drinks are consumed, the concentration of carbohydrate should not exceed 10%, so that fluid absorption is not delayed. Most sport drinks and fluid replacement products currently available are formulated at this level, but fruit juice must be diluted to half-strength to achieve the appropriate concentration. Heat acclimation is another important protective factor, and this occurs in older as well as younger athletes who exercise regularly in warm ambient temperatures.

IV. PRACTICAL CONSIDERATIONS AND APPROACHES

A. NUTRITIONAL ASSESSMENT

Nutritional assessment of the older athlete is hampered by the fact that the majority of the normative data and standards available are based on observations of younger subjects or have been extrapolated from those data. Another problem is that historically, the older age groups studied have had a functional capacity that is substantially lower than is likely to be found in the older trained athlete. Thus, changes associated with chronological age have been confused with changes due to chronic physical inactivity. Also, as aging progresses, there is an increased likelihood of disease, so that physiologic and metabolic characteristics of disease are represented in most collective data from older age groups. Over the past few years, nationally representative reference data have been collected from the noninstitution-alized older age groups in NHANES III, so these data may improve the comparability of standards available.[60]

Specific nutritional issues in the older athlete can be addressed by obtaining a comprehensive diet history, which includes exploring the reasons for food choices and patterns. For example, some older athletes consume inadequate amounts of water because they suffer mild incontinence when exercising, which requires a practical solution if fluid needs are to be met. Gastroesophageal reflux is more likely to be problematic in the older (vs younger) athlete, which may occur with exercise even if minimal amounts of low-fat foods are consumed before the activity.[61] Symptoms of gastroesophageal reflux can be confused with chest pain and other sensations indicative of impaired myocardial function, which is particularly an issue for the older athlete at risk of (or diagnosed with) coronary heart disease. Solutions to minimize the uncomfortable symptoms of reflux include avoidance of pre-exercise meals and modifications in the intensity or type of exercise (if this option is acceptable to the individual), but pharmacologic management may need to be considered. As is true of athletes of all ages, recognizing the importance of individual preference and tolerance is crucial in providing meaningful dietary guidance.

Serum albumin is the most commonly available biochemical measure that may reflect overall nutritional status, although the concentration of this visceral protein is strongly influenced by numerous non-nutritional variables, such as level of hydration and posture when the blood sample is collected. Although it has been suggested that serum albumin concentration declines as part of the aging process, any age-related reduction appears to be minimal.[62] Many of the micronutrients are transported nonspecifically by albumin in the circulation, so any changes in the level of this or any other transport protein affects interpretation of circulating micronutrient concentrations. Vitamin E and the carotenoids are transported in the circulation nonspecifically by the cholesterol-carrying lipoproteins, so lipoprotein levels are a major determinant of these micronutrient concentrations.[63]

Among the anthropometric approaches to evaluating nutritional status, multiple skinfold fat measures are useful for estimating percent body fat of older athletes, but calculation formulas or tables that are used should be age-specific.[64] Body composition estimates that are derived from measuring the fat-free compartment may be more difficult to interpret in the older athlete because of the changes in body composition associated with aging.[65] Changes in skeletal mass, which can be anticipated in the older individual, will affect density of fat-free tissues and the interpretation of body composition estimates using mathematical models derived from data on younger individuals. Height should always be measured in the older athlete rather than obtained by self-report, because stature decline occurs over the lifespan. Based on data collected from men and women aged 60–80 years, the rate of decrease in stature is estimated to be up to 0.5 cm/year.[65]

Older athletes with comorbid disease (i.e., diabetes mellitus) or multiple medication use are likely to benefit from an individualized diet prescription from a registered dietitian.[66] Assistance with meal planning that is specific for the lifestyle of the individual can be crucial to enable the older athlete to eat a healthy diet. For example, older individuals are more likely to live alone or in a two-person household when compared with younger age groups, so convenience foods may form the basis of the food choices. Convenience food choices range from health-promoting to nutritionally lacking, so strategies such as food label reading can be useful.

B. CURRENT TRENDS

In a balanced exercise program for the older athlete, both endurance and resistance training are likely to be helpful components: endurance exercise to promote aerobic fitness and increase the cardiovascular capacity and resistance or weight training to increase skeletal mass and strength. Results from numerous studies have demonstrated that older individuals can improve VO₂max with either low or high intensity aerobic exercise,[7] which also improves metabolic changes such as delayed glucose clearance. More recently, high-intensity resistance training, as a specific strategy to increase muscle size and strength, has been demonstrated to have a substantial favorable effect in subjects 60 years of age and older, as reviewed by others.[7,47,67] For example, a 10-week high-intensity resistance training program involving progressive training of the hip and knee extensors 3 days/week was shown to increase muscle size, strength, and ambulation capabilities in a group of 100 very frail elderly (average age 87 years).[68] Clearly, an increase in muscle mass and strength can occur at any age.

Combined exercise approaches can also have synergistic effects. Following a 12-week resistance training program, a group of 24 community-dwelling, nondisabled older individuals (65–79 years old) increased both leg strength and submaximal walking endurance.[69] As reviewed elsewhere,[7] both aerobic and resistance exercise approaches may influence nutritional needs: adequate energy and protein intake is necessary to enable protein synthesis and increased muscle mass, and protein requirements increase during endurance exercise due to utilization of amino acids as substrates for energy production.

In studies of the cohorts that currently comprise the older age groups, substantial gender differences are usually evident in strength and fitness measures, with women having markedly lower baseline (and sometimes post-training) muscle strength and peak aerobic capacity. This difference reflects leisure-time physical activity patterns during the adult years, which have been observed to decrease with increasing age more markedly among women than men.[3] The socialization of women has traditionally not involved any encouragement to exercise and has made older women feel uncomfortable with normal aspects of exercise, such as sweating. Social support and opportunities for women to participate in athletic activities, especially among mature adults, is a relatively recent phenomenon. With the trend for increasing acceptability of women to achieve and maintain athletic abilities throughout adulthood, a reduction in gender differences may be evident as new generations enter the older age groups.

V. SUMMARY AND CONCLUSIONS

The older age groups are an increasing proportion of the population, notable for both physiologic heterogeneity and overall changing nature due to shifts in demographic and sociocultural patterns in the United States.[1] In general, aging is associated with reductions in lean body mass and bone mineral density and an increased proportion of abdominal fat,[10] although changes in body composition and metabolic features that have been assumed to be age-related may be modifiable by regular physical activity.[16-18] Both endurance and resistance training are helpful components of a balanced exercise program for the older athlete. Increased likelihood of disease and medication use in the older age groups also influences the nutritional needs and the nature of the dietary guidance that is provided.[30,33] A lower level of energy intake is usually required for weight maintenance in the older adult, so that healthful weight-control behaviors may need to be encouraged. Specific considerations of nutrient density and dietary characteristics that may prevent disease need to be addressed in the eating plan. Fluid replacement and dietary intake of adequate amounts of several micronutrients, such as vitamin D, vitamin B₁₂, and calcium, may be important issues in the nutritional care of the older athlete.[48,52] An important practical consideration is that dietary advice should be individualized to accomodate lifestyle, tolerance, and preferences.

REFERENCES

1. Manton, K. G., Corder, L. S., and Stallard, E., Estimates of change in chronic disability and institutional incidence and prevalence rates in the U.S. elderly population from the 1982, 1984, and 1989 National Long Term Care Survey, *J. Gerontol.*, 48, S153, 1993.
2. Chernoff, R., Baby boomers come of age: nutrition in the 21st century, *J. Am. Diet. Assoc.*, 95, 650, 1995.
3. Crespo, C. J., Keteyian, S. J., Heath, G. W., and Sempos, C. T., Leisure-time physical activity among US adults, *Arch. Intern. Med.*, 156, 93, 1996.
4. Lipschitz, D. A., Preface: nutrition, aging, and age-dependent diseases, *Clin. Geriatr. Med.*, 11, xi, 1995.
5. Food and Nutrition Board, Commission on Life Sciences, National Research Council, *Recommended Dietary Allowances*, 10th ed., National Academy Press, Washington, D.C., 1989.
6. Sipila, S., Viitasalo, J., Era, P., and Suominen, H., Muscle strength in male athletes aged 70–81 years and a population sample, *Eur. J. Appl. Physiol.*, 63, 399, 1991.
7. Evans, W. J., Exercise, nutrition, and aging, *Clin. Geriatr. Med.*, 11, 725, 1995.
8. Aniansson, A. and Gustafsson, E., Physical training in elderly men with special reference to quadriceps muscle strength and morphology, *Clin. Physiol.*, 1, 87, 1981.
9. Viitasalo, J., Era, P., Leskinen, A.-L., and Heikkinen, E., Muscular strength and anthropometry in random samples of men aged 31–35, 51–55, and 71–75 years, *Ergonomics*, 28, 1563, 1985.
10. Forbes, G. B., The adult decline in lean body mass, *Hum. Biol.*, 48, 162, 1976.
11. Munro, H. H., Nutrition and aging, *Br. Med. Bull.*, 37, 83, 1981.
12. Pratley, R. E., Hagberg, J. M., Rogus, E. M., and Goldberg, A. P. Enhanced insulin sensitivity and lower waist-to-hip ratio in master athletes, *Am. J. Physiol.*, 31, E484, 1995.
13. Kendrick, Z. V., Nelson-Steen, S., and Scafidi, K., Exercise, aging, and nutrition, *Southern Med. J.*, 87, S50, 1994.
14. Nelson, M. E., Fiatarone, M. A., Morganti, C. M., Trice, I., Greenberg, R. A., and Evans, W. J., Effects of high-intensity strength training on multiple risk factors for osteoporotic fractures, *J. Am. Med. Assoc.*, 272, 1909, 1994.
15. Astrand, I., Aerobic work capacity in men and women with special reference to age, *Acta Physiol. Scand.*, 169 (Suppl.), 1, 1960.
16. Pollock, M. L., Foster, C., Knapp, D., Rod., J. L., and Schmidt, D. H., Effect of age and training on aerobic capacity and body composition of master athletes, *J. Appl. Physiol.*, 62, 625, 1987.
17. Rogers, M. A., Hagberg, J. M., Martin, W. H., Ehsani, A. A., and Holloszy, J. O., Decline in VO_2max with aging in master athletes and sedentary men, *J. Appl. Physiol.*, 68, 2195, 1990.
18. Marti, B. and Howald, H., Long-term effects of physical training on aerobic capacity: controlled study of former elite athletes, *J. Appl. Physiol.*, 69, 1452, 1990.
19. Stevenson, E. T., Davy, K. P., and Seals, D. R., Maximal aerobic capacity and total blood volume in highly trained middle-aged and older female endurance athletes, *J. Appl. Physiol.*, 77, 1691, 1994.
20. Grassi, B., Cerretelli, P., Narici, M. V., and Marconi, C., Peak anaerobic power in master athletes, *Eur. J. Appl. Physiol.*, 62, 394, 1991.
21. Hartley, A. A. and Hartley, J. T., Age differences and changes in sprint swimming performances of masters athletes, *Exp. Aging Res.*, 12, 65, 1986.
22. Lowenthall, D. T., Kirschner, D. A., Scarpace, N. T., Pollock, M., and Graves, J., Effects of exercise on age and disease, *Southern Med. J.*, 87, S5, 1994.
23. Lindeman, R. D., Tobin, J., and Shock, N. W., Longitudinal studies on the rate of decline in renal function with age, *J. Am. Geriatr. Soc.*, 33, 278, 1985.
24. Davidson, M. B., The effect of aging on carbohydrate metabolism: a review of the English literature and a practical approach to the diagnosis of diabetes mellitus in the elderly, *Metab. Clin. Exp.*, 28, 687, 1979.
25. Hagberg, J. M., Seals, D. R., Yerg, J. E., Gavin, J., Gingerich, R., Premachandra, B., and Holloszy, J. O., Metabolic responses to exercise in young and older athletes and sedentary men, *J. Appl. Physiol.*, 65, 900, 1988.
26. Forman, M. D., Malamet, R., and Kaplan, D., A survey of osteoarthritis of the knee in the elderly, *J. Rheumatol.*, 10, 282, 1983.
27. Lampman, R., Evaluating and prescribing exercise for elderly patients, *Geriatrics*, 42, 63, 1987.
28. Kovar, P. A., Allegrante, J. P., MacKenzie, C. R., Peterson, M. G., Gutin, B., and Charlson, M. E., Supervised fitness walking in patients with osteoarthritis of the knee: a randomized controlled trial, *Ann. Intern. Med.*, 116, 529, 1992.
29. Wenger, N. K., Guidelines for exercise training of elderly patients with coronary artery disease, *Southern Med. J.*, 87, S66, 1994.
30. Roe, D., Drug and nutrient interactions in the elderly diabetic, *Drug-Nutrient Interactions*, 5, 195, 1988.
31. Subar, A. F. and Block, G., Use of vitamin and mineral supplements: demographics and amounts of nutrients consumed, *Am. J. Epidemiol.*, 132, 1091, 1990.

32. Blumberg, J., Nutrient requirements of the healthy elderly — should there be specific RDAs?, *Nutr. Rev.*, 52, S15, 1994.
33. Chernoff, R., Effects of age on nutrient requirements, *Clin. Geriatr. Med.*, 11, 641, 1995.
34. Dallosso, W. M., Morgan, K., Bassey, E. J., Ebrahim, S. B., Fentem, P. H., and Arie, T. H., Levels of customary physical activity among the old and the very old living at home, *J. Epidemiol. Comm. Health*, 42, 1221, 1988.
35. Hagberg, J. M., Graves, J. E., Limacher, M., Woods, D. R., Leggett, S. H., Cononie, C., Gruber, J. J., and Pollock, M. L., Cardiovascular responses of 70–79 year old men and women to endurance and strength training, *J. Appl. Physiol.*, 66, 2589, 1989.
36. Kaplan, J. P., Powell, K. E., Sikes, R. K., Shirley, R. W., and Campbell, C. C., Epidemiologic study of the benefits and risks of running, *J. Am. Med. Assoc.*, 248, 3118, 1982.
37. Hogan, D. B. and Cape, R. D., Marathoners over sixty years of age: results of a survey, *J. Am. Geriatr. Soc.*, 34, 121, 1984.
38. Kannus, P., Niittymaki, S., Jarvinen, M., and Lehto, M., Sports injuries in elderly athletes: a three-year prospective, controlled study, *Age Ageing*, 18, 263, 1989.
39. Williamson, D. F., Serdula, M. K., Anda, R. F., Levy, A., and Byers, T., Weight loss attempts in adults: goals, duration, and rate of weight loss, *Am. J. Pub. Health*, 82, 1251, 1992.
40. Rock, C. L., Nutrition of the older athlete, *Clin. Sports Med.*, 10, 445, 1991.
41. Harris, J. A. and Benedict, F. G., *A Biometric Study of Basal Metabolism in Man*, The Carnegie Institute, Washington, D.C., 40, 1919.
42. Owen, O. E., Kavle, E., Owen, R. S., Polansky, M., Caprio, S., Mozzoli, M. A., Kendrick, Z. V., Bushman, M. C., and Boden, G., A reappraisal of caloric requirements in healthy women, *Am. J. Clin. Nutr.*, 44, 1, 1986.
43. Owen, O. E., Holup, F. L., D'Alessio, D. A., Craig, E. S., Polansky, M., Smalley, K. J., Kavle, E. C., Bushman, M. C., Owen, L. R., Mozzoli, M. A., Kenrick, Z. V., and Boden, G. H., A reappraisal of the caloric requirements of men, *Am. J. Clin. Nutr.*, 46, 875, 1987.
44. Coulston, A. M. and Rock, C. L., Popular diets and use of moderate calorie restriction for the treatment of obesity, in *Obesity: Pathophysiology, Psychology and Treatment*, Blackburn, G. L. and Kanders, B. S., Eds., Chapman Hall, North Potomac, MD, 1994, 185.
45. Expert Panel on Detection, Evaluation, and Treatment of High Blood Cholesterol in Adults, *Second Report of the Expert Panel on Detection, Evaluation, and Treatment of High Blood Cholesterol in Adults*, NIH Publication no. 93-3095, National Institutes of Health, Bethesda, MD, 1993
46. Human Nutrition Information Service, U.S. Department of Agriculture, *The Food Guide Pyramid*, Home and Garden Bulletin no. 252, U.S. Government Printing Office, Washington, D.C., 1992.
47. Evans, W. J., Exercise, nutrition, and aging, *J. Nutr.*, 122, 796, 1992.
48. Russell, R. M. and Suter, P. M., Vitamin requirements of elderly people: an update, *Am. J. Clin. Nutr.*, 48, 4, 1993.
49. Krall, E. A., Sahyoun, N., Tannenbaum, S., Dallal, G. E., and Dawson-Hughes, B., Effects of vitamin D intake on seasonal variations in parathyroid hormone secretion in postmenopausal women, *New Eng. J. Med.*, 321, 1777, 1989.
50. MacLaughlin, J. and Holick, M. F., Aging decreases the capacity of human skin to produce vitamin D_3, *J. Clin. Invest.*, 76, 1536, 1985.
51. Ribaya-Mercado, J. D., Russell, R. M., Sahyoun, N., Morrow, F. D., and Gershoff, S. N., Vitamin B-6 requirements of elderly men and women, *Am. J. Clin. Nutr.*, 121, 1062, 1991.
52. Dawson-Hughes, B., Dallal, G. E., Krall, E. A., Sadowski, L., Sahyoun, N., and Tannenbaum, S., A controlled trial of the effect of calcium supplementation on bone density in postmenopausal women, *New Eng. J. Med.*, 323, 878, 1990.
53. Heaney, R. P., Recker, R. R., and Saville, P. D., Menopausal changes in calcium balance performance, *J. Lab. Clin. Med.*, 92, 953, 1978.
54. Weaver, C. M. and Rajaram, S., Exercise and iron status, *J. Nutr.*, 122, 782, 1992.
55. Salonen, J. T., Nyyssonen, K., Korpela, H., Tuomilehto, J., Seppanen, R., and Salonen, R., High stored iron levels are associated with excess risk of myocardial infarction in Eastern Finnish men, *Circulation*, 86, 803, 1992.
56. Chernoff, R., Thirst and fluid requirements, *Nutr. Rev.*, 52, S3, 1994.
57. Meischer, E. and Forney, S. M., Responses to dehydration and rehydration during heat exposure in young and older men, *Am. J. Physiol.*, 257, R1050, 1989.
58. Kenney, W. L., Control of heat-induced vasodilation in relation to age, *Eur. J. Appl. Physiol.*, 57, 120, 1988.
59. Kenney, W. L. and Hodgson, J. L., Heat tolerance, thermoregulation and aging, *Sports Med.*, 4, 446, 1987.
60. National Center for Health Statistics, Plan and operation of the Third National Health and Nutrition Examination Survey, 1988–94, *Vital Health Stat.*, 1(32), 1, 1994.
61. Clark, C. S., Kraus, B. B., Sinclair, J., and Castell, D. O., Gastroesophageal reflux induced by exercise in healthy volunteers, *J. Am. Med. Assoc.*, 261, 3599, 1989.
62. Campion, E. W., DeLabry, L. O., and Glynn, R. J., The effect of age on serum albumin in healthy males: report from the Normative Aging Study, *J. Gerontol.*, 43, M18, 1988.

63. Rock, C. L., Jacob, R. A., and Bowen, P. E., Biological characteristics of the antioxidant micronutrients, vitamin C, vitamin E, and the carotenoids: an update, *J. Am. Diet. Assoc.*, 96, 693, 1996.

64. Durnin, J. V. and Wormersley, J., Body fat assessed from total body density and its estimation from skinfold thickness: measurements of 481 men and women aged from 16 to 72 years, *Br. J. Nutr.*, 32, 77, 1974.

65. Chumlea, W. C. and Baumgartner, R. N., Status of anthropometry and body composition data in elderly subjects, *Am. J. Clin. Nutr.*, 50, 1158, 1989.

66. Position of the American Dietetic Association: nutrition recommendations and principles for people with diabetes mellitus, *J. Am. Diet. Assoc.*, 94, 504, 1994.

67. Graves, J. E., Pollock, M. L., and Carroll, J. F., Exercise, age, and skeletal muscle function, *Southern Med. J.*, 87, S17, 1994.

68. Fiatarone, M. A., O'Neill, E. F., Ryan, N. D., Clements, K. M., Solares, G. R., Nelson, M. E., Roberts, S. B., Kehayias, J. J., Lipsitz, L. A., and Evans, W. J., Exercise training and nutritional supplementation for physical frailty in very elderly people, *New Eng. J. Med.*, 330, 1769, 1994.

69. Ades, P. A., Ballor, D. L., Ashikaga, T., Utton, J. L., and Sreekumaran, K., Weight training improves walking endurance in healthy elderly persons, *Ann. Int. Med.*, 124, 568, 1996.

Chapter 20

THE DIABETIC ATHLETE

Eric Small
Elliott Rayfield
Doron Aaronson

CONTENTS

0-8493-8560-1/97/$0.00+$.50
© 1998 by CRC Press LLC

I. INTRODUCTION

Diabetes, a complex disease that in its terminal stages may affect almost every organ system, affects up to seven million U.S. children and adults. For the sake of this chapter, one can assume that Type I Diabetes (insulin dependent — IDDM) is reserved for children, adolescents, and young adults while Type II Diabetes (non-insulin dependent — NIDDM) refers to adults. It is the purpose of this chapter to discuss the interplay of nutrition and exercise on the individual with diabetes. Wherever possible the benefits and risks of exercise in addition to the types of appropriate activities will be discussed.

II. TYPE I DIABETES

Type I Diabetes affects approximately one million U.S. children and adolescents. Several key factors have been attributed to its occurrence including genetic predisposition, autoimmune factors, and environmental conditions.[1,2] Individuals with Type I Diabetes often demonstrate an association with inherited histocompatibility antigen types and with cell-mediated and serologic autoimmunity.[3] The nature of the disease requires a keen knowledge of one's dietary intake and anticipated activities. Open communication and consultation with others knowledgeable about the disease is a necessity.

A. EXERCISE AND THE TYPE I DIABETIC

The diabetic youngster who partakes in athletics must be able to handle a diet regimen, exercise, and insulin administration (Figure 1). All of these factors are independent variables yet, when one is affected the others are altered as well.

By first defining the intensity and duration of exercise one can further elucidate both the dietary and insulin requirements. Aerobic exercise can be divided into short (less than 20 min), intermediate (20–60 min), and endurance exercise (greater than 60 min). The intensity of the exercise (mild — <50% VO_2max; moderate — 50–60% VO_2max; severe 70–80% VO_2max) must also be taken into account when deciding on the proper nutritional requirements and insulin treatment.

B. METABOLIC CONTROL OF BLOOD GLUCOSE

It is necessary to compare the control of serum glucose in healthy individuals to those with Type I diabetes during exercise. General factors and hormones affect metabolic fuel utilization during exercise as well as glucose homeostasis.

Exercise intensity and duration, physical training and diet affect the proportion of carbohydrate and free fatty acids utilized during exercise. During moderate exercise intensity (50–60% VO_2max) 50% of energy comes from carbohydrate oxidation and 50% from free fatty acids (FFA). At 70–75% VO_2max carbohydrate is the predominant energy source; at 100% VO_2max almost all energy is derived from carbohydrate oxidation.[4] At low to moderate

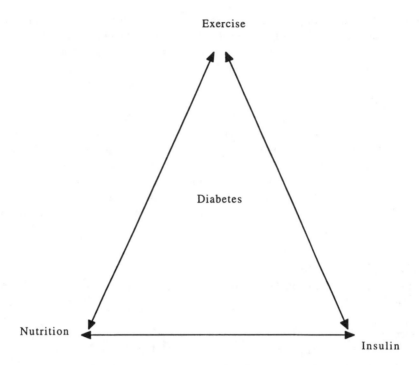

FIGURE 1 Management of Diabetes.

intensity exercise that is continuous in nature, carbohydrate oxidation is the main energy source up to two hours. Beyond two hours FFA becomes the primary metabolic fuel.

The aerobic physical fitness of an individual affects the metabolic fuel preferentially used during exercise. More fit individuals exercising at the same VO_2max use less carbohydrate and more FFA than the untrained. This physiologic fact leads to less depletion of glycogen stores and therefore better endurance.

C. DIET

The pre-exercise diet plays a role in substrate utilization during exercise. Over the years investigators have analyzed the effect of a high carbohydrate diet[5,6] on carbohydrate oxidation and endurance. Success on high intensity cycling exercise is correlated with pre-exercise muscle glycogen content.[6]

The effects of feeding supplemental drinks or snacks on glucose homeostasis prior to exercise has received much attention.[7-12] One study revealed increased utilization of muscle glycogen and a fall in blood glucose to hypoglycemic levels after administration of sugar sweetened drink 45 min prior to exercise.[7] Other studies found no effect on glycogen use during exercise when given pre-exercise glucose.[8,13]

One study[10] showed maintenance of glycogen stores while another two[8,13] showed signs of glycogen depletion when given a fructose preparation prior to exercise. Finally, Devlin et al.[14] showed that a snack (candy bar preparation) with a fat, carbohydrate, and protein mixture showed a superior maintenance of exercise glucose homeostasis when compared to noncaloric placebo drink. This leads to the conclusion that a mixed snack may be preferable to glucose preparation in maintaining glucose levels during and after exercise. Finally the form of carbohydrate (complex or simple) consumed during exercise[11,12] seems not to make a difference on glucose homeostasis.

The regulatory hormones (epinephrine, norepinephrine, insulin, glucagon, cortisol, and growth hormone) may also affect metabolic fuel utilization. The sympathetic nervous system plays a key role in glucose metabolism during exercise. In general, plasma norepinephrine plays a more important role during low and moderate intensity exercise while epinephrine plays a more substantial role in high intensity exercise. In a state of insulin-induced hypoglycemia, children demonstrate greater increases in plasma epinephrine than adults.[15]

Insulin secretion is suppressed during physical activity in response to alpha-adrenergic inhibitory effects on the pancreatic beta cells.[16,17] Insulin is the major inhibitor of hepatic glucose production.

Glucagon plays a key role in high intensity or prolonged exercise,[18] while cortisol and growth hormone may play roles in glucose homeostasis during prolonged exercise.[4]

Type I diabetics may experience untoward consequences during exercise for several reasons. Berger[19-21] states that insulin levels generally do not decrease during exercise and may even increase if exercise is undertaken within one hour of the insulin injection. Some patients with Type I Diabetes have deficient responses to hypoglycemia.[22] Epinephrine, growth hormone, and cortisol may not act in usual fashion when blood glucose falls to 50 mg/dl[23] resulting in hypoglycemia.

D. BENEFITS OF EXERCISE

Numerous studies have investigated the benefits of exercise on Type I Diabetes.[24-34] Proved benefits include:

1. increased insulin sensitivity,[24,25]
2. improved glucose transport,[26-29]
3. decreased heart rate and blood pressure at rest, and
4. maintenance of lean body mass with weight reduction.

Some possible beneficial effects are decreased fasting blood glucose,[30] decreased hemoglobin A1,[31-34] development of an improved lipid profile, and reduced coronary risk. These benefits will be explained in more detail in the section on Type II Diabetes.

One other benefit not usually addressed is the psychological benefit of increased self-esteem and self-confidence.[35] These positive feelings are especially important at the initial diagnosis of diabetes where the patient feels hopeless. Exercise gives the diabetic a sense of control over himself and the disease.

E. ADVERSE EFFECTS OF EXERCISE ON TYPE I DIABETICS

Hypoglycemia represents the most common adverse consequence while hyperglycemia and ketosis are less frequent events. Hypoglycemia, defined as a blood glucose less than 60 mg/dl, may occur during, immediately after, or up to 48 hours after a sporting event.[3] It is of paramount importance to know the individual's response to a particular exercise. Hypoglycemia occurs in a Type I Diabetic who is exercising because of a hyperinsulinemic state. A failure to reduce insulin before exercise results in hyperinsulinemia. Exercising muscles utilize the glucose while the extra insulin blocks glucose production by the liver and fatty acid release from adipose tissue.

The athlete must be aware of certain subtle and obvious signs which may signal upcoming hypoglycemia. Fatigue, dizziness, nausea, and sluggishness are subjective symptoms while tremors and even seizures are more overt signs. A decrease in athletic performance in the middle or toward the end of a competition may occur. Inability to concentrate may be a sign which may go unnoticed by the athlete but aware by the coach, parent, or teammate.

Hyperglycemia occurs in patients who demonstrate poor metabolic control who are deprived of insulin. In such cases peripheral glucose uptake lags behind hepatic glucose production; ketogenesis results because of increased release of lipolytic hormones.[36]

Exercise-induced ketosis occurs when the exercising individual has severe insulin deficiency. In this metabolic condition, plasma insulin concentration is low or absent and hyperglycemia and ketosis are present. With exercise, peripheral glucose utilization is impaired, lipolysis is enhanced, and hepatic glucose production and ketogenesis are stimulated. This sets up a rapid rise in the already high blood glucose and induces ketosis.[37] The mechanism for the development of ketosis is not clear. Fery[38] suggests that there is a defect in peripheral ketone clearance rather than a marked increase in ketogenesis during exercise in hypoinsulinemic individuals.

III. THE CHILD WITH DIABETES

Like the healthy child, the child with diabetes in most cases should be encouraged to exercise. A contraindication to exercise is poor metabolic control and signs of autonomic neuropathy. A position statement by the American Academy of Pediatrics in 1994[39] recommended that an assessment of a child's physical activity should be ascertained by the pediatrician at age three and each subsequent year at health care maintenance. This same activity should be performed for the diabetic by the primary care provider and diabetologists at routine health visits.

The parent must play an active role in monitoring the child's physical activities. It is the parent who must alter the insulin dosage and provide appropriate food sources for the child. The child cannot take full responsibility by himself. It is important for the parent to join support groups and that the child be associated with other older children and adults who have diabetes.

IV. THE ADOLESCENT WITH DIABETES

The diabetic adolescent poses a challenging problem to manage because of the physical, physiological, and psychological changes that occur over a short period of time. The physical changes are characterized by a rapid growth spurt which induces an increased caloric intake. This increased caloric intake may necessitate an increased insulin requirement. Hormonal changes may also account for changes in insulin requirement. The adolescent faced with these changes must come to terms with his or her "new body."

V. MANAGEMENT OF TYPE I DIABETES

A. NUTRITIONAL REQUIREMENT

The diabetic's diet should consist of 55–65% complex carbohydrate, 20% fat, and less than 15% protein. The protein requirement will vary depending upon the nature of the athletic training and growth status. For a maintenance diet, 0.8 g/kg/day is sufficient while 1.2–1.5 g/kg/day are required for growth and strength training.[40] These recommendations are similar to the maintenance diet for the healthy child (60% carbohydrate, <30% fat, and 10–15% protein). The difference in the fat component is related to the abnormal lipid profile and premature atherosclerosis that Type I Diabetics demonstrate after 10–15 years with the disease.[41]

B. HYDRATION DURING SPORTING EVENTS

Children are not "miniature" adults, and they should not be treated as such. Children's thirst mechanisms are not as sophisticated as adults; they dissipate heat more quickly and have a higher surface area to body weight than adults.[42] During prolonged exercise the athlete should drink one extra glass of fluid after he or she no longer feels thirsty. This recommendation is especially important in diabetics who demonstrate autonomic neuropathy as they do not tolerate heat well.[4] The child should drink a beverage that he finds palatable. A child will drink more of a preferred liquid.[43]

C. RECOMMENDATIONS DURING EXERCISE

At any sporting event or recreational activity the diabetic should always have carbohydrate snacks (fruit, bread, or candy) available. The amount of carbohydrate will vary according to body size. There is no consensus as to the standard caloric equivalence of exercise. The concept of "exercise exchange" analogous to carbohydrate exchange has been proposed.[4]

Exercise intensity plays a major role in determining the carbohydrate intake. Etzwiler et al.[44] makes the following recommendations: exercise of low to moderate intensity and glucose above 100 mg/dl (no increase of carbohydrate intake); exercise of moderate intensity and blood glucose 100–180 mg/dl (10–15 g of carbohydrate per hour of exercise), with blood glucose 180–250 mg/dl (no carbohydrate); exercise of high intensity and blood glucose 180–250 mg/dl (10–15 g of carbohydrate per hour of exercise). If blood glucose is greater than 250 mg/dl urine must be tested for ketones and insulin administered.

D. INSULIN TREATMENT

Proper insulin treatment varies according to the individual but must account for exercise intensity, daily insulin requirement and sensitivity, degree of glycemic control, and pubertal development. In mild to moderate intensity exercise insulin requirements drop 10–50%.[3,36] For high intensity or endurance events (cycling marathon) insulin dose may have to be lowered by up to 90%.[45]

The insulin preparation (porcine or human) may affect glucose metabolism. At rest, human insulin is absorbed more rapidly than porcine; during exercise this difference disappears, both types being absorbed more rapidly than the resting state.[4]

The timing of insulin as well as site of insulin injection are key factors to consider. The diabetic should not plan to exercise at the peak onset of insulin action to avoid hypoglycemia.[3] Insulin should be injected away from exercising muscles[46] as this could stimulate increased release of insulin at the injection site. For example, a runner should not inject insulin in the thigh while a rower should avoid injection in the arm.

Some patients are more sensitive to insulin than others. Highly trained diabetics have demonstrated greater insulin sensitivity than untrained. It is not wise to begin exercise if in poor metabolic control. A diabetic must take into account the onset of a viral illness as this may upset the glycemic control and undoubtedly affect the insulin requirement.

Insulin requirements may change during puberty because of increased caloric consumption and hormonal changes.

When exercise is planned in advance, athletic performance is optimized and there are less frequent bouts of hypoglycemia. With planned exercise insulin dosage can be adjusted. For the diabetic who takes only a single dose of intermediate acting insulin the dose may be lowered by 30–35% the morning before exercise; another alternative is to split the dose, taking two thirds in the morning and one third before dinner, if it is needed.[46] Some individuals take a combination of short- and intermediate-acting insulin. The short-acting insulin may be reduced to 50% or eliminated.[3] For those taking multiple doses of short-acting insulin the pre-exercise doses may be lowered by 30–50% and post-exercise dose adjusted according to glucose reading.[3] These are only guidelines; the most important concept is for the athlete to be familiar with all of his responses during exercise.

E.   RECOMMENDED ACTIVITIES

There are no activities that are not recommended for diabetic children as there is no fear of nephropathy, neuropathy, or hypertension. The importance of exercise should be instilled by all adults dealing with the child (parents, health teachers, physical educators, recreation specialists, physicians). They should be monitored regularly. At each contact with a physician, physical activity should be encouraged. Activities that are easier to manage are those that are progressive in nature with a known energy expenditure — cycling, running, and swimming.[36,46] Activities with an unknown energy expenditure where access to glucose monitoring and carbohyrate supplementation is difficult (sky diving, mountaineering, scuba diving, auto or motor cycle racing, and hanggliding) are not recommended.[46] Young diabetics should be reminded that their disease should not be an impediment to athletic success. There are world class athletes with the disease.[45]

VI.   TYPE II DIABETES

Patients with Type II Diabetes account for 90% of diabetics. Type II Diabetics generally do not require insulin and therefore may rely heavily on diet, exercise, and oral hypoglycemics to manage their disease.

A.   NUTRITIONAL THERAPY IN TYPE II DIABETES

Medical nutrition therapy is an essential component of successful diabetes management, especially for Type II Diabetes patients. A significant proportion of patients with Type II Diabetes who comply with their diet will not require any additional therapy. The nutritional emphasis in diabetic patients aims not only at achieving near-normal blood glucose levels but also at achieving an optimal lipid profile in an attempt to reduce the risk for cardiovascular disease (CVD).[47]

1.   Protein

The recommended dietary allowance (RDA) for normal adults is 0.8 g/kg/day or ~10% of calories ingested. Recent surveys indicate that the average protein intake is 14–18% of total energy requirements,[48] and diabetics also have protein intake in this range. Thus, on average, daily protein consumption is more than necessary to meet known nutritional needs. Insulin deficiency increases both whole-body protein synthesis and protein breakdown.[49,50] However, presently there is no compelling evidence to suggest that protein requirements are increased in diabetes.[51] Accordingly, current recommendation for protein intake in diabetic patients is 10–20% of the daily caloric intake derived primarily from plant and lean animal sources.[47,51]

Use of hypocaloric weight loss diet for the treatment of NIDDM requires an increase in the proportion of calories derived from protein to preserve lean body mass.[51,52] During exercise, a small amount of protein is needed for muscle growth that is achieved by chronic exercise conditioning. High protein intake increases glomerular filtration rate and may accelerate the progression of diabetic nephropathy. Conversely, a low protein diet may impede renal function loss. In patients with diabetic nephropathy protein intake should be restricted to 0.8 g/kg body wt/day (~10% of daily calories).[51] Based on current consumption data, this recommendation translates to a significant reduction in protein intake in the majority of patients.

2.   Fats

As will be discussed below, the most common and serious complications of diabetes result from accelerated atherosclerosis. The dyslipidemia associated with insulin resistance in Type II Diabetes is common and contributes to the excess of CVD. The salutary effect of low fat diet on the risk for CVD are the main reason why current recommendations for dietary macronutrient composition have shifted toward a higher carbohydrate intake and lower fat intake in patients with diabetes. In addition, since fat is the most energy-rich of all macronutrients, reduction of dietary fat may be associated with a reduction in caloric intake and weight loss. For individuals (nondiabetic or diabetic) who have normal lipid levels the recommended calories from fat is ≤30% of total calories (≤10% from saturated fat, 10% polyunsaturated fats, 10–15% mono-unsaturated fats, and daily cholesterol <300 mg/day).[47,53] In the presence of hyperlipidemia saturated fat should be cut to <7% of total calories and dietary cholesterol to <200 mg/day. In most patients, the largest and most important reduction will be the reduction in saturated fatty acids.[53] This requires an isocaloric increase of either unsaturated fatty acids or carbohydrates.

In several Mediterranean countries mono-unsaturated fatty acids, mostly from olive oil, form a significant proportion of dietary intake and is associated with low rates of dietary intake. Omega-3 fatty acids also have considerable beneficial effect in primary and secondary prevention of CVD.[54] The primary effect of fish oil on lipid metabolism is to lower very low density lipoprotein (VLDL) levels by inhibiting hepatic triglyceride and VLDL synthesis.[55] In most IDDM and NIDDM subjects, fish oil therapy markedly reduces triglyceride and VLDL concentrations.[56,57] The effects of fish oils on low density lipoprotein (LDL) and high density lipoprotein (HDL) cholesterol are highly variable. However, a significant increase in LDL and apoprotein B can be observed, especially in patients who were initially hypertriglyceridemic.[57,58] In some cases, the increased LDL level may warrant pharmacological intervention.

Omega-3 fatty acids may decrease insulin secretion and increase hepatic glucose output resulting in increased hyperglycemia in subjects with NIDDM.[58,59] However, this has not been a significant problem in recent studies.[54,57]

In conclusion, the incorporation of fish per se in the diet of diabetic patients is not known to have deleterious effects. However, supplementation of pharmacological doses of ω-3 fatty acids (e.g., for treatment of severe hypertriglyceridemia) requires medical supervision and cannot be recommended routinely for diabetics.[52]

3. Carbohydrates

If dietary fat contributes up to 30% of total caloric content, then 50–60% remain for carbohydrates. Based on the assumption that sugars are more rapidly digested and absorbed than starches, the traditional thinking has been that "simple" sugars should be avoided and replaced with complex carbohydrates. However, when fed as a single nutrient, sucrose produces a glycemic response similar to that of bread, rice, and potatoes.[60] Studies comparing the glycemic effects of meals containing different amounts of sucrose and starch have found no adverse effect of glucose on glycemic control.[61,62]

The main obstacle to high carbohydrate intake is that it may lead to hyperglycemia and hypertriglyceridemia. Several studies have shown that increasing carbohydrate content from 40% to 60% of total calories resulted in higher plasma glucose and VLDL triglyceride levels.[63,64] Thus, a prudent course of action is to follow glucose and triglyceride levels on a liberal carbohydrate intake since some patients will require lowering carbohydrate levels and higher fat diet. Increased consumption of dietary fiber (particularly soluble fiber) has a mild hypoglycemic and hypolipidemic (reducing LDL and VLDL) effects and may prevent these problems when incorporated into a high carbohydrate diet.[53]

Dietary fructose (fruits, vegetables, honey) produces a smaller rise in plasma glucose than sucrose or starch.[62] An additional benefit of fruit and vegetables is also recommended in diabetics, because they contain antioxidants required to protect against polysaturated fatty acids oxidation.[53] However, because fructose in large amounts may increase serum cholesterol, the use of added fructose as a sweetening agent in the diabetic diet is not recommended.[52]

4. Diet and Weight Reduction

Obesity is present in as many as 75–85% of NIDDM patients and contributes to the insulin resistance and dyslipidemia.[65] The increased caloric consumption during exercise may facilitate weight loss. However, since the caloric expenditure induced by moderate exercise is not large, patients must also adhere to caloric restriction in order to achieve weight loss. Nonetheless, weight loss programs that incorporate exercise are more likely to be successful in maintaining weight reduction.[66]

Although weight loss is a major focus of the dietary management of Type II Diabetes, current dietary strategies are often not effective.[52] A recent review on the treatment of Type II Diabetes stated that "obese people expend more calories than lean and so can only remain overweight if they eat more than lean people; any claims to be eating next to nothing must be firmly but sympathetically rejected."[65] However, it has been pointed out that only if one is fat can one be said to have overeaten.[67]

Indeed, obese individuals do not necessarily consume more calories than lean individuals. The two components of the energy balance equation, energy intake and expenditure, are linked and are not independent variables.[68] Under normal conditions, when food intake increases, so does energy expenditure, and vice versa.[69] For example, resting metabolic rate (which is the most important component of energy expenditure) declines during caloric restriction or weight loss.[70]

The body has complex mechanisms for regulating its fat stores. These mechanisms conserve calories when food is deprived and prevent obesity when excess food is ingested. This is accomplished by exerting a powerful influence on eating, physical activity, and the efficiency of metabolic processes (Figure 2).[67,69]

In several single-gene autosomal recessive disorders, such as *ob/ob* or *db/db* mice, in which the normal protection against obesity is lost, the increase in the size of fat cells occurs before the onset of hyperphagia, suggesting that the primary defect resides in the fat cell itself. Some of the mechanisms involved in the regulation of adipocyte mass have been recently elucidated following the cloning of the *ob* gene.[71] The *ob* gene encodes for a protein, leptin,[72,73] that is expressed and found in adipose tissue (Figure 2). An autosomal recessive

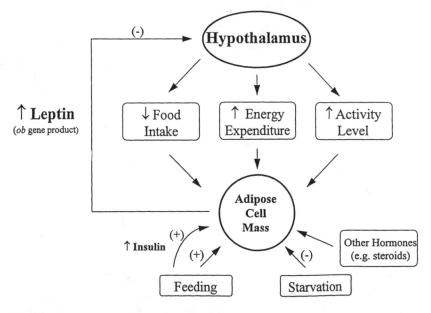

FIGURE 2 Metabolic processes that affect fat stores.

mutation known as *ob/ob* leads to the expression of a dysfunctional protein, which phenotypically manifests as severe obesity together with marked hyperphagia and diminished energy expenditure. Leptin exerts its powerful effects on appetite and body weight via direct binding to a specific receptor (OB-R) in the central nervous system.[74-77]

Studies with mice indicate that the *db/db* phenotype may results from a defective leptin receptor. Normalization of body weight was exhibited by *ob/ob* mice whose peripheral circulation was joined surgically with control mice. By contrast, *db/db* mice, when linked to their lean controls, did not exhibit weight loss.[78] A recently discovered mutation in the gene encoding the OB-R protein in *db/db* mice results in a receptor that can bind leptin but cannot initiate intracellular signal transduction.[79] This explains the apparent resistance of these animals to exogenous administration of leptin.[73,76,77]

Although the size of adipose depot is an important determinant of leptin levels, acute changes in energy stores also influence the expression of the *ob* gene. Leptin levels fall with caloric restriction and rise with feeding before any significant change in fat cell mass occurs.[80] In fact, the *ob* gene exhibits diurnal variation that corresponds to changes in daily food intake.[81]

An important mediator of the effect of food intake on *ob* expression is insulin, which increases *ob* mRNA in adipocytes. Insulin deficiency in streptozotocin-induced diabetes causes a marked suppression of leptin MRNA, which can be readily reversed with insulin administration.[82] Recent studies have suggested that obese rodents (other than *ob/ob* mice) and humans are not defective in their ability to produce leptin and generally produce higher levels than lean individuals.[74,83] These data suggest that resistance to normal or elevated levels of leptin rather than inadequate leptin production is more important as a pathogenic mechanism in human obesity.

The foregoing discussion has practical implications for the clinical management of the obese diabetic. The scale of anticipated benefit from low-calorie diets may not entirely depend on patient compliance but on inherited defects in mechanism that regulate fat stores and energy balance or by the interaction of insulin deficiency or insulin resistance with these mechanisms. It should be emphasized, however, that mild to moderate weight loss has been shown to improve glycemic control even if desirable body weight is not attained.[52] Therefore, persistent efforts at weight reduction and maintenance of reduced body weight is justified in the management of diabetic patients.

B.   BENEFIT OF EXERCISE IN NIDDM

Exercise exerts a beneficial effect on glycemic control and cardiovascular risk profile. Cardiovascular disease is the leading cause of death among patients with NIDDM, accounting for virtually 80% of all deaths among North American diabetic patients.[84] Therefore, a major focus of treatment in NIDDM is the prevention of the atherosclerotic process.

In NIDDM the atherosclerotic process is accelerated through multiple potential mechanisms. NIDDM usually occurs in association with a cluster of other atherogenic risk factors including hyperinsulinemia, hypertension, an atherogenic lipoprotein profile, and a procoagulant state. The increasing evidence for the association between insulin resistance, hypertension, dyslipidemia, and CHD led to the description of the insulin resistance syndrome or "syndrome X" by Reaven.[85] Regular exercise usually ameliorates all the atherogenic abnormalities associated with this syndrome (Table 1), thereby decreasing the risk for cardiovascular disease.[86]

C.   GLYCEMIC CONTROL AND INSULIN SENSITIVITY

Several studies have demonstrated that regular exercise improves glycemic control in middle-aged NIDDM patients[87-89] and that this improvement is associated with increased insulin sensitivity in skeletal muscle.[90,91] The greatest improvement in glycemic control occurs in patients with mild diabetes (fasting blood glucose <200 mg/dl).[89,92] These individuals are

TABLE 1   Exercise Recommendations

Pre-Exercise

1. Eat a meal 2–3 hours prior to competition.
2. Measure blood glucose prior to exercise.
3. Eat a mixed snack 30–60 min prior to exercise
4. Alter insulin dose according to expected duration and intensity.

During Exercise

1. Monitor glucose every 30 min during exercise.
2. Have carbohydrate on hand.
3. Exercise with a partner if possible.

Post Exercise

1. Measure glucose immediately after exercise and at regular
   intervals according to previous experience.
2. Consume a meal 2–3 hours after exercise to replenish glycogen
   stores.

more hyperinsulinemic than diabetic patients with less severe hyperglycemia, and their insulin levels decrease during training.[89] However, the long-term beneficial effects of physical training on metabolic control is less clear. First, the enhanced insulin sensitivity associated with physical training is lost if exercise is not continued on a regular basis.[87] Indeed, insulin sensitivity deteriorates rapidly following discontinuation of an exercise program before aerobic fitness decreases. Second, a number of studies have questioned the efficacy of training programs in the treatment of NIDDM.[93]

In summary, NIDDM patients most likely to derive significant benefit from regular exercise with regard to glycemic control and insulin sensitivity are young, relatively healthy patients in the early stage of the disease (i.e., hyperinsulinemic).[87]

D. CARDIOVASCULAR DISEASE

In two large prospective studies of middle-aged men at high risk of atherosclerosis (diabetics and nondiabetics), moderate physical conditioning was associated with a 30–50% decrease in cardiovascular mortality.[94,95] In the Multiple Risk Factor Intervention Trial (MRFIT), patients who performed regular, moderate physical activity had 30% lower fatal cardiac events and a significant decrease in total mortality compared with less active patients.[94] In a study of almost 17,000 healthy subjects of diverse ages, adoption of moderate physical sporting activity during a 4-year interval correlated with lower mortality over a subsequent 9-year follow up and demonstrated that regular exercise is associated with longevity independent of the age at which it is begun.[96] Exercise is also beneficial in secondary prevention of CVD. An intensive physical training program in association with moderate diet intervention has been shown to favorably affect the progression of coronary atherosclerotic lesions and stress-induced myocardial ischemia in patients with stable angina pectoris.[97]

The effects of regular exercise on coronary risk factors are multifactorial (Table 2). Although most of the experimental evidence has been obtained in nondiabetic subjects, it is commonly believed that these findings apply also to patients with NIDDM.[86] In fact, much of the reported benefit of exercise in the general population is mediated through the amelioration of metabolic risk factor associated with insulin resistance.[98,99]

E. LIPOPROTEIN PROFILE

As mentioned above, dyslipidemia is commonly associated with NIDDM and is an integral part of the insulin resistance syndrome. Dyslipidemia is thought to promote the accelerated

TABLE 2   Beneficial Effects of Exercise on
Cardiovascular Risk Factors

Benefit	Exercise Intensity	Ref.
Improved glycemic control		
Weight loss	Moderate	
Enhance insulin sensitivity	Low–Moderate	
Improved lipoprotein profile		
Increased HDL	Moderate–High	102
Decrease triglycerides	Moderate	87, 101
Decrease small, dense LDL	Moderate	103
Reduction in blood pressure	Low–Moderate	105, 122
Corrects coagulation abnormalities	Moderate	124

Note: High: 75–90% of VO$_2$max. Moderate: 60–75% of VO$_2$max.
Low: 40–60% of VO$_2$max.

atherosclerosis that characterizes NIDDM. The typical lipoprotein profile in NIDDM consists of increased triglyceride levels, decreased high density lipoprotein-cholesterol (HDL-C) levels, and a preponderance of small, dense LDL particles. These particles have a higher atherogenic potential due to an increased susceptibility to oxidative modification.[100]

Endurance-trained subjects consistently demonstrate lower triglyceride and higher HDL-C concentrations. The improvement in lipoprotein profile is more evident with endurance-type exercise than in power or speed-type training. Endurance exercise training decreases plasma triglyceride concentrations particularly when pre-training values are elevated.[87,101] Within the general population, HDL-C correlates with the level of physical activity. However, the effect of exercise training on HDL-C levels was shown to be inconsistent. Only part of the studies could demonstrate increased HDL-C levels,[102] presumably because a higher training intensity is required to decrease HDL-C levels.

Exercise, without a change in body composition or diet, has no significant impact on plasma LDL-C concentrations. However, LDL composition is shifted from the small, dense LDL particle to the large, buoyant LDL, which has a lower atherogenic potential.[103]

F. HYPERTENSION

After regularly repeated aerobic exercise, the resting blood pressure is lowered independent of weight loss.[104,105] Certain individuals experience an exaggerated rise in both systolic and diastolic blood pressure during acute exercise, and this phenomenon may be more frequent in NIDDM.[106] Although the degree of rise in blood pressure during exercise is blunted after regular physical training, restricting the intensity of exercise may be required in some patients to prevent further end-organ damage (e.g., in the presence of diabetic nephropathy).

G. EXERCISE IN THE PREVENTION OF DIABETES

In genetically prone individuals insulin resistance and compensatory hyperinsulinemia are the earliest detectable defects and can occur 15–25 years or more before the clinical onset of overt Type II Diabetes.[107] Impaired glucose tolerance is present in 23% of adults aged 40–74 who are overweight and have a family history of diabetes.[108] Of these individuals, 5–15% are expected to progress to Type II Diabetes each year. Furthermore, macrovascular disease and its risk factors are already present in subjects at high risk for Type II Diabetes.[109] Since exercise improves insulin resistance and its associated metabolic abnormalities that predict future NIDDM,[96,98,99] an obvious question is whether exercise (or other interventions aimed at reducing insulin resistance) could be beneficial in delaying the onset of Type II Diabetes.

Indirect evidence for a protective role of exercise derives from studies demonstrating a lower prevalence of Type II Diabetes among active rural populations compared with sedentary urban populations. In cross-sectional studies the prevalence of Type II Diabetes was lower in active than in sedentary individuals.[110] Prospective studies of physical activity have also provided substantial support for the protective effect of exercise.[111,112] In the Nurses' Health Study, a reduced incidence of Type II Diabetes was observed among women who engaged in regular exercise.[111] In the Physicians' Health Study, regular vigorous exercise was associated with a decreased incidence of Type II Diabetes in a dose-response manner.[112]

H. RISKS OF EXERCISE

Because many patients with NIDDM have preexisting CHD at the time diabetes is diagnosed, all NIDDM patients should be screened for silent ischemia, previously undiagnosed hypertension, neuropathy, retinopathy, and nephropathy before beginning an exercise program.

1. Hypoglycemia

NIDDM patients treated with sulfonylureas and/or insulin are prone to develop exercise-induced hypoglycemia. Post-exercise hypoglycemia is usually less common in patients taking sulfonylureas, compared with patients on insulin.[113] However, hypoglycemia may develop when such patients have normal glucose levels at the onset of exercise. Although exercise is associated with a decrease in circulating insulin levels, exercise is not able to blunt pancreatic insulin secretion during sulfonylurea treatment.[113] The hyperinsulinemia induced by the sulfonylurea can prevent an adequate rise in hepatic glucose production, and hypoglycemia may ensue. NIDDM patients on sulfonylurea treatment may need to decrease the dose or omit the drug altogether before exercise.

2. Retinopathy

The risk of exercise aggravating proliferative retinopathy is not known.[114] However, exercise-induced blood pressure excursions result in increased blood flow into the ophthalmic circulation.[115] Thus, intensive exercise may result in viteroretinal hemorrhage in patients with proliferative retinopathy. In one study, 10% of hemorrhages occurred with a temporal relationship to strenuous activity or Valsalva-type maneuvers.[115] Laser therapy may be required prior to the initiation of an exercise program.

3. Nephropathy

Exercise exacerbates hypertension and proteinuria in patients with nephropathy. In diabetic patients with normal resting glomerular filtration and urinary albumin excretion, a substantial increase in urinary albumin excretion occurs following exercise.[116] This phenomenon can be observed during a 15–30 min graded exercise period arriving at a total amount of 450–600 kg/min.[117,118] The mechanism is related to the superimposition of elevated intraglomerular pressure upon the evolving glomerulopathy[119] and can be corrected either by intensive insulin therapy or ACE inhibitors.[120] Although nonstimulated microalbuminuria predicts future overt diabetic nephropathy, there is no long-term study to suggest that strictly normoalbuminuric patients with exercise-induced microalbuminuria are at higher risk for future diabetic nephropathy. The impact of regular exercise on the progression of overt diabetic nephropathy is also unknown.

4. Cardiovascular Disease

Patients with NIDDM are usually diagnosed at >40 years of age and frequently already have clinical evidence of CHD. A thorough medical history and physical examination should be performed to rule out cardiovascular disease. Most patients should probably undergo an exercise stress test before participating in a training program. The presence of ischemia or arrhythmias require specific precautions. It should be emphasized however that exercise is beneficial as secondary prevention in patients with documented CHD. For example, a structured exercise program as part of cardiac rehabilitation in patients following myocardial infarction significantly lowers total and cardiac mortality, fatal reinfarction, and sudden cardiac death.[117] Regular exercise training also has a favorable effect on the walking capacity of patients with intermittent claudication.[119]

5.   Diabetic Neuropathy/Lower Extremity Injury

Diabetic peripheral neuropathy results in decreased pain sensation and predisposes patients to foot ulceration. Exercise that traumatizes the feet (e.g., jogging) should be limited in patients with diabetic neuropathy, especially if repeated foot trauma is involved. Non-weight-bearing activities are most appropriate (e.g., cycling, swimming). Proper footwear and other protective equipment should be used, and feet should be inspected daily and after exercise. Exercise tolerance in patients with diabetic autonomic neuropathy may be substantially limited because of impaired sympathetic and parasympathetic reflexes that normally increase cardiac output and redistribute blood flow to muscles.

I.   RECOMMENDED SPORTS/ACTIVITIES

Exercise training for most patients with diabetes is similar to that recommended for the general population. To improve glycemic control and insulin sensitivity and achieve optimal cardiovascular benefit, exercise is recommended at least 3 days a week for 20–45 min (with a 5–10 min warm-up and cool-down period) at 70–85% of maximal heart rate or 50-70% of maximal oxygen uptake. If weight reduction is a major goal, exercise ≥5 days/week is probably necessary.

To promote compliance with an exercise program, patients should choose the type of exercise that they enjoy. In addition, the type of exercise program should fit into the patient's lifestyle and daily schedule. Aerobic training, including brisk walking, running, swimming, bicycling, tennis, gardening, and yoga, are preferred to resistance training, such as weight-lifting, which can put undue stress on the cardiorespiratory system.[120]

Since diabetic patients have increased prevalence of foot problems, osteoarthritis of knee joint and lumbosacral spine, and peripheral vascular disease, non-weight-bearing exercise such as stationary biking, swimming, upper body exercise, and yoga may be preferred. Similarly, it is preferable to avoid exercise that involves Valsalva maneuvers, actvities that increase intrathoracic pressure (e.g., heavy weightlifting), which can result in a large increase in blood pressure. Sports where hypoglycemia may be dangerous (e.g., diving, climbing) should be avoided.

As already mentioned, exercise is beneficial also for patients with established CHD. These patients can be classified by risk based on characteristics of the clinical evaluation.[121] Exercise training technique has been developed for such patients and has been reviewed elsewhere.[122]

When deciding on an exercise program, the patient should gradually increase his duration and intensity. A good rule of thumb is not to increase exercise volume or intensity by more than 10% per week.[123] A drastic increase in exercise results in an increased risk of overuse injury (tendinitis, stress fracture). Another tip when beginning an exercise program is to rest for 24 hours to give the body time to heal.

VII.   CONCLUSION

Diet and exercise play key roles in the management of patients with Type I and Type II Diabetes. Careful planning must be made before exercise regarding exercise intensity and duration,[44] site and timing of insulin injection and dosage,[3,36,45,46] and food intake.[40,41,47,48,53]

Regular aerobic exercise may help with metabolic control in patients with Type I and II Diabetes. A common sense approach to nutritional intake with the importance of low fat diet can help diabetics gain some control over their disease. A clear plan during and after exercise is necessary in terms of carbohydrate administration. Precautions must be made to avoid adverse consequences during exercise: hypoglycemia, hyperglycemia. Plans should be made to combat these problems in case they occur. Particular activities and sports must be taken into account.

A support team of peers, family members, physicians, nurses, and others helps the diabetic achieve optimal health and functioning.

REFERENCES

1. Rimoin, D.L. and Roiter, J.I., Genetic heterogeneity in diabetes mellitus and diabetic microangiopathy, *Hormone,* 7 (Suppl. Series), 63, 1981.
2. Rotier, J.I. and Rimoin, D.L., The genetics of the glucose intolerance disorders, *Am. J. Med.,* 70, 116, 1981.
3. Campaigne, B.N. and Lampman, R.M., *Exercise in the Clinical Management of Diabetes*, Human Kinetics Publisher, Champaign, IL, 1994, 39.
4. Horton, E., Exercise and Diabetes in Youth, in *Perspectives in Exercise Science and Sports Medicine. Volume 2. Youth, Exercise, and Sport,* Gisolfi, C.V. and Lamb, D.R., Eds., Benchmark Press, Indianapolis, IN, 1989.
5. Christensen, E.H. and Hansen, O., Zur methodik der respiratorischen quotient-bestim-mungen in ruhe und bei arbeit. II. Untersuchungen ueber die verbrennungsvorgaenge bei langdaurnder, schwerer muskelarbeit: Arbeits faehigkeit und ernahrung, *Skandinavisches Archiv fur Physiologie,* 81, 138, 1939.
6. Bergstrom, J., Hermansen, L., Hultman, E., and Saltin, B., Diet, muscle glycogen and physical performance, *Acta Physiol. Scand.,* 71, 140, 1967.
7. Costill, D.L., Coyle, E., Dalsky, G., Evans, W., Fink, W., and Hoopes, D., Effects of elevated plasma FFA and insulin on muscle glycogen usage during exercise, *Appl. Physiol.,* 43, 695, 1977.
8. Fielding, R.A., Costill, D.L., Fink, W.J., King, D.S., Kovaleski, J.E., and Kirwan, J.P., Effects of pre-exercise carboyhdrate feedings on muscle glycogen use during exercise in well trained runners, *Eur. J. Appl. Physiol.,* 55, 225, 1987.
9. Koivisto, V.A., Harkonen, M., Karonen, S.L., Groop, P.H., Elovainio, R., Ferrannini, E., Sacca, L., and DeFronzo, R.A., Glycogen depletion during prolonged exercise: influence of glucose, fructose and placebo, *J. Appl. Physiol.,* 58, 731, 1985.
10. Levine, L., Evans, W.J., Cadarette, B.S., Fisher, E.C., and Bullen, B.A., Fructose and glucose ingestion and muscle glycogen use during submaximal exercise, *J. Appl. Physiol.,* 55, 1767, 1983.
11. Coyle, E.F., Hagberg, J.M., Hurley, B.F., Mardin, W.H., Ehsani, A.A., and Holloszy, J.O., Carbohydrate feeding during prolonged strenuous exercise can delay fatigue, *J. Appl. Physiol.,* 55, 230, 1983.
12. Ivy, J.F., Miller, W., Power, V., Goodyear, L.G., Sherman, W.M., Farrell, S., and Williams, H., Endurance improved by ingestion of a glucose polymer supplement, *Med. Sci. Sports Exer.,* 15, 466, 1983.
14. Devlin, J.T., Calles-Escandon, J., and Horton, E.S., Effects of pre-exercise snack feeding on endurance cycle exercise, *J. Appl. Physiol.,* 60, 980, 1986.
15. Amiel, S.A., Tamborlan, W.V., Sacca, L., and Sherwin, R.S., Hypoglycemia and glucose counterregulation in normal and insulin-dependent diabetic subjects, *Diabetes/Metab. Rev.,* 4, 71, 1988.
16. Hartley, L.H., Mason, W.J., Hogan, R.P., Jones, L.G., Kotchen, T.A., Mougey, E.H., Pennington, L.L., and Ricketts, T., Multiple hormonal responses to graded exercise in relation to physical training, *J. Appl. Physiol.,* 33, 602, 1972.
17. Hermansen, L., Pruett, E.D.R., Osnes, J.B., and Giere, F.A., Blood glucose and plasma insulin in response to maximal exercise and glucose infusion, *J. Appl. Physiol.,* 29, 13, 1970.
18. Bjorkman, O., Felig, P., Hagenfeldt, L., and Wahren, J., Influence of hypoglucagonemia on splanchnic glucose output during leg exercise in man, *Clin. Physiol.,* 1, 43, 1981.
19. Berger, M., Halban, P.A., Muller, W.A., Offer, R.E., Renold, A.E., and Vranic, A., Mobilization of subcutaneously injected tritiated insulin in rats: effects of muscular exercise, *Diabetolgia,* 15, 133, 1978
20. Berger, M., Halban, P.A., Assal, J.P., Offord, R.E., Vranic, M., and Renold, A.E., Pharmokinetics of subcutaneously injected tritiated insulin: effects conference on diabetes and exercise, *Diabetes,* 28 (Suppl. 1), 53, 1979.
21. Berger, M., Cuppers, H.J., Hegner, H., Jorgens, V., and Berchtold, P., Absorption kinetics and biologic effects of subcutaneously injected insulin preparations, *Diabetes Care,* 5, 77, 1982.
22. Gerich, J.E., Langloise, M., Noacco, C., Karam, J.H., and Forsham, P.H., Lack of a glucagon response to hypoglycemia in diabetes: evidence for an intrinsic pancreatic alpha-cell defect, *Science,* 182, 171, 1973.

23. Simonson, D.C., Tamborlane, W.V., DeFronzo, R.A., and Sherwin, R.S., Intensive insulin therapy reduces the counterregulatory hormone responses to hypoglycemia in patents with Type I diabetes, *Ann. Int. Med.,* 103, 184, 1985.

24. Richter, E.A., Turcotte, L., and Hespel, P., Metabolic responses to exercise, *Diabetes Care,* 15, 1767, 1992.

25. Sane, T., Helve, E., Pelkonen, R., and Koivisto, V.A., The adjustment of diet and insulin dose during long-term endurance exercise in Type I (insulin-dependent diabetic men), *Diabetologia,* 31, 35, 1988.

26. Goodyear, L.J., Hirshman, M.F., and Valyou, P.M., Glucose transporter number, function and subcellular distribution in rat skeletal muscle after exercise training, *Diabetes,* 41, 1091, 1992.

27. Houmard, J.A., Egan, P.C., Neufer, P.D., Friedman, J.E., Wheeler, W.S., Israel, R.G., and Dohm, G.L., Elevated skeletal muscle glucose transporter levels in exercise-trained middle-aged men, *Am. J. Physiol.,* 261, 437, 1991.

28. Ploug, T., Stallknaecht, B.M., Pederson, O., Kahn, B.B., Ohkuwa, T., Vinten, J., and Galbo, H., Effect of endurance training on glucose transport capacity and glucose transporter expression in rat skeletal muscle, *Am. J. Physiol.,* 259, E778, 1990.

29. Wake, S.A., Sowden, J.A., Storlien, L.H., James, D.E., Clark, P.E., Shine, J., Chisholm, D.J., and Kraegen, W.E., Effects of exercise training and dietary manipulation on insulin-regulatable glucose-transporter mRNA in rat muscle, *Diabetes,* 40, 275, 1991

30. Campaigne, B.N., Gilliam, T.B., Spencer, M.L., Lampman, R.M., and Schork, M.A., Effects of a physical activity program on metabolic control and cardiovascular fitness in children with insulin-dependent diabetes mellitus, *Diabetes Care,* 7, 57, 1984.

31. Dahl-Jorgensen, K., Meen, H.D., Hanssen, K.R.F., and Genaes, O.A.A., The effect of exercise on diabetic control and hemoglobin A (hbA1) in children, *Acta Paediatrica Scandinavica,* 283, 53, 1980

32. Landt, K.W., Campaigne, B.N., James, F.W., and Sperling, M.A., Effects of exercise training on insulin sensitivity in adolescents with Type I diabetes, *Diabetes Care,* 8, 461, 1985.

33. Larsson, Y., Persson, B., Sterky, G., and Thoren, C., Functional adaptation to rigourous training and exercise in diabetic and non-diabetic adolescents, *J. Appl. Physiol.,* 19, 629, 1964.

34. Rowland, T.W., Swadba, L.A., Biggs, D.E., Burke, E.J., and Ritter, E.O., Glycemic control with physical training in insulin-dependent diabetes mellitus, *Am. J. Dis. Child,* 139, 307, 1985.

35. Landry, G.L. and Allen, D.B., Diabetes mellitus and exercise, *Clin. Sports Med.,* 11, 403, 1992.

36. Dorchy, H. and Poortmans, J., Sport and the diabetic child, *Sports Med.,* 7, 248, 1989.

37. Berger, M., Berchtold, P., Cuppers, H.J., Drost, H., Kley, H.K., Muller, W.A., Wiegelmann, W., Zimmermann-Telschow, H., Gries, F.A., Kruskemper, H.L., and Zimmerman, H., Metabolic and hormonal effect of muscular exercise in juvenile type diabetics, *Diabetolgia,* 13, 355, 1977.

38. Fery, F., de Maertelaer, V., and Balasse, E.O., Mechanism of the hyperketonaemic effect of prolonged exercise in insulin-deprived type 1 (insulin-dependent) diabetic patients, *Diabetologia,* 30, 298, 1987.

39. American Academy of Pediatrics, Committee on Sports Medicine and Fitness, Assessing physical activity and fitness in the office setting, *Pediatrics,* 93, 686, 1994.

40. Hough, D.O., Diabetes mellitus in sports, *Med. Clin. N. Am.,* 78, 423, 1994.

41. Ganda, O.P., Pathogenesis of macrovascular disease in the human diabetic, *Diabetes,* 29, 931, 1980.

42. Bar-Or, O., *Pediatric Sports Medicine for the Practicioner: Physiological Principles to Clinical Applications,* Springer Verlag, New York, 1983.

43. Wilk, B. and Bar-Or, O., Effect of drink flavor and NaCl on voluntary drinking and hydration in boys exercising in the heat, *J. Appl. Physiol.,* 41, 1112, 1996.

44. Etzwiler, D.D., Franz, M.J., Hollander, P. et al., *Learning to Live Well with Diabetes,* Chronimed Publishing, Park Nicollet Medical Center, Minnentonka, MN, 1987, 58.

45. Thurm U. and Harper P.N., I'm running on insulin, *Diabetes Care,* 15, 1811, 1992.

46. Horton, E.S., Role and management of exercise in diabetes mellitus, *Diabetes Care,* 11, 201, 1988.

47. Position statement: nutrition recommendations and principles for people with diabetes mellitus, *Diabetes Care,* 18 (suppl), 16, 1995.

48. National Research Council, Recommended Dietary Allowance. 10th ed. National Academy Press, Washington, D.C., 1989, 521.

49. Nair, K.S., Garrow, J.S., Ford, C., Mahler, R.F., and Halliday, D., Effect of poor diabetic control on whole body protein metabolism in man, *Diabetologia,* 25, 400, 1983.

50. Luzi, L., Castellino, P., Simonson, D.C., Petrides, A.S., and DeFronzo, R.A., Leucine metabolism in IDDM, *Diabetes,* 39, 38, 1990.

51. Henry, R.R., Protein content of the diabetic diet, *Diabetes Care,* 17, 1502, 1994.

52. Franz, M.J., Horton, E.S., Bantle, J.P., Beeke, C.A., Brunzell, J.D., Coulston, A.M., Henry, R.R., Hoogwerf, B.J., Stacpoole, P.W., et al., Nutrition principles for the management of diabetes and related complications, *Diabetes Care,* 17, 490, 1994.

53. Nutrition Sub-Committee of the British Diabetic Association's Professional Advisory Committee, Dietary recommendations for people with diabetes: an update for the 1990's, *Diabet Med.,* 9, 189, 1992.

54. Israel, D.H. and Gorlin, R., Fish oils in the prevention of atherosclerosis, *J. Am. Coll. Cardiol.,* 19, 174, 1991.
55. Malasanos, T.H. and Stacpoole, P.W., Biological effects of ω-3 fatty acids in diabetes mellitus, *Diabetes Care,* 14, 1160, 1991.
56. Connor, W.E., Prince, M.J., Ullmann, D., Riddle, M., Hatcher, L., Smith, F.E., and Wilson, D., The hypotriglyceridemic effect of fish oil in adult-onset diabetes without adverse glucose control, *Ann. N.Y. Acad. Sci.,* 683, 337, 1993.
57. Westerveld, H.T., Sixma, J.J., de Graph, J.C., Van Brengel, H.H., Akkerman, J.W., Erkelens, F., and Tchobroutsky, G., Effect of low dose EPA-E on glycemic control, lipid profile, lipoprotein(a), platelet aggregation, viscosity, and platelet and vessel wall interactions, *Diabetes Care,* 16, 683, 1993.
58. Glauber, H., Wallace, P., Griver, K., and Brechtel, G., Adverse metabolic effects of omega-3 fatty acids in non-insulin dependent diabetes mellitus, *Ann. Intern. Med.,* 108, 663, 1988.
59. Kasim, S.E., Dietary marine fish oils and insulin action in type 2 diabetes, *Ann. N.Y. Acad. Sci.,* 683, 250, 1993.
60. Jenkins, D.J.A., Wolever, T.M.S., Junkins, A.L., Josse, R.J., and Wong, G.S., The glycemic response to carbohydrate and food, *Lancet,* 2, 388, 1984.
61. Slama, G., Haardt, M.J., Jean-Joseph, P., Costagliola, D., Joicolea, I., Bornet, F., Elgrably, F., and Tchobroutsky, G., Sucrose taken during mixed meal has no additional hyperglycemic action over isocaloric amounts of starch in well-controlled diabetics, *Lancet,* 2, 122, 1984.
62. Bantle, J.P., Laine, D.C., Castle, G.W. et al., Postprandial glucose and insulin responses to meals containing different carbohydrates in normal and diabetic subjects, *N. Engl. J. Med.,* 309, 7, 1983.
63. Chen, Y.D.I., Coulstone, A.M., Zhou, M.Y., Hollenbeck, C.B., and Reaven, G.M., Why do low-fat high-carbohydrate diets accentuate postprandial lipemia in patients with NIDDM, *Diabetes Care,* 18, 10, 1995.
64. Garg, A., Bantle, J.P., Henry, R.R., Coustan, A.M., Driver, K.A., Raatz, S.K., Brinkley, L., Chen, Y.D., Grundy, S.M., Hinet, B.A. et al., Effects of varying carbohydrate content of diet in patients with non-insulin-dependent diabetes mellitus, *J. Am. Med. Assoc.,* 271, 1421, 1994.
65. Williams, G., Management of non-insulin-dependent diabetes mellitus. *Lancet,* 343, 95, 1994.
66. Paternostro-Bayles, M., Wing, R.R., and Robertson, R.J., Effect of life-style activity of varying duration on glycemic control in type II diabetic women, *Diabetes Care,* 12, 34, 1989.
67. Bennet, W.I., Beyond overeating, *N. Engl. J. Med.,* 332, 673, 1995.
68. Flier, J.S., The adipocyte: storage depot or node on the energy information highway, *Cell,* 80, 15, 1995.
69. Leibel, R.L., Rosenbaum, M., and Hirsch, J., Changes in energy expenditure resulting from altered body weight, *N. Engl. J. Med.,* 332(10), 621, 1995.
70. Wadden, T.A., Foster, G.D., Letizia, K.A., and Mullen, J.L., Long-term effects of dieting on resting metabolic rate of obese outpatients, *J. Am. Med. Assoc.,* 264, 707, 1990.
71. Zhang, Y. et al., Positional cloning of the mouse obese gene and its human homologue, *Nature,* 372, 425, 1994.
72. Halaas, J.L., Gajiwala, K.S., Maffei, M., Cohen, S.L., Chait, B.T., Kapinowitz, D., Lallone, R.L., Burley, S.K., and Friedman, J.M., Weight-reducing effects of plasma protein encoded by the *obese* gene, *Science,* 269, 543, 1995.
73. Maffei, M., Halaas, J., Ravussin, E., Pratley, R.E., Lee, G.H., Zhang, Y., Fei, H., Kim, S., Lallone, R., Ranganathau, S. et al., Leptin levels in human and rodent: measurement of plasma leptin and *ob* RNA in obese and weight-reduced subjects, *Nature Med.,* 11, 1155, 1996.
74. Frederich, R.C., Hamann, A., Anderson, S., Lollmann, B., Lowell, B.B., and Flier, J.S., Leptin levels reflect body lipid content in mice: evidence for diet-induced resistance to leptin action, *Nature Med.,* 12, 1131, 1995.
75. Pelleymounter, M.A., Cullen, M.J., Baker, M.B., Hecht, R., Winters, D., Boche, T., and Collins, F., Effects of the obese gene product on body regulation in *ob/ob* mice, *Science,* 269, 540, 1995.
76. Campfield, L.A., Smith, F.J., Guisez, Y., Daves, R., and Burn, P., Recombinant mouse OB protein: evidence for a peripheral signal linking adiposity and central neural networks, *Science,* 269, 546, 1995.
77. Tartaglia, L.A., Dembski, M., Weng, X., Deng, N., Culpepper, J., Devas, K., Richards, G.J., Campfield, L.A., Clark, F.T., Deeds, J. et al., Identification and expression cloning of a leptin receptor, OB-R, *Cell,* 83, 1263, 1995.
78. Coleman, D.L., Obese and diabetes: two mutant genes causing diabetes-obesity syndrome in mice, *Diabetologia,* 14, 141, 1978.
79. Chen, H., Charlat, O., Tartaglia, L., Woulf, E.A., Weng, X., Ellis, S.J., Lakey, N.D., Culpepper, J., Moore, K.J., Breitbart, R.E., Duyk, G.M., Tepper, R.I., and Morgenstern, J.P., Evidence that the diabetes gene encodes the leptin receptor: identification of a mutation in the leptin receptor gene in *db/db* mice, *Cell,* 84, 491, 1996.
80. Frederich, R.C. et al., Expression of *ob* mRNA and its encoded protein in rodents: impact of nutrition and obesity, *J. Clin. Invest.,* 96, 1658, 1995.
81. Saladin, R., De Vos, P., Guerre-Millo, M., Leturque, A., Giraud, J., Staels, B., and Auwert, J., Transient increase in *obese* gene expression after food intake or insulin administration, *Nature,* 377, 527, 1995.
82. MacDougald, O.A., Hwang, C.S., Fan, H., and Lane, D., Regulated expression of the obese gene product (leptin) in white adipose tissue and 3T3-L1 adipocytes, *Proc. Natl. Acad. Sci. USA,* 92, 9034, 1995.
83. Lonnqvist, F., Arner, P., Nordfors, L., and Shalling, M., Overexpression of the obese (*ob*) gene in adipose tissue of human obese subjects, *Nature Med.,* 1, 950, 1995.

84. American Diabetes Association, Consensus statement: role of cardiovascular risk factors in prevention and treatment of macrovascular disease in diabetes, *Diabetes Care*, 16, 72, 1993.

85. Reaven, G.M., Role of insulin resistance in human disease, *Diabetes*, 37, 1595, 1988.

86. Ruderman, N.B. and Schneider, S.H., Diabetes, exercise, and atherosclerosis, *Diabetes Care*, 15, 1787, 1992.

87. American Diabetes Association, Exercise and NIDDM: technical review, *Diabetes Care*, 13, 785, 1990.

88. Schneider, S.H., Amorosa, L.F., Khachadurian, A.K., and Ruderman, N.B., Studies on the mechanism of improved glucose control during regular exercise in type 2 (non-insulin dependent) diabetes, *Diabetologia*, 26, 353, 1984.

89. Rogers, M.A., Yamamoto, C., King, D.S., Hagberg, J.M., Ehsani, A.A., and Holloszy, J.D., Improvement in glucose tolerance after 1 week of exercise in patients with mild NIDDM, *Diabetes Care*, 11, 613, 1988.

90. Reitman, J.S., Vasques, B., Klimes, I., and Nagulesparan, M., Improvement of glucose homeostasis after exercise training in non-insulin-dependent diabetes, *Diabetes Care*, 7, 434, 1984.

91. Bogardus, C., Ravussin, E., Robbins, D.C., Wolfe, R.R., Horton, E.S., and Sims, E.A.H., Effects of physical training and wet therapy on carbohydrate metabolism in patients with glucose intolerance and non-insulin dependent diabetes mellitus, *Diabetes*, 7, 416, 1984.

92. Barnard, R.J., Jung, T., and Inkeles, S.B., Diet and exercise in the treatment of NIDDM. The need for early emphasis, *Diabetes Care*, 17, 1469, 1994.

93. Skarfors, E.T., Wegener, T.A., Lithell, H., and Selinus, I., Physical training as treatment for Type 2 (non-insulin-dependent) diabetes in elderly men. A feasibility study over 2 years, *Diabetologia*, 30, 930, 1987.

94. Leon, A., Connett, J., Jacobs, D.R., and Rauramaa, R., Leisure-time physical activity level and risk of coronary artery disease and death: the multiple risk factor intervention trial, *J. Amer. Med. Assoc.*, 258, 2388, 1987.

95. Kohl, H.W., Villegas, J.A., Gordon, N.F., and Blair, S.N., Cardiorespiratory fitness, glycemic status, and mortality risk in man, *Diabetes Care*, 15, 184, 1992.

96. Paffenbarger, R.S. Jr., Hyde, R.T., Wing, A.L., Lee, I.M., Jung, D.L., and Kampert, J.B., The association of changes in physical-activity level and other lifestyle characteristics with mortality among men, *N. Engl. J. Med.*, 328, 538, 1993.

97. Schuler, G., Hambrecht, R., Schlierf, G., Niebauer, J., Hauer, K., Neumann, J., Hogberg, E., Drinkmann, A., Bacher, F., Emaze, M. et al., Regular physical exercise and low-fatiet. Effects on progression of coronary artery disease, *Circulation*, 86, 1, 1992.

98. Rodriguez, B.L., Curb, J.D., Burchfiel, C.M., Abbott, R.D., Petrovitch, H., Masaki, K, and Chin, D., Physical activity and 23-year incidence of coronary heart disease morbidity and mortality among middle-aged men. The Honolulu Heart Program, *Circulation*, 89, 2540, 1994.

99. Després, J.P., Pouliot, M.C., Moorjani, S. et al., Loss of abdominal fat and metabolic response to exercise training in obese women, *Am. J. Physiol.*, 261, E159, 1991.

100. Tribble, D.L., Vandenberg, J.J.M., Motchnik, P.A., Ames, B.N., Lewis, D.M., Chait, A., and Krauss, R.M., Oxidative susceptibility of low-density lipoprotein subfractions is related to their ubiquinol-10 and α-tocopherol content, *Proc. Natl. Acad. Sci. U.S.A.*, 91, 1183, 1994.

101. Holloszy, J.O., Skinner, G., Toro, G., and Cureton, T.K., Effects of six-month program for endurance exercise on serum lipids in middle-aged men, *Am. J. Cardiol.*, 14, 753, 1964.

102. Tran, Z.V. and Weltman, A., Differential effects of exercise on serum lipid and lipoprotein levels seen with changes in body weight, *J. Am. Med. Assoc.*, 254, 919, 1985.

103. Houmard, J.A., Bruno, N.J., Bruner, R.K., McCammon, M.R., Israel, R.G., Barakat, H.A. et al., Effects of exercise training on the chemical composition of plasma LDL, *Arteriosclr Thromb.*, 14, 325, 1994.

104. Arroll, B. and Beaglehole, R., Does physical activity lower blood pressure? A critical review of the clinical trials, *J. Clin. Epidemiol.*, 45, 439, 1992.

105. Arroll, B. and Beaglehole, R., Exercise for hypertension, *Lancet*, 341, 1248, 1993.

106. Black, G.A., Levin, S.R., and Koyal, S.N., Exercise-induced hypertension in normotensive patients with NIDDM, *Diabetes Care*, 13, 799, 1990.

107. Kahn, C.R., Insulin action, diabetogenes, and the cause of type II diabetes, *Diabetes*, 43, 1066, 1994.

108. Harris, M.I., Hadden, W.C., Knowler, W.C., and Bennett, P.H., Prevalence of diabetes and impaired glucose tolerance and plasma glucose levels in US population aged 20–74, *Diabetes*, 36, 532, 1987.

109. McPhillips, J.B., Barrett-Connor, E., and Wingard, D.L., Cardiovascular disease risk factors before the diagnosis of impaired glucose tolerance and non-insulin-dependent diabetes mellitus in a community of older adults, *Am. J. Epidemiol.*, 131, 443, 1990.

110. Helmrich, S.P., Ragland, D.R., Leung, R.W., and Paffenbarger, R.S., Physical activity and reduced occurrence of non-insulin-dependent diabetes mellitus, *N. Engl. J. Med.*, 325, 147, 1991.

111. Manson, J.E., Rimm, E.B., Stampfer, M.J., Colditz, G.A., Willett, W.C., Krolewski, H.J., Rosner, B., Hennekens, C.H., and Speizer, F.E., Physical activity and incidence of non-insulin-dependent diabetes mellitus in women, *Lancet*, 338, 774, 1991.

112. Manson, J.E., Nathan, D.M., Krolewski, A.S., Stampfer, M.J., Willett, W.C., and Hennekens, C.H., A prospective study of exercise and incidence of diabetes among US male physicians, *J. Am. Med. Assoc.*, 268, 63, 1992.

113. Kemmer, F.W., Tacken, M., and Berger, M., Mechanisms of exercise-induced hypoglycemia during sulfonyl-urea treatment, *Diabetes*, 36, 1178, 1987.
114. Albert, S.G. and Bernbaum, M., Exercise for patients with diabetic retinopathy, *Diabetes Care,* 18, 130, 1995.
115. Anderson, B., Jr., Activity and diabetic vitreous hemorrhages, *Ophthalmology*, 87, 173, 1980.
116. Vittinghus, E. and Mogensen, C.E., Graded exercise and protein excretion in diabetic men and the effect of insulin treatment, *Kidney Int.,* 21, 725, 1982.
117. O'Connor, G.T., Buring, J.E., Yusuf, S., Goldhafer, S.Z., Olmstead, E.M., Paffenbarger, R.S. Jr., and Henneken, C.H., An overview of randomized trials of rehabilitation with exercise after myocardial infarction, *Circulation*, 80, 234, 1989.
118. The Expert Panell II, Summary of the second report of the National Cholesterol Education Program (NCEP) Expert Panel on detection, evaluation, and treatment of high blood cholesterol in adults, *J. Am. Med. Assoc.,* 269, 3015, 1993.
119. Larsen, O.A. and Lassen, N.A., Effect of daily muscular exercise in patients with intermittent claudication, Lancet, 2, 1093, 1966.
120. Inserra, F., Daccordi, H., Ippolito, J.L., Romano, L., Zelechower, H., and Farder, L., Decrease of exercise-induced microalbuminuria in patients with type I diabetes by means of an angiotensin-converting enzyme inhibitor, *Am. J. Kidney Dis.*, 27, 26, 1996.
121. Fletcher, G.F., Balady, G., Froelicher, V.F., Hartley, L.H., Haskell, W.L., Polloch, M.L., Hartley, L.H., Haskell, W.L., and Pollock, M.L., Exercise standards, *Circulation*, 91, 580, 1995.
122. Fletcher, G.F., The antiatherosclerotic effect of exercise, *Cardiol. Clin.,* 14, 85, 1996.
123. Outerbridge, R. and Micheli, L.J., Overuse injuries, *Clin. Sports Med.,* 14, 3, July 1995.
124. Stratton, J.R., Chandler, W.L., and Schwartz, R.S., Effects of physical conditioning on fibrinolytic variables and fibrinogen in young and old healthy adults, *Circulation*, 83, 1692, 1991.

Chapter **21**

NUTRITION AND THE PHYSICALLY DISABLED ATHLETE

_____ Jayanthi Kandiah

CONTENTS

I. INTRODUCTION

Athletes who train regularly and compete for one or more hours per day have nutritional needs that go beyond those of a recreational athlete. An athlete's ability to perform is dictated not only by the type of sport, duration of the activity, and type of muscles utilized, but also by the diet. In recent years, competitions have been designed for not only the able-bodied athlete but for the athlete with disabilities. Like the Olympics, the Special Olympics provides an array of competitive sports for mentally retarded athletes, while the Paralympic Games caters international competitions for physically disabled athletes. Though extensive research has been conducted on able-bodied athletes and the role of nutrients in athletic performance[1-8] limited nutrition research is available on disabled athletes.[9-11] Thus, the present review will deal concisely with health and nutritional considerations of physically disabled athletes and nonathletes, with particular emphasis placed on my research with Paralympic athletes.

II. HEALTH CONSIDERATIONS FOR THE DISABLED

Individuals who experience a physical disability are faced with many obstacles. Some of these originate from their functional inabilities to perform tasks and others may be related

0-8493-8560-1/97/$0.00+$.50
© 1998 by CRC Press LLC

to the environment, such as the inaccessibility to grocery stores. Together these hurdles have a negative impact on their health and well being.[12-15]

Research evidence indicates the prevalence of cardiovascular disease,[16-19] obesity,[20] osteoporosis,[13,14] and malnutrition[21] is significantly higher in amputees, the blind, the spinally injured, and those with cerebral palsy (CP). The occurrence of these chronic diseases places this population at a higher risk of mortality than the physically abled population. De Vivo et al.[22] noted a 10% reduction in the life expectancy of the spinal cord-injured (SCI) population than in their able-bodied counterparts. This was associated with smaller amount of active muscle mass induced by the disability and/or physical inactivity.

According to the National Research Council, composition of dietary intake for a healthy individual should be 55–60% for carbohydrates, 12–15% for protein, and no greater than 30% for fat.[23] Trauma to the body increases the need for a larger intake of protein. In people with immobilizing physical disabilities, fat intake should be limited to less than 20% of total caloric intake.[13] Nutrient deficiencies commonly observed among the SCI population are iron, calcium, vitamin C, beta carotene, thiamin, folate, and copper.[24-26]

Adults who are affected with CP have a broad spectrum of health problems. Severity of the illness is dependent upon the type of disorder — spastic or athetosis CP. Obesity is often an issue with nonambulatory spastic individuals, while increase in energy requirement is observed in athetoid CP.[15,20] Continuous involuntary movement in athetosis has been shown to increase resting metabolic rate by approximately 500 kcal/day (2100 kJ).[15] Nutritional inadequacies in adults with CP resemble that of nondisabled adults, with high intake of fat and protein and low intake of fiber. Males' diet met the recommendation for all nutrients except calcium, while females were deficient in calcium, iron, and niacin.[27] The increased susceptibility to nutrient deficiencies is attributed to low nutrient intake, drug nutrient interaction, type and severity of the physical disability, and health complications, e.g., gastrointestinal problems, infections.

III. PARALYMPIC GAMES

The philosophy guiding the Paralympic Games is that elite athletes with physical disabilities around the world should have opportunities and experiences equivalent to nondisabled athletes. In 1948, Sir Ludwig Guttman, an English neurosurgeon at Stroke-Mandeville Hospital in Aylesbury, England, organized the International Wheelchair Games to coincide with the London Olympics. The first attempt to connect the Olympics and the Paralympics was not made until 1960, when the first Paralympic Games were held in Rome, just a few weeks after the 1960 Rome Olympics. Since then, the Paralympic Games are hosted in the same country and city that hosts the Olympics.[28]

In the first Paralympics held in 1960, wheelchair athletes were the only participants. Currently competitors represent four international federations namely: the blind, paraplegics and quadriplegics with CP, amputees, and others (spinal-cord injuries, dwarfism, etc.). To create an equal starting point for competition, all athletes are evaluated and classified by disability and/or functional ability. Based on their classification, the athletes then compete in a variety of sports — aquatic, track and field.

IV. MEDICAL BENEFITS AND CONCERNS OF DISABLED ATHLETES

Participation in sports by the physically disabled has been associated with decreased obesity,[29] improved endurance,[30,31] better mobility,[31,32] higher self-esteem,[14,31] and diminished depression.[14] Ten hours a week of sports participation by spinal cord-injured athletes resulted in fewer infections, rehospitalizations, and medical complications when compared to the nonathlete group. The competitive athlete group had an average of 2.4 visits to the doctor per year compared to 6.7 visits by the nonathletes.[33]

Results from studies reveal the common injuries among physically disabled athletes are shoulder muscle strains, abrasions, upper respiratory infections, and elbow tendinitis.[33-34] These injuries could be reduced by using proper equipment and wearing appropriate attire (e.g., padded gloves to prevent carpal tunnel syndrome frequently observed in wheelchair athletes).[37]

Prevalence of other injuries can be avoided through good nutrition. Athletes with spinal cord injury experience hypo- and hyperthermia during moderate temperature variations (between 50–60°F or 10–15.5°C). Adequate hydration and protection of the athletes from extremes of temperature are recommended.[37] Plenty of water or cool fluid replacement beverages (16 oz or 471 ml for every pound of water lost) before, during, and after exercise will prevent dehydration. Alcoholic and caffeinated beverages should be avoided because of their diuretic properties. In addition, hydration will reduce the incidence of bladder infection in athletes with cerebral palsy and spinal cord injury.[38] Since long-term immobilization of the lower extremities is a risk factor for fractures and osteoporosis, calcium is highly recommended in the diets of wheelchair athletes.[37]

V. NUTRITION AND PARALYMPIC ATHLETES

Though there are no specific U.S. Recommended Dietary Allowances (RDA) and no minimum requirements for athletes in training, the distribution of nutrients composing the athletes' diet are similar to the recommendations for the general population. With the advent of the Paralympic Games, there has been a rise in the participation of disabled athletes at various competitions. Since diet plays a vital role in athletic performance, and since disabled athletes have multifactorial complications, investigations on their nutritional status would help educate and prevent the occurrence of chronic diseases.

Three-day diet records of 33 Paralympics athletes (19 CP and 14 vision impaired) were analyzed for calcium.[9] Sixty-four percent of the visually impaired (VI) and 53% CP athletes consumed an average of less than 800 mg calcium/day. All the female CP athletes had calcium intake ranging from 446–638 mg/day. These findings are similar to a more recent study by Kandiah,[10] where 12 female CP athletes who had participated in the Paralympics had a mean intake of 364 mg calcium/day. Unlike the earlier study, where milk and dairy products were the major contributors of calcium, in this research, 9 of the 12 female athletes drank less than two cups of milk per day and none took any kind of calcium supplements.

In addition to calcium, female CP athletes had a daily mean intake of 10.3 mg iron, 8.4 mg zinc, and 0.9 mg folate. Though not statistically significant, males had higher intake of cholesterol. Dietary fiber intake in 78% of the men and 75% of the women was less than 12 gm/day. A pattern exists between this and the previous study, where females are deficient in calcium and iron that is of utter importance to their gender and athletic performance.[10] Although none of the female athletes were vegetarians, they generally consumed <3 oz (<85 grams) of meat, fish, or poultry per day; thus absorption of the readily available heme iron was limited. However, nutrition considerations should be given to the overall nutritional status of these athletes as a deficiency of one nutrient could stimulate the deficiency of another because of overlapping of similar food sources.

Preventive nutrition is a new concept currently used in dietetics. Like their normal counterparts, the disabled athletes have numerous deficiencies.[9,10] When the general nutrition knowledge of 101 Paralympic athletes (40 VI and 61 CP) was evaluated, VI athletes received significantly (p <0.05) higher scores than athletes with CP. Type of competition, age, sex, and educational level of the athletes did not significantly influence their nutrition knowledge. However, a contradictory result was found that in spite of the VI athletes having a higher score in nutrition knowledge, more than 50% of the athletes had higher intake of fat and cholesterol and lower intake of zinc and fiber.[11]

VI. CONCLUSION

With an increasing number of physically disabled athletes in competitive sports, inferences from studies cited here will be helpful to health professionals and coaches working with this population. Future studies should investigate the diets of other Paralympic athletes, and longitudinal nutrition studies are urgently required to promote better health, which will enhance athletic performance.

REFERENCES

1. Roberts, K.M., Nobel, E.G., Hayden, D.B., and Taylor, A.W., Simple and complex carbohydrate rich diets and muscle glycogen content of marathon runners, *Eur. J. Appl. Physiol.*, 57, 70, 1988.
2. Wright, E.D. and Paige, D.M., Lipid metabolism and exercise, *J. Clin. Nutr.*, 7, 28, 1988.
3. Wolinsky, I. and Hickson, J.F., Jr., *Nutrition in Exercise and Sport*, 2nd ed., CRC Press, Boca Raton, FL, 1994.
4. Bernardot, D., Schwarz, M., and Heller, D.W., Nutrient intake in young, highly competitive gymnasts, *J. Am. Diet. Assoc.*, 89, 401, 1989.
5. Dressendorfer, R.H. and Sockolov, R., Hypozincemia in runners, *Phys. Sports. Med.*, 8, 97, 1980.
6. Gerster, H., The role of vitamin C in athletic performance, *J. Am. Col. Nutr.*, 8, 636, 1989.
7. Murray, R., The effects of consuming carbohydrate-electrolyte beverages on fluid absorption during and following exercise, *Sports Med.*, 4, 322, 1987.
8. Barr, S. and Costill, D., Water: can the endurance athlete get too much of a good thing?, *J. Am. Diet. Assoc.*, 89, 1629, 1989.
9. Kandiah, J., Calcium and iron intakes of disabled elite athletes, in *Sports Nutrition — Mineral and Electrolytes*, Kies, C. and Driskell, J.A., Eds., CRC Press, Boca Raton, FL, 1995, chap. 9.
10. Kandiah, J., Nutritional assessment of paralympic athletes with cerebral palsy, *FASEB J.*, A489, 1996.
11. Kandiah, J., Dietary intake and nutrition knowledge of elite disabled athletes, *INFORM-AOCS*, #94, Denver, CO, 1993.
12. Santiago, M.C., Coyle, C.P., and Kinney, W.B., Aerobic exercise effect on individuals with physical disabilities, *Arch. Phys. Med. Rehabil.*, 74, 1192, 1993.
13. Rice, H.B., Ponichtera-Mulcare, J.A., and Glaser, R.M., Nutrition and the spinal cord injured individual, *Clin. Kinesiol.*, 54, 20, 1994.
14. Shepard, R.J., Benefits of sport and physical activity for the disabled: implications for the individual and for society, *Scand. J. Rehab. Med.*, 23, 51, 1991.
15. Johnson, R.K., Goran, M.I., and Ferrara, M.S., Athetosis increases resting metabolic rate in adults with cerebral palsy, *J. Am. Diet. Assoc.*, 95, 145, 1995.
16. Geisler, W.O., Jousse, A.T., Wynne-Jones, M., and Breithaupt, D., Survival in traumatic spinal cord injury, *Paraplegia*, 21, 364, 1983.
17. LaPorte, R.E., Brenes, G., and Dearwater, S., HDL cholesterol across a spectrum of physical activity from quadriplegia to marathon running, *Lancet*, 1, 1212, 1983.
18. Lee, C.T. and Price, M., Survival from spinal cord injury, *J. Chronic. Dis.*, 35, 487, 1982.
19. United States Committee on Veterns Administration Affairs, Relationship between the amputation of an extremity and the subsequent development of cardiovascular disorders, U.S. Government Printing Office, Washington, D.C., 1979.
20. Taylor, S.B. and Shelton, J.E., Caloric requirements of a spastic immobile cerebral palsy patient: a case report, *Arch. Phys. Med. Rehabil.*, 76, 281, 1995.
21. Lee, B.Y., Agarwal, N., Corcoran, A., Thoden, W.R., and Guercio, A.D., Assessment of nutritional and metabolic status of paraplegics, *J. Rehabil. Res. Dev.*, 22, 11, 1985.
22. De Vivo, M.J., Fine, P.R., Maetz, H.M., and Stover, S.L., Prevalence of spinal cord injury: a re-estimation of employing life table techniques, *Arch. Neurol.*, 37, 239, 1980.
23. Committee on Diet and Health, Diet and Health: Implications for Reducing Chronic Disease Risk, National Academy Press, Washington, D.C., 1989.
24. Huang, L.T., Devivo, M.J., and Stover, S.L., Anemia in acute phase of spinal cord injury, *Arch. Phys. Med. Rehabil.*, 71, 3, 1990.

25. Naftchi, N.E., Viau, A.T., Sell, G.H., and Lowman, E.W., Mineral metabolism in spinal cord injury, *Arch. Phys. Med. Rehabil.,* 61, 139, 1980.
26. Laven, G.T., Huang, C.T., Devivo, M.J., Stover, S.L., Kuhleimer, K.V., and Fine, P.R., Nutritional status during acute stage of spinal cord injury, *Arch. Phys. Med. Rehabil.,* 70, 277, 1989.
27. Ferrang, T.M., Johnson, R.K., and Ferrara, M.S., Dietary and anthropometric assessment of adults with cerebral palsy, *J. Am. Diet. Assoc.,* 92, 1083, 1992.
28. United States Olympics Committee, Atlanta, GA, 1996.
29. Mardorsky, B.J.G. and Mardorsky, A., Wheelchair racing: important modality in acute rehabilitation after paraplegia, *Arch. Phys. Med. Rehabil.,* 64, 186, 1983.
30. Jackson, R.W. and Fredrickson, A., Sports for the physically disabled: 1976 Olympiad (Toronto), *Am. J. Sports Med.,* 7, 293, 1979.
31. Small, E. and Bar-Or, O., The young athlete with chronic disease, *Clin. Sports Med.,* 14, 709, 1995.
32. Weiss, M. and Beck, J., Sports as part of therapy and rehabilitation of paraplegics, *Paraplegia,* 11, 166, 1973.
33. Curtis, K.A., McClanahan, S., Hall, K.M., Dillon, D.D., and Brown, K.F., Health, vocational, and functional status in spinal cord injured athletes and nonathletes, *Arch. Phys. Med. Rehabil.,* 67, 862, 1986.
34. Ferrara, M.S., Buckely, W.E., and McCann, B.C., The injury experience of the competitive athletes with a disability: prevention implications, *Med. Sci. Sports Exer.,* 24, 184, 1992.
35. Burnham, R., Newell, E., and Steadward, R., Sports medicine for the physically disabled: the Canadian team experience at the 1988 Seoul Paralympics games, *Clin. J. Sports Med.,* 1, 193, 1991.
36. Ritcher, K.E., Hyman, S.C., and Mushett-Adams, C.A., Injuries in world class cerebral palsy athlete of the 1988 South Korea Paralympics, *J. Osteo. Sports Med.,* 1, 15, 1991.
37. Peck, D.M. and Mckeag, D.B., Athletes with disabilities, *Phys. Sports Med.,* 22, 59, 1994.
38. Fike, S., Kanter, M., and Markely, E., Fluid and electrolyte requirements of exercise, in *Sports Nutrition,* 2nd ed., Benardot, D., Ed., American Dietetic Association, Chicago, IL, 1992, p 38.

Chapter 22

NUTRIENT REQUIREMENTS FOR COMPETITIVE SPORTS

Robert Murray
Craig A. Horswill

CONTENTS

0-8493-8560-1/97/$0.00+$.50
© 1998 by CRC Press LLC

I. INTRODUCTION

The overviews presented in other sections of this volume provide the scientific *backdrop* against which recommendations can be made regarding the nutritional practices of athletes. This chapter will focus on the nutrient requirements for specific sports, taking into consideration the demands of training and competing in a variety of team and individual sports. Although it is impossible to make precise recommendations regarding the nutritional practices of an individual athlete in a specific sport, there is more than ample scientific information

TABLE 1   Categories of Sport-Specific Events Referred to Within This Chapter

Category	Examples
team sports	soccer, basketball, football, ice hockey, rugby, field hockey, and lacrosse
short-duration, high-intensity sports	track and field, wrestling, swimming, rowing, and gymnastics
long-duration, moderate-intensity sports	running, cycling, triathlon, and cross-country skiing

available to draw general recommendations that can be tailored to suit the needs of individual athletes. In addition to the information in this chapter, there are many other resources that coaches, trainers, and athletes can turn to for excellent scientific and practical information.[1-14]

The subsections in this chapter that refer to team sports; short-duration, high-intensity sports; and long-duration, moderate-intensity sports, provide a convenient means of giving sport-specific examples of athlete's nutrient requirements (see Table 1). Soccer, basketball, football, ice hockey, rugby, field hockey, lacrosse, and similar activities fall under the *team-sports* categories. *Short-duration, high-intensity sports* include track and field, wrestling, swimming, rowing, and gymnastics. Sports such as running, cycling, triathlon, and cross-country skiing have been categorized as *long-duration, moderate-intensity sports*. Obviously, these lists are not all-inclusive, nor should the categories be viewed too stringently. Many characteristics, habits, and requirements of team-sport athletes apply to athletes in individual sports, and vice versa. Likewise, the nutrient requirements of athletes training for competition in sprint-type activities are not all that dissimilar from athletes involved in endurance sports.

II.   ENERGY REQUIREMENTS FOR ATHLETES

A.   FUNDAMENTAL CONCEPTS
1.   Energy Intake
The appropriate energy requirement for an athlete is one that strikes a balance between energy intake and energy expenditure such that body mass and body composition are maintained at a level consistent with good health and optimal athletic performance. For example, it is possible that an energy intake of only 1800 kcal (7535 J) might be appropriate in a small athlete if body mass, body composition, health, and performance are *all* maintained at acceptable levels. Violation of one or more of these tenets signals that energy intake is not appropriate. A female gymnast who desires to restrict energy intake to maintain a small, lean figure for the purpose of optimizing performance, risks good health (and performance) in the process. On the other end of the spectrum, a football player who ingests excess calories in a desire to gain body mass, also jeopardizes health and performance.

2.   Resting Energy Expenditure
To maintain body weight, energy intake must balance the sum of the energy expended at rest, during physical activity, and for thermogenesis. The thermic effect of food intake is small, representing only 5–10% of energy intake,[15] exists for only a few hours following a meal,[16] and will be disregarded in this analysis. Resting energy expenditure (REE) is proportional to lean body mass and can be estimated by the following equations:[17]

$$\text{In males 10–18, REE} = (17.5 \times \text{BW}) + 651$$
$$\text{In males 18–30, REE} = (15.3 \times \text{BW}) + 679$$
$$\text{In males 30–60, REE} = (11.6 \times \text{BW}) + 879$$

$$\text{In females } 10\text{--}18, \text{ REE} = (12.2 \times \text{BW}) + 746$$
$$\text{In females } 18\text{--}30, \text{ REE} = (14.7 \times \text{BW}) + 496$$
$$\text{In females } 30\text{--}60, \text{ REE} = (8.7 \times \text{BW}) + 829$$

where BW = body weight in kg.

3. Exercise Energy Expenditure

The daily energy requirements of athletes vary widely, depending upon body size and activity level.[18] For example, a small female tennis player training for 60 min a day may require only 20 kcal/kg BW/day (84 joules/kg/day) to meet her energy requirements, whereas a male triathlete may require in excess of 75 kcal/kg BW/day (314 joules/kg/day) to meet the energy needs induced by 3 h of daily training. As a general guideline, Economos et al.[19] recommend that male athletes ingest >50 kcal/kg/day (>209 joules/kg/day) and females consume 45–50 kcal/kg/day (188–209 joules/kg/day) to meet the energy needs of training for 90 or more minutes per day. Based upon these figures, a 40-kg (88-lb) female gymnast training for 2 h each day would require approximately 2000 kcal (8372 kJ) to maintain body weight, an 85-kg (187-lb) soccer player would need more than 4250 kcal (17,790 kjoules), and a 127-kg (280-lb) football lineman might ingest in excess of 6000 kcal (25,116 kJ).

Dietary energy intake fluctuates daily to reflect an individual's overall energy expenditure, which varies day to day according to the intensity and duration of physical activity. A long, difficult training session may require an energy expenditure of 2000 kcal (8372 kJ), but the same athlete could expend considerably less than 1000 kcal (4186 kJ) on an easy training day. For less-active athletes, the energy allowance for physical activity may range between about 1.6 to 2.4 × REE.[15] For an 18-year-old, 63.6-kg (140-lb) female volleyball player training for 1 h each day, an intake of about 2500 kcal (10,465 kJ) might be enough to satisfy her energy requirements on days of fairly light training (1.6 × REE), but she may need more than 3500 kcal (14,651 kJ) on days of heavy training (2.4 × REE).

Without sophisticated methods of estimating daily energy expenditure (e.g., doubly labeled water, activity monitors, indirect calorimetry, etc.), it is impossible to do more than estimate an athlete's daily energy expenditure. For example, the estimated energy requirements of a 19-year-old college football lineman weighing 108 kg (about 240 lb) might range from 3728 kcal (15,605 kJ) (1.6 × REE) to more than 5500 kcal (23,023 kJ) (2.4 × REE) per day. Hickson et al.[20] measured the food choices of football athletes and determined that their mean energy intake over three consecutive days of training (2 h per day) was approximately 3600 kcal (15,070 kJ), or only 33 kcal/kg BW (138 kJ/kg). While it is possible that these measurements underestimated the actual energy intake of the football players, it is also possible that the data were accurately reflective of a relatively modest level of energy expenditure during training.

Regardless of the manner in which energy requirements are estimated, the athlete's appetite (and associated factors) ultimately determine daily energy intake. The adequacy of energy intake is most accurately reflected by changes in the athlete's body weight and body composition, two measures that have seen unfortunate misuse by well-intentioned coaches who place too much emphasis upon the importance of these values. There is no doubt that both measures should be monitored in athletes who are attempting to gain or lose weight, but for the vast majority of athletes for whom body weight is not an issue, the most important reason to keep track of body weight is to detect and prevent dehydration.

B. TEAM SPORTS

The energy expenditure during training and competition for team sports varies substantially by sport and by position. For example, a midfielder in soccer might cover an average of 10 km per game while a defensive player covers far less ground.[21] The same, of course, is true for all team sports where there often exist substantial differences in the body sizes, and exercise intensity and durations among players on the same team. Consequently, there are wide variations in the energy expenditure and, therefore, the energy requirements of athletes in team sports.

C. SHORT-DURATION, HIGH-INTENSITY SPORTS

Proper nutrition is just as valuable for athletes who compete in sports that require explosive movements of comparatively short duration as it is for athletes who train and compete in endurance events. The primary exception is that, for endurance athletes, nutrition is important *during* both training and competition. For athletes involved in sports requiring high-intensity efforts of short duration (e.g., <20 min), the primary value of proper nutrition is to help sustain hard training and promote rapid recovery. This is most effectively achieved by assuring adequate energy and carbohydrate intake.[22]

Track runners, swimmers, sprint cyclists, rowers, gymnasts, wrestlers, and weight lifters engage in sports requiring high energy expenditures during both training and competition. Consequently, these athletes also have correspondingly high requirements for energy, principally in the form of carbohydrate. The adequate intake of calories and carbohydrate assures the complete restoration of muscle and liver glycogen stores and is an important factor in sparing cellular proteins from catabolism.[23]

D. LONG-DURATION, MODERATE-INTENSITY SPORTS

Athletes who train and compete in endurance sport require large caloric intakes to match their equally large caloric expenditures. For example, a marathon runner who completes a 10-mile (16.1 km) run at a 6 min/mile pace in the morning and 8 miles (12.9 km) of interval training on the track in the afternoon, would require an intake of at least 3000 calories (12,558 kJ) in addition to his or her REE to cover daily energy requirements and assure restoration of glycogen stores.

Failure to ingest enough energy will result in weight loss, an undesirable response in athletes who are normally quite lean.[24] This presents quite a nutritional challenge for athletes such as cross-country skiers who may expend 4000 kcal (16,744 kJ) during a 50-km race and 6000–8000 kcal/day (25,116–33,488 kJ/day) during training camp.[25] For triathletes training 19 h/week, Burke et al.[26] recorded an average energy intake of 60 kcal/kg BW/day (251 kJ/kg/day). For triathletes training 11 h/week, energy intake dropped to 37–40 kcal/kg BW/day (155–167 kJ/kg/day).

E. OTHER CONSIDERATIONS
1. Monitoring Dietary Intake

Consumption of foods and beverages must provide more than 40 nutrients required to maintain health and assure optimal athletic performance. Proper diet planning can help remove some of the mystery and confusion that often accompanies dietary recommendations. Using a tool such as the *Sports Food Swap*[27] or similar approach,[28,29] can be effective with both meat-eating and vegetarian athletes. Diet planning notwithstanding, athletes who train more than 2 h each day often find it difficult to ingest the volume of food needed to meet their caloric requirements. In these cases, effective alternatives include eating small meals and snacks throughout the day, and ingesting commercially available supplements that provide nutritionally balanced and calorically dense sources of energy.

2. Weight Reduction

Certain athletes will restrict energy intake as a part of their preparation for competition. Such athletes include those who must attain a specific body weight classification to be eligible to compete (boxers, wrestlers, weight lifters, and light-weight rowers) or those whose performance may be enhanced by being lighter (gymnasts, distance runners) or appearing to be leaner (figure skaters, body builders). Short and Short[30] reported that within one individual athlete who practiced weight reduction for competition, energy intake varied from 78 kcal (326 kJ) during the day just prior to competition to 11,000 kcal (46,046 kJ) when attempting to recover after "making weight." Adolescent athletes attempting to lose weight for competition may experience an average decrease in energy intake of 38%, from 42 kcal/kg to 26 kcal/kg (176 kJ/kg to 109 kJ/kg), between the pre-season intake and intake during the competitive season.[31]

Several recommendations can be made for athletes who must restrict energy intake to lose weight.[32] First, an assessment of the amount of reasonable weight loss is warranted to allow the athletes to maintain good health and performance. The determination of body fatness will help establish the amount of stored energy that can be reduced by creating a daily energy deficit and yet allow the athlete to eat properly for quality training and good performance. For males, the suggested minimum body fat is 5–7% of body weight; for females the ranges is 12–14% body fat.[32] Knowing the amount of weight that can be lost safely, the athlete should then maintain a diet that creates an energy deficit of 500–1000 kcal/day (2093–4186 kJ/day). This is usually accomplished by modifying both the diet and volume of training. An energy deficit in this range will allow a reduction of 0.5–1.0 kg/week, and in theory, will minimize the loss of body protein. Finally, once the desired weight is attained, the athlete can then increase energy intake to an isocaloric level to maintain the target weight and level of body fatness, and to provide enough energy to meet the demands of training.

3.   Weight Gain

Many athletes attempt to gain weight for their sport. Most of these athletes attempt to increase muscle mass in hopes of simultaneously increasing their power. Other athletes might be less particular and will accept an overall increase in mass, which could translate into greater momentum and resistance to opponents' movements on the athletic field. The overall increase in mass would include an increase in body fat as often seen in Olympic lifters and wrestlers in the heavy weight classes, football lineman, and field athletes (shot putters and the throwers).

Regardless of the compositional change, energy intake in excess of that needed to simply maintain weight is required for increasing the body mass. For most athletes, the desirable outcome of increasing energy intake and undertaking a properly designed resistance training program would be to gain 0.5–0.7 kg of muscle weight per week.[33] The diet component of a weight-gain program would require an increase in the daily energy intake by as much as 23% to provide energy to meet the demands of intense training and to allow for the synthesis of additional muscle protein. In some unique cases, such as the female athlete who suffers amenorrhea and the loss of the bone component of the lean body mass, a decrease in training may need to accompany the increase in energy intake to increase body weight and to improve nutritional status.[34]

III.   FLUID REQUIREMENTS OF ATHLETES

A.   FUNDAMENTAL CONCEPTS

The fluid requirements of athletes generally reflect sweat and urine losses, a volume that may exceed 10 l/day in athletes exercising in warm environments.[35] Fluid losses for individual athletes vary widely and are dependent upon the athlete's genetic predisposition for sweating, the athlete's level of fitness and acclimation, the prevailing environmental conditions, the amount and type of clothing and headgear, and the intensity at which the athlete is exercising.[36]

During low-intensity exercise in cool, dry environments, sweat loss may be less than 500 ml/h but may exceed 3 l/h during intense exercise in hot, humid conditions in athletes who are profuse sweaters.[37]

1. Dehydration and Performance

Voluntary fluid intake also varies widely among athletes, but generally approximates about 50% of sweat loss.[38] This mismatch of fluid ingestion vs. loss results in varying amounts of dehydration, often exceeding 3% of body weight.[39] Under such circumstances, the resulting dehydration will compromise cardiovascular and thermoregulatory response and will result in performance impairment.[40]

Even small amounts of dehydration have a detrimental effect on performance during high-intensity exercise. The research of Walsh et al.[41] underscores the impact that slight dehydration can have on performance. Athletes in this experiment were dehydrated by only −1.8% of body weight during 60 min of exercise before they cycled to exhaustion at 90% VO_2max. When the subjects prevented dehydration by ingesting fluids during the 60-min exercise bout, they cycled for nearly 10 min before exhaustion occurred. When mildly dehydrated, the subjects lasted only about 6 min.

2. Preventing Dehydration

The preponderance of scientific evidence that underscores the impairment in physiological and performance response and the benefits of adequate fluid replacement prompted the American College of Sports Medicine (ACSM) to issue a position stand on exercise and fluid replacement.[42] The ACSM position stand recognizes that dehydration has a negative impact upon both physiological and performance response, and recommends that athletes — regardless of sport — pay close attention to their hydration status. This includes entering training and competition well hydrated; the ACSM recommends that athletes ingest at least 500 ml (about 16 oz) of fluid (water, fruit juice, sports drink) 2 h prior to exercise. This will allow time for urine formation, providing the athlete a valuable indication of hydration status. If the urine is small in volume and darkly colored, it is likely that the athlete is still dehydrated and should consume more fluid. To help assure adequate hydration in preparation for training and competition in a warm environment (indoors or outdoors), athletes should consider ingesting an additional 250–500 ml of fluid in the 30 min prior to exercise.

Other considerations noted in the ACSM position stand are:

1. educate athletes about the absolute necessity of remaining well hydrated before and during exercise;
2. make certain that cool fluid is conveniently available at all times to make it easy for athletes to drink;
3. the fluid should be flavored and sweetened to encourage fluid intake;
4. to help maintain training intensity, the fluid should contain carbohydrate;
5. to stimulate rapid and complete rehydration, the beverage should contain sodium chloride.

Some commercially available sports beverages meet these qualifications and can be used effectively for the purposes noted above.[43]

B. TEAM SPORTS

Competitors in team sports are well advised to take advantage of any opportunity to ingest fluids. Substitutions, time-outs, and half-time breaks all present occasions for fluid ingestion. In some sports, such as soccer, fluid intake is often limited to the half-time break, a less-than-optimal scenario for maintaining hydration. However, in the practice setting, there is rarely an excuse for limiting fluid intake. To the contrary, every effort should be made to make fluid freely available and to encourage athletes to drink.

1.   Practical Tips

On the basis of research conducted on elite Australian athletes, Broad[44] makes a number of suggestions to help assure proper hydration for athletes in team sports. Most of these suggestions also apply to athletes in other sports.

- Make certain that fluid is always nearby. Making fluid easy to obtain is an important way of increasing fluid intake.
- Assign individual squeeze bottles to each player. This emphasizes the importance of drinking and enables athletes, coaches, and trainers to better gauge how much fluid is being consumed.
- Encouragement from coaches provides an important endorsement for the value of fluid ingestion. Coaches must also be willing to design practices to include frequent opportunities for their athletes to drink.
- Coaches, trainers, and athletes should be aware of individual sweat rates so that fluid-replacement regimens can be designed accordingly. Particular attention should be paid to those athletes with above-average sweat rates to assure that they are drinking appropriately.
- Train athletes to drink. Fully replacing sweat loss is a goal that most athletes are unaccustomed to achieving. It takes both time and practice for athletes to increase their ability to ingest large volume of fluids.

The relatively large variation in sweat rates among players in team sports[45] limits the effectiveness of making general recommendations for fluid intake. For example, advising athletes to ingest 1 l of fluid an hour would be inappropriate for both the female basketball player who sweats at 600 ml/hour and the male soccer player who sweats at 1.8 l/h. For this reason, it is imperative that the sweat rates of each athlete are calculated by recording changes in pre- and postexercise body weight during a typical training session.

There is also value in encouraging athletes to increase their fluid intake between practices to help assure adequate hydration (euhydration). Soccer players were able to increase their total body water when required to ingest an average of 4.6 l of fluid a day for one week, as opposed to a week when they voluntarily ingested 2.7 l/day. The latter volume proved insufficient for total rehydration; the players' total body water was approximately 1 l lower than when euhydrated.[46] To help achieve normal hydration status, athletes should be encouraged to eat their meals slowly, providing added time and impetus for increased fluid intake.

C.   SHORT-DURATION, HIGH-INTENSITY SPORTS

There is little doubt that maintaining euhydration will also benefit athletes who train and compete at high intensities. It is important to keep in mind that although the amount of dehydration incurred by a 400-meter run or a single gymnastics' routine may be very slight, such athletes often warm up and compete a number of times each day, making it likely that substantial dehydration can occur by day's end. In addition, these athletes complete training sessions — often in warm environments — that require repeated, high-intensity efforts that provoke profuse sweating.

Swimmers can also experience dehydration during training sessions due to modest sweat losses coupled with increased urine losses stimulated by the diuretic effect of supine posture and water immersion.[47] Unfortunately, there is a dearth of scientific information regarding fluid homeostasis in swimmers and the effects of fluid ingestion upon physiological and performance responses during swim training.[48]

Wrestlers often experience significant, planned dehydration as a means of losing body weight in preparation for competition. Depending upon the level of competition (e.g., high school, collegiate, international), wrestlers can have from 30 min to 20 h between weigh-in and competition, allowing for varying degrees of rehydration and restoration of related physiological responses.[49] Interestingly, most research indicates that performance in tasks requiring less than 30 sec is not significantly affected by dehydration.[50] However, in tasks requiring greater than 30 sec, performance is reduced by rapid weight loss.[51] Although research indicates that rehydration does not appear to impact competitive wrestling performance,[52] the chronic dehydration experienced by many wrestlers undoubtedly diminishes their capacity to train hard and recover quickly.[53] There is no reason to believe that wrestlers cannot enjoy the same benefits of adequate hydration as other athletes. For this reason, wrestlers should prevent dehydration during training by ingesting water or sports beverages as often as their weight-loss regimen allows.

Dehydration can also be problematic for rowers. As with wrestling, rowing competition lasts only 5–8 min, but lingering dehydration during two-a-day practices in warm weather can reduce the athlete's ability to train and can increase the possibility of heat-related problems. As Hagerman[54] points out, this is particularly true for lightweight rowers who dehydrate to attain weight-class standards.

There are minimal opportunities for ingesting fluid during sprint- and track-cycling competition, but the day-long format of many of these events and the demands of training necessitate adequate fluid intake if peak performance is a goal. The same is true of track runners for whom fluid intake during competition is virtually unheard of, even during events as long as 10,000 m. Regardless of what athletes currently do, all practical steps should be taken to assure that athletes enter competition well hydrated and have unrestricted access to fluids during the course of the competitive event.

D. LONG-DURATION, MODERATE-INTENSITY SPORTS

The detrimental influence of dehydration on exercise performance has been known for decades.[55] It can safely be said that dehydration knows no boundaries; regardless of the sport or activity, dehydration will have a marked, negative effect on performance. Conversely, euhydration will improve the chances for optimal performance. This is particularly true during all types of prolonged exercise, even when conducted in cold weather. Holm et al.[56] reported losses of 2–4% of body weight during cross-country ski races.

Most of the research that demonstrates the performance impairment experienced by dehydrated subjects has employed running or cycling as the mode of activity. For example, in 1985, Armstrong et al.[57] reported that dehydration of 2% of body weight can impair exercise performance during competitive runs as short as 1500 m (as well as in 5000 and 10,000 m runs). More recently, the negative influence of dehydration and the positive effect of euhydration on cycling performance has been clearly established.[58]

Athletes who compete in events lasting greater than 30 min (e.g., 10-km road races, triathlons, road cycling, cross-country skiing, etc.) often have the advantage of having access to fluids at regular intervals during the event. In the case of cyclists and triathletes, the ability to be able to replenish their bike bottles provides them the opportunity to drink comparatively large volumes at regular intervals. For this reason, cyclists generally ingest substantially greater amounts of fluid than do runners.[59]

Fluid ingestion during road races presents some unique problems for runners, not the least of which is the logistical challenge of drinking from a paper cup while running. Many runners have learned to crumple the top of the cup to prevent spilling and form a small spout to make drinking easier. Even so, the amount of fluid that can be ingested in this fashion is usually well less than optimal. Runners who wear bottle belts that allow for fluid to be easily transported have the advantage of immediate access to ample fluid, provided the bottle can be replenished when necessary. Elite runners often enjoy the benefit of having their own squeeze bottle of fluid waiting for them at each aid station.

Runners and other athletes tend to restrict fluid intake in response to developing gastrointestinal distress (e.g., stomach fullness or bloating, mild nausea, fluid "sloshing," etc.), a response that may be due more to dehydration[60] than to the actual act of drinking. Regardless of the cause of gastrointestinal distress, it is in the athlete's best interest to develop good drinking skills for competition by making drinking a regular habit during training.[61]

E.   OTHER CONSIDERATIONS
1.   Glycerol Ingestion

Glycerol ingestion has been recommended as a possible method of hyperhydrating before exercise, in an attempt to provide a physiological and performance advantage during exercise in the heat. Ingestion of glycerol along with large volumes of fluid (e.g., 1.5 l) an hour or so before exercise will result in decreased urine production and the temporary retention of fluid.[62] This effect is attributable to the lingering osmotic influence of the glycerol molecules, which are cleared slowly from the body water. Glycerol ingestion increases the osmolality of intra- and extracellular fluid compartments (the aqueous humor and the cerebral-spinal fluid being two notable exceptions), resulting in a temporary decrease in urine production.

Theoretically, hyperhydration might provide some cardiovascular and thermoregulatory advantages during physical activity in the heat. In this regard, lower core temperature and greater sweat loss in response to glycerol-enhanced hydration were noted in one study.[63] However, another study[64] demonstrated no such changes but did report an improvement in time to exhaustion during steady-state cycling. Interestingly, the only physiological difference between the glycerol and water-placebo trials in this study appeared to be a slightly lower heart rate during exercise.

It should be noted that the weight gain that goes hand-in-hand with glycerol-enhanced hydration (~0.5–1.0 kg) may be problematic for athletes, who pay a metabolic — and perhaps a performance — cost for carrying extra body weight. All things considered, it is premature to recommend glycerol-enhanced hydration to athletes, in no small part because the possible side effects of ingesting glycerol can range from mild sensations of bloating and lightheadedness to more-severe symptoms of headaches, dizziness, nausea, and vomiting.[65,66]

IV.   CARBOHYDRATE REQUIREMENTS OF ATHLETES

A.   FUNDAMENTAL CONCEPTS

Carbohydrate (CHO) is the macronutrient required in greatest amounts by athletes during training and competition. The importance of adequate carbohydrate ingestion is made apparent by the realization that muscle and liver glycogen levels are relatively small (compared to triglyceride stores) and are substantially lowered during many forms of training and competition.[67] For example, cross-country skiers have extremely low glycogen levels in arm and leg muscles following training and competition.[68] It is also important to bear in mind that glycogen depletion is not a phenomenon solely of endurance exercise but can occur during high-intensity exercise as well.[69]

1.   Maximizing Carbohydrate Availability

In terms of increasing the chances for optimal performance, the overall goal of carbohydrate ingestion before, during, and following exercise is to maximize the amount of carbohydrate available to muscles late in the exercise bout. When carbohydrate availability is reduced, exercise intensity will inevitably decrease and complete fatigue will eventually ensue. For that reason, it is recommended that athletes ingest 9–10 g CHO/kg BW/day (~4.0–5.0 g CHO/lb BW/day) to restore and maintain muscle glycogen levels.[70] The relevance of this recommendation is well illustrated in the study of Sherman et al.[71] who studied runners and cyclists over seven days of run or cycle training. Each day, the subjects completed 70 min of intense interval training on the treadmill or cycle ergometer. The runners and cyclists who ingested 10 g CHO/kg/day maintained their muscle glycogen stores at significantly higher levels than the subjects who consumed 5 g CHO/kg/day. The practical significance of such a difference in daily carbohydrate intake was noted by Hagerman[54] who studied a female rower who was having difficulty maintaining her training intensity. The athlete thought that she might be anemic, but diet analysis revealed that she was ingesting only 36% of her total kcal intake as carbohydrate.

2. Daily Carbohydrate Intake

It is often recommended that athletes consume a diet in which at least 60% of the total energy is supplied by carbohydrate.[72] However, the effectiveness of this recommendation depends upon the total energy intake of the athlete. For example, consider the case of a female runner who restricts caloric intake because of concern about body weight. If this individual ingested a 1500-kcal (6279 kJ) diet in which 60% of the energy came from carbohydrate, she would be consuming only 225 g of carbohydrate, too little to effectively restore muscle glycogen. Walberg-Rankin[73] noted the disparity between carbohydrate intake as a percent of total energy intake and carbohydrate intake expressed relative to body weight in a wide range of athletes involved in aerobic (e.g., swimmers, cyclists, runners, triathletes) and anaerobic (e.g., soccer players, gymnasts, bodybuilders) sports. For example, female cyclists who consumed 60% of their total caloric intake as carbohydrate ingested only 4.4 g CHO/kg of body weight.

It is best to make recommendations for daily carbohydrate intake in terms of the grams of carbohydrate to be consumed on the basis of body weight (e.g., 4 g CHO/lb BW/day). By reading the nutrition labels on food products, athletes can quickly learn how much food to ingest to meet their daily goals for carbohydrate intake. Table 2 contains recommended carbohydrate intakes over a range of body weights for athletes involved in rigorous training for at least 2 h a day. Maximum benefits appear to occur when athletes in hard training ingest between 500 and 600 g of carbohydrate each day.[74] Table 3 includes a list of the amounts of common foods equivalent to 100 g of carbohydrate.

TABLE 2   Recommended Carbohydrate Intakes on the Basis of Body Weight[a]

Body Weight		Daily CHO Intake	Energy as CHO	
lb	kg	g CHO	kcals	kJ
100	45	400	1600	6698
125	57	500	2000	8372
150	68	600	2400	10,046
175	80	700	2800	11,721
200	91	800	3200	13,395
225	102	900	3800	15,907

[a]   Based upon 4 g CHO/lb/day. Athletes training for less than 2 h/day can moderate their carbohydrate intake accordingly.

Recommendations adapted from References 2, 9, 14, 22, 27, 28, 70, 71, 72, and 112.

TABLE 3   The Number of Servings of
Common Foods Equivalent to
100 g of Dietary Carbohydrate[a]

Food	Servings
Grains	
Bread	8 slices
Pancakes	6 medium
Cereal	2.5 cups
Rice (cooked)	2 cups (400 g)
Pasta (cooked)	2.5 cups (350 g)
Fruit	
Bananas	4 medium
Apples	5 medium
Grapefruit	5 medium
Oranges	6 medium
Strawberries	10 cups (1490 g)
Fast Food	
Chicken nuggets	7 servings
Cheeseburger	3.5
French fries	4 regular servings
Beverages	
Beer	96 oz (2880 ml)
Soft drink	30 oz (900 ml)
Apple juice	28 oz (840 ml)
Cranberry juice	21 oz (630 ml)
Orange juice	30 oz (900 ml)
Milk	67 oz (2010 ml)
Desserts	
Brownies	8 medium
Cheesecake	4 slices
Pound cake	7 slices
White cake	2.5 pieces
Choc. chip cookies	13 small
Doughnut	6 regular
Sherbet (orange)	1.5 cups (100 g)
Ice cream (vanilla)	3 cups (400 g)

[a] Meat is not included because meat contains little
to no carbohydrate.

Data from Pennington.[182]

3.   Pre-Exercise Carbohydrate Feeding

Although it was once thought that pre-exercise carbohydrate ingestion would impair performance, recent research indicates that such is not the case. In fact, carbohydrate ingested before exercise has been shown to improve exercise performance,[75] with the greatest performance benefits resulting from a combination of pre-exercise and during-exercise feedings.[76] Athletes should ingest between 200 and 350 g of carbohydrate in the 3–6 h preceding exercise; the carbohydrate can be ingested as part of a meal or in the form of liquid supplement.[77]

B. TEAM SPORTS

Although team sports have traditionally been the bastion of the steak-and-eggs approach to sports nutrition, there is no doubt that these athletes can benefit from ingesting adequate amounts of carbohydrate energy each day. The intermittent, high-intensity nature of team-sport activity can quickly diminish muscle glycogen stores.[78] In 1969, Karlsson[79] noted that the glycogen concentration in the vastus lateralis muscles of soccer players was essentially depleted by the end of a match. Similar findings were reported by Jacobs et al.,[80] who also noted that the relatively low-carbohydrate content of the players' diets prevented full restoration of muscle glycogen stores even 48 h after the match.

Carbohydrate ingestion during training and competition also has beneficial effects for soccer players and ostensibly for other team-sport athletes as well. Players who ingested a carbohydrate beverage before and during a soccer match used less muscle glycogen than when just water was consumed.[81] Glycogen sparing has also been reported in ice-hockey players who ingested carbohydrate during exercise.[82] Under similar circumstances, other research has demonstrated that soccer players covered 25% more ground during a game when a carbohydrate beverage was ingested.[83] Ice-hockey players who consumed a carbohydrate supplement (360 g/day for 3 days) in addition to their diet before a championship series had muscle glycogen levels that were twice as high as players who were not given the supplement.[84]

Athletes who participate in team sports rely heavily upon muscle glycogen stores to provide the energy required for the rapid and explosive movements required by these activities. Rapid and complete restoration of muscle glycogen depends upon adequate carbohydrate intake, a fact that applies to all athletes, regardless of sport.

C. SHORT-DURATION, HIGH-INTENSITY SPORTS

Although the dietary intakes of sprint athletes are not particularly well documented, it is likely that these athletes consume less-than-recommended quantities of carbohydrate.[85] This is certainly true for wrestlers who are not only notorious for restricting energy intake, but often ingest only about 45–50% of total energy as carbohydrate (e.g., <4 g/lb BW/day).[31,86] It may be to the advantage of wrestlers, sprinters, and similar athletes — especially during periods of intense training — to ingest a high-carbohydrate diet. Williams[87] noted that sprinters who simulated a 90-min training session that included a mixture of sprints were able to reproduce their performances the next day only when they ingested 10 g CHO/kg BW during the 24 h of recovery.

A high-carbohydrate diet should also enable higher training intensities, a response noted in a study performed on basketball, field hockey, and soccer players.[88] The athletes completed a series of 30, 6-s, all-out sprints on a treadmill; the sprints were interspersed with walking and jogging for a total test duration of 1 h. When the power output of the first 9 of the 30 sprints were compared among groups, the performances of the low-carbohydrate group (12% of kcal from CHO for one day) and the normal-carbohydrate group (47% of kcal as CHO) declined 3.4% to 7.6% while the performance of the high-carbohydrate group (79% kcal as CHO) improved 3.5%. There were no differences in performance among diets across the 30 sprints. The authors attributed the performance benefit in the initial stages of the test to a greater reliance on carbohydrate oxidation in accordance with the carbohydrate content of the diet. Although these data provide some indication that the carbohydrate content of the diet may affect high-power performance, it would be foolish to make any sweeping conclusions on the basis of one study. There is a clear need for additional research that explores the possible link between dietary carbohydrate content and high-intensity exercise performance, particularly under circumstances of repeated days or weeks of training.

Interestingly, the rate of glycogen resynthesis following high-intensity exercise is considerably faster than that following prolonged exercise. The same appears to be true for recovery from strength-training exercise. The reasons for the greater rate of glycogenesis likely include higher plasma glucose and insulin concentrations, greater levels of metabolic intermediates (including lactate), and the higher activity of glycogen synthase in fast-twitch muscle cells. In fact, the rate of muscle glycogen resynthesis provoked by carbohydrate feeding can be two to four times greater following short-term, high-intensity exercise than following prolonged exercise.[89]

Swimmers often train in excess of 2 h per day, relying upon high-intensity interval training mixed with longer-duration swims. This type of training places great demands upon muscle glycogen as a fuel source. It would be logical to assume that swimmers will benefit from consuming a high-carbohydrate diet to allow for greater training intensities. However, Lamb et al.[90] failed to see an effect of diet on training times, due perhaps to the fact that, even on the low-carbohydrate diet, the swimmers still ingested more than 500 g of carbohydrate per day. Costill et al.[91] did note that swimmers who ate slightly less than 400 g of carbohydrate per day were unable to maintain increased training loads, in contrast to those swimmers who consumed about 600 g of carbohydrate per day.

Although the effect of carbohydrate feeding before and during high-intensity, intermittent exercise has not received a lot of scientific attention, the results of recent studies indicate that performance can be improved, even in events lasting less than 1 h. For example, carbohydrate feeding during resistance training,[92] intermittent running,[93] intermittent cycling,[94] and continuous cycling[95,96] (~50 min) resulted in improved performance compared to ingestion of a water placebo. These results should be confirmed by additional research before a consensus opinion can be developed, but the preliminary evidence does look positive.

D. LONG-DURATION, MODERATE-INTENSITY SPORTS

There is little doubt that carbohydrate feeding during prolonged exercise (i.e., >1 h) can benefit performance. Carbohydrate ingestion maintains blood glucose and insulin concentrations, stimulating glucose uptake by active muscle and increasing carbohydrate oxidation.[97] Various types and combinations of carbohydrate, including glucose, sucrose, maltodextrins, and fructose, are effective at improving performance.[98] Beverages containing mostly or only fructose should be avoided because fructose is slowly absorbed and metabolized, eliminating the performance benefit and increasing the risk of gastrointestinal distress.[99]

During training and competition, endurance athletes often have the opportunity to ingest carbohydrate in solid or liquid form. Both forms provoke similar metabolic[100] and performance[101] responses, but carbohydrate solutions provide the added benefit of helping assuring proper hydration. Research indicates that ingesting carbohydrate at the rate of 45–75 g/h is sufficient to provoke an improvement in exercise performance.[102] This consumption rate is consistent with the finding that the maximal oxidation rate for exogenous carbohydrate is approximately 60 g/h.[103] This is the equivalent of ingesting 1 l (1 qt) of sports drink per hour.

It is not uncommon for cyclists, triathletes, and ultradistance runners to ingest a combination of liquid and solid forms of carbohydrate during prolonged training and competition. Part of this practice undoubtedly arises from the desire to eat as well as drink during training sessions that may last 6 h or longer.[104] Unfortunately, little is known about how the ingestion of carbohydrate at rates greater than 60 g/h may affect performance during prolonged exercise (e.g., >4 h). Athletes often report that they experience a "lift" after ingesting concentrated sources of carbohydrates (i.e., an energy bar, carbohydrate gel, etc.) during prolonged exercise, even when they have been consuming carbohydrate throughout. Coyle et al.[105] showed that a large dose of carbohydrate ingested about 30 min prior to when fatigue occurred on a placebo trial extended cycling time to exhaustion by about 35 min. However, numerous investigators[106-108] have demonstrated that increasing the rate of carbohydrate ingestion beyond 60 g/h does not further improve exercise performance, at least for exercise lasting 4 h or less.

To maximize the chances for peak performance during both training and competition, the endurance athlete must balance the need for carbohydrate energy against the need for fluids. Ingesting too much carbohydrate in either solid or liquid form along with too little fluid will delay gastric emptying.[109]

E. OTHER CONSIDERATIONS

1. Postexercise Carbohydrate Intake

The rate at which glycogen is resynthesized following exercise depends upon the timing of ingestion, the amount and type of carbohydrate consumed, and the extent of existing muscle damage (which slows resynthesis).[110] Eating carbohydrates with a high glycemic index at an average rate of about 50 g (200 kcal, or 837 kJ) every 2 h until the next meal will help maximize the rate of glycogenesis in liver and muscle.[111] High-glycemic index foods are those that enter the bloodstream rapidly, provoking a spike in blood glucose and insulin levels. Potatoes, breakfast cereals, bread, and white rice are examples of foods with high glycemic indices. Food with a high- or moderate-glycemic index stimulates rapid glycogen resynthesis and, for that reason, should be ingested by athletes soon after exercise.[112]

V. FAT REQUIREMENTS OF ATHLETES

A. FUNDAMENTAL CONCEPTS

As with their sedentary counterparts, athletes require relatively little dietary fat. In fact, the need for essential fatty acids (primarily linoleic acid) can be met by a daily intake of only 1–2% of total dietary calories[15] (e.g., less than 10 g of fat in a 4000 kcal, or 16,744 kJ, diet.) In the vast majority of cases, athletes ingest considerably more fat than is required. In a comprehensive review of the literature on the dietary habits of athletes, Short[113] described the large and varied amount of fat intake among athletes in different sports; suffice to say that intake of adequate amounts of dietary fat is rarely a problem among athletes. For example, athletes on calorically restricted diets (e.g., 1800 kcal/day, or 7535 kJ/day) would ingest sufficient fat even if fat intake represented only 10% of total calories. Wrestlers, gymnasts, and other athletes in weight-class sports who consume <1000 kcal/day (4186 kJ/day) may find it difficult — but certainly not impossible — to ingest >15 g of fat per day. In all likelihood, the weekly or monthly fat intake of these athletes is adequate in terms of providing ample quantities of linoleic acid. However, fat intake is also essential in assuring the adequate intake of fat-soluble vitamins. Theoretically, athletes who ingest diets low in fat over a period of months or years may run the risk of inadequate intakes of fat-soluble vitamins.

In terms of protecting cardiovascular health, there is no question that a diet low in fat (e.g., <30% of total calories) should be the standard for athletes and nonathletes alike. However, as Short[113] noted, "it would be difficult to eat over 10,000 kcals, or 41,860 kjoules (as the men on the football line frequently did) on a low-fat diet." It may well be that, in terms of performance, fat intake is not a critical concern for athletes provided that their carbohydrate intake meets the needs for muscle and liver glycogen resynthesis. Table 4 contains estimates of dietary fat intake among athletes of varying body size and caloric intake. These values indicate that limiting fat intake to 1 g fat/kg/day (~0.5 g fat/lb/day) will be more than sufficient to meet the needs for dietary fat and assure that carbohydrate intake is also adequate.

B. TEAM SPORTS

A football player who weighs 100 kg (220 lb) and is only 8% body fat has more than 70,000 kcal (293,020 kJ) of fat energy stored as triglycerides in adipose tissue, enough to fuel continuous, moderate-intensity exercise for days. Although we store ample amounts of energy as fat, the contribution of fat to energy production during exercise is limited by the

TABLE 4   Examples of Dietary Fat Intake Over a Range of
Body Weights and Caloric Intakes[a]

Body Weight		Energy Intake		Fat Intake (g)
				0.5 g fat/lb BW/day or
lb	kg	kcal	kJ	1.1 g fat/kg BW/day
100	45.4	2000	8372	50
125	56.8	2500	10,465	63
150	68.2	3000	12,558	75
175	79.5	3500	14,651	88
200	90.9	4000	16,744	100
225	102.3	4500	18,837	113
250	113.6	5000	20,930	125

[a]   The values for energy intake are based upon an assumed caloric requirement of 20 kcals/lb (186 kJ/kg) of body weight. In all cases, 23% of the
total energy intake would come from fat.

Adapted using the information presented in References 2, 7, 15, 17, and 27.

relative slowness with which fat can be mobilized, transported, taken up, and oxidized by active muscle. For these reasons, the oxidation of fatty acids contributes only about 25% of the total energy required for exercise at 85% VO_2max.[114]

C.   SHORT-DURATION, HIGH-INTENSITY SPORTS

Fatty acids are continually oxidized to provide energy for cellular functions, including that of muscle contraction. For this reason, even sprinters benefit from fat oxidation, particularly during the rest or low-intensity phases of interval training. In fact, the extremely lean body type of most sprinters indicates a reliance upon fat metabolism; even though fat is not the predominant fuel during high-intensity exercise, the large overall caloric expenditure during training dictates that substantial amounts of fat will be oxidized during rest.

D.   LONG-DURATION, MODERATE-INTENSITY SPORTS

The relative contribution of fat to energy metabolism increases as exercise intensity decreases, but even many marathoners can sustain an intensity of 85% VO_2max,[115] an intensity at which the vast majority of energy is provided by muscle glycogen and blood glucose. During ultraendurance exercise, fat metabolism becomes increasingly important, but the virtually inexhaustible stores of fat in the body negate the need for fat supplementation during exercise.[116]

E.   OTHER CONSIDERATIONS
1.   Fat Loading

Some individuals[117] are currently promoting the intake of a higher-fat and -protein diet (the 40-30-30 diet; i.e., 40% carbohydrate, 30% fat, 30% protein) in place of a high-carbohydrate diet under the mistaken contention that alterations in dietary macronutrient intake can provoke hormonal changes that will result in increased fat oxidation during exercise. However, there is little-to-no scientific support for this contention. Although increased fat oxidation is a well-established response to aerobic training, there is a paucity of scientific evidence in support of the notion that manipulating the macronutrient content of the diet will have a similar effect.[118] Athletes are well advised to make carbohydrate the primary macronutrient in their diets.

VI. PROTEIN REQUIREMENTS FOR ATHLETES

A. FUNDAMENTAL CONCEPTS

Dietary protein serves the same functions in the nutrition of the athletes as it does in the sedentary individual. Protein derived from food contributes the amino acids necessary for the body to assimilate proteins that comprise the skeletal structures and hormones; that generate colloid osmotic pressure for fluid balance and that facilitate the transport of other nutrients in the plasma; that function as receptors in cell membranes; and that may provide energy.

For the latter function, relatively small amounts of protein are used as a percentage of the total energy requirement. For example, only 5–10% of the energy produced during exercise is thought to originate from protein.[119] One group of researchers has argued that the contribution may go as high as 18%.[120] Interestingly, whereas the rate of protein degradation has been shown to increase during prolonged, low-intensity exercise,[121] protein breakdown is suppressed and synthesis is stimulated at the cessation of the prolonged activity.[122] The cumulative effect would appear to be no net change in the protein balance. The exception to this might be for the situation in which the athlete's energy or carbohydrate intake is inadequate. In such a case, the breakdown of protein (cellular or dietary) and amino acid oxidation for energy may be accelerated[118,123] or gluconeogenesis may increase to maintain blood glucose levels.[124]

B. TEAM SPORTS

Protein intake will vary depending on the needs or goals of the athlete. General recommendations for protein intake are listed in Table 5 in accordance with the athlete's body mass and training regiments.[23,125] To sustain lean body mass when training at an accustomed intensity the recommended dietary allowance (RDA) of 0.8 g/kg/day is adequate.[15] If the athlete desires to change his or her current weight (either gain or reduce body weight) or if training intensity and/or volume are dramatically increased, the protein needs should be adjusted accordingly, i.e., increasing the intake to twice that of the RDA. Because most team-sport athletes attempt to maintain if not increase body mass, adequate protein intake is rarely a dietary limitation. In the next section, we discuss the needs of the strength athlete who often competes in team sports in which efforts are of short-duration, high-intensity.

C. SHORT-DURATION, HIGH-INTENSITY SPORTS

Similar to many team sport athletes, athletes participating in sports of short-duration and high-intensity often emphasize large intakes of protein on a daily basis. The reason is that

TABLE 5 Recommended Daily Protein Intake (g/day) According to Body Weight and Demands of Training[a]

| Body Weight | | | Heavy, Intense Training, or |
lb	kg	Normal Training	Modifying Body Weight
100	45.4	36	73
125	56.8	45	91
150	68.2	54	109
175	79.5	64	127
200	90.9	73	145
225	102.3	82	164
250	113.6	91	182

[a] Based on recommendations of Butterfield,[23] Lemon,[125] and Williams.[126]

power and force are key to success in such sports (e.g., shot put, javelin throw, sprints, weight lifting). Many athletes undergo extensive resistance training and may ingest extra dietary protein in hopes of promoting muscle hypertrophy that will translate into increased force production and power in their sport.[126] However, the relationship between increases in lean body mass and increases in strength is not as consistent as many athletes believe,[127] and the association between protein intake and strength gains may be more nebulous.[128,129]

Recent research by Tarnopolsky and colleagues[130] shows that a moderately high protein intake of 1.4 g/kg body weight may be needed to keep strength trained athletes in a positive protein balance. A discrepancy does exists between their recent findings and the same investigators' previous research,[131] which showed that body builders may require only 0.82 g/kg to maintain nitrogen balance. The authors could not completely reconcile this difference, but the discrepancy could have been due to the normal variability between the different groups of subjects who were studied or perhaps, that in the latest study, the energy intake of the experimental diets more closely meet the actual requirements of the athletes.

Lemon et al.[129] provide similar findings that support a requirement of 1.5 g of protein/kg body weight to maintain a positive nitrogen balance. The authors recommended an intake of 1.7 g/kg for subjects who are just beginning a strength training program. However, whether the subjects received a high protein diet that produced a positive nitrogen balance or a low protein diet that created a negative nitrogen balance, both groups had similar gains in strength and muscle hypertrophy. It remains to be determined whether athletes who have resistance-trained for long periods would also acquire gains in strength on a low protein diet.

For athletes who restrict nutrient intake to lose weight for competition (e.g., wrestlers, boxers, figure skaters, gymnasts), inadequate protein intake could become a limiting factor in maintaining good nutritional status. Research indicates that these athletes may not consume the RDA for protein during their competitive seasons.[30,86,132] If the low intake is sustained for prolonged periods, overall nutritional status, including muscle mass could be adversely affected. Adolescent wrestlers who decreased protein intake during a weight loss of about 6% of body weight showed significant decreases in rapid-turnover plasma proteins, indicating a decrease in overall protein nutritional status.[31] Estimates of their lean body mass determined from body weight and skinfold thickness indicated a significant decrease in lean body mass during 12 weeks of the competitive season. It is unclear, though, whether dietary protein restriction alone produced the diminished protein nutritional status. Inadequate intake of energy or carbohydrate could also contribute to a decrease in the visceral proteins and lean body mass, independent of the level of dietary protein.[133,134]

D. LONG-DURATION, MODERATE-INTENSITY SPORTS

In contrast to sprint athletes, less focus is typically placed on dietary protein for the endurance athlete. This may be due to a greater emphasis on obtaining adequate carbohydrate as the major source of energy and the potential for displacement of protein from the diet. Also, the endurance athlete tends to de-emphasize the practices that might increase body size (e.g., resistance training and ingesting compounds that stimulate muscle hypertrophy) and have a potentially negative effect of endurance performance. Despite the reasons to de-emphasize dietary protein consumption, most endurance athletes seem to obtain at least the recommended dietary allowance of 0.8 g protein per kg of body weight per day.[30,132,135-138]

Research during the past 10 years indicates that contrary to what seems logical, the endurance-trained athlete might have a higher protein requirement to maintain nitrogen balance than the requirements of the resistance-trained athlete. Tarnopolsky et al.[131] found that endurance-trained individuals needed 1.7 times that of sedentary person, or 1.37 g/kg, which was also higher than that required to maintain nitrogen balance in the body builders who were also studied. Friedman et al.[139] provide supportive data for a protein requirement that is higher than previously recommended for endurance athletes, e.g., the distance runner.

A requirement above the RDA could be due to the tremendous volume of energy expended during training[25,140] and the trauma of repeated muscular contractions, particularly the eccentric contractions, in the endurance athlete.[141,142]

E. OTHER CONSIDERATIONS

1. Actual Protein Intake in Athletes

The findings from the experimental research studies reported above offer value in discriminating the protein needs of various athletes, but the debate over whether athletes need more than the RDA might be considered academic. Most research suggests that athletes generally have daily intakes that surpass the RDA for protein.[23,125,132,143] Furthermore, when one considers that surveys typically underestimate the actual dietary intake,[144] it is likely that true intakes are well in excess of the needs and that dietary protein is not a limiting factor in the nutrition of the athlete. Again, this is with the possible exception of athletes who attempt to lose weight for competition.

2. Excess Protein

It has been suggested that protein intake in excess of twice the RDA (i.e., >1.6 g/kg/day) could increase the risk of renal degeneration and chronic diseases such as heart disease and cancers.[23,125] In general, amino acids are renal vasodilators that can elevate the pressure in the glomerular capillary and eventually lead to glomerulosclerosis.[145] High protein diets have been linked to renal degeneration in patients with certain pre-existing renal pathology,[145] and low protein diets have been used as part of the therapy for chronic renal disease.[146]

It is unclear whether the association between protein intake and heart disease or certain cancers are a direct effect of the protein *per se* or the effects of a high intake of fat, which typically accompanies a high protein diet. Identification of foods containing a high quality of protein, i.e., adequate levels of essential amino acids, but a low fat content will permit the athlete to minimize fat intake and still obtain adequate amounts of protein. Table 6 furnishes examples of foods to use. Whereas there are no data to confirm that athletes on high protein diets have a greater incidence of kidney disease or other aliments later in life, it does behoove the athlete or those who counsel the athlete to take these matters into consideration before embarking on protein or amino acid supplementation in the diet.

Finally, a high protein diet can produce diuresis, and thereby contribute to subsequent dehydration in the athlete. When protein intake is increased, urea production will also be increased.[23] The osmotic load of urea excreted by the kidney will draw additional fluid into the urine. Such an effect might explain why, anecdotally, some individuals have observed a decrease in body weight on diets high in protein and low in carbohydrate (e.g., the 40-30-30 diet previously described under the fat loading, V.E.1.).

VII. MINERAL REQUIREMENTS OF ATHLETES

A. FUNDAMENTAL CONCEPTS

Macrominerals, which are found in amounts of at least 5 g in the body, serve important functions that include maintaining the mass of certain body compartment (identified in Table 7). For example, fluid balance is dependent, in part, on sodium, chloride, and potassium levels in the body. Bone mass is largely dependent on the amount of calcium and, to a lesser extent, phosphorous (as phosphate) that are absorbed and retained in the body. Macrominerals are also involved in the physiological events that ultimately allow the athlete to move. In particular, sodium, potassium, and chloride are critical in producing the action potentials and propagating nerve impulses. These same minerals, along with calcium and magnesium, also contribute to intramuscular events that lead to force generation. Phosphorous and magnesium

TABLE 6   Sources of Protein with Corresponding Fat
and Calorie Content[a]

	Protein, g	Fat, g	Energy	
			kcal	J
Chicken, 100 g roasted				
dark with skin	26	16	253	1059
dark, no skin	27	10	205	858
light with skin	29	11	222	929
light, no skin	31	4	173	724
Ground beef, 100 g				
lean	24	18	268	1122
regular	23	21	287	1201
Lamb chop, 1				
lean	14	4	92	385
regular	16	21	255	1067
Ham, 100 g roasted				
lean	21	6	145	607
regular	20	15	226	946
Pork Loin, 100 g	29	22	350	1465
Fish				
salmon, 3 oz or 85 g	17	3	99	414
shrimp, 3 oz or 85 g	17	1.5	90	377
sole, 1 fillet	18	1	80	335
Egg, 1 large				
fried	5	6	83	347
boiled	6	6	79	331
Milk, 8 oz or 240 mL				
skim	8	0.4	90	377
milk	8	0.8	150	628
Pinto beans, 1 cup or 171 g				
boiled	14	0.9	235	984

Note: 100 g meat or poultry = 3.5 oz.

[a]   Data from Pennington.[182]

serve respectively, to form and stabilize high-energy phosphates that provide fuel for the muscle contraction. Calcium and magnesium are necessary for the crossbridge formation that precedes the actual contraction.

In contrast to macrominerals, each micromineral contributes to less than 5 g of the mass of the body (see list, Table 7). Nonetheless, each makes a substantial contribution to physiological functions in the body. For example, the presence of chromium is necessary to produce the insulin action that promotes glucose uptake into cells; iron must be bound to hemoglobin for the erythrocyte to transport oxygen in the blood; and zinc is a critical cofactor for the enzymes that include alkaline phosphatase, lactate dehydrogenase, and carbonic anhydrase, to name a few.

With the exceptions of sodium and chloride, the primary route of loss of most minerals from the body is usually in the excretion of urine.[147] Depending upon the athlete's volume of sweat and the electrolyte concentration in the sweat, sodium and chloride losses via sweat can be tremendous whereas losses of other minerals are relatively minor.[148] This is an important consideration for athletes who are often under the impression that they may experience a mineral deficiency, for example a potassium deficiency, due to sweat loss. Costill et al.[149] demonstrated that at least for short periods (4 days) on a low potassium diet and heavy exercise that induced high sweat volumes, a significant decrease in total body potassium did not occur. As another example, using the recent data of Waller and Haymes,[150] we can extrapolate to total iron losses for the period of exercise. We find that losses are quite low

TABLE 7 Recommended Dietary Allowance for Minerals for Athletes Who Are At Least 15 Years of Age

	Male	Female
Macrominerals		
sodium	1100–3300 mg[a]	1100–3300 mg[a]
potassium	1875–5625 mg[a]	1875–5625 mg[a]
chloride	1700–5100 mg[a]	1700–5100 mg[a]
calcium	1200 mg	1200 mg
magnesium	350–400 mg	280–300 mg
phosphorus	1200 mg	1200 mg
Microminerals		
iron	10–12 mg	15 mg
iodine	150 μg	150 μg
fluoride	1.5–4.0 mg[a]	1.5–4.0 mg[a]
zinc	15 mg	12 mg
copper	2.0–3.0 mg[a]	2.0–3.0 mg[a]
selenium	50–70 μg	50–55 μg
manganese	2.5–5.0 mg[a]	2.5–5.0 mg[a]
molybdenum	0.15–5.0 mg[a]	0.15–5.0 mg[a]
chromium	50–200 μg[a]	50–200 μg[a]
tin	ne[b]	ne
silicon	ne	ne
vanadium	ne	ne
boron	ne	ne
nickel	ne	ne
bromine	ne	ne
aluminum	ne	ne
sulfur	ne	ne
arsenic	ne	ne

[a] Indicates a safe intake, as no RDA has been established.[182]
[b] ne: no established RDA or safe level, despite each of these having a known function in the body.

relative to the RDA for iron (Table 8), regardless of whether exercise was performed in a hot or a neutral environment. Noteworthy is the observation that the concentration of iron in sweat decreased during the exercise session such that minerals seemed to be conserved by the body as exercise continued.[150]

TABLE 8 Estimated Sweat Rates and Total Iron Loss Via Sweating During Exercise[a]

	Sweat Loss, l/h	Fe Loss, mg	% RDA
Males			
Exercise in heat	1.4	0.26	1.7
Exercise, neutral	0.9	0.26	1.8
Females			
Exercise in heat	0.8	0.08	0.4
Exercise, neutral	0.6	0.08	0.5

[a] Calculated using the body surface area, iron sweat concentration, and sweat rates data of Waller and Haymes.[150]

Adequate intake of the macro- and microminerals (Table 7) from daily food consumption is often of minor concern to many athletes. Yet, the use of mineral supplements can receive a disproportionate focus among athletes. In the next sections, we will examine several examples of minerals that:

- may deviate inappropriately from the RDA in the athlete's diet;
- have been proposed to have ergogenic effects in supplemental dosages; and
- have been taken in conjunction with a multimineral supplement in hopes of enhancing performance.

B. TEAM SPORTS

In general, most male athletes in team sports consume a diet adequate in energy, so that the micronutrient content, including the mineral intake, is also adequate.[30,188] A small percentage of low intakes of calcium or iron among some team-sport athletes has been observed, but the frequency is relatively low among males in contrast to that of female athletes.[30] Issues related to low intake of specific microminerals in female athletes will be discussed under the long-duration, moderate-intensity section.

Of arguable concern is the intake of sodium by athletes in football and basketball, and its relation to blood pressure in these athletes. Short and Short[30] reported that several of the athletes studied were diagnosed with high blood pressure (defined as systolic pressures above 140 mm Hg and diastolic pressured above 90 mm Hg) and appeared to be consuming sodium in excess of what is considered normal and safe. Unfortunately, dietary sodium is often identified as the cause of the problem, when in fact, it may be an accomplice to the cause. Research indicates that insulin resistance and subsequent hyperinsulinemia may stimulate the reabsorption of sodium by the kidney; this consequence would then contribute to an elevation in blood pressure.[151,152] Because insulin resistance is more likely to occur in those with abdominal obesity,[153] which may exist in lineman in football, and possibly at different frequencies depending on the race (Native American vs. Negro vs. Caucasian), a more comprehensive medical exam is justified for athletes to determine the cause of hypertension and to administer the most appropriate treatment.

A clear understanding of the relationship between sodium intake and blood pressure in these athletes is further confounded by 1) the use of tobacco in these athletes,[30] and 2) the extent that the daily loss does not exceed the daily intake. It is possible for some team athletes to lose up to 4 g of sodium per practice sessions. With two practice sessions per day, the sodium intake would need to be at least double that which is considered safe in order to meet the athletes' needs. Future research should attempt to account for all contributory or causative factors that may be present when hypertension is present in the athlete and not focus only on the sodium intake.

In contrast to male athletes, female athletes often exhibit deficient intakes of minerals, particularly calcium, iron, and zinc, even when the sport does not demand weight control or the restriction of nutrient intake. These nutrients will be addressed under long-duration, moderate-intensity sports. Previous reports have done an excellent job of reviewing these mineral requirements for athletes, and we would encourage the reader to peruse those summaries as well.[154-156]

C. SHORT-DURATION, HIGH-INTENSITY SPORTS

With the exception of sports in which weight control is an issue, most athletes in short-duration, power sports consume adequate levels of minerals.[30,157] Also, athletes within the groups that attempt to build muscle mass for power are more likely than other athletes to consume mineral and vitamin supplements, which would contribute to achieving the adequate intake.[158] Within high intensity sports in which weight control is prevalent, intakes of magnesium, zinc, and iron are more likely to be low.[30,86] This would seem to support the argument for athletes in weight control sports to consume a multimineral supplement during their competitive season. However, the deficiencies appeared to persist in the off-season, at a time when the athletes were not attempting to control their body weight.[86] Thus, it is possible that these athletes simply do not recognize, at any time, how to establish a proper diet to obtain adequate amounts of all micronutrients.

Supplementation of individual and specific minerals is more prevalent among athletes in sports such as body building, field events, weight lifting, and football.[158] Two trace minerals that we'll address here are chromium and magnesium because of the association that has developed between these minerals and the anabolism of muscle. Chromium supplements, in particular, are currently marketed to the athletic population with claims that additional dietary chromium can increase lean body mass and decrease body fat. The theory behind the claims is that chromium interacts with insulin to augment insulin's actions.[159] Insulin exhibits a strong anabolic effect by inhibiting the breakdown of protein[160] and possibly by stimulating protein synthesis.[161] Thus, hypothetically, an enhanced insulin action via the presence of additional chromium in the plasma might increase lean body mass.

The claims used to market chromium supplements are largely based on two unpublished studies, which have only been reported within a review article.[162] In both studies, the subjects consumed 200 µg of chromium picolinate per day during a weight training program that lasted approximately 6 weeks. In comparison to groups receiving a placebo treatment during the weight training, those on chromium appeared to gain between 1.5 and 2 kg of lean body mass. In one of the studies, the lean body mass increase was enough to produce a decrease in percent body fat, although it is unclear whether the absolute fat mass actually decreased.

On the surface, these results appear impressive. However, a critical evaluation of these studies[162] reveals a weakness in the research methods that were employed. The method for determining the change in body composition was estimated using measurements of skinfold thickness, not one of the criterion methods typically required for research purposes. Since this initial report,[162] several other fully published studies have failed to find a similar anabolic effect of chromium in humans.[163-165] In one of these studies, an accepted, criterion method of determining body composition (hydrostatic weighing) was used.[163] The results of this recent study showed no increase in fat-free weight for the placebo group or the group receiving 200 µg of chromium per day. Because the resistance training was conducted in conjunction with the treatments, both groups, placebo and chromium-treated, showed significant and similar increases in strength.

Before leaving the chromium issue, it is important to note that certain health risks may be associated with the intake of a mineral, or specific forms of the mineral. Chromium supplementation has been described as offering minimal risks of side-effects, and studies have been successfully conducted with dosages of up to four-times the safe, upper limit per day (i.e., 800 µg/day) without side-effects.[166] There has been some debate over which form of chromium is most readily absorbed and has the greatest physiologic effects.[167,168] Recent research suggests that the form most widely marketed, chromium picolinate, might cause damage to the DNA of cells.[169] Using a cell culture model, exposure to chromium picolinate significantly increases the frequency of aberrations in the chromosomes of ovarian cells from Chinese hamsters. Whereas it may be difficult to accept inferences from this model to the intact human, it should be noted that equivalent doses of other forms of chromium (chromium chloride, chromium nicotinate) did not damage cell DNA. Subsequent research is needed to confirm whether chromium picolinate truly puts the athlete at risk.

In the future, if not already, athletes will likely hear about similar potential benefits of other mineral supplements, those being vanadium and molybdenum. Both vanadium and molybdenum mimic the effects of insulin, i.e., stimulating glucose uptake, in animal models of diabetes.[170,171] Currently, no data are available to show that either mineral has an anabolic effect or that either mineral mimics insulin in humans who have normal insulin sensitivity.

However, implications for such use in the athlete will likely be created by those who unscrupulously market mineral supplements to athletes.

Magnesium is another trace mineral to receive recent attention as an ergogenic element for the strength athlete. One research report has indicated that strength gains from resistance training may be enhanced with supplementation of this mineral. Brilla and Haley,[172] using a between-group comparison in which one group received a placebo and the other received a supplement of magnesium oxide, found that the magnesium treated group had twice the increase in strength for leg extension as did the placebo group. Presently, this is the only study to show an ergogenic effect of magnesium on strength performance in combination with resistance training. At this time, there is no explanation to support why magnesium supplementation would have enhanced strength development. It should be noted, though, that the placebo group in this study had an average daily intake of magnesium that was below the RDA. Therefore, the findings may actually represent the effects of inadequate intake as opposed to supplemental effects. In addition, inadequate magnesium intake in the placebo group might indicate that the intake of other nutrients was also inadequate, and this could also have impeded the placebo group's gain in strength.

D. LONG-DURATION, MODERATE-INTENSITY SPORTS

Previous publications have reviewed mineral needs, in particular the micromineral requirements, of athletes.[154-156,173,174] We will briefly summarize information on a few of these minerals, but we refer the reader to previous reviews for more details.

Athletes who train for long duration each day may lose substantial amounts of specific minerals in their sweat. As presented earlier, sodium and chloride are the key minerals that can be lost in substantial amounts via this route. Estimates made from the data on sodium sweat content in the acclimatized athletes and the sweat volume per day[175] show that a marathoner training in the heat could conceivable lose up to 10 g of sodium per day. The safe upper level of sodium intake for a sedentary individual in the United States is about 3 g (Table 7). Thus, athletes in this situation could experience hyponatremia if they did not supplement the diet. Loss of electrolytes in the sweat during exercise has been associated with overall fatigue and muscle cramps,[175,176] although the losses induced by moderate dehydration do not, in theory, appear to be a limiting factor for nerve function or for the recruitment of motor units.[149] Nevertheless, severe sodium depletion over a matter of days of training and inadequate intake can impair cardiovascular function and can contribute to heat exhaustion.[175]

Two minerals of particular interest to the female endurance athlete include calcium and iron. An emphasis on adequate calcium intake is needed in female endurance athletes. It is not so much that they have increased losses or requirements with training. Rather, due to their tendency to restrict energy intake, female athletes may not consume enough minerals such as calcium and iron.[177,178] Recent data suggest that the peak bone mass achieved during adolescence might be a critical factor in minimizing the occurrence of osteoporosis among females later in life.[179] It should be recognized, though, that proper calcium balance and optimal bone mineral mass may be just as dependent on hormonal status (eumenorrhea) and overall nutrient intake (calories, protein, and fat), as they are on calcium intake.[34,180,181]

To achieve the RDA for calcium[15] (800–1200 mg/day depending on the age), the athlete may need up to four servings of food from the category of milk and dairy products. This volume of one food group may seem excessive especially to smaller athletes who attempt to control body weight or to female athletes in general. However, by using low fat dairy products, the total calorie contribution can be kept to a minimum and thus, make this goal more achievable by the athlete. For example, four, eight-ounce (240 ml) servings of skim milk affords 100% of the RDA for calcium (1200 mg) and only a total of 1.6 g of fat (less than 18 kcal, or 75 kJ).[182] In addition, this volume of low fat milk would provide nearly 34 g of protein (over one-half the protein RDA for many females) and 364 kcal (1524 kJ) of energy to the daily diet.

The issue of iron intake in the female endurance athlete is just as critical as that of calcium intake. Female athletes frequently do not meet the RDA for iron due to overall restriction of energy intake and a lower consumption of foods that are good sources of iron, in particular, red meat. Also, the female has a relatively greater loss of iron due to the menstrual period. One approach to remedying this is to have the female athlete consume an iron source (multimineral supplement) with a glass of orange juice, and then delay drinking caffeinated beverages at the time of supplement ingestion.[183] The vitamin C in the orange juice reduces the iron from the ferric form (+3 valence) to ferrous iron (+2 valence state), which is the form most readily absorbed. The presence of vitamin C can double the amount of iron that is absorbed,[184] whereas caffeine may bind with the iron and prevent the absorption. The approach of using a multimineral is not the exclusive answer, though, to poor iron status. The athletes are still encouraged to obtain an adequate iron intake from a variety of foods that include red meat, organ meat, legumes, dark-green leafy vegetables, and dried fruits.

With the increasing interest in maximizing antioxidant capacities in athletes, athletes might begin to experiment with supplemental intakes of minerals such as copper, zinc, manganese, and selenium.[185] Presently, little research exists to document the value of supplementation of these minerals and their actions in the athlete. However, because selenium has received some recent attention, we will discuss this particular micromineral. Selenium is recognized as a coenzyme in the glutathione antioxidant enzyme system.[186] Interestingly, epidemiological studies show that intake of selenium is inversely related to the incidence of cancer.[187]

Decreasing the risk of cancer is seldom a concern of the young and otherwise healthy athlete, but sport scientists and athletes are curious as to whether selenium supplementation could enhance antioxidant capacities to assist in recovery of muscle tissues following intense competition and training. Tessier et al.[188] recently investigated whether the effects of selenium supplementation had an interactive effect with physical training on antioxidant capacity and physical performance. The subjects were randomized into either a placebo treatment or a selenium treatment (180 µg selenomethionine/day). As part of a 10 week treatment, subjects trained 3 days per week at various intensities that averaged 65% of peak VO_2. The results showed that blood glutathione peroxidase activity was increased with training, and there appeared to be an interactive effect of training and selenium supplementation. Nearly twice the increase in blood glutathione peroxidase activity occurred in those receiving selenium compared to those receiving placebo. Under either treatment, peak VO_2 and maximal aerobic capacity increased similarly, by 10% and about 30%, respectively. Thus, selenium supplementation did not produce an ergogenic effect, but it might play a role in boosting the athlete's antioxidant systems.

E.   OTHER CONSIDERATIONS
1.   Multimineral Supplementation in Athletes

Several studies have been conducted to determine the effects of multimineral supplementation on athletic performance.[189-191] In most, if not all, cases, the supplement also contained multiple vitamins besides the minerals. Depending on the study, the treatment periods ranged from 3 to 9 months. Among others, some of the key minerals that were contained in the supplement included zinc, calcium, and magnesium. In two studies, the supplement additionally provided iron, chromium, manganese, selenium, or copper.[192,193] In both of these studies, the results showed that the athletes consumed at least 97% of the RDA for all minerals supplemented within the respective study; the third study[189] did not assess dietary intake. Two of the three studies determined how physical performance was affected by the supplementation program by including a placebo group.[189,190] Whether performance was assessed using laboratory methods (e.g., VO_2max, endurance time, isokinetic strength) or field assessment (vertical jump, shuttle run, or coach's evaluation of improvement in training and competition), with one exception (vertical jump in female basketball players), no differences between mineral-supplemented and placebo-treated groups. Thus, while the multimineral supplement might have ensured the athletes' maintenance of nutritional status, i.e., adequate intake of the minerals that were supplemented, there were no ergogenic effects on performance because of the supplementation program.

VIII. VITAMIN REQUIREMENTS OF ATHLETES

A. FUNDAMENTAL CONCEPTS

Dietary vitamins serve the same important functions in the athlete as they do in the nonathlete. The functions include everything from serving as a cofactor with specific enzymes that regulate metabolic pathways (e.g., pyridoxine interacting with glycogen phosphorylase) to assisting in the production of synthesis of specific tissues such as connective tissue (e.g., vitamin C promoting crosslinkage of the collagen). The water-soluble and fat-soluble vitamins and their corresponding recommended daily allowance[15] are listed in Table 9.

To date there is little evidence to suggest that the vitamin requirements are increased for athletes.[192-197] Studies that have demonstrated a benefit or need for increasing the intake of a particular vitamin also show that the athletes or subjects who participated in the research were initially deficient in terms of the intake.[194,196] It should be emphasized then, that recommendations or encouragement for increasing the vitamin intake in athletes is due to a pre-existing inadequate intake, not an increased requirement due to the physical training. Possibly, the only exceptions to this might be the requirements for riboflavin, thiamin, and niacin. However, an increased intake of these three has been recommended based on daily energy intake.[15] For most athletes, energy intake naturally follows their daily energy expenditure, so with possibly a few exceptions, supplementation outside of the normal diet would not be mandatory.

TABLE 9   Recommended Dietary Allowance for
Vitamins for Athletes Who Are At Least 15
Years of Age

	Male	Female
Water Soluble		
B_1, thiamin	1.5 mg	1.1 mg
B_2, riboflavin	1.7–1.8 mg	1.3 mg
B_3, niacin	19–20 mg	15 mg
B_6, pantothenic acid	2.0 mg	1.5–1.6 mg
	4–7 mg[a]	4–7 mg[a]
biotin	100–200 mg[a]	100–200 mg[a]
folic acid	200 μg	180 μg
B_{12}, cobalamine	2.0 μg	2.0 μg
Ascorbate, vitamin C	60 μg	60 μg
Fat Soluble		
Vitamin A	1000 μg retinol or	800 μg retinol or
	6000 μg β-carotene	4800 μg β-carotene
Vitamin D	10 mg	10 mg
	400 IU	400 IU
Vitamin E	10 mg (IU) of	8 mg (IU) of
	α-tocopherol	α-tocopherol
Vitamin K	70–140 μg[a]	70–140 μg[a]

[a]   Indicates a safe intake, as no RDA has been established.[182]

Regardless of the lack of supportive research, vitamin requirements and the effects of vitamin supplementation on athletic performance remain of great interest. Some of the interest or concern has been driven by the notion that fluid losses through sweating increase the loss of the water-soluble vitamins, ascorbic acid, and the B-vitamin complex, or that the high metabolic demands of heavily training athletes, increase the vitamins requirements. However, available research indicates that sweat is not a significant route of loss of these vitamins.[147] Nor can an increase in carbohydrate metabolism be demonstrated by supplementing an adequate diet with certain vitamins.[197] Research shows that with one exception, treatment with a multivitamin, multimineral supplement has not improved physical performance or athletic performance in athletes.[190] The exception will be discussed in more detail below.

The next sections will focus on practices within each category of sport. In particular, we present data indicating where deficiencies might occur. Also, we summarize current supplementation practices of certain athletes and the theory behind the supplementation.

B. TEAM SPORTS

Several studies have examined nutrient intake of athletes in team sports such as football, basketball, soccer, and women's lacrosse and volleyball.[30,198,199] Most of the participants studied consumed adequate levels of all vitamins. Possibly, because they do not need to reduce body weight and in fact might attempt to gain weight, athletes in most team sports are unlikely to show deficiencies in diet. One exception to this appears to be Vitamin A. Up to 70% of football players and 17% of all female athletes studied consumed a diet low in vitamin A in one report.[30]

Research on diet supplementation practices among team sport athletes reveals that a substantially high percentage use vitamin and/or mineral supplements.[158] Approximately 46% of athletes take supplements to increase vitamin and/or mineral intake. In contrast, to prevalence among athletes, a frequency of supplementation of 35–40% has been observed in the general population.

As mentioned above, supplementation has never been shown conclusively to improve performance of athletes. Interestingly, though, an improvement in overall nutritional status could account for cases in which a vitamin supplementation program was associated with enhanced performance. This confounding influence can be demonstrated in the data of Telford et al.[190] An improvement in one performance task (vertical jump) out of the five conducted tests was detected in female basketball players. These athletes also showed an increase in body weight and skinfold thickness. Thus, a coincidental improvement in overall nutritional status, as reflected in the increase in body weight, skinfold thickness, and possibly lean body mass, would more likely have contributed to the increased vertical jump than simply the effect of the multivitamin, multimineral supplements alone. The authors concluded, though, that supplementation with the multiple micronutrients did not seem to enhance athletic performance.[190]

C. SHORT-DURATION, HIGH-INTENSITY SPORTS

As we've seen with other micronutrients, athletes who participate in short-duration, high-intensity sports and who consume a varied diet, which meets their energy needs, do not experience shortfalls in vitamin intake. The exception to this is those athletes, such as wrestlers, who control food intake in order to maintain or reduce their body weight.[30,86] The vitamins identified as deficient in the diet of these athletes have included vitamin A, vitamin C, the B-vitamins, thiamin, pyridoxin (B_6), riboflavin, and niacin. Research also indicates that biochemical evaluations indicate that gradual weight loss in weight-class athletes may increase their susceptibility to a diminished status for B_6.[200] The diminished status, though, did not impair physical performance of these athletes.

It is possible that inadequate intake of select vitamins over an extended period of the athletic season could compromise performance. In one study designed to examine this, the intakes of B_6, thiamin, and riboflavin were experimentally restricted to 55% of the Dutch recommended dietary intake (RDI) for 11 weeks.[201] The results revealed a reduction in maximum oxygen uptake of nearly 12% and a decrease in anaerobic power of 7% (average power) to 9% (peak power) at the end of the 11 week treatment period. Because the subjects also showed a decrease in body weight and exhibited adverse changes in serum iron status, it was difficult to conclude unequivocally that the deficient intake of these B-vitamins was the cause. Furthermore, the investigators were not able to demonstrate a decrement in performance when any one of the vitamins was deficient in the diet; only combined inadequacies of all three produced decrements in physical performance. The subjects did not exhibit overt symptoms of vitamin deficiencies.

Whereas no data exist to demonstrate that fat oxidation is increased at rest or during exercise as a result of ingesting more B-vitamins, some have speculated, without scientific evidence, that such supplementation might help athletes to reduce body fat during the course of weight loss for competition.[202] Depending on which B-vitamins are supplemented, quite the opposite effect could occur. For example, niacin at high intakes may suppress the release of fatty acids from adipocytes at rest or during exercise.[203,204] This effect and its impact on performance are discussed in more detail in the next section.

Contrary to the concept that supplements are benign if not helpful to the athlete, there is reason to speculate that high levels of supplementation of certain vitamins could have adverse consequences in the certain athletes. For example, those who might experience dehydration to "make weight" could be at risk for renal calculi. High intakes of vitamin C, in this case, could theoretically elevate the production of calcium oxalate, a key substrate for the formation of kidney stones.[205] In theory, high production levels of calcium oxalate in combination with reduced fluid intake and urine production during weight loss might precipitate kidney stones in these athletes. To date, there are no reports to substantiate that this specific complication has ever occurred. However, this example reinforces the potential for adverse outcomes in the athlete's health as a consequence of the imbalance that can develop with nutrition supplementation (vitamin C in this case) and nutrition inadequacy (fluids in this case).

Ideally, athletes in any power sport, but particularly those who restrict nutrient intake, might focus their efforts on increasing the intake of whole grain cereals and breads, fruits, and vegetables. Such an approach will assist the athlete in maintaining a low fat diet that sustains gradual weight loss and yet provides all vitamins at the necessary levels (Table 9). Alternatively, there might be a happy medium for moderate vitamin supplementation in athletes in the weight-control sports so that impaired health and performance do not occur over the course of the competitive season.

D. LONG-DURATION, MODERATE-INTENSITY SPORTS

Based on available data, it appears that most male endurance athletes consume adequate levels of both fat and water soluble vitamins.[135-137] It would appear that as long as the athlete is meeting his or her energy needs by eating a wide variety of foods, intake of vitamins will be in sufficient levels.

Yet, many endurance athletes remain fascinated by the reputed enhancement in work capacity that certain vitamins in extra dosages might provide. For example, early research was suggestive of an enhancement in endurance as a result of wheat germ consumption, presumably because of the extra dietary vitamin E and octacosanol that the wheat germ provided.[206] Since that time, research has refuted that either compound is an ergogenic aid.[207]

In a similar way, nicotinic acid has been investigated for potential ergogenic effects. When ingested in large dosages, niacin will increase skin blood flow and possibly enhance thermoregulatory capability.[208] Metabolically, niacin suppresses the mobilization of free fatty acids and thus shifts the demand for energy production to the oxidation of carbohydrate, potentially allowing for exertion at higher intensities than if fatty acids were present.[204] To date, though, the research indicates that if anything, niacin supplementation has an adverse effect on endurance performance. Niacin in large dosages eliminates the carbohydrate-sparing effect that plasma-free fatty acids have when the fatty acids are available as substrate and can be oxidized during moderately high intensities of exercise.[114,209,210] Despite the scientific evidence, the unfounded notion that vitamin supplements offer a performance advantage still exists in the minds of many present-day athletes.

One of the most intriguing issues among endurance athletes is the potential benefit of using of antioxidants to reduce the risk of illness and to speed the recovery time following intense training. Previously published reviews[185,211] and other chapters within this volume provide more background and details on the antioxidants; however, we will briefly examine recent research on the role of vitamin E as an antioxidant. High rates of energy metabolism combined with repetitive eccentric contractions may elevate the production of oxygen free radicals and lipid peroxidation, which may indicate or facilitate damage to skeletal muscle.[212,213] Meydani et al.[214] recently showed that with approximately seven weeks of supplementation of vitamin E (800 IU/day), exercise-induced lipid peroxidation was significantly decreased. Supplementation increased muscle levels of the vitamin, but levels were reduced to normal (placebo levels) following stressful exercise. Vitamin E appeared to provide an alternative substrate for lipid peroxidation such that a decrease in muscle levels of fatty acids was attenuated, and the urinary excretion of thiobarbituric acid adducts (an index of oxidative damage) was reduced compared to that of the placebo group. Further research is needed to confirm whether vitamin E supplementation would be beneficial to the athlete's recovery. However, as discussed in the next section, at least one influential organization has issued a recommendation to athletes.

E. OTHER CONSIDERATIONS
1. Multivitamin Supplementation Studies

As discussed under mineral requirements for athletes, studies involving multivitamin, multimineral supplementation treatment have been conducted for periods of up to nine months.[189-191] Where the experimental treatment may have allowed the athletes to consume nearly 100% of the RDA for the supplemented vitamins, the supplementation did not translate into an improvement of performance, whether the performance relied on primarily anaerobic or aerobic metabolism for energy production. Also worth noting was the observation in one study that only two of the seven supplemented vitamins, those being riboflavin and pyridoxine, showed a significant increase in the blood levels of the subjects.[191] The authors of that study explained that possibly the lack of deficiencies in their subjects or the interactive negative effects between the micronutrients on their absorption may have prevented the expected elevations in the blood levels of all supplemented vitamins and minerals. Based on the available data, multivitamin supplements are not ergogenic agents. Possibly multivitamin supplementation could assist the athlete in obtaining adequate intakes on a daily basis, but only if the vitamins are bioavailable.

2. Antioxidant Recommendations

In light of the recent research on vitamin E and potential reductions in exercise-induced muscle damage,[214] the putative beneficial effects of a combination of antioxidants on

TABLE 10 U.S. Olympic Committee's Recommended Upper Levels for Antioxidant Supplementation[a]

Antioxidant	Dosage
β-carotene	3000–20,000 μg or 5000–33,340 IU
Vitamin C	250–1,000 mg
Vitamin E	100–400 IU as α-tocopherol

[a] Presented at the 1996 Sports and Cardiovascular Nutritionists (SCAN) Symposium on Nutrition, Exercise and Fitness by Evans, W.: The protective role of antioxidants on exercise induced oxidative stress. Levels established by Task Force on Guidelines for Dietary Supplementation, USOC, 1993.

reducing lipid peroxidation during exercise,[215] and some evidence that additional vitamin C intake may decrease the risk of upper respiratory tract infection in athletes,[216] the U.S. Olympic Committee (USOC) has issued a position stand on the recommended intakes of the antioxidants, vitamin C, vitamin E, and beta-carotene for those athletes desiring to take supplements (Table 10). The USOC's position for offering the recommendation is to help guide athletes to safe intakes that, while being supplemental, are in moderation compared to the dosages that some of the athletes actually consume. However, a two-fold risk exists in the recommendation. First, many athletes might interpret the USOC's recommendation as an endorsement or an obligation to supplementation. With many athletes, the "more-is-better" philosophy persists, so actual intakes may be higher than those recommended. This could increase the possibility of some athletes reacting to intakes that induce adverse side-effects. The second concern is that by isolating three micronutrients, the position stand might cause the athlete to disregard adequate intakes of other micronutrients. Having met the suggested levels by taking a supplement, the athlete might presume that it is then safe to skip meals and not attend to other aspects of the diet. Regardless of supplement use, athletes are strongly encouraged to rely first on acquiring their micronutrient requirements from whole foods from a wide variety of categories as suggested in the U.S. Department of Agriculture's food pyramid.[27]

IX. SUMMARY

Within this chapter, we have identified the nutrient needs of athletes in team sports; short-duration, high-intensity sports; and long-duration, moderate-intensity sports. In general, the nutrients demonstrating the most profound depletion as a consequence of the athlete's high intensity and volume of training are water (fluids) and carbohydrate.[37,39,70,72,75] Consequently, the athlete should develop a nutrition plan that ensures the complete replacement of fluids and body glycogen stores and, at the same time, meets the requirements for all other nutrients.[2,8,15,27] Such a diet strategy will help maintain the athlete's nutritional status and health,[15,17,32,42] which are prerequisites for optimal training and sports performance. To provide guidelines for creating such a plan, Table 11 presents recommendations for nutrient intake in athletes training for 90 min or more each day. These guidelines were developed for broad populations of athletes and may not be suitable on an individual basis. Recommendations for specific athletes must be made on a case-by-case basis.

TABLE 11 Recommended Nutrient Intake for Athletes Training 90 Min or More Each Day

Category	Recommendations
Energy	• 1.6–2.4 × resting energy expenditure or ... • 188–209 kJ/kg BW/day for females (20–23 kcal/lb BW/day) • >209 kJ/kg BW/day for males (>23 kcal/lb BW/day)
Fluid	• 500 ml (~16 oz) 2 h before exercise • Drink frequently (e.g., every 10–15 min) to replace sweat loss during exercise; if not possible, drink as much as is tolerable • Replace weight loss before next training session
Carbohydrate	• >60% total caloric intake • 500–600 g/day or ... • 9–10 g/kg BW/day (4 to 5 g/lb BW/day)
Fat	• <1 g/kg BW/day (<0.45 g/lb BW/day) • <30% of total caloric intake
Protein	• ≤1.6 g/kg BW/day • 10–15% of total caloric intake • sources to include meat (beef, chicken, fish, pork) and dairy products as well as vegetables, cereals, and grains
Minerals	• levels as indicated in Table 7 • acquire from cereals and grains (6–11 servings/day), vegetables (3–5 servings/day), fruits (2–3 servings /day), dairy products (2–3 servings/day), and meat/protein foods (2–3 servings/day) • with heavy sweat losses, consume additional electrolytes, sodium, chloride, and possibly potassium, with fluid replacement and meals • mineral supplements may be warranted to meet iron and calcium needs in female athletes
Vitamins	• levels as indicated in Table 9 • acquire from cereals and grains (6–11 servings/day), vegetables (3–5 servings/day), fruits (2–3 servings/day), dairy products (2–3 servings/day), and meat/protein foods (2–3 servings/day) • supplementation of antioxidants not to exceed levels identified in Table 10

Based on recommendations from References 1, 4, 7, 9, 12, 15, 17, 27, 28, and 33.

REFERENCES

1. *Clinical Sports Nutrition,* Burke, L. and Deakin, V., Eds., McGraw-Hill, New York, 1995.
2. Coleman, E., *Eating for Endurance*, Bull Publishing Co., Palo Alto, CA, 1989.
3. Tribole, E., *Eating on the Run*, Leisure Press, Champaign, IL, 1992.
4. Williams, M. H., *Nutrition and Fitness for Sport*, 4th ed., William C. Brown, Dubuque, IA, 1995.
5. Brouns, F., *Nutritional Needs of Athletes*, John Wiley and Sons, Inc. New York, 1993.
6. Clark, N., *The New York City Marathon Cookbook*, Rutledge Hill Press, Nashville, 1994.
7. *Sports Nutrition: a Guide for the Professional Working With Active People*, 2nd ed., Bernadot, D., Ed., American Dietetic Association, Chicago, 1994.
8. Houtkooper, L., *Winning Sports Nutrition: Training Manual*, University of Arizona, Tucson, 1994.
9. Burke, L., *The Complete Guide to Food for Sports Performance*, Allen and Unwin, Sydney, Australia, 1992.
10. *Perspectives in Exercise Science and Sports Medicine: Ergogenics: Enhancement of Performance in Exercise and Sport*, Lamb, D. R. and Williams, M. H., Eds., Brown and Benchmark, Indianapolis, IN, 1991.
11. *Perspectives in Exercise Science and Sports Medicine: Physiology and Nutrition for Competitive Sport*, Lamb, D. R., Knuttgen, H. G., and Murray, R., Eds., Cooper Publishing, Indianapolis, IN, 1994.
12. *Sports Nutrition for the 90s: The Health Professional's Guidebook*, Berning, J. and Nelson-Steen, S., Eds., Aspen Publishing, Gaithersburg, MD, 1991.
13. Clark, N., *Nancy Clark's Sports Nutrition Guidebook*, 2nd ed., Human Kinetics, Champaign, IL, 1996.
14. Peterson, M. and Peterson, K., *Eat To Compete: A Guide to Sports Nutrition*, Year Book Medical Publishers, Chicago, 1988.

15. Food and Nutrition Board, *Recommended Dietary Allowances*, 10th ed., National Academy of Sciences, Washington, D.C., 1989, 30.

16. Garrow, J. S., *Energy Balance and Obesity in Man, 2nd edition*, Elsevier/North-Holland Biomedical Press, New York, 1978, 243.

17. World Health Organization, Energy and protein requirements, *Report of a Joint FAO/WHO/UNU Expert Consultation*, Technical Report Series 724, WHO, Geneva, Switzerland, 1985, 206.

18. Brotherhood, J., Nutrition and sports performance, *Sports Med.*, 1, 350, 1984.

19. Economos, C. D., Bortz, S. S., and Nelson, M. E., Nutritional practices of elite athletes, *Sports Med.*, 16, 383, 1993.

20. Hickson, J., Wolinsky, I., Pivarnik, J., Neuman, E., Itak, J., and Stockton, J., Nutritional profile of football athletes eating from a training table, *Nutr. Res.*, 7, 27, 1987.

21. Ekblom, B., Applied physiology of soccer, *Sports Med.*, 3, 50, 1986.

22. Sherman, W. M., Recovery from endurance exercise, *Med. Sci. Sports Exer.*, 24, S336, 1992.

23. Butterfield, G., Amino acids and high protein diets, in *Perspectives in Exercise Science and Sports Medicine: Ergogenics — Enhancement of Performance in Exercise and Sport*, Lamb, D. R. and Williams, M. H., Eds., Brown and Benchmark, Indianapolis, IN, 1990, 4, 87.

24. Pate, R. R. and Branch, J. D., Training for endurance sport, *Med. Sci. Sports Exer.*, 24, S340, 1992.

25. Ekblom, B. and Bergh, U., Physiology and nutrition for cross-country skiing, in, *Perspectives in Exercise Science and Sports Medicine: Physiology and Nutrition for Competitive Sport*, Lamb, D., Knuttgen, H., and Murray, R., Eds., Benchmark Press, Indianapolis, IN, 1994, 373.

26. Burke, L., Gollan, R., and Read, R., Dietary intakes and food use of groups of elite Australian male athletes, *Int. J. Sports Nutr.*, 1, 378, 1991.

27. Houtkooper, L., Food selection for endurance sports, *Med. Sci. Sports Exer.*, 24, S349, 1992.

28. Hoffman, C. J. and Coleman, E., An eating plan and update on recommended dietary practices for the endurance athlete, *J. Am. Diet. Assoc.*, 91, 325, 1991.

29. Moses, K. and Manore, M. M., Development and testing of a carbohydrate monitoring tool for athletes, *J. Am. Diet. Assoc.*, 91, 962, 1991.

30. Short, S. and Short, W., Four-year study of university athletes' dietary intake, *J. Am. Diet. Assoc.*, 82, 632, 1983.

31. Horswill, C., Park, S., and Roemmich, J., Changes in the protein nutritional status of adolescent wrestlers, *Med. Sci. Sports Exer.*, 22, 599, 1990.

32. American Collge of Sports Medicine, Position stand: weight loss in wrestlers, *Med. Sci. Sports Exer.*, 28, ix, 1996.

33. Williams, M.H., *Nutritional Aspects of Human Physical and Athletic Performance*, C.C. Thomas, Springfield, IL, 1985, 399.

34. Dueck, C., Matt, K., Manore, M., and Skinner, J., Treatment of athletic amenorrhea with a diet and training intervention program, *Int. J. Sports Med.*, 6, 24, 1996.

35. Armstrong, L., Considerations for replacement beverages: fluid-electrolyte balance and heat illness, in *Fluid Replacement and Heat Stress*, Marriott, B. and Rosemont, C., Eds., National Academy Press, Washington, D.C., 1991, IV 1–IV26.

36. Sawka, M. N. and Wenger, C. B., Physiological responses to acute exercise-heat stress, in *Human Performance Physiology and Environmental Medicine at Terrestrial Extremes*, Pandolf, K. B., Sawka, M. N., and Gonzalez, R. R., Eds. Benchmark Press, Indianapolis, IN, 1988, 153.

37. Sawka, M. N. and Pandolf, K. B., Effects of body water loss in physiological function and exercise performance, in *Perspectives in Exercise Science and Sports Medicine: Fluid Homeostasis During Exercise*, Lamb, D. R. and Gisolfi, C. V., Eds. Benchmark Press, Indianapolis, IN, 1990, 1.

38. Noakes, T. D., Adams, B. A., Myburgh, K. H., Greeff, C., Lotz, T., and Nathan, M., The danger of an inadequate water intake during prolonged exercise, *Eur. J. Appl. Physiol.*, 57, 210, 1988.

39. Maughan, R. J., Shirreffs, S. M., Galloway, D. R., and Leiper, J. B., Dehydration and fluid replacement in sport and exercise, *Sports Exer. Inj.*, 1, 145, 1995.

40. Hargreaves, M., Physiological benefits of fluid ingestion during exercise, in *Exercise and Thermoregulation*, Sutton, J., Thompson, M., and Torode, M., Eds., University of Sydney, Sydney, Australia, 1995, 175.

41. Walsh, R. M., Noakes, T. D., Hawley, J. A., and Dennis, S. C., Impaired high-intensity cycling performance time at low levels of dehydration, *Int. J. Sports. Med.*, 15, 392, 1994.

42. American College of Sports Medicine, Position stand on exercise and fluid replacement, *Med. Sci. Sports Exer.*, 28, i, 1996.

43. Murray, R., The effects of consuming carbohydrate-electrolyte beverages on gastric emptying and fluid absorption during and following exercise, *Sports Med.*, 4, 322, 1987.

44. Broad, E., Fluid requirements of team sport players, *Sports Coach*, 20–23, Summer 1996.

45. Broad, E. M., Burke, L. M., Cox, G. R., Heeley, P., and Riley, M., Body weight changes and voluntary fluid intakes during training and competition sessions in team sports, *Int. J. Sports Nutr.*, 6, 307, 1996.

46. Rico-Sanz, J., Frontera, W. R., Rivera, M. A., River-Brown, A., Mole, P. A., and Meredith, C. N., Effects of hyperhydration on total body water, temperature regulation and performance of elite young soccer players in a warm climate, *Int. J. Sports Med.*, 17, 85, 1996.

47. Boening, D., Ulmer, H. V., Meier, U., Skipka, W., and Stegemann, J., Effects of a multi-hour water immersion on trained and untrained subjects: I. Renal function and plasma volume, *Aerospace Med.*, 43, 300, 1972.

48. Troup, J. P., Strass, D., and Trappe, T. A., Physiology and nutrition for competitive swimming, in *Perspectives in Exercise Science and Sports Medicine: Physiology and Nutrition for Competitive Sport*, Lamb, D. R., Knuttgen, H. G., and Murray R., Eds., Benchmark Press, Indianapolis, IN, 1994, 99.

49. Horswill, C. A., Physiology and nutrition for wrestling, in *Perspectives in Exercise Science and Sports Medicine: Physiology and Nutrition for Competitive Sport*, Lamb, D. R., Knuttgen, H. G., and Murray R., Eds., Benchmark Press, Indianapolis, IN, 1994, 146.

50. Horswill, C. A., Does rapid weight loss by dehydration adversely affect high-power performance?, *Sports Sci. Exch.*, 4, 1, 1991.

51. Horswill, C. A., Physiology and nutrition for wrestling, in *Perspectives in Exercise Science and Sports Medicine: Physiology and Nutrition for Competitive Sport*, Vol. 7, Lamb, D. R., Knuttgen, H. G., and Murray R., Eds., Benchmark Press, Indianapolis, IN, 1994, 150.

52. Horswill, C. A., Scott, J. R., Dick, R. W., and Hayes, J., Influence of rapid weight gain after the weigh-in on success in collegiate wrestlers, *Med. Sci. Sports Exer.*, 26, 1290, 1994.

53. Horswill, C. A., Physiology and nutrition for wrestling, in *Perspectives in Exercise Science and Sports Medicine: Physiology and Nutrition for Competitive Sport*, Lamb, D. R., Knuttgen, H. G., and Murray R., Eds., Benchmark Press, Indianapolis, IN, 1994, 163.

54. Hagerman, F. C., Physiology and nutrition for rowing, in *Perspectives in Exercise Science and Sports Medicine: Physiology and Nutrition for Competitive Sport*, Lamb, D. R., Knuttgen, H. G., and Murray R., Eds., Benchmark Press, Indianapolis, IN, 1994, 281.

55. Rothstein, A., Adolph, E., and Willis, J., Voluntary dehydration, in, *Physiology of Man in the Desert*, Adolph, E. and associates, Eds., Interscience Publishers, New York, 1947, 254.

56. Holm, I., Sjodin, B., Nilsson, J., and Forsberg, A., Changes in muscle functions during long distance skiing, the Vasa race, *Svensk Skidsport*, 8, 27, 1976.

57. Armstrong, L. E., Costill, D. L., and Fink, W. J., Influence of diuretic-induced dehydration on competitive running performance, *Med. Sci. Sports Exer.*, 17, 456, 1985.

58. Murray, R., Intra-race fluid replacement, in, *Exercise and Thermoregulation*, Sutton, J., Thompson, M., and Torode, M., Eds., University of Sydney, Sydney, Australia, 1995, 329.

59. Burke, E. R., Physiology and nutrition for cycling, in *Perspectives in Exercise Science and Sports Medicine: Physiology and Nutrition for Competitive Sport*, Lamb, D. R., Knuttgen, H. G., and Murray R., Eds., Benchmark Press, Indianapolis, IN, 1994, 315.

60. Rehrer, N. J., Beckers, E. J., Brouns, F., Ten Hoor, F., and Saris, W. H. M., Effects of dehydration on gastric emptying and gastrointestinal distress while running, *Med. Sci. Sports Exer.*, 22, 790, 1990.

61. Broad, E., Fluid requirements of team sport players, *Sports Coach*, 20, Summer 1996.

62. Riedesel, M. L., Allen, D. Y., Peake, G. T., and Al-Qattan, K., Hyperhydration with glycerol solutions, *J. Appl. Physiol.*, 63, 2262, 1987.

63. Lyons, T. P., Riedesel, M. L., Meuli, L. E., and Chick, T. L., Effects of glycerol induced hyperhydration prior to exercise in the heat on sweating and core temperature, *Med. Sci. Sports Exer.*, 22, 477, 1990.

64. Montner, P., Stark, D. M., Riedesel, M. L., Murata, G., Robergs, R., Timms, M., and Chick, T. L., Pre-exercise glycerol hydration improves cycling endurance time, *Int. J. Sports Med.*, 17, 27, 1996.

65. Murray, R., Eddy, D. E., Paul, G. L., Seifert, J. G., and Halaby, G. A., Physiological responses to glycerol ingestion during exercise, *J. Appl. Physiol.*, 71, 144, 1991.

66. Tourtellotte, W. W., Reinglass, J. L., and Newkirk, T. A., Cerebral dehydration action of glycerol, *Clin. Phar. Therap.*, 13, 159, 1972.

67. Coggan, A. and Coyle E. F., Carbohydrate ingestion during prolonged exercise: effects on metabolism and performance, in *Exercise and Sports Science Reviews*, Vol. 19, Holloszy, J. O., Ed., Williams and Wilkins, Baltimore, 1991, 1.

68. Tesch, P., Forsberg, A., and Karlsson, E., Selective muscle glycogen depletion during cross-country skiing, *J. U.S. Ski Coaches Assoc.*, 2, 12, 1978.

69. Boobis, L., Williams, C., and Wootton, S., Human muscle metabolism during brief maximal exercise, *J. Physiol.*, 338, 21, 1982.

70. Costill, D. L., Carbohydrates for exercise: dietary demands for optimal performance, *Int. J. Sports Med.*, 9, 1, 1988.

71. Sherman, W. M., Doyle, J. A., Lamb, D. R., and Strauss, R. H., Dietary carbohydrate, muscle glycogen, and exercise performance during 7 d of training, *Am. J. Clin. Nutr.*, 57, 27, 1993.

72. Costill, D. L., Carbohydrate nutrition before, during, and after exercise, *Fed. Proc.*, 44, 364, 1985.

73. Walberg-Rankin, J., Dietary carbohydrate as an ergogenic aid for prolonged and brief competitions in sport, *Int. J. Sports Nutr.*, 5, S13, 1995.

74. Ivy, J. L., Muscle glycogen synthesis before and after exercise, *Sports Med.*, 11, 6, 1991.
75. Sherman, W. M., Metabolism of sugars and physical performance, *Am. J. Clin. Nutr.*, 62, 228S, 1995.
76. Wright, D., Sherman, W. M., and Dernbach, A. R., Carbohydrate feedings before, during, or in combination improve cycling endurance performance, *J. Appl. Physiol.*, 71, 1082, 1991.
77. Coggan, A. R. and Swanson, S. C., Nutritional manipulations before and during endurance exercise: effects on performance, *Med. Sci. Sports Exer.*, 24, S331, 1992.
78. Fitts, R., Substrate supply and energy metabolism during brief high intensity exercise: importance in limiting performance, in *Perspectives in Exercise Science and Sports Medicine: Energy Metabolism in Exercise and Sport*, Lamb, D.R. and Gisolfi, C.V., Eds., Brown and Benchmark, Indianapolis, IN, 1992, 53.
79. Karlsson, H. G., Kolhydratomsattning under en fotbollsmatch, *Report Department of Physiology III*, reference 6, Karolinska Institute, Stockholm, Sweden, 1969.
80. Jacobs, I., Westlin, N., Rasmusson, M., and Houghton, B., Muscle glycogen and diet in elite soccer players, *Eur. J. Appl. Physiol.*, 48, 297, 1982.
81. Leatt, P. B. and Jacobs, I., Effect of glucose polymer ingestion on glycogen depletion during a soccer match, *Can. J. Sports Sci.*, 14, 112, 1989.
82. Simard, J., Effects of carbohydrate intake before and during an ice hockey game on blood and muscle energy substrates, *Res. Quart. Exer. Sport*, 59, 144, 1988.
83. Kirkendall, D., Foster, C., Dean, J., Grogan, J., and Thompson, N., Effect of a glucose polymer supplementation on performance of soccer players, in *Science and Football*, Reilly, T., Lees, A., David, K., and Murphy, W., Eds., E&FN SPON, London, England, 1988, 33.
84. Rehunen, S. and Littsola, S., Modification of the muscle-glycogen level of ice-hockey players through a drink with high carbohydrate content, *Z. Sportsmed.*, 2, 15, 1978.
85. Williams, C., Carbohydrate needs of elite athletes, in *Nutrition and Fitness for Athletes*, Simopolous, A.P. and Pavlou, K.N., Eds., Karger Publishing, New York, 1993.
86. Steen, S. and McKinney, S., Nutrition assessment of college wrestlers, *Physician Sportsmed.*, 14, 100, 1986.
87. Williams, C., Physiology and nutrition for sprinting, in *Perspectives in Exercise Science and Sports Medicine: Physiology and Nutrition for Competitive Sport*, Lamb, D., Knuttgen, H., and Murray, R., Eds., Benchmark Press, Indianapolis, IN, 1994, 55.
88. Nevill, M. E., Williams, C., Roper, D., Slater, C., and Nevill, A. V., Effect of diet on performance during recovery from intermittent sprint exercise, *J. Sports Sci.*, 11, 119, 1993.
89. Pascoe, D. D. and Gladden, L. B., Muscle glycogen resynthesis after short term, high intensity exercise and resistance exercise, *Sports Med.*, 21, 98, 1996.
90. Lamb, D., Rinehardt, K., Bartels, R., Sherman, W. M., and Snook, J., Dietary carbohydrate and intensity of interval swim training, *Am. J. Clin. Nutr.*, 52, 1058, 1990.
91. Costill, D., Flynn, M., Kirwan, J., Houmard, J., Mitchell, J., Thomas, R., and Park, S., The effects of repeated days of intensified training on muscle glycogen and swimming performance, *Med. Sci. Sports Exer.*, 20, 249, 1988.
92. Lambert, C. P., Flynn, M. G., Boone, J. B., Michaud, T. J., and Rodriguez-Zayas, J., Effects of carbohydrate feeding on multiple-bout resistance exercise, *J. Appl. Sports Sci. Res.*, 5, 192, 1991.
93. Nicholas, C. W., Williams, C., Phillips, G., and Nowitz, A., Influence of ingesting a carbohydrate-electrolyte solution on endurance capacity during intermittent, high intensity shuttle running, *J. Sports Sci.*, 1996.
94. Jackson, D. A., Davis, J. M., Broadwell, M. S., Query, J. L., and Lambert, C. L., Effects of carbohydrate feedings on fatigue during intermittent high-intensity exercise in males and females, *Med. Sci. Sports Exer.*, 27, S223, 1995.
95. Below, P. R., Mora-Rodriguez, R., Gonzalez-Alonso, J., and Coyle, E. F., Fluid and carbohydrate ingestion independently improve performance during 1 h of intense exercise, *Med. Sci. Sports Exer.*, 27, 200, 1995.
96. Ball, T. C., Headley, S. A., Vanderburgh, P. M., and Smith, J. C., Periodic carbohydrate replacement during 50 min of high-intensity cycling improves subsequent sprint performance, *Int. J. Sports Nutr.*, 5, 151, 1995.
97. Maughan, R., Carbohydrate-electrolyte solutions during prolonged exercise, in *Perspectives in Exercise Science and Sports Medicine: Ergogenics — Enhancement of Performance in Exercise and Sport*, Lamb, D. and Williams, M., Eds., Brown and Benchmark, Indianapolis, IN, 1991, 35.
98. Murray, R., Paul, G. L., Seifert, J. G., Eddy, D. E., and Halaby, G. A., The effects of glucose, fructose, and sucrose ingestion during exercise, *Med. Sci. Sports Exer.*, 21, 1989.
99. Murray, R., The effects of consuming carbohydrate-electrolyte beverages on gastric emptying and fluid absorption during and following exercise, *Sports Med.*, 4, 322, 1987.
100. Mason, W. L., McConell, G., and Hargreaves, M., Carbohydrate ingestion during exercise: liquid vs solid feedings, Med. Sci. Sports Exer., 25, 966, 1993.
101. Lugo, M., Sherman, W. M., Wimer, G. S., and Garleb, K., Metabolic responses when different forms of carbohydrate energy are consumed during cycling, *Int. J. Sports Nutr.*, 3, 398, 1993.
102. Sherman, W. M. and Lamb, D. R., Nutrition and prolonged exercise, in *Perspectives in Exercise Science and Sports Medicine: Prolonged Exercise*, Lamb, D. R. and Murray, R., Eds., Benchmark Press, Indianapolis, IN, 1988, 213.

103. Hawley, J., Dennis, S., and Noakes, T., Oxidation of carbohydrate ingested during prolonged endurance exercise, *Sports Med.*, 14, 27, 1992.

104. Brouns, F., *Food and Fluid Related Aspects in Highly Trained Athletes*, Uitgeverji De Vrieseborch, Haarlem, Netherlands, 1988.

105. Coyle, E. F., Coggan, A. R., Hemmert, M. K., and Ivy, J. L., Muscle glycogen utilization during prolonged strenuous exercise when fed carbohydrate, *J. Appl. Physiol.*, 61, 165, 1986.

106. Maughan, R. J., Fenn, C. E., and Leiper, J. B., Effects of fluid, electrolyte, and substrate ingestion on endurance capacity, *Eur. J. Appl. Physiol.*, 58, 481, 1989.

107. Mitchell, J., Costill, D., Houmard, J., Flynn, M., Fink, W., and Beltz, J., Effects of carbohydrate dosage on exercise performance and glycogen metabolism, *J. Appl. Physiol.*, 67, 1843, 1989.

108. Murray, R., Paul, G., Seifert, J., and Eddy, D., Responses to varying rates of carbohydrate ingestion during exercise, *Med. Sci. Sports Exer.*, 23, 713, 1991.

109. Costill, D. L., Gastric emptying of fluids during exercise, in *Perspectives in Exercise Science and Sports Medicine: Fluid Homeostasis During Exercise*, Gisolfi, C. V. and Lamb, D. R., Eds., Benchmark Press, Indianapolis, IN, 1990, 97.

110. Costill, D. L. and Hargreaves, M., Carbohydrate nutrition and fatigue, *Sports Med.*, 13, 86, 1992.

111. Coyle, E. F., Timing and method of increased carbohydrate intake to cope with heavy training, competition, and recovery, *J. Sports Sci.*, 9, 29–51, 1991.

112. Coyle, E. F. and Coyle, E., Carbohydrates that speed recovery from training, *Phys. Sports Med.*, 21, 111, 1993.

113. Short, S. H., Surveys of dietary intake and nutrition knowledge of athletes and their coaches, in *Nutrition in Exercise and Sport, 2nd edition*, Wolinsky, I. and Hickson, J.F., Jr., Eds., CRC Press, Boca Raton, FL, 1989.

114. Romijn, J. A., Coyle, E. F., Sidossis, L. S., Gastaldelli, A., Horowitz, J. F., Endert, E., and Wolfe, R. R., Regulation of endogenous fat and carbohydrate metabolism in relation to exercise intensity and duration, *Am. J. Physiol.*, 265, E380, 1993.

115. Wells, C. L. and Pate, R. R., Training for performance of prolonged exercise, in *Perspectives in Exercise Science and Sports Medicine: Prolonged Exercise*, Lamb, D. R. and Murray, R., Eds., Benchmark Press, Indianapolis, IN, 1988, 75.

116. Bjorntorp, P., Importance of fat as a support nutrient for energy: metabolism of athletes, *J. Sports Sci.*, 9, 71, 1991.

117. Sears, B., Hormonal dangers of carbohydrate loading, *Triathlete*, 136, 54, 1995.

118. Sherman, W. M. and Leenders, N., Fat loading: the next magic bullet?, *Int. J. Sports Nutr.*, 5, S1, 1995.

119. Lemon, P. and Mullin, J., Effect of initial muscle glycogen levels on protein catabolism during exercise, *Med. Sci. Sports Exer.*, 48, 624, 1980.

120. Dohm, G., Williams, R., Kasperek, G., and van Rij, A., Increased excretion of urea and N-methylhistidine by rats and humans after a bout of exercise, *J. Appl. Physiol.*, 52, 27, 1982.

121. Wolfe, R., Goodenough, R., Wolfe, M., Royle, G., and Nadel, E., Isotopic analysis of leucine and urea metabolism in exercising humans, *J. Appl. Physiol.*, 52, 458, 1982.

122. Carraro, F., Stuart, C., Hartl, W., Rosenblatt, J., and Wolfe R., Effect of exercise and recovery on muscle protein synthesis in human subjects, *Am. J. Physiol.*, 259, E470, 1990.

123. Knapik, J., Meredith, C., Jones, B., Fielding, R., Young, V., and Evans, W., Leucine metabolism during fasting and exercise, *J. Appl. Physiol.*, 70, 43, 1991.

124. Felig, P., Amino acid metabolism in exercise, *Ann. N.Y. Acad. Sci.*, 301, 56, 1977.

125. Lemon, P., Do athletes need more dietary protein and amino acids?, *Int. J. Sports Nutr.*, 5, S39, 1995.

126. Williams, C., Macronutrients and performance, *J. Sports Sci.*, 13, S1, 1995.

127. Bartels, R., The relationship between strength and lean body mass: a rational for strength improvement, in *Muscle Development: Nutritional Alternatives to Anabolic Steroids,* Ross Laboratories, Columbus, OH, 1988, 7.

128. Frontera, W., Meredith, C., O'Reilly, K., Knuttgen, H., and Evans, W., Strength conditioning in older men: skeletal muscle hypertrophy and improved function, *J. Appl. Physiol.*, 64, 1038, 1988.

129. Lemon, P., Tarnopolsky, M., MacDougall, J., and Atkinson, S., Protein requirements and musclemass/strength changes during intensive training in novice bodybuilders, *J. Appl. Physiol.*, 73, 767, 1992.

130. Tarnopolsky, M., Atkinson, S., MacDougall, J., Chesley, A., Philips, S., and Schwarcz, H., Evaluation of protein requirements in trained strenght athletes, *J. Appl. Physiol.*, 73, 1986, 1992.

131. Tarnopolsky, M., MacDougall, J., and Atkinson, S., Influence of protein intake and training status on nitrogen balance and lean body mass, *J. Appl. Physiol.*, 66, 187, 1988.

132. Grandjean, A., Macronutrient intake of US athletes compared with the general population and recommendations made for athletes, *Am. J. Clin. Nutr.,* 49, 1070, 1989.

133. Shettty, P., Jung, R., Watrasiewicz, K., and James, W., Rapid-turnover transport proteins: an index of subclinical protein-energy malnutrition, *Lancet*, 2, 230, 1979.

134. Kelleher, P., Phinney, S., Sims, E., Bogardus, C., Horton, E., Bistrian, B., Amatruda, J., and Lockwood, D., Effects of carbohydrate-containing and carbohydrate-restricted hypocaloric and eucaloric diets on serum concentrations of retinol-binding protein, thyroxine-binding prealbumin and transferrin, *Metabolism,* 32, 95, 1983.

135. Nieman, D., Butler, J., Pollet, L., Dietrich, S., and Lutz, R., Nutrient intake of marathon runners, *J. Am. Diet. Assoc.,* 89, 1273, 1989.

136. Niekamp, R. and Baer, J., In-season dietary adequacy of trained male cross-country runners, *Int. J. Sport Nutr.,* 5, 45, 1995.

137. Gabel, K., Aldous, A., and Edington, C., Dietary intake of two male cyclists during 10-day, 2,050-mile ride, *Int. J. Sport Nutr.,* 5, 55, 1995.

138. Hawley, J., Dennis, S., Lindsay, F., and Noakes, T., Nutritional practices of athletes: are they sub-optimal?, *J. Sports Sci.,* 13, S75, 1995.

139. Friedman, J. and Lemon, P., Effect of chronic endurance exercise on the retention of dietary protein, *Int. J. Sport Med.,* 10, 118, 1989.

140. Meredith, C., Zachin, M., Frontera, W., and Evans, W., Dietary protein requirements and protein metabolism in endurance-trained men, *J. Appl. Physiol.,* 66, 2850, 1989.

141. Fielding, R., Meredith, C., O'Reilly, K., Frontera, W., Cannon, J., and Evans, W., Enhanced protein breakdown after eccentric exercise in young and older men, *J. Appl. Physiol.,* 71, 674, 1991.

142. Evans, W., Meredith, C., Cannon, J., Dinarello, C., Frontera, W., Hughes, V., Jones, B., and Knuttgen, H., Metabolic changes following eccentric exercise in trained and untrained men, *J. Appl. Physiol.,* 61, 1864, 1986.

143. Walberg-Rankin, J., A review of nutritional practices and needs of bodybuilders, *J. Strength Cond. Res.,* 9, 116, 1995.

144. Edwards, J., Lindeman, A., Mikesky, A., and Stager, J., Energy balance in highly trained female endurance runners, *Med. Sci. Sports Exer.,* 25, 1398, 1993.

145. Brenner, B. M., Meyer, T. W., and Hostetter, T. H., Protein intake and the progressive nature of kidney disease: the role of hemodynamically mediated glomerular sclerosis in aging, renal ablation, and intrinsic renal disease, *New Eng. J. Med.,* 307, 652, 1982.

146. Klahr, S., Levey, A., Beck, G., Caggiula, A., Hunsiker, L., Kusek, J., and Striker, G., The effects of dietary protein restriction and blood-pressure control on the progression of chronic renal disease, *New Eng. J. Med.,* 330, 877, 1994.

147. Altman, P. and Dittmer, D., *Blood and Other Body Fluids,* FASEB, Bethesda, MD, 1961.

148. Costill, D., Water and electrolyte requirements during exercise, *Clinics Sports Med.,* 3, 639, 1984.

149. Costill, D., Cote, R., and Fink, W., Dietary potassium and heavy exercise: effects on muscle water and electrolytes, *Am. J. Clin. Nutr.,* 36, 266, 1982.

150. Waller, M. and Haymes, E., The effects of heat and exercise on sweat iron loss, *Med. Sci. Sports Exer.,* 28, 197, 1996.

151. DeFronzo, R. and Ferrannini, E., Insulin resistance: a multifaceted syndrome responsible for NIDDM, obesity, hypertension, dyslipidemia, and atherosclerotic cardiovascular disease, *Diab. Care,* 14, 173, 1991.

152. Daly, P. and Landsberg, L., Hypertension in obesity and NIDDM: role of insulin and sympathetic nervous system, *Diab. Care,* 14, 240, 1991.

153. Peiris, A., Mueller, R., Smith, G., Struve, M., and Kissebah, A., Splanchnic insulin metabolism in obesity: impact of body fat distribution, *J. Clin. Invest.,* 78, 1648, 1986.

154. Clarkson, P. and Haymes, E., Exercise and mineral status of athletes: calcium, magnesium, phosphorus, and iron, *Med. Sci. Sports Exer.,* 27, 831, 1995.

155. Clarkson, P. and Haymes, E., Trace mineral requirements for athletes, *Int. J. Sport Nutr.,* 4, 104, 1994.

156. McDonald, R. and Keen, C., Iron and magnesium nutrition and athletic performance, *Sports Med.,* 5, 171, 1988.

157. Faber, M. and Spinnler Benade, A., Mineral and vitamin intake in field athletes (discus-, hemmer-, javelin-throwers and shotputters), *Int. J. Sports Med.,* 12, 324, 1991.

158. Sobal, J. and Marquart, L., Vitamin/mineral supplement use among athletes: a review of the literature, *Int. J. Sport Nutr.,* 4, 320, 1994.

159. Mertz, W., Chromium in human nutrition: a review, *J. Nutr.,* 123, 626, 1993.

160. Gelfand, R. and Barrett, E., Effect of physiologic hyperinsulinemia on skeletal muscle protein synthesis and breakdown, *J. Clin. Invest.,* 80, 1, 1987.

161. Welle, S., Thornton, C., Statt, M., and McHenry, B., Postprandial myofibrillar and whole body protein synthesis in young and old human subjects, *Am. J. Physiol.,* 267, E599, 1994.

162. Evans, G., The effect of chromium picolinate on insulin controlled parameters in humans, *Int. J. Biosocial Med. Res.,* 11, 163, 1989.

163. Hallmark, M., Reynolds, T., DeSouza, C., Dotson, C., Anderson, R., and Rogers, M., Effects of chromium and resistance training on muscle strength and body composition, *Med. Sci. Sports Exer.,* 28, 139, 1996.

164. Hasten, D., Rome, E., Franks, B., and Hested, M., Effects of chromium picolinate on beginning weight training students, *Int. J. Sport Nutr.,* 2, 343, 1992.

165. Trent, L. and Thieding-Cancel, D., Effects of chromium picolinate on body composition, *J. Sports Med. Phys. Fit.,* 35, 273, 1995.

166. Lefavi, R., Wilson, D., Keith, R., Anderson, R., Blessing, D., Hames, C., and McMillan, J., Lipid-lowering effect of a dietary chromium (III)-nicotinic acid complex in male athletes, *Nutr. Res.,* 13, 239, 1993.

167. Evans, G., Chromium picolinate is an efficacious and safe supplement (Letter to the editor), *Int. J. Sports Nutr.,* 3, 117, 1993.

168. Lefavi, R., Response to letter to editor: chromium picolinate is an efficacious and safe supplement, *Int. J. Sports Nutr.,* 3, 120, 1993.

169. Stearns, D., Wise, J., Patierno, S., and Wetterhahn, Chromium (III) picolinate produces chromosome damage in Chinese hamster ovary cells, *FASEB J.,* 9, 1643, 1995.

170. Cam, M.C., Faun, J., and McNeill, J.H. Concentration-dependent glucose-lowering effects of oral vanadyl are maintained following treatment withdrawal in streptozotocin-diabetic rats, *Metabolism,* 44, 332, 1995.

171. Ozcelikay, A., Becker, D., Ongemba, L., Pottier, A., Henquin, J., and Brichard, S., Improvement of glucose and lipid metabolism in diabetic rats treated with molybdate, *Am. J. Physiol.,* 270, E344, 1996.

172. Brilla, L. and Haley, T., Effect of magnesium supplementation on strength training in humans, *J. Am. Coll. Nutr.,* 11, 326, 1992.

173. Clarkson, P., Micronutrients and exercise: antioxidants and minerals, *J. Sports Sci.,* 13, S11, 1995.

174. Clarkson, P., Vitamins and trace minerals, in *Perspectives in Exercise Science and Sports Medicine: Ergogenics — Enhancement of Performance in Exercise and Sport,* Lamb, D. R. and Williams, M. H., Eds., Brown and Benchmark, Indianapolis, IN, 1990, chap. 4.

175. Hubbard, R., Szlyk, P., and Armstrong, L., Influence of thirst and fluid palatability on fluid ingestion during exercise, in *Perspectives in Exercise Science and Sports Medicine Vol. 3 Fluid Homeostasis During Exercise,* Gisolfi, C. and Lamb, D., Benchmark Press, Carmel, IN, 1990, 56.

176. Bergeron, M., Heat cramps during tennis: a case report, *Int. J. Sports Nutr.,* 6, 62, 1996.

177. Moffatt, R., Dietary status of elite female high school gymnasts: inadequacy of vitamin and mineral intake, *J. Am. Diet. Assoc.,* 84, 1361, 1984.

178. Moen, S., Sanborn, C., and DiMarco, N., Dietary habits and body composition in adoelscent female runners, *Women Sport Phys. Activity J.,* 1, 85, 1992.

179. Matovic, V., Fontana, D., Tominac, C., Goel, P., and Chestnut, C., Factors that influence peak bone mass formation: a study of calcium balance and inheritance of bone mass in adolescent females, *Am. J. Clin. Nutr.,* 52, 878, 1990.

180. Nelson, M., Fisher, E., Catsos, P., Meredith, C., Turksoy, R., and Evans, W., Diet and bone mass in amenorrheic runners, *Am. J. Clin. Nutr.,* 43, 910, 1986.

181. Marcus, R., Cann, C., Madvig, P., Minkoff, J., Goddard, M., Bayer, M., Martin, M., Gaudiani, A., Haskell, W., and Genant, H., Menstrual function and bone mass in women distance runners, *Ann. Int. Med.,* 102, 158, 1985.

182. Pennington, J., *Bowes and Church's Food Values of Portions Commonly Used,* 15th ed., Harper and Row Publishers, New York, 1989.

183. Eichner, E. R., Sports anemia, iron supplements, and blood doping, *Med. Sci. Sports Exer.,* 24, S315, 1992.

184. Cook, J. and Monsen, E., Vitamin C, the common cold, and iron absorption, *Am. J. Clin. Nutr.,* 30, 235, 1977.

185. Kanter, M., Antioxidants, carnitine, and choline as putative ergogenic aids, *Int. J. Sports Nutr.,* 5, S120, 1995.

186. Rotruck, J., Pope, A., Ganther, H., Swanson, A., Hafeman, D., and Hoekstra, W., Selenium, biochemical role as a component of glutathione peroxidase, *Science,* 179, 588, 1973.

187. Scott, M., The selenium dilemma, *J. Nutr.,* 103, 803, 1973.

188. Tessier, F., Margaritis, I., Richard, M. J., Moynot, C., and Marconnet, P., Selenium and training effects on the glutathione system and aerobic performance, *Med. Sci. Sports Exer.,* 27, 390, 1995.

189. Singh, A., Moses, F., and Deuster, P., Chronic multivitamin mineral supplementation does not enhance physical performance, *Med. Sci. Sports Exer.,* 24, 726, 1992.

190. Telford, R. D., Catchpole, E. A., Deakin, V., Hahn, A. G., and Plank, A. W., The effect of 7 to 8 months of vitamin/mineral supplementation on athletic performance, *Int. J. Sports Nutr.,* 2, 135, 1992.

191. Weight, L., Noakes, T., Labadarious, D., Graves, J., Jacobs, P., and Berman, P., Vitamins and mineral status of trained athletes including the effects of supplementation, *Am. J. Clin. Nutr.,* 47, 186, 1988.

192. van der Beek, E., Vitamins and endurance training: food for running or faddish claims?, *Sports Med.,* 2, 175, 1985.

193. Haymes E., Vitamin and mineral supplementation to athletes, *Int. J. Sports Med.,* 1, 146, 1991.

194. Belko, A., Vitamins and exercise — an update, *Med. Sci. Sports Exer.,* 19, S191, 1987.

195. Manore, M. and Leklem, J., Effect of carbohydrate and vitamin B_6 on fuel substrates during exercise in women, *Med Sci. Sports Exer.,* 20, 233, 1988.

196. Belko, A., Obarzanek, E., Roach, R., Rotter, M., Urban, G., Weinberg, S., and Roe, D., Effects of aerobic exercise and weight loss on riboflavin requirements of moderately obese, marginally deficient young women, *Am. J. Clin. Nutr.,* 40, 553, 1984.

197. Fogelholm, M., Ruokonen, I., Laakso, J., Vuorimaa, T., and Himberg, J., Lack of association between indices of vitamin B_1, B_2, and B_6 status and exercise-induced blood lactate in young adults, *Int. J. Sport Nutr.,* 3, 165, 1993.

198. Hickson, J., Schrader, J., Pivarnik, J., and Stockton, J., Nutritional intake from food sources of soccer athletes during two stages of training, *Nutr. Rep. Int.,* 34, 85, 1986.

199. Welch, P., Zager, K., Endres, J., and Poon, S., Nutrition education, body composition, and dietary intake of female college athletes, *Phys. Sportsmed.,* 15, 63, 1987.

200. Fogelholm, G., Koskinen, R., Laakso, J., Rankinen, J., and Ruokonen, I., Gradual and rapid weight loss: effects on nutrition and performance in male athletes, *Med. Sci. Sports Exer.,* 25, 371, 1993.

201. van der Beek, E., van Dokkum, W., Wedel, M., Schrijver, J., and van den Berg, H., Thiamin, riboflavin, and vitamin B_6: impact of restricted intake on physical performance in man, *J. Am. Coll. Nutr.,* 13, 629, 1994.

202. Henson, S., The problem of losing weight encountered by young wrestlers, *J. Sports Med. Phys. Fit.,* 10–11, 49, 1971.

203. Carlson, L., Havel, R., Ekelund, L., and Holmgren, A., Effect of nicotinic acid on turnover rate and oxidation of the free fatty acids of plasma in man during exercise, *Metabolism,* 12, 837, 1963.

204. Bergstrom, J., Hultman, E., Jorfeldt, L., Pernow, B., and Wahren, J., Effect of nicotinic acid on physical working capacity and on metabolism of muscle glycogen in man, *J. Appl. Physiol.,* 26, 170, 1969.

205. Baker, E., Saari, J., and Talbert, B., Ascorbic acid metabolism in man, *Am. J. Clin. Nutr.,* 19, 371, 1966.

206. Ershoff, B. and Levin, E., Beneficial effect of an unidentified factor in wheat germ oil on the swimming performance of guinea pigs, *Fed. Proc.,* 14, 431, 1955.

207. Consolazio, C., Matoush, L., Nelson, R., Isaac, G., and Hursh, L., Effect of octacosanol, wheat germ oil, and vitamin E on performance of swimming rats, *J. Appl. Physiol.,* 19, 265, 1964.

208. Stephenson, L. and Kolka, M., Cardiovascular and thermoregulatory effects of niacin, in *Thermal Physiology,* Mercer, J., Ed., Excerpta, New York, 1989, 279.

209. Murray, R., Bartoli, W., Eddy, D., and Horn, M., Physiological and performance responses to nicotinic-acid ingestion during exercise, *Med. Sci. Sports Exer.,* 27, 1057, 1995.

210. Pernow, B. and Saltin, B., Availability of substrates and capacity for prolonged heavy exercise in man, *J. Appl. Physiol.,* 31, 416, 1971.

211. Kanter, M., Free radicals, exercise, and antioxidant supplementation, *Int. J. Sport Nutr.,* 4, 205, 1994.

212. Maughan, R., Donnelly, A., Gleeson, M., Whiting, P., Walker, K., and Clough, P., Delayed-onset muscle damage and lipid peroxidation in man after a downhill run, *Muscle Nerve,* 12, 332, 1989.

213. Gee, D. and Tappel, A., The effect of exhaustive exercise on expired pentane as a marker of *in vivo* lipid peroxidation in the rat, *Life Sci.,* 28, 2425, 1981.

214. Meydani, M., Evans, W. J., Handelman, G., Biddle, L., Fielding, R. A., Meydani, S. N., Burrill, J., Fiatarone, M. A., Blumberg, J. B., and Cannon, J. G., Protective effect of vitamin E on exercise-induced oxidative damage in young and older adults, *Am. J. Physiol.,* 264, R992, 1993.

215. Kanter M., Nolte, L., and Holloszy, J., Effects of an antioxidant vitamin mixture on lipid peroxidation at rest and postexercise, *J. Appl.Physiol.,* 74, 965, 1993.

216. Peters, E., Goetzsche, J., Grobbelaar, B., and Noakes, T., Vitamin C supplementation reduces the incidence of postrace symptoms of upper-respiratory-tract infection in ultramarathon runners, *Am. J. Clin, Nutr.,* 57, 170, 1993.

Chapter 23

NUTRITION KNOWLEDGE OF ATHLETES AND THEIR COACHES AND SURVEYS OF DIETARY INTAKE

Leonard F. Marquart
Elyse A. Cohen
Sarah H. Short

CONTENTS

I. INTRODUCTION

The goals of this chapter are to investigate the nutritional knowledge of coaches and those who supervise the training of athletes; investigate the nutritional knowledge of those involved in physical activity and athletic performance; discuss nutritional surveys; and consider dietary intake of athletes.

Athletes need and want correct nutrition information. "There is still no sphere of nutrition in which faddism and ignorance are more obvious than in athletics."[1] Misinformation spreads through electronic and print media to the players, their coaches, and trainers. "There is a growing need for sports nutrition counseling and education to help athletes improve their eating habits."[2]

Too few involved in sports and fitness know that there are qualified sports nutritionists and dietitians in the practice of sports and cardiovascular nutrition. These specialists are organized to promote the integration of nutrition, exercise, and respiratory fitness to achieve and maintain optimal health.[3] A registered dietitian (RD) or licensed nutritionist (LN) is an essential part of the sports medicine team.

In many cases, advice for athletes is presented as if all athletes had the same needs. Nutrition advice must be individualized. When providing nutritional information, it is necessary to know the duration and intensity of an athletic event, body composition and age of an athlete, length of time spent practicing and training, and whether or not an athlete is training for a meet/match/tournament lasting one day or held on successive days. General nutrition advice for an all-inclusive group of athletes makes little sense since athletes' nutritional needs encompass a wide range. "Although coaches, trainers and athletes usually understand the principles of physical training, they often neglect the equally well-developed principles of nutrition."[4]

In order to best serve athletes, it is also necessary to know something about what coaches are telling players, what athletes know about nutrition, and what athletes are actually eating. Surveys of nutrition knowledge provide the starting point for nutrition education of athletes, coaches, and other professionals caring for athletes. Dietary surveys provide information on nutrient intake and serve as a basis for sports nutrition education for coaches and athletes at all levels of competition.

II.   NUTRITION KNOWLEDGE

A.   NUTRITION KNOWLEDGE OF COACHES, TRAINERS, AND OTHERS

It is important to investigate the nutrition knowledge of coaches, trainers, and others who influence athletes, since they can greatly affect all aspects of the athlete's life including their eating habits. Coaches, however, may have learned about nutrition from their coaches, thereby promulgating many nutrition myths. This section will address nutrition knowledge of coaches of high school and college athletes along with nutrition knowledge of college, high school, recreational, and child athletes.

1.   Coaches of High School and College Athletes

A nutrition knowledge survey of 348 coaches, 179 athletic trainers, and 2977 athletes in high school and college settings throughout the United States reported that more than 70% of athletic trainers certified by the National Athletic Trainers Association had taken nutrition courses and felt they should provide athletes with nutrition information.[5] Despite the fact that only 27% of coaches had taken a formal nutrition course, half of them stated that they should provide nutrition education to athletes. Noncertified athletic trainers (81%) believed they should counsel athletes on diet, although more than 25% had little nutrition education. Coaches and certified and uncertified trainers all reported fluids as the prime nutritional concern for athletes. On the other hand, athletes ranked fluid intake third, after concerns about body weight and vitamins. Sources of nutrition information reported by athletes were parents (ranked first or second by 77%), followed by print or electronic media. Athletes were asked about their familiarity with, and daily use of, three nutritional guidelines. Most (68%) athletes were very familiar with daily food guides, and 71% used a guide daily. Since athletes were not asked to define their nutritional guides, it is difficult to judge if these guidelines were actually being used. Additionally, these guidelines were not formulated for athletes. Athletes were not identified by their event except to state that wrestlers and swimmers relied more on coaches for nutrition information, while football and baseball players relied on trainers.

2.   Coaches of College Athletes

More than 100 college coaches in North Carolina were surveyed to measure nutrition knowledge, identify recommendations for dietary practices, and to discover sources of coaches' nutrition information.[6] A true/false nutrition test was answered correctly by 70% of coaches, but only one-third of coaches were certain their answers were correct. Most (82%) coaches never took a college nutrition course but 48% planned pre-game meals. These coaches (80%) knew little about the amounts of carbohydrate, fat, and protein appropriate for an athlete's diet. The majority of coaches reported that eating "junk food" was the worst dietary problem. Three coaches urged their athletes to enroll in a college nutrition course. Coaches' recommendations of vitamin/mineral supplements (60%), carbohydrate loading (40% of male coaches), protein supplements (20%), fluid restriction (12% of male coaches), and milk restriction (24% of male coaches) all indicated that more nutrition education was needed. Coaches indicated that their nutrition information came from books, physician's advice, professional journals, and the popular press. Dietitians or nutritionists were consulted by only 2% of coaches. The authors recommended special nutrition workshops to increase the depth of coaches' nutrition information.

3.   Coaches of High School Athletes

A nutrition knowledge survey of 342 high school coaches from Alabama found that 69% could not recommend a correct diet for athletes, 32% recommended protein supplements, 20% recommended salt tablets, and 62% told athletes to take vitamin and mineral supplements.[7]

The Iowa Dairy Council, Iowa High School Athletic Association, and an area hospital held a conference for high school coaches to learn about sports nutrition.[8] Coaches indicated that they would use nutrition information for their athletes, but no follow-up was reported.

Texas high school coaches were studied using a questionnaire.[9] More than half of all coaches suggested that athletes supplement with vitamins or multivitamins with minerals. Water was recommended by the majority of coaches, but schedules were not set for drinking water. Twelve percent of coaches recommended salt tablets to athletes.

A survey of 303 North Carolina high school coaches and trainers found that trainers knew more about 15 nutrition questions than coaches and that trainers more frequently recommended better nutrition procedures for athletes.[10] Trainers may be more knowledgeable because those certified by the National Athletic Trainers Association must have passed a nutrition course or equivalent and the state of North Carolina requires an additional nutrition course. Coaches believed they should provide nutrition information to athletes, while trainers believed the responsibility should be shared between coaches and trainers. Nutrition information was obtained from professional publications, meetings, workshops, and textbooks. The professionals most frequently consulted for nutrition information were physicians. However, trainers usually consulted with other trainers, while coaches asked other coaches or trainers for advice.

High school football, basketball, and track coaches in Texas were surveyed to determine their nutrition knowledge.[11] Only 11% had taken a separate college course in nutrition, but 86% provided athletes with nutrition information on a monthly basis. A majority (73%) indicated that their preparation for advising athletes was sufficient, but almost all of them stated that a nutrition course or workshop would be beneficial. Coaches indicated that their source of nutrition information came mainly from professional journals and popular magazines. They believed that a coach is responsible for nutrition as it relates to athletic performance.

Zuniga et al.[12] assessed nutrition knowledge, attitude, and weight loss behavior among 33 high school wrestlers from 2 high schools. Significant differences existed between the two teams in the use of dieting, binge-eating, fluid restriction, spitting, weight loss to meet weight classification, and weight loss per week before a match. Greater differences in nutrient intake occurred during the season vs. after the season in wrestlers from a school where improper weight loss techniques were encouraged. The study suggests that coaches can strongly influence eating behaviors of their athletes.

Sossin et al.[13] examined beliefs and attitudes of 311 New York state high school wrestling coaches and their use of nutrition resources. Most coaches (82%) considered themselves very knowledgeable about wrestling but less informed about sports nutrition, weight loss, and vitamin supplements. Only 36% of coaches attended a nutrition workshop. More experienced coaches attended nutrition workshops and felt more informed about weight loss and sports nutrition. Mean scores for correct responses to questions about weight loss were 64%, training diets 59%, dehydration 57%, body composition 52%, eating disorders 80%, and mean scores for positive attitudes about weight loss were 69%, training diets 34%, dehydration 29%, body composition 70%, and eating disorders 69%. Most coaches believed that rapid weight loss had an effect on endurance, strength, performance, and health. About 91% of coaches believed wrestlers should not limit their intake of bread, rice, and potatoes as opposed to fats. Most coaches (93%) believed correctly that flushing, cramps, headaches, rapid pulse, weakness, and fainting are signs of dehydration. Many coaches (67%) believed wrestlers used their weight loss advice. Binge-eating is a concern among coaches (75%) while 95% believe it is unacceptable for wrestlers to use this practice during the season.

Weissinger et al.[14] explored knowledge, attitudes, and practices of high school wrestling coaches relative to weight loss in their wrestlers. Coaches did not recommend methods if they were perceived as dangerous, even if the methods were also perceived as effective for weight loss. Coaches viewed most weight loss methods as detrimental to wrestling performance and had a realistic sense of inherent danger associated with some methods. Despite these findings, a majority of coaches reported that wrestlers, not coaches or parents, should be allowed to make final decisions about wrestling weight. This belief is a concern since research has shown that wrestlers are poor judges of their minimal wrestling weight.[15] Coaches appear to have a strong influence on the weight management practices of wrestlers. Wrestlers rate coaches as the most important source of weight control information.[16]

Many recommendations can be made based on the results of these studies. There is a need for local training programs on specific topics and interests for school administrators, coaches, parents, nutritionists, physicians, and nurses. Newsletters, manuals, and handbooks tailored to the needs of coaches can be disseminated. For example, guidelines for coaches regarding information about appropriate percent body fat and weight loss are available through the Wisconsin Wrestling Minimum Weight (WWMW) Project.[17] The WWMW Project provides a model for other states to emulate.

B. NUTRITION KNOWLEDGE OF ATHLETES

What do athletes know about general or sports nutrition, and from what source is this information obtained? It is difficult to sort out sources when the public is being bombarded by the media and athletes are surrounded by older players with their ideas of nutrition "facts." Some studies have been reported which attempt to discover nutrition knowledge of athletes. More studies are needed to describe methods of providing correct information and encouraging athletes to change their diets for enhanced health and performance.

1. College Athletes

A study of nutrition knowledge and food practices of 115 college athletes compared to 55 nonathletes found that nonathletes and females had significantly higher nutrition knowledge scores and lower nutrient intakes (from a 24-h recall) than athletes and male subjects.[18] Nutrition knowledge was not related to better dietary intakes.

Most of the 171 college athletes questioned about their nutritional beliefs, indicated that a high-protein diet would improve athletic performance and increase muscle mass.[19] More than 75% felt that athletes need a larger quantity of vitamins as compared to nonathletes and that natural vitamin supplements are better than synthetic supplements. Half of the athletes thought water was the best fluid for athletes, but only 13% strongly agreed athletes need more water than thirst dictates. Almost half thought athletes should use salt tablets in hot weather.[20]

One study examined bone densities of 13 female college track team members, 14 college dancers, 14 nonathletic college women, and 18 postmenopausal women.[21] Scores from a nutrition knowledge and attitude test administered to participants were not significantly correlated with one another. All of the nonathletic group had taken a college nutrition course and earned higher scores on the nutrition test. The knowledge scores of the dancers were the lowest. Nutrition knowledge was positively correlated with age and milk drinking and negatively correlated with the use of carbonated beverages. Sources of nutrition education for dancers were parents and friends and then media. Track team members gained nutrition information from media, followed by parents and friends. Only one dancer and two track team members had consulted a registered dietitian.

A study of 75 male members of college track, baseball, and football teams questioned athletes about their nutrition knowledge sources and found that less than half could define glycogen loading, list good food sources of carbohydrates, recommend a healthy pre-game meal, or knew major functions of vitamins.[22] More than half, however, were aware of fluid intake for athletes, food sources of fat, functions of carbohydrates, and how muscle mass is increased. The major sources of nutrition information for these men were parents first, followed by high school physical education/health courses. Only about 10% of athletes on all three teams cited nutritionists/dietitians as sources of their nutrition information, yet most believed nutrition can influence performance. Few thought they had current nutrition information, but up to 70% of team members believed they had adequate knowledge.

Division I football and basketball players at the University of Southern Mississippi were given a nutrition test resulting in a mean score of 57%.[23] The conclusion from the test and dietary assessment was that these athletes should be provided with information about increasing complex carbohydrates in the diet and decreasing simple sugar, total fat, and saturated fat.

Self- and group-instruction for teaching sports nutrition to college athletes was developed to assess athletes' basic diet, pre-game meal, fluids, and ergogenic aids.[24] The mean gain in post-test scores was 23 for self-instruction and 17 for group-instruction, possibly due to the self-instruction group receiving review questions while the other group had no review. This is certainly a step in the right direction, since athletes knew only about half the information before they started.

The U.S. Military Academy at West Point provided 1040 cadets with two 2-h lessons on sports nutrition, which included worksheets on energy expenditure and fluid replacement during exercise.[25] Students also receive 3-h nutrition education, but it was not stated if this was 3 credit hours or 3 clock hours of study.

Since the relationship between nutrition and sports has become of increasing interest in college athletics, a study at Florida International University found that nutrition education during six weekly small group lectures improved nutrition knowledge for female athletes, but little difference was noted for male athletes.[26]

A family health history, as well as physical and blood measurements, were taken for 49 male athletes at the University of Nevada-Reno.[27] A nutrition knowledge exam on dietary sodium and fat found 43% of the sample scored below 70%.

A study of nutrition knowledge of 70 female varsity athletes and 129 university students found test scores averaging 34% for both groups.[28] Sources of nutrition information for both groups came mainly from magazines, books, and teammates or friends. The most useful sources were listed as magazines or books, followed by school courses. Coaches were listed at the bottom of the most useful list but were listed as a source by 30% of varsity athletes.

McReynolds et al.[29] conducted a nutrition education program consisting of information about the four food groups/food guide pyramid, weight control, precompetition meals, and eating disorders for 60 women's softball and men's and women's track athletes at Texas A & M University. Based on pre- and post-assessments, athletes realized they were not eating as well as they could be, and knowledge about a healthy fat intake improved the most. Athletes believed their top five dietary changes should be: decreasing fat intake, eating less fast food, increasing fruit and vegetable intake, eating fewer snacks, and decreasing total calories.

Investigators looking at the nutrition knowledge of two college wrestling teams concluded that "the wrestlers lacked a good understanding of basic nutrition and were prone to common food fallacies."[30] It was found that 32% of wrestlers avoided breads, pasta, and potatoes and preferred high-protein foods. They believed that protein was non-fattening. Only 8% of these men thought fluids were essential for training or performance.

Keller-Grubbs et al.[31] assessed changes in nutrition knowledge and dietary intake among university female cross-country runners before and after a nutrition education program. A small group format was used to communicate the following topics through presentations, handouts, and group discussions: carbohydrates, fat, protein, five food groups, iron status, fluids and dehydration, amenorrhea, calcium intake and its effect on bone mass, and pathogenic weight control. Nutrition knowledge increased significantly among the experimental group (n = 9) from a mean pre-test score of 11.22 to 15.44 post-test compared to controls. No significant change occurred for 21 nutrients except thiamin, dietary fiber, and saturated fat.

Nutrition knowledge, attitudes, and dietary practices of female college athletes (dancers and track team) and nonathletic college women along with postmenopausal women were measured.[32] The nonathletic group earned a higher score on a knowledge test than did dancers or track team members, and their score was slightly higher than the postmenopausal women. All four groups showed no significant difference in attitude scores. Nonathletes took a college nutrition course. The source of nutrition information reported the most frequently by the track team was the media. Dancers relied on parents, nonathletes learned most from their college nutrition course, while postmenopausal women most frequently listed friends, physicians, and media as nutrition information sources.

Clark[33] suggests that athletic departments at college and university levels are beginning to recognize the importance of sports nutritionists in providing nutrition counseling to athletes and nutrition education to teams, coaches, and trainers. Sports nutritionists can relieve coaches and trainers of having to address issues of weight management, nutrition supplementation, eating disorders, and body composition. The establishment of sports nutrition positions at major universities is increasing.

2. High School Athletes

Although millions of adolescents take part in school sports in the United States, less than 45% of 179 secondary schools surveyed in one state had health intervention nutrition programs for athletes.[34] More than 60% of respondents (health teachers, nurses, and coaches) stated coaches were qualified to supervise intervention programs, although no nutritional qualifications were presented.

Adolescents may know more about nutrition than they apply to their own diets. While investigating conceptual relationships between training and eating in high school distance runners, it was concluded that nutrition knowledge was poor (52% on test scores) and that educators should make nutrition messages more meaningful to individual adolescents.[35]

Competitive adolescent female gymnasts (age 11 to 17) practicing at least 9-h /week did poorly on nutrition questions about fuel for energy and food sources of carbohydrate.[36] Half of the girls could not describe complex carbohydrates, and they knew little about the role of carbohydrates as a fuel during exercise.

National male and female elite adolescent swimmers who train between 10,000 and 16,000 m a day at 85–90% of VO_2max were given a nutrition test.[37] Swimmers performed well on basic knowledge, but poorly on choosing foods high in specific nutrients such as carbohydrates or proteins. If they were unable to answer questions on food sources, it seems improbable that they would be able to choose an appropriate diet.

Less than half of 31 female volleyball team members age 13 to 17 correctly answered general nutrition or sports nutrition questions.[38] These volleyball players knew little about dietary protein, carbohydrate loading, sodium levels, or energy needed during exercise. Subjects were knowledgeable about reducing diets, vitamin supplements, plant oils vs. animal fats, and the value of eating a variety of foods. Less than one third believed that nutrition was a coach's responsibility, but they did not state who should have that responsibility. Scores on nutrition knowledge and attitude tests did not correlate with dietary intakes, indicating other forces shaped their dietary habits. These forces might include a desire to be thin or easily accessible high-caloric foods.

Nutrition knowledge and weight control practices of 317 high school wrestlers and 81 national Junior Olympic boxing competitors were compared.[39] These adolescent athletes had similar nutrition knowledge and agreed fasting was dangerous and weight should be lost by proper dieting and exercise. However more than 90% of both groups were losing weight and many were using techniques such as saunas, rubber suits, and vomiting. Both groups considered their coaches to be the most important source of nutrition information about weight control, with their fellow team members rated second.

Marquart and Sobal[16] examined weight loss beliefs and practices among 197 high school wrestlers. Personal desire to win, coaches, and teammates were reported to have the greatest influence on weight-loss efforts. The percentage of wrestlers who thought the following were "very accurate" sources of weight loss advice was: coaches (60%), doctors (59%), teammates (20%), teachers (9%), and TV/radio (5%). This suggests physicians could become more involved in educating coaches and athletes about safe weight management. Unfortunately, 42% of wrestlers indicated nobody helped plan their weight-loss program. A majority of wrestlers (88%) were receptive to receiving nutrition information. Only 9% of wrestlers indicated that they used commercial diets to make weight. About 93% of wrestlers endorsed exercise as the best way to lose weight.

Wisconsin was the first state to have mandatory body composition testing for wrestlers in high schools.[40] Dietitians dispensed sports nutrition education in 158 high schools in 1990, providing hope that sports nutrition education is viewed as important.

A test of nutritional knowledge and food practices of 943 male and female high school athletes showed a mean score of 55% on nutrition questions.[41] Of the 18 different sports teams in this study, members of the cross-country team and track-and-field participants scored higher on nutrition knowledge than the high school athletes in other sports. Athletes who participated in their sport for a longer period of time had higher nutrition knowledge scores. When asked to rate their sources of nutrition information besides school, most ranked parents first, then popular books and magazines. Only 10% ranked medical personnel first. At school, science courses and home economics classes were ranked first as sources of nutrition information by 50% of students. Only 15% of students ranked coaches as a major source of information about sports nutrition.

A survey of nutrition knowledge of 101 competitive swimmers (age 13 to 20) in the areas of general and sports nutrition found a low level of nutrition knowledge.[42] The majority believed a well- balanced meal was necessary at all times, a balanced diet without supplements was adequate for top performance, eating steak did not provide extra strength before competition, and not everyone should take iron supplements (41%). Almost half, however, stated everyone should take supplements, extra energy is derived from vitamin B supplements, vitamin E supplements improve performance, drinking milk the day of the event decreased performance, and protein supplements improved performance.

Massad et al.[43] assessed knowledge and factors that influence nutrition supplement use among 509 high school athletes. Mean knowledge scores were higher for females. One-third of subjects believed protein drinks offered nutritional advantages over protein found in food. Contrary to scientific evidence, about 50% of athletes believed arginine increased human growth hormone production. About one-third of athletes believed B-vitamins were a source of energy while one-half did not know that vitamins A and D could be harmful. About one-third of athletes believed that athletes could not get enough iron or calcium from diet alone. Approximately one-half of subjects believed animal glandular material (bull testicles) provide significant amounts of testosterone, and nutritional supplements sold at health food stores are scientifically tested and safe for use. Greater nutrition knowledge about supplements was associated with less use.

Marquart and Sobal[44] examined the beliefs and sources of information regarding muscle development among 742 high school athletes. A majority (73%) believed protein supplements were important in muscle development, and many believed carbohydrates (71%) and vitamin supplements (61%) were important. Most athletes (84%) believed that good nutrition could prevent disease later in life. More than 40% believed that steroids were more important than nutrition for muscle development. These athletes believed that the following sources provide accurate information: doctors (86%), coaches (76%), trainers (68%), parents (38%), teachers (33%), and other athletes (33%).

When 416 high school football players were asked: where do you get information or advice about nutritional supplements, 25% reported from friends, 23% from coaches, 17% from magazines, 16% from television, 15% from doctors, 14% from parents, and 14% from trainers.[45] About 25% of athletes reported eating greater amounts of food to improve muscle size and strength.

Hornick et al.[46] evaluated the effects of a 2-month nutrition education program on sports nutrition knowledge and ergogenic aid usage among 68 male and female adolescents, 15–18 years of age, enrolled in a physical education class. No significant changes occurred in nutrition education. There was a significant decrease in use of vitamin/minerals, muscle building products, protein and amino acid supplements, and salt tablets after the sports nutrition education program. Family (35%) was the most frequently reported source of nutrition information followed by coach/teacher (24%) and friends (14%). The author concluded that there is a need for more sports nutrition education strategies involving parents, teachers, and coaches.

3. Recreational Athletes

To determine if exercising adult members of a university wellness center have greater nutrition knowledge and better eating habits, 240 subjects were interviewed by a mail survey.[47] It was found that exercisers were significantly better informed and had better eating patterns than nonexercisers.

The majority of 104 female marathon runners and 105 fitness club members obtained their nutrition information from magazines and books.[48] Runners found books most useful, while fitness women found books and their fitness class most useful. The mean for general nutrition knowledge and sports nutrition tests was slightly higher for runners than for the fitness class. Dietetic interns completing the same test scored well on general nutrition knowledge, but low on sports nutrition. These findings suggest dietetic programs need to include more information on sports nutrition in course work.

A nutrition knowledge survey of 120 males and females who participated in either private or commercial, corporate, community, or a cardiac rehabilitation facility found higher scores on health and fitness than on nutrient functions.[49] Those exercising for 20–45 min had higher mean scores than those exercising for only 20 min.

Learning nutrition information from their families may not be the best source for accuracy. Investigating more than 2300 members of the public, health-care workers, university graduate students, and health club attendees, it was found that 90% did not know recommendations for calcium, salt, vitamin A, and fiber.[50] The majority of subjects with college degrees or higher were ignorant of nutrition information needed to use the dietary guidelines.

As part of a study to investigate dietary patterns and gastrointestinal complaints of recreational triathletes, researchers administered a nutrition knowledge test.[51] There was no significant difference in scores between triathletes (21 women and 50 men) and controls, but female athletes scored higher on the test than male athletes. Their nutrition information was mostly derived from newspapers and sports magazines. However, many athletes were misinformed since they believed that spinach is a good source of iron and peanut butter is high in cholesterol. Many athletes used nutritional supplements and had atypical eating patterns.

A survey of 100 adult male and female runners indicated that 68% believed 8 glasses of water or more per day were recommended; however, only 28% reported actually drinking more than 8 glasses.[52] A statistically significant correlation was found between the daily amount of water believed to be recommended by sports nutritionists and the daily amount consumed by recreational runners. This study is consistent with other research on runners suggesting that runners across all age groups scored higher on sports-related knowledge tests than participants in other sports.

Walsh studied the health beliefs and practices of 77 runners and 66 nonrunners using a mailed questionnaire, one section of which covered nutrition.[53] Results of the nutrition test were not presented, but it was stated that because of the runners' emphasis on leanness and strict weight control, "nutrition counseling often is indicated."

4. Child Athletes

Young athletes in community sports programs are often entrusted to inexperienced and untrained coaches.[54] Several organizations in the United States and Canada are attempting to remedy this situation. Nutrition information is included in some of the guides published by such organizations as Little League.[55] However, too many supervisors of young athletic teams leave the children to pick up sports nutrition information from their families or the media. Others have found that nutrition education in an extra-curricular setting over a two month period was an effective method of providing nutrition information to Little League cheerleaders.[56]

Sossin et al.[57] developed a nutrition program for parents, coaches, and 400 children 7–10 years of age participating in a youth soccer league. The objectives were to increase awareness and knowledge about sports nutrition in parents, coaches, and children and to encourage families to use easy-to-prepare recipes on game and practice days. A series of nutrition booklets and refrigerator fact sheets were effective in increasing awareness and knowledge about sports nutrition and encouraged positive dietary practices by some parents and children.

Additional emphasis needs to be placed on nutrition education of child and adolescent athletes. The American Dietetic Association (ADA) has recently released statements regarding nutrition guidance for these athletes.[58,59] Also, ADA has sponsored a book entitled *Play Hard Eat Right* to help parents, coaches, and health professionals promote healthy diets among children involved in sports.[60] The American Academy of Pediatrics Committee on Sports Medicine and Fitness released a statement on "Promotion of healthy weight control practices in young athletes."[61]

C. CONCLUSIONS

Over the past 10–15 years, knowledge of the relationship between nutrition and sports has grown dramatically. Great strides have been made as to the ergogenic effects and health benefits of certain dietary practices. Despite this knowledge, efforts to effectively and systematically promote positive dietary practices among the majority of athletes, for both performance and health reasons, has lagged behind.

Although nutritionists have developed numerous educational resources for athletes, coaches, parents, and administrators, there is no specific model or framework upon which to base decisions when developing and implementing nutrition education programs. In addition, little research has been conducted to explore the psycho-socio-cultural aspects of nutrition and sports. There is a lack of understanding about influences that affect the athlete from inside and outside the sporting world as it relates to food.

To further explore the relationship between nutrition and sport, a practical model needs to be developed to provide a framework for: understanding influences that affect athletes' food choices; educating coaches and athletes about healthful nutrition and dietary practices; implementing group nutrition education programs and individual counseling for athletes; and questioning our understanding of what influences athletes' knowledge and food selection.

III. DIETARY SURVEYS AND STANDARDS

A. OVERVIEW OF SURVEYS

Reports of survey methods for populations and for individuals are numerous. Methods of nutritional assessment, including body composition and assessment of specific nutrients, are covered extensively by Gibson.[62] The usefulness of dietary surveys depends on certain areas: (a) method of collecting dietary intake data of athletes, (b) nutrient comparison standard, (c) data base of nutrients and food composition, and (d) how to provide athletes with feedback from dietary assessments.

1. Methods of Quantifying Dietary Intake

A 50-year history of methods used to collect individual dietary intake data has been reviewed[63] and so have guidelines for the use of dietary intake data.[64] Individual food intake information may be obtained from a variety of methods including a 24-h recall, records of various lengths (commonly 1 d, 3 d, or 7 d), diet history, food frequency list, weighed food intake, electronic monitoring, or a combination of methods. There are advantages and disadvantages to the use of any of these methods.

Regardless of the method used, the number of days the diet is monitored is important since usual intake varies for an individual.[65] Food habits change over a lifetime, food intake changes from season to season, some foods are eaten everyday while others are eaten rarely. Diets should be assessed for both weekends and weekdays since there are significant differences in the number of meals and snacks eaten and type of food/nutrient intake when collecting intake data. For accurate results, intake for different nutrients needs to be monitored for different lengths of time;[66] however, the exact length of time necessary for a dietary survey is unknown. Another difficult aspect of collecting dietary information is estimating food portion sizes. Using food models or household measures increased the accuracy of estimating the amount of food eaten.[67]

2. Weighed Intake of Food

A weighed food intake report is costly, time consuming, and it can be difficult to achieve desired accuracy. This method may interfere with a subject's typical eating patterns.

The method of duplicate food collection, collecting duplicate amounts of all food and beverages consumed for analysis, may not represent habitual levels of intake at other times throughout the year.[68] A computer program technique for quantifying individual dietary intake enables individuals to self-weigh and identify all foods ingested to ensure complete food records may be valuable.[69]

3. 24-Hour Recall of Daily Food Intake

A 24-h recall of food intake requires an accurate memory and may not truly represent foods and portions consumed during one day. The subject may change the intake information in an effort to please the interviewer. An advantage of this method is that the interviewer may ask for more details about the intake and its logistical simplicity.[70] Increasing to three recalls at 6-week intervals improves the reliability of the estimate for all nutrients.

According to Woteki, a report[71] from the National Center for Health Statistics stated that the 24-h recall method provides accurate and reproducible estimates of the mean intakes of population groups, but multiple days' information is necessary for characterizing an individual's usual nutrient intake. Others agree that the validity of the 24-h dietary recall is unsatisfactory on the individual level.[72] Some call one-day data meaningless[73] and valueless for individual dietary intakes.[74]

4. Written Diet Record

Diet records require subject cooperation. Validity decreases with the length of time the record is kept and may depend on the time of the week or season.[75] Some researchers state that there is a greater stability of mean nutrient intakes from 3-d than from 1-d dietary records,[76] while others prefer a 4-d record (Friday through Monday) since weekend intakes are the most variable for individuals.[77]

A 7-d dietary record was deemed sufficiently precise to describe dietary intake and show relationships of intake to serum nutritional indicators.[78] Underreporting of food consumption data can be a potential problem according to Mertz et al.[79]

Records based on detailed food descriptions with portion sizes estimated using household measures and standardized photographs were almost as reliable as weighed records and were more convenient, which may increase compliance.[80]

Nutrient intake is more variable in children (age 5 to 14) than in adults.[81] The minimum number of days of food records needed to estimate energy intake was 7 d for boys and 8 d for girls with more than 20 d required for an estimate of vitamin intake. Validation of mother's reports of dietary intake by four- to seven-year-old children was reported to be useful for classifying children by intake of calories, macronutrients, and micronutrients but is a less accurate measure of actual food eaten, portion sizes, and nutrient levels consumed.[82]

5. Dietary History

A dietary history is an interview that may take an hour or longer by a trained dietitian and may include a 24-h recall, a 3-d record, and a questionnaire. The interviewer collects information about the subject's eating habits and patterns, food likes and dislikes, frequency and size of intake portions, and other diet and health-related questions.[83] This method takes time and expertise but allows for follow-up questions to be asked.

6. Food Frequency Questionnaires

Food frequency questionnaires provide information about the quality of the diet but require a good memory since the subject is required to remember both frequency and amount of various food categories eaten over a period of time. Dietary changes during the time between questionnaires contributes to poor reproducibility and validity.[84]

Questionnaires are useful in categorizing individuals and groups by food intake characteristics.[71] Food frequency questionnaire validity is limited by the adequacy of the food list and the ability of respondents to report usual intake patterns. It can only place individuals into broad categories.[85]

A food behavior checklist consisting of yes/no questions about food consumed in the previous 24 h is a simple dietary assessment tool to evaluate intervention programs or to monitor dietary change.[86] Questionnaires are inexpensive, valid, and reliable tools for rapid assessment of eating habits and diet composition.[87]

An advantage is that questionnaires can be adapted for computer use. A data collection and nutrient analysis computer program may permit modification of questionnaires[88] and can check for unusual or omitted answers.

A problem with using a food frequency questionnaire is the need to know portion size consumed. The use of a standard portion size can reduce interview time. However, results of a comparison using reported and standard portion sizes indicated that this leads to different results.[89] People do not always eat standard portions.

7. Other Methods of Quantifying Dietary Intake

The selection of an appropriate dietary method depends on the level of measurement required. The dietary assessment method should be validated to ensure it is measuring what it claims to measure.[90] Intake assessment should be viewed only as an estimate of habitual intake and interpretations based on such data should be made with caution. In long-term studies, continuous monitoring is needed since current intake may not be a good estimator of past intake for most nutrients.[91]

Direct observation of children's consumption of bag lunches brought from home and eaten in school was reported to be a reliable method for assessing energy and nutrient intake of children.[92] One observer could only watch two children and required many hours of training.

One study reported use of an *ad libitum* automated food-selection system with two vending machines containing a large variety of foods to measure intake in volunteers on a metabolic ward.[93] This automated system allowed entrees, snacks, and beverages to be freely accessible to the subjects with continuous monitoring by the computer.

A photographic procedure for measurement of individual food consumption could predict the actual weight of a food item better than a recall.[94] Analysis of daily nutrient intakes estimated from photographs via computer program compared well with those obtained from a weighed record.[95] Computer graphics were used to simulate actual food size on the screen to increase the accuracy of serving size estimates.[96]

8. Survey Concerns and Limitations

A review of dietary assessment techniques by Bingham makes many important points.[97] Asking people to estimate the weight of food as opposed to actually weighing the food may produce a variation of about 50% for foods and 20% for nutrients. Differences in nutrient intake from a 24-h recall compared with direct observation may range from 4 to 400%. Sources of error include food tables used, coding errors, incorrect food weights, reporting errors, variation with time, incorrect consumption frequency, change in diet, response bias, and sampling bias. All results from dietary surveys are dependent on the quality of the food tables unless food is analyzed in the laboratory. Errors in estimating portion weights of food can reach 90%.

The 24-h recall is prone to reporting error, and overall average energy intake may be underestimated by 21%. When subjects are asked to keep a record of everything they eat, there is a risk they will change their normal dietary habits. "Categorically, a single 24-h record or recall should never be used to assess dietary status or to test associations between diet and some other variable such as blood cholesterol or serum lipids."[97] If energy and energy-yielding nutrients are to be investigated, a 7-d record would be sufficient if an accuracy of plus or minus 10% standard error is acceptable. Vitamins, minerals, and fiber require longer periods of observation, at least 14 d, which does not have to be obtained over a single period of time. This could be 4-d periods of records over several months.

Pennington states that using food records, weighed intakes, and duplicate portions to assess dietary status distorts the usual eating patterns.[98] The concern with diet histories, food frequencies, and 24-h recalls is the ability to remember food and quantities consumed.

Food intake survey reports in the literature should include: information about the type of intake record used, instructions to athletes for collecting information, forms for athletes to complete, and methods of measuring (or estimating) intake using food models, especially for foods that vary greatly by portion size.

B. STANDARDS USED FOR COMPARISONS
1. Recommended Dietary Allowances

After accumulating the results of a dietary analysis, a decision must be made about the standard to be used for a comparison. Comparing individual intake to the Recommended Dietary Allowance is open to criticism.

"The Recommended Dietary Allowances (RDAs) are the levels of intake of essential nutrients that, on the basis of scientific knowledge, are judged by the Food and Nutrition Board to be adequate to meet the known nutrient needs of practically all healthy persons."[99] In the past these RDAs were presumed to be acceptable for group applications. However the present RDA states that "a comparison of individual intakes, averaged over a sufficient length of time, to the RDA allows an estimate to be made about the probable risk of deficiency for that individual."[99]

RDA recommendations are for "reference" people and may require adjustments for athletes with increased physical activity, varying body size, increased sweat losses of salt, and other essential nutrients. Athletes' heights and weights may vary substantially from reference people upon which the RDAs are calculated.

Intake of nutrients, such as protein, are based on body weight.[100] Various sports medicine scientists have suggested that athletes need from 1 to 3 g of protein per kg body weight per day.[101] The RDA for protein is 0.8 g protein per kg body weight per day.[99] Calculations for protein requirements should be presented in diet analysis results to enable those trained to judge if RDA protein intake is adequate for certain athletes. Inadequate protein intake can occur when recommendations for protein consumption are the same for individuals with different amounts of body fat and lean muscle tissue. Perhaps nutrients calculated on a body weight basis should be calculated according to lean body mass or estimated lean body mass of reference persons of normal body weight.

2.   Nutrient Intakes Considered Low

A cut-off point for low or poor intake of a nutrient is usually indicated in nutritional surveys. Except for calories, the RDA has set two standard deviations above the mean to cover the needs of almost all individuals within the group. The RDA for caloric intake was set at the mean population requirement for each age group. "Since a wide margin of safety is incorporated in the Recommended Dietary Allowances, the average intake of a group does not have to equal the recommended allowance."[99] Using the value of a mean intake below 70% of the RDA, problem nutrients were identified in the Nationwide Food Consumption Survey of 1977–78.[102] Other nutritional studies have classified nutrient intakes below two-thirds of the RDA as low.[103]

3.   Data Bases and Dietary Analysis

When selecting nutrient-calculation software packages, the quality of the nutrient data base is important.[104] Data base concerns include: completeness of foods and nutrients of interest to researchers, specificity in order to accurately assess nutrients, current information on nutrients and foods including reformulations of existing products, and quality control procedures to ensure accuracy. If the described food is not in the data base, a loss of dietary information results. If a specific food were not found, substitutions made could cause errors resulting in inaccurate diagnostic information and guidance.[105]

The U.S. Department of Agriculture (USDA) Nutrient Data Base contains data for energy and 28 components for more than 5000 food items.[106] Data are based on the latest information from Handbook No. 8. However, "there are substantial gaps in the tables of food composition."[71] And only a small amount of information may be available for some nutrients.

It has been suggested that dietary survey reports publish the following information: the type of computer and computer program used and data base and method of indicating incomplete data in the foods and nutrient information. After considering these points, an expert is needed to translate the computer output into dietary advice. One problem with computer dietary analysis is the hazard of "having an unqualified individual interpret the data."[107]

IV.   SURVEYS OF ATHLETES' DIETARY INTAKES

Evaluating sports nutrition research is difficult because of the variety of sports and individual variation in athletes competing in those sports. Attempts to use survey data for comparison of athletes' intake must consider the sport, specific event, times (minutes, hours, or days to complete the event), climate, number of subjects surveyed, age, experience in the sport, supplements, and freedom of food choices. It is even difficult to compare the nutrient intake of members of the same team, especially if they play different positions. Sweeping statements about "all athletes" add little to sports nutrition research. "Dietary surveys of athletes are useful not to set standards of nutrition but rather to discover deficiencies and thus to know what dietary corrections are needed."[108]

A. SURVEYS OF TEAMS

Grandjean studied the macronutrient intake of 237 Division I athletes, those participating in the U.S. Olympic Committee-sponsored competitions and professional athletes which were compared with a sample of the U.S. general population from a large government nationwide survey.[109] These 237 athletes were competing in a variety of sports: wrestling, figure skating, distance running, judo, weightlifting, football, swimming, basketball, cycling, and baseball. Of the male athletes, baseball players had the highest mean caloric intake and wrestlers the lowest. Of three female teams surveyed, figure skaters were lowest in caloric intake while cyclists were the highest. Wrestlers consumed the highest percentage of calories from carbohydrates (54%) and the lowest protein (12%). Figure skaters consumed the lowest percentage of calories from fat (34%). Baseball players and weight lifters had the highest percentage of calories from protein (18%), and basketball players had the highest percentage of calories from fat (41%). Grandjean points out that it is very difficult to calculate amounts of macronutrients needed for sports. She states that "either the majority of athletes are consuming less than desirable diets, the recommendations are not on target, or the recommendations are too unspecific."

Short and Short[110] collected data for 4 years on 554 athletes involved with 10 men's and 6 women's athletic teams at Syracuse University. At various times during this period, 3-d records, (14-d records for wrestlers), 24-h records, and weighed intakes were used to analyze men's basketball, body builders, crew, football, gymnastics, lacrosse, mountain climbers, soccer, track and field, and wrestling teams as well as women's basketball, crew, dancing, lacrosse, swimming, and volleyball teams. Diet records were kept by the football teams every semester, six different semesters by the wrestling teams, and less frequently by members of other teams. The diets including snacks were analyzed using a computer data base of 6076 foods and 37 nutrients. The mean caloric intake for fall football team members was 5270 with a maximum intake of 14,000 kcal (58,520 J) per day. On the other hand, the minimum for wrestling and gymnastic teams was very low (400 kcal [1672 J]). Wrestlers cutting weight may eat no food the day before a match. During a season, this practice may lead to nutritional deficits. All athletes, with the exception of wrestlers and gymnasts with minimum caloric intakes, received enough protein when intake was calculated on a per kg body weight basis, compared to the RDA, or on a per 1,000 kcal (4180 J) basis. More than one-third of the teams surveyed had at least 20% of its members with low intakes of vitamin A. Athletes frequently had diets low in potassium. Wrestlers' diets were poor in calories, thiamin, riboflavin, vitamin A, niacin, and fiber. Women's teams were low in iron intake. A high proportion of calories in the football players diets came from fat (ranging from 38 to 61%) often necessary to amass more than 10,000 kcal (41,800 J) which would be difficult on a low-fat diet. Cholesterol intake of football teams was from 800 to 1,200 mg cholesterol with a maximum of more than 3400 mg per day. More than half of the men ate over three times the RDA for protein. Excluding the wrestling team, half of the men and more than one-fourth of the women were eating over three times the RDA for vitamin C. For all teams surveyed, mean percent of calories from fat was about 36% over four years. Snacks or additional meals for some teams provided a large amount of calories. The ADA recommends that the "distribution of nutrients composing the athlete's diet should be about 15% protein, less than 30% fat, and 60% to 65% carbohydrate."[111]

Burke et al.[112] reported on the dietary intake of Australian male triathletes, marathon runners, football players, and weightlifters in four separate articles. Authors examined the food-use patterns of the four groups. Endurance athletes had a higher carbohydrate intake from breads, cereals, and starchy vegetables. The weightlifters consumed more protein from meat, eggs, and dairy products. Football players and weightlifters amassed a higher percentage of fat calories from fats and oils. Endurance athletes were most conscious of the importance of nutrition to their sport. Triathletes modified their eating habits to meet their specialized needs but in so doing became unnecessarily restrictive and focused on single nutrients. Football players were uninterested in nutrition and did not believe it affected their performance except in a specific case, such as the pregame meal.

Midway through their competitive season and 2 weeks post-season, diet records of 24 college females from diverse sports such as field hockey (9), golf (5), cross-country (6), and tennis (4) were grouped together to compare to records of 24 nonathletes.[113] Dietary intake changed very little across this time span. The athletes' diet was very similar to that of the nonathletes. All were low in calories, iron, and calcium. It was suggested that the female athletes' wish to be thinner may influence their eating habits more than their exercise regimen.

Welch studied 39 female athletes (age 17 to 22) participating on intercollegiate teams including basketball, cross-country running, field hockey, golf, softball, swimming, tennis, track and field, and volleyball.[114] Women were divided into two groups. One group of 10 women had nutritional problems (such as weight, anemia, spastic colon), and the others served as a control. The first group was given two to five counseling sessions. Each athlete kept a 7-d diet record, and interviewers obtained a 24-h diet recall from each athlete before and after the season. The counseled group improved their protein and vitamin A intake but not their iron. Calcium intake was only slightly improved. The average caloric intake of both groups was between 1700 and 1800 kcal (7106 and 7524 J). The counseled group increased calories from protein and carbohydrate. Also, the counseled group decreased fat calories significantly by increasing foods from the bread/cereal and dairy groups while decreasing foods high in fats, oils, and sweets.

In The Netherlands, 4- or 7-d food diaries were obtained from 418 endurance, strength, and team athletes.[115] Mean energy intake for males ranged from 2868 to 5975 calories (11,988 to 24,976 J) and for females from 1673 to 3107 calories (6993 to 12,987 J). Thirty-five percent of endurance athletes and 52% of strength athletes had energy intakes less than the World Health Organization standard for light activity. Carbohydrate contributed from 40 to 63% of energy. Athletes need an energy intake of at least 3107 kcal (12,987 J) in order to meet the RDA for iron (18 mg). When energy intake of athletes was more than 4063 kcal (16,983 J), thiamin intake was insufficient for the athletes' needs.

A 122-item food frequency questionnaire was used to assess nutrient intake of 427 male athletes who competed on a national or international level.[116] Athletes were grouped according to their energy expenditure (moderate; high) and body weight (light ≤75 kg; heavy >75 kg). Mean energy intake was significantly higher for athletes with high (3260 kcal [13,627 J]/day) vs. moderate (2805 kcal [11,725 J/day]/day) energy expenditure. Calcium and riboflavin intakes were significantly higher for athletes with high-energy expenditure. Calcium and riboflavin intakes were significantly higher for athletes with high-energy expenditure. Athletes tended to have a high mean intake of micronutrients (>150% of RDA). Athletes with high-energy expenditure derived 55–57% calories from carbohydrate and 29–31% from fat. Supplements containing amino acids were regularly consumed by 37–59% of athletes. Supplements were most frequently consumed by heavy, moderate-energy expenditure athletes (mainly weight lifters, body builders, and throwers) and light, high-energy expenditure athletes (mainly endurance athletes).

1. Supplement Use

Sobal and Marquart[117] reviewed the prevalence, patterns, and explanations for vitamin and mineral supplement use among athletes. Based on 51 studies (1969–1994) providing quantitative prevalence data for 10,274 male and female athletes in more than 15 sports, 46% reported supplement use. Elite athletes (59%) used supplements more than college (43%) or high school athletes (47%). Women (57%) used supplements more often than men (47%). The weighted mean prevalence for a variety of sports was weightlifters (100%), speed skaters (71%), body builders (69%), swimmers (59%), dancers (55%), triathletes (48%), football players (43%), runners (42%), cyclists (42%), gymnasts (42%), wrestlers (39%), field athletes (33%), basketball players (33%), and mixed sports (46%). The authors suggest that health professionals should actively counsel athletes about proper usage of vitamin and mineral supplements.

A study investigating factors influencing the use of nutritional supplements by college athletes found no relationship between exercise level and supplement use.[118] All men in the weightlifting group were taking megavitamins (more than 1000% of the USRDA) and/or other unorthodox products. Runners supervised by a coach used fewer supplements than runners who were unsupervised.

While surveying 2977 athletes in high school and college, Parr found that 42% of college athletes and 46% of high school athletes took multivitamin supplements.[5] They also took single vitamin supplements of vitamins A, C, E, or B-complex. Nine-percent of college athletes and 15% of high school athletes took mineral supplements, mostly iron, but some took zinc, multi-mineral, or calcium tablets. Only six percent of college students and 10% of high school players took protein supplements.

As part of a questionnaire sent to 943 high school athletes, Douglas and Douglas asked how often foods in each of the four food groups were consumed.[41] Males had higher scores (indicating better diets) than did females. Athletes in cross-country, football, lacrosse, soccer, swimming, and track and field had higher scores than did athletes in other sports. Field hockey players and gymnasts earned the lowest scores. Replies to questions about vitamin supplementation elicited the information that 36% took vitamin pills; 19% regularly took vitamins while 3% took vitamin supplements only during season. The authors found that the higher food practice scores could not be attributed to increased knowledge but were attributed to the fact that they ate more food and were, therefore, more likely to consume the recommended number of servings in each of the food groups.

The frequency of daily to weekly nutritional supplement use among 509 high school athletes included fluid replacement drinks (43%), multi-vitamins or multi-minerals (42%), vitamin C (25%), protein drinks (22%), carbohydrate loading drinks (21%), calcium (15%), and iron (15%).[43] Less frequently consumed items included: vitamins A and E (13%), amino acids (9%), weight-loss (10%) and weight-gain formulas (7%), selenium (5%), and royal jelly (3%). Males reported greater supplement use compared to females. Supplement use varied by sport category with higher supplement use for participants in contact sports (football, boxing, wrestling) than other groups. The authors concluded that emphasis placed on greater muscle mass may contribute to increased use of protein powders, amino acids, and steroid alternatives. Few harmful side-effects may be attributed to the types of supplements used by tennis players, swimmers, runners, and golfers.

Sobal and Marquart[119] found that 38% of 742 high school athletes used vitamin and mineral supplements. The prevalence of supplement use did not vary by gender or grade in school. Athletes who expected to compete in college sports were more likely to use supplements. A variety of supplements were consumed: vitamin C (25%), multivitamins (19%), iron (11%), calcium (9%), vitamin A (9%), B-vitamins (8%), vitamin E (8%), and vitamin D (5%). Healthy growth was the most important reason for supplement use followed by treating illness and enhancing sports performance. Sixty-two percent of athletes believed supplementation increased athletic performance. Athletes who believed supplements improve performance were more likely to consume them. Fifty-nine percent of wrestlers used supplements while 76% believed they increased performance.

2. Eating Disorders

A study of pathogenic weight-control behavior in 182 university varsity female athletes (age 17 to 23 years) found that about one-third of athletes used at least one pathogenic weight control behavior such as vomiting (14%), use of laxatives (16%), diet pills (25%), diuretics (5%), and food binges (20%).[120] Almost 75% of gymnasts and almost half of distance runners practiced some of these behaviors. The authors concluded that these patterns of eating were mainly an attempt to increase athletic performance not to enhance body image.

Sundgot-Borgen[121] assessed nutrient intake and eating behavior of 92 Norwegian female elite athletes who met criteria for anorexia nervosa, anorexia athletica, and bulimia nervosa. Three-d and 24-h food records indicated that anorexia nervosa and anorexia athletica athletes have diets too low in energy, carbohydrate, calcium, and vitamin D. Anorexia nervosa athletes consumed less than the Nordic Nutrition Recommended Daily Intake for all reported nutrients. The low energy and nutrient inadequacies combined with various purging techniques is a major concern for these athletes.

In another study, 20% of female athletes in activities defined as emphasizing leanness including ballet dancers, bodybuilders/weight trainers, cheerleaders, and gymnasts were pre-occupied with weight concerns or had tendencies toward eating disorders.[122]

B. BASKETBALL PLAYERS

National Basketball Association (NBA) players on an all-star team were compared to those playing professional basketball but not yet named an all-star.[123] A 24-h recall was used to determine dietary intake with only 5 males per group. The superstars were found to eat more carbohydrate and less fat and protein on game days than did the regular NBA players.

Hickson et al.[124] surveyed female intercollegiate basketball and gymnastic teams for dietary intake during their competitive seasons. Basketball players had higher mean energy intakes (1995 kcal [8339 J]) than gymnasts (1827 kcal (7637 J)), but the basketball players were heavier. If energy intake is expressed as kcal per d divided by kg body weight (BW), mean intake is 30 kcal (125 J)/kg BW for basketball and 32 kcal (134 joules)/kg BW for gymnasts. Researchers found no significant difference in nutritional intake between the two teams. Marginal intakes (less than 70% of the RDA) for pyridoxine and magnesium, and intakes below 60% of the RDA for iron and zinc were reported. Only 5% of the 22 subjects consumed more than 70% of the RDA for all nutrients. Hickson et al.[124] concluded that exercise-enhanced energy intake will not necessarily prevent occurrence of marginal nutrient intake as is commonly believed.

In a study of basketball players, caloric intakes of 16 males averaged twice that of 10 female players.[125] All nutrient intakes except vitamins A and D were higher for male than for female players.

C. CYCLISTS

Competitive cycling is a lengthy endurance exercise which demands high energy consumption. A high carbohydrate intake is critical. Food and beverage intake was recorded for 10 d for two elite cyclists traveling 2050 miles over dirt trails and highway.[126] Caloric intake averaged 7195 kcal (30,075 J) with 10% from protein, 26% from fat, and 64% from carbohydrate, of which 44% came from cookies, sugar drinks, and candy. Total fluid intake averaged 14.5 oz (411 g) per h of riding time, of which 54% was water. It was noted that when planning menus for endurance athletes, it is necessary to plan according to the athletes' food preferences.

An example of ultra-endurance cycling is the Race Across America (RAAM) starting from the west coast and finishing on the east coast. This was a nonstop multiple-day race allowing for no rest time. Lindeman studied one 39-year-old male who finished this race in 10 d, 7 h.[127] Averaging dietary intake over time spent cycling, produced 8429 kcal (35,233 J) (78% from carbohydrate, 13% from protein, and 9% from fat). All other nutrient intake was very high. Glucose electrolyte solutions were consumed as well as high-fiber "sports bars." The cyclist had major gastrointestinal complaints which may be attributed to chronic hyperhydration, very high fiber intake (57 g/d), large doses of ascorbic acid (3300 mg/d), a high concentration of the glucose electrolyte drink (23% diluted to 17%), and/or a high protein and amino acid intake from the glucose electrolyte drink.

Slavin and McNamara[128] investigated the nutritional practices of 36 elite women racing cyclists (average age 27) and 76 recreational bicycle riders (average age 32). Only eight racers submitted a 3-d food intake record. More tourists than racing cyclists reported carbohydrate loading, but this was described as just "eating more carbohydrate." About one-third of each group described themselves as moderate vegetarians (avoided red meat). More racers than tourists consumed megadoses of supplements including vitamin C (58% of racers), multivitamins (64%), iron (47%), and B-complex vitamins (56%). About one-third of the tourists took vitamin C supplements. The racers who completed diet records had excellent nutrient intakes. Only 10% of tourists and 8% of racers consulted a dietitian or nutritionist (qualifications not stated). About one-third of racers were amenorrheic, all of whom were also vegetarians. However, some women racers with normal menstrual cycles were also vegetarians. Diet "histories" for racers indicated they ate more than 2000 kcal (8360 J)/d. Iron was the only nutrient that was marginally low. The authors "believe that nutrition educators should familiarize themselves with these issues if they wish to provide nutrition counseling to athletes."

D. DANCERS

Dancers involved in ballet, jazz, and modern dance were mailed a brief (13 foods) food frequency (amount per week) questionnaire.[129] Of the 106 dancers who responded, 89 were female and 17 were male. More than half the dancers consumed two servings of dairy food per day. Mean intake of dancers who drank milk was one cup per day. Among the 77% who reported eating fresh fruit, mean intake was 1.8 pieces per day. Almost the same percentage ate vegetables. When asked about fiber cereals and whole-grain bread, almost half (46%) reported eating less than one serving per day. Most dancers ate some animal protein averaging 3 oz (85g)/d ranging from 0–10 oz (0–284 g)/d. The majority of dancers indicted that they ate more when not dancing. Many dancers (60%) took supplements including multivitamin supplements, vitamin C, calcium, vitamin E, B-complex vitamins, and iron plus other supplements such as potassium, yeast, and protein products. Ballet dancers averaged more than four caffeinated beverages per day, and almost 75% of dancers drank alcoholic beverages, some as much as 20 drinks per week.

Ballet dancers from national ballet companies in the United States (49) and China (17) were surveyed to discover eating problems.[130] Dancers from companies that were highly selective in choosing dancers were more likely to have eating disorders than companies that were moderately selective. Ballet dancers from Utah completed food frequency and injury questionnaires.[131] No significant differences were found among three groups: (1) those with nutrient intakes less than 70% of the RDA who were given vitamin/supplements, (2) those with similar intakes who were given a placebo, and (3) dancers with adequate intakes.

Calabrese et al.[132] studied the nutritional habits and menstrual abnormalities of 34 female classical ballet dancers. Dancers kept a 3-d record of food, drink, and nutritional supplements. Mean caloric intake was 1358 calories ranging from 550 to 2115 calories (2299 to 8841 J). Mean protein intake of these dancers was 99% of the RDA. Their diets were of low nutrient density "being deficient in many water- and fat-soluble vitamins and minerals." Intake of vitamins A, D, pyridoxine, and folic acid were low as was iron, calcium, and phosphorus. Nutritional supplements, typically large doses of one or two nutrients, were taken by 40% of the subjects. Nutritional histories and 1-d recalls were evaluated one year later with similar results. The authors concluded that these subjects knew little about basic nutritional concepts and were involved with a significant number of food fads. Mean percent body fat was found to be 16.9% by hydrostatic weighing. Half of these women age 15 to 31 had menstrual abnormalities.

Brooks-Gunn et al.[133] surveyed 55 dancers performing in national and regional ballet companies in America and Western Europe. One-third of these professionally trained dancers had eating disorders.

Cohen et al.[134] studied nutrition and hematologic assessment of 22 men and women who were American Ballet Theater dancers (mean age 25). All of the men and 10 of the 12 women completed a 6-d food diary. Mean caloric intake was almost 3000 kcal (12,540 J) for men and nearly 1700 kcal (7106 J) for women. Protein intake averaged 122 g for men and 60 g for women. Percent of calories from carbohydrate was 38% for men and 50% for women. Intakes below 25% of the RDA were most frequently noted for pyridoxine, folic acid, biotin, and vitamin D. For females, mean iron intake was low (13.5 mg) as was calcium intake. All deficiencies were calculated to be more severe and more frequent among women than men. Except for four dancers, all took daily multiple megavitamin supplements. The dancers' diets were judged to be monotonous and unbalanced. Factors contributing to low nutrient intakes among these female dancers were low caloric intake, lack of correct nutrition information, avoidance of red meat and milk, and low carbohydrate intake as a percentage of total calories.

Evers measured and evaluated dietary intake and anorexia nervosa symptoms of 21 female students in university dance classes and compared them with 29 nondance class students.[135] Based on 3-d food records, there was no significant difference between the two groups except for caloric and vitamin A intake. The control group had a mean caloric intake of 1931 kcal (8072 J) while the dancers were eating 1775 kcal (7420 J). The percent of subjects consuming less than two-thirds of the RDA for energy was significantly higher in the dance group than in controls. Dancers consumed more vitamin A (6166 IU) than did controls (5294 IU). Members of both dancers and control groups were low in calcium (24 and 35, respectively) and iron (67 and 62%, respectively). Almost half of the subjects consumed some type of supplements. Evers concluded that almost half of the women were consuming iron poor diets and were not taking supplements. More dancers (33%) than controls (13.8%) scores indicated symptoms of anorexia nervosa on the Eating Attitudes Test.

Benson et al.[136] analyzed diets of 92 female adolescent ballet dancers (age 12 to 17) enrolled in six different professional schools. Results of 3-d diet records of dancers, analyzed with a data base program of 700 foods, indicated that many dancers were consuming less than two-thirds of the RDA for folacin, calcium, iron, and zinc. About 50% of dancers had iron intakes less than two-thirds of the RDA. Other low intake nutrients included vitamin E, pyridoxine, and magnesium. Average caloric intake was 1890 kcal (7900 J)/d, but 50% of dancers ate less than 1800 kcal (7524 J)/d, and 11% ate less than 1200 kcal (5016 J)/d. Caloric intake was 15.6% from protein, 34.6% from fat, and 49.8% from carbohydrate. Over half of these girls derived more than 20% of their calories from protein and one-fourth derived more than 40% of calories from fat. About 60% of subjects took mineral or vitamin supplements but rarely did the supplement cover the dancers' nutritional deficiencies. Many dancers took supplements providing more than twice the RDA for vitamins A, B, and C when no deficiencies were evident.

E. FIELD HOCKEY PLAYERS

Ready evaluated 19 athletes from the Canadian women's Olympic field hockey team (average age 13 years).[137] A 3-d dietary record was analyzed by computer and compared to the 1983 Recommended Nutrient Intake (RNI) for Canadians.[138] Mean energy intake was 1967 kcal (8222 J); 42% as carbohydrate, 39% as fat, and 15% as protein. A significant number of field hockey players did not meet the recommendations for vitamin A, B_{12}, pyridoxine, and folate. Only five women met the RNI for iron. Fiber intake was also low.

More than 25% of caloric intake came from high calorie fats, sweets, and alcohol. About 50% of athlete's intake was consumed during the evening. Ready recommended that players receive regular dietary evaluation, counseling and education.

F. FOOTBALL PLAYERS

Gorman and Berning described a nutrition program used with the Denver Broncos professional football team.[139] Informal nutrition education seminars were presented to players, coaching staff, and players' wives. Individual football players were provided with dietary counseling after a 3-d food record was analyzed and diets were designed to fit specific needs of each player.

Hickson and colleagues[140] studied 16 intercollegiate football athletes (19.6 years old) at training table over three consecutive weekdays during winter conditioning. Food items and plate waste were weighed or estimated at the dining hall. Snacks were reported by recall at the next meal. Dinner provided 70% more energy than breakfast or lunch. Caloric intake ranged from 2053 to 5464 kcal (8582 to 22,839 J) with a mean of 22% from protein, 39% from fat, and 39% from carbohydrate. Meat consumption provided one-third of calories, two-thirds of protein, and 45% of fat intake. The major source of carbohydrate came from fats, sweets, and alcohol. Mean intake of 10 vitamins and minerals exceeded the RDA except for magnesium, folacin, and pyridoxine which were low but not less than 70% of the RDA.

Zallen and Fitterhof[141] compared nutrient intakes of 33 East Carolina University football players with that of 35 male students. Both groups mailed completed 24-h records on three nights in successive weeks. The athletes consumed close to 5000 kcal (20,900 J) with 165g protein, 190 g fat, and 637 g carbohydrate. Fluid intake was 370 oz (10,490 g); all other nutrients were within 87% of recommendations. Since mail-in responses are difficult to check for poor memory or lack of information, methods used to verify the data should be stated.

Members of the Syracuse University football team who regularly played most games (33 men) were surveyed about their use of 23 different supplements.[142] A multivitamin pill (containing no more than the RDA for vitamins) was the most used supplement used by 50% of those surveyed. Single vitamin use included vitamin E (used by 30%) and vitamin C (used by 20%). Twenty-four percent of men took calcium supplements and 15% took iron pills. Only two men consumed protein supplements. Caffeine intake was extensive (88% of those surveyed drank two to three cans of soft drinks containing caffeine per day and 40% regularly drank coffee).

Hickson et al.[143] surveyed food intake (using 24-h recalls) of 134 high school football players (age 12–18 years) during training in August. Mean caloric and nutrient intakes for senior high (15–18 years) students met or exceeded the RDA and were greater than junior high (12–14 years) students except for vitamin A. Junior high school boys met or exceeded the RDA for nutrients analyzed except they were low in calories and slightly low in zinc (87% RDA). Mean caloric intake for these boys was 2523 kcal (10,546 J)/d while that of the high school boys was 3365 kcal (14,066 J)/d. Distribution of energy was similar for both groups with about 14% of caloric intake from protein, about 45% from carbohydrate, and roughly 40% from fat. Football players ate more from the dairy and fats, sweets and alcohol groups than did a sample of same-age boys from a national survey. Meals were frequently skipped by these football players: 19% missed breakfast, 13% skipped lunch, and 3% did not eat dinner. The authors stated that the body weight of senior high students indicated that they consumed enough fluid to prevent dehydration. However, during days six through nine of training, the temperature reached 97°F (36°C) in the morning with relative high humidity.

As part of a larger series of investigations that examined nutritional practices of high school athletes, a questionnaire was designed to assess nutritional supplement use among 416 high school football players from a rural county in New York state.[45] When asked about a list of 14 different supplements that athletes used over the past year, those most frequently consumed were: sports drinks (53%), caffeine (38%), protein powders (18%), vitamin and mineral supplements (17%), amino acid supplements (14%), energy bars (13%), honey (13%), and carbohydrate loaders (11%). Nutritional supplements that were consumed less frequently included gelatin (5%), weight loss supplements (4%), wheat germ (3%), bee pollen (1%) and brewers yeast (1%). When athletes were asked whether they thought muscle size or strength increased due to use of nutritional supplements, 14% reported yes, 22% no, and 61% "I don't use nutritional supplements." When asked about where they bought nutritional supplements, 16% reported purchases from a nutrition store, 15% from a drug or grocery store, 3% from friends or teammates, 3% from fitness or health clubs, and 2% by mail order.

G. GYMNASTS

The nutritional habits of 97 competitive female adolescent (11–17 years) gymnasts from six different gymnastic schools were evaluated by Loosli et al.[36] using 3-d diet records. Average caloric intake was low (1838 kcal) and 40% or more consumed diets low (less than two-thirds of the RDA) in calcium, folate, vitamin E, pyridoxine, iron, and zinc. Forty percent of gymnasts were low in calcium and 53% were low in iron intake. Average caloric intake from protein was 15%, from fat 36%, and from carbohydrate 49%. These athletes chose diets low in fiber (3.6 g/d) but type of fiber was not reported. Gymnasts used vitamin or mineral supplements (43%) but rarely did usage compensate for low nutrient intake. According to Loosli et al., "gymnasts and their coaches would benefit from a nutrition education program."

Moffatt[144] examined the dietary status of 13 elite female high school gymnastic team members (age 15) by analyzing two 3-d food records collected over a three week period using 1963 food composition tables. Between 30 and 60% of gymnasts consumed less than 50% of the RDA for pyridoxine, folic acid, calcium, iron, and zinc. Only three girls used supplements. Gymnasts had 10% less body fat (13%) than nonathletic girls of the same age, height, and body weight (23.5%). About 44% of the girls' caloric intake was provided by cakes, candy, soft drinks, butter, jelly, and jams.

Huber et al.[145] studied the nutritional status of eight female collegiate gymnasts and seven female collegiate cross-country runners using 3-d diet intakes, activity records, underwater weighing, and treadmill tests. Gymnasts had caloric intakes of 1357 kcal (5672 J)/d while the runners ate 1661 kcal (6943 J)/d. It was calculated that gymnasts used 2855 kcal (11,934 J)/d and the runners used 2651 kcal (11,081 J)/d. For both groups, diets were composed of more than 25% fat. Only 12.5% consumed more than 60% carbohydrates. More than 50% of both groups were low (less than 75% of the RDA) in calcium, iron, and vitamin A. Gymnasts were also low in thiamin and riboflavin. Both gymnasts and runners had low percentages of body fat, serious caloric deficiencies, and inadequate nutritional intake.

Calabrese[146] reviewed the nutritional and medical aspects of gymnastics and reported on his study of the nutritional habits and menstrual patterns of 20 club level A gymnasts. These girls (average age 14.8 years) recorded all food, drink, and supplements during a 3-d training period. Diets were found to be low (less than 85% RDA) for vitamins A, D, folic acid, calcium, phosphorus, magnesium, and zinc. Vitamin supplements were used by one-fourth of the group. Mean intake of calories was 1744 kcal (7290 J)/d, with 56 g protein, 75 g fat, and 218 g carbohydrate. Calabrese noted that although the female gymnasts were taking in 122% of the RDA for protein, caloric input was low compared to energy expended.

H. ICE SKATERS

Competitive figure skaters, 17 males and 23 females, were studied to assess the relationship between body image and dietary intake.[147] Results indicated that there was more pressure on females than males to be thin. Females' diets were low in energy, iron, vitamin B$_{12}$, and calcium. Dietary intake for men was adequate in energy and most nutrients.

I. OUTDOOR, COLD WEATHER EXERCISE AND SPORTS

Energy intakes and physical performance of eight men were studied for 31 d at moderate altitudes.[148] The authors developed a lightweight, energy-dense ration modified after one used in sustained military field operations. Temperatures ranged from 5 to 35°C, and men climbed to 14,104 ft (4300 m). Mean energy intake averaged 2354 kcal (9840 J)/d before the expedition, 3430 kcal (14,337 J)/d during a 3-d expedition, and 3384 kcal (14,145 J)/d after their return. Reduction in body fat was significant at 18.9%, and energy deficit was estimated at between 473 to 963 kcal (1977 to 4025 J)/d. It was concluded that when using dehydrated rations, weight loss and gastrointestinal distress may be minimized by substituting some fat in place of carbohydrate, at approximately 67% of calories.

A study comparing energy balances of men on long and short sledding journeys in Antarctica found that men could tolerate energy imbalances for short trips of 8–14 d; but during the Antarctic crossing of 74 d, men had to increase their energy intake to keep body weight constant.[149] Standard British Antarctic Survey rations provide 48% of caloric content from fat.

The Leningrad Scientific Research Institute for Physical Culture conducted surveys of athletes.[150] They reported on more than 1000 athletes (age 11–25 years) involved in winter sports. They concluded that the younger (11–14 years) group had lower intakes of thiamin, riboflavin, and vitamin C. A significant number of athletes were also iron deficient.

Ellsworth et al.[151] investigated the nutrient intake of 13 male (age 18–28 years) and 14 female (15–31 years) members of the U.S. Nordic Ski Team. Four sets of 3-d records were collected at 3–4 month intervals during a year of training and competition (cross-country skiing for females and 9 men; and combined Nordic events for 4 men). Food intake, weighed and measured at the third session, indicated they consumed a diet high in fat, low in carbohydrate, and averaged more than the RDA for vitamin C, thiamin, riboflavin, niacin, and calcium. Females had low iron intakes for three out of the four recording sessions. Although the female skiers' mean calcium intake met the RDA, 40% of skiers at the last session ate less than 800 mg calcium. Caloric intake was high (49–76 kcal [205–318 J]/kg BW) for men and (42–71 kcal [176–297 J]/kg BW) for women. Caloric needs for skiers have been calculated to be 90 kcal (376 J)/kg BW but only two men consumed calories at that level. The percentage of calories from energy nutrients ranged between 13 and 14% for protein for both men and women, 34–43% calories from fat for men, and 34–41% for women, and 40–52% of calories from carbohydrate for men and 42–50% for women. Alcohol provided up to 3% of calories for men and 4.5% for women. Intake ranged from 655 to 1210 mg cholesterol for men and from 369 to 736 mg cholesterol for women which is far above any dietary guidelines. Fat consumption increased and carbohydrate intake decreased at training table as compared to at-home eating habits suggesting that training table menus need to be revised.

J. ROWERS

Collegiate rowers (12 men and 10 women) were studied for four weeks to determine if dietary carbohydrate would affect muscle glycogen and power output.[152] Ohio State University researchers found that a diet high in carbohydrate (10 g carbohydrate/kg BW/d which was 70% of energy intake) increased muscle glycogen levels and resulted in better time trials than diets containing 5 g carbohydrate/kg BW/d in these rowers training twice a day for four weeks. However, the lower carbohydrate diet maintained normal muscle glycogen and power during the same time period.

K. RUNNERS

The term runner covers many types of events and a wide variety of energy expenditures from sprints to ultramarathons and triathlons. Dietary intakes, obviously, will differ.

Dietary intake, energy expenditure, and anthropometric characteristics of 44 junior high and high school female cross-country runners were studied in central New York state.[153] Pyridoxine, magnesium, and zinc intakes were below 76% of the RDA while iron and calcium intakes were about 80% of the RDA. Mean energy intake was 84% of calculated mean caloric needs although there was not a progressive weight loss. It is not mandatory that students have a lunch period in New York state and eight of the athletes did not have time for lunch.

Amenorrheic and eumenorrheic (six each) adolescent runners completed 7-d dietary records and a questionnaire about health and exercise habits.[154] Amenorrheic runners ran more miles per week, consumed an average of 1912 kcal (7992 J)/d (15% protein, 50% carbohydrate, 35% fat), and less than 70% of the RDA for calcium, iron, magnesium, and zinc.

Some elite runners with low caloric intake seem to be able to maintain their weight and still run well. This was investigated with 8 runners with a deficit of 1260 calories (5267 J) over a 3-month period and 7 runners on a balanced energy diet.[155] Weights of both groups of runners were similar and did not change. The low calorie intake group ate 2585 kcal (10,805 J)/d which was 47% carbohydrate, 34% fat, and 1.7 g protein per kg BW/d. The balanced intake group ate 3833 kcal (16,021 J), of which 50% was carbohydrate, 34% fat, and 2 g protein/kg BW/d. Low intake runners were "compromising carbohydrate intake" according to study conclusions.

Elite male distance runners (80) were questioned by mail about their nutritional practices.[156] More than 50% reported never restricting food intake and never (78%) exercising to control weight. Most men had breakfast, lunch, and dinner, although more skipped lunch than any other meal. Red meat was restricted by 35%, and 12% restricted milk intake. Stress fractures occurred in 29% of the 41% who had restricted red meat. It was concluded that elite male runners do not report eating disorders frequently seen in female runners.

Three-day diet records collected from 103 distance runners and compared with 74 age-matched inactive women showed that the runners consumed more carbohydrate, magnesium, thiamin, and fiber but less fat, protein, and cholesterol than the less active women.[157]

Nutrient intakes and iron status were studied in 10 female (average age 34 years) long distance runners during nine weeks of training.[158] Three-day diet records collected during weeks one, four, and nine, revealed that caloric intake went from 2272 to 1786 kcal/d (9497 to 7465 J/d). Percent of calories from protein (14%), carbohydrate (48–50%), and fat (36–38%) remained similar over time. Dietary intakes of iron, pyridoxine, vitamin B_{12}, and folacin were low but blood tests were normal. It was suggested that if these deficiencies continued over a long period of time, the women would show deficiency symptoms.

The diets of 15 male distance runners (age 25 to 47) were evaluated during eight consecutive days in the middle of the 1982 Great Hawaiian Footrace (500 km).[159] Each runner kept his own daily intake record. Of the 8-d recorded intake, six were race days (averaged 28 km/d) and two were rest days. The average body weight and body fat (by skinfold calipers) increased by the end of the race, which seems unusual. Caloric intake averaged 4400 kcal (18,392 joules)/d (10% protein, 49% carbohydrate, 26% fat, 15% alcohol) and 4336 kcal (18,124 joules)/d for rest days. All nutrient intakes met or exceeded the RDA except zinc and magnesium. Twelve of the runners took nutrition supplements. This evidence does "not support excessive (e.g. twice the RDA) supplementation need for a male distance runner's diet."

Earlier, some of the same scientists studied the 1979 Great Hawaiian Footrace.[160] Twelve men (age 23 to 60) kept daily records of their dietary intakes. Caloric intakes were estimated to average 4800 kcal (20,064 J)/d while they were running 28 km/d. Their morning body weight and percent body fat did not change significantly during the race. Blood samples were taken on eight different days to analyze for nine different minerals. All nine mineral blood values were within normal clinical values, although they changed at various times during the race. It was unclear how the diet records were analyzed. The authors stated that "according to the basic four food plan, the reported diets on all subjects should have provided the essential nutrient requirements." The authors concluded that using the daily food plan might be all that is required to prevent mineral deficiency in healthy athletes.

Three-day diet records, blood tests and skinfold thickness were used by Deuster et al.[161] to assess the nutritional intake and status of 51 women (age 19–43) who had trained and qualified for the First Women's Olympic Marathon Trials. Mean caloric intake was 2397 kcal (10,019 J)/d (range of 1067–4271 kcal [4460–17,852 J]/d) which was low for their activity level (running 48–158 km per week). Caloric intake averaged 13% from protein, 32% from fat, and 55% from carbohydrate. Mean intake of crude fiber was 7.5 g. Mean intakes of calcium, magnesium, iron, and copper met or exceeded the RDA or suggested range. However, 23% of women had lower than recommended amounts of calcium and magnesium, 43% were consuming less than the RDA for iron, more than 62% were consuming less copper than the lower suggested range, and 76% were low in zinc. The concentration of serum ferritin and plasma zinc indicated marginal iron and zinc status. Assuming that less than 12 ng/ml serum ferritin concentration indicated absent iron stores, 35% of these women had low iron stores. Nutrition supplements taken by 53% of runners contributed more to total intake than did nutrients from food.

Female runners (93) who had competed nationally answered survey questions about their eating habits and nutrition knowledge.[162] More than 40% of women did not eat red meat and many were amenorrheic, anemic, and consumed inadequate protein, iron, and zinc. Nutrition education needs of this group were listed.

Barr[48] found that 75% of 104 female marathon runners and 65% of 105 fitness class women reported using an average of two to three supplements per day. These were mainly multivitamin/mineral supplements, followed by iron and vitamin C. Supplement use was most common among 38% of women who described themselves as semi-vegetarians.

Snyder et al.[163] studied the dietary patterns and iron parameters of middle-aged (average approximately 38 years) female runners. They used 3-d dietary intake analyses to compare nine women who consumed a modified vegetarian diet with nine women who ate red meat. In the vegetarian women, researchers found a marked decrease in ferritin which they felt was due to low dietary iron bioavailability.

Haymes and Spillman[164] analyzed 3-d food diaries of 11 women distance runners, 12 sprinters, and 11 moderately active women. Differences in dietary iron, hemoglobin, plasma iron, and transferrin were not significant among the three groups. Almost half of the distance runners had ferritin levels suggestive of iron depletion. The authors concluded that low ferritin levels were more common among women distance runners than sprinters and that this difference was not due to differences in dietary iron intake. Authors also reported that caloric intake of middle distance runners (1823 kcal [7620 J]), sprinters (2018 kcal [8435 J]), and field event university female athletes (1731 kcal [7236 J]) was not significantly different from controls (1845 kcal [7712 J]).[165] Sprinters' diets were highest in fat (85 g) but lowest in carbohydrates (220 g). Sprinters had low thiamin intake and riboflavin and niacin intakes were less than the RDA for runners. All groups were low in iron, and all athletes except the runners had low calcium intakes. Athletes' intake of sodium was less than controls.

Besenfelder et al.[166] studied iron status of five long distance female runners during a nine-week training period. Three-day diet records were collected at week one, four, and nine. Mean caloric intake ranged from 2073 to 2513 kcal/d (8665 to 10,504 J/d), protein ranged from 83 to 110 g, vitamin C from 164 to 199 mg, and iron from 17 to 21 mg. Although iron intake was satisfactory according to the RDA, blood iron status decreased from week one to week four and then stabilized, independent of iron intake and decreased physical performance.

Thompson et al.[167] reported that 10 male distance runners (16 km/d) ate 3587 kcal (14,993 J)/d of which 53% was carbohydrate, 15% protein, and 32% fat for 21 d. HDL-cholesterol decreased 6 mg/dl during the first two weeks, and then there was no change in HDL.

Bassler, a former member of Pritikin's advisory board, reported on the hazards of restrictive diets for runners.[168] He cited cases of 14 men (ages 18–60) whose death was associated with low body fat, high training mileage, and dietary restriction. Eleven of these men were restricting an average of six of the following foods: beef, eggs, milk, other animal protein, salt, sugar, alcohol, caffeine, and vegetable oil. Bassler proposed the term "nutritional arrhythmia" for cases of diet restriction and unexplained sudden death in runners. He pointed out that those who advocate such diets should be aware of the possible dangers and stated that "cachectic vegetarian athletes should be encouraged to eat a balanced diet including ample foods from all food groups."

Lampe et al.[169] evaluated iron status in nine female marathon runners (ages 27–34) during 11 weeks of training for a marathon and following the race. Results of a 3-d food diary recorded midway in the training indicated that average consumption for energy, protein, and vitamin C, were all near or above the RDA. Mean intake of iron, however, was 14 mg (78% of the RDA) ranging from 7 to 20 mg. Three subjects took iron and vitamin C supplements. The authors noted that although the iron status was poor, serum ferritin levels were elevated for 3 d after the marathon and may not adequately reflect iron stores.

Grace and Jeffrey[170] measured trace mineral intakes for 13 members of a college women's track team (age 18–22 years) and 13 sedentary female college students of the same age. Iron, zinc, and copper intakes were measured by analysis of 1-d duplicate-portion composites, 4-d weighed food records, and 24-h recalls. The iron and zinc intakes were lowest in the duplication-portion analysis. Copper intake means were higher by analysis and by 24-h dietary recall than by other methods. Calculated average caloric intake of athletes was 1668 kcal (6972 J)/d. Almost half (46%) of the athletes and 85% of nonathletes consumed less than two-thirds of the RDA for iron and zinc.

Four-d food records were used to assess usual and pre-race dietary intake of 17 ultra-marathoners registered to compete in the Old Dominion 100-Miler.[171] Runners were 40 years of age and ran 68 miles (109 km) per week (range 25–123 miles per week [40–198 km per week]). Usual and pre-race energy, carbohydrate, and fat intake were not significantly different. Energy provided by carbohydrate rose from the usual intake of 54–60% in the pre-race period. Protein and alcohol intake were significantly lower during the pre-race period vs. the usual recording period. Twelve subjects reported vitamin/mineral supplement use. Vitamin and mineral intake from food alone did not differ for the usual or pre-race period; however, vitamin A, calcium, and phosphorus were significantly higher during the usual recording period.

Eden and Abernethy[172] assessed food and fluid intake of a 38-year-old male ultraendurance runner competing in an Australian 1005 km race from Sydney to Melbourne over a 9-d period. A diet history method revealed a mean energy intake of 5961 kcal (24,917 J)/d (range 4031–7779 kcal/d; 16,849–32,516 J/d) with 62% of energy from carbohydrate, 27% from fat, and 11% from protein. Carbohydrate and protein intake were estimated at 16.8 g/kg BW/d and 2.9 g/kg BW/d, respectively. Water intake was 11 l/d. The author concluded that athletes can successfully complete ultraendurance events if guidelines for prolonged exercise are followed.

A food frequency questionnaire was used to assess dietary intake among 100 adult recreational runners.[173] The percentage of total energy from carbohydrate (52%), fat (28%), and protein (15%) compared favorably to the National Cholesterol Education Program (NCEP) Step I Guidelines. Only 6% of runners had greater than 10% of calories from saturated fat. Dietary fiber intake was 33 g, considerably higher than the National Cancer Institute recommendation of 25–35 g fiber per day. The authors concluded that these recreational runners more closely met the NCEP Step I Guidelines than did the general U.S. population.

L. SOCCER PLAYERS

Dietary analysis of the Puerto Rico National Soccer Team for two 6-d periods showed a dietary intake close to 4000 kcal (16,720 J)/d.[174] Protein intake averaged 2.3 g/kg BW/d, carbohydrates were 53% of calories, fat contributed 32% of total energy, and cholesterol intake was 591 mg. All micronutrients exceeded the RDA for these adolescents (age 17) with the exception of calcium. It was recommended that these athletes increase carbohydrate and reduce fat intake.

Hickson et al.[175] investigated 18 members of a men's intercollegiate soccer team during preseason conditioning and fall competition season. The athletes' preseason intake was observed and recorded at the university cafeteria training table over three consecutive weekdays. During the competitive season, players kept food intake records over two to three weekdays. Caloric intake for preseason was 4492 kcal (18,777 J)/d and 3346 kcal (13,986 J)/d during season. During preseason, percent of total calories from protein was 14%, from fat 33%, and from carbohydrate 52%. During the competitive season, caloric intake was divided 17% protein, 37% fat, and 46% carbohydrate. Mean intake of six vitamins and four minerals exceeded the RDA during preseason and during competitive season except that zinc was 97% of the RDA. The carbohydrate intake may have been below optimal level recommended for sports performance. Since the team won the NCAA Division I championships, the authors believe that a high carbohydrate intake is not the only factor in winning soccer competitions.

Tater et al.[176] reported on lipoprotein status after vacation in professional soccer players and then again, one month after start of intensive training. A 7-d diet recall was taken by a dietitian on day 1 and a month later. Athletes were consuming more than 3900 kcal (16,302 J)/d, 130 g protein, 482 g carbohydrates, 163 g fat, and 675 g cholesterol and had a P/S ratio of 0.33. LDL-cholesterol was constant throughout this period and was lower than controls. The HDL-cholesterol which was higher than controls decreased after intensive training.

M. SWIMMERS

The dietary intakes of 14 members of a collegiate women's swim team were studied.[177] They completed a 3-d food intake record and trained for a minimum of 2 h/d. The swimmers' diets met the RDA for all nutrients evaluated except calcium. Energy intake ranged from 1576 to 3131 kcal (6588 to 13,087 J)/d, and carbohydrate and fat intake was close to recommendations. No significant relationship was found between eating attitudes and caloric intake.

United States Swimming, International Center for Aquatic Research selected 22 male swimmers and 21 female swimmers (ages 14–18) to participate in a training camp.[178] Swimmers 5-d dietary records showed a caloric intake of 5221 kcal (21,824 J)/d for males and 3572 kcal (14,931 J)/d for females. Their diets were high in fat and low in carbohydrate. Female swimmers did not meet the RDA for calcium and iron. The authors point out that, although a group of athletes may have adequate diets, individual athletes may have poor intakes.

All members of a university men's (13) and women's (16) swim teams provided 7-d dietary records before and at the end of a competitive season as part of a study of copper, iron, and zinc status.[179] Caloric intake increased post-season for both men and women. It was found that copper, iron, and zinc status was not adversely affected by intensive training when dietary intakes were adequate.

Earlier, the same authors studied copper, zinc, and iron status of 12 female university swim team members before and at the end of a competitive season.[180] Self-reported 7-d records were used for dietary analysis. Caloric intake increased during training because of an increase in dietary carbohydrate. As long as dietary intake was adequate, trace mineral status was not affected by strenuous training. Average energy intake at the start of the season was 2030 kcal (8485 J)/d and at the end, the athletes were eating 2269 kcal (9484 J)/d.

Berning[37] surveyed the dietary intake of male (mean age 16) and female (mean age 15) elite national swimmers. The total number of subjects was not stated. It was found that these swimmers ate 46–48% kcal from carbohydrate, 12–13% kcal from protein, and 41–43% kcal from fat. These athletes were more than meeting the requirements for vitamins A, C, thiamin, riboflavin, and niacin. Vitamin A intake was high: 294% of the RDA for males and 239%

for females. Average calcium and iron intakes met the RDAs, but 50% of girls were low in calcium and iron, while 14% of boys were low in calcium only. The majority (63%) took vitamin/mineral supplements, most commonly vitamin C, followed by multivitamin pills, iron, and calcium pills. Consumption of lecithin, amino acids, bee pollen, RNA, and DNA was noted. The timing of the pre-event meal varied. Eleven-percent of swimmers ate up to 30 min before swimming, 12% ate 31–60 min prior, and 77% of the subjects ate 1–1.5 h before swimming. The meals were composed mostly of complex carbohydrate foods.

Campbell and MacFadyen[181] assessed the dietary practices of 101 Canadian adolescent male and female competitive swimmers. They divided these swimmers into groups: 15- to 16-year-olds, 16- to 18-year-olds, and 20-year-olds who could meet time standards set in two events of 100 m or over and in one event of 50 m or greater. Three-day food records were collected and compared to the 1975 Canadian Dietary Standard Committee for revision of the Canadian Dietary Standard.[182] The 3-d mean intake of calories and nutrients met the Canadian Dietary Standard recommendations for all ages and for both boys and girls, however some swimmers ate less than recommended amounts of calories, iron, and vitamin A. A higher percentage of calories and nutrients were consumed at home than away from home by all age and sex groups. Evening snacks provided almost the same percentage of calories and nutrients as breakfast. In some cases, this was also true of lunch. About 40% or more of total calorie and nutrient intake was provided by dinner and evening snack. More swimmers took supplements during training than before competition. These supplements included vitamin C, vitamin E, iron, and the B-complex vitamins. The most frequently eaten foods for pre-game meals were cereals and carbohydrate foods.

N. TRIATHLETES

The triathlon may refer to a combination of any three athletic events but usually combines swimming, cycling, and running. The Ironman World Triathlon Championship is a race consisting of a 3.9 km swim, a 180 km bicycle course, and a 42 km (26.2-mile) run. A half-triathlon involves 1.9 km swimming, 90 km bicycling, and 21.1 km running.

A study of the dietary habits of 52 triathletes at various times during competition indicated that almost half of survey respondents had no dietary change 1–3 d before the event.[183] The last meal before the event for 60% of subjects was breakfast, most drank water 1 h before the event, 98% drank fluids during the event (mostly water), and after the event all drank fluids (mostly water) and 73% ate a high carbohydrate meal. During this short course triathlon, only 19% reported eating solid food during the event, although 30% said they ate solid food in longer triathlons. Traditional carbohydrate loading (with depletion phase) was rarely practiced, but more than 40% used a modified carbohydrate loading (70% calories from carbohydrate or more). Prior to competition, 58–76% of triathletes omitted foods from their diets including dairy, meat and meat substitutes, sweets, fats, convenience foods, snacks, supplements, and beverages such as carbonated drinks, alcohol, coffee, and tea.

Triathletes were studied to determine gastrointestinal complaints and dietary patterns.[51] All 21 females and 50 males studied finished the triathlon (1.5 km swim, 40 km bike, 10 km run). The 3-d dietary intake was self-recorded during a training period within 6 weeks after the triathlon. The average caloric intake was 2590 kcal (10,826 J)/day with 54% from carbohydrate, 30% from fat, 15% from protein, and 3.4% from alcohol. Protein intake averaged 1.4 g/kg BW/d. Mean intakes for vitamins, except vitamin E, were above the RDA, but some individuals were low. Almost 40% of athletes took a vitamin-mineral supplement daily, but even with supplements, more than half were low in folacin and vitamin E. Mean intake of minerals from food was above the RDA, but more than 40% consumed less than the RDA for magnesium and zinc. Copper intake was also low. Even when iron from supplements was calculated, 43% of women and 2% men were below the RDA for iron. Most athletes preferred water as a beverage, but glucose-polymer drinks were used by 29%

of women when biking and 19% when running and by more than 50% of men while biking and running.

Nutritional problems confronting ultraendurance athletes (including triathletes) were discussed in two articles by the same author.[184,185] Carbohydrate intake is of prime importance for these athletes. In order to meet carbohydrate needs, low intake of protein may result especially in women athletes with low caloric intakes. It was stated that protein intake should be from 15–18% of total calories.

Gastrointestinal complaints in relation to dietary intakes in triathletes (half-triathlon) were studied in The Netherlands and Belgium.[186] More gastrointestinal problems were reported by 55 male athletes during the running part of the event than during swimming or cycling. Those athletes who ate diets with higher amounts of protein, fat, and increased beverage osmolality had more gastrointestinal problems, probably since these substances have all been reported to delay gastric emptying time. All athletes who vomited had eaten in the last half-hour before the event. Solid foods and beverages were self-reported as those eaten before, during, and after competition. Diets were analyzed, but nutrient content was not reported. Researchers concluded that increased intake of fat, protein, dietary fiber, and hypertonic beverages (more than 325 mOsm/kg BW) should be discouraged, while low-fiber, low-fat, low-protein, and high-carbohydrate diets should be encouraged.

Burke and Read[187] described the self-reported diets of 25 Australian male triathletes (age 19–46). During training, diet histories, and food frequency techniques were used to collect dietary intake information. Twenty subjects completed 7-d food diaries. Skinfold and other anthropometric measurements were performed and blood samples were taken to measure iron status. Athletes indicated that foods they used during triathlons lasting from an average of 3 h to completion to those events lasting 9–17 h to completion (e.g., Ironman) were fresh and dried fruit, cookies, sandwiches, water, electrolyte drinks, soft drinks, 2–5% glucose/fructose-polymer drinks during the cycling phase, and cookies with the same liquids during the running phase. Foods used during a training week included (per day): 18 servings of breads/cereals, nine servings of fruit/starchy vegetables, five servings of high-sugar foods, and from one to three servings from other food groups. More than 80% of men reported carbohydrate loading 2–4 d before the race. Mean energy intake of the training diet was 4095 kcal (17,117 J)/d (59 kcal [247 J]/kg BW/d) with 59.5% from carbohydrate, 13% from protein (2 g/kg BW), 27% from fat, and 0.5% from alcohol. Intake of five vitamins and two minerals was above the Australians' nutrient recommendations. Intake of iron was calculated to be 30 mg (three times the recommendation), and all iron status measurements were normal. These triathletes had frequent snacks and multiple meals to increase caloric intake. At the pre-event meal, all triathletes reported drinking extra liquids and all but two men had high carbohydrate meals. All subjects recognized the importance of fluids before and during triathlons.

Bazzarre et al.[188] evaluated the nutritional status of 32 men and 5 women triathletes, 17 men and 11 women endurance athletes (runners, swimmers, and/or cyclists), and 12 men and 16 women controls (age 14–51 years) using 7-d food records. Males had a greater intake of calories and 17 out of 28 nutrients than did females. Mean intake of male subjects was greater than the RDA for all nutrients except zinc and folic acid. Females in all groups were low in iron, zinc, pyridoxine, folic acid, and magnesium. Blood measurements indicative of nutritional status showed that females had poor iron levels but acceptable levels of zinc, copper, and vitamin C. Female triathletes and endurance athletes reported more cases of fatigue than did other groups.

Novak[189] of Czechoslovakia described studies performed with ten males competing in a super Ironman event involving swimming 5 km, bicycling 103 km, and running 50 km. Subjects did not use carbohydrate loading techniques and consequently their carbohydrate stores were depleted by the end of the event. The author reported that in another study of an Ironman competition, it was determined that the food intake could never cover the endurance performance calorie requirements of approximately 40,000 kcal (167,200 J).

O. VOLLEYBALL PLAYERS

Perron and Endres[38] used a 24-h recall and 48-h record to evaluate diets of 31 female adolescent volleyball players. They found that these athletes' diets were low in energy, calcium, and iron. These young women ate an average of five times per day consuming 13 servings of food daily. The largest percent of total servings came from the other food groups, composed of desserts, beverages, sugar, and salty snacks.

P.   WRESTLERS

Because wrestlers believe that food intake has little effect on performance, good nutritional practices may be overlooked.[190] Nutrition advice comes, not from sports nutritionists, but from fellow wrestlers who may recommend from 0–500 kcal (0–2090 J)/d. Wrestlers may need from 1500 to 2200 kcal/d (6270 to 9196 J/d). Food restriction and fluid restriction are all too frequent weight-loss techniques.[191]

Steen and McKinney collected data from two college wrestling teams (42 wrestlers age 18–23 years) using 24-h diet recall preseason, 4-d food record midseason, and a 1-d report three to four weeks after the last match.[30] Thirty-seven percent of wrestlers did not meet the RDA for calories for an "average person" and 15% had low protein intakes. Including supplements, 25% of men consumed less than two-thirds of the RDA for vitamin C, thiamin, and iron. Almost half were low in vitamin A, while more than half were below two-thirds of the RDA for pyridoxine, zinc, and magnesium. Percentages of calories from protein and fat were higher than that recommended for athletes while carbohydrate consumption was lower than recommended. All but five percent of subjects used alcohol during the season. Food and fluid intake was low and sometimes nothing was taken by mouth for two days before a match.

Schwarzkopf and Jensen[192] reported on the effects of dietary control on making weight in seven collegiate wrestlers. Varsity wrestlers were given food containing 60% carbohydrate, 1 g protein/kg BW/d, and a caloric deficiency (equal to, or more than 1200 kcal [5016 J]/d) to reach a target weight in six weeks. Teammates (11 men) were assigned a target weight but given no dietary guidance. Wrestlers provided with the diet lost 6 lbs (13.2 kg); the control group lost 1.4 lbs (3.1 kg), reached target weight, and decreased lean weight one pound (controls lost 1.4 lbs [3.1 kg]). There was a trend for greater improvement in performance by wrestlers given dietary guidance.

It is difficult to follow college athletes after they graduate, but researchers persuaded 51 ex-wrestlers and 39 nonwrestlers to return questionnaires about their health.[198] Ex-wrestlers were found to have a greater incidence of weight gain and obesity than nonwrestlers. Although not significant, ex-wrestlers had greater incidences of hypertension and hypercholesterolemia than did nonwrestlers indicating that some practices of wrestlers may increase their risk of developing heart disease in later life.

V.   CONCLUSIONS

Coaches, trainers, and physical education teachers provide nutrition education for athletes and even dispense nutrition supplements with little, or no, knowledge of sports nutrition. Williams states that "the education of modern coaches should include nutrition among other subjects … ."[194] He indicates that without valid information, myths and misconceptions will continue.

Athletes often cite coaches as a major source of nutrition information.[16] Coaches, trainers, and especially athletes need more effective nutrition education. Not only do they need to know more about diet for fitness and sports, but they need to be warned about buying useless or even dangerous pills and other products. Very few athletes realize that fad products sold as food supplements are not monitored for efficacy or safety. Athletes should be warned about nutrition information presented by unqualified people attempting merely to sell a product. More emphasis is needed on scientifically based nutrition education.

Concerns are raised when dietary intake is collected.[63-67] A standard form should be used to survey athletic teams. Investigators need to be more precise about methods used such as data bases, computer procedures, nutrient intake standards, cut-off points for low intakes, etc., so that survey information can be of more use to teams in other areas.

Recommended Dietary Allowances probably should be used as a minimum. At least some of the B-vitamins might be better reported on a per 1000 kcal (4180 J) basis, and protein should be calculated on a g protein/kg BW basis. A major problem is interpreting diet analysis figures based on computer programs. A registered dietitian or licensed nutritionist specializing in sports nutrition must translate these figures into actual needs for specific foods and then provide acceptable menus and diets for the individual. It would be ideal to have nutrient intake data along with blood tests and physiological test results and enough time with each athlete to work out the optimum diet. It is impossible to make specific recommendations for all athletes. Even for a specific sport, dietary intakes vary and advice must be individualized.

Teams or groups having to "make weight" (i.e., gymnasts, wrestlers, dancers) are at greatest risk for nutritional problems.[30,110,133] Members of other teams may consume sufficient amounts of energy to adequately meet nutrient needs. Some athletes may be low in nutrients even if slightly high in calories due to poor food choices. Typically, if a diet is very high in calories, nutrient intake may meet most standards.

Surveys indicate that those taking supplements are not the athletes who are low in these nutrients.[119] There seems to be no conclusive evidence from well-defined studies to indicate that marginal intake decreases performance. There is room for more research to clarify whether marginally low nutrient intake affects athletic performance.

What constitutes an optimum diet for an athlete? Advice probably should include lowering the percentage of fat in the diet, but this is difficult for athletes requiring large amounts of calories simply to make up for those burned during intensive exercise. Higher percentages of carbohydrates are being recommended for most athletes, but this may be necessary for all-out events lasting more than an hour but not for other events. All experts agree that athletes should be well hydrated; although in actual practice, they may consume less water than is desirable. The optimum requirement for protein for athletes seems to be changing, as more research is reported.

In summary, there is no answer to the question of an optimal diet for an athlete since each diet must be individualized for the sport, position played, body composition, and many other factors. Devising the diet best suited for any athlete or team should be left to a registered dietitian or licensed nutritionist specializing in sports nutrition.

Nutritional adequacy is not going to make an Olympian from someone who has not trained, but good nutrition is an essential part of all athletes' training. Elite teams have physicians, coaches, trainers, strength coaches, and sport psychologists yet ignore the nutritional practices used by athletes. All health professionals, including qualified sports nutritionists, must work together for the good of each individual athlete.

REFERENCES

1. Durnin, J.V.G.A., The influence of nutrition, *Can. Med. Assoc. J.,* 96, 715, 1967.
2. Storlie, J., Nutrition assessment of athletes: a model for integrating nutrition and physical performance indicators, *Int. J. Sport Nutr.,* 1, 192, 1991.
3. Council on Practice, The American Dietetic Association, 216 W. Jackson Boulevard, Chicago, IL, 60606-6995.
4. McCutcheon, M.L., The athlete's diet: a current view, *J. Am. Diet. Assoc.,* 16, 529, 1983.
5. Parr, R.B., Porter, M.A., and Hodgson, S.C., Nutrition knowledge and practice of coaches, trainers, and athletes, *Phys. Sportsmed.,* 12, 127, 1984.

6. Corely, G., Demarest-Litchford, M., and Bazzarre, T. L., Nutrition knowledge and dietary practices of college coaches, *J. Am. Diet. Assoc.*, 90, 705, 1990.

7. Spear, B.A., Lummis, B., and Craig, C.B., Nutrition knowledge survey of high school coaches in Alabama, *J. Am. Diet. Assoc.*, 91, A-45, 1991.

8. Pelzer, M.K., Hemmersbach, L.M., Valencic, C.A., and Vokaty, L.L., Implementing nutrition education with coaches of adolescents, *J. Am. Diet. Assoc.*, 91, A-96, 1991.

9. Lapin, C.S., Cashman, L.K., Wright, D.E., and Stone, K.A., Nutrition recommendations made by Texas high school coaches to athletes, *J. Am. Diet. Assoc.*, 90, 774 , 1990.

10. Graves, K.L., Farthing, M.C., Smith, S.A., and Turchi, J.M., Nutrition training, attitudes, knowledge, recommendations, responsibility and resource utilization of high school coaches and trainers, *J. Am. Diet. Assoc.*, 91, 321, 1991.

11. Bedgood, B.L. and Tuck, M.B., Nutrition knowledge of high school athletic coaches in Texas, *J. Am. Diet. Assoc.*, 83, 672, 1983.

12. Zuniga, M.E., Spear, B.A., and Craig, C.B., A comparison of knowledge, attitudes, behavior, weight loss methods and dietary intake of two high school wrestling teams, *J. Am. Diet. Assoc.*, 93, A-78, 1993.

13. Sossin, K., Gizis, F., Marquart, L.M., and Sobal, J., Nutrition beliefs, attitudes and resource use among high school wrestling coaches. Presented at Sports and Cardiovascular Nutritionists Annual Meeting, Baltimore, MD, 1995.

14. Weissinger, E., Housh, T.J., and Johnson, G.O., Coaches' attitudes, knowledge and practices concerning weight loss behaviors in high school wrestling, *Pediatr. Exer. Sci.*, 5, 145, 1993.

15. Housh, D.J., Housh, T.J., Johnson, G.O., and Hughes, R.J., The validity of high school wrestlers' estimations of minimal wrestling weight, *Pediatr. Exer. Sci.*, 2, 124, 1990.

16. Marquart, L.F. and Sobal, J., Weight loss beliefs, practices and support systems for high school wrestlers, *J. Adoles. Health,* 15, 410, 1994.

17. Oppliger, R.A., Harms, R.D., Herrmann, D.E., Streich, C.M., and Clark, R.R., The Wisconsin Wrestling Minimum Weight Project: a model for weight control among high school wrestlers, *Med. Sci. Sports Exer.,* 27, 1220, 1995

18. Leeds, M.J. and Denegar, C., Nutrition knowledge and food practices of collegiate athletes compared to nonathletes, *J. Am. Diet. Assoc.*, 91, A-13, 1991.

19. Grandjean, A.C., Hursh, L.M., Majure, W.C., and Hanley, D.F., Nutrition knowledge and practices of college athletes, *Med. Sci. Sports Exer.,* 13, 82, 1981.

20. Grandjean, A.C., Profile of nutritional beliefs and practices of the elite athlete, *The Elite Athlete,* Butts, N.K., Gushiken, T.T., and Zarins, C., Eds., Spectrum Publications, 1985.

21. Frederick, L. and Hawkins, S.T., A comparison of nutrition knowledge and attitudes, dietary practices, and bone densities of postmenopausal women, female college athletes, and nonathletic college women, *J. Am. Diet. Assoc.*, 92, 299, 1992.

22. Shoaf, L.R., McClellan, P.D., and Birskovich, K.A., Nutrition knowledge, interests and information sources of male athletes, *J. Nutr. Educ.*, 18, 243, 1986.

23. Shearer, J.D., Yadrick, M.K., Loudreaux, L.J., and Norris, P.A., Nutritional assessment of college freshman athletes, *J. Am. Diet. Assoc.*, 91, A-110, 1991.

24. Potter, G.S. and Wood, O.B., Comparison of self- and group instruction for teaching sports nutrition to college athletes, *J. Nutr. Educ.*, 23, 288, 1991.

25. Walantas, S.D., Implementing a sports nutrition education program for the corps of cadets at the United States Military Academy, West Point, NY, *J. Am. Diet. Assoc.*, 90, A-129, 1990.

26. Bermudez, M.G., Keane, M.W., Curry, K.R., and Lopez, R., The effect of nutrition education on the nutrition knowledge of college athletes, *J. Am. Diet. Assoc.*, 91, A-47, 1991.

27. Reed-Wiesner, A.K. and Read, M.H., Health beliefs, nutrition knowledge and nutrient intake of university athletes, *J. Am. Diet. Assoc.*, 90, A-103, 1990.

28. Barr, S.I., Nutrition knowledge of female varsity athletes and university students, *J. Am. Diet. Assoc.*, 87, 1660, 1987.

29. McReynolds, C.J., Collen, J.W., Gambrell, K.M., and Dirks, K.R., Nutrition education with Texas A & M athletes, *J. Am. Diet. Assoc.*, 93, A-56, 1993.

30. Steen, S.N. and McKinney, S., Nutrition assessment of college wrestlers, *Phys. Sportsmed.*, 14, 100, 1986.

31. Keller-Grubbs, G.A., Landis, W., Lowe, J., and Finn, A., Differences in nutrition knowledge and dietary intake among female runners upon completion of a nutrition education program, *J. Am. Diet. Assoc.*, 94, A-86, 1994.

32. Frederick, L. and Hawkins, S.T., A comparison of nutrition knowledge and attitudes, dietary practices, and bone densities of postmenopausal women, female college athletes, and nonathletic college women, *J. Am. Diet. Assoc.*, 92, 299, 1992.

33. Clark, K.L., Working with college athletes, coaches and trainers at a major university, *Int. J. Sport Nutr.*, 4, 135, 1994.

34. Auld, G.W., Smiciklas-Wright, H., and Shannon, B.M., School health interventions for adolescents at nutritional risk: a survey of health teachers, nurses, and coaches, *J. Nutr. Educ.*, 20, 319, 1988.

35. Updegrove, N.A. and Achterberg, C.L., The conceptual relationship between training and eating in high school distance runners, *J. Nutr. Educ.*, 23, 18, 1990.

36. Loosli, A.R., Benson, J., Gillien, D.M., and Bourdet, K., Nutrition habits and knowledge in competitive adolescent female gynmasts, *Phys. Sportsmed.*, 14, 118, 1986.

37. Berning, J., Swimmers' nutrition knowledge and practice, *Sports Nutr. News*, 4, 1, 1986

38. Perron, M. and Endres, J., Knowledge, attitudes, and dietary practices of female athletes, *J. Am. Diet. Assoc.*, 85, 573, 1985.

39. Landry, R.V., Oppliger, R.A., Estwanik, J., and Landry, G.L., Nutrition knowledge and weight control practices in adolescent wrestlers and boxers: a comparative study, *Med. Sci. Sports Exer.*, 23, S-52, 1991.

40. Holler, H.J. and Hilliker, M.L., Nutrition education for high school wrestlers, *J. Am. Diet. Assoc.*, 91, A-79, 1991.

41. Douglas, P.D. and Douglas, J.G., Nutrition knowledge and food practices of high school athletes, *J. Am. Diet. Assoc.*, 84, 1198, 1984.

42. Campbell, M.L. and MacFadyen, K.L., Nutritional knowledge, beliefs and dietary practices of competitive swimmers, *Can. Home Econ. J.*, 34, 47, 1984.

43. Massad, S.J., Shier, N.W., Koceja, D.M., and Ellis, N.T., High school athletes and nutritional supplements: a study of knowledge and use, *Int. J. Sport Nutr.*, 5, 232, 1995.

44. Marquart, L.F. and Sobal, J., Beliefs and information sources of high school athletes regarding muscle development, *Pediatr. Exer. Sci.*, 5, 377, 1993.

45. English, G. and Marquart, L.M., Nutritional supplement use among high school footbal players, Presented at American Association of Health, Physcial Education, Recreation and Dance Annual Meeting, 1995.

46. Hornick, T.M., Kopel, B.H., Hermann, J., and Forbes, S., Impact of nutrition education on adolescents' sports nutrition knowledge and use of ergogenic products, *J. Am. Diet. Assoc.*, 93, 51, 1994.

47. Gollman, B.S. and Carlyle, T.L., Nutrition knowledge and eating practice survey of exercising adults, *J. Am. Diet. Assoc.*, 90, A-121, 1990.

48. Barr, S.I., Nutrition knowledge and selected nutritional practices of female recreational athletes, *J. Nutr. Educ.*, 18, 167, 1986.

49. Day, P.J. and Arnold, R.K., Nutrition knowledge among male and female participants of four distinct health/fitness facilities, *J. Am. Diet. Assoc.*, 90, A-18, 1990.

50. Schapira, D.V., Kumar, N.B., Lyman, G.H., and McMillan, S.C., The value of current nutrition information, *Prev. Med.*, 19, 45, 1990.

51. Worme, J.D., Doubt, T.J., Singh, A., Ryan, C.J., Moses, F.M., and Deuster, P.A., Dietary patterns, gastrointestinal complaints, and nutrition knowledge of recreational triathletes, *Am. J. Clin. Nutr.*, 51, 690, 1990.

52. Cumming, C.M., Brevard, P.B., and Pearson, J.M., Recreational runners' beliefs and practices concerning water intake, *J. Nutr. Educ.*, 26, 195, 1994.

53. Walsh, V.R., Health beliefs and practices of runners versus nonrunners, *Nursing Res.*, 34, 353, 1985.

54. Murphy, P., Youth sports coaches: using hunches to fill a blank page, *Phys. Sportsmed.*, 13, 136, 1985.

55. Jobe, F.W. and Moynes, D., *The Official Little League Fitness Guide,* Simon and Schuster, New York, 1984.

56. Furtado, M.M., Keane, M.W., Curry, K.R., and Johnson, P.M., The effect of nutrition education on nutrition knowledge and body composition of Little League cheerleaders, *J. Am. Diet. Assoc.*, 90, A-19, 1990.

57. Sossin, K., Marquart, L.F., O'Neil, N., and Travis, S., Community-based sports nutrition program, *J. Am. Diet. Assoc.*, 93, A-63, 1993.

58. American Dietetic Association, Timely statement of the American Dietetic Association: nutrition guidance for adolescent athletes in organized sports, *J. Am. Diet. Assoc.*, 96, 611, 1986.

59. American Dietetic Association, Timely statement of the American Dietetic Association: nutrition guidance for child athletes in organized sports, *J. Am. Diet. Assoc.*, 96, 610, 1996.

60. Jennings, S.D. and Steen, S.N., *Play Hard Eat Right: A Parents' Guide to Sports Nutrition,* Chronimed Publishing, Minneapolis, MN, 1995.

61. American Academy of Pediatrics, Promotion of healthy weight control practices in young athletes, *Pediatrics,* 752, 1996.

62. Gibson, R.S., *Principles of Nutritonal Assessment,* Oxford University Press, New York, 1990.

63. Medlin, C. and Skinner, J.D., Individual dietary intake methodology: a 50-year review of progress, *J. Am. Diet. Assoc.*, 88, 1250, 1988.

64. Anderson, S.A., Guidelines for use of dietary intake data, *J. Am. Diet. Assoc.*, 88, 1258, 1988.

65. Basiotis, P.P., Welsh, S.O., Cronin, F.J., Kelsay, J.L., and Mertz, W., Number of days of food intake records required to estimate individual and group nutrient intakes with defined confidence, *J. Nutr.*, 117, 1638, 1987.

66. Thompson, F.E., Larkin, F. A., and Brown, M.B., Weekend-weekday differences in reported dietary intake: the nationwide food composition survey, 1977–78, *Nutr. Res.*, 6, 647, 1986.

67. Bolland, J.E., Yuhas, J.A., and Bolland, T.W., Estimation of food portion sizes: effectivess of training, *J. Am. Diet. Assoc.*, 88, 817, 1988.

68. Kim, W.W., Mertz, W., Judd, J.T., Marshall, M.W., Kelsay, J.L., and Prather, E.S., Effect of making duplicate food collections on nutrient intakes calculated from food records, *Am. J. Clin. Nutr.,* 40, 1333, 1984.

69. Kretsch, M.J. and Fong, A.K.H., Validation of a new computerized technique for quantitating individual dietary intake: the Nutrition Evaluation Scale System (NESS) vs. the weighed food record, *Am. J. Clin. Nutr.,* 51, 477, 1990.

70. Ahluwalia, N. and Lammi-Keefe, C.J., Estimating the nutrient intake of older adults: components of variation and the effect of varying the number of 24-hour dietary recalls, *J. Am. Diet. Assoc.,* 91, 1438, 1991.

71. Woteki, C.E., Methods for surveying food habits: how do we know what Americans are eating?, *Clin. Nutr.,* 5, 9, 1986.

72. Karvetti, R. and Knuts, L., Validity of the 24-hour dietary recall, *J. Am. Diet. Assoc.,* 85, 1437, 1985.

73. Todd, K.S., Hudes, M., and Calloway, D.H., Food intake measurement: problems and approaches, *Am. J. Clin. Nutr.,* 37, 139, 1983.

74. Guthrie, H.A. and Crocetti, A.F., Variability of nutrient intake over a 3-day period, *J. Am. Diet. Assoc.,* 85, 325, 1985.

75. Gersovitz, M., Madden, J.P., and Smiciklas-Wright, H., Validity of the 24-h dietary recall and seven-day record for group comparisons, *J. Am. Diet. Assoc.,* 73, 48, 1978.

76. Pao, E.M., Mickle, S.J., and Burk, M.C., One-day and 3-day intakes by individuals — Nationwide Food Consumption Survey, findings, Spring 1977, *J. Am. Diet. Assoc.,* 85, 313, 1985.

77. St. Jeor, S.T., Guthrie, H.A., and Jones, M.B., Variability in nutrient intake in a 28-day period, *J. Am. Diet. Assoc.,* 83, 155, 1983.

78. Payette, H. and Gray-Donald, K., Dietary intake and biochemical indices of nutritional status in an elderly population with estimates of the precision of the 7-d food record, *Am. J. Clin. Nutr.,* 54, 478, 1991.

79. Mertz, W., Tsui, J.C., Judd, J.T., Reiser, S., Hallfrisch, J., Morris, E.R., Steele, P.D., and Lashley, E., What are people really eating? The relation between energy intake derived from estimated diet records and intake determined to maintain body weight, *Am. J. Clin. Nutr.,* 54, 291, 1991.

80. Edington, J., Thorogood, M., Geekie, M., Ball, M., and Mann, J., Assessment of nutritional intake using dietary records with estimated weights, *J. Human Nutr. Diet.,* 2, 407, 1989.

81. Miller, J.Z., Kimes, T., Hui, S., Andon, M.B., and Johnson, C.C., Jr., Nutrient intake variability in a pediatric population: implications for study design, *J. Nutr.,* 121, 265, 1991.

82. Basch, C.E., Shea, S., Arliss, R., Contento, I.R., Rips, J., Gutin, B., Irigoyen, M., and Zybert, P., Validation of mothers' reports of dietary intake by four to seven-year-old children, *Am. J. Public Health,* 81, 134, 1990.

83. Burke, B.S., The dietary history as a tool in research, *J. Am. Diet. Assoc.,* 23, 1041, 1947.

84. Block, G. and Hartman, A.M., Issues in reproducibility and validity of dietary studies, *Am. J. Clin. Nutr.,* 50, 1133, 1989.

85. Horwath, C.C., Food frequency questionnaires: a review, *Aust. J. Nutr. Diet.,* 47, 71, 1990.

86. Kristal, A.R., Abrams, B.F., Thornquist, M.D., Disogra, L., Croyle, R. T., Shattuck, A.L., and Henry, H.J., Development and validation of a food use checklist for evaluation of community interventions, *Am. J. Public Health,* 80, 1318, 1990.

87. Connor, S.L., Gustafson, J.R., Sexton, G., Becker, N., Aaartaud-Wild, S., and Connor, W.E., The diet habit survey: a new method of dietary assessment that relates to plasma cholesterol changes, *J. Am. Diet. Assoc.,* 92, 41, 1992.

88. Smucker, R., Block, G., Coyle, L., Harvin, A., and Kessler, L., A dietary and risk factor questionnaire and analysis system for personal computers, *Am. J. Epidemiol.,* 129, 445, 1989.

89. Clapp, J.A., McPherson, R.S., Reed, D.B., and Hsi, B.P., Comparison of a food frequency questionnaire using reported vs. standard portion sizes for classifying individuals according to nutrient intake, *J. Am. Diet. Assoc.,* 91, 316, 1991.

90. Gibson, R.S., Validity in dietary assessment: a review, *J. Am. Diet. Assoc.,* 51, 275, 1990.

91. Heaney, R.P., Davies, K.M., Recker, R.R., and Packard, P.T., Long-term consistency of nutrient intakes in humans, *J. Nutr.,* 120, 869, 1990.

92. Simons-Morton, B.G., Forthofer, R., Huang, I.W., Baranowski, T., Reed, D., and Fleishman, R., Reliability of direct observation of schoolchildren's consumption of bag lunches, *J. Am. Diet. Assoc.,* 92, 219, 1992.

93. Rising, R., Alger, S., Boyce, V., Seaagle, H., Ferraro, R., Fontvielle, A.M., and Ravussin, E., Food intake measured by an automated food-selection system: relationship to energy expenditure, *Am. J. Clin. Nutr.,* 55, 343, 1992.

94. Sevenhuysen, G.P. and Zacharias, E., Comparison of food intake assessments obtained with recall interviews and photographic records, *Nutr. Rep. Int.,* 40, 49, 1989.

95. Sevenhuysen, G.P., Staveren, W.V., Dekker, K., and Spronck, E., Estimates of daily intakes obtained by food image processing, *Nutr. Res.,* 10, 965, 1990.

96. Gines, D.J., Computer graphics increase accuracy of estimates of sizes of servings of food in dietary assessment, *J. Am. Diet. Assoc.,* 91, A-19, 1991.

97. Bingham, S.A., The dietary assessment of individuals: methods, accuracy, new techniques and recommendations, *Nutr. Abs. Rev.,* 57, 1, 1987.

98. Pennington, J.A.T., Associations between diet and health: the use of food consumption measurements, nutrient data bases, and dietary guidelines, *J. Am. Diet. Assoc.,* 88, 1221, 1988.

99. Subcommittee on the Tenth Edition of the RDAs, Food and Nutrition Board, Commission on Life Sciences, National Research Council, *Recommended Dietary Allowances,* 10th ed., National Academy Press, Washington, D.C., 1989.

100. Johnston, J.L. and Morin, L., Limitations of nutrient requirement estimates based on body weight, *J. Can. Diet. Assoc.,* 51, 33, 1990.

101. Williams, M.H., *Nutritional Aspects of Human Physical and Athletic Performance,* 2nd ed., Charles C. Thomas, Springfield, IL, 1985.

102. Pao, E.M. and Mickle, S.J., Problem nutrients in the United States, *Food Tech.,* 35, 58, 1981.

103. Stuff, J.E., Garza, C., Smith, E.O., Nichols, B.L., and Montandon, C.M., A comparison of dietary methods in nutritional studies, *Am. J. Clin. Nutr.,* 37, 300, 1983.

104. Buzzard, I.M., Price, K.S., and Warren, R.A., Considerations for selecting nutrient-calculation software: evaluation of the nutrient data base, *Am. J. Clin. Nutr.,* 54, 7, 1991.

105. Hoover, L.W., Dowdy, R.P., and Hughes, K.V., Consequences of utilizing reduced nutrient data bases for estimating dietary adequacy, *J. Am. Diet. Assoc.,* 85, 298, 1985.

106. Perloff, B.P., Rizek, R.L., Haytowitz, D.B., and Reid, P.R., Dietary intake methodology II. USDAs nutrient data base for nationwide dietary intake surveys, *J. Nutr.,* 120, 1530, 1990.

107. Guthrie, H.A., *Introductory Nutrition,* 7th ed., C.V. Mosby Co., St. Louis, MO, 1989.

108. Leaf, A. and Frisa, K.B., Eating for health or for athletic performance?, *Am. J. Clin. Nutr.,* 49, 1066, 1989.

109. Grandjean, A.C., Macronutrient intake of U.S. athletes compared with the general population and recommendations made for athletes, *Am. J. Clin. Nutr.,* 49, 1070, 1989.

110. Short, S.H. and Short, W.R., Four-year study of university athletes' dietary intake, *J. Am. Diet. Assoc.,* 82, 632, 1983.

111. American Dietetic Association, Position of the American Dietetic Association and the Canadian Dietetic Association: nutrition for physical fitness and athletic performance for adults, *J. Am. Diet. Assoc.,* 93, 691, 1993.

112. Burke, L.M., Gollan, R.A., and Read, R.S.D., Dietary intakes and food use of groups of elite Australian male athletes, *Int. J. Sport Nutr.,* 1, 378, 1991.

113. Nutter, J., Seasonal changes in female athletes' diets, *Int. J. Sport Nutr.,* 1, 395, 1991.

114. Welch, P.K., Zager, K.A., Endres, J., and Poon, S.W., Nutrition education, body composition, and dietary intake of female college athletes, *Phys. Sportsmed.,* 15, 63, 1987.

115. Van Erp-Baart, A.M.J., Saris, W.H.M., Binkhorst, R.A., Voos, J.A., and Brouns, F., A nation-wide survey on nutritional habits in athletes, *Med. Sci. Sports Exer.,* 19, S21, 1987.

116. Fogelholm, G.M., Himberg, J.J., Alopaesus, K., Gref, C.G., Laakso, J.T., Lehto, J.J., and Rauhamaa, H.M., Dietary and biochemical indices of nutritional status in male athletes and controls, *J. Am. Coll. Nutr.,* 11, 181, 1992.

117. Sobal, J. and Marquart, L.F., Vitamin/mineral supplement use among athletes: a review of the literature, *Int. J. Sport Nutr.,* 4, 320, 1994.

118. Minessale, R.A. and Schulz, L.O., Factors influencing the use of nutritional supplements by college athletes, *Am. J. Clin. Nutr.,* 46, 529, 1987.

119. Sobal, J. and Marquart, L.F., Vitamin/mineral supplement use among high school athletes, *Adolescence,* 29, 835, 1994.

120. Rosen, L.W., McKeag, D.B., Hough, D.O., and Curley, V., Pathogenic weight-control behavior in female athletes, *Phys. Sportsmed.,* 14, 79, 1986.

121. Sundgot-Borgen, J., Nutrient intake of female elite athletes suffering from eating disorders, *Int. J. Sport Nutr.,* 3, 431, 1993.

122. Sundgot-Borgen, J. and Corbin, C.B., Eating disorders among female athletes, *Phys. Sportsmed.,* 15, 89, 1987.

123. Fujioka, K., Kain, D., Mackenzie, R.B., and Gray, D.S., Increased carbohydrate intake of National Basketball Association superstar athletes, *Am. J. Clin. Nutr.,* 54, S-32, 1991.

124. Hickson, J.F., Schrader, J., and Trischler, L.C., Dietary intakes of female basketball and gymnastic athletes, *J. Am. Diet. Assoc.,* 86, 251, 1986.

125. Nowak, R.K. and Schulz, L.O., Body composition and nutrient intakes of college men and women basketball players, *J. Am. Diet. Assoc.,* 88, 575, 1988.

126. Gabel, K.A. and Aldous, A., Dietary and hematological assessment of elite cyclists during ten day 2050 mile ride, *J. Am. Diet. Assoc.,* 90, A-107, 1990.

127. Lindeman, A.K., Nutrient intake of an ultraendurance cyclist, *Int. J. Sport Nutr.,* 1, 79, 1991.

128. Slavin, J.L. and McNamara, E.A., Nutritional practices of women cyclists, including recreational riders and elite racers, in *Sport, Health and Nutrition,* Vol. 2, Human Kinetics Publishing Inc., Champaign, IL, 1986.

129. Stensland, S.H. and Sobal, J., Dietary practices of ballet, jazz and modern dancers, *J. Am. Diet. Assoc.,* 92, 319, 1992.

130. Hamilton, L.H., Brooks-Gunn, J., Warren, M.P., and Hamilton, W.G., The role of selectivity in the pathogenesis of eating problems in ballet dancers, *Med. Sci. Sports Exer.*, 20, 560, 1988.

131. Benson, J.E., Geiger, C.J., Eiserman, P.A., and Wardlaw, G.M., Relationship between nutrient intake, body mass index, menstrual function and ballet injury, *J. Am. Diet. Assoc.*, 89, 58, 1989.

132. Calabrese, L.H., Kirkendall, D.T., Floyd, M., Rapoport, S., Williams, G.W., Weiker, G.G., and Bergfeld, J.A., Menstrual abnormalities, nutritional patterns, and body composition in female classical ballet dancers, *Phys. Sportsmed.*, 11, 86, 1983.

133. Brooks-Gunn, J., Warren, M.P., and Hamilton, L.H., The relation of eating problems and amenorrhea in ballet dancers, *Med. Sci. Sports Exer.*, 19, 41, 1987.

134. Cohen, J.L., Potosnak, L., Frank, O., and Baker, H., A nutritional and hematologic assessment of elite ballet dancers, *Phys. Sportsmed.*, 13, 43, 1985.

135. Evers, C.L., Dietary intake and symptoms of anorexia nervosa in female university dancers, *J. Am. Diet. Assoc.*, 87, 66, 2987.

136. Benson, J., Gillien, D.M., Bourdet, K., and Loosli, A.R., Inadequate nutrition and chronic calorie restriction in adolescent ballerinas, *Phys. Sportsmed.*, 13, 79, 1985.

137. Ready, A.E., Nutrient intake of the Canadian women's Olympic field hockey team (1984), *Can. Home Econ. J.*, 37, 29, 1987.

138. Bureau of Nutritional Sciences, Recommended Nutrient Intake for Canadians, 4th ed., Ottawa: Health and Welfare, Canada, 1983.

139. Gorman, I. and Berning, J., Nutrition education in a strength and conditioning program?, *Natl. Strength Cond. Assoc. J.*, 7, 68, 1985.

140. Hickson, J.F., Wolinksy, I., Pivarnik, J.M., Neuman, E.A., Itak, J.F., and Stockton, J.E., Nutritional profile of football athletes eating from a training table, *Nutr. Res.*, 7, 27, 1987.

141. Zallen, E.M. and Fitterhof, W.F., Nutrition knowledge and nutrient intake of football players in training compared to male students not in training, *J. Am. Diet. Assoc.*, 87, 144, 1987.

142. Stoeppel, C., Survey of supplement use by Syracuse University football team members, Unpublished paper, Syracuse University, Fall, 1986.

143. Hickson, J.F., Duke, M.A., Risser, W.L., Johnson, C.W., Palmer, R., and Stockton, J.E., Nutritional intake from food sources of high school football athletes, *J. Am. Diet. Assoc.*, 87, 926, 1987.

144. Moffatt, R.J., Dietary status of elite female high school gymnasts: inadequacy of vitamin and mineral intake, *J. Am. Diet. Assoc.*, 84, 1361, 1984.

145. Huber, L.H., Zeigler, P., Congdon, K., Lindholm, S., and Manfredi, T.G., Nutritional status of college female gynmasts and cross-country runners, *Med. Sci. Sports Exer.*, 18, S-64, 1986.

146. Calabrese, L.H., Nutritional and medical aspects of gymnastics, *Clinic Sports Med.*, 4, 23, 1985.

147. Rucinski, A., Relationship of body image and dietary intake of competitive ice skaters, *J. Am. Diet. Assoc.*, 89, 98, 1989.

148. Worme, J.D., Lickteig, J.A., Reynolds, R.D., and Deuster, P.A., Consumption of a dehydrated ration for 31 days at moderate altitudes: energy intakes and physical performance, *J. Am. Diet. Assoc.*, 91, 1543, 1991.

149. Duncan, R., A comparison between the energy blance of men on long and short sledding journeys, *Nutrition*, 4, 357, 1988.

150. Morozov, V.I., Priyatkin, S.A., Rogozkin, V.A., Shishina, N.N., and Fedorova, G.P., Vitamin supply, iron status and the state of the nonspecific resistance system in athletes of different ages and sexes, *Soviet Sports Rev.*, 23, 152, 1988.

151. Ellsworth, N.M., Hewitt, B.F., and Haskell, W.L., Nutrient intake of the elite male and female Nordic skiers, *Phys. Sportsmed.*, 13, 79, 1985.

152. Simonsen, J.C., Sherman, W.M., Lamb, D. R., Dernbach, A.R., Doyle, J.A., and Strauss, R., Dietary carbohydrate, muscle glycogen, and power output during rowing training, *J. Appl. Physiol.*, 70, 1500, 1991.

153. Bergen-Cico, D.K. and Short, S.H., Dietary intakes, energy expenditures, and anthropometric characteristics of adolescent female cross-country runners, *J. Am. Diet. Assoc.*, 92, 611, 1992.

154. Baer, J.T. and Taper, L.J., Amenorrheic and eumenorrheic adolescent runners: dietary intake and exercise training status, *J. Am. Diet. Assoc.*, 92, 89, 1992.

155. Manore, M.M., Thompson, J.L., and Skinner, J.S., Nutrient intakes in elite male runners with low and balanced (BAL) energy intakes, *Med. Sci. Sports Exer.*, 23, S-75, 1991.

156. Clark, N. and Snyder, A., Nutritional practices of elite male runners, *J. Am. Diet. Assoc.*, 90, A-31, 1990.

157. Pate, R.R., Sargent, R.G., Baldwin, C., and Burgess, M.L., Dietary intake of women runners, *Int. J. Sport Med.*, 11, 461, 1990.

158. Manore, M.M., Basenfelder, P.D., Carroll, S.S., and Hooker, S.P., Nutrient intakes and iron status in female long distance runners during training, *J. Am. Diet. Assoc.*, 89, 257, 1989.

159. Peters, A.J., Dressendorfer, R.H., Rimar, J., and Keen, C.L., Diets of endurance runners competing in a 20-day road race, *Phys. Sportsmed.*, 14, 63, 1986.

160. Dressendorfer, R.H., Wade, C.E., Keen, C.L., and Scaff, J.H., Plasma mineral levels in marathon runners during a 20-day road race, *Phys. Sportsmed.*, 10, 113, 1982.

161. Deuster, P.A., Kyle, S.B., Moser, P.B., Vigersky, R.A., Singh, A., and Schoomaker, E.B., Nutritional survey of highly trained women runners, *Am. J. Clin. Nutr.,* 44, 954, 1986.

162. Clark, N., Nelson, M., and Evans, W., Nutrition education for elite female runners, *Phys. Sportsmed.,* 18, 124, 1988.

163. Snyder, A.C., Dvorak, L.L., and Roepke, J.B., Dietary patterns and iron parameters of middle aged female runners, *Med. Sci. Sports Exer.,* 19, S-38, 1987.

164. Haymes, E.M. and Spillman, D.M., Iron status of women distance runners, sprinters, and moderately active women, *Med. Sci. Sports Exer.,* 19, S-20, 1987.

165. Spillman, D.M. and Haymes, E.M., Nutrient intake of an elite collegiate women's track team, *J. Am. Diet. Assoc.,* 87, 91, 1987.

166. Besenfelder, P.D., Manore, M.M., and Wells, C.L., Effect of training on iron status in female long-distance runners, *J. Am. Diet. Assoc.,* 86, 122, 1986.

167. Thompson, P.D., Culliname, E., Eshleman, R., and Herbert, P.N., Lipoprotein changes when a reported diet is tested in distance runners, *Am. J. Clin. Nutr.,* 39, 368, 1984.

168. Bassler, T.J., Hazards of restrictive diets, *J. Am. Diet. Assoc.,* 252, 483, 1984.

169. Lampe, J.W., Slavin, J.L., and Apple, F.S., Poor iron status of women runners training for a marathon, *Int. J. Sport Med.,* 7, 111, 1986.

170. Grace, S.J. and Jeffrey, D.M., Iron, zinc and copper intakes of women track team members, *Fed. Proc.,* 42, 803, 1983.

171. Singh, A., Evans, P., Gallagher, K.L., and Deutster, P.A., Dietary intakes and biochemical profiles of nutritional status of ultramarathoners, *Med. Sci. Sports Exer.,* 25, 328, 1992.

172. Eden, B.D. and Abernethy, P.J., Nutritional intake during an ultraendurance running race, *Int. J. Sport Nutr.,* 4, 166, 1994.

173. Cummings, C.M., Brevard, P.B., and Pearson, J.M., Recreational runners' diets compare favorably with Step I Diet, *Int. J. Sport Nutr.,* 3, 349, 1993.

174. Rico, J., Frontera, W.R., Rivera, M.A., Mole, P.A., and Meredith, C.N., Nutritional habits and body composition of elite soccer players, *Med. Sci. Sports Exer.,* 24, S-288, 1992.

175. Hickson, J.F., Schrader, J.W., Pivarnik, J.H., and Stockton, J.E., Nutritional intake from food sources of soccer athletes during two stages of training, *Nutr. Rep. Int.,* 34, 85, 1986.

176. Tater, D., Leglise, D., Person, B., Lambert, D., and Bercovici, J.P., Lipoproteins status in professional football players after period of vacation and one month after a new intensive training program, *Horm. Metab. Res.,* 19, 24, 1987.

177. Barr, S.I., Relationship of eating attitudes to anthropometric variables and dietary intakes of female collegiate swimmers, *J. Am. Diet. Assoc.,* 91, 976, 1991.

178. Berning, J.R., Troup, J.P., VanHandel, P.J., Daniels, J., and Daniels, N., The nutritional habits of young adolescent swimmers, *Int. J. Sport Nutr.,* 1, 240, 1991.

179. Lukaski, H.C., Hoverson, B.S., Gallagher, S.K., and Bolonchuk, W.W., Physical training and copper, iron and zinc status of swimmers, *Am. J. Clin. Nutr.,* 51, 1093, 1990.

180. Lukaski, H.C., Hoverson, B.S., Molne, D.B., and Bolonchuk, W.W., Copper, zinc, and iron status of female swimmers, *Nutr. Res.,* 9, 493, 1989.

181. Campbell, M.L. and MacFadyen, K.L., Nutritional knowledge, beliefs and dietary practices of competitive swimmers, *Can. Home Econ. J.,* 34, 47, 1984.

182. Bureau of Nutritional Sciences, Dietary Standards of Canada, Ottawa: Health and Welfare, Canada, 1975.

183. Lindeman, A.K., Eating and training habits of triathletes: a balancing act, *J. Am. Diet. Assoc.,* 90, 991, 1990.

184. Applegate, E.A., Nutritional concerns of the ultraendurance triathlete, *Med. Sci. Sports Exer.,* 21, S-205, 1989.

185. Applegate, E.A., Nutritional considerations for ultraendurance performance, *Int. J. Sport Nutr.,* 1, 118, 1991.

186. Rehrer, J.J., van Kemenade, M., Meester, W., Brouns, F., and Saris, W.H.M., Gastrointestinal complaints in relation to dietary intake in triathletes, *Int. J. Sport Nutr.,* 2, 48, 1992.

187. Burke, L.M. and Read, R.S.D., Diet patterns of elite Australian male triathletes, *Phys. Sportsmed.,* 15, 140, 1987.

188. Bazzarre, T.L., Marquart, L.F., Izurieta, M., and Jones, A., Incidence of poor nutritional status among triathletes, endurance athletes and control subjects, *Med. Sci. Sports Exer.,* 18, S-90, 1986.

189. Novak, J., Super iron-man competitions, *Natl. Strength Cond. Assoc. J.,* 7, 66, 1985.

190. Barnes, L., How physicians can help high school wrestlers control weight, *Phys. Sportsmed.,* 15, 166, 1987.

191. Tipton, C.M., Commentary: physicians should advise wrestlers about weight loss, *Phys. Sportsmed.,* 15, 160, 1987.

192. Schwarzokopf, R. and Jensen, D., The effects of dietary control on making weight in collegiate wrestlers, *Med. Sci. Sports Exer.,* 19, S-69, 1987.

193. Gunderson, H.K. and McIntosh, M.K., An increased incidence of overweight, obesity, and indicators of chronic disease among ex-collegiate wrestlers, *J. Am. Diet. Assoc.,* 90, A-121, 1990.

194. Williams, M.H., *Nutrition for Fitness and Sport,* 4th ed., William C. Brown, Dubuque, IA, 1995.

Chapter 24

NUTRITION AND PERFORMANCE IN HOT, COLD, AND HIGH ALTITUDE ENVIRONMENTS

_____ Eldon W. Askew

CONTENTS

I.   INTRODUCTION

Humans are remarkably adaptive, surviving and even thriving in physical environments outside their normal "comfort" zone. Man accomplishes these adaptations through metabolic and behavioral changes. Environments that threaten to overwhelm the ability of humans to adjust their metabolism and/or change behavioral strategies have been referred to as "hostile" environments.[1] This terminology is somewhat of a misnomer, since man can function safely and effectively in extremes of environments, provided adequate behavioral precautions (e.g., clothing, shelter, food, water) are taken. The environment becomes "hostile" only when man has entered it unprepared or the environment is so severe that it threatens to surpass man's ability to adapt or respond appropriately to its challenges.

Although humans are "remarkably adaptive," they have limitations. One of these limitations is homeothermy. Shephard[2] described humans as being " ... metabolic hostages of the homeothermic condition." This means regardless of the environmental temperatures, man must defend the normal body temperature of 37°C (98.5°F) within a relative narrow range of temperatures. We have several physiologic defense mechanisms at our disposal (e.g., shivering, sweating, vasodilation, or vasoconstriction) to help maintain homeothermy. When the capability of these physiological defense mechanisms and compensating behavioral mechanisms are exceeded and body core temperature drops below 35°C (95°F) or rises above 41°C (106°F), the human body functions at such reduced efficiency that both physical and mental performance deteriorates rapidly. Left unchecked, hypothermia and hyperthermia can be life threatening. Hypoxia associated with high-altitude environments can also impose severe restrictions on physical performance and jeopardize survival. High altitudes are usually accompanied by cold temperatures, compounding environmental stress and metabolic challenge.

The body's metabolic response to heat, cold, and hypoxia can also be impaired by inadequate nutrition. This is depicted schematically in Figure 1. Appetite and thirst responses are frequently inappropriate in these environmental extremes, leading to inadequate calorie or fluid intakes. The availability of water and food is often limited due to logistical constraints. Backpackers, mountaineers, and explorers are usually limited to the food they can carry with them in their packs. The weight of these packs is critical; often food and water are sacrificed to make room for essential equipment, clothing, and gear. Inadequate dietary energy (particularly carbohydrate and protein) can result in glycogen depletion and loss of lean body mass. A chronic deficiency of energy (and in particular carbohydrate) will lead to the mobilization and oxidation of body fat which in turn leads to increased ketone body production. If ketone body production exceeds the kidneys' capacity to produce bicarbonate to buffer the ketone bodies (ketoacids), ketoacidosis can develop. Left unchecked, ketoacidosis can have detrimental metabolic consequences. As blood pH drops, the efficiency of the body's metabolic processes is reduced. This, in turn can result in impaired thermoregulation and impaired muscle strength, coordination, and endurance. Inadequate fluid intakes coupled with increased sweating, loss of lung-humidified air to an arid environment or altitude, or cold-induced diuresis can lead to dehydration and compromised thermoregulation and endurance. The usual increased energy and fluid demands for work in environmental extremes can be exacerbated by anorexia (hypophagia) and inappropriate thirst response (hypodipsia). The effects of hypophagia and hypodipsia can be further complicated by the general lack of food and water in cold, arid, or high-altitude settings. Persistent negative energy and fluid balances can combine to cause substantial decreases in physical performance capacities.[3-7]

Expeditionary or recreational outdoor activities are frequently conducted in hot, cold, high-altitude, or rugged-terrain environments. Mountaineering, cross-country skiing, snowshoeing, sledging, and backpacking can be as physically demanding as more conventional sporting events, plus there is an added element of danger. The wilderness is much less forgiving of mistakes than an urban environment where medical care is just minutes away. A miscalculation of physical ability or inadequate preparation can be life threatening in environmental extremes. Proper education, planning, preparation, equipment, and training are essential for work in the heat, cold, and high altitudes.

Proper nutrition is an often-overlooked but critical component of planning to support effective work under these conditions. The information in this chapter may be useful to individuals planning nutritional support for work or recreation in hot (greater than 30°C/86°F), cold (less than 0°C/32°F), or at high-altitude (greater than 3050 m/10,000 ft elevation) environments.

II. ENVIRONMENT, METABOLISM, AND NUTRIENT REQUIREMENTS

Extremes in the external environment can influence the requirements for certain nutrients[8] and may have implications for people who live, work, or recreate, and athletes who train or compete, under these conditions. The reader is referred to recent publications of workshop proceedings by the Institute of Medicine on nutritional needs in hot, cold, and

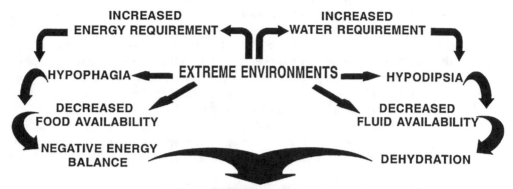

**CASCADE EFFECT OF ENVIRONMENTAL EXTREMES
ON WORK PERFORMANCE**

FIGURE 1 Schematic representation of the influence of extreme environments upon energy balance, hydration status, and resultant consequences of inadequate food or fluid intake. This generalized diagram illustrates the influence of heat, cold, and/or high altitude on the cascade of events that can lead to physiological consequences and impaired performance. (From Askew, E. W., in *Nutrition in Exercise and Sport*, 2nd ed., CRC Press, 1994, p 457. With permission.)

high-altitude environments for detailed discussions of the influence of the physical environment on nutrient requirements.[9,10] The need for additional vitamins and minerals may be influenced by certain environments, but the two nutrients most often in short supply are energy (more specifically carbohydrate) and water.[8] Achieving energy and fluid balance is often difficult in environmental extremes, for the reasons illustrated in Figure 1. Consolazio[11] estimated energy requirements for work in temperate, hot, cold, and high-altitude environments. These guidelines are shown in Table 1. More precise determinations of energy requirements utilizing the doubly labeled water technique (DLW) have been made in recent

TABLE 1 Energy Requirements for Physical Activity in Temperate, Cold, and Hot Environments

Physical Activity	Environment (kcal/kg)[b]		
	Temperate[a]	Cold	Hot
Light	32–44	35–46	40–54
Moderate	45–52	47–55	55–61
Heavy	53–63	56–68	62–75

[a] Altitude energy requirements are similar to temperate environment energy requirements. From Consolazio, C. F., *Army Research and Development Newsmagazine*, November 1966, p. 24. With permission.

[b] 1 kJ = 239 kcal.

years, eliminating some of the inherent inaccuracies of estimating food intakes. While the actual caloric requirement depends upon both the environment and the activity, energy expenditures measured over extended time periods by DLW are quite high, generally greater than 4000 kcal/d (16.74 MJ/d).[8] Extremely high energy expenditure levels (approaching 6700 kcal/d (28 MJ/d) have been reported for high altitude climbing expeditions[12] and manhauling sledges on an Arctic expedition.[13]

Athletes can sustain a high-level work output only when they manage to maintain energy balance.[14] Prolonged caloric underconsumption has adverse effects on lean body mass, physical performance, and host defense against infection.[3,15,16] However, moderate intensity work is not necessarily severely impaired following hypocaloric diets for relatively short durations.[6,17] More commonly, the upper limit of power output during endurance exercise with intensity greater than 60% VO_2max is limited during energy deficiency[14] and the ability of muscles to resist fatigue may be reduced.[18,19] Energy (more specifically carbohydrate) deficiency results in reduced muscle glycogen stores[20] and an increased reliance upon body fat stores to support work output.[3]

Trekkers often take along high-fat foods to increase the energy density of their diets. Under most circumstances, relying upon dietary or body fat stores to meet energy requirements in high energy expenditure activities in the heat, cold, or at high altitude is not advisable. Given a sufficient period for adaptation, muscles are able to shift their substrate utilization from carbohydrate to lipid,[21] this permits maintenance of only a relatively low intensity work load. High-fat diets are not generally recommended for environmental extremes where high power outputs are necessary (due to the requirement of carbohydrate by muscles for maximum power output).[14] High-fat diets may not be well tolerated (reduced appetite appeal or digestibility) in hot or high-altitude settings; however, they may be tolerated relatively well in cold environments close to sea level.

Exposures to extreme heat, cold, or high altitude alters muscle metabolism by a variety of factors, including muscle temperature, pH, O_2 tension, as well as cofactor and substrate availability.[22] As an example, unacclimatized individuals generally exhibit greater muscle glycogen breakdown, glycolytic flux, and lactate accumulation in extreme environments compared to temperate conditions at sea level.[22] (The "lactate paradox" of diminished blood lactate following *maximal* exercise at altitude compared to sea level is an exception to this generalization.[23])

III. NUTRIENT REQUIREMENTS FOR WORK IN HOT ENVIRONMENTS

Adequate fluid replacement overshadows all other considerations of nutrient requirements for work in a hot environment.[24] Drinking adequate water for work in the heat prevents dehydration, heat illness, and reduced performance.[4,25] Heat acclimation can reduce sodium requirements for work in the heat,[5] but water requirements remain relatively unaffected.[4,26] Thirst is a poor indicator of hydration status.[25] Intense thirst is usually noticed at 5–6% body weight loss due to dehydration. By this time physical performance is compromised. Vague discomfort, lethargy, weariness, sleepiness, and apathy, as well as elevated body core temperature, heart rate, and muscular fatigue are noted as body water loss reaches the 3–5% level. The magnitude of the increase in body core temperature and heart rate elicited by dehydrating exercise is linearly related to the level of body water deficit.[27]

Severe hypohydration can lead to decreased blood volume and increased plasma osmolality, which can decrease sweating and heat dissipation.[27,28] Approximately eighty percent of the energy metabolized during exercise in a hot environment is liberated as heat (20% is utilized for mechanical work) and 80–90% of heat dissipation during exercise in a hot-dry

TABLE 2   Water Requirements (l/h) for Rest and Work in the Heat as Influenced by Solar Load and Temperature

Temperature and Relative Humidity (°F @ % rh)	Indoors (No Solar Load)				Outdoors (Clear Sky)			
	Rest	Light	Medium	Heavy	Rest	Light	Medium	Heavy
85 @ 50	0.2	0.5	1.0	1.5	0.5	0.9	1.3	1.8
96 @ 30	0.3	0.9	1.3	1.9	0.8	1.2	1.7	2.0
105 @ 30	0.6	1.0	1.5	2.0	0.9	1.3	1.9	2.0
115 @ 20	0.8	1.2	1.7	2.0	1.1	1.5	2.0	2.0
120 @ 20	0.9	1.3	1.9	2.0	1.3	1.7	2.0	2.0

Note: The values for water requirements in l/h were calculated according to the prediction model of Shapiro et al.[32] courtesy of L. A. Stroschein, Biophysics and Biomedical Modeling Division, U.S. Army Research Institute of Environmental Medicine, Natick, MA. The following conditions were assumed in these calculations: clothing, tropical fatigues; heat-acclimatized subjects; wind speed 2 m/s.

environment is accomplished by the evaporation of sweat.[29,30] Water consumed during exercise in the heat can move to the sweat glands within 9–18 min of ingestion, where it is available for cooling the body.[29] Each milliliter of sweat evaporated from the skin will lead to a heat loss or dissipation of approximately 0.6 kcal (2.5 kJ).[30] Sweat rates are highly variable between individuals, but can reach 2l/h for prolonged time periods.[31] Dehydration depends in large part upon sweat loss, which is in turn determined by exercise intensity and duration, as well as environmental factors such as temperature, solar load, wind speed, and relative humidity and clothing. The influence of these factors on water requirements for work in the heat is illustrated in Table 2.[32,33]

It is important to note under certain environmental conditions a 10°F (5.6°C) increase in temperature can cause a 50–60% increase in water requirements at *rest*. Superimposing an increased work load at high temperatures greatly increases fluid requirements. The solar load, relative humidity, clothing, wind speed, and prior acclimation to heat all interact in determining sweat rates, insensible water loss, and water requirements at any given workload.[33] Consolazio[11] recommended up to 12 l of water per day for soldiers engaged in heavy physical activity in 100°F (37.8°C) weather. While this level of water intake may be necessary to replenish fluid losses in a hot environment, it may be difficult to ingest such a large volume. As an example, it would be necessary to consume 1 l of water upon arising in the morning, 1 l with each of three meals, and 1 l for each hour during an 8-h work day to achieve a daily intake of 12 l. This rate of fluid consumption is possible but requires conscious effort. The U.S. military refers to planned or programmed water drinking as "water discipline"[34] and credits this doctrine for the relatively low incidence of U.S. heat casualties in the 1990–1991 Desert War in Iraq and Kuwait. It is best to "force" water intake in a regular and planned drinking program in advance of, during, and after a period of work in the heat. Research has shown that acute water loading (1.5–2 l of water drunk 1 h before exercise) is of little or no benefit to work performance in the heat compared to chronic forced water intake (double the quantity normally consumed over a 1 week time period)[35] and may even be detrimental due to "uncomfortable feelings" in the stomach following acute water loading.[36]

As a general rule, salt supplements are not necessary for work in the heat unless water is available but food is not.[37] Since the typical daily American diet[38] contains 6–18 g of NaCl, replacement of sodium lost during exercise in the heat can usually be met by consuming normally salted food in proportion to caloric requirements.[11,37] This is usually an adequate amount of sodium to replace that lost in sweat in a hot environment. Armstrong et al.[39] demonstrated that humans could successfully acclimate to work in the heat on as little as 6 g of NaCl/d although higher levels of sodium intake (8 g/d) reduced some of the adverse symptoms associated with this period of heat acclimation.

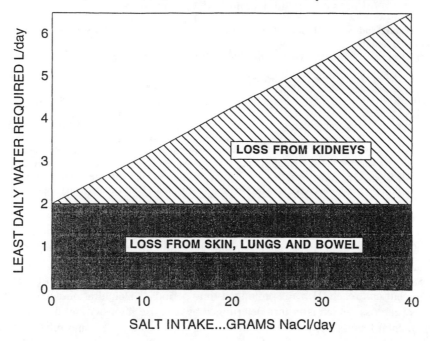

Influence of salt intake on water requirements

FIGURE 2 Estimated minimum daily water requirement of a sedentary man weighing 70 kg at an ambient temperature of 75°F, relative humidity of 19%, consuming 0–30 g of NaCl/day. (From Baker, E. M., Plough, I. C., and Allen, T. H., *Am. J. Clin. Nutr.*, 12, 394, 1963. With permission.)

Sodium losses can, however, be quite high at sustained moderate work rates in a hot environment. Sweat losses amounting to 12 l/24 h can result in the loss of 11,000–16,500 mg of Na[+] per day.[40] Under these conditions sodium replacement will require liberal salting of food, drinking water that contains 1.0 g of NaCl/l[11] (390 mg Na[+]), or consuming sodium containing "sports" beverages in place of a portion of the 12 l/d water requirement. Sodium supplementation should be given consideration only when fluid replacement is adequate. Barr et al.[41] found that sodium replacement during exercise in the heat does not appear necessary for moderate-intensity work up to 6 h duration. Excess salt consumption can place an added burden on water requirements in all environments (Figure 2).[42] In addition to increasing water requirements, high salt intake (without adequate water intake) can elevate plasma osmolality, which can lead to decreased sweating and as a result, increase thermal strain during work.[26]

Some sports drinks are promoted as enhancing water and/or glucose absorption due to their sodium content. There seems to be little basis for this claim. Gisolfi et al.[43] found that sodium concentrations of 0, 25, or 50 meq/l in a 6% carbohydrate solution had similar effects on water and glucose absorption from the gut. Likewise, Hargreaves et al.[44] found no effect of the sodium content of beverages on glucose bioavailability during exercise. The lack of effect of sodium upon water or glucose absorption from the gut may be due to the rapid mixing of ingested beverages with the sodium of intestinal secretions leading to similar osmotic concentrations of sodium along the gut. Whereas supplemental sodium in sports beverages is relatively ineffective in promoting fluid absorption, glucose in the sports drink does promote fluid absorption.[43] Murray[45] emphasized that complete rehydration following work in the heat is dependent upon the ingestion of both adequate fluid and sodium chloride. Salt plays a critical role in rehydration because the osmotic properties of Na[+] and Cl[-] ions assist in retaining fluid in the extracellular space.

Although water and sodium replenishment are the primary nutrients of concern in a hot environment, consideration should also be given to providing adequate energy. Food and water intakes are closely related; food intake is reduced during water deprivation and water intake is reduced during starvation.[46] Energy requirements for work in the heat may be elevated 0.5% for each 1°F increase as the ambient temperature increases from 86 to 104°F.[11] Below temperatures of 86°F (30°C), temperature has little influence on energy requirements until cold temperatures (requiring additional clothing to prevent excessive heat loss) are reached. The relatively small increase in energy requirements for work at high temperatures is believed to be attributable to increased cardiovascular work needed to dissipate heat, increased sweat gland activity, and metabolic rate. Consolazio et al.[47] found approximately a 10% increase in metabolic cost for work at 100°F (38°C) compared to work at 70°F (21°C). Sawka et al.[48] subsequently demonstrated that heat acclimation can lower the rate of metabolism during exercise in the heat by as much as 3%, indicating that the actual increase in energy requirements for work at high ambient temperatures may vary with the degree of heat acclimation of the individual.

Work in the heat has implications with regard to muscle glycogen synthesis and utilization.[20] Fink et al.[49] found that exercise in the heat increased muscle glycogen utilization, although this has not been observed in all studies.[28,50] Hargreaves[20] speculated that a reduction in muscle blood flow, increased muscle temperature, and elevated catecholamines may contribute to stimulation of muscle glycogenolysis during exercise in the heat. These observations indicate that exercise in the heat may increase glycogen utilization, although Febbraio et al.[51] found that the greater reliance upon carbohydrate as a fuel during exercise in the heat appears to be at least partially reduced after acclimation. Surprisingly, hypohydration comprising up to 5% body weight loss does not seem to impair muscle glycogen synthesis after exercise,[52] although hypohydration may lower resting metabolic rate.[53]

Sustained heavy sweat rates increase the loss of sodium and a number of other nutrients, including chloride, potassium, calcium, magnesium, iron, and nitrogen.[40] There is little evidence to suggest these nutrients cannot be replaced adequately by a normal diet.[31] Relying upon the diet to replace sodium chloride lost in the sweat does require a conscious effort to maintain food intake and hence sodium chloride intake. Murray[45] has calculated that a 2% body weight loss via sweating for an 80 kg individual will require the ingestion of 1.8 g of Na^+ (approximately 4.5 g of NaCl). This amount of dietary sodium replacement can easily be achieved by diet provided a diligent effort is made to eat to energy requirements.

Vitamin supplementation for work in the heat is also unnecessary, with two possible exceptions.[54] Vitamin C has been reported to facilitate heat acclimation,[55] and multiple B vitamins have been reported to lessen fatigue during work in the heat.[56] Generally speaking, vitamin and mineral supplements will be advantageous only for those with extremely poor dietary habits. Water supplementation during work in the heat is more critical than even carbohydrate supplementation,[31] since performance will be impacted sooner by heat and dehydration than depletion of muscle glycogen. Hence, the provision of water should take precedence over carbohydrate and electrolytes during exercise in the heat,[31] although carbohydrate-containing beverages may be more effective than plain water in the support of continuous exercise lasting longer than 50 min.[29] The key to carbohydrate and water provision during work in the heat is to administer both simultaneously to ensure complete rehydration.[45] Commercial carbohydrate/electrolyte or "sports" drinks containing 5–10% carbohydrate and ~20 meq Na^+/l are appropriate. If it is not feasible to use a carbohydrate/electrolyte drink, concentrate on rehydration with plain water accompanied by adequate food salted a bit more than normal.

Hydration solutions designed to deliver 1 g of glycerol/kg body weight prior to work in temperate, hot, or cold environments may help maintain a better hydration status than plain water alone.[57-60] This effect is believed to be due to glycerol's hyperhydrating properties. Glycerol may provide an osmotic force helping to maintain a fluid reservoir in the interstitial spaces of body tissues or influence reabsorption of water by the kidney.[57,59] The ingestion of a glycerol solution and water compared to water alone results in decreased urine output, decreased body temperature, increased sweat rate, and lower heart rate during moderate work in the heat.[57] Glycerol-induced hyperhydration appears to be a promising method of reducing the acute thermal burden during moderate exercise in the heat and may have application in cold or high altitude environments.[60]

IV. NUTRIENT REQUIREMENTS FOR WORK IN COLD ENVIRONMENTS

Energy requirements are the major consideration for providing nutritional support in a cold environment.[61] Energy expenditure in hot and high-altitude environments is usually limited by the rate of heat buildup and hypoxia, respectively, whereas in a cold environment the rate of energy expenditure (with proper clothing ventilation) is usually not restricted by the heat burden or hypoxia. In addition, high rates of energy expenditure in the cold (~29.3 MJ/d or ~7000 kcal/d) have been attributed to the high degree of motivation of cold-weather expedition team members.[62] Energy requirements in a cold environment are influenced by the intensity of the cold, windspeed, physical difficulties associated with working under winter conditions (preparing shelters, melting snow, locomotion on icy or snow-covered surfaces, etc.), and the light-dark cycle in arctic areas.[63-66] At the same time that energy requirements are high, energy intakes may be reduced by such factors as monotony of the diet and the difficulty of preparing food for consumption under adverse conditions.

People in a cold climate normally eat more than those in a warm climate. This observation agrees with the widely held belief that cold exposure increases energy requirements. This is generally true, but there are several caveats. Gray et al.[67] suggested that increased energy requirements were primarily due to a "hobbling" effect of the weight of the clothing and associated inefficiencies of locomotion. Teitlebaum and Goldman[68] subsequently demonstrated that the energy expenditure increase attributable to the weight of arctic clothing (24.6 lbs. or 11.2 kg) was greater than that which could be accounted for by the weight of the clothing alone and attributed it to "friction drag" between the multiple layers of arctic clothing. The weight of cold-weather clothing has decreased as technology has improved; however, clothing is still a considerable burden contributing to caloric expenditure.

Properly outfitted, modern cold-weather clothing ensembles now weigh 15–20 lbs. (6.8–9.0 kg) and still account for the major part of the additional energy expenditure in cold not attributed to discernable work such as skiing, snowshoeing, sledging, etc. Mechanical inefficiencies associated with "hobbling" and "clothing friction" combine with small energy requirements to heat and humidify inspired air and air "pumped" into and out of clothing sleeves and seams. These factors contribute to a 10–15% increase in the metabolic cost of working in the cold compared to unencumbered work in a temperate environment.[47,68,69]

Energy requirements for activities in a cold environment are considerably higher than the previously mentioned 10–15% increase when accompanied by heavy work. However, provided that adequate clothing is worn and allowances are made for the increased weight of the clothing, increases in energy requirements are usually comparable to those for similar activities in a temperate environment.[70,71] (However, energy requirements for an activity may be higher in certain cold environments if the terrain is inefficient for locomotion due to ice or snow.) Cold-weather energy expenditures can range from approximately 3200 kcal/d (13.4 MJ/d) in low-activity situations to 5000 kcal/d (20.9 MJ/d) during sledging and manhauling activities.[1] Although considerably higher rates of energy expenditure have been reported,[62] recent measurements of U.S. and Canadian military cold-weather energy expenditures have confirmed that 4000–5000 kcal/d (16.8–20.9 MJ/d) will usually meet cold weather energy requirements.[65,72,73] 4500 kcal/d (18.8 MJ/d) is a reasonable target figure for planning cold weather energy needs.[65]

The dietary patterns of natives of arctic and subarctic regions and their obvious success in coping with harsh environments have influenced arctic explorers to embrace diets high in fat and led to the general belief that diets high in fat impart a special advantage for work in the cold. Such information is largely anecdotal and probably relates more to the availability of local foods (seal, fish, whale, caribou) and the familiarity of indigenous natives with these foods than any real nutritional advantage. Indeed, many Alaskan natives (Eskimos, Indians, and Aleuts) currently consume diets containing 38% of the energy from fat, which is similar to that of the general U.S. population (37%).[74] This change toward lower-fat diets probably reflects the availability of a changing supply of local foods rather than any conscious or unconscious choice influenced by cold weather. Swain et al.[75] reported the caloric consumption distribution pattern of military troops stationed in cold, temperate, and tropical areas was similar across these environments.

Few studies in the literature deal specifically with nutrient requirements in the cold. These limited studies support the concept that cold does not cause a greater demand for any nutrients other than calories.[66,76,77] Anecdotal reports of "craving" classes of food such as fat or carbohydrate have not been substantiated,[76] yet the idea persists that high-fat diets are especially appropriate for cold-weather operations. Humans can adapt over a period of time to a high-fat diet[21,78] and much of the submaximal endurance type of work in the cold such as cross-country skiing, snowshoeing, and sledging can be supported by VO_2max efforts of less than 60%. These moderate sustained power outputs can be supported relatively well by high levels of lipid oxidation.[14,78]

The question next arises: "Does the consumption of a high-fat diet in the cold increase cardiovascular health risk?" It would be irresponsible to recommend a chronically high-fat diet; however, it appears that cardiovascular risk is minimized by the high rate of caloric expenditure associated with work in the cold. An example of this is provided by Ekstedt et al.[79] Despite consuming a diet containing twice the fat and cholesterol of the low-fat group, cross-country skiers fed the high-fat diet decreased their cholesterol, very-low-density lipoproteins (VLDL), and triglycerides over an 8-d period of cross-country skiing in the cold. The observed decreases were similar to those of the low-fat group and suggests that, in the short run, at least, hard physical work can lessen the normally adverse effect of a high-fat diet on blood lipids. In addition to the anecdotal, historical, and scientific evidence that high-fat diets are well tolerated in the cold, there is also evidence to suggest that high-fat diets may improve cold tolerance provided that meals are fed at regular intervals during cold exposure.[80]

Despite the arguments that can be made for high-fat diets in the cold, there is evidence suggesting that carbohydrates are more important than fat in fueling metabolic heat production during cold exposure.[22,81] The effect of cold exposure on the utilization of metabolic substrates is illustrated in Figure 3. Vallerand and Jacobs[81] studied the contribution of protein, carbohydrate, and fat to energy expenditure during 2-h exposures of semi-nude men to warm (29°C or 84°F) or cold (2°C or 36°F) environments. Cold exposure elevated energy expenditure almost 2.5 times over that observed for subjects in the warm environment. This increase in energy expenditure resulted in an increase in carbohydrate oxidation of 588% and a 63% increase in fat oxidation. Protein oxidation was unaffected. These results demonstrate that cold exposure causes a much greater increase in carbohydrate utilization than lipid. They also suggest that both fat and carbohydrate fuel the shivering response in humans, with carbohydrate (presumably glycogen) being the more important of the two fuel sources. Shivering is impaired by fasting and hypoglycemia.[82,83] Light exercise in the cold results in lower muscle glycogen levels than similar exercise at normal temperature.[84] These observations, coupled with the observation that low muscle glycogen levels are associated with a more rapid body cooling during cold exposure,[85] suggests that muscle glycogen and blood

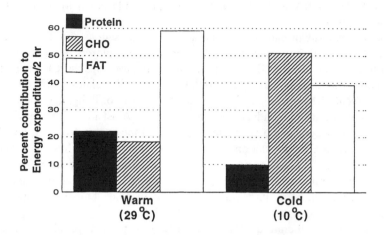

FIGURE 3 Influence of cold exposure on the calorie source for energy expenditure in resting male subjects. Seven subjects were exposed to both warm (29°C) and cold (10°C) conditions for 2 h while they rested (clothed in shorts). Cold exposure induced a body heat debt of 825.9 ± 63.3 kJ, whereas warm exposure produced a heat gain of 92.4 ± 19.2 kJ. Energy expenditure in the cold was 1519.4 ± 150.6 kJ, whereas in the warm it was 617.8 ± 28 kJ. (Data from Vallerand, A. L. and Jacobs, I., *Eur. J. Appl. Physiol.*, 58, 873,1989. With permission.)

glucose are important, if not critical, fuels for thermogenesis from shivering.[86] Fat can potentially contribute to thermogenesis by fueling the shivering response and/or through triglyceride-fatty acid cycling.[87] The relative importance of these two cycles in humans is not known.[88] Young et al.[88] have reported that metabolic heat production was not significantly affected by dietary lowering of muscle glycogen stores prior to cold exposure, indicating either that fat can adequately fuel cold-induced thermogenesis under reduced muscle glycogen concentrations or that a critical level of muscle glycogen depletion had not been reached. Martineau and Jacobs[89] were unable to alter the thermal responses to cold exposure by simultaneously lowering muscle glycogen and plasma-free fatty acids, leading them to suggest that thermal and metabolic responses in the cold can rapidly adjust to compensatory utilization of alternative fuels. Although the increase in metabolic rate secondary to cold exposure is dependent upon an adequate supply of metabolic substrates, the relationship between cold stress and substrate utilization remains poorly understood. Glickman-Weiss et al.[90] suggested that the metabolic responses to cold exposure is multifactorial and is related to the intensity of the cold stress, the intensity of the shivering response, diet composition, amount of food consumed prior to cold exposure, amount and pattern of fat deposition, and the overall rate of heat loss. Despite an early study by Keeton et al.[91] that indicated that high carbohydrate diets were superior to high protein diets with respect to cold tolerance and accumulated evidence that carbohydrate is closely related to heat generation via the shivering response,[81] recent studies of supplementary carbohydrate provision during cold exposure have failed to demonstrate a beneficial effect of carbohydrate feeding on cold tolerance during 120 min exposure to 8, 12, or 27°C temperatures.[92,93] Since the degree of cold exposure and subsequent shivering was of relatively low intensity in these studies,[92,93] Glickman-Weiss el al.[92] did not rule out an effect of diet on thermoregulatory and metabolic responses to cold exposure under different cold exposure conditions. Although the lowering of carbohydrate stores does not necessarily result in reduced heat production,[88,89] there is evidence to suggest that a stimulation of carbohydrate oxidation by the ingestion of ephedrine-caffeine mixtures or ephedrine-xanthine mixtures can improve cold tolerance in humans.[94,95] Ephedrine/xanthine mixtures are currently one of the most promising pharmacological means to enhance thermoregulatory thermogenesis in the cold.[96]

Water requirements for work in cold environments are similar to those for temperate environments.[97] Roberts et al.[98] suggested that it is possible to remain adequately hydrated in the cold (at low activity levels) on a minimum of 3 l of water per day. Edwards et al.[99,100] and King et al.[101] reported water consumption rates of 3.5–5 l/d for U.S. Army solders engaged in arctic cold-weather training. An allowance of 4–6 l/d will usually cover increased fluid requirements for humidifying inspired air and a certain degree of sweating that may accompany moderate to heavy work levels in the cold.[102] Although water requirements are not as high in the cold as in the heat, the consequences of dehydration are still important. Exposure to cold can cause a reduction in the sense of thirst and consequently reduced water consumption.[99,103] This relationship was observed by Edwards and Roberts,[99] who noted that elevated urine specific gravities (>1.030) were associated with the consumption of less than 2 l of water per day by soldiers working in the cold. When forced drinking was initiated, water consumption in these soldiers doubled and urine specific gravities rapidly decreased to the normal range of 1.020. They also found that water consumption and food intake were strongly correlated (r = 0.76).[99] Dann et al.[103] observed marked voluntary dehydration in a control group during a 4.5-h, 1700-m, cold-weather (0°C) march. The control group exhibited evidence of dehydration, decreased glomerular filtration rate, osmotic clearance, and urine volume compared to the imposed drinking discipline group. Dann et al.[103] calculated that a fluid intake of 150 ml/h during exercise in the cold would be required to maintain a urinary flow rate of about 1 ml/kg/h necessary for a good state of hydration.

Hypohydration in the cold can reduce food consumption, efficiency of physical and mental performance, and resistance to cold exposure.[60,104] While adequate fluid intake is paramount in preventing hypohydration in the cold, it is also prudent to consider the temperature of fluid and food provided for work in the cold. Warm fluids and heated foods are generally recommended in the cold, whenever possible, to impart a feeling of warmth and well-being.[104] The warming effect of a hot beverage in the cold is probably related to its effect upon subsequent vasodilation and increased blood flow to cold extremities rather than to the actual quantity of heat contained in the ingested fluid. Wilson and Culik[105] have provided the thought-provoking suggestion that the real advantage to providing warm food in the cold is the net heat savings that results to the body compared to ingesting ambient temperature (cold) food. Their calorimetric calculations based upon observations conducted with penguins fed warm or cold krill (arctic crustaceans) suggest that up to 13% of the daily energy expenditure of the penguin may be devoted to heating cold ingested food to body temperature. The lesson for human sojourners in the cold is apparent and is probably applicable even in the absence of similar human studies.

It is clear that in a cold environment, humans must adapt their behavior to minimize cold exposure and achieve homeothermy; failure to do so will result in rapid performance decrements and even death. The energy costs of performing any task under extreme cold conditions is higher than performing the same task under temperate conditions because of the difficulties in working in heavy clothing and traveling in snow. Working in cold environments does not lead to an increased requirement for any nutrient other than energy and perhaps antioxidants.[8] Carbohydrate intake may be of concern if high power output (>50% VO$_2$max) is required for extended periods of time. Replenishment of muscle glycogen stores will assure the availability of this fuel during exercise and shivering to support thermogenesis and aid the body in fighting hypothermia. Caloric demands for moderate to high activity levels in arctic and subarctic areas are usually adequately supported by 4000–5000 kcal/d (16.8–20.9 MJ/d).

Weight loss is common during cold-weather field expeditions, often due to the monotony of the diet and difficulty in preparing food, coupled with increased energy expenditures. Water requirements are not increased in cold-weather operations, but intakes may be decreased due to the difficulty of melting snow and ice and the tendency of cold weather travelers to utilize dry foods that will not freeze and can be eaten without thawing. Inadequate hydration may decrease the body's ability to adjust to cold stress.

V. NUTRIENT REQUIREMENTS FOR WORK AT HIGH ALTITUDE

Abrupt exposure to altitudes greater than 10,000 ft (3050 m) elevation is frequently associated with symptoms of altitude sickness.[106] Altitude sickness is a generalized term referring to a combination of symptoms, including headaches, anorexia, nausea, vomiting, and malaise. Gradual acclimation to progressively higher altitude exposure is the best preventive medicine for high-altitude sickness. Gradual ascent over a period of days from sea level to high altitude is accompanied by a number of simultaneous physiologic adaptations that permit the accomplishment of significant work with minimal physical symptoms other than an increased perceived exertion. Unfortunately, it is not always practical or possible to delay ascent to altitude. Soldiers and rescue workers frequently must travel abruptly to high altitudes to perform critical missions. Prior acclimation is not possible. Abrupt transportation from sea level to high altitude is usually accompanied by debilitating altitude sickness influencing symptoms, mood, and performance.[107] These uncomfortable symptoms usually increase in intensity for periods of up to 48 h after altitude exposure and then gradually lessen.[108] Unfortunately, it is usually during the first 48 h at altitude that critical work must be accomplished. Although there is some debate as to whether altitude exposure causes an absolute increase in energy requirements above that of similar work performed at sea level,[71,109] the usual activities associated with missions at altitude and the lack of adequate food intakes almost invariably result in an initially negative energy balance.[12,110-113] Altitude exposure (and the accompanying hypoxia) is associated with approximately a 17% increase in basal metabolic rate which raises energy requirements above sea level[114] (Figure 4). However, altitude exposure may be accompanied by a decrease in voluntary energy expenditure which may cancel the new effect of an increase in basal metabolic rate.[114] Energy expenditures in experienced and motivated climbers who are acclimated can be quite high[12] and depend upon the activity level achievable under hypoxic conditions.

Food intakes are typically reduced 10–50% during acute altitude exposure depending upon the individual and rapidity of ascent.[110-112] Rose et al.[115] observed depressed food intakes and weight loss at altitude even under the controlled chamber conditions of Operation Everest II. In this study, work requirements were relatively low and a thermoneutral hypobaric environment with an adequate quantity and variety of palatable food was provided. Reduced food intake under these conditions indicated that hypoxia by itself was a major factor reducing appetite and food intake. Adequate food intake can be achieved at altitude but it requires a concerted conscious effort of dietary management and forced eating.[112,114] The usual combination of anorexia and reduced food intake can potentially exert a negative effect on work performance at even moderate altitude.[71]

Numerous pharmacological attempts to reduce acute mountain sickness have been investigated, with limited success. High carbohydrate diets have been recommended as a "nonpharmacological" method to reduce the symptoms associated with acute mountain sickness.[1] To be effective, these diets should be fed prior to and during the initial 3- to 4-d critical period of acute altitude exposure. It should be noted that only a limited number of investigators have studied high-carbohydrate diets or carbohydrate supplements for the relief of acute mountain sickness and performance enhancement. Most, but not all, have reported some beneficial effects upon symptoms, mood, and performance. Consolazio et al.[116] conducted a study at 14,000 ft (4300 m) elevation with two groups of young sea-level natives transported

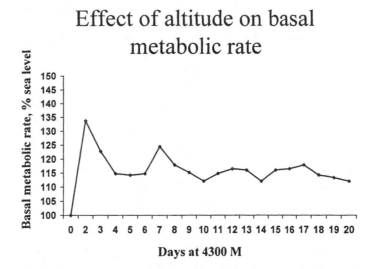

FIGURE 4 Basal metabolic rate at sea level (day 0) and 4300 m elevation (days 1–20). Basal oxygen consumption values expressed as a percent of sea level control (sea level control = 100% = 302 ml O_2/min). Values are means for seven subjects. (Adapted from Butterfield, G. E., Gates, J., Fleming, S., Brooks, G. A., Sutton, I. R., and Reeves, J. T., *J. Appl. Physiol.*, 72, 1741, 1992. With permission.)

abruptly to altitude. One group consumed a normal diet containing 35% of the calories in the form of carbohydrate. The second group consumed a diet containing approximately 70% of the calories from carbohydrate. The normal carbohydrate group was more nauseated, less energetic, and more depressed than the group consuming the high-carbohydrate diet. The normal carbohydrate group also experienced greater heart pounding, was more irritable, more tired, and less happy than the high carbohydrate group. They also felt less lively and experienced greater shortness of breath. Both groups experienced dizziness, cramping, headaches, and trouble sleeping to approximately the same degree. Work performance was compared in a relatively high-exertion, short-duration protocol consisting of walking on a treadmill at 3.5 mph on an 8% grade carrying a 20-kg pack. During the sea level control period all men completed the 15-min walk but, at altitude, the normal carbohydrate group averaged only 4.5 min, while the high-carbohydrate group averaged 9.8 min until exhaustion. Askew et al.[1,110] studied exercise at high altitude under conditions designed to stress muscle glycogen stores. They abruptly transported three groups of soldiers from sea level to 13,500 ft (4100 m) elevation (summit of Mauna Kea, Hawaii). One group of soldiers remained sedentary and consumed a normal military field ration (45% carbohydrate) during 4 d at this elevation. The other two groups were paired according to their VO_2 max determined at sea level and exercised for 2 h/d at altitude by running on a cross-country course at an exertion level of 70% of their maximum heart rate. One of the exercise groups consumed the same 45% carbohydrate ration as the sedentary group. The other exercise group consumed the same basal diet as the other two groups but received approximately 200 g of carbohydrate supplement per day through glucose polymer-supplemented beverages (approximately 40 g of carbohydrate per 8-oz (227 g) beverage). The nonsupplemented groups consumed similar beverages sweetened with a non-nutritive sweetener. All beverages were provided *ad libitum*. The nonsupplemented group consumed an average of 190 g of carbohydrate per day, whereas the group receiving the carbohydrate supplement consumed an average of 400 g of carbohydrate per day during the 4 d at altitude. Total voluntary mileage covered during the 2 h/d running period was recorded daily. The carbohydrate-supplemented group logged a significantly greater (p <0.05) 12% total miles covered over the course of this 4-d study. In addition to improving energy balance, carbohydrate supplementation also improved nitrogen balance in the initial phase of acute altitude exposure. Butterfield et al.[114] have confirmed that the negative nitrogen balances encountered at altitude is not due to any decrease in protein digestibility or absorption, but primarily due to negative energy balances.

The exact mechanism by which carbohydrate exerts a beneficial effect on relieving symptoms of altitude sickness and prolongs endurance at altitude is not known. Hansen et al.[117] showed that blood oxygen tension is increased by a high-carbohydrate diet, and Dramise et al.[118] reported that carbohydrate can increase lung pulmonary diffusion capacity at altitude. The energy production per liter of oxygen uptake is greater when carbohydrate is the energy source compared to fat (carbohydrate, 5.05 kcal/l (0.0211 kJ)/l O_2; fat, 4.69 kcal/l (0.0196 kJ)/l O_2) regardless of the oxygen tension in the inspired air.[119] Taken together, these different lines of evidence suggest that carbohydrate is a more efficient energy source for work at reduced oxygen tension.[120] The beneficial effect of high-carbohydrate diets on physical performance at sea level is well known.[7] Carbohydrate can prolong endurance by its effect on muscle glycogen stores which are in turn closely related to endurance. It is unlikely that the ergogenic effect of the high carbohydrate diets at altitude reported by Consolazio et al.[116] was related to a specific muscle glycogen effect, since the short exercise time periods (<10 min) should not have been limited by glycogen stores, but may have been related to the provision of blood glucose to the working hypoxic muscles. Caffeine has also been reported to enhance relatively short-term, high-intensity work at simulated high altitude,[121] perhaps via a similar influence upon blood glucose availability. Catecholaminergic agonists such as tyrosine may also be beneficial in reducing the stress of altitude exposure.[122]

There is little evidence that chronic or acute altitude exposure increases the requirement for any specific nutrient other than possibly vitamin E and iron.[123] Reviews of the effects of cold, energy expenditure, UV light exposure, and the reductive atmosphere at altitude indicates that supplementation of vitamins having an antioxidant function may be desirable at high altitude.[8,124,125] Supplemental vitamin E (2 × 200 mg daily) during a prolonged stay at high altitude prevented a "deterioration" of blood flow and a decrease in physical performance associated with free radical damage to cellular antioxidant defense systems.[126,127] Simon-Schnass[128] theorized that the "oxidative stress" during hypoxia is a consequence of alterations in the oxidation-reduction potential leading to lipid peroxidation and free radical production and subsequent oxidative injury to tissue and blood. Manipulations that improve oxygen delivery to tissues under the conditions of hypoxia are generally beneficial to work performance.[129] In general, dietary treatments that preserve or enhance the fluidity or deformability of red blood cell (RBC) membranes at altitude are beneficial to oxygen delivery to tissues. Exposure to hypoxia reduces red cell deformity (ability of RBC to bend or flex as they pass through a capillary bed).[130,131] This change in RBC membrane fluidity can be achieved by either exercise and altitude exposure[132] or exercise induced hypoxemia[133] at sea level. RBCs are also more fragile and susceptible to exercise-induced hemolysis at altitude.[134] The improvement of RBC membrane fluidity (increased ability to deform) can be achieved by two dietary mechanisms: supplementing the diet with polyunsaturated fatty acids[132,133] or protecting existing membrane polyunsaturated fatty acids from oxidizing by supplementing the diet with antioxidant(s) such as vitamin E.[126,127]

The suggestion that supplementary dietary iron may be beneficial at altitude stems from the observation that there is an increased erythropoietic response to altitude exposure as the oxygen delivery system of the body attempts to support increased hemoglobin synthesis at high altitude.[129] Although Hornbein[135] concluded that normal dietary iron intakes are adequate to support increased hemoglobin synthesis for males at high altitude, Hannon[136] suggested that females exposed to high altitude may benefit from a dietary iron supplement, and Stray-Gundersen et al.[137] have demonstrated that iron deficient runners regardless of sex fail to exhibit a normal hematopoietic response upon exposure to altitude. Although Berglund[129] recommended oral supplement iron (ferrous sulfate, 200–300 mg/d) for 2–3 weeks before ascent and continuation of iron supplementation for 2–4 weeks while at altitude, he cautioned that a simultaneous free radical production might be enhanced by excess free iron.

One of the inevitable consequences of work at high altitudes is weight loss, specifically of lean body mass.[113] Muscle wasting while at high altitudes has been noted by many expeditions and thought to be attributed to inadequate energy[114] and/or protein[138] intakes to support energy expenditure levels. Other investigators have noted the importance of the branched chain amino acids (BCAA) — leucine, isoleucine, valine — to oxidative pathways of energy generation at altitude[139,140] leading to the suggestion that BCAA supplementation in diets at altitude may help conserve body protein stores.[141] The effectiveness of BCAA supplementation during work at high altitude is controversial.[142,143] Some investigators believe BCAA supplementation may benefit the conservation of muscle mass,[141,143] while others hypothesize that an increase in oxidation of BCAA from exogenous or endogenous sources would put a drain on the carbon flux of the TCA cycle during prolonged exercise at altitude leading to glycogen depletion and might even lead to early fatigue.[142] Despite the lack of agreement on BCAA supplementation at altitude, most investigators agree that there is a lack of compelling indication for BCAA supplements in healthy well-nourished subjects at altitude or in any particular environmental condition.[143] Wagenmakers[139] has proposed a mechanistic model illustrating how BCAA metabolism and glutamine production is influenced by metabolic scenarios resulting in reduced muscle glycogen and subsequently reduced TCA cycle intermediates (Figure 5). BCAA may have a regulatory function on carbon flux in the TCA cycle and consequently alter levels of glutamine production by skeletal muscle.

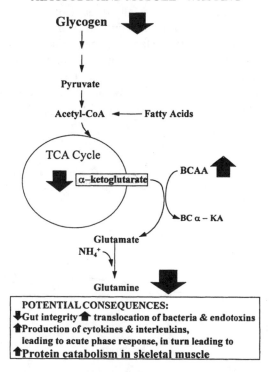

**PROPOSED MECHANISM:
ALTITUDE AND MUSCLE "WASTING"**

FIGURE 5 Proposed mechanism for the loss of lean body mass at high altitude. Glycogen stores are rapidly depleted by hypoxic work and reduced carbohydrate consumption at the same time that fat oxidation is reduced due to hypoxia. This leads to reduced replenishment of TCA cycle intermediates which are "siphoned" off by increased BCAA from muscle protein breakdown combining with α-ketoglutarate to form glutamate which accepts NH_4^+ from protein deamination to form glutamine. The potential consequences of reduced glutamine formation secondary to reduced TCA cycle intermediates could lead to an increased protein catabolism in skeletal muscle. (After Wagenmakers, A. J. M., *Int. J. Sports Med.*, 13, (Suppl. 1), S110, 1992. With permission.)

Wagenmakers[139] proposed that a reduced rate of glutamine synthesis at altitude secondary to reduced TCA cycle intermediates could lead to increased muscle protein catabolism. The same sequence of metabolic events that is observed for sea level patients with trauma or sepsis might explain the inability of high altitude mountaineers to curtail muscle wasting.

Water requirements at altitude may be greater than those at sea level, due to the low humidity of the atmosphere at altitude and hyperventilation associated with altitude exposure.[144] Normal water consumption and normal to slightly reduced urine outputs at altitude (compared to sea level) can still lead to dehydration when accompanied by an increased rate of insensible water loss. The risk of dehydration is high at altitude due to diuresis, water loss in breath, and sweat coupled with the difficulty of obtaining adequate water.[144,145] An inappropriate thirst response coupled with an increase in insensible water loss and a transient diuresis during the initial hours of altitude exposure, can result in rapid dehydration if adequate fluid is either unavailable or neglected.[25] Based upon the equations and assumptions of Ferrus et al.,[146] Milledge[145] has estimated that the rate of respiratory water loss is probably less than 1 1/d. This is still about twice the rate of respiratory water loss for an equivalent activity at sea level. Milledge[145] has calculated theoretical 24-h respiratory water loss at rest and at work at sea level and at high altitude. These predictions are shown in Figure 6.

High altitude and cold environments are often similar with respect to the thermal challenge, tempting one to categorize work in the cold at sea level with work under similar conditions at altitude. There are some distinct differences, however, which should be considered when planning nutritional support at high altitude. Fat, while tolerated relatively well in the cold at sea level, may not be as well tolerated in diets at high altitude. The symptoms of acute altitude exposure may worsen, especially if fat displaces carbohydrate from the diet. Although high-fat foods are energy dense and reduce the weight/calorie aspect of food carried on climbs, fat requires more oxygen for metabolism than carbohydrate and will place a small, but added, burden upon the already overtaxed oxygen economy of the climber. Fat absorption may also be reduced as the climber exceeds elevations above 6300 m;[147] however, elevations commonly reached by recreational skiers, snowshoers, and backpackers are usually not associated with impaired fat or protein absorption.[114] Carbohydrate absorption is relatively

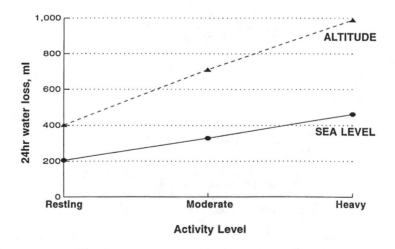

FIGURE 6   Calculation of 24-h respiratory water loss at three activity levels, at sea level, and at altitude. Resting and moderate estimations are at sea level and 5570 m. The estimation for heavy activity is at sea level (hill walking) and ~8000 m (climbing). Detailed information on the equations and assumptions involved in the calculation of these values can be found in Milledge.[145] (After Milledge, J., *Newsl. Int. Soc. Mountain Med.,* 2, 5, 1992. With permission.)

unaffected by altitude,[114] but studies at 5730 m by Dinmore et al.[148] have indicated that the absorption of the marker 3-0-methyl-D-glucose is reduced despite normal intestinal permeability, indicating that high altitude hypoxia may reduce the absorption of certain carbohydrates that are absorbed via an actively mediated intestinal transport system.

One other difference between cold exposure at sea level and high altitude is the calorigenic response to cold. Cold exposure during hypoxia results in an increased reliance upon shivering for thermogenesis due to a reduction in nonshivering thermogenesis at altitude.[149-151] Robinson and Haymes[150] suggested that this is due to a reduction in aerobic catabolism of free fatty acids during hypoxia. Other workers have speculated that impaired thermogenesis at altitude involves an alteration in the neural-hormonal axis thermogenic response.[151,152]

Inappropriate thirst and appetite responses, together with increased insensible water loss, transient diuresis, and increased energy expenditures can lead to rapid dehydration and glycogen depletion and weight loss at altitude if adequate food and fluid is neglected. Dehydration may intensify the symptoms of altitude sickness and result in even lower food intakes. One of the most effective and practical performance-sustaining measures that can be adopted upon arrival at high altitude is to consume a minimum of 3–4 l of fluid per day containing 200–300 g of carbohydrate in addition to that contained in the diet. This should prevent dehydration, improve energy balance, improve the oxygen delivery capability of the circulatory system, replenish muscle glycogen, and conserve body protein levels.

VI. SUMMARY

The challenge of providing adequate nutrition in environmental extremes is one of furnishing a palatable diet generally high in carbohydrate in sufficient quantity to meet high energy demands. Even the best larder of provisions is for naught if water needs are not first attended. Adequate fluid replacement is critical in any environment. Dehydration can reduce appetite, compromise thermoregulation, and impair performance in any environment. Practical dietary recommendations can be made to optimize performance in environmental extremes. Some practical guidelines for recreational or expedition meal planning in environmental extremes are shown in Table 3. Proper nutrition can prevent or minimize performance

TABLE 3   Guidelines for Recreational and Expedition Meal Planning

DO provide group/hot meals whenever possible. People will generally eat more when warm meals are consumed "socially."

DON'T assume that everyone is eating adequately in group feeding situations. A meal prepared is not necessarily a meal eaten.

DO schedule breaks for meals and snacks even when individual food will be consumed for the meal or snack. Left to their own initiative people will frequently skip or shorten meals to accomplish tasks they feel are more "important."

DON'T allow snack food to substitute for meals. Snacks should augment or supplement daily meals, primarily as a means to increase total daily energy or carbohydrate intake. Snacks should be a morale and performance booster, not an obsession.

DO observe what food items are being consumed. Picky dietary habits can lead to imbalances of vitamins, minerals, or energy. Vitamin and mineral supplements are usually not needed; a multivitamin supplement can provide some "insurance" for finicky eaters.

DON'T permit individuals to use the expedition as a "crash" weight loss program. Dehydrated, ketotic, and weak team members jeopardize the safety of others as well as themselves.

DO encourage water consumption with meals. Meal time is often a major fluid consumption point due to the opportunity to prepare beverages, soups, and other water-containing food items. Encourage drinking during periods of strenuous work and during breaks.

DON'T permit food and personal hygiene to slip just because you are in the field. Clean hands, clean utensils, and disinfected water are requisite for safe food preparation, especially in temperate or hot environments.

decrements that often accompany environmental stress and help to make a challenging environment a bit less "hostile."

ACKNOWLEDGMENTS

The assistance of Sharon L. Askew in the preparation of this manuscript is gratefully acknowledged.

REFERENCES

1. Askew, E. W., Nutrition and performance under adverse environmental conditions, in *Nutrition in Exercise and Sport,* Hickson, J. F., Jr. and Wolinsky, 1., Eds., CRC Press, Boca Raton, FL, 1989, 367.
2. Shepherd, R. J., Adaptation to exercise in the cold, *Sports Med.,* 2, 59, 1985.
3. Moore, R. J., Friedl, K. E., Kramer, T. R., Martinez-Lopez, L. E., Hoyt, R. W., Tulley, R. E., Delany, J. P., Askew, E. W., and Vogel, J. A., Changes in soldier nutritional status and immune function during the ranger training course, Technical Report No. T13-92, U.S. Army Research Institute of Environmental Medicine, Natick, MA, September, 1992.
4. Gisolfi, C. V., Impact of limited fluid intake on performance, in *Predicting Decrements in Military Performance Due to Inadequate Nutrition,* National Academy Press, Washington, D.C., 1986, 17.
5. Hubbard, R. W., Armstrong, L. E., Evans, P. K., and DeLuca, J. P., Long-term water and salt deficits — a military perspective, in *Predicting Decrements in Military Performance Due to Inadequate Nutrition,* National Academy Press, Washington, D.C., 1986, 29.
6. Johnson, H. L., Practical military implications of fluid and nutritional imbalances for performances, in *Predicting Decrements in Military Performance Due to Inadequate Nutrition,* National Academy Press, Washington, D.C., 1986, 55.
7. Askew, E. W., Effect of protein, fat and carbohydrate deficiencies on performance, in *Predicting Decrements in Military Performance Due to Inadequate Nutrition,* National Academy Press, Washington, D.C., 1986, 189.
8. Askew, E. W., Environmental and physical stress and nutrient requirements, *Am. J. Clin. Nutr.,* 61(suppl), 6315, 1995.
9. Marriott, B. M., Ed., *Nutritional Needs in Hot Environments,* National Academy Press, Washington, D.C., 1993.
10. Marriott, B. M. and Carlson, S. J., Eds., *Nutritional Needs in Cold and in High-Altitude Environments,* National Academy Press, Washington, D.C., 1996.
11. Consolazio, C. F., Nutrient requirements of troops in extreme environments, *Army Research and Development Newsmagazine,* November 1966, p. 24.
12. Reynolds, R. D., Howard, M. P., Deuster, P., Lickteig, J. A., Conway, J., Rumpler, W., and Seale, J., Energy intakes and expenditures on Mt. Everest, *FASEB J., 6,* A1084, 1992.
13. Stroud, M. A., Coward, W. A., and Sawyer, M. B., Measurements of energy expenditure using isotope-labeled water ($^2H_2{}^{18}O$) during an Arctic expedition, *Eur. J. Appl. Physiol.*, 67, 375, 1993.
14. Westerterp, K. R. and Saris, W. H. M., Limits of energy turnover in relation to physical performance, achievement of energy balance on a daily basis, *J. Sports Sci., 9, 1,* 1991.
15. Phinney, S., The functional effects of carbohydrate and energy underconsumption, in *Not Eating Enough,* Marriott, B.M., Ed., National Academy Press, Washington, D.C., 1995, 303.
16. Shippee, R. L., Friedl, K. E., Kramer, T., Mays, M., Popp, K., Askew, E. W., Fairbrother, B., Hoyt, R., Vogel, J., Marchitelli, L., Frykman, P., Martinez-Lopez, L., Bernton, E., Kramer, M., Tulley, R., Rood, J., DeLany, J., Jezior, D., and Arsenault, J., Nutritional and immunological assessment of ranger students with increased caloric intake, Technical Report, No. T95-S, U.S. Army Research Institute of Environmental Medicine, Natick, MA, 1994.
17. Friedl, K. E., When does energy deficit affect soldier physical performance?, in *Not Eating Enough,* Marriott, B. M., Ed., National Academy Press, Washington, D.C., 1995, 253.
18. Barclay, C. J. and Loiselle, D. S., Dependence of muscle fatigue on stimulation protocol: effect of hypocaloric diet, *J. Appl. Physiol.,* 72, 2278, 1992.
19. Askew, E. W., Munro, 1., Sharp, M. A., Siegel, S., Popper, R., Rose, M. S., Hoyt, R. W., Martin, J. W., Reynolds, K., Lieberman, H. R., Engell, D., and Shaw, C. P., Nutritional status and physical and mental performance of special operations soldiers consuming the ration, lightweight, or the meal, ready-to-eat military field ratio during a 30-day field training exercise, Technical Report No. T7-87, U.S. Army Research Institute of Environmental Medicine, Natick, MA, March, 1987.

20. Hargreaves, M., Carbohydrates and exercise, *J. Sports Sci., 9,* 17, 1991.
21. Phinney, S. D., Bistrian, B. R., Evans, W. J., Gervino, E., and Blackburn, G. L., The human metabolic response to chronic ketosis without caloric restriction: preservation of submaximal exercise capability with reduced carbohydrate oxidation, *Metabolism, 32,* 769, 1983.
22. Young, A. J., Energy substrate utilization during exercise in extreme environments, in *Exercise and Sport Sciences Reviews, Vol. 18,* Pandolf, K. B., Ed., Williams & Wilkins, Baltimore, 1990, 65.
23. Brooks, G. A., Wolfel, E. E., Groves, B. M., Bender, P. R., Butterfield, G. E., Cymerman, A., Mazzeo, R. S., Sutton, J. R., Wolfe, R. R., and Reeves, J. T., Muscle accounts for glucose disposal but not blood lactate appearance during exercise after acclimatization to 4,300 m, *J. Appl. Physiol., 72,* 2435, 1992.
24. Askew, E. W., Water: more than just a nutrient, in *Present Knowledge of Nutrition,* 7th ed., Filer, L. J., Jr. and Ziegler, E. E., Eds., International Life Sciences Press, Washington, D.C., 1996, 98.
25. Sawka, M. N. and Neufer, P. D., Interaction of water bioavailability, thermoregulation and exercise performance, in *Fluid Replacement and Heat Stress,* Marriott, B. M. and Rosemont C., Eds., National Academy Press, Washington, D.C., 1989, VII-I.
26. Sawka, M. N., Francesconi, R. P., Young, A. J., and Pandolf, K. B., Influence of hydration level and body fluids on exercise performance in heat, *J. Am. Med. Assoc., 252,* 1165, 1984.
27. Sawka, M. N., Young, A. J., Francesconi, R. P., Muza, S. R., and Pandolf, K. B., Thermoregulatory and blood response during exercise at graded hypohydration levels, *J. Appl. Physiol., 59,* 1394, 1985.
28. Young, A. J., Sawka, M. N., Levine, L., Cadarette, B. S., and Pandolf, K. B., Skeletal muscle metabolism during exercise is influenced by heat acclimation, *J. Appl. Physiol., 59,* 1929, 1985.
29. Armstrong, L. E., Is fluid intake important in the control of body temperature? If yes, which fluid is best in a hot environment?, *Natl. Strength Cond. Assoc. J., 13,* 68, 1991.
30. Brouns, F., Heat-sweat-dehydration-rehydration a praxis oriented approach, *J. Sports Sci., 9,* 143, 1991.
31. Maughan, R. J., Fluid and electrolyte loss and replacement in exercise, *J. Sports Sci., 9,* 117, 1991.
32. Shapiro, Y., Pandolf, K. B., and Goldman, R. F., Predicting sweat loss response to exercise, environment and clothing, *Eur. J. Appl. Physiol., 48,* 83, 1982.
33. Pandolf, K. B., Stroschein, L. A., Drolet, L. L., Gonzalez, R. R., and Sawka, M. N., Prediction modeling of physiological responses and human performance in the heat, *Comput. Biol. Med., 16,* 319, 1986.
34. Glenn, J. F., Burr, R. E., Hubbard, R. E., Mays, M. Z., Moore, R. I., Jones, B. H., and Krueger, G. P., Sustaining Health and Performance in the Desert: Environmental Medicine Guidance for Operations in Southwest Asia, Technical Note No. 91-1, U.S. Army Research Institute of Environmental Medicine, Natick, MA, December, 1990.
35. Kristal-Boneh, E., Glusman, J. G., Shitrit, R., Chaemovitz, C., and Cassuto, Y., Physical performance and heat tolerance after chronic water loading and heat acclimation, *Aviat. Space Environ. Med., 66,* 733, 1995.
36. Robinson, T. A., Hawley, J. A., Palmer, G. S., Wilson, G. R., Gray, D. A., Noakes, T. D., and Dennis, S. C., Water ingestion does not improve 1-h cycling performance in moderate ambient temperatures, *Eur. J. Appl. Physiol., 71,* 153, 1995.
37. Hubbard, R. W., Mager, M., and Kerstein, M., Water as a tactical weapon: a doctrine for preventing heat casualties, *Proc. Army Sci. Conf., 2,* 125, 1982.
38. Beauchamp, G. K., The human preference for excess salt, *Am. Sci., 75,* 27, 1987.
39. Armstrong, L. E., Hubbard, R. W., Askew, E. W., DeLuca, J. P., O'Brian, C., Pasqualicchio, A., and Francesconi, R. P., Response to moderate and low sodium diets during exercise-heat acclimation, *Int. J. Sports Nutr., 3,* 207, 1994.
40. Costill, D. L., Sweating: its composition and effects on body fluids, in *The Marathon: Physiological, Medical, Epidemiological and Psychological Studies,* Milvy, R., Ed., New York Academy of Sciences, New York, 1977, 160.
41. Barr, S. I., Costill, D. L., and Fink, W. J., Fluid replacement during prolonged exercise: effects of water, saline, or no fluid, *Med. Sci. Sports Exer., 23,* 811, 1991.
42. Baker, E. M., Plough, I. C., and Allen, T. H., Water requirements of men as related to salt intake, *Am. J. Clin. Nutr. 12,* 394, 1963.
43. Gisolfi, C., Summers, R. D., Schedl, H. P., and Bleiler, T. L., Effect of sodium concentration in a carbohydrate-electrolyte solution on intestinal absorption, *Med. Sci. Sports Exer., 27,* 1414, 1995.
44. Hargreaves, M., Costill, D., Burke, L., McConell, G., and Febbraio, M., Influences of sodium on glucose availability during exercise, *Med. Sci. Sports Exer., 26,* 365, 1994.
45. Murray, R., Fluid needs in hot and cold environments, *Int. J. Sports Nutr., 5,* S62, 1995.
46. Greenleaf, J. E., Environmental issues that influence intake of replacement beverages, in *Fluid Replacement and Heat Stress,* Marriott, B. M. and Rosemont, C., Eds., National Academy Press, Washington, D.C., 1989, 15.
47. Consolazio, C. F., Matoush, L. O., Nelson, R. A., Torres, J. B., and Isaac, G. J., Environmental temperature and energy expenditures, *J. Appl. Physiol., 18,* 65, 1963.
48. Sawka, M. N., Pandolf, K. B., Avellini, B. A., and Shapiro, Y., Does heat acclimation lower the rate of metabolism elicited by muscular exercise?, *Aviat. Space Environ. Med., 54,* 27, 1983.

49. Fink, W. J., Costill, D. L., and van Handel, P. J., Leg muscle metabolism during exercise in the heat and cold, *Eur. J. Appl. Physiol.*, 34, 183, 1975.
50. Nielsen, B., Savard, G., Richter, E. A., Hargreaves, M., and Saltin, B., Muscle blood flow and muscle metabolism during exercise and heat stress, *J. Appl. Physiol.*, 69, 1040, 1990.
51. Febbraio, M. A., Snow, R. J., Hargreaves, M., Stathis, C. G., Martin, I. K., and Carey, M. F., Muscle metabolism during exercise and heat stress in trained men: effect of acclimation, *J. Appl. Physiol.*, 76, 589, 1994.
52. Neufer, P. D., Sawka, M. N., Young, A. J., Quigley, M. D., Latzka, W. A., and Levine, L., Hypohydration does not impair skeletal muscle glycogen resynthesis after exercise, *J. Appl. Physiol.*, 70, 1490, 1991.
53. Woodland, K. K., Benson, J. E., Luetkemeier, M. J., Bullough, R. C., Barton, R. G., and Askew, E. W., Dehydration: Does it influence resting metabolic rate?, *Med. Sci. Sports Exer.*, 28, S43, 1996.
54. Clarkson, P. M., The effect of exercise and heat on vitamin requirements, in *Nutritional Needs in Hot Environments*, Marriott, B. M., Ed., National Academy Press, Washington, D.C., 1993, 137.
55. Strydhom, N. B., Kotze, M. E., van der Walt, W. H., and Rogers, G. G., Effect of ascorbic acid on rate of heat acclimation, *J. Appl. Physiol.*, 41, 202, 1976.
56. Early, R. G. and Carlson, B. R., Water-soluble vitamin therapy in the delay of fatigue from physical activity in hot climatic conditions, *Int. Z. Angew. Physiol.*, 27, 43, 1969.
57. Lyons, T. P., Riedesel, M. L., Meuli, L. E., and Chick, T., Effects of glycerol-induced hyperhydration prior to exercise in the heat on sweating and core temperature, *Med. Sci. Sports Exer.*, 22, 477, 1990.
58. Murray, R., Eddy, D. E., Paul, G. L., Seifert, J. G., and Halaby, G. A., Physiological responses to glycerol ingestion during exercise, *J. Appl. Physiol.*, 7, 144, 1991.
59. Freund, B. J., Montain, S. J., Young, A. J., Sawka, M. N., DeLuca, J. P., Pandolf, K. B., and Valeri, C. R., Glycerol hyperhydration: hormonal, renal and vascular fluid responses, *J. Appl. Physiol.*, 79, 2069, 1995.
60. Freund, B. J. and Sawka, M. N., Influence of cold stress on human fluid balance, in *Nutritional Needs in Cold and in High-Altitude Environments*, Marriott, B. M., Ed., National Academy Press, Washington, D.C., 1996, 161.
61. Askew, E. W., Nutrition for a cold environment, *Physician Sportsmed.*, 17, 77, 1989.
62. Stroud, M. A., Effects on energy expenditure of facial cooling during exercise, *Eur. J. Appl. Physiol.*, 63, 376, 1991.
63. Henschell, A., Energy balance in cold environments, in *Cold Injury*, Horvath, S. M., Ed., Josiah Macy Foundation, New York, 1960, 303.
64. Campbell, I. T., Nutrition in adverse environments. II. Energy balance under polar conditions, *Hum. Nutr. Appl. Nutr.*, 36A, 165, 1982.
65. Edwards, J. S. A., Askew, E. W., and King, N., Rations in cold Arctic environments — recent American military experiences, *Wilderness Environ. Med.*, 6, 407, 1995.
66. Johnson, R. E. and Kark, R. M., Environment and food intake in man, *Science*, 105, 378, 1947.
67. Gray, E. L., Consolazio, C. F., and Kark, R. M., Nutritional requirements for men at work in cold, temperate and hot environments, *J. Appl. Physiol.*, 4, 270, 1951.
68. Teitlebaum, A. and Goldman, R. F., Increased energy cost with multiple clothing layers, *J. Appl. Physiol.*, 32, 743, 1972.
69. Romet, T. T., Shephard, R. J., Frim, J., and Goode, R. C., The metabolic cost of exercising in cold air (−20°C), *Arctic Med. Res.*, 47 (Suppl. 1), 280, 1988.
70. Consolazio, C. F., Energy metabolism and extreme environments (heat, cold, high altitude), *Proc. 8th Int. Congr. Nutr.*, Excerpta Medica Int. Cong. Ser. Amsterdam, No. 213, 1969.
71. Buskirk, E. R. and Mendez, J., Nutrition, environment and work performance with special reference to altitude, *Fed. Proc.*, 26, 1760, 1967.
72. Delany, J. P., Moore, R. J., and Hoyt, R. W., Use of doubly labeled water for energy expenditure of soldiers during training exercises in a cold environment, *Int. J. Obesity*, 15, 48, 1991.
73. Jones, P. J. H., Jacobs, I., Morris, A., and Ducharme, M. B., Adequacy of food rations in soldiers during an Arctic exercise measured using doubly labeled water, *J. Appl. Physiol.*, 75, 1790, 1993.
74. Nobmann, E. D., Byers, T., Lanier, A. P., Hankin, J. H., and Jackson, M. Y., The diet of Alaska native adults: 1987–1988, *Am. J. Clin. Nutr.*, 55, 1024, 1992.
75. Swain, H. L., Toth, F. M., Consolazio, C. F., Fitzpatrick, W. H., Allen, D. J, and Koehn, C. J., Food consumption of soldiers in a subarctic climate (Port Churchill, Manitoba, Canada, 1947–1948), *J. Nutr.*, 38, 63, 1949.
76. Rodahl, K., Nutritional requirements in cold climates, *J. Nutr.*, 53, 575, 1954.
77. Rodahl, K., Horvath, S. M., Birkhead, N. C., and Issekutz, B., Jr., Effects of dietary protein on physical work capacity during severe cold stress, *J. Appl. Physiol.*, 17, 763, 1962.
78. Bjorntorp, P., Importance of fat as a support nutrient for energy metabolism of athletes, *J. Sports Sci.*, 9, 71, 1991.

79. Ekstedt, B., Johnson, E., and Johnson, O., Influence of dietary fat, cholesterol and energy on serum lipids at vigorous physical exercise, *Scand. J. Clin. Lab. Invest.*, 51, 437, 1991.

80. Mitchell, H. H., Glickman, N., Lambert, E. H., Keeton, R. W., and Fahnestock, M. K., The tolerance of man to cold as affected by dietary modification: carbohydrate versus fat and the effect of the frequency of meals, *J. Physiol.*, 146, 84, 1946.

81. Vallerand, A. L. and Jacobs, I., Rates of energy substrates utilization during human cold exposure, *Eur. J. Appl. Physiol.*, 58, 873, 1989.

82. Haight, J. S. I. and Keating, W. R., Failure of thermoregulation induced by exercise and ethanol, *J. Physiol.*, 229, 87, 1973.

83. MacDonald, I. A., Bennett, T., and Sainsburg, R., The effect of a 48 hour fast on the thermoregulatory responses to graded cooling in man, *Clin. Sci.*, 67, 445, 1984.

84. Jacobs, I., Romet, T. T., and Kerrigan-Brown, D., Muscle glycogen depletion during exercise at 9°C and 21°C, *Eur. J. Appl. Physiol.*, 54, 35, 1985.

85. Martineau, L. and Jacobs, I., Muscle glycogen availability and temperature regulation in humans, *J. Appl. Physiol.*, 66, 72, 1989.

86. Martineau, L. and Jacobs, I., Muscle glycogen utilization during shivering thermogenesis in humans, *J. Appl. Physiol.*, 65, 2046, 1988.

87. Wolfe, R. R., Klein, S., Carraro, F., and Weber, J. M., Role of triglyceride-fatty acid cycle in controlling fat metabolism in humans during and after exercise, *Am. J. Physiol.*, 258, E382, 1990.

88. Young, A. J., Sawka, M. N., Neuter, P. D., Muza, S. R., Askew, E. W., and Pandolf, K. B., Thermoregulation during cold water immersion is unimpaired by low muscle glycogen levels, *J. Appl. Physiol.*, 66, 1809, 1989.

89. Martineau, L. and Jacobs, I., Effects of muscle glycogen and plasma FFA availability on human metabolic responses in cold water, *J. Appl. Physiol.*, 71, 1331, 1991.

90. Glickman-Weiss, E. L., Nelson, A. G., Hearon, C. M., Vasanthakumar, S. R., Stringer, B. T., and Shulman, S., Does feeding regime affect physiologic and thermal responses during exposure to 8, 20 and 27°C?, *Eur. J. Appl. Physiol.*, 67, 30, 1993.

91. Keeton, R. W., Lambert, E. H., Glickman, N., Mitchell, H. H., Last, J. H., and Fahnestock, M. K., The tolerance of man to cold as affected by dietary modifications: protein versus carbohydrates and the effect of variable protective clothing, *Am. J. Physiol.*, 146, 66, 1946.

92. Glickman-Weiss, E. L., Nelson, A. G., Hearon, C. M., Windhauser, M., and Heltz, D., The thermogenic effect of carbohydrate feeding during exposure to 8, 12, and 27°C, *Eur. J. Appl. Physiol.*, 68, 291, 1994.

93. Glickman-Weiss, E. L., Nelson, A. G., and Hearon, C. M., Effect of body composition on metabolic responses to carbohydrate feeding in males during exposure to 8, 12 and 27°C, *J. Wilderness Med.*, 6, 173, 1995.

94. Vallerand, A. L., Jacobs, I., and Kavanagh, M. F., Mechanism of enhanced cold tolerance by an ephedrine-caffeine mixture in humans, *J. Appl. Physiol.*, 67, 438, 1989.

95. Vallerand, A. L., Effects of ephedrine/xanthines on thermogenesis and cold tolerance, *Int. J. Obesity*, 17(Suppl. 1), S53, 1993.

96. Vallerand, A. L., Drug-induced delay of hypothermia, in *Nutritional Needs in Cold and in High-Altitude Environments*, Marriott, B. M. and Carlson, S. J., Eds., National Academy Press, Washington, D.C., 1996, 257.

97. Welch, B. E., Buskirk, E. R., and Iampietro, P. F., Relation of climate and temperature to food and water intake in man, *Metabolism*, 7, 141, 1958.

98. Roberts, D. E., Patton, J. F., Pennycook, J. W., Jacey, M. J., Tappan, D V., Gray, P., and Heyder, E., Effects of restricted water intake on performance in a cold environment, Technical Report No. T21-84, U.S. Army Research Institute of Environmental Medicine, Natick, MA, 1984.

99. Edwards, J. S. A. and Roberts, D. E., The influence of a calorie supplement on the consumption of the meal, ready-to-eat in a cold environment, *Military Med.*, 156, 466, 1991.

100. Edwards, J. S. A., Roberts, D. E., and Mutter, S. H., Rations for use in a cold environment, *J. Wilderness Med.*, 3, 27, 1992.

101. King, N., Mutter, S. H., Roberts, D. E., Sutherland, M. R., and Askew, E. W., Cold weather field evaluation of the 18-man arctic tray pack ration module, the meal, ready-to-eat and the long life ration packet, *Military Med.*, 158, 458, 1993.

102. Thomas, C. D., Askew, E. W., Baker-Fulco, C. J., Jones, T. E., King, N., Jezior, D. A., and Fairbrother, B. N., Nutrition for health and performance: nutrition guidance for military operation in temperate and extreme environments, Technical Note No. T93-3, U.S. Army Research Institute of Environmental Medicine, Natick, MA, 1993.

103. Dann, E. J., Gillis, S., and Burstein, R., Effect of fluid intake on renal function during exercise in the cold, *Eur. J. Appl. Physiol.*, 61, 133, 1990.

104. Young, A. J., Roberts, D. E., Scott, D. P., Cook, J. E., Mays, M. Z., and Askew, E. W., Sustaining health and performance in the cold environmental medicine guidance for cold-weather operations, Technical Note No. 92-2, U. S. Army Research Institute of Environmental Medicine, Natick, MA, 1992.

105. Wilson, R. P. and Culik, B. M., The cost of a hot meal: facultative specific dynamic action may ensure temperature homeostasis in post-ingestive endotherms, *Comp. Biochem. Physiol.,* 100A, 151, 1991.

106. Cymerman, A., The physiology of high-altitude exposure, in *Nutritional Needs in Cold and in High-Altitude Environments,* Marriott, B. M. and Carlson, S. J., Eds., National Academy Press, Washington, D.C., 1996, 295.

107. Shukitt-Hale, B. And Lieberman, H. R., The effect of altitude on cognitive performance and mood states, in *Nutritional Needs in Cold and in High-Altitude Environments,* Marriott, B. M. and Carlson, S. J., Eds., National Academy Press, Washington, D.C., 1996, 435.

108. Carson, R. P., Evans, W. O., Shields, J. L., and Hannon, I. P., Symptomatology, pathophysiology, and treatment of acute mountain sickness, *Fed. Proc.,* 28, 1085, 1969.

109. Johnson, H. L., Consolazio, C. F., Krzywicki, H. J., and Isaac, G. J., Increased energy requirements of man after abrupt altitude exposure, *Nutr. Rep. Int.,* 4, 77, 1971.

110. Askew, E. W., Claybaugh, J. R., Hashiro, G. M., Stokes, W. S., Sato, A., and Cucinell, S. A., Mauna Kea III Metabolic effects of dietary carbohydrate supplementation during exercise at 4100 m altitude, Technical Report No. T12-87, U.S. Army Research Institute of Environmental Medicine, Natick, MA, May 1987.

111. Edwards, J. S. A., Askew, E. W., King, N., Fulco, C. S., Hoyt, R. W., and DeLany, J. P., An assessment of the nutritional intake and energy expenditure of unacclimatized U. S. Army soldiers living and working at high altitude, Technical Report No. T/10-91, U. S. Army Research Institute of Environmental Medicine, Natick, MA, June 1991.

112. Butterfield, G. E., Maintenance of body weight at altitude: in search of 500 kcal/day, in *Nutritional Needs in Cold and in High-Altitude Environments,* Marriott, B. M. and Carlson, S. J., Eds., National Academy Press, Washington, D.C., 1996, 357.

113. Kayser, B., Nutrition and energetics of exercise at altitude. Theory and possible practical implications, *Sports Med.,* 17, 309, 1994.

114. Butterfield, G. E., Gates, J., Fleming, S., Brooks, G. A., Sutton, I. R., and Reeves, J. T., Increased energy intake minimizes weight loss in men at high altitude, *J. Appl. Physiol.,* 72, 1741, 1992.

115. Rose, M. S., Houston, C. S., Fulco, C. S., Coates, G., Sutton, J. R., and Cymerman, A., Operation Everest. II. Nutrition and body composition, *J. Appl. Physiol.,* 65, 2545, 1988.

116. Consolazio, C. F., Matoush, L. O., Johnson, H. L., Krzywicki, H. J., Daws, T. A., and Isaac, G. J., Effects of high-carbohydrate diets on performance and clinical symptomatology after rapid ascent to high altitude, *Fed Proc.,* 28, 937, 1969.

117. Hansen, J. E., Hartley, L. H., and Hogan, R. P., Arterial oxygen increase by high- carbohydrate diet at altitude, *J. Appl. Physiol.,* 33, 441, 1972.

118. Dramise, J. G., Inouye, C. M., Christensen, B. M., Fults, R. D., Canham, J. E., and Consolazio, C. F., Effects of a glucose meal on human pulmonary function at 1600 m and 4300 m altitudes, *Aviat. Space Environ. Med.,* 46, 365, 1975.

119. Durnin, J. V. G. A. and Passmore, R., Eds., *Energy, Work and Leisure,* Heinemann, London, 1967, 16.

120. Maher, J. T., Nutrition and altitude acclimatization, in *Handbook of Nutritional Requirements in a Functional Context,* Vol. 2, Rechcigl, M. R., Jr., Ed., CRC Press, Boca Raton, FL, 1981, 549.

121. Fulco, C. S., Rock, P. B., Trad, L. A., Rose, M. S., Forte, V. A., Young, P. M., and Cymerman, A., The effect of caffeine on endurance time to exhaustion at high altitude, Technical Report No. T1789, U. S. Army Research Institute of Environmental Medicine, Natick, MA, 1989.

122. Lieberman, H. R. and Shukitt-Hale, B., Food components and other treatments that may enhance mental performance at high altitudes and in the cold, in *Nutritional Needs in Cold and in High-Altitude Environments,* Marriott, B. M. and Carlson, S. J., Eds., National Academy Press, Washington, D.C., 1996, 453.

123. Committee on Military Nutrition Research, Review of the physiology and nutrition in cold and in high-altitude environments, in *Nutritional Needs in Cold and in High-Altitude Environments,* Marriott, B. M. and Carlson, S. J., Eds., National Academy Press, Washington, D.C., 1996, 3.

124. Simon-Schnass, I., Risk of oxidative stress during exercise at high altitude, in *Exercise and Oxygen Toxicity,* Sen, C. K., Packer, L., and Hänninen, O., Eds., Elsevier, Amsterdam, 1994, 191.

125. Simon-Schnass, I., Oxidative stress at high altitudes and effects of vitamin E, in *Nutritional Needs in Cold and in High-Altitude Environments,* Marriott, B. M. and Carlson, S. J., Eds., National Academy Press, Washington, D.C., 1996, 393.

126. Simon-Schnass, I. and Pabst, H., Influence of vitamin E on physical performance, *Int. J. Vit. Nutr. Res.,* 58, 49, 1988.

127. Simon-Schnass, I. and Korniszewski, L., The influence of vitamin E on rheological parameters in high altitude mountaineers, *Int. J. Vit. Nutr. Res.,* 60, 26, 1990.

128. Simon-Schnass, I. M., Nutrition at high altitude, *J. Nutr.,* 122, 778, 1992.

129. Berglund, B., High-altitude training. Aspects of haematological adaptation, *Sports Med.,* 14, 289, 1992.

130. LaCelle, P. L. and Weed, R. I., Low oxygen pressure: a cause of erythrocyte membrane rigidity, *J. Clin. Invest.,* 49, 52, 1970.

131. Palareti, G., Coccheris, P. M., Tricarico, M. G., Magelli, M., and Cavazzuti, F., Modifications des propriétés rheologiques de sang aprés une expédition en haute altitude, *Angiology,* 35, 451, 1984.

132. Guezennec, C. Y., Naudaud, J. F., Satabin, P., Leger, F., and LaFargue, P., Influence of polyunsaturated fatty acid diet on the hemorrheological response to physical exercise in hypoxia, *Int. J. Sports Med.,* 10, 286, 1989.

133. Acuilaniu, B., Flore, P., Perrault, H., Page, J.E., Payan, E., and Lacour, J. R., Exercise-induced hypoxaemia in master athletes: effects of a polyunsaturated fatty acid diet, *Eur. J. Appl. Physiol.,* 72, 44, 1995.

134. Bigard, X., Satabin, P., Leger, C., Louisy, F., and Guezennec, C., Effects of polyunsaturated fatty acids on physical performance at high altitude, in *Proceedings from Second IOC World Congress on Sports Sciences,* Barcelona, 1991, 260.

135. Hornbein, T. F., Evaluation of iron stores as limiting high-altitude polycythemia, *J. Appl. Physiol.,* 17, 243, 1962.

136. Hannon, J. P., Nutrition at high altitude, in *Environment Physiology: Aging. Heat and Altitude,* Horvath, S. M. and Yousef, M. K., Eds., Elsevier, Amsterdam, 1980, 309.

137. Stray-Gundersen, J., Alexander, C., Hochstein, A., deLomos, D., and Levine, B. D., Failure of red cell volume to increase to altitude exposure in iron deficient runners, *Med. Sci. Sports Exer.,* 24(Suppl.), S90, 1992.

138. Kayser, B., Acheson, K., DeCombaz, J., Fern, E., and Cerretelli, P., Protein and energy digestibility at high altitude, *J. Appl. Physiol.,* 73, 2425, 1992.

139. Wagenmakers, A. J. M., Amino acid metabolism, muscular fatigue and muscle wasting. Speculation on adaptations at high altitude, *Int. J. Sports Med.,* 13(Suppl. 1), s110, 1992.

140. Bigard, A. X., Satabin, P., Lalier, P., Canon, F., Taillandier, D., and Guezennec, C. Y., Effects of protein supplementation during prolonged exercise at moderate altitude on performance and plasma amino acid pattern, *Eur. J. Appl. Physiol.,* 66, 5, 1993.

141. Schena, F., Guerrini, F., Tregnaghi, P., and Kayser, B., Branched-chain amino acid supplementation during trekking at high altitude, *Eur. J. Appl. Physiol.,* 65, 394, 1992.

142. Wagenmakers, A. J. M., Branched-chain amino acid supplementation during trekking at altitude. The effects on loss of body mass, body composition and muscle power, *Eur. J. Appl. Physiol.,* 67, 92, 1993. (Letter to the editor.)

143. Schena, F., Guerrini, F., Tregnaghi, P., and Kayser B., Branched-chain amino acid supplementation during trekking at high altitude. The effects on loss of body mass, body composition and muscle power, *Eur. J. Appl. Physiol.,* 67, 94, 1993. (Letter to the editor.)

144. Hoyt, R. W. and Honig, A., Body fluid and energy metabolism at high altitude, in *Handbook of Physiology, Section 4: Environmental Physiology,* Blatteis, C. M. and Frealy, M. J., Eds., Oxford University Press, New York, 1996, 1277.

145. Milledge, J., Respiratory water loss at altitude, *Newsl. Int. Soc. Mountain Med.,* 2 (No. 3), 5, 1992.

146. Ferrus, L., Commenges, D., Gire, J., and Varene, P., Respiratory water loss as a function of ventilatory or environmental factors, *Res. Physiol.,* 56, 11, 1984.

147. Boyer, S. J. and Blume, F. D., Weight loss and changes in body composition at high altitude, *J. Appl. Physiol.,* 57, 1580, 1984.

148. Dinmore, A. J., Edwards, J. S. A., Menzies, I. S., and Travis, S. P. L., Intestinal carbohydrate absorption and permeability at high altitude (5,730 m), *J. Appl. Physiol.,* 76(5), 1903, 1994.

149. Blatteis, C. M. and Lutherer, L. O., Effect of altitude exposure on thermoregulatory response of man to cold, *J. Appl. Physiol.,* 41, 848, 1976.

150. Robinson, K. A. and Haymes, E. M., Metabolic effects of exposure to hypoxia plus cold at rest and during exercise in humans, *J. Appl. Physiol.,* 68, 720, 1990.

151. Gautier, H., Bonora, M., Scholtz, S. A., and Remmens, J. E., Hypoxia-induced changes in shivering and body temperature, *J. Appl. Physiol.,* 77, 726, 1994.

152. Giesbrecht, G. G., Fewell, J. E., Megirian, D., Brant, R., and Remmers, J. E., Hypoxia similarly impairs metabolic responses to cutaneous and core cold stimuli in conscious rats, *J. Appl. Physiol.,* 77, 726, 1994.

Chapter 25

BODY COMPOSITION IN EXERCISE AND SPORT

Henry C. Lukaski

CONTENTS

I.   INTRODUCTION

Physically active individuals generally have an appearance and a body composition profile that distinguishes them from their sedentary counterparts. One might deduce that physical activity is associated with a relatively angular appearance characterized by modest amounts of body fat and perhaps increased amounts of muscle. This generalization can be misleading because differences in the type of activity pursued may be associated with different body types and body composition. Characterizations of physical appearance of the body have been summarized in the general description of body build or physique which is termed somatotype.[1-4] A summary of the body builds of male and female athletes participating in the gamut of sports at the Olympic Games has been published.[5] For example, ectomorphy (e.g., tall, lean appearance) is dominant while endomorphy (e.g., body rotundness) is minimal in long-distance runners as compared to dominant mesomorphy (e.g., muscularity) and minimal ectomorphy in hammer throwers. These descriptions suggest that specific body builds or somatotypes apparently dominate certain types of physical activities. Thus, body structure is one factor that impacts body function during physical activity.

This chapter will address the interaction between body structure and physical activity. It will review the different models used to describe human composition and the methods used to measure these components, describe body composition characteristics by physical activity or sport, and examine the relationship between body composition and performance in some activities including sport and military tasks. A final topic, estimation of minimal weight for performance, also will be discussed.

II.   HUMAN BODY COMPOSITION ASSESSMENT

A.   MODELS OF BODY COMPOSITION

A systematic approach has been developed to describe the components of the body.[6] If one views the human body in terms of increasing stages of complexity, then five levels of body composition can be envisioned (Figure 1). Each of these levels is distinct and inclusive. At each level, the sum of the components equals the body mass.

1.   Atomic Level

The fundamental components of the body are described in the atomic level. Although more than 50 different atoms are found in the body, the vast majority located in various tissues and organs are oxygen, carbon, hydrogen, nitrogen, calcium, and phosphorus, which constitute about 98% of body mass.[7] One element, oxygen, represents more than 60% of body weight.[7] The remaining 44 elements, of which the predominant are potassium, sulfur, sodium, chloride, and magnesium, only make up about 2% of body mass.

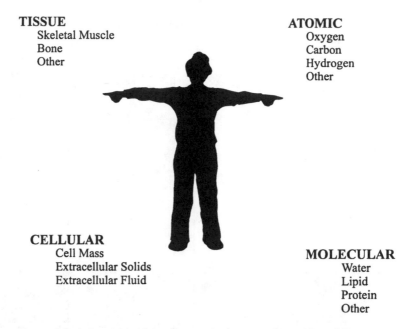

TISSUE
Skeletal Muscle
Bone
Other

ATOMIC
Oxygen
Carbon
Hydrogen
Other

CELLULAR
Cell Mass
Extracellular Solids
Extracellular Fluid

MOLECULAR
Water
Lipid
Protein
Other

FIGURE 1 Chemical and physical models of human body composition. Adapted from Wang et al.[6]

2.   Molecular Level

The 11 principal elements in the body are incorporated into compounds that represent the molecular level of body composition. These essential molecules include water, lipid or fat, protein, mineral, and glycogen. The molecular level is important because it provides the conceptual basis for subsequent levels of organization that follow, and a link with biochemistry and energy metabolism which relate body structure and function.

The molecular level of body composition is emphasized because its components are most frequently measured in studies of physical activity. The major molecular level components and models are summarized in Figure 2. The classical cadaver analysis, which serves as the basis for this level of body composition, reveals five major components of the body: fat, water, protein, bone minerals, and nonbone or soft tissue minerals. Although another component, glycogen, may be included, its limited amount precludes its determination.

This molecular model can be further divided into functional components (Figure 2). The fat-free mass, which represents the metabolically active tissue, is distinct from fat because of chemical and physical characteristics. Fat has a lower density (0.900 vs 1.100 g/cc) than the fat-free body and does not contain water or potassium.[8-13] The individual components of the fat-free body (water, bone mineral, and cell mass) can be determined with appropriate methods.

3.   Cellular Level

The cellular level of body composition assembles the components of the molecular level into the cells that comprise the human body. Four groups of cells can be characterized: muscle, nerve, connective, and epithelial cells. The connective cells constitute a multi-functional group which includes adipocytes, osteocytes and blood cells. There are also extracellular components, fluid and solids, in this compositional model. The extracellular fluid is the nonmetabolizing fluid that surrounds all cells. It contains about 95% water and is distributed between the plasma and the interstitial fluid which are estimated to be about 5 and 20% of body mass, respectively.[7] The extracellular solids also are nonmetabolizing components of the body. They include organic compounds, such as collagenous, reticular, and elastic fibers, and inorganic compounds, principally dry bone matrix or calcium hydroxyapatite, magnesium, sodium, citrate, and bicarbonate.

Component Models

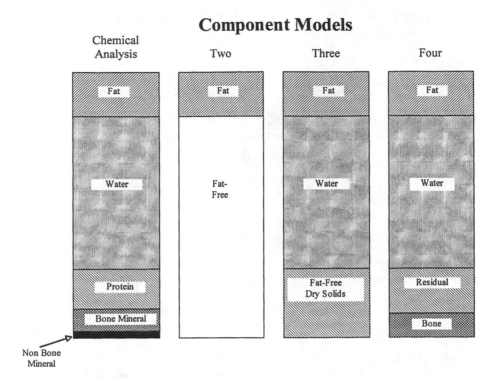

FIGURE 2 General molecular models of body composition and their components.

4. Tissue-Systems Level

The combination of cells and extracellular components combine to form the tissue and systems level of body composition. The tissues are categorized as muscular, nervous, connective, and epithelial. Importantly, bone, muscle, and adipose tissue constitute more than 75% of body mass.[7] The systems component also includes multiple organs that share an integrated function (e.g., the digestive, excretory, reproductive, and respiratory systems).

5. Whole-Body Level

The combination of the components of these four levels culminates in the whole-body or the fifth level of body composition. The body is characterized by size (stature and mass), shape, and its various dimensions (limb and trunk lengths and their circumferences). Importantly, biological and genetic processes impact all levels of body composition. Therefore, functional adaptations associated with physical activity are manifest in structural changes or alterations in the components at all levels of body composition.

B. METHODS OF BODY COMPOSITION ASSESSMENT

Assessment of human body composition may be performed by using a variety of methods.[14-17] All methods of body composition assessment are indirect; they rely on chemical or physical characteristics of a body component to determine that component. This review will describe the physical bases of methods for determination of the components of the molecular models of body composition that can be useful in applications with physically active people.

1. Body Fat

Fat is a compositional variable that is generally viewed as a detrimental component of the body because of its negative image with regard to appearance and the adverse effects it

TABLE 1   Indirect Methods of Assessment of Human Body Composition

Fat Mass — *Fat-Free Mass*

Fat Mass	Fat-Free Mass
Densitometry	Water
Skinfold thickness	Isotope dilution
	Bioelectrical impedance

Skeletal Muscle Mass

Radiologic techniques
   Computed tomography
   Magnetic resonance imaging
   Dual x-ray absorptiometry

may have on health and, in some cases, physical performance. Assessment of body fat may be undertaken with different types of methods (Table 1). One approach uses techniques that utilize a characteristic of fat to estimate its content in the body while another determines the fat-free mass and calculates fat by difference from body mass.

a.   Densitometry

The term *densitometry* refers to the procedure of estimating body composition by determining the density of the body. This method uses the principle that the density (D) of a material can be determined from measurements of mass (M) and volume (V): D = M/V. The density of the human body (D_B) is calculated from measurements of mass in air (M_A) and mass in water (M_W) along with some other corrections. Body density is calculated from apparent body volume, ($M_A - M_W$) corrected for water density (D_W), and residual lung volume (V_R): $D_B = M_A/\{[(M_A - M_W)/D_W] - V_R\}$. From body density, percent body fat can be calculated by using either the two component model of Brozek et al.[12] or Siri[10] (Table 2).

The density of any heterogenous material depends on the proportions and densities of its components. Early applications of densitometry assumed that the body consisted of two components: fat (F) and fat-free mass (FFM). This classic model stated that $1/D_B = F/D_F +$ FFM/D_{FEM}. This two-component model has been used for the majority of all densitometric assessments of body composition of physically active people. Recognition that the density of the fat-free body is variable because of inter-individual differences in bone mineral density and the ratio of muscle (protein) to bone[18] has stimulated the use of multicomponent models to determine body fatness by using measurement of body density which is corrected for water content (W), bone mineral content (M), or W and M. Examples of some commonly used prediction models are shown in Table 2. Use of multicomponent models permits an individualized determination of body fatness based on the specific chemical composition of the fat-free body. This approach enables body composition assessment in children and the elderly with the same model when measurements of body density, total body water, and bone mineral content are available.[19]

TABLE 2   Equations for Estimating Body Fatness (%BF) from Densitometric and other Measurements

Components	Equation	Reference
2	%BF = [(4.95/D_B) − 4.5] × 100	Siri[10]
	%BF = [(4.57/D_B) − 4.142] × 100	Brozek et al.[12]
3	%BF = [(2.118/D_B) − 0.78W − .354] × 100	Siri[10]
4	%BF = [2.749/D_B) − 0.727W + 1.146M − 2.053] × 100	Lohman[19]

Note: D_B = body density; W and M = total body water and bone mineral expressed as a percentage of body mass.

Traditionally, body density measurements have been made with underwater weighing procedures.[20] In addition, body volume measurements of infants and small children have used air[21] and helium displacement[22] techniques. Inaccuracies in volume determinations because of thermodynamic problems have limited the use of these methods. Acoustic plethysmography, a technique which uses the principle of the Helmholtz resonator to measure the volume of an object, has yielded improved accuracy (<2% error) in infants and children, but its application has not been developed.[23] A recent revision of an air displacement plethysmograph has rekindled interest in this technique because it eliminates many problems associated with hydrodensitometry and has shown good correspondence with hydrodensitometry.[24]

b.   Anthropometry

The use of simple measurements of regions of the body with inexpensive devices has promoted the routine assessment of body composition. Measurements of skinfold thicknesses and body circumferences are used to predict body density and to calculate body fatness. The basic assumptions are that the thickness of subcutaneous adipose tissue (fat and connective tissues) reflects a constant proportion of the total body fat and the sites selected for measurement represent the average thickness of the subcutaneous adipose tissue mass.[14] Neither of these assumptions have been proven to be true. Nevertheless, the use of skinfold thicknesses and some body circumferences has gained wide acceptance in epidemiological surveys of children and adults.[25]

The anthropometric method also has been used to develop generalized prediction equations. These equations rely on a curvilinear relationship between anthropometric measurements (e.g., skinfold thicknesses) and body density (Table 3). Although one might speculate that sport-specific equations might be needed, research has shown that the generalized equations for athletes are valid for groups of athletes. Cross-validation studies by Sinning et al.[26] indicated that the general equations of Jackson and Pollock[28] gave acceptable estimates of average body fatness among male athletes. Whether these equations are accurate for prediction of body fatness for individual athletes has not been evaluated. The use of multicomponent models as reference will be needed to re-examine this question.

c.   Dual X-Ray Absorptiometry

The dual X-ray absorptiometry (DXA) method relies on the principle that the attenuation of x-rays exiting the body reflects the amount of bone and soft tissue (lean and fat) composition. Briefly, the body is exposed to collimated x-rays at two discrete energy levels. The attenuation of the high and low energy x-rays reflects the amount of bone, fat, and fat-free, mineral-free mass (FFMF).[30,31] Radiation exposure is minimal with DXA, less than 1 mrem[31] with current instrumentation.

An advantage of the DXA method is the lack of reliance on assumptions regarding the determination of body fat. Because fat is determined from the soft tissue attenuation in each

TABLE 3   Generalized Anthropometric Equations for Prediction of Body Density (BD)

Gender	Equation	Ref.
M & F	BD = C – M (X1)	Durnin and Womersley[27]
M	BD = 1.15737 – 0.02288 (X2) – 0.00019 (X3) – 0.0075 (X4) + 0.0223 (X5)	Jackson and Pollock[28]
F	BD = 1.096095 – 0.0006952 (X6) + 0.0000011 (X6)^2 – 0.0.0000714 (X3)	Jackson et al.[29]

Note: M, F = male, female; C = intercept; M = slope; X1 = log (biceps + triceps + subscapular + supra-iliac skinfolds); X2 = ln (pectoral + abdominal + thigh skinfolds); X3 = age; X4 = abdominal circumference; X5 = forearm circumference; X6 = triceps + abdominal + suprailiac + thigh skinfolds.

pixel in individual regions of the scan and the soft tissue attenuation factors for lean and fat have been established by calibration from a series of phantoms of known composition,[32] the proportion of fat and lean in each pixel is determined.[33] The validity of DXA to estimate body fat has been shown to be acceptable in large animals[34] but questionable in small animals[35,36] based on comparisons between chemical analysis of animals and DXA estimates of body fat.

Some physical factors influence the validity of the DXA technique. Changes in body hydration influence estimates of FFMFM without affecting the estimated fat mass.[37,38] Body thickness (e.g., anteroposterior distance) impacts the validity of DXA determinations of soft tissue composition. Studies using anthropometric phantoms and *in vitro* models found that body thickness less than 20 cm or exceeding 25 cm result in increasing variability in soft tissue composition determinations.[39,40] Another issue is the validity of the assumption that the composition of soft tissue anterior to bone is similar to the fat and FFMF tissue posterior to the bone.[38]

The DXA method offers promise for routine assessment of body composition of physically active individuals. High precision measurements with minimal radiation exposure make this an attractive method for longitudinal studies of physically active individuals. However, concerns about physical factors that influence the validity of DXA estimates of FFMF mass may limit its use in some groups of individuals.

2. Fat-Free Mass

Reliance on the two-component model of body composition resulted in an emphasis in determination of FFM. Methods for assessment of FFM, other than densitometry, utilize the measurement of a component of the fat-free body and calculation of FFM based on the assumption that the component represents a relatively constant proportion of the FFM.

a. Total Body Water

Although water is the most abundant constituent of the body, it is found only in the fat-free component of the body. It is distributed between the intracellular and extracellular components that are in a relatively constant proportion of total body water (TBW) in healthy individuals. Because the water content of the fat-free body is 72–74%[12] based on direct measurements in animals, determination of TBW represents an indirect measure of FFM. Measurement of TBW in humans relies on indirect determinations.

i. isotope dilution

The use of hydrogen (deuterium and tritium) and oxygen (^{18}O) isotopes permits the determination of TBW by the dilution method.[41] It is assumed that the isotopic tracer is only distributed in TBW; it is equally distributed in all anatomic water compartments; there is a rapid rate of equilibration of tracer in TBW; and the tracer is not metabolized. In general, these assumptions are valid with the exception that all tracers used for TBW determination are metabolized and excreted in the urine. Briefly, a volunteer ingests a small quantity of tracer, waits a fixed duration for equilibration to occur (about 4 hr), collects all urine passed during the equilibration period, and undergoes a phlebotomy before and after the equilibration.[42] The concentration of the tracer is determined in the pre- and post-dose blood sample and the amount of tracer lost in the urine is measured. Total body water is calculated as: TBW = [(amount of tracer given – amount excreted in urine)/(post – pre plasma tracer concentration)].

The estimated TBW is influenced by the tracer used. Based on desiccation studies of animals, deuterium and tritium overestimate TBW by 4% whereas ^{18}O only overestimates TBW by 1%.[41] Reported errors exceeding these values represent measurement errors and not biological influences including nonaqueous hydrogen exchange and oxygen lost in exhaled air.

Determinations of TBW are used to calculate FFM assuming that TBW/FFM is relatively constant.[14] Use of isotope dilution methods to assess FFM in athletic populations is very

TABLE 4   Hydration of the Fat-Free Body in Athletes

Group	n	Body Mass, kg	TBW, kg	FFM, kg	TBW/FFM, %
			Swimmers		
Female	43	63.8 ± 6.7	34.9 ± 3.9	47.7 ± 4.8	73.3 ± 1.4
Male	31	76.1 ± 5.0	48.4 ± 3.8	65.3 ± 4.8	74.1 ± 1.3
			Football		
Male	24	98.9 ± 4.6	63.8 ± 4.9	84.7 ± 3.5	75.3 ± 1.4

Note: TBW = total body water; FFM = fat-free mass by densitometry. Values are mean ± SE.

limited because densitometry and anthropometry are routinely used for body composition assessment. However, some recent data suggest that isotope dilution may be useful in some groups of athletes because the hydration of the fat-free body is constant within a sport-specific group (Table 4). Apparently, the TBW/FFM ratio increases, albeit slightly, from female to male swimmers and to male football players. One might speculate that as muscular development increases, the hydration of the fat-free body also increases to a slight degree.

ii.   bioelectrical impedance analysis

An alternative method for determining FFM is tetrapolar bioelectrical impedance analysis (BIA). A radiofrequency, alternating current is administered into an individual and the impedance to the flow and distribution of the current is measured.[43] Because water and electrolytes influence the impedance to the flow of the applied current, BIA measures TBW and indirectly determines FFM.

The single-frequency BIA method has been used for body composition assessment in the field. Chapman et al.[44] used a 50 kHz BIA device to monitor the body composition of 17 participants in the 1992 Iditarod Sled Dog Race and reported no change in FFM but a loss of 2.1 and 1.0 kg of fat in male and female competitors, respectively. The accuracy of these estimates was not evaluated because of the lack of availability of a reference method.

Comparisons of BIA estimates of body composition have yielded contradictory results. In a survey of 46 female and 58 male collegiate athletes, FFM determined by BIA and densitometry was similar.[45] In contrast, body fatness determined in adolescent female speed skaters and gymnasts was significantly greater with BIA models derived in adults than skinfold measurements.[46] This finding suggests the need for age- and sport-specific BIA models to account for apparent differences in the chemical composition of the fat-free body (e.g., hydration and bone mineral density) of the adolescent as compared to the more mature, adult athlete.

Additional evidence indicates that differences in the chemical composition of the fat-free body will impact the validity of the BIA method. Studies of African-American football players found that BIA overestimates body fatness compared to densitometry or anthropometry.[47,48] This discrepancy is explained by the recent report of Wang et al.[49] who showed that although similar correlations exist between BIA resistance and FFM, the regression coefficients differ for Caucasian, African-American, and Asian adults; the authors report a similar finding for BIA measures and TBW.

When using BIA to determine body composition of athletes, it is important to standardize the measurement conditions. The body composition of athletes measured under standardized conditions to minimize alterations in skin temperature and fluid imbalance was similar to densitometric estimates.[45] However, BIA measurements made without regard to controlled conditions yielded significant increases in body fatness.[45] Thus, use of the BIA method in physically active individuals requires attention to measurement conditions and the use of race-specific prediction models.

Alternative BIA approaches use multiple-frequency instruments that are proposed to delineate TBW and extracellular fluid and thus permit determination of FFM. Bioelectrical impedance spectroscopy utilizes signal frequencies ranging from 5 to about 600 kHz to construct a complex spectrum or plot of reactance (Xc) and resistance (R). These data are fitted to the Cole-Cole suspension model using non-linear curve fitting to determine the frequency at which reactance is maximal, termed the critical frequency (F_C), and the apparent resistances of the extracellular water (ECW) and intracellular water (ICW). Based on general mixture theory,[50] equations are developed to predict ECW and ICW. Although this approach has been used to monitor changes in fluid distribution during human pregnancy,[51] it has not been routinely used to evaluate FFM, particularly among athletic populations.

Another multiple-frequency model has been proposed. Cornish et al.[52] determined impedance and phase angle (arc tangent of Xc/R) at frequencies ranging from 4 kHz to 1 MHz, used the Cole-Cole model to derive a spectrum of Xc plotted against R, and determined the F_C and R at zero frequency (R_0). The authors hypothesize that F_C and R_0 relate to TBW and ECW, respectively. This approach has not been applied to assessment of FFM.

3. Skeletal Muscle Mass

Although skeletal muscle represents the largest mass in the body (30 and 40% body mass of a woman and man, respectively) and its importance in metabolism and work performance is well known, there is a conspicuous lack of methods for its assessment. One reason for this limitation is the deficit of information on skeletal muscle masses from direct dissection studies.[53] Therefore, development and validation of new methods rely on the use of indirect reference methods.

a. Anthropometry

The use of measurements of the body to predict either regional or whole-body skeletal muscle mass requires selection of appropriate measurements and measurement sites. Thus, a muscle group is selected with the assumptions that site-specific physical measurements reflect the mass of the muscle and the mass of the estimated muscle group is proportional to the whole-body skeletal muscle mass.

Limb measurements have been used as indices of nutritional status in developing countries and in hospitalized patients. Estimates of upper arm muscle circumference have served as a functional indicator of protein-energy malnutrition.[54] Measurements of the lower leg have been less frequently used to diagnose hospital malnutrition.[55] The use of arm circumference has been superceeded by estimates of upper arm muscle area.[56] Use of this anthropometric indicator assumes that the upper, mid-arm is circular; the triceps skinfold thickness is twice the average of the adipose tissue distributed in the upper arm, the mid-arm muscle circumference is circular; and bone responds similarly to muscle and adipose during periods of caloric restriction and repletion.[57] Although the attraction of this anthropometric approach is high, attempts to validate estimates of upper-arm muscle area have indicated errors of 15–25% in adults ranging from 60–120% of ideal body weight.[53] Subsequent attempts to revise prediction equations have not been successful, particularly in obese adults.[58]

Anthropometric models also have been proposed to estimate whole-body skeletal muscle mass.[59] Briefly, these approaches used regional limb circumference measurements, corrected for skinfolds thickness determinations, and stature. As compared to skeletal muscle mass estimated from endogenous creatinine excretion, errors ranged from 5–9%.[60] In contrast, Martin et al.[53] used anthropometric measurements and tissue mass determinations from human cadavers to develop another prediction model: MM = S (0.0553 CTG^2 + 0.0987 FG^2 + 0.0331 CCG^2) – 2445, where MM = total skeletal muscle mass; S = stature; CTG = thigh circumference corrected for anterior skinfold thickness; FG = uncorrected forearm circumference; and CCG = calf circumference corrected for skinfold thickness. Values of skeletal muscle mass were predicted using this and other anthropometric models in another group of cadavers.

Martin et al.[53] found that the model yielded reduced errors (measured – predicted) of 2 kg whereas other models had significantly greater bias ranging from 5 to 10 kg.

b.   Radiographic Techniques

In contrast to other methods that indirectly assess skeletal muscle mass, radiographic techniques offer an opportunity for direct visualization and measurement of muscle, as well as other anatomical structures. These methods rely on the differing responses among tissues, based on their unique chemical composition, as the tissue reacts with electromagnetic energy to determine the amount of specific tissue in a segment or the whole-body.

i.   computed tomography

As x-rays pass through the tissues of the body their intensity is reduced or attenuated based on the differences in chemical composition and physical density. This attenuation is expressed as the linear attenuation coefficient or computed tomography (CT) number; the units of measure are Hounsfield units. For example, air, adipose tissue, and muscle have average CT numbers of –1000, –70 and +20, respectively.

The use of CT has provided unique measurements of changes in regional body composition. Fiatarone et al.[61] used CT scans of the mid-thigh to identify significant increases in quadriceps (9%) and adductor areas (8.4%) of elderly men in response to physical training. No changes were found in subcutaneous or intramuscular adipose. Densitometry was unable to detect any changes in whole-body composition. Similarly, Lonn et al.[62] used CT to determine a significant increase (2.4 kg) in skeletal muscle mass in 10 adults with complete pituitary deficiency after receiving recombinant human growth hormone treatment. Thus, CT has the ability to determine small, but biologically significant, changes in regional and whole-body skeletal muscle mass.

ii.   magnetic resonance imaging

Nuclear magnetic resonance (NMR) is a potentially useful technique that provides both images (magnetic resonance imaging [MRI]) and chemical composition (NMR spectroscopy) of tissues *in vivo*. In contrast to CT which uses x-rays, MRI does not expose an individual to ionizing radiation. The MRI technique uses an external magnetic field to induce a temporary dipole moment or realignment of atomic nuclei either in parallel or antiparallel to the induced magnetic field. When the magnetic field is turned off, the nuclei realign themselves by a process termed relaxation which enables a determination of the chemical composition of the body segment under study.

The MRI method has been used to determine human body composition. Ross et al.[63] used transverse slices of 10 mm thickness acquired at 50 mm distances from head to foot to determine the fat-free and fat masses of men and women, respectively. Compared to anthropometric predictions, MRI estimates of FFM had a variability of 3.6 and 6.5% for men and women. The effects of caloric restriction alone or in combination with exercise on skeletal muscle mass was examined with MRI.[64] The MRI method distinguished small (4%) but significant changes in whole-body FFM and significant decreases (about 1 l) in appendicular skeletal muscle volume. These findings indicate the potential important role that MRI can play in detecting biologically important changes in skeletal muscle mass.

iii.   dual x-ray absorptiometry

The dual x-ray absorptiometry (DXA) method also offers important opportunities to measure regional skeletal muscle mass. Heymsfield et al.[65] demonstrated good reproducibility in determining skeletal muscle mass in the arms, legs, and total muscle of adults (7, 2, and 3% variability, respectively). Significant correlations were also reported for DXA-determined total appendicular skeletal muscle mass and total body potassium ($r = 0.94$). Changes in appendicular skeletal muscle mass have also been documented by DXA in men in response to resistance training.[66]

One potential limitation of DXA to measure regional skeletal muscle mass is altered fluid distribution. As shown by Horber et al.,[37] DXA determinations of regional skeletal muscle mass in patients with chronic renal failure were increased in the arms (5.5%), legs (30%), and trunk (60%) before as compared to after dialytic treatment.

III. BODY COMPOSITION PROFILES OF SELECTED GROUPS OF ATHLETES

For many athletes, the term *body composition* is synonymous with body fatness because most descriptions of groups of athletes by sporting activity emphasize the fatness of the participants. While this approach may be informative for the general public, it probably is not useful to an individual athlete. The use of group body composition values as standards for individual athletes rests on some weak assumptions: the mean body fatness for a representative group of athletes reflects optimal physiological and biomechanical function, and the average body fatness is characteristic of the best performing athletes in a particular sport. Summaries of body composition profiles of men and women participating in a variety of sports have been presented.[67,68] In contrast to the previous compilations which have used predominantly anthropometric assessments, the present synopsis (Figure 3) only includes determinations made with densitometry or hydrometry and emphasizes ranges of body fatness based on 90% confidence intervals calculated from the original reports.

A. RUNNING AND THROWING EVENTS

Participants in track and field events have a wide range of body fatness. Competitive and collegiate female distance runners[69,70] and sprinters[67] had similar levels of body fatness (14.3 ± 3.3 [mean ± SE] and 10.9 ± 3.6%) as do pentathletes[71] and long jumpers[72] (11.0 ± 3.3 and 12.9 ± 2.5%). Among female athletes studied, javelin throwers had the greatest body fatness but with the largest range of values (27.0 ± 8.8%).[67] Male distance runners[73] tended to be leaner (4.7 ± 3.1 vs 8.3 ± 5.2%) than sprinters and hurdlers[74] who also had a large variability in body fatness. Male decathletes[74] and long and high jumpers[72] had similar levels of body fatness (8.4 ± 5.1 and 8.5 ± 2.1%, respectively). Among male field event participants, body fatness was greatest among shot putters (16.5 ± 4.3%) and discus throwers (16.4 ± 4.3%).[67,75]

B. RESISTANCE TRAINING ACTIVITIES

There is an apparent specificity in the body composition characteristics of female participants in different types of resistance training. Among women, body builders are leaner (13.5 ± 1.5 vs 21.5 ± 1.3%) than power lifters.[76] Men, however, do not exhibit a similar response. Body fatness is quite similar among Olympic (9.9 ± 1.9%) and power lifters (9.1 ± 1.2%) and body builders (9.3 ± 0.8%).[77,78] It has been suggested that differences in training and dietary habits might explain the observed range in body fatness in the resistance training with body builders regulating food intake more than Olympic or power lifters.[79] While this hypothesis may be true for the women studied by Johnson et al.,[76] it apparently is not valid for the observations in the various studies of men.

C. GYMNASTICS

Body composition has been assessed in collegiate gymnasts. Male gymnasts were leaner (6.5 ± 2.4 vs 15.3 ± 4.0 and 14.5%) than their female counterparts.[80,81] Among high school female gymnasts aged 15–17 yr, body fatness was 13.1%.[82,83] Because a majority of these

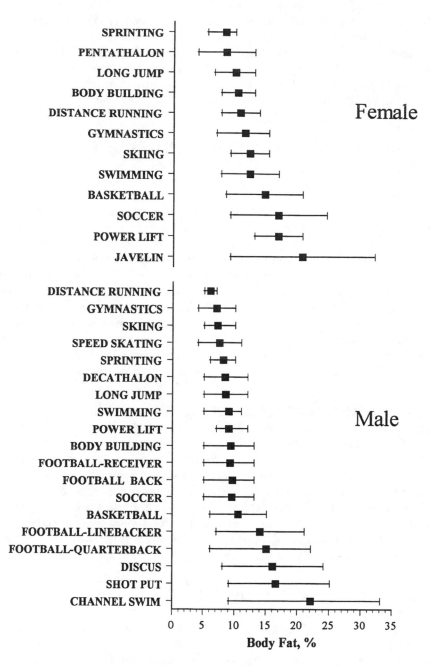

FIGURE 3 Survey of body fatness among various groups of athletes. Values are means with 90% confidence intervals.

girls had not reached menarche, it is questionable if the densitometric determinations reflect actual body fatness because their bone mineral density was probably compromised.

D. SKIING

Data from Olympic Nordic skiers indicate that these athletes are as lean as long distance runners which indicates the endurance requirement of these activities. U.S. male and female Olympians had body fatness levels of 7.2 ± 1.9 and 16.1 ± 1.6%, respectively.[84] The data for the male Nordic skiers are similar to previous results of a mean value of 8.9% reported by Hanson.[85] These values are consistent with survey results of anthropometric determinations among European male (9.4–14.1%) and female (16.2–20%) Alpine skiers.[86]

E. SOCCER

Male collegiate soccer players in the U.S.[67] had body fat levels (9.5 ± 4.9%) that were similar to those found in European club players (9.7%) reported by Withers et al.[74] Among international caliber male players, however, body fat levels were only 6.9 ± 1.5%.[87] Limited data for female soccer players[74] indicate higher body fatness (22 ± 6.8%).

F. BASKETBALL AND FOOTBALL

Women from four U.S. universities provide the largest database of body composition data for female basketball players.[88] Body fatness was 19.2 ± 4.6% which is very similar to data reported by other investigators.[74,81,89] Male collegiate basketball players tend to be leaner (10.5 ± 3.4%);[81] professional players have slightly less body fatness (9–10.6%).[90] Withers et al.[74] reported 10.3% body fatness in national caliber Australian basketball players.

The consistency of body fatness among basketball players is not found among members of football teams. Surveys of professional[91] and collegiate football players[92,93] at different levels of competition indicate position-specific body composition characteristics. Offensive (15.6 ± 3.8%) and defensive (18.2 ± 5.4%) lineman weighing more than 120 kg have the greatest body burden of fat. Although linebackers (14.0 ± 4.6%) and quarterbacks (14.4 ± 6.5%) have similar body fatness to linemen, their body masses are much less (90–100 kg). Body fatness is least among running backs (9.4 ± 4%) and defensive backs (9.6 ± 4.2%).

G. SWIMMING

Representative data for national caliber female swimmers indicate body fatness of 16.4 ± 4.4%[94] while female collegiate swimmers had higher body fatness (25.0 ± 1%).[95] Among male collegiate swimmers, body fatness ranged from 14 ± 0.5%[95] to 9±3.2%[26] at different universities. An unusual and demanding aquatic competition is swimming the English channel. Participants in this competition, on the average, tend to have the greatest body fatness (22.4 ± 7.5%) because of the demands for temperature regulation in the cold water and the long duration of the swim.[96]

IV. BODY COMPOSITION AND PERFORMANCE

There is continuing interest among coaches and athletes to determine a body composition profile that is associated with optimal physical performance.[97] Attempts to delineate a relationship between body composition and performance have been hampered by the lack of discrimination between the strict components of performance (endurance, power and speed, and combined power and endurance). This section reviews the experimental evidence indicating that body composition variables are related to different types of physical performance.

A. ATHLETIC PERFORMANCE

In general, a significant negative relationship between body weight, or body fatness, and performance, including running for speed or endurance and jumping for height or distance, has been demonstrated.[97] This finding suggests that, in general, body fat per se rather than body weight limits athletic performance that requires the body be moved in space for prolonged, uninterrupted periods of time.

TABLE 5   Body Weight and Body Fatness
As Predictors of Physical
Fitness Test Results

Performance Test	Body Mass	% Body Fat
Sit-ups	−0.09	−0.29
Standing long jump (sum of 3 trials)	−0.13	−0.61
75-yd (22.7 m) dash	−0.22	−0.52
220-yd (66.7 m) dash	−0.38	−0.68

Note: Values are correlation coefficients.

Adapted from Riendeau et al.[99]

Kireillis and Cureton[98] related the body fatness, estimated by skinfold thickness measurements, and performance to standardized physical fitness tests of 113 male collegians. Body fatness was significantly correlated with the time for the mile (1600 m) run (r = 0.40), the 100-yd (30.3 m) run (r = 0.34), and the long jump (r = −0.33) distance; this suggests that body fatness adversely affected the performance of these activities. The effects of body weight and densitometrically determined body fatness on physical performance of men also emphasized the deleterious role of body fat.[99] Although body mass and fatness were predictors of poor performance, percent body fat was the stronger (e.g., significant) predictor of adverse performance (Table 5). Furthermore, as body fatness increased, fitness test performances decreased (Table 6). In a sample of college students (55 men and 55 women), Cureton et al.[100] found gender-dependent differences in body fatness and physical performance test results; the men were leaner and performed better than the women. When the data were combined, body fatness was significantly correlated with distance achieved in a 12-min run (r = −0.58), total time to complete a 50-yd (15.3 m) dash (r = 0.73), and total height jumped in a vertical jump test (r = −0.67). Other studies in children and adolescents[101,102] confirmed that body fatness was a significant, negative factor in isolated activities requiring endurance, speed, and jumping.

An early attempt to examine the effect of body fatness on running performance utilized the addition of external weight to mimic the body burden of fat.[103] Men performed a series of submaximal and maximal treadmill tests, then repeated the tests while carrying weight added to the trunk, which when combined with the individual's body fatness approximated the body fatness of a matched female runner. With the added weight, the oxygen uptake of the submaximal test was increased and the maximal test time was decreased. These findings indicate that the increased body burden of simulated excess fat impaired running performance. Pate et al.[104] matched male and female competitive runners on the basis of 15-mile road race performance times. Interestingly, they found similar body fatness between the women and men (17.8 vs 16.3%, respectively).

TABLE 6   Specificity of Body Fatness Levels As
Predictors of Physical Fitness Measures

| Fitness Measure | Body Fatness | | |
	<10%	10–15%	>15%
Sit-ups in 2 min	43.4	41.6	36.2
Standing long jump (sum of 3 trials), ft (m)	23.8 (7.2)	22.7 (6.9)	20.2 (6.1)
75-yd (22.7 m) dash, s	9.8	10.1	10.7
220-yd (66.7 m) dash, s	29.3	31.6	35.0

Adapted from Riendeau et al.[99]

In contrast to these studies in which noncompetitive athletes were studied, there are relatively few reports that examine the relationship between competitive performance and body composition. Wilmore[97] reported relationships between body compositional variables and an endurance measure (1.75 mile run) in professional football players during training camp. The men ranged in body mass from 75 to 120 kg with a densitometrically determined percent body fat of 3–24%, FFM ranged from 68 to 99 kg, and run times of 10.5–13.9 min. Run times were correlated with body mass (r = 0.73), FFM (r = 0.56), and percent fat (r = 0.71). These results confirm the previous findings that body mass and body fatness negatively impact endurance running performance.

Although the majority of research has focused on the adverse effects of body fatness of specific aspects of physical performance, there is evidence of a beneficial role of FFM in athletic competition. Stager and Cordain[105] determined relationships between body composition, determined by densitometry, and swimming performance of competitive female swimmers aged 12–17 yr. Swim performance, defined as the individual's best time in the 100-yd (30.3 m) freestyle, was unrelated to body fatness (r = 0.18) but significantly correlated with FFM (r = –0.26). Siders et al.[95] also found that FFM was an important predictor of swimming performance. In collegiate swimmers, early season 100-yd (30.3 m) swim times were significantly related to body fatness (r = 0.351) and FFM (r = –0.32). At the end of the season, when performance (swim times) was improved, only FFM was a significant predictor of 100-yd (30.3 m) performance (r = –0.657). These findings emphasize that body composition variables may be sport-specific predictors of performance.

B. MILITARY PERFORMANCE

The relationship of body composition to performance of physical tasks is a concern of the military. It encompasses the basis for decisions on acceptance or rejection of recruits for military service and has implications for individual decisions on retention and advancement for active duty personnel. In addition, there are financial concerns because of the costs of training replacement personnel when individuals are discharged for failure to meet established weight-for-height standards. The discharge of trained and experienced specialists has further potential ramifications concerning military readiness and performance.

Physical standards are used to evaluate candidates for accession and retention in the military. In general, weight-for-height is determined and compared to acceptable standards that differ among the various branches of the military based on perceived needs of each service branch. If an individual is identified as not meeting the acceptable standard of weight-for-height, an assessment of body composition by the anthropometric technique is performed. The Army uses a combination of stature, body mass, and circumferences of the neck and wrist in men and of stature, body mass, and circumferences of neck, forearm, wrist, and hips in women.[106] The Navy uses stature, mass, and circumferences of neck and waist, for men[107] and stature, mass, and circumferences of neck, waist, and hips in women.[108] The Marine Corps uses measurements of stature, mass, and neck circumference for men[109] and measurements of stature, mass, flexed biceps, forearm, neck, waist, and thigh circumferences for women.[110] The Air Force uses stature, mass, and biceps measurement for men[111] and stature, mass, and forearm circumference for women.[112] For retention, military personnel are evaluated on a regular basis for stature, mass, and/or body circumferences and are required to perform a test of aerobic fitness. For the Army and Navy, the standards for admission permit a greater degree of overweight persons than do the standards for retention. It is assumed that the high levels of physical activity during basic training result in a general loss of body fat and a gain in FFM in overweight individuals. For the Marine Corps and the Air Force, retention standards are similar to accession standards.

Maintenance of an acceptable body composition is emphasized in the military. This emphasis originates from three concerns: body composition is an integral part of physical

TABLE 7   Correlations Between U.S. Navy Physical Readiness Test Measures and Body Composition Variables with Materials Handling Tasks

	Box-Lift Maximum Weight	Box-Carry Power
Sit-reach distance	–0.21	0.01
Sit-ups in 2 min	–0.00	0.31
Push-ups in 2 min	0.63	0.56
1.5 mile (2400 m) run time	–0.34	–0.67
Percent fat	–0.36	–0.43
Fat-free mass	0.84	0.44

Adapted from Beckett and Hodgdon.[115]

fitness and hence combat-readiness; control of body fat is necessary to maintain appropriate military appearance; and control of body fat is necessary to maintain the health and well-being of military personnel.[113] It is assumed that body composition, more appropriately body fatness, is related to the performance of military-specific tasks.

Although it has been demonstrated that body fatness adversely impacts running performance of military personnel,[114] there is limited evidence that fatness impairs the performance of service-related duties. Beckett and Hodgdon[115] evaluated the performance of 64 male and 38 female Naval personnel in standard physical readiness test and materials handling tasks that are common aboard ship, the maximum weight of a box that could be lifted to elbow height (box-lift maximum weight), and the total distance that a 34 kg box could be carried (box carry power). Physical fitness measures, such as flexibility and aerobic endurance, accounted for no more than 45% of the variability in materials handling tasks (Table 7). Body fatness, although significantly correlated with these tasks, was only modestly correlated with these materials handling tasks. Body fatness would not be a useful predictor of Navy-specific task performance, as less than 20% of functional capacity in materials handling could be attributed to body fatness. Importantly, FFM was a strong, significant predictor (70%) of maximum weight lifted.

There is increasing evidence that FFM, as compared to fatness, is a key predictor of function in specific military tasks. The most common physically demanding tasks in the U.S. Army are lifting and carrying (e.g., load carriage). Relationships between speed of carrying a constant mass over varying distances indicate a benefit of FFM (Table 8). Soldiers with greater FFM perform the load carriage faster than soldiers with less FFM. Also, increased fatness is associated with slower times to traverse the same distance.

Additional evidence of the importance of FFM for performance of military tasks is the positive relationship between FFM and lifting ability (Table 9). Importantly, FFM explains more of the variance in lifting performance (20–41%) than does body fatness (up to 6%). The low positive correlations of percent body fat with lifting ability suggest a weak trend for

TABLE 8   Correlations of Load Carriage Performance and Body Composition in Male Soldiers

Distance, km	Load, kg	% Body Fat	Fat-Free Mass	Ref.
2	46	0.00	–0.54	Mello et al.[116]
4	46	0.38	–0.39	
8	46	0.48	–0.45	
12	46	0.29	–0.55	
20	46	0.05	–0.26	
16	18	0.15	–0.30	Dziados et al.[117]

TABLE 9   Correlations Between Lifting Performance and Body Composition

Lift Type	Men		Women		Ref.
	% Body Fat	Fat-Free Mass	% Body Fat	Fat-Free Mass	
Maximal	0.06	0.45	0.10	0.26	Teves et al.[118]
Maximal	0.26	0.64	−0.03	0.45	Meyers et al.[119]

fatter soldiers to lift more effectively because fatter individuals tend to have increased amounts of FFM. The weaker correlations for women than men between FFM and lifting performance are apparently related to a lack of experience among women with lifting. Myers et al.[119] showed that the relationship between FFM and lifting increased after basic training from 0.45 to 0.58.

In addition to the positive relationships with load carriage and lifting, FFM is related to the performance of other military tasks. For assignments that require pushing, carrying, and torque development, FFM is a better predictor of performance than is body fatness (Table 10). Similarly, individuals with greater FFM would be expected to perform lifting assignments better than soldiers with lesser amounts of FFM. These findings also suggest a weaker trend for fatter people to push and exert torque better apparently because they could use their fat mass to generate momentum. Overall, FFM is a better predictor of physical performance in task-related military duties than is body fatness.

V.   MINIMUM WEIGHT

Every competitor would like to attain a body mass that minimizes body fat and maximizes FFM and muscle mass without adverse effects on health and physical performance. This goal is termed *minimum weight*. Unfortunately, there is no absolute standard of minimum weight for an individual. One sport, wrestling, has developed a program for the attainment of a generalized minimum weight for its participants. The objective of this program is to avoid the potentially hazardous side effects of rapid weight loss that has been a practice used by high school wrestlers to attain a specific weight category.

Minimum weight may be described as the body mass at which fat content is minimal without alternation of physiological function and growth. Determination of minimum weight for an individual assumes that body fat be limited to essential fat or the fat found in cell membranes, central nervous system, bone marrow, and certain organs.[120] The proposed essential fat levels are 3–5% for men and 14% for women.

TABLE 10   Relationships Between Physical Performance Measures and Body Composition after Physical Training

Task	Percent Body Fat		Fat-Free Mass	
	Men	Women	Men	Women
Weight pushed	0.20	0.17	0.52	0.37
Torque	0.18	0.14	0.35	0.30
Push work	0.09	0.10	0.23	0.26
Carry work	0.03	0.17	0.27	0.02

Note: Values are correlation coefficients.

Adapted from Myers et al.[119]

In 1989, the state of Wisconsin implemented a minimum weight policy for high school wrestlers with the goal of minimizing adverse effects of weight loss on the health and well-being of the participants.[121] This program assumes a relationship between subcutaneous adipose tissue and body fat and establishes 7% body fat as the lower limit for safe and normal growth. Minimum weight is defined as the body mass at which the athlete will be allowed to compete. There is no competition until the minimum weight has been established.

Minimum weight is determined by anthropometry before the start of wrestling season. A certified health care professional measures skinfold thickness at three sites (triceps, subscapular, and abdominal). The sum of these measurements is transformed into body density;[19] body fatness is calculated with the Brozek model.[12] Minimum weight (M_W) is calculated at the 7% body fat level: $M_W = \{[1 - (\%BF/100)] \times \text{current body mass}\}/0.93$.

The effects of the minimum weight program recently have been examined. Opplinger et al.[122] surveyed the weight reducing and eating behaviors of some Wisconsin high school wrestlers in 1990 (n = 713), one year prior to the implementation of the minimum weight program, and in 1993 (n = 368), two years after enforcement of the mandatory rules restricting weight loss for competition. Implementation of the minimum weight rule resulted in some beneficial behavioral changes; these included significant decrease in the use of weight loss methods, such as food and fluid restriction and forced dehydration, most weight lost, and most weight lost to qualify at a weight class, and the frequency of cutting weight. In addition, the number of wrestlers expressing bulimic eating behaviors significantly decreased by about 11%. These findings suggest that a mandatory minimum weight rule significantly reduced unhealthy weight loss behaviors.

VI. CONCLUSIONS

Body composition is one factor that impacts physical performance. Although many diverse methods are available to assess body composition, they all rely on a chemical or physical characteristic to determine fatness. Studies in athletes and military personnel demonstrate that body fatness, rather than body weight, negatively affects cardiovascular endurance, balance, agility, speed, and jumping ability. Whereas increased fat-free mass promotes performance involving strength, power, and muscular endurance, it may limit endurance activities in which the body must be moved for prolonged periods of time. Thus, sport- and activity-specific profiles in body composition are characteristic within specific groups of athletes.

Skeletal muscle is an important component of the body that has not been intensively studied in response to physical activity. Investigations are needed to delineate relationships between changes in skeletal muscle mass, both regional and whole-body, and physical performance.

Excessive weight loss in athletes may be hazardous to health and function. An important new approach to establishing minimum weight for participation in wrestling offers an opportunity for application in other sports. By assuming a specific level of body fatness appropriate for growth, development, and physiological function, it is possible to calculate an appropriate body weight. Preliminary experience indicates that this approach may lead to a reduction in aberrant weight loss practices in some athletes.

Body composition assessment of an individual remains the first step in the evaluation of appropriate body weight for health and performance. Studies have routinely relied on methods based on the two component model of body composition: fat and fat-free mass. Use of this approach can lead to errors in body composition measurement because changes in the chemical composition of the fat-free body, such as alterations in hydration and in bone mineral density which can bias estimates of body fat, are not determined. Ethnicity also can influence the chemical composition of the fat-free body. Future studies of the interaction between physical activity and body composition should utilize multicomponent models of body composition to account for subtle differences in muscle, bone and water.

Optimal physical performance is multifactorial; it is the result of the interaction of genetics, biomechanics, training, body composition, and nutrition. The emphasis of body fatness alone is inappropriate and may predispose an individual to disordered eating behavior.

REFERENCES

1. Parnell, R. W., Somatotyping by physical anthropometry, *Am. J. Phys. Anthropol.,* 12, 209, 1954.
2. Heath, B. H. and Carter, J. E. L., A comparison of somatotype methods, *Am. J. Phys. Anthropol.,* 24, 87, 1966.
3. Wilmore, J. H., Validation of the first and second components of the Heath-Carter somatotype method, *Am. J. Phys. Anthropol.,* 32, 369, 1970.
4. Hartl, E. M., Monnelly, E. P., and Elderkin, R. D., *Physique and Delinquent Behavior: A Thirty-Year Follow-Up of William H. Sheldon's Varieties of Delinquent Behavior,* Academic Press, New York, 1989, 5.
5. De Garay, A. L., Levine, L., and Carter, J. E. L., *Genetic and Anthropological Studies of Olympic Athletes,* Academic Press, New York, 1974, 27.
6. Wang, Z.-M., Pierson, R. N., and Heymsfield, S. B., The five-level model: a new approach to organizing body composition research, *Am. J. Clin. Nutr.,* 56, 19, 1992.
7. Snyder, W. S., Cook, M. J., Nasset, E. S., Karhausen, L. R., Howells, G. P., and Tipton, I. H., *Report of the Task Group on Reference Man,* Pergamon Press, Oxford, 1984.
8. Behnke, A. R., Feen, B. G., and Welham, W. C., Specific gravity of healthy men, *J. Am. Med. Assoc.,* 118, 495, 1942.
9. Keys, A. and Brozek, J., Body fat in adult men., *Physiol. Rev.,* 33, 245, 1953.
10. Siri, W. B., The gross composition of the body, in *Advances in Biological and Medical Physics,* Vol. 4, Tobias, C.A. and Lawrence, J.H., Eds., Academic Press, New York, 1956, 239.
11. Mendez, J., Keys, A., Anderson, J. T., and Grande, F., Density of fat and mineral of mammalian body., *Metabolism,* 9, 472, 1960.
12. Brozek, J., Grande, F., Anderson, J. T., and Keys, A., Densitometric analysis of body composition: revision of some quantitative assumptions, *Ann. N. Y. Acad. Sci.,* 110, 113, 1963.
13. Boddy, K., King, P. C., Womersley, J., and Durnin, J. V. G. A., Body potassium and fat-free mass, *Clin. Sci.,* 44, 622, 1973.
14. Lukaski, H. C., Methods for the assessment of human body composition: traditional and new, *Am. J. Clin. Nutr.,* 46, 537, 1987.
15. Forbes, G. B., *Human Body Composition: Growth, Aging, Nutrition, and Physical Activity,* Springer-Verlag, New York, 1987.
16. Roche, A. F., Heymsfield, S. B., and Lohman, T. G., Eds., *Human Body Composition,* Human Kinetics, Champaign, IL, 1996.
17. Forbes, G. B., Body Composition, in *Present Knowledge in Nutrition,* 7th ed., Ziegler, E. E. and Filer, L.J., Eds., International Life Sciences Institute, Washington, D.C., 1996, 7.
18. Womersley, J., Durnin, J. V. G. A., Boddy, K., and Mahaffy, M., Influence of muscular development, obesity, and age on the fat-free mass of adults, *J. Appl. Physiol.,* 41, 223, 1976.
19. Lohman, T. G., Applicability of body composition techniques and constants for children and youth, in *Exercise and Sport Sciences Reviews,* Vol. 14, Pandolf, K. B., Ed., Macmillan, New York, 1986, 325.
20. Buskirk, E. R., Underwater weighing and body density: a review of procedures, in *Techniques for Measuring Body Composition,* Brozek, J. and Henschel, A., Eds., National Academy of Sciences, National Research Council, Washington, D.C., 1961, 90.
21. Falkner, F., An air displacement method for measuring body volumes in babies: a preliminary communication, *Ann. N. Y. Acad. Sci.,* 110, 75, 1963.
22. Fomon, S. J., Jensen, R. L., and Owen, G. M., Determination of body volume of infants by a method of helium displacement, *Ann. N. Y. Acad. Sci.,* 110, 80, 1963.
23. Sheng, H.-P., Dang, T., Adolph, A. L., Schanler, R. J., and Garzr, C., Infant body volume measurement by acoustic plethysmography, in *In Vivo Body Composition Studies,* Ellis, K. J., Yasumura, S., and Morgan, W. D., Eds., Institute of Physical Sciences in Medicine, London, 1987, 415.
24. McCrory, M. A., Gomez, T. D., Bernauer, E. M., and Mole, P. A., Evaluation of a new air displacement plethysmograph for measuring human body composition, *Med. Sci. Sports Exer.,* 27, 1686, 1995.
25. Norgan, N. G., Anthropometric assessment of body fat and fatness, in *Anthropometric Assessment of Nutritional Status,* Himes, J. H., Ed., Wiley-Liss, New York, 1991, 197.

26. Sinning, W. E., Dolny, D. E., Little, K. D., Cunningham, L. N., Racaniello, A., Siconolfi, S. F., and Sholes, J. L., Validity of generalized equations for body composition analysis in male athletes, *Med. Sci. Sports Exer.*, 17, 124, 1985.

27. Durnin, J. V. G. A. and Womersley, J., Body fat from total body density and its estimation from skinfold thickness: measurements on 481 men and women aged from 16 to 72 years, *Brit. J. Nutr.*, 32, 77, 1974.

28. Jackson, A. S. and Pollock, M. L., Generalized equations for predicting body density of men, *Brit. J. Nutr.*, 40, 497, 1978.

29. Jackson, A. S., Pollock, M. L., and Ward, A., Generalized equations for predicting body density of women, *Med. Sci. Sports Exer.*, 12, 175, 1980.

30. Lukaski, H. C., Soft tissue composition and bone mineral status: evaluation by dual energy x-ray absorptiometry, *J. Nutr.*, 123, 438, 1993.

31. Laskey, M. A., Dual-energy x-ray absorptiometry and body composition, *Nutrition*, 12, 45, 1996.

32. Mazess, R. B., Barden, H. S., Bisek, J. P., and Hanson, J., Dual energy x-ray absorptiometry for total body and regional bone mineral and soft tissue composition, *Am. J. Clin. Nutr.*, 51, 1106, 1990.

33. Gotfredsen, A., Jensen, J., Borg, J., and Christiansen, C., Measurement of lean body mass and total body fat using dual photon absorptiometry, *Metabolism*, 35, 88, 1986.

34. Svendsen, O. L., Haarbo, J., Hassager, C., and Christiansen, C., Accuracy of measurements of total body soft tissue composition by dual energy x-ray absorptiometry *in vivo*, *Am. J. Clin. Nutr.*, 57, 605, 1993.

35. Ellis, K. J., Shypailo, R. J., Pratt, J. A., and Pond, W. G., Accuracy of dual energy x- ray absorptiometry for body composition measurements of children, *Am. J. Clin. Nutr.*, 60, 660, 1994.

36. Jebb, S. A., Garland, S. W., Jennings, G., and Elia, M., Dual energy x-ray absorptiometry for the measurement of gross body composition in rats, *Br. J. Nutr.*, 75, 803, 1996.

37. Horber, F. F., Thomi, F., Casez, J. P., Fonteille, J., and Jaeger, P., Impact of hydration status on body composition as measured by dual energy x-ray absorptiometry in normal volunteers and patients on hemodialysis, *Br. J. Radiol.*, 65, 895, 1992.

38. Nord, R. H. and Payne, R. K., Body composition by dual energy x-ray absorptiometry — a review of the technology, *Asia Pacific J. Clin. Nutr.*, 4, 167, 1995.

39. Laskey, M. A., Lyttle, K. D., Flarman, M. E., and Barber, R. W., The influence of tissue depth and composition on the performance of the Lunar dual energy x-ray absorptiometer whole-body scanning mode, *Eur. J. Clin. Nutr.*, 46, 39, 1992.

40. Jebb, S. A., Goldberg, G. R., and Elia, M., DXA measurements of fat and bone mineral density in relation to depth and adiposity, in *Human Body Composition*, Ellis, K. J. and Eastman J. D., Eds., Plenum Press, New York, 1993, 115.

41. Schoeller, D. A. and Jones, P. J. H., Measurement of total body water by isotope dilution: a unified approach to calculation, in In Vivo *Body Composition Studies*, Ellis, K. J., Yasumura, S., and Morgan, W. D., Eds., Institute of Physical Sciences in Medicine, London, 1987, 131.

42. Lukaski, H. C. and Johnson, P. E., A simple, inexpensive method for determining total body water using a tracer dose of D_2O and infrared absorption of biological fluids, *Am. J. Clin. Nutr.*, 41, 363, 1985.

43. Lukaski, H. C., Johnson, P. E., Bolonchuk, W. W., and Lykken, G. I., Assessment of fat-free mass using bioelectrical impedance measurements of the human body, *Am. J. Clin. Nutr.*, 41, 810, 1985.

44. Chapman, R., Tibbetts, G., Case, S., Evans, D., and Mills, W. J., Body composition testing of athletes in the field using bioelectrical impedance analysis, *Alaska Med.*, 34, 87, 1992.

45. Lukaski, H. C., Bolonchuk, W. W., Siders, W. W., and Hall, C. B., Body composition assessment of athletes using bioelectrical impedance measurements, *J. Sports Med. Phys. Fitness*, 30, 434, 1990.

46. Webster, B. L. and Barr, S. I., Body composition analysis of female adolescent athletes: comparing six regression equations, *Med. Sci. Sports Exer.*, 25, 648, 1992.

47. Hortobagyi, T., Israel, R. G., Houmand, J. A., O'Brien, K. F., Johns, R. A., and Wells, J. A., Comparison of four methods to assess body composition in black and white athletes, *Int. J. Sports Nutr.*, 2, 60, 1992.

48. Clark, R. R., Kuta, J. M., and Sullivan, J. C., Cross-validation of methods to predict body fat in African-American collegiate football players, *Res. Q. Exer. Sport*, 65, 21, 1994.

49. Wang, J., Thornton, J. C., Burastero, S., Heymsfield, S. B., and Pierson, R. N., Bioimpedance analysis for estimation of total body potassium, total body water, and fat-free mass in White, Black, and Asian adults, *Am. J. Human Biol.*, 7, 33, 1995.

50. Hanai, T., Electrical properties of emulsions, in *Emulsion Science*, Sherman, P. H., Ed., Academic Press, London, 1968, 354.

51. Van Loan, M. D., Kopp, L. E., King, J. C., Wong, W. W., and Mayclin, P. L., Fluid changes during pregnancy: use of impedance spectroscopy, *J. Appl. Physiol.*, 78, 1037, 1995.

52. Cornish, B. H., Ward, L. C., Thomas, B. J., Jebb, S. A., and Elia, M., Evaluation of multiple frequency bioelectrical impedance and Cole-Cole analysis for assessment of body water volumes in healthy humans, *Eur. J. Clin. Nutr.*, 50, 159, 1996.

53. Martin, A. D., Spenst, L. F., Drinkwater, D. T., and Clarys, J. P., Anthropometric estimation of muscle mass, *Med. Sci. Sports Exer.*, 22, 729, 1990.

54. Jelliffe, D. B., *The Assessment of Nutritional Status of the Community*, WHO Monograph Series No. 53, World Health Organization, Geneva, 1966.

55. Heymsfield, S. B., Olafson, R. P., Kutner, M. H., and Nixon, D. W., A radiographic method of quantifying protein-calorie undernutrition, *Am. J. Clin. Nutr.*, 32, 693, 1979.

56. Frisancho, A. R., New standards of weight and upper arm muscle size for assessment of nutritional status, *Am. J. Clin. Nutr.*, 27, 1052, 1974.

57. Gurney, L. M. and Jelliffee, D. B., Arm anthropometry in nutritional assessment: nomogram for rapid calculation of muscle circumference and cross-sectional muscle and fat areas, *Am. J. Clin. Nutr.*, 26, 912, 1973.

58. Heymsfield, S. B., McMannus, C., Stevens, V., and Smith, J., Muscle mass: reliable indicator of protein-energy malnutrition severity and outcome, *Am. J. Clin. Nutr.*, 35, 1192, 1982.

59. Lukaski, H. C., Estimation of muscle mass, in *Human Body Composition Assessment,* Roche, A.F., Heymsfield, S.B., and Lohman, T.G., Eds, Human Kinetics, Champaign, IL, 1996, 109.

60. Heymsfield, S. B., McMannus, C., Smith, J., Stevens, V., and Nixon, D. W., Anthropometric measurement of muscle mass: revised equations for calculating bone-free arm muscle area, *Am. J. Clin. Nutr.*, 36, 680, 1982.

61. Fiatarone, M. A., Marks, E. C., Ryan, N. D., Meredith, C. N., Lipsitz, L. A., and Evans, W. J., High-intensity strength training in nonagenarians, *J. Am. Med. Assoc.*, 263, 3029, 1990.

62. Lonn, L., Kvist, H., Grangard, U., Bengtsson, B. A., and Sjostrom, L., CT-determined body composition changes in recombinant human growth hormone treatment to adults with growth hormone deficiency, in *Human Body Composition:* In Vivo *Methods, Models and Assessment*, Ellis, K. J. and Eastman J. D., Eds., Plenum Press, New York, 1993, 229.

63. Ross, R., Shaw, K. D., Rissanen, J., Martel, Y., de Guise, J., and Avruch, L., Sex differences in lean and adipose tissue distribution by magnetic resonance imaging: anthropometric relationships, *Am. J. Clin. Nutr.*, 59, 1277, 1994.

64. Ross, R., Pedwell, H., and Rissanen, J., Effects of energy restriction and exercise on skeletal muscle and adipose tissue in women as measured by magnetic resonance imaging, *Am. J. Clin. Nutr.*, 61, 1179, 1995.

65. Heymsfield, S. B., Smith, R., Aulet, M., Bensen, B., Lichtman, S., Wang, J., and Pierson, R. N., Appendicular skeletal muscle mass: measurement by dual-photon absorptiometry, *Am. J. Clin. Nutr.*, 52, 214, 1990.

66. Lukaski, H. C., Bolonchuk, W. W., Siders, W. A., and Milne, D. B., Chromium supplementation and resistance training: effects on body composition, strength and trace element status of men, *Am. J. Clin. Nutr.*, 63, 954, 1996.

67. Wilmore, J. H., The application of science to sport: physiological profiles of male and female athletes, *Can. J. Appl. Sport Sci.*, 4, 103, 1979.

68. Lamb, D. B., Knuttgen, H. G., and Murray, R., Eds., *Physiology and Nutrition for Competitive Sport*, Perspectives in Exercise Science and Sports Medicine, Vol. 7, Cooper Publishing Group, Carmel, IN, 1994.

69. Graves, J. E., Pollock, M. L., and Sparling, P. B., Body composition in elite female distance runners, *Int. J. Sports Med.*, 8, 96, 1987.

70. Wilmore, J. H., Brown, C. H., and Davis, J. A., Body physique and composition of the female distance runner, *Ann. N. Y. Acad. Sci.*, 301, 764, 1977.

71. Krahenbuhl, G. S., Wells, C. L., Brown, C. H, and Wood, P. E., Characteristics of national and world class female pentathletes, *Med. Sci. Sports Exer.*, 11, 20, 1979.

72. Thorland, W. G., Johnson, G. O., Fagot, T. G., Tharp, G. D., and Hammer, R.W., Body composition and somatotype of Junior Olympic athletes, *Med. Sci. Sports Exer.*, 13, 332, 1981.

73. Pollock, M. L., Gettman, L. R., Jackson, A., Ayers, J., Ward, A., and Linnerud, A. C., Body composition of elite distance runners, *Ann. N.Y. Acad. Sci.*, 301, 361, 1977.

74. Withers, R. T., Craig, N. P., Bourdon, P. C., and Norton, K. I., Relative body fat and anthropometric prediction of body density of male athletes, *Eur. J. Appl. Physiol.*, 56, 191, 1987.

75. Fahey, T. D., Akka, L., and Ralph, R., Body composition and VO$_2$max of exceptional weight trained athletes, Alpine skiers, *J. Appl. Physiol.*, 39, 559, 1975.

76. Johnson, G. O., Housh, T. J., Powell, D. R., and Ansorge, C. J., A physiological profile comparison of female body builders and power lifters, *J. Sports Med. Phys. Fitness*, 30, 361, 1990.

77. Spitler, D. L., Diaz, F. J., Horvath, S. M., and Wright, J. E., Body composition and maximal aerobic capacity of body builders, *J. Sports Med. Phys. Fitness*, 20, 181, 1980.

78. Katch, V. L., Katch, F. I., Moffatt, R., and Gittleson, M., Muscular development and lean body weight in body builders and weight lifters, *Med. Sci. Sports Exer.*, 12, 340, 1980.

79. Newton, L. E., Hunter, G., Bammon, M., and Roney, R., Changes in psychological state and self-reported diet during various phases of training in competitive body builders, *J. Strength Cond. Res.*, 7, 153, 1993.

80. Sinning, W. E., Anthropometric estimation of body density, fat, and lean body weight in women gymnasts, *Med. Sci. Sports Exer.*, 10, 243, 1978.

81. Johnson, G. O. and Nebelsick-Gullett, L. I., The effect of a competitive season on the body composition of university female athletes, *J. Sports Med. Phys. Fitness*, 29, 314, 1989.

82. Novak, L. P., Woodward, W. A., Bestit, C., and Mellerowicz, H., Body composition and physiological function of athletes, *J. Am. Med. Assoc.*, 205, 764, 1977.

83. Moffatt, R. J., Surina, B., Golden, B., and Ayers, N., Body composition and physiological characteristics of female high school gymnasts, *Res. Q. Exer. Sports,* 55, 80, 1984.

84. Sinning, W. E., Cunningham, L. N., Racaniello, A. P., and Sholes, J. L., Body composition and somatotype of male and female Nordic skiers, *Res. Q.,* 48, 741, 1977.

85. Hanson, J. S., Maximal exercise performance in members of the U.S. Nordic ski team, *J. Appl. Physiol.,* 35, 592, 1973.

86. Orvanova, E., Physical structure of winter sports athletes, *J. Sports Sci.,* 5, 197, 1987.

87. Farmosi, I., Apor, P., Meceki, S., and Haasz, S., Body composition of notable soccer players, *Hung. Rev. Sports Med.,* 25, 91, 1984.

88. Walsh, F. K., Heyward, V. H., and Schau, C. G., Estimation of body composition of female intercollegiate basketball players, *Physician Sports Med.,* 12, 74, 1984.

89. Siders, W. A., Bolonchuk, W. W., and Lukaski, H. C., Effects of participation in a collegiate sport season on body composition, *J. Sports Med. Phys. Fitness,* 31, 571, 1991.

90. Parr, R. B., Wilmore, J. H., Hoover, R., Bachman, D., and Kerlan, R., Professional basketball players: athletic profiles, *Physician Sports Med.,* 6, 77, 1976.

91. Wilmore, J. W., Parr, R. B., Haskell, W. L., Costill, D. L., Millburn, L. J., and Kerlan, R. K., Athletic profile of professional football players, *Physician Sports Med.,* 4, 45, 1976.

92. Smith, J. F. and Mansfield, E. R., Body composition prediction in university football players, *Med. Sci. Sports Exer.,* 16, 398, 1984.

93. White, J., Mayhew, J. L., and Piper, F. C., Prediction of body composition in college football players, *J. Sports Med. Phys. Fitness,* 20, 317, 1980.

94. Melesky, B. W., Shoup, R. F., and Malina, R. M., Size, physique and body composition of competitive female swimmers 11 through 20 years of age, *Human Biol.,* 54, 609, 1982.

95. Siders, W. A., Lukaski, H. C., and Bolonchuk, W. W., Relationships among swimming performance, body composition and somatotype in competitive collegiate swimmers, *J. Sports Med. Phys. Fitness,* 33, 166, 1993.

96. Pugh, L. G. C. E., Edholm, O. G., Fox, R. H., Wolff, H. S., Hervey, G. R., Hammond, W. H., Tanner, J. M., and Whitehouse, R. H., A physiological study of channel swimmers, *Clin. Sci.,* 19, 257, 1960.

97. Wilmore, J. H., Body weight and body composition, in *Eating, Body Weight and Performance in Athletes: Disorders of Modern Society,* Brownell, K. D., Rodin, J., and Wilmore, J. H., Eds., Lea and Febiger, Philadelphia, 1992, 77.

98. Kireillis, R. W. and Cureton, T. K., The relationships of external fat to physical education activities and fitness tests, *Res. Q.,* 18, 123, 1947.

99. Riendeau, R. P., Welch, B. E., and Crisp, C. E., Relationships of body fat to motor fitness test scores, *Res. Q.,* 29, 200, 1958.

100. Cureton, K. J., Hensley, L. D., and Tiburzi, A., Body fatness and performance differences between men and women, *Res. Q.,* 50, 333, 1979.

101. Cureton, K. J., Boileau, R. A., and Lohman, T. G., Relationship between body composition measures and AAHPER test performance in young boys, *Res. Q.,* 46, 218, 1975.

102. Boileau, R. A. and Lohman, T. G., The measurement of human physique and its effect on physical performance, *Orthop. Clin. N. Am.,* 8, 563, 1977.

103. Cureton, K. J. and Sparling, P. B., Distance running performance and metabolic responses to running in men and women with excess weight experimentally equated, *Med. Sci. Sports Exer.,* 12, 288, 1980.

104. Pate, R. R., Barnes, C. H., and Miller, W., A physiological comparison of performance-matched female and male distance runners, *Res. Q. Exer. Sport,* 56, 245, 1985.

105. Stager, J. M. and Cordain, L., Relationship of body composition to swimming performance in female swimmers, *J. Swim. Res.,* 1, 21, 1984.

106. Vogel, J. A., Kirkpatrick, J. W., Fitzgerald, P. I., Hodgdon, J. A., and Harman, E. A., Derivation of anthropometry-based body fat equations for the Army's weight control program, Report No. T17/88, U.A. Army Research Institute of Environmental Medicine, Natick, MA, 1988.

107. Hodgdon, J. A. and Beckett, M. B., Prediction of body fat for U.S. Navy men from body circumferences and height, Report No. 84-11, Naval Health Research Center, San Diego, CA, 1984.

108. Hodgdon, J. A. and Beckett, M. B., Prediction of body fat for U.S. Navy women from body circumferences and height, Report No. 84-29, Naval Health Research Center, San Diego, CA, 1984.

109. Wright, H. G., Dotson, C. D., and Davis, P. D., Simple techniques for measurement of percent body fat in men, *U.S. Navy Med.,* 72, 23, 1981.

110. Wright, H. G., Dotson, C. D., and Davis, P. D., An investigation into assessment techniques for body composition of women Marines, *U.S. Navy Med.,* 71, 15, 1980.

111. Fuchs, R. J., Their, C. F., and Lancaster, M. C., A nomogram to predict lean body mass in men, *Am. J. Clin. Nutr.,* 31, 673, 1978.

112. Brennan, E. H., Development of binomial involving anthropometric measurements for predicting lean mass in young women, M.S. Thesis, Incarnate Word College, San Antonio, TX, 1974.

113. U.S. Department of Defense, *Physical Fitness and Weight Control*, Directive No. 1308.1, June 29, 1981, Washington, D.C.

114. Harman, E. A. and Frykman, P. N., The relationship of body size and composition to the performance of physically demanding military tasks, in *Body Composition and Physical Performance: Applications for the Military Services*, Marriott, B. M. and Grumstrup-Scott, J., Eds., National Academy Press, Washington, D.C., 1992, 105.

115. Beckett, M. B. and Hodgdon, J. A., Lifting and carrying capacities relative to physical fitness measures, Report No. 87-26, Naval Health Research Center, San Diego, CA, 1987.

116. Mello, R. P., Damokosh, A. I., Reynolds, K. L., Witt, C. E., and Vogel, J. A., The physiological determinants of load bearing performance at different march distances, Technical Report T15-88, U.S. Army Research Institute of Environmental Medicine, Natick, MA, 1988.

117. Dziados, J., Damokosh, A., Mello, R., Vogel, J., and Farmer, K., The physiological determinants of load carriage, Technical Report T19-87, U.S. Army Research Institute of Environmental Medicine, Natick, MA, 1987.

118. Teves, M. A., Wright, J. E., and Vogel, J. A., Performance on selected candidate screening test procedures before and after Army basic and advanced individual training, Technical Report T13-85, U.S. Army Research Institute of Environmental Medicine, Natick, MA, 1985.

119. Myers, D. C., Gebhardt, D. L., Crump, C. E., and Fleishman, E. A., Validation of the military enlistment physical strength capacity test, Technical Report 610, U.S. Army Research Institute for the Behavioral Sciences, Natick, MA, 1983.

120. Behnke, A. R., Comment on the determination of whole-body density and a resume of body composition data, in *Techniques for Measuring Body Composition*, Brozek, J. and Henschel, A., Eds., National Academy of Science, National Research Council, Washington, D.C., 1961, 118.

121. Opplinger, R. A., Harms, R. D., Herrman, D. E., Streich, C. M., and Clark, R. R., The Wisconsin wrestling minimum weight project: a model for weight control among high school wrestlers, *Med. Sci. Sports Exer.*, 27, 1220, 1995.

122. Opplinger, R. A., Landry, G. L., Foster, S. W., and Lambrecht, A. C., Wisconsin minimum weight rule curtails weight cutting practices in high school wrestlers, *Med. Sci. Sports Med.*, 27, S12, 1995.

Chapter 26

IMMUNOCOMPETENCE IN PHYSICAL ACTIVITY AND SPORT

Laurie Hoffman-Goetz*

CONTENTS

I. INTRODUCTION

The idea that exercise modulates immunological response comes primarily from three types of observations. First, acute physical stressors in animals (e.g., rotational, restraint, handling) and in humans (e.g., surgical, hypoxia, hyperthermia, head-up tilt) influence a variety of immune parameters. Second, neuroendocrine changes elicited by these acute physical stressors, including increased sympathetic activation and elevated blood levels of epinephrine, cortisol, and endogenous opioids, also occur during intense exercise. Third, increased episodes of infectious disease, especially of the upper respiratory tract, have been reported clinically and epidemiologically in athletes during intense training and with over-training. Additionally, psychologically stressful events have been correlated with an increased incidence of various infections.[1,2] Competitive exercise involves pronounced stress, and immunological changes may occur due to the psychosocial factors surrounding sport.

In contrast, the biological rationale for linking exercise conditioning and fitness with persistent changes in immune function stems from reports of reduced growth of experimental tumors in animals given long-term exercise training.[3-6] Reduced experimental tumorigenesis in animals forced to participate in vigorous exercise has been related to a variety of potential mechanisms. These include reduced energy availability,[7,8] increased antioxidant enzyme activities,[9] and significant reductions in circulating insulin levels.[10] Other potentially important mechanisms implicated in exercise-tumor interactions are decreased growth rate and production

---

* Work was done while at the National Cancer Institute, National Institutes of Health, Bethesda, Maryland.

of growth factors[11] and increased natural immune effector components involved in the control of tumor growth and metastases.[12-15]

This review focuses on the effects of physical conditioning and exercise on the immune system and in particular on cellular and natural immune mechanisms. The term *cellular immunity* refers to immunological effects mediated by specifically sensitized lymphocytes. *Natural immunity* involves that aspect of host defense that does not display specificity to antigens (or only partial specificity) and includes natural killer (NK) cells, macrophages, other phagocytic cells, and the cytokine or nonantibody secretory products of these cells.

Wherever possible, the immunological responses of humans involved in exercise and sport is described. However, since much of the mechanistic work on exercise and immunity has been done in animal models, examples of these are given with a view of what might occur in humans. The clinical relevance of exercise-mediated changes in immune functions will also be discussed in relation to risk of infections in the athlete. Finally, the potential role of physical conditioning in reducing the risk of chronic diseases, such as cancer and autoimmune diseases, are considered. The nutritionist who is monitoring changes in dietary consumption during athletic training and evaluating health risks needs these relationships defined. Therefore, it is appropriate to review various areas of the research literature that relate to physical fitness and immune function within the context of a monograph on nutrition in exercise and sport. For the interested reader, recent reviews on general aspects of exercise and immunity, of exercise and cancer, and of psychoneuroimmunology are available.[16-20]

II. ACUTE EXERCISE AND IMMUNE FUNCTIONS

The most widely utilized model to assess the impact of exercise on immunity has been that of a single aerobic exercise session. Despite variations in the type, duration, and intensity of the exercise, the timing of the immune assessments, and differences in initial fitness levels of the subjects, several consistent patterns emerge regarding leukocyte and lymphocyte circulation patterns. First, physical exercise results in a transient leucocytosis which quickly returns to pre-exercise values.[21-27] These transient changes in leukocyte and lymphocyte numbers follow a biphasic pattern with an initial post-exercise increase and then decrease, with eventual recovery to pre-exercise levels within 2–6 h (depending on the intensity and duration of the exercise). Further, most studies show that this leukocytosis is not uniform among all leukocyte subsets, with the largest increase due to a pronounced neutrophilia. The biological basis for the neutrophilia of exercise involves a number of coordinated responses including demargination from intravascular pools, increased mobilization from bone marrow, and/or decreased efflux from the circulation. The hormonal contribution to this neutrophilia has been linked to increased growth hormone levels. Kappel et al.[28] reported that an intravenous bolus injection of growth hormone at levels comparable to that observed during exercise induced a marked neutrophilia without accompanying lymphocytosis.

Second, the transient increase in leukocyte number includes a striking lymphocytosis with a significant portion due to an increase in the absolute (and relative) numbers of NK cells.[9,29,30] A recent study showed that the post-exercise lymphocytosis (and especially the increase in NK cells) was not altered by a signal dose of glucocorticoid administered before high-intensity intermittent treadmill running in men.[31] Exercise-associated increases in epinephrine levels likely contribute to increased circulating NK cell numbers. Selective administration of epinephrine at physiologic levels observed during concentric exercise results in increased natural killer cell numbers,[32] and exercise stimulates an up-regulation of β-adrenergic receptors on NK cells.[33]

Third, the absolute or relative numbers of circulating T-lymphocyte subsets, defined by monoclonal antibodies, vary with acute exercise although circulating CD3[+] lymphocytes (pan T cells) tend to increase after acute aerobic exercise. Some studies report an increase in cytotoxic/suppressor (CD8+) phenotypes[26,34] whereas others report no changes in this subset after exercise.[35,36] These lymphocyte subset responses accompanying intense aerobic exercise occur with exhaustive resistance exercise. Nieman et al.[37] reported a marked CD3+ lympho-cytosis in male adult body builders given an exhaustive resistance exercise protocol (sets of 10 repetitions at 65% 1-RM of the parallel leg squat, with one repetition every 6 s until muscular fatigue). The observed lymphocytosis immediately after exercise was followed by a drop of between 30–60% in CD3+ lymphocyte counts compared with pre-exercise values.

The *in vitro* proliferative response of lymphocytes to mitogenic or antigenic stimuli is a commonly used technique to describe functional status. A number of studies have assessed the proliferative responses of human and rodent lymphocytes isolated after acute exercise. Most reports indicate that lymphocyte responses to T-cell mitogens are reduced after a single episode of exercise.[38-41] Exercise studies with human subjects show that the ability of lym-phocytes to proliferate to the plant T cell lectins, Concanavalin A (ConA) and phytohemag-glutinin (PHA), transiently decreases after exercise. The proliferative response to pokeweed mitogen (PWM), lipopolysaccharide (LPS), and interleukin-2 (IL-2) increases after exer-cise.[16,42-45] The decrease in proliferative responses to T-cell mitogens is on the order of 30–40%, most consistently occurs after high intensity exercise, and recovers within 2 h after exercise.

There are several factors which appear to be involved in the decreased T-cell mitogen response with a single bout of acute exercise. These factors are given below.

1. Decreased mitogenesis may reflect the shift in the proportion of subsets following exercise. Randall Simpson et al.[46] reported an increased percentage of cytotoxic and suppressor T cells in cultures from mice given exhaustive exercise relative to controls. Hoffman-Goetz et al.[47] described the redistribution patterns of murine lymphocyte subsets in spleen, thymus, and lymph nodes and hypothesized that tissue compartment changes could lead to spurious differences in mitogen responses attributed to exercise (i.e., a type of measurement bias due to the tissue sampling site). The shift may also reflect the large increase in lymphocytes with the natural killer cell phenotype which are not normally responsive to T-cell mitogens.
2. Exercise-associated increases in endogenous opioids may contribute to the immuno-suppression since subcutaneous injection of naltrexone before an acute swim session in rats blocks the expected immunosuppression to mitogen.[40] Exercise-associated increases in central opioid receptors have been associated with increased NK cell cytotoxicity *in vivo* (but not T-cell mitogenesis).[48]
3. Acute exercise is associated with increased *in vitro* monocyte/macrophage production of prostaglandins E (PGE) during and for 2 h after an exercise session.[49] PGE is thought to have down-regulatory effects on various functions of macrophages, including inter-leukin-1β (IL-1β) release.[50] It is possible that a reduction in IL-1β release attenuates the early signalling events in CD4+ lymphocytes which are responsive to mitogens. However, most studies fail to detect IL-1β in plasma obtained during or after exercise.[51-53]

The effects of acute exercise on immunoregulatory cytokines have been the subject of many studies; a recent, comprehensive review on exercise and cytokines is available.[54] Gen-erally, exercise results in a pattern of cytokine response that is small and rather transient; the exception to this occurs when the exercise is accompanied by concurrent inflammation. IL-6, and to a lesser extent IL-1β, TNFα, and IFNα, are the predominant cytokines observed after acute exercise. The blood levels of these cytokines tend to increase particularly with eccentric exercise and associated skeletal muscle damage.

Short, vigorous exercise enhances several aspects of neutrophil and macrophage phago-cytic activity.[55] Neutrophil activation, as measured by myeloperoxidase concentration (an enzyme involved in oxygen-dependent killing of phagocytosed particles), increased after extremely short (<10 min), vigorous ergometry exercise. Fehr et al.[56] found an enhancement of phagocytic activity and enzyme release from connective tissue macrophages after a single session of exhaustive endurance running. Whether the exercise-associated enhancement in phagocytic activities of granulocytes is due to an increase specifically in the C3bi receptor or other surface constituents that act as intracellular adhesion molecules is not known.

Because natural killer cells play an important role in host-nonspecific defense responses in viral infections and cancer[57,58] the impact of acute exercise on this immune cell has been the topic of numerous reports. The frequency of human blood lymphocytes positive for monoclonal antibodies against NK-cell surface markers (e.g., CD16, CD56) increases dramatically after exercise.[59-61] The increase in NK cell numbers in peripheral circulation during exercise is on the order of a two- to fivefold increase above pre-exercise levels. For humans at rest, NK cells account for <15% of peripheral blood mononuclear cells (PBMC) although there is an additional small fraction of NK cells sequestered in splenic and pulmonary tissue reservoirs. During exercise the percentage of NK cells can reach 25–30% of PBMCs.[62] The kinetic pattern of NK cells has been described by Gabriel et al.[30,63] and Shinkai and associates.[64] NK cell numbers increase significantly during the first 10 min of exercise followed by a plateau or a decline during the final 30 min of moderately intense exercise.

Work by Carroll et al.[65] suggests that there is a limiting duration of exercise beyond which increased NK cell numbers in peripheral circulation is not observed. A minimal threshold of 30% of VO$_2$max appears to be necessary to induce an increase in blood NK cell numbers. The dynamic source of these NK cells has not been determined with tracer studies. However, animal studies using static measures of lymphocyte distribution suggest that the increase in NK cells in the circulation is due to a concurrent demargination from other tissue compartments, such as the spleen,[66] and entry into the circulating pool. Iversen et al.[67] have shown that the post-exercise redistribution of leukocytes occurs even in splenectomized individuals. Hence, it remains unclear whether the spleen is the source of NK cell recruitment during exercise.

Natural killer cytotoxic activity (NKCA) increases during acute exercise irrespective of whether the exercise is brief submaximal, brief maximal, or long submaximal.[32,49,59,62,68,69] This increase in NKCA is transient however, followed by a decrease anywhere from 30 min to 2 h post-exercise.[59,61] The increase in NKCA at the end of exercise is likely due to a concurrent increase in NK cell numbers. However, the delayed reduction in NKCA cannot be easily explained by changes in NK cell numbers since, typically, this parameter has already returned to the baseline. The delayed reduction in NKCA may well reflect fluctuations in neuroendocrine factors during the exercise session. For example, Kappel et al.[32] found the increase and subsequent decreases in natural killer cytolytic in response to physical activity also occurred after an infusion of epinephrine. The role of other neuroendocrine and hormonal mediators (e.g., serotonin, cytokines, endorphins, eicosanoids) in the post-exercise suppression of NKCA has not been well studied.

III. EXERCISE TRAINING, FITNESS, AND IMMUNE RESPONSES

In contrast to the evidence that an acute exercise bout (of either maximal or submaximal intensity) modulates immune responses, far less is known about the impact of chronic exercise, exercise training, or physical conditioning on immune parameters. The impact of chronic exercise and training on leukocyte and lymphocyte numbers is variable. An older study[70] reported the absolute numbers of blood leukocytes and lymphocytes obtained at rest to be low in some marathoners. Papa et al.[71] reported the absolute number of lymphocytes and the percentage of T lymphocytes to be lower in water-polo players relative to untrained controls in blood samples obtained at rest. In contrast, body builders and trained swimmers did not differ in baseline numbers of leukocytes, lymphocytes, or neutrophils relative to sedentary individuals.[72] At rest, the percentage of T cells (determined by the "E-rosetting" technique) was increased among ballet dancers compared with controls.[73] In women assigned to a walking training program for 15 weeks, the total number of lymphocytes and T cells was reduced at 6 weeks but not at 15 weeks relative to pretraining levels.[74] This apparent inconsistency in the reported effects of exercise training on baseline leukocyte numbers may well be due to the timing of blood sample collections in relation to the last exercise session and training protocol.

Lymphocyte proliferation to mitogens is a well-established technique to determine general lymphocyte responsiveness *in vitro*; it is thought to mimic *in vivo* lymphocyte responses to antigens. The studies in humans on the effects of long-term exercise conditioning on lymphocyte function at rest tend to suggest no differences relative to nonathletes.[75-77] In response to intense exercise, however, most studies show that mitogen-induced lymphocyte proliferative responses are reduced.[78-80] MacNeil, Hoffman-Goetz, and colleagues[44] found reduced lymphocyte blastogenesis in response to mitogen stimulation after cycle ergometry exercise undertaken at intensities up to 75% of max. In contrast, spontaneous blastogenesis (i.e., without mitogen stimulation) was increased in marathoners following a 3 h run to exhaustion.[81] However, urinary neopterin (an indirect *in vivo* marker of lymphocyte cellular function) in elite male oarsmen did not change in 19 out of 27 subjects comparing pretraining with 4 weeks of hard training in anticipation of the Barcelona Olympic Games.[82] This discrepancy between the results from the lymphocyte proliferation studies vs the study using neopterin excretion may be due to differences in test sensitivity between *in vitro* and *in vivo* measures.

In general, the results from numerous small clinical studies indicate that highly conditioned subjects experience a suppression in lymphocyte function following an acute bout of exercise, which is qualitatively (but not quantitatively) similar to the response observed in untrained subjects after acute exercise. Although it is possible that training may blunt the magnitude of the lymphocyte suppression, it is not surprising that the stability of this exercise-stress response holds across fitness groups. In response to acute exhaustive exercise, swim-trained rats[41] and treadmill-trained mice[39] had suppressed splenic-lymphocyte proliferative responses to T cell mitogens. Physical conditioning, apart from the immediate effects of exercise, appears to augment splenic-lymphocyte responses to mitogens in rodents.[83,84]

The impact of exercise conditioning on NKCA has not been well characterized. A recent study by Nieman and collaborators[69] indicates an enhanced NKCA in blood samples obtained at rest from athletes as compared with nonathletes. In contrast, two studies suggest that at rest there is no difference in NKCA between athletes and nonathletes.[59,85] Of course, it is not known whether observed differences at rest among athletes reflects confounding due to sample bias (i.e., that individuals who excel at athletics are inherently more fit physiologically or immunologically). Moderate exercise training at levels has not been shown to induce any increase in blood NKCA obtained at rest.[85,86] Taken together these data suggest that intense (but not moderate) exercise conditioning is associated with an elevation in resting NKCA in humans. Thus, while there is experimental evidence to support a training-mediated enhancement of NKCA, the confidence in this effect is weak due to the limited number of studies. Further, even if there is an augmentation of NKCA, the physiological mechanisms have not been well studied. For example, in studies with experimental animal models, Hoffman-Goetz[87] found that moderate exercise increased NKCA and this was not due to a corresponding increase in the activity of proteolytic enzymes (serine esterases) within NK cells. However, these types of mechanistic links between NK cell activation and exercise (e.g., changes in perforin activity) have not been undertaken with NK cells or macrophage samples from human subjects during exercise.

IV. EXERCISE, IMMUNITY, AND DISEASE

Over the last several decades, there has been increasing experimental, epidemiological, and clinical evidence on the impact of exercise and/or physical conditioning on risk reduction for coronary heart disease,[56] noninsulin dependent diabetes mellitus,[88] and osteoporosis.[89,90] Less information is available regarding possible associations between physical activity and other common diseases, including acute infections, cancer, and autoimmune disorders. In this section, relationships between exercise and two chronic diseases which have strong immunological components, autoimmunity and cancer, are reviewed. In addition, because of the importance of acute self-limiting infections (which nevertheless impair athletic performance) the relationship between exercise and infectious disease risk is considered in detail.

Links between extreme exertion and infection has been the focus of epidemiological, clinical, and experimental studies. An early report of health concerns of Olympic athletes noted that upper respiratory tract infections were common.[91] More recent experiences of elite athletes are further anecdotal support of the notion that higher risk of infection and heavy exertion interact.[92] In contrast, many individuals engage in exercise because of a belief that regular exercise improves resistance and reduces risk of infection. Thus, understanding the link between infection and physical activity has important implications for health promotion. For the athlete, this relationship is critical since performance may be compromised by infectious sequelae.

The impact of exercise on infectious disease risk can be considered by intensity of exercise and/or duration of exercise. For example, Peters and Bateman[93] reported that an increased incidence of self-reported upper respiratory tract infections in 150 runners participating in a 56-km Cape Town (South Africa) race compared with individuals who did not run. Greater symptomatology of infections occurred in runners compared with nonrunners in the 2 weeks after the race. In later studies Peters et al.[94,95] confirmed reports of a greater number of minor upper respiratory infection symptoms in individuals participating in ultra marathon events (the 56-km Milo Korkie Ultra marathon and the 90-km Comrades Ultra marathon). Linde[96] found that elite orienteers followed for more than 1 year experienced greater numbers of infectious episodes than did age and sex matched nonorienteers. Nieman et al.[97] surveyed more than 2000 marathoners who reported retrospectively training activities and infectious disease episodes and symptomatology for 2 months prior to and 1 week after the 1987 Los Angeles marathon. This group reported 12.9% upper respiratory tract infections in marathoners after the race compared with 2.2% upper respiratory tract infections in nonrunners. During an 8 week competitive season, 86% of men participating in intercollegiate sports developed at least one upper respiratory tract infection, with the point of prevalence being highest during the initial 5 weeks.[98] Budgett and Fuller[99] reported that among 30 international caliber oarsmen, 83% reported recurrent upper respiratory tract infections with a frequency of 1.4 episodes per year. Although these epidemiological studies suggest an association between extreme exertion and post-exercise infection, it is important to stress that they are characterized by a number of methodological weaknesses. These studies' limitations include lack of clinical verification of infection (for example, reliance on self-report only), sample selection bias (for example, nonrespondents are not typically followed in these studies), and a number of reporting biases (for example, differences in recall due to one's ranking in the marathon or exercise event).

Few studies have addressed whether there is a dose-response association between exercise intensity and infectious disease risk. Nieman and colleagues,[97,100] who have contributed substantially to this literature, found that physical activity was associated with fewer episodes of upper respiratory infections than in sedentary conditions. For example, walking briskly for 45 min, 5 d a week over a 15 week training period for moderately overweight women was associated with 5.1 ± 1.2 symptom d compared with 10.8 ± 2.3 symptom d in sedentary women. Schouten et al.[101] found a negative correlation between the incidence of upper respiratory tract infections and moderate intensity physical activity (as measured in multiples of resting metabolic rate or METs/week) in female but not male study participants. Based on this type of evidence, several investigators have suggested a "J"-shaped model to explain the association between exercise and infectious disease risk.[102,103] The model suggests that

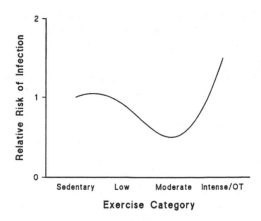

FIGURE 1 Schematic representation of relative risk of infection plotted against increasing levels of physical exertion. The model proposes that during periods of intense physical activity, exhaustive exercise, or overtraining (OT), a transient reduction occurs in some parameters of immune function. The combination of intense physical demands and immunosuppression may be associated with a higher risk of occurrence of upper respiratory tract infections. (Modified from Nieman, D. C. and Nehlsen-Cannarella, S. L., in *Exercise and Disease*, CRC Press, Boca Raton, FL, 1992, chap. 8. With permission.)

overtraining or a single bout of extreme exercise increases the risk whereas moderate exercise lowers the risk of upper respiratory tract infections. This model is presented diagrammatically in Figure 1. A related model, the "open window" model, to explain exercise-infection links has been described by Hoffman-Goetz and Pedersen.[16,104] Both the open window model and J-shaped curve propose that following a period of heavy or intense physical exertion, a transient immunosuppression occurs. During this window of risk, opportunistic infections are more likely to develop than at other times when immune functions are not compromised. During this period, then, a transition from healthy to subclinical disease state or from subclinical to the clinical horizon for disease occurs.

Under selected conditions, exercise may alter immune function or cell location resulting in increased death or damage.[105] For example, during Coxsackie B3 infection in mice, T cells migrate to the heart; of significance is the finding that T cell migration is accompanied by myocardial calcification. Mice infected with the virus and forced to swim had four times the number of sensitized T cells which were redirected to the heart from other parts of the body. Furthermore, more severe myocardial calcification occurred. Ilbäck and colleagues[106] found that the increased inflammatory and necrotic lesions seen in exercised mice with Coxsackie B viral myocarditis was associated with decreased mobilization of macrophages, followed by increased tissue destruction likely due to activation of cytotoxic T lymphocytes. Other experimental studies testing the hypothesis that exercise modulates response to infection showed that rodents physically trained before infection with *Salmonella typhimurium*[107] had a higher survival rate than sedentary animals. These data, then, point to the importance of timing of exercise in relation to infection: exercise training before exposure to infectious agents may be protective whereas exercise training after exposure to infectious agents may be deleterious for the host.

In summmary, there are some epidemiological studies suggestive that an increase in risk of upper respiratory tract infection occurs in athletes who overtrain or participate in extremely demanding exercise bouts. Athletic competition places an additional burden since there are the associated psychological stress effects of the competitive event. Despite the anecdotal appeal of an association between extreme exertion and increased risk of infection, there are no controlled clinical trials to test this in a systematic and methodologically rigorous fashion (e.g., with biological validation, attention to quality control, inclusion of a sufficient sample size). Moreover, although there are studies linking exercise with immune function, causal inference to infectious disease has not been demonstrated. While it is comparatively easy to show experimentally an augmentation or suppression of immune responses to exercise, it has been more difficult to establish clinical relevance. Part of the difficulty in evaluating the causal nature of exercise-induced changes in immune parameters with risk for infection is due to methodological limitations in measuring physical activity and fitness in large populations, the factor of clustering of positive health behaviors (such as the absence of tobacco use by athletes), and the multifactorial etiology of chronic diseases including those with an immunological component. With respect to infectious disease episodes, there is no clear consensus as to whether the exercise-mediated immune changes are protective, detrimental, or neutral for disease occurrence, magnitude, or progression.

The potential role for exercise in modifying risk for cancer has been known since the beginning of the century. Early studies suggested that intense physical activity reduced the occurrence of experimental tumors in animals.[3,108] More recently, there have been some epidemiological and experimental studies demonstrating reasonably consistent associations between lifetime physical activity and risk of colon and breast cancers.[18,19,109-115] The biological mechanisms involved in this risk reduction are thought to include changes in lifetime exposure to growth factors and steroid hormones (such as estrogen) for breast cancer, changes in fecal transit time and secondary bile acid formation for colon cancer, exercise-associated reduction in body fat and obesity for both colon and breast cancer, and changes in natural immune function. Experimental studies show, for example, that exercise in rodents alters the expression of cell adhesion molecules which have a role in tumor metastasis[116] and that training is associated with increased clearance of tumors from the lungs more effectively than sedentary controls.[12,117] Nevertheless, the strength and clinical significance of these studies on the long term impact for cancer risk and progression remain unclear.

Far fewer studies have been conducted to test the nature and magnitude of relationships between exercise and the development or course of autoimmune diseases. Ferry et al.[118,119] reviewed the literature on a variety of autoimmune conditions including rheumatoid arthritis, multiple sclerosis, and experimental autoimmune encephalitis (EAE). There was little evidence to conclude one way or the other the role of exercise in the acceleration of autoimmunity in experimental autoimmune encephalitis or the exacerbation of pre-existing autoimmunity.

V. SUMMARY

On the basis of experimental studies involving humans and animals, it appears that intense exercise and/or overtraining depresses and regular, moderate exercise enhances certain cellular immune functions. The biological basis for this immunomodulation likely involves the neuroendocrine and cardiorespiratory responses of exercise. This review emphasized that many of the immunological changes occurring with exercise also occur during periods of physical (and psychological) stress. In a practical sense, exercise immunology can be viewed as a subset of stress immunology.[16]

These comments notwithstanding, the clinical relevance of the immunological changes with exercise remains open. This is largely because the magnitude of the effects are small and transient.[120,121] Moreover, the majority of the exercise-associated changes in immune parameters fall well within the range of "normal" values. Other limitations arise due to difficulties in accurately measuring physical activity in populations, the lack of standardization in exercise-immunology protocols, and the failure to follow subjects for a sufficient period of time to ascertain clinical outcomes. However, given the public health importance of regular physical activity in reducing chronic disease risk,[122] it is appropriate to ask whether any of this risk reduction is mediated by changes in immune function.

REFERENCES

1. Kemeny, M., Zegans, L., and Cohen, F., Stress, mood, immunity, and recurrence of genital herpes, *Ann. N.Y. Acad. Sci.*, 494, 735, 1987.
2. Zarski, J., Hassles and health: a replication, *Health Psychol.*, 3, 243, 1984.
3. Rusch, H.P. and Kline, B.E., The effect of exercise on the growth of a mouse tumor, *Cancer Res.*, 4, 116, 1944.
4. Thompson, H.J., Ronan, A.M., Ritacco, K.A., Tagliaferro, A.R., and Meeker, L.D., Effect of exercise on the induction of mammary carcinogenesis, *Cancer Res.*, 48, 2720, 1988.
5. Cohen, L.A., Meschter, C., and Zang, E., Inhibiton of rat mammary tumorigenesis by voluntary exercise, *Proc. Am. Assoc. Cancer Res.*, 32, 125, 1991.
6. Ikuyama, T., Watanabe, T., Minegishi, Y., and Osanai, H., Effect of voluntary exercise on 3'-methyl-4-dimethylaminoazobenzene-induced hepatomas in male Jc1:Wistar rats, *Proc. Soc. Exp. Biol. Med.*, 204, 211, 1993.
7. Tannenbaum, A., The genesis and growth of tumors. II. Effects of caloric restriction per se. *Cancer Res.*, 2, 460, 1942.
8. Kritchevsky, D., The effect of over- and undernutrition on cancer, *Eur. J. Cancer Prev.*, 4, 445, 1995.
9. Djuric, Z. and Kritschevsky, D., Modulation of oxidative DNA damage levels by dietary fat and calories, *Mutat. Res.*, 295, 181, 1993.
10. Ruggeri, B.A., Klurfeld, D.M., Kritchevsky, D., and Furlanetto, R.W., Growth factor binding to 7,12-dimethylbenz(a)anthracen-induced mammary tumors from rats subject to chronic caloric restriction, *Cancer Res.*, 49, 4135, 1989.
11. Klurfeld, D.M., Welch, C.B., Einhorn, E., and Kritchevsky, D., Inhibition of colon tumor promotion by caloric restriction or exercise in rats, *FASEB J.*, 2, A433, 1988.
12. MacNeil, B. and Hoffman-Goetz, L., Chronic exercise enhances *in vivo* and *in vitro* cytotoxic mechanisms of natural immunity in mice, *J. Appl. Physiol.*, 74, 388, 1993.
13. Jadeski, L. and Hoffman-Goetz, L., Exercise and *in vivo* natural cytotoxicity against tumour cells of varying metastatic capacity, *Clin. Exp. Metastasis*, 14, 138, 1996.
14. Woods, J.A., Davis, J.M., Mayer, E.P., Ghaffar, A., and Pate, R.R., Effects of exercise on macrophage activation for anti-tumor cytotoxicity, *J. Appl. Physiol.*, 76, 2177, 1994.
15. Jonsdottir, I.H., Asea, A., Hoffmann, P., Dahlgren, U.I., Andersson, B., Hellstrand, K., and Thorén, P., Voluntary chronic exercise augments *in vivo* natural immunity in rats, *J. Appl. Physiol.*, 80, 1799, 1996.
16. Hoffman-Goetz, L. and Pedersen, B.K., Exercise and the immune system: a model of the stress response?, *Immunol. Today*, 15, 382, 1994.
17. Pedersen, B.K., Immune responses to acute exercise, in *Exercise and Immune Function*, Hoffman-Goetz, L., Ed., CRC Press, Boca Raton, FL, 1996, 79.
18. Hoffman-Goetz, L. and Husted, J., Exercise, immunity, and colon cancer, in *Exercise and Immune Function*, Hoffman-Goetz, L., Ed., CRC Press, Boca Raton, FL, 1996, 179.
19. Sternfeld, B., Cancer and the protective effect of physical activity: the epidemiological evidence, *Med. Sci. Sports Exerc.*, 24, 1195, 1992.
20. Blalock, J.E., The syntax of immune-neuroendocrine communication, *Immunol. Today*, 15, 504, 1994.
21. Andersen, K.L., Leukocyte response to brief, severe exercise, *J. Appl. Physiol.*, 7, 671, 1955.
22. McCarthy, D.A. and Dale, M.M., The leukocytosis of exercise: a review and a model, *Sports Med.*, 6, 333, 1988.
23. Galun, E., Burstein, R., Assia, E., Tur-Kaspa, I., Rosenblum, J., and Epstein, Y., Changes of white blood cell count during prolonged exercise, *Int. J. Sports Med.*, 8, 253, 1987.
24. Gimenez, M., Mohan-Kumar, T., Humbert, J.C., DeTalance, N., and Buisine, J., Leukocyte, lymphocyte and platelet response to dynamic exercise, *Eur. J. Appl. Physiol.*, 55, 465, 1986.
25. Oshida, Y., Yamanouchi, Y., Hayamizu, S., and Sato, Y., Effect of acute physical exercise on lymphocyte subpopulations in trained and untrained subjects, *Int. J. Sports Med.*, 9, 137, 1988.
26. Ferry, A., Picard, F., Duvallet, A., Weill, B., and Rieu, M., Changes in blood leukocyte populations induced by acute maximal and chronic submaximal exercise, *Eur. J. Appl. Physiol.*, 59, 435, 1990.
27. Keast, D., Cameron, K., and Morton, A.R., Exercise and the immune response, *Sports Med.*, 5, 248, 1988.
28. Kappel, M., Hansen, M.B., Diamant, M., Jorgensen, J.O., Gyhrs, A., and Pedersen, B.K., Effects of an acute bolus growth hormone infusion on the human immune system, *Hormone Metab. Res.*, 11, 593, 1993.
29. Kendall, A., Hoffman-Goetz, L., Houston, M., MacNeil, B., and Arumugam, Y., Exercise and blood lymphocyte subset responses: intensity, duration and subject fitness effects, *J. Appl. Physiol.*, 69, 251, 1990.
30. Gabriel, H., Schwarz, L., Steffens, G., and Kindermann, W., Immunoregulatory hormones, circulating leucocyte and lymphocyte subpopulations before and after endurance exercise of different intensities, *Int. J. Sports Med.*, 13, 359, 1992.
31. Singh, A., Zelazowska, E.B., Petrides, J.S., Raybourne, R.B., Sternberg, E.M., Gold, P.W., and Deuster, P.A., Lymphocyte subset response to exercise and glucocorticoid suppression in healthy men, *Med. Sci. Sports Exerc.*, 28, 822, 1996.

32. Kappel, M., Tvede, N., Galbo, H., Haahr, P.M., Kjær, M., Linstow, M., Klarlund, K., and Pedersen, B.K., Evidence that the effect of physical exercise on NK cell activity is mediated by epinephrine, *J. Appl. Physiol.*, 70, 2530, 1991.

33. Maisel, A.S., Harris, T., Rearden, C.A., and Michel, M.C., β-adrenergic receptors in lymphocyte subsets after exercise. Alterations in normal individuals and patients with congestive heart failure, *Circulation*, 82, 2003, 1990.

34. Nieman, D.C., Nehlsen-Cannarella, S.L., Donohue, K.M., Chritton, D.B.W., Haddock, B.L., Stout, R.W., and Lee, J.W., The effects of acute moderate exercise on leukocyte and lymphocyte subpopulations, *Med. Sci. Sports Exerc.*, 23, 578, 1991.

35. Field, C.J., Gougeon, R., and Marliss, E.B., Circulating mononuclear cell numbers and function during intense exercise and recovery, *J. Appl. Physiol.*, 71, 1089, 1991.

36. Tvede, N., Heilmann, C., Halkjær-Kristensen, J., and Pedersen, B.K., Mechanisms of B-lymphocyte suppression induced by acute physical exercise, *J. Clin. Lab. Immunol.*, 30, 169, 1989.

37. Nieman, D.C., Henson, D.A., Sampson, C.S., Herring, J.L., Suttles, J., Conley, M., Stone, M.H., Butterworth, D.E., and Davis, J.M., The acute immune response to exhaustive resistance exercise, *Int. J. Sports Med.*, 16, 322, 1995.

38. Eskola, J., Russkanen, O., Soppi, E., Viljanen, M., Jarvinen, M., and Toivonen, H., Effect of sport stress on lymphocyte transformation and antibody formation, *Clin. Exp. Immunol.*, 32, 339, 1978.

39. Hoffman-Goetz, L., Keir, R., Thorne, R., Houston, M., and Young, C., Chronic exercise stress in mice depresses splenic T lymphocyte mitogenesis *in vitro*, *Clin. Exp. Immunol.*, 66, 551, 1986.

40. Ferry, A., Weill, B., Amiridis, I., Laziry, F., and Rieu, M., Splenic immunomodulation with swimming-induced stress in rats, *Immunol. Lett.*, 29, 261, 1991.

41. Mahan, M.P. and Young, M.R., Immune parameters of untrained or exercise-trained rats after exhaustive exercise, *J. Appl. Physiol.*, 66, 282, 1989.

42. Beatson, D.G., On the treatment of inoperable cases of carcinoma of the mamma: suggestions for a new method of treatment with illustrative cases, *Lancet*, 2, 104, 1896.

43. Pedersen, B.K., Influence of physical activity on the cellular immune system: mechanisms of action, *Int. J. Sports Med.*, 12, S23, 1991.

44. MacNeil, B., Hoffman-Goetz, L., Kendall, A., Houston, M., and Arumugam, Y., Lymphocyte proliferation responses after exercise in men: fitness, intensity, and duration effects, *J. Appl. Physiol.*, 70, 179, 1991.

45. Tvede, N., Kappel, M., Klarlund, K., Duhn, S., Halkjær-Kristensen, J., Kjær, M., Galbo, H., and Pedersen, B.K., Evidence that the effect of bicycle exercise on blood mononuclear cell proliferative responses and subsets is mediated by epinephrine, *Int. J. Sports Med.*, 15, 100, 1994.

46. Randall Simpson, J.A., Hoffman-Goetz, L., Thorne, R., and Arumugam, Y., Exercise stress alters the percentage of splenic lymphocyte subsets in response to mitogen but not in response to interleukin-1, *Brain Behav. Immun.*, 3, 119, 1989.

47. Hoffman-Goetz, L., Thorne, R., Randall Simpson, J., and Arumugam, Y., Exercise stress alters murine lymphocyte subset distribution in spleen, lymph nodes and thymus, *Clin. Exp. Immunol.*, 76, 307, 1989.

48. Jonsdottir, I.H., Asea, A., Hoffmann, P., Hellstrand, K., and Thorén, P., Natural immunity and chronic exercise in rats. The involvement of the spleen and the splenic nerves, *Life Sci.*, 1996.

49. Pedersen, B.K., Tvede, N., Klarlund, K., Christensen, L.D., Hansen, F.R., Galbo, H., Kharazmi, A., and Halkjær-Kristensen, J., Indomethacin *in vitro* and *in vivo* abolishes post-exercise suppression of natural killer cell activity in peripheral blood, *Int. J. Sports Med.*, 11, 127, 1990.

50. Bloom, E.T. and Babbitt, J.T., Prostaglandin E_2, monocytes adherence and interleukin-1 in the regulation of human natural killer cell activity by monocytes, *Nat. Immun. Cell Growth Regul.*, 9, 36, 1990.

51. Cannon, J.G., Meydani, S.N., Fielding, R.A., Fiatarone, M.A., Meydani, M., Farhangmehr, M., Orencole, S.F., Blumberg, J.B., and Evans, W.J., Acute phase response in exercise. II. Associations between vitamin E, cytokines, and muscle proteolysis, *Am. J. Physiol.*, 260, R1235, 1991.

52. Smith, B.K. and Kluger, M.J., Human IL-1 receptor antagonist partially suppresses LPS fever but not plasma levels of IL-6 in Fischer rats, *Am. J. Physiol.*, 263 (3 pt 2), R653, 1992.

53. Ullum, H., Haahr, P.M., Diamant, M., Palmo, J., Halkjær-Kristensen, J., Kjær, M., Galbo, H., and Pedersen, B.K., Bicycle exercise enhances plasma IL-6 but does not change IL-1α, IL-1β, or TNF-α pre-mRNA in BMNC, *J. Appl. Physiol.*, 77, 93, 1994.

54. Bagby, G.J., Crouch, L.D., and Shepherd, R.E., Exercise and cytokines: spontaneous and elicited responses, in *Exercise and Immune Function*, Hoffman-Goetz, L., Ed., CRC Press, Boca Raton, FL, 1996, 55.

55. Pincemail, J., Camus, G., Roesgen, A., Dreezen, E., Bertrand, Y., Lismonde, M., Deby-Dupont, G., and Deby, C., Exercise induces pentane production and neutrophil activation in humans. Effect of propranolol, *Eur. J. Appl. Physiol.*, 61, 319, 1990.

56. Fehr, H.G., Lötzerich, H., and Michna, H., Human macrophage function and physical exercise: phagocytic and histochemical studies, *Eur. J. Appl. Physiol.*, 58, 613, 1989.

57. Herberman, R.B. and Ortaldo, J.R., Natural killer cells: their role in defense against disease, *Science*, 214, 24, 1981.

58. Lotzová, E., Effector immune mechanisms in cancer, *Nat. Immun. Cell Growth Regul.*, 4, 293, 1985.

59. Brahmi, Z., Thomas, J.E., Park, M., and Dowdeswell, I.R.G., The effect of acute exercise on natural killer cell activity of trained and sedentary human subjects, *J. Clin. Immunol.*, 5, 321, 1985.

60. Fiatarone, M.A., Morley, J.E., Bloom, E.T., Benton, D., Makinodan, T., and Solomon, G.F., Endogenous opioids and the exercise-induced augmentation of natural killer cell activity, *J. Lab. Clin. Med.*, 112, 544, 1988.

61. Kotani, T., Aratake, Y., Ishiguro, R., Yamamoto, I., Uemura, Y., and Tamura, K., Influence of physical exercise on large granular lymphocytes, leu-7 bearing mononuclear cells and natural killer activity in peripheral blood-NK-cell and NK-activity after physical exercise, *Acta Haematol. Jap.*, 50, 1210, 1987.

62. Pedersen, B.K., Tvede, N., Hansen, F.R., Andersen, V., Bendix, T., Bendixen, G., Galbo, H., Haahr, P.M., Klarlund, K., Sylvest, J., Thomsen, B.S., and Halkjœr-Kristensen, J., Modulation of natural killer cell activity in peripheral blood by physical exercise, *Scand. J. Immunol.*, 27, 673, 1988.

63. Gabriel, H., Schwarz, L., Born, P., and Kindermann, W., Differential mobilization of leucocyte and lymphocyte subpopulations into the circulation during endurance exercise, *Eur J. Appl. Physiol.*, 65, 529, 1992.

64. Shinkai, S., Shore, S., Shek, P.N., and Shephard, R.J., Acute exercise and immune function, *Int. J. Sports Med.*, 13, 452, 1992.

65. Carroll, K.K., Flynn, M.G., Brolinson, P.G., Kooiker, B.A., Freeman, S., and Brickman, T.M., Natural cell-mediated cytotoxicity and lymphocyte proliferation following a 24 hour road race, *Med. Sci. Sports Exer.*, 26 (Suppl. 1), S34, 1994(Abstract).

66. Randall Simpson, J. and Hoffman-Goetz, L., Exercise stress and murine natural killer cell function, *Proc. Soc. Exp. Biol. Med.*, 195, 129, 1990.

67. Iversen, P.O., Arvesen, B.L., and Benestad, H.B., No mandatory role for the spleen in exercise-induced leucocytosis in man, *Clin. Sci.*, 86, 505, 1994.

68. Berk, L.S., Nieman, D.C., Youngberg, W.S., Arabatzis, K., Simpson-Westerberg, M., Lee, J.W., Tan, S.A., and Eby, W.C., The effect of long endurance running on natural killer cells in marathoners, *Med. Sci. Sports Exerc.*, 22, 207, 1990.

69. Nieman, D.C., Miller, A.R., Henson, D.A., Warren, B.J., Gusewitch, G., Johnson, R.L., Davis, J.M., Butterworth, D.E., and Nehlsen-Cannarella, S.L., Effects of high- vs moderate-intensity exercise on natural killer cell activity, *Med. Sci. Sports Exerc.*, 25, 1126, 1993.

70. Green, R.L., Kaplan, S.S., Rabin, B.S., Stanitski, C.L., and Zdziarski, U., Immune function in marathon runners, *Ann. Allergy*, 47, 73, 1981.

71. Papa, S., Vitale, M., Mazzotti, G., Neri, L.M., Monti, G., and Manzoli, F.A., Impaired lymphocyte stimulation induced by long-term training, *Immunol. Lett.*, 22, 29, 1989.

72. Lewicki, R., Tchorzewski, H., Denys, A., Kowalska, M., and Golinska, A,. Effect of physical exercise on some parameters of immunity in conditioned sportsmen, *Int. J. Sports Med.*, 8, 309, 1987.

73. Xusheng, S., Yugi, X., Yongguang, Z., and Li, S., Effect of ballet on immunity in young people, *J. Sports Med. Phys. Fitness*, 30, 397, 1992.

74. Nehlsen-Cannarella, S.L., Nieman, D.C., Balk-Lamberton, A.J., Markoff, P.A., Chritton, D.B.W., Gusewitch, G., and Lee, J.W., The effects of moderate exercise training on immune response, *Med. Sci. Sports Exerc.*, 23, 64, 1991.

75. Baj, Z., Kantorski, J., Majewska, E., Zeman, K., Pokoca, L., Fornalczyk, E., Tchorzewski, H., Sulowka, Z., and Lewicki, R., Immunological status of competitive cyclists before and after the training season, *Int. J. Sports Med.*, 15, 319, 1994.

76. Tvede, N., Steensberg, J., Baslund, B., Kristensen, J.H., and Pedersen, B.K., Cellular immunity in highly trained elite racing cyclists and controls during periods of training with high and low intensity, *Scand. J. Sports Med.*, 1, 163, 1991.

77. Nieman, D.C., Brendle, D., Henson, D.A., Suttles, J., Cook, V.D., Warren, B.J., Butterworth, D.E., Fagoaga, O.R., and Nehlsen-Cannarella, S.L., Immune function in athletes versus nonathletes, *Int. J. Sports Med.*, 16, 329, 1995.

78. Gmünder, F.K., Lorenzi, G., Bechler, B., Joller, P., Muller, J., Ziegler, W.H., and Cogoli, A., Effect of long-term physical exercise on lymphocyte reactivity: similiarity to spaceflight reactions, *Aviat. Space Environ. Med.*, 59, 146, 1988.

79. Nieman, D.C., Simandle, S., Henson, D.A., Warren, B.J., Suttles, J., Davis, J.M., Buckley, K.S., Ahle, J.C., Butterworth, D.E., Fagoaga, O.R., and Nehlsen-Cannarella, S.L., Lymphocyte proliferation response to 2.5 hours of running, *Int. J. Sports Med.*, 16, 404, 1995.

80. Shinkai, S., Kurokawa, Y., Hino, S., Hirose, M., Torii, J., Watanabe, S., Shiraishi, S., Oka, K., and Watanabe, T., Triathlon competition induced a transient immunosuppressive change in the peripheral blood of athletes, *J. Sports Med. Phys. Fitness*, 33, 70, 1993.

81. Nieman, D.C., Berk, L.S., Simpson-Westerberg, M., Arabatzis, K., Youngberg, S., Tan, S.A., Lee, J.W., and Eby, W.C., Effects of long-endurance running on immune system parameters and lymphocyte function in experienced marathoners, *Int. J. Sports Med.*, 10, 317, 1989.

82. Jakeman, P.M., Weller, A., and Warrington, G., Cellular immune activity in response to increased training of elite oarsmen prior to Olympic competition, *J. Sports Med.*, 13, 207, 1995.

83. Ferry, A., Rieu, P., Laziri, F., Guezennec, C.Y., El Habazi, A., Le Page, C., and Rieu, M., Immunomodulation of thymocytes and splenocytes in trained rats, *J. Appl. Physiol.*, 71, 815, 1991.

84. Tharp, G.D. and Preuss, T.L., Mitogenic responses of T-lymphocytes to exercise training and stress, *J. Appl. Physiol.*, 70, 2535, 1991.

85. Nieman, D.C., Buckley, K.S., Henson, D.A., Warren, B.J., Suttles, J., Ahle, J.C., Simandle, S., Fagoaga, O.R., and Nehlsen-Cannarella, S.L., Immune function in marathon runners versus sedentary controls, *Med. Sci. Sports Exer.*, 27, 986, 1995.

86. Nieman, D.C., Prolonged aerobic exercise, immune response, and risk of infection, in *Exercise and Immune Function*, Hoffman-Goetz, L., Ed., CRC Press, Boca Raton, FL, 1996, 143.

87. Hoffman-Goetz, L., Serine esterase (BLT-esterase) activity in murine splenocytes is increased with exercise but not training, *Int. J. Sports Med.*, 16, 94, 1995.

88. Manson, J.E., Nathan, D.M., Krolewski, A.S., Stampfer, M.J., Willett, W.C., and Hennekens, C.H., A prospective study of exercise and incidence of diabetes among U.S. male physicians, *J. Am. Med. Assoc.*, 268, 63, 1992.

89. Drinkwater, B.L., Physical activity, fintess, and osteoporosis, in *Physical Acitivity, Fitness, and Health: International Proceedings and Consensus Statement*, Bouchard, C., Shephard, R.J., and Stephens, T., Eds., Human Kinetics Press, Champaign, IL, 1994, 724.

90. Smith, E.L., Smith, K.A., and Gilligan, C., Exercise, fitness, osteoarthritis, and osteoporosis, in *Exercise, Fitness and Health: A Consensus of Current Knowledge*, Bouchard, C., Shephard, R.J., Stephens, T., Sutton, J.R., and McPherson, B.D., Eds., Human Kinetics Press, Champaign, IL, 1990, 517.

91. Hanley, D.F., Medical care of the U.S. Olympic team, *J. Amer. Med. Assoc.*, 12, 147, 1976.

92. Nieman, D.C. and Nehlsen-Cannarella, S.L., The immune response to exercise, *Seiminars Hematol.*, 31, 166, 1994.

93. Peters, E.M. and Bateman, E.D., Respiratory tract infections: an epidemiological survey, *S. A. Med. J.*, 64, 582, 1983.

94. Peters, E.M., Altitude fails to increase susceptibility of ultramarathon runners to post-race upper respiratory tract infections, *S. A. Med. J.*, 5, 4, 1990.

95. Peters, E.M., Goetzche, J.M., Grobbelaar, B., and Noakes, T.D., Vitamin C supplementation reduces the incidence of postrace symptoms of upper respiratory tract infection in ultramarathon runners, *Am. J. Clin. Nutr.*, 57, 170, 1993.

96. Linde, F., Running and upper respiratory tract infections, *Scand. J. Sport Sci.*, 9, 21, 1987.

97. Nieman, D.C., Johanssen, L.M., Lee, J.W., and Arabatzis, K., Infectious episodes in runners before and after the Los Angeles marathon, *J. Sports Med. Phys. Fit.*, 30, 316, 1990.

98. Strauss, R.H., Lanese, R.R., and Leizman, D.J., Illness and absence among wrestlers, swimmers, and gymnasts at a large university, *Am. J. Sports Med.*, 16, 653, 1988.

99. Budgett, R.G. and Fuller, G.N., Illness and injury prevention in international oarsmen, *Clin. Sports Med.*, 1, 57, 1989.

100. Nieman, D.C., Nehlsen-Cannarella, S.L., Markoff, P.A., Balk-Lamberton, A.J., Yang, H., Chritton, D.B.W., Lee, J.W., and Arabatzis, K., The effects of moderate exercise training on natural killer cells and acute upper respiratory tract infections, *Int. J. Sports Med.*, 11, 467, 1990.

101. Schouten, W.J., Verschuur, R., and Kemper, H.C.G., Physical activity and upper respiratory tract infections in a normal population of young men and women: the Amsterdam growth and health study, *Int. J. Sports Med.*, 9, 451, 1988.

102. Nieman, D.C. and Nehlsen-Cannarella, S.L., Exercise and infection, in *Exercise and Disease*, Watson, R.R. and Eisinger, M., Eds., CRC Press, Boca Raton, FL, 1992, 121.

103. Heath, G.W., Ford, E.S., Craven, T.E., Macera, C.A., Jackson, K.L., and Pate, R.R., Exercise and the incidence of upper respiratory tract infections, *Med. Sci. Sports Exerc.*, 23, 152, 1991.

104. Hoffman-Goetz, L. and Pedersen, B.K., Exercise and immune response, in *Encyclopedia of Immunology*, Delves, P.J. and Roitt, I., Eds., W.B. Saunders, London, 1996.

105. Reyes, M.P., Smith, F.E., and Lerner, A.M., An enterovirus-induced murine model of an acute dilated-type cardiomyopathy, *Interviol.*, 22, 146, 1984.

106. Ilbäck, N.-G., Fohlman, J., and Friman, G., Exercise in Coxsackie B3 myocarditis: effects on heart lymphocyte subpopulations and the inflammatory reaction, *Am. Heart J.*, 117, 1298, 1989.

107. Cannon, J.G. and Kluger, M.J., Exercise enhances survival rate in mice infected with *Salmonella typhimurium*, *Proc. Soc. Exp. Biol. Med.*, 175, 518, 1984.

108. Hoffman, S.A., Paschkis, K.E., DeBias, D.A., Cantarow, A., and Williams, T.L., The influence of exercise on the growth of transplanted rat tumors, *Cancer Res.*, 22, 597, 1962.

109. Hoffman-Goetz, L. And Husted, J., Exercise and cancer: do the biology and epidemiology correspond?, *Ex. Immunol. Rev.*, 1, 81, 1995.

110. Bernstein, L., Henderson, B.E., Hanisch, R., Sullivan-Halley, J., and Ross, R.K., Physical exercise and reduced risk of breast cancer in young women, *J. Natl. Cancer Inst.*, 86, 1403, 1994.

111. Bernstein, L., Ross, R.K., and Henderson, B.E., Prospects for the primary prevention of breast cancer, *Am. J. Epidemiol.*, 135, 142, 1992.

112. Frisch, R.E., Wyshak, G., Albright, N.L., Albright, T.E., Schiff, I., Jones, K.P., Witschi, J., Shiang, E., Koff, E., and Marguglio, M., Lower prevalence of breast cancer and cancers of the reproductive system among former college athletes compared to non-athletes, *Br. J. Cancer*, 52, 885, 1985.

113. Wyshak, G., Frisch, R.E., Albright, N.L., Albright, T.E., and Schiff, I., Lower prevalence of benign diseases of the breast and benign tumours of the reproductive system among former college athletes compared to non-athletes, *Br. J. Cancer*, 54, 841, 1986.

114. Vena, J.E., Graham, S., Zielezny, M., Brasure, J., and Swanson, M.K., Occupational exercise and risk of cancer, *Am. J. Clin. Nutr.*, 45, 318, 1987.

115. Hoffman-Goetz, L., Exercise, natural immunity, and experimental tumor metastasis, *Med. Sci. Sports Exerc.*, 26, 157, 1994.

116. Hoffman-Goetz, L., Effect of acute treadmill exercise on LFA-1 antigen expression in murine splenocytes, *Anticancer Res.*, 15, 1981, 1995.

117. Hoffman-Goetz, L., May, K.M., and Arumugam, Y., Exercise training and mouse mammary tumour metastasis, *Anticancer Res.*, 14, 2627, 1994.

118. Ferry, A., LePage, C., and Rieu, M., Sex as a determining factor in the effect of exercise on an *in vivo* autoimmune response, adjuvant arthritis, *J. Appl. Physiol.*, 76, 1172, 1994.

119. Ferry, A., Exercise and autoimmune diseases, in *Exercise and Immune Function*, Hoffman-Goetz, L., CRC Press, Boca Raton, FL, 1996, 163.

120. Hoffman-Goetz, L. and MacNeil, B., Exercise, natural immunity, and cancer: causation, correlation, or conundrum, in *Exercise and Disease*, Watson, R.R. and Eisinger, M., Eds., CRC Press, Boca Raton, FL, 1992, pp. 37–62.

121. Cannon, J.G., Exercise and resistance to infection, *J. Appl. Physiol.*, 74, 973, 1993.

122. Surgeon General's Report. Physical Activity and Health, USDHHS, CDC, Washington, D.C., 1996.